Atlas
of
Pediatric Physical Diagnosis

Atlas
of
Pediatric Physical Diagnosis

Edited by

BASIL J. ZITELLI, MD

Professor of Pediatrics,
University of Pittsburgh,
School of Medicine;
University Pediatric Diagnostic Referral Service,
Children's Hospital of Pittsburgh,
Pittsburgh, Pennsylvania

HOLLY W. DAVIS, MD

Associate Professor of Pediatrics,
University of Pittsburgh,
School of Medicine;
Director,
Pediatric Emergency Medicine,
Children's Hospital of Pittsburgh,
Pittsburgh, Pennsylvania

THIRD EDITION

with 2248 illustrations

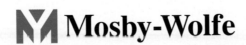 **Mosby-Wolfe**

St. Louis Baltimore Boston Carlsbad Chicago Naples New York Philadelphia Portland
London Madrid Mexico City Singapore Sydney Tokyo Toronto Wiesbaden

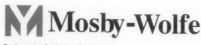

Mosby-Wolfe

Dedicated to Publishing Excellence

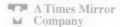

A Times Mirror
Company

Vice President and Publisher: Anne S. Patterson
Editor: Laura DeYoung
Senior Developmental Editor: Sandra Clark Brown
Project Manager: Carol Sullivan Weis
Senior Production Editor: Christine Carroll Schwepker
Manufacturing Manager: David Graybill
Designer: Renee Duenow

Printed in Singapore
Composition by Graphic World, Inc.
Printing/binding by Imago

Mosby–Year Book, Inc.
11830 Westline Industrial Drive
St. Louis, Missouri 63146

Library of Congress Cataloging-in-Publication Data
Atlas of pediatric physical diagnosis / edited by Basil J. Zitelli,
  Holly W. Davis. — 3rd ed.
      p.   cm.
    Includes bibliographical references and index.
    ISBN 0-8151-9930-9
    1. Children—Diseases—Diagnosis.   2. Physical diagnosis.
  3. Children—Medical examinations.   I. Zitelli, Basil J. (Basil
  John), 1946–   . II. Davis, Holly W., 1945–   .
    [DNLM: 1. Diagnosis—in infancy & childhood—atlases.   2. Physical
  Examination—in infancy & childhood—atlases.   WS 17 A881 1997]
  RJ50.A86   1997
  618.92'00754—dc21
  DNLM/DLC
  for Library of Congress   96-46308
                                                              CIP

97 98 99 00 /9 8 7 6 5 4 3 2

Contributors

Michael J. Balsan, MD
Associate Professor of Pediatrics,
Northeastern Ohio Universities College of Medicine;
Tod Children's Hospital,
Youngstown, Ohio

Roberta E. Bauer, MD
Associate Professor of Pediatrics,
Northeastern Ohio Universities College of Medicine;
Director, Division of Developmental Pediatrics,
Children's Hospital Medical Center of Akron,
Akron, Ohio

Lee B. Beerman, MD
Professor of Pediatrics,
Division of Pediatric Cardiology,
University of Pittsburgh School of Medicine,
Pittsburgh, Pennsylvania

Mark F. Bellinger, MD
Professor of Surgery, Division of Urology,
University of Pittsburgh School of Medicine;
Chief, Pediatric Urologic Surgery,
Children's Hospital of Pittsburgh,
Pittsburgh, Pennsylvania

Albert W. Biglan, MD
Adjunct Associate Professor,
University of Pittsburgh School of Medicine;
Director, Department of Ophthalmology,
Children's Hospital of Pittsburgh,
Pittsburgh, Pennsylvania

Greg Bisignani, MD
Resident, Department of Orthopedics,
University of Pittsburgh School of Medicine,
Pittsburgh, Pennsylvania

Julie Blatt, MD
Professor of Pediatrics,
Division of Hematology/Oncology,
University of Pittsburgh School of Medicine;
Member, Division of Hematology/Oncology,
Children's Hospital of Pittsburgh,
Pittsburgh, Pennsylvania

Mary M. Carrasco, MD
Associate Professor of Pediatrics,
University of Pittsburgh School of Medicine;
Director, Section of Community Health,
Children's Hospital of Pittsburgh,
Pittsburgh, Pennsylvania

Kenneth P. Cheng, MD
Clinical Instructor, Ophthalmology,
Division of Pediatric Ophthalmology,
University of Pittsburgh School of Medicine;
Member, Division of Pediatric Ophthalmology,
Children's Hospital of Pittsburgh,
Pittsburgh, Pennsylvania

Bernard A. Cohen, MD
Associate Professor of Pediatrics and Dermatology,
Johns Hopkins University School of Medicine;
Director, Pediatric Dermatology,
Johns Hopkins Children's Center,
Baltimore, Maryland

Holly W. Davis, MD
Associate Professor of Pediatrics,
University of Pittsburgh School of Medicine;
Director,
Pediatric Emergency Medicine,
Children's Hospital of Pittsburgh,
Pittsburgh, Pennsylvania

Demetrius Ellis, MD
Professor of Pediatrics and Nephrology,
University of Pittsburgh School of Medicine;
Director of Nephrology,
Children's Hospital of Pittsburgh,
Pittsburgh, Pennsylvania

Heidi Feldman, MD, PhD
Associate Professor of Pediatrics,
University of Pittsburgh School of Medicine;
Director, Division of General Academic Pediatrics,
Children's Hospital of Pittsburgh,
Pittsburgh, Pennsylvania

Jonathan D. Finder, MD
Assistant Professor of Pulmonology,
University of Pittsburgh School of Medicine;
Member, Division of Pulmonology,
Children's Hospital of Pittsburgh,
Pittsburgh, Pennsylvania

David Finegold, MD
Professor of Pediatrics,
University of Pittsburgh School of Medicine;
Member, Division of Endocrinology,
Children's Hospital of Pittsburgh,
Pittsburgh, Pennsylvania

Philip Fireman, MD
Professor of Pediatrics and Medicine,
Director, Section of Allergy and Immunology,
University of Pittsburgh School of Medicine;
Children's Hospital of Pittsburgh,
Pittsburgh, Pennsylvania

F. Jay Fricker, MD
Professor of Pediatric Cardiology,
University of Florida College of Medicine,
Gainesville, Florida

J. Carlton Gartner, Jr., MD
Professor of Pediatrics,
University of Pittsburgh School of Medicine;
Vice Chairman, Department of Pediatrics,
Children's Hospital of Pittsburgh,
Pittsburgh, Pennsylvania

Melissa Hamp, MD, MPH
Associate Professor of Pediatrics and Human Development,
Program Director of Pediatric Education,
Michigan State University College of Human Medicine–Flint Campus,
Flint, Michigan

Edward N. Hanley, Jr., MD
Clinical Professor of Surgery,
University of North Carolina;
Chairman, Department of Orthopedic Surgery,
Carolinas Medical Center,
Charlotte, North Carolina

David A. Hiles, MD
Private Practice,
Scottsdale, Arizona

Ian R. Holzman, MD
Professor of Pediatrics, Obstetrics, and Gynecology,
City University of New York;
Director, Division of Newborn Medicine,
Mount Sinai Medical Center,
New York, New York

Raymond B. Karasic, MD
Associate Professor of Pediatrics,
University of Pittsburgh School of Medicine;
Pediatric Emergency Medicine,
Member, Division of General Academic Pediatrics,
Children's Hospital of Pittsburgh,
Pittsburgh, Pennsylvania

Cora C. Lenox, MD
Professor Emeritus,
University of Pittsburgh School of Medicine;
Division of Pediatric Cardiology,
Children's Hospital of Pittsburgh,
Pittsburgh, Pennsylvania

Aldo Vincent Londino, Jr., MD
Associate Professor of Medicine and Pediatrics,
University of Pittsburgh School of Medicine;
Chief of Rheumatology,
Children's Hospital of Pittsburgh,
Pittsburgh, Pennsylvania

J. Jeffrey Malatack, MD
Professor of Pediatrics,
Temple University School of Medicine;
Director, Diagnostic Referral Center,
St. Christopher's Hospital for Children,
Philadelphia, Pennsylvania

Susan B. Mallory, MD
Associate Professor of Medicine (Dermatology) and Pediatrics,
Washington University School of Medicine;
Director, Pediatric Dermatology,
St. Louis Children's Hospital,
St. Louis, Missouri

Timothy P. McBride, MD
Private Practice,
Fairfax, Virginia

David H. McKibben, DMD
Member, Dental Department,
Children's Hospital of Pittsburgh,
Pittsburgh, Pennsylvania

Pamela J. Murray, MD, MHP
Assistant Professor of Pediatrics,
University of Pittsburgh School of Medicine;
Director, General Academic Pediatrics/Adolescent Medicine,
Children's Hospital of Pittsburgh,
Pittsburgh, Pennsylvania

Don K. Nakayama, MD
Professor of Surgery and Pediatrics,
University of North Carolina at Chapel Hill School of Medicine,
Chapel Hill, North Carolina

Mamoun M. Nazif, DDS, MDS
Director, Dental Services,
Dental Department,
Children's Hospital of Pittsburgh,
Pittsburgh, Pennsylvania

Blakeslee E. Noyes, MD
Assistant Professor of Pediatrics,
St. Louis University;
Director, Pulmonary Medicine,
Cardinal Glennon Hospital,
St. Louis, Missouri

David M. Orenstein, MD
Professor of Pediatric Pulmonology,
University of Pittsburgh, School of Medicine;
Pulmonary Disease Center,
Children's Hospital of Pittsburgh,
Pittsburgh, Pennsylvania

Sang C. Park, MD
Professor of Pediatric Cardiology,
University of Pittsburgh School of Medicine;
Member, Division of Cardiology,
Children's Hospital of Pittsburgh,
Pittsburgh, Pennsylvania

Lila Penchansky, MD
Professor of Pathology,
University of Pittsburgh School of Medicine;
Member, Department of Pathology,
Children's Hospital of Pittsburgh,
Pittsburgh, Pennsylvania

Mary Ann Ready, DMD
Public Health Service,
Crow Agency, Montana

James S. Reilly, MD
Professor of Otolaryngology and Pediatrics,
Jefferson Medical College of Thomas Jefferson University,
Philadelphia, Pennsylvania;
Chief, Division of Pediatric Otolaryngology,
Alfred I. duPont Institute Children's Hospital,
Wilmington, Delaware

David P. Skoner, MD
Associate Professor of Pediatrics,
Division of Allergy, Immunology, and Rheumatology,
University of Pittsburgh School of Medicine;
Children's Hospital of Pittsburgh,
Pittsburgh, Pennsylvania

Mark W. Steele, MD
Associate Professor of Pediatrics,
Department of Medical Genetics,
University of Pittsburgh School of Medicine;
Former Chief, Department of Genetics,
Children's Hospital of Pittsburgh,
Pittsburgh, Pennsylvania

Andrew H. Urbach, MD
Associate Professor of Pediatrics,
University of Pittsburgh School of Medicine;
Member, Diagnostic Referral Service,
Children's Hospital of Pittsburgh,
Pittsburgh, Pennsylvania

W. Timothy Ward, MD
Associate Professor, Orthopaedic Surgery,
University of Pittsburgh School of Medicine;
Division of Pediatric Orthopaedic Surgery,
Member, Division of Pediatric Orthopedics,
Children's Hospital of Pittsburgh,
Pittsburgh, Pennsylvania

Henry B. Wessel, MD
Associate Professor of Pediatric Neurology,
University of Pittsburgh School of Medicine;
Member, Division of Neurology,
Children's Hospital of Pittsburgh,
Pittsburgh, Pennsylvania

John A. Zitelli, MD
Private Practice,
Shadyside Hospital,
Pittsburgh, Pennsylvania

Basil J. Zitelli, MD
Professor of Pediatrics,
University of Pittsburgh School of Medicine;
University Pediatric Diagnostic Referral Service,
Children's Hospital of Pittsburgh,
Pittsburgh, Pennsylvania

Foreword

Sir William Osler once wrote, "There is no more difficult art to acquire than the art of observation." Doctors Basil Zitelli and Holly Davis have done a great deal of observing and recording to assist you in acquiring the skills necessary to become a better than average clinician.

The more you see, the more you will know. Although there is no true substitute for experience, the superb collection of photographs and drawings in the *Atlas of Pediatric Physical Diagnosis* is the next best thing to being there.

Spending time with more than 2200 illustrations will result in your heightened capacity to make a prompt and correct diagnosis. Look, read, and enjoy, secure in your knowledge that you are learning some valuable pediatric lessons.

Frank A. Oski, MD
Given Professor of Pediatrics,
The Johns Hopkins University,
School of Medicine,
Baltimore, Maryland

In memorium

Dr. Frank Oski was a giant of pediatrics. His contributions to pediatric hematology, pediatric education, and child health care policy were visionary and paved the road for bringing children's care into a new era. We were honored to have Dr. Oski contribute the Foreword to the *Atlas*. We will miss him, and children the world around will be poorer because of his loss.

Basil J. Zitelli, MD

Holly W. Davis, MD

Preface

For many disorders, visual recognition is the major factor in making a correct diagnosis. The experienced clinician who has seen a wide spectrum of different disorders carries a wealth of information for diagnosis and for teaching.

This book was envisioned by teachers and developed to aid students, residents, nurses, and practitioners who care for children in the diagnosis of pediatric disorders. Our goal is to broaden the visual experience of the student and clinician through rapid visual examination or review of simple laboratory tests.

The enthusiastic response to the previous editions led us to believe that a third edition was not only possible but necessary. Many readers offered helpful suggestions for photos and topics to be included. Every chapter has been reviewed, revised, and updated. New information and diagnostic techniques have been included. Emphasis on physical examination techniques has been stressed in each chapter. Additional contributors have provided greater depth and dimension to the *Atlas*. The *Atlas* is by no means encyclopedic, but rather presents an overview of clinical disorders that lend themselves to visual diagnosis. The accompanying text deliberately emphasizes pertinent historical factors, examination techniques, visual findings, and diagnostic methods rather than therapy. We firmly believe that a careful history and physical examination provide the foundation for any clinical assessment. We have attempted to select disorders that are common and/or important, and where relevant, to describe the spectrum of clinical findings. It is our hope that this *Atlas* will continue to serve as a useful and practical reference for anyone who cares for children.

Acknowledgments

The *Atlas* is the product of the unstinting efforts of many dedicated people over the course of three editions. The authors devoted much time, effort, and expertise and gathered photographs largely from their patient populations and clinical material at Children's Hospital of Pittsburgh. Most of these were taken and produced by our Medical Media Department. Norman Rabinovitz, Norman Snyder, Russell Weleski, Laura Dugan, William Winstein, Jr., Douglas Sellers, Kathleen Muffie, and Dino Bovo aided by Eric Jablonowski and Suzanne Mikesell, deserve credit for being at our beck and call.

Cynthia Vogt, past coordinator of the Neuroradiology teaching file; Maureen McKay of Pediatric Neurosurgery; Bernadette Marshalek, Sandra Williams, and Barbara Glaneman, coordinators of the Radiology teaching files; along with Georgette Babbit, Theresa Buffo, Jeanette Ference, Tracy Fisher, Bruce Gyms, Jodie Henrickson, Linda Jacobs, William Thomas, and Christine Tuttle of the Radiology file room deserve high praise for scouring their files to find the numerous radiographs, CT, MRI, and bone scans we needed.

Nancy Dunn, Dolores Blumstein, Nancy Spears, and Colleen Lako of the Blaxter Medical Library at Children's Hospital of Pittsburgh were most helpful in locating and double-checking the many references we used.

We thank the staff at Mosby–Year Book who have logged countless hours in the process of design, layout, and production of the final product.

We also appreciate the work of Darlene Chiponis, Joy Harris, and Marian Michaels in proofreading.

Special acknowledgement is due to Diane Weidner and Sandra Eddy for their tireless work on nearly half of the manuscripts for the third edition; to David Kazimer for comparable work on the second edition and for his care and talent in helping design many of the tables; to Helen Shorner for her work on the first edition; and to Susan Gelnett who made major secretarial contributions to the first two editions. Further, we must acknowledge the assistance provided by all the other secretaries who prepared manuscripts for individual authors.

We would also like to express our gratitude to numerous colleagues at Children's Hospital of Pittsburgh and around the country who generously shared clinical photographs and radiographs with us and to the many patients and families who graciously allowed us to include their pictures.

Finally, we would like to thank the many thousands of people who have found the first and second editions of the *Atlas* so useful for their praise, support, and suggestions. We hope their thoughts and our labors have resulted in an improved text that will be of help to all who care for children.

Basil J. Zitelli, MD

Holly W. Davis, MD

Contents in Brief

Contents

Atlas
of
Pediatric Physical Diagnosis

1

Common Chromosomal Disorders

MARK W. STEELE

General Principles

The Nature of Chromosomes

Human hereditary factors are located in genes (the genome); 10% (about 100,000) are structural genes that code for proteins (such as enzymes), and the other 90% have functions that are not clear. The genes are composed of deoxyribonucleic acid (DNA) and are stored in intranuclear cell organelles called *chromosomes.* Each chromosome contains one linear DNA molecule folded over onto itself several times, as well as ribonucleic acid (RNA) and proteins. Because all genes exist in pairs, all chromosomes must likewise exist in pairs. The members of each pair of genes are called *alleles,* and the members of each pair of chromosomes are known as *homologues.* The conventional depiction of the constitution of homologues in the nucleus is called the cell's karyotype (Fig. 1-1). If at any gene locus the alleles are identical, that gene locus is homozygous. If the alleles are not identical, the gene locus is heterozygous.

Except for gametes, normal human cells contain 23 pairs of chromosomes, 46 in all. One of these pairs is concerned in part with inducing the primary sex of the embryonic gonads. These sex chromosomes are called the *X and Y chromosomes,* and they are not genetically homologous except in a few areas. Women have two X chromosomes, whereas men have an X and a Y chromosome. The remaining 22 pairs are called *autosomes* and determine non–sex-related (somatic) characteristics.

During most of a cell's life cycle, chromosomes are diffusely spread throughout the nucleus and cannot be morphologically identified. Only when the cell divides does chromosome morphology become apparent (Fig. 1-2). The in vitro life cycle and the cellular division, or mitosis, of a somatic cell are illustrated in Figs. 1-3 and 1-4, respectively. The life cycle and divisions, or meiosis, of a germ cell are much more complex and are not suitable for ordinary clinical evaluation.

Any somatic cell that can divide in tissue culture can be used for chromosomal (cytogenetic) analyses. The most convenient tissue source is peripheral blood from which lymphocytes can be stimulated to divide during 2 or 3 days of incubation in tissue culture media. After death, lung tissue is the best tissue to culture for chromosomal analyses, although the process requires a 4- to 6-week incubation pe-

riod. When a treatment decision requires urgency, preliminary chromosomal evaluation can be made within 4 to 24 hours using uncultured bone marrow aspirate.

An abnormality in chromosome number less than an even multiple of 23 (the haploid number) is called *aneuploidy* (Fig. 1-5). Usually, in aneuploidy there are 45 or 47 chromosomes; rarely, multiples of the X or Y chromosome result in individuals with 48 or 49 chromosomes. If aneuploidy occurs in a gamete as a result of a chromosomal division error (nondisjunction or anaphase lag) during meiosis, all cells are affected in the fertilized embryo. With subsequent pregnancies, the risk for another chromosomally abnormal offspring is increased to approximately 1% to 2% overall. The reason for this increased risk is obscure, but such couples should seek antenatal diagnostic counselling. About half of such abnormal infants have a chromosomal abnormality different from that of the proband.

If the one-celled embryo (zygote) is chromosomally normal and aneuploidy occurs after fertilization in an embryonic somatic cell because of a division error during mitosis, only one or two lines of embryonic cells are affected. The remaining embryonic cells are chromosomally normal. This mixed chromosomal state is called *mosaicism* and cannot be inherited because it occurred after conception. However, with a mosaic child the parents' recurrent risk still may be increased over that of the general population (to 1% to 2% as mentioned previously), since the zygote may have been aneuploid to start with. In the latter case the chromosomally normal cell line resulted from a division error during somatic cell mitosis.

Chromosomes can be normal in number (diploid) but still be abnormal in structure. Inversions (Fig. 1-6), deletions (Fig. 1-7), and translocations (Fig. 1-8) are examples of structural chromosomal abnormalities. These abnormalities can arise as new (sporadic) mutations in the egg or sperm from which the embryo was formed, in which case the parents' recurrent risk for another chromosomally abnormal offspring is again 1% to 2%. However, the abnormality also may be inherited from a phenotypically normal carrier parent (Fig. 1-9).

About 1 in 500 normal individuals carries a balanced, structurally abnormal set of chromosomes. *Balanced* here means that on cytogenetic analysis the structural abnormality does not appear to have resulted in any net loss or gain of genetic material. If the balanced chro-

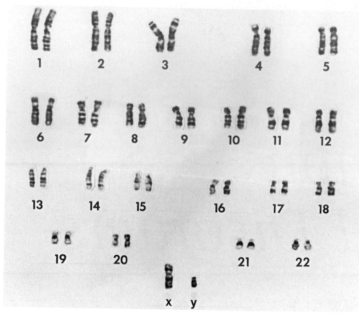

FIG. 1-1 Photomicrographs show that this is a G-banded male karyotype (a female would have two X chromosomes and no Y chromosome). The horizontal banding produced by the Giemsa staining technique allows for precise identification of homologous chromosomes.

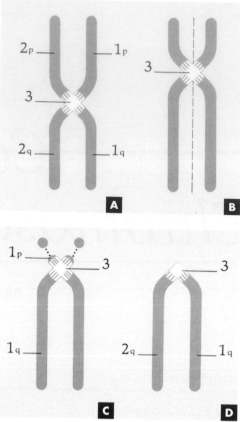

FIG. 1-2 Morphology of a chromosome during metaphase. *A*, Metacentric chromosome with centromere *(3)* in middle. *B*, Submetacentric chromosome with centromere off center. *C*, Acrocentric chromosome with centromere near one end. *D*, Telocentric chromosome (not found in humans) with centromere at one end. The DNA of the chromosome has replicated to form two chromatids: *1p* and *1q* represent one complete chromatid, *2p* and *2q* the other complete chromatid. The chromosome will then divide longitudinally, as shown in *B*.

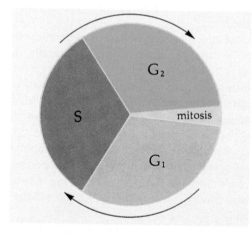

FIG. 1-3 The in vitro life cycle of a somatic cell. The interphase lasts 21 hours and can be divided into the following three stages: G_1 (7 hours)—cell performs its tasks; S (7 hours)—DNA replicates; G_2 (7 hours)—cell prepares to divide. Then mitosis occurs.

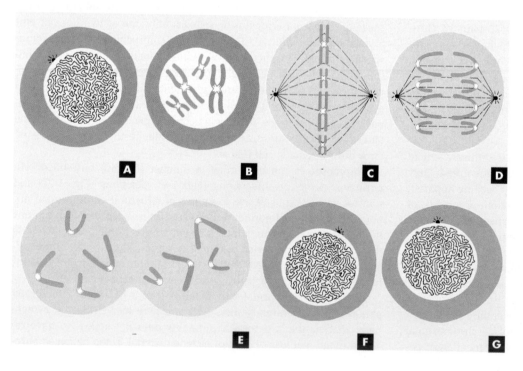

FIG. 1-4 Mitosis lasts about 1 hour, during which time the cell divides. *A*, Interphase cell at end of G_2. *B*, Prophase—replicated DNA condenses and is visible. *C*, Metaphase—46 duplicated chromosomes align randomly on spindle and can be photographed for karyotyping. *D*, Anaphase—chromosomes divide longitudinally, and half of each one moves to the opposite pole of the cell. *E*, Telophase—cell wall divides. *F* and *G*, Interphase at G_1—two daughter cells each with 46 chromosomes.

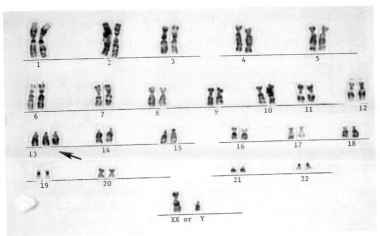

FIG. 1-5   Karyotype of a patient with trisomy 13 demonstrates aneuploidy. Note the extra chromosome 13, causing the cell to have 47 instead of 46 chromosomes.

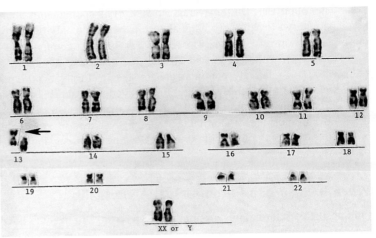

FIG. 1-6   Pericentric inversion (*arrow*) of chromosome 13.

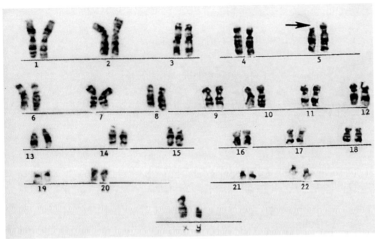

FIG. 1-7   Deletion (*arrow*) of the p arm of chromosome 5 (cri du chat syndrome).

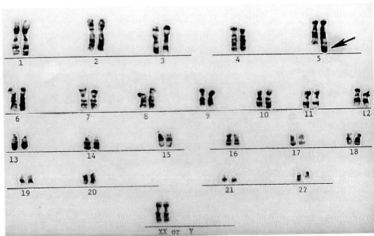

FIG. 1-8   Unbalanced translocation. The additional DNA was translocated onto the q arm of chromosome 5. The abnormality was inherited from a normal carrier father (Fig. 1-9) with a balanced reciprocal translocation between the q arms of chromosome 3 and chromosome 5. The patient died of multiple birth defects and in essence had a partial trisomy of the distal portion of the q arm of chromosome 3.

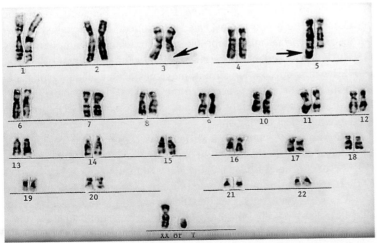

FIG. 1-9   A "balanced" reciprocal translocation from chromosomes 3 to 5 in a normal man (the father of the chromosomally defective newborn in Fig. 1-8).

mosomal abnormality runs in the family (i.e., is inherited from a normal parent), the carrier is usually phenotypically normal; but, though still controversial, there may be about a 1% to 3% increased risk for mental retardation and/or major birth defects. However, if the carrier state resulted from a new mutation, there is about a 6% risk that the carrier will have some degree of mental retardation and/or other major congenital anomalies. Presumably these abnormalities result from submicroscopic chromosomal defects.

Incidence of Chromosomal Abnormalities

At least 25% and perhaps as many as 40% of all pregnancies terminate in spontaneous abortion. Most such abortions are so early in gestation that pregnancy is not recognized. The earlier the abortion, the more probable it is that the fetus had a chromosomal abnormality. Of first trimester abortuses, 62% are chromosomally abnormal, compared with

5% of later abortuses. On the average, in 50% of all spontaneous abortions the embryo is chromosomally abnormal, with triploidy (69 chromosomes), trisomy 16, and 45XO being by far the most common findings (Table 1-1). Although the former two are not found among liveborns, 45XO is relatively common and results in Turner syndrome. Nevertheless, 98% of embryos with Turner syndrome abort. Because most chromosomally abnormal embryos abort spontaneously, the incidence of chromosomal abnormalities among liveborns in general is only about 6 in 1000 and about 50 in 1000 among stillborns and other perinatal deaths.

When to Suspect a Chromosomal Abnormality

Chromosomal abnormalities, in number or structure, are likely to have a detrimental effect on the phenotype. Aneuploidy of an autosome is lethal or interferes significantly with physical and mental development. However, aneuploidy of an X or Y chromosome may have little effect on the phenotype. Aneuploidy is not an entirely random event, and familial clustering is common.

Carriers of an inherited, or *de novo*, reciprocal translocation are usually genetically balanced and are subsequently normal. Their conceptions are likely to be genetically unbalanced and may abort spontaneously or be born with major congenital anomalies. A history of unexplained infertility, multiple spontaneous abortions (three or more), and particularly the prior birth of an abnormal baby to the couple or to a close relative is an indication that one of the parents carries a balanced chromosomal translocation. A chromosome study on the couple is thus indicated, and if translocation is found, they should seek antenatal diagnostic counseling.

A normal person who carries a balanced reciprocal translocation commonly can produce six chromosomal types of gamete. On fertilization, these gamete types result in a normal conceptus, a carrier conceptus like the normal carrier person, two types of immediately lethal conceptus resulting from gross chromosomal imbalances (i.e., too much or too little DNA), or two types of abnormal conceptus caused by lesser chromosomal imbalances. Whether or not the latter two types abort spontaneously or come to term as defective liveborns cannot be predicted in advance solely on theoretical grounds. Therefore genetic counseling in such situations simply depends on knowledge of what has happened in similar situations. Rarely, other types of chromosomal imbalances are found in conceptuses of such carrier parents.

Experience suggests the following: if a carrier has already produced a chromosomally defective liveborn, it is known that such defective fetuses can come to term. Consequently, that carrier's recurrent risk for another defective liveborn is about 20%. However, if a carrier has produced only spontaneous abortuses, it is less likely that such defective fetuses can come to term. Consequently, that person's risk for producing a chromosomally abnormal liveborn is only about 4%. Finally, if a couple of whom one spouse is a carrier has not yet experienced any pregnancies, their risk for a chromosomally defective liveborn is estimated to be about 10%. The sex of the carrier parent does not affect these risks.

FISH Technology

Fluorescent in situ hybridization (FISH) is a dramatic new laboratory technology developed over the past 5 years. Although it is still pending formal approval by the Food and Drug Administration, FISH technology has revolutionized the diagnostic capabilities of clinical laboratory cytogenetics.

TABLE 1-1

Incidence of Chromosomal Abnormalities

Among spontaneous abortuses	%
1st trimester	62
After 1st trimester	5
Type of Abnormality	
Trisomy 16	8
Other trisomies	18
Triploidy	8
45XO	9
Miscellaneous	7
Overall Incidence	**50**

Among liveborns	Per 1000
Abnormality of Autosomes (males and females)	4.0
Trisomies	1.4
Balanced rearrangements	2.0
Unbalanced rearrangements	0.6
Abnormality of Sex Chromosomes (males and females)	2.2
In males (XXY, XYY, mosaics)	3.0
In females	1.4
45XO (0.1)	
XXX, mosaics (1.3)	
Overall Incidence	**6.2**

About one quarter of all conceptuses are chromosomally abnormal. About 50 in 1000 stillborns have a chromosomal abnormality.

In this technique a DNA probe is tagged with a label that fluoresces when viewed under a special microscope. The probe is applied to slides of metaphase chromosomes, to which it binds, but the probe also binds to interphase nuclei on the slide (Fig. 1-10, *A* to *J*). The probe can be a cosmid probe for a small segment of single-copy DNA, such as part of a specific gene or an anonymous bit of chromosomal DNA. The probe can be an alpha or beta satellite probe for repetitive DNA sequences, such as those found in the centromeric area of a chromosome, or it can be a probe specific for repetitive DNA at the telomeric end of a chromosome. Finally, a cocktail of many repetitive DNA probes blanketing a specific chromosome from end to end can be obtained. This is called a *FISH paint*. Using special microscope filters, a clinician can simultaneously FISH a slide with probes fluorescing in two or three different colors.

FISH paints specific for all chromosomes are available. Alpha and beta satellite FISH probes specific to the X and Y chromosomes and all but two autosomes also are available, and telomeric FISH probes are available for select chromosomes.

With respect to chromosomal deletions, cosmid FISH probes are available specific for the following malformations: Angelman syndrome (46, XX or XY, del 15q12), cri du chat syndrome (46, XX or XY, del 5p15.2), DiGeorge sequence or its variant velocardiofacial syndrome (46, XX or XY, del 22q11.2), Miller-Dieker syndrome (46, XX or XY, del 17p13.3), Prader-Willi syndrome (46, XX or XY, del 15q12), Smith-Magenis syndrome (46, XX or XY, del 17p11.2), Williams syndrome (46, XX or XY, del 7q11.23), and Wolf-Hirschhorn syndrome (46, XX or XY, del 4p16.3). DiGeorge sequence is detailed in Chapter 4; Williams

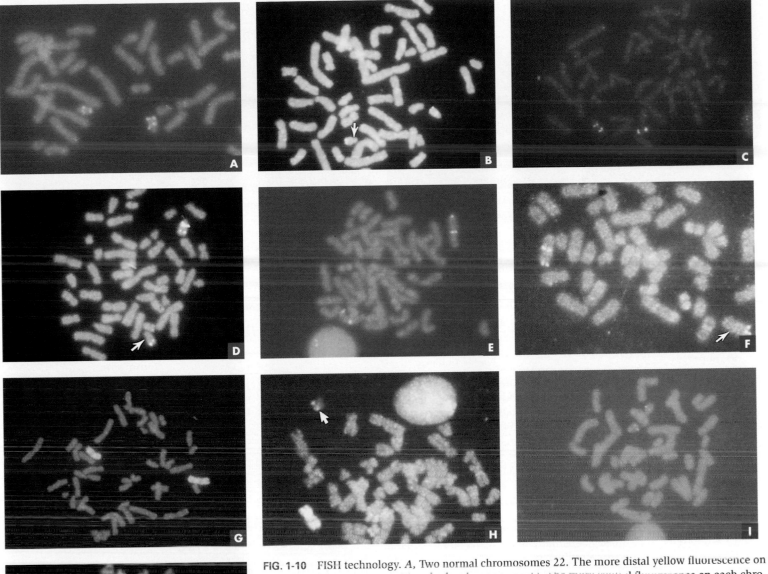

FIG. 1-10 FISH technology. *A,* Two normal chromosomes 22. The more distal yellow fluorescence on each chromosome is a cosmid probe for chromosome 22. The more central fluorescence on each chromosome is a cosmid probe for the DiGeorge sequence critical region. The general chromosome-DNA background stains orangish-red. *B,* Patient with DiGeorge sequence. The normal chromosome 22 is at 4 o'clock. The arrow points to the chromosome 22 with deleted DiGeorge critical region. *C,* Two normal chromosomes 15. The lower fluorescence on each chromosome is a cosmid probe for chromosome 15. The upper fluorescence on each chromosome is a cosmid probe for the Prader-Willi syndrome critical region. *D,* Patient with Prader-Willi syndrome. The normal chromosome 15 is at 1 o'clock. The arrow points to the chromosome 15 with deleted Prader-Willi syndrome critical region. *E,* Two normal chromosomes 7. The more distal fluorescence on each chromosome is a cosmid probe for chromosome 7. The more central fluorescence on each chromosome is a cosmid probe for the William syndrome critical region. *F,* Patient with William syndrome. The normal chromosome 7 is at 9 o'clock. The arrow points to the chromosome 7 with deleted William syndrome critical region. *G,* Two normal X chromosomes each fluorescing end to end with an X-chromosome FISH paint in a normal female. *H,* Male patient with a pericentric inversion of the Y chromosome determined by FISH and molecular analyses. An X chromosome FISH paint fluoresces the normal X chromosome at 7 o'clock. The arrow points to a fluorescence on the p arm end of the Y chromosome, which fluoresces because the p arm ends of the X and Y chromosomes normally are genetically homologous. *I,* Two normal chromosomes 21. The fluorescence on each chromosome is a cosmid probe for the Down syndrome critical region. *J,* Patient with Down syndrome caused by a cryptic translocation involving the Down syndrome critical region. The two normal 21 chromosomes are at 10 o'clock. The small arrow points to a chromosome 12 with fluorescence from the Down syndrome critical region on its end. The large arrow points to a nearby interphase nucleus with three fluorescent areas because of the trisomy for the Down syndrome critical region. The patient's conventional chromosome test (karyotype) on both blood and cultured skin fibroblasts was normal. (Courtesy Dr. Sharon L. Wenger and Mr. James H. Cummins, Children's Hospital of Pittsburgh.)

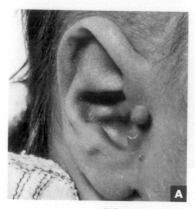
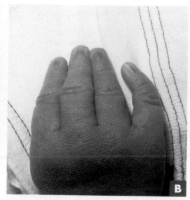
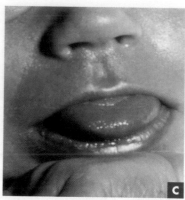
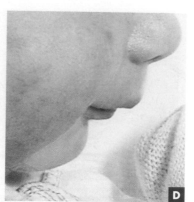

FIG. 1-11 Clinical photographs show several minor anomalies seen at birth. *A,* Preauricular skin tag. *B,* Clinodactyly of the fifth finger. *C,* Macroglossia. *D,* Micrognathia. (Courtesy Dr. Christine L. Williams, New York Medical College.)

TABLE 1-2

Some Syndromes Diagnosable by FISH Probes

Syndrome	Major findings	Comments
Cri du chat 46, XX or XY, del 5p15.2	High-pitched, shrill (catlike) cry and round face in young infants; downward-slanting wide-spaced eyes with epicanthal folds; broad nasal bridge; micrognathia; premature graying hair; microcephaly; severe mental retardation; CHD (30%)	Incidence—approximately 1 in 20,000 live births; about 15% result from a chromosome imbalance inherited from a normal carrier parent and tend to be more severe; facial features ameliorate with age; life span to 60 years possible
Miller-Dieker 46, XX or XY, del 17p13.3	Type I lissencephaly; microcephaly; high, wrinkled forehead with bitemporal hollowing; epicanthal folds; small nose with broad nasal bridge and upturned nares; growth and severe mental retardation; seizures; FTT; death usually by 5 years	Incidence—rare; chromosome deletion often submicroscopic, detected only by FISH probe; can be inherited from a normal carrier parent
Smith-Magenis 46, XX or XY, del 17p11.2	Brachycephaly; flat, broad face with prominent forehead; short, broad hands; growth delay; mental retardation with speech and hearing problems; hyperactive, self-destructive behavior	Incidence—rare; all cases sporadic; can live to 60 years
Velocardiofacial 46, XX or XY, del 22q11.2	Cleft palate or submucous cleft with hypernasal speech and conductive hearing loss; prominent nose with large squared root and narrow alar base; long face and philtrum; small ears; slender hands with tapering fingers; CHD (VSD, right aortic arch, tetralogy of Fallot); mild microcephaly and developmental delay; small stature	Incidence—over 150 cases reported; infants may have features of DiGeorge sequence; the chromosomal abnormality is usually submicroscopic, requiring a FISH probe; can segregate in families like an autosomal dominant trait
Wolf-Hirschhorn 46, XX or XY, del 4p16.3	Resembles cri du chat but without the cat cry and with low birth weight; cleft lip or palate; iris coloboma; hypospadias in males; seizures	Incidence—approximately 1 in 50,000 live births; about 10% result from a chromosome imbalance inherited from a normal carrier parent; one-third die by age 2 years, but survival to adulthood is possible

CHD, Congenital heart disease; *FTT,* failure to thrive; *VSD,* ventricular septal defect; *FISH,* fluorescent in situ hybridization.

syndrome is covered in Chapter 5; and Angelman and Prader-Willi syndromes are discussed later in this Chapter. The remaining syndromes are outlined briefly in Table 1-2.

Approach to Dysmorphology

Structural anomalies at birth are categorized as minor or major (Table 1-3 and Figs. 1-11 and 1-12). Minor anomalies, such as epicanthal folds (in whites), simian creases, and raised hemangiomas, are of little physiologic significance, and each one occurs in less than 4% of the popula-

tion. In contrast, major anomalies, such as coloboma of the iris (see Chapter 19), polydactyly, myelomeningocele, congenital heart defects, and cleft lip, have a greater adverse effect on the individual.

Among newborns, 2% to 3% have at least one major anomaly, and this number rises to about 6% by 5 years of age, when more anomalies are recognized. Major anomalies are more likely in premature than full-term newborns. The incidence of any specific major anomaly is less than 1%. Minor anomalies are found in about 15% of newborns and again are more likely in prematures. The probability of an infant having a major anomaly increases with the number of minor anomalies found. If a newborn has no minor anomalies, the probability of finding

TABLE 1-3

Examples of Congenital Anomalies

Category	Minor	Major
Craniofacial	Bony occipital spur Flat occiput Slight micrognathia (3)*	Choanal atresia Severe scapho- cephaly Cleft lip and/or palate (1.5)
Eye	Inner epicanthal folds (4) Short palpebral fissures	Coloboma of iris Cataract
Auricle	Sinus Skin tags (2)	Severely malformed Rudimentary
Skin	Raised hemangioma Café au lait spots	Multiple heman- giomas Posterior webbed neck
Hand	Simian crease (20) Duplication of thumbnail Rudimentary poly- dactyly Clinodactyly of the fifth digit (10)	Polydactyly Absence of thumbs Complete cutaneous syndactyly Absence of all metacarpals
Foot	Partial syndactyly of second and third toes (2) Recessed fifth toes	Absence of nails Equinovarus
Other skeletal regions	Shieldlike chest Cubitus valgus	Short thoracic cage Absence of radius
Miscellaneous	Diastasis recti (>3 cm) Ectopic femoral testes	Neural tube defects Severe hypospadias

*Except as noted in parentheses, the incidence of each is 1 in 1000 liveborns.

a major anomaly is about 1%; with one minor anomaly (14% of new-borns) it is about 3%; with two minor anomalies (0.8% of newborns) it is about 10%; and with three or more minor anomalies (0.5% of newborns) it is about 20%.

The etiology of major congenital anomalies can be divided into three main categories. Disruptions and deformations are mainly the consequence of adverse forces that interfere with normal morphogenesis. Malformations, on the other hand, represent abnormal morphogenesis usually resulting from genetic, chromosomal, or teratogenic influences.

Disruptions and deformations differ mainly in degree. With disruptions, vascular problems or adverse mechanical forces destroy normal morphogenesis, producing severe defects, particularly if this occurs early during embryogenesis. The resulting birth defects usually are too bizarre to represent the orderly progression of morphogenesis; examples include limb reduction defects and/or severe facial clefts. A common cause of disruptions is amniotic bands caused by early amnion rupture. About 1 in 5000 liveborns is affected by amniotic bands to some extent, but the incidence is much higher among spontaneous abortuses. A hallmark of this disruption is constriction bands around various body parts (see Fig. 2-43). Almost all disruptions are sporadic.

Deformations usually are the effect of less severe mechanical forces on morphogenesis; body parts are abnormally molded rather than de-stroyed. This usually is the result of increased uterine pressure on the fetus in whole or in part. For example, a transverse lie or face presentation of the fetus can result in retrognathia or micrognathia and a squashed nose. Premature and prolonged descent of the fetal head into the pelvis can result in sagittal synostosis. Uterine abnormalities, such as fibroma or bicornuate uterus, can decrease the uterine cavity volume available to the fetus, and the same relative problem can result in a normal uterus with relatively large or multiple fetuses.

Oligohydramnios can result in a particularly severe fetal deformation—compression of the thorax, leading to pulmonary hypoplasia and neonatal death. Potter sequence, in which the fetus usually has agenesis of the kidneys or polycystic kidneys, is an example. Because fetal urine output contributes to the volume of amniotic fluid later in gestation, their failure to produce urine or low urine output results in oligohydramnios and the fetus is fatally deformed by uterine pressure (see Fig. 13-36).

Most deformations, however, allow a relatively good prognosis for general growth and development of the newborn, and most are sporadic with a low recurrent risk. However, uterine abnormalities could increase the recurrent risk if not corrected, and conditions like fetal polycystic kidneys, an autosomal recessive condition, have a 25% recurrence risk at each conception for the couple.

Malformations represent abnormal embryonic morphogenesis and are the subject of most of this chapter. A malformation can be a single localized major anomaly or a connected sequence of major anomalies. An isolated cleft palate is an example of a single localized major anomaly. Severe micrognathia, leading secondarily to glossoptosis, leading in turn to U-shaped cleft palate (Pierre Robin syndrome) is an example of a connected sequence of major anomalies. The micrognathia is the primary defect, with the glossoptosis and cleft palate being sequentially secondary to it (see Fig. 22-63).

These localized malformations or sequences, representing a single primary defect in morphogenesis, are usually multifactorial in etiology. That is, they are the result of polygenic influences interacting with the in utero environment. Usually the specifics of the latter are unknown. However, if the polygenic predisposition for clubfoot is inherited, this malformation is more likely to occur if the fetus is in the breach position. Single localized malformations or sequences comprise the majority of major birth defects.

In contrast to single localized malformations or sequences, syndromes of congenital anomalies or recognizable patterns of childhood malformations constitute a group of medical entities that share only the presence at birth of at least two different primary developmental anomalies that individually tend to be rare, are usually genetic in origin, and are variable in degree of expression. The constellation of anomalies defines the syndrome.

Most such malformation syndromes represent the effects of simple mendelian (single genic) inheritance; a few represent the effect of environmental teratogens on the fetus in utero (e.g., rubella, maternal alcohol ingestion, antiepileptic medication). About 10% of these syndromes represent the effect of unique or known chromosomal abnormalities.

The approach to a dysmorphic child is basically the same as with any other medical problem. Of particular importance are good family and pregnancy histories with special emphasis on the possibility of genetic, teratogenic, and environmental problems. The Look at Parents (LAP) test is most important. That is, in taking a history, the parents' statements are particularly unsatisfactory respecting relatively benign birth defects (such as camptodactyly) segregating through a family. Parents often consider such defects "normal" and respond accordingly. If considering Waardenburg syndrome (white forelock, premature graying of hair, hearing loss, iris heterochromia, characteristic facies, au-

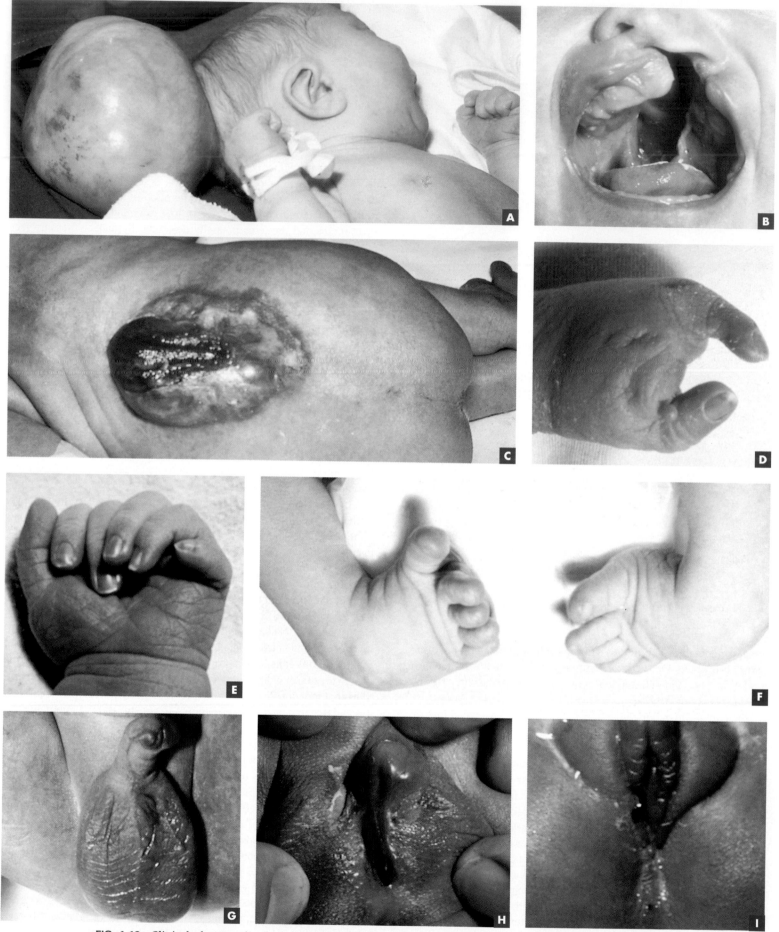

FIG. 1-12   Clinical photographs show several major anomalies seen at birth. *A,* Encephalocele. *B,* Cleft lip and palate. *C,* Meningomyelocele. *D,* Lobster-claw hand. *E,* Polydactyly (postaxial). *F,* Bilateral clubfoot. *G,* Hypospadias. *H,* Fused labia with enlarged clitoris. *I,* Imperforate anus. (Courtesy Dr. Christine L. Williams, New York Medical College.)

tosomal dominant inheritance), the proband's parents (diplomatically) should be asked if they dye their hair. Children resemble their parents, so if the patient has a small head, the parents' head circumferences should be measured. If menses or puberty is late, the onset of this in the mother and father, respectively, should be noted. In examining the patient, minor and major anomalies should be identified. Sometimes a limited but focused examination of the proband's parents and siblings is also helpful.

If the history and physical examination eliminate disruptions, deformations, and single localized major anomalies or sequences, a syndrome of congenital anomalies may be present. For a differential diagnosis of the latter it is helpful to seek a "hallmark" history or physical finding that may define a relatively small diagnostic ballpark. For this purpose, relatively common or amorphous findings, such as mental retardation, mild micrognathia, congenital heart disease, abnormally shaped ears, vertebral defects, and syndactyly, should be avoided. Some specific major anomalies or problems, such as polydactyly, craniosynostosis, microphthalmos, iris coloboma, macrosomia, arachnodactyly, tracheoesophageal fistula, anal defects, hypothyroidism, hypocalcemia, and familial hearing loss, are useful for defining a diagnostic ballpark. Minor anomalies can be as useful as major anomalies in defining a diagnostic ballpark (for example, synophrys, ear tags, short palpebral fissures, raised hemangioma, and café au lait spots).

Having defined a diagnostic ballpark, differential discriminators within the history and physical findings should be sought. For example, if the patient has synophrys (the ballpark): is it simply familial; if not, did the mother take trimethadione during pregnancy; if not, is there microbrachycephaly, small nose with anteverted nostrils, hirsutism, micromelia, or mental retardation, all of which suggest de Lange syndrome; or is there coarse facies with mental retardation, suggesting Sanfilippo syndrome; and so on. Finally, radiographs and laboratory tests likely to confirm the diagnosis should be ordered and followed by appropriate genetic counseling.

A chromosome study should be considered on every child with a syndrome of congenital anomalies. Such a study may establish or confirm the diagnosis of a chromosomal disorder and its hereditary potential and possibly help map the chromosomal location of genes for those syndromes known to be simple mendelian disorders.

Finally, there are several commercial computer programs designed to help diagnose dysmorphology. The medical data are entered and a differential diagnosis is given. However, such computer programs are more likely to be helpful to those already fairly expert in the field.

Abnormalities of Autosomes

Down Syndrome

The worldwide incidence of Down syndrome among liveborns is 1 in 700, with 45% of affected individuals being born to women over 35 years of age. In the United States the incidence is somewhat lower: about 1 in 1100 liveborns, and only 20% are born to women over age 35. This difference represents the effect of elective infertility among older US women and to a lesser extent the impact of antenatal diagnosis leading to selective abortion of Down syndrome fetuses. The incidence of Down syndrome among conceptuses is three times greater than among liveborns, because about two thirds of Down syndrome fetuses spontaneously abort.

There is no single physical stigma of Down syndrome; rather, the clinical diagnosis rests on a gestalt of many minor and a few major anomalies. Although any one of the minor anomalies may be found in a normal person, it is the constellation of several anomalies in one individual that characterizes Down syndrome (Fig. 1-13). The minor anomalies include brachycephaly, inner epicanthal folds, upward slant-

ing eyes, Brushfield spots, small ears, a small upturned nose with saddle bridge, a small mouth with protruding tongue that fissures with age, a short neck with redundant skin folds, simian creases, clinodactyly of the fifth fingers, with single digital crease caused by hypoplasia of the middle phalanx, and a wide space between the first and second toes. The number of such anomalies varies in any particular case.

Other features of Down syndrome are infection-prone dry skin; relatively short stature; rapid aging with premature graying of hair; hypotonia during infancy; wide, flat iliac wings; and a narrow acetabular angle on radiographs. Adult men have reduced libido and are usually impotent (or perhaps sterile). Adult women may have normal libido and are fertile; about one third of their liveborns may have Down syndrome; the rest should be normal. In both genders, puberty is delayed.

Several major anomalies are commonly associated with Down syndrome. Congenital heart disease is found in 45% of cases, particularly atrioventricular communis and ventricular septal defects. All newborns with Down syndrome should undergo cardiac evaluation with echocardiogram. About 7% have a gastrointestinal anomaly, most often duodenal atresia. There is also an increased incidence of thyroid disorders (particularly of the autoimmune type) in Down syndrome individuals, their mothers, and their close relatives. Individuals with Down syndrome should have their thyroid function checked annually by blood T_4 and TSH testing. Acute and neonatal leukemias occur 15 times more frequently in people with Down syndrome than in the general population. In newborns, much of this is represented by transient leukemoid reactions (with complete remission likely) rather than true leukemia. Quantitative abnormalities are found in many enzyme systems. However, the most consistent major anomaly is mental retardation.

With rare exceptions, Down syndrome individuals are mentally retarded. The degree of retardation varies, with ultimate intelligence quotients (IQs) ranging from 20 to 80, and is significantly related to the environment in which the Down syndrome child is raised. A warm, accepting, stimulating upbringing with early special education maximizes the child's intellectual potential. With such an upbringing, over 95% are highly trainable to educable and as adults should be capable of a semi-independent existence within the parents' home or a sheltered workshop. This is facilitated by the fact that their social quotients (SQs) are relatively higher than their IQs. Additionally, mosaic Down syndrome individuals tend to be somewhat brighter than their nonmosaic counterparts, given a comparably positive rearing. There may even be a slight positive correlation between parental IQ and that of the Down syndrome child, but whether this reflects genetic or environmental influences is not known. With rare exceptions, institutionalization is contraindicated because it has an extremely negative effect on the patient's mental development.

The apparent decline in both IQ and SQ with age in Down syndrome individuals may be largely an artifact of testing, particularly in children younger than 12 years. Most Down syndrome children should be tested between the ages of 6 and 8 years for the best estimate of their intellectual potential. Given proper rearing, most Down syndrome children have an IQ between 45 and 55, though there are rare cases with IQ scores between 60 and 85. Autopsy analyses of brains from Down syndrome persons revealed the neuropathologic changes of Alzheimer disease in 1.6% of 20- to 38-year-old individuals and in 100% of those older than 40 years. In the 42- to 69-year-old group the Alzheimer pathologic findings were considered severe in 60% of the cases. Nevertheless, only about 25% of older individuals with Down syndrome exhibit clinical manifestations of Alzheimer disease. The reason for the clinical-pathologic discordance is not known. The life span of Down syndrome individuals is less than that of the general population but about 44% survive to age 60 years and 14% to age 68 years.

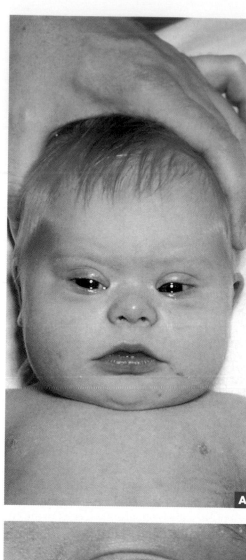

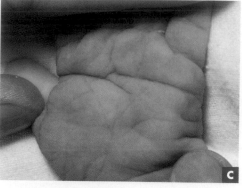

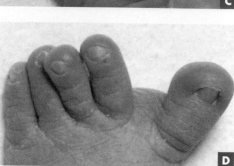

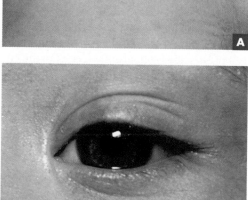

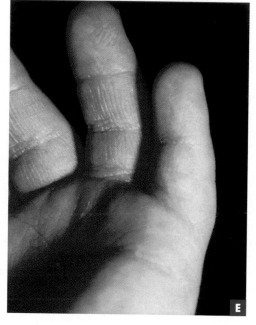

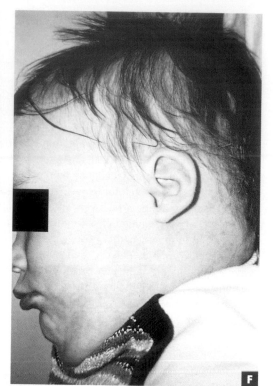

FIG. 1-13 Clinical photographs show several minor anomalies associated with Down syndrome. *A,* Typical facies with upward-slanting eyes, epicanthal folds, small upturned nose with saddle bridge, and protruding tongue. *B,* Brushfield spots. *C,* Simian crease. *D,* Wide space between first and second toes. *E,* Short fifth finger. *F,* Small ears and flat occiput.

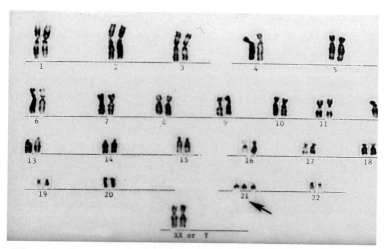

FIG. 1-14   Karyotype of a Down syndrome patient indicates trisomy 21.

The cause of Down syndrome is trisomy 21 (Fig. 1-14). In 95% of cases this is a consequence of meiotic nondisjunction. The extra chromosome 21 is maternally derived in 95% of instances and paternally derived in 5 percent. Aneuploidy in offspring increases with maternal but not paternal age. Consequently a couple's risk of having a liveborn child with Down syndrome is directly correlated with maternal age (Table 1-4). However, once a couple has had a trisomy 21 child, their recurrent risk for a child with some chromosomal abnormality (Down syndrome in half of the cases) is about 1% to 2% overall. In 25% of instances where a normal couple has had a second child with trisomy 21, one of the parents is found to be a low-level mosaic for trisomy 21 cells.

About 1% of Down syndrome cases are chromosomal mosaics with a mixture of normal and trisomy 21 cells. Although mosaicism represents a chromosomal division error occurring after conception, recurrent risk for the couple is still 1% to 2% because 80% of mosaics represent trisomy 21 zygotes.

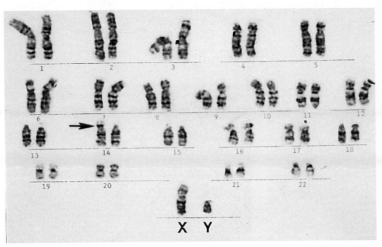

FIG. 1-15 Karyotype of a Down syndrome patient shows 14/21 centric fusion translocation.

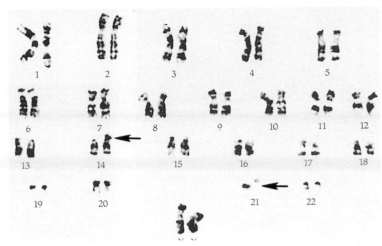

FIG. 1-16 Karyotype of a normal female 14/21 centric fusion translocation carrier (the mother of the Down syndrome patient in Fig. 1-15).

TABLE 1-4

Risk of Down Syndrome in Liveborns (By Maternal Age)

Age (years)	Risk factor
<25	1 in 1600
25-29	1 in 1100
30-34	1 in 700
35-39	1 in 250
40-42	1 in 80
>42	1 in 40

Risk for any chromosomal abnormality in liveborns: maternal age <35 years—1 in 400; 35 to 40 years—1 in 100; >40 years—1 in 50.

About 4% of Down syndrome cases represent a centric fusion translocation between the long arm of a chromosome 21 and those of a 14, 15, 13 (Fig. 1-15) or a 21/22 acrocentric chromosome. Of these, about one third are inherited from a clinically normal, balanced carrier (Fig. 1-16); the remainder are sporadic. Chromosome studies should therefore be performed on the parents and siblings of a translocation Down syndrome individual. If a parent carries a 21/21 translocation, all liveborns will have Down syndrome; for the remaining 21/centric fusion translocations, the empiric recurrent risk for a Down syndrome liveborn is less than 2% if the father is the carrier and 15% if the mother is the carrier. In the United States, Canada, and other highly industrialized Western nations, 20% of Down syndrome individuals die by age 5 (most from congenital heart disease), 56% die by age 60, and 86% die by age 68. The improved longevity in Down syndrome means that a significant proportion of affected individuals will survive both their parents. Consequently, contingency care plans for the Down syndrome child should be made early.

Rarely an individual with the clinical gestalt of Down syndrome has normal chromosomes. Many of these cases represent a cryptic (i.e., submicroscopic) chromosomal rearrangement resulting in three copies of the DNA located in chromosomal area 21q22.2-22.3. Called the *Down syndrome critical region*, triplication of the 50 to 100 genes here accounts for many but not all of Down syndrome features. For exam-

ple, hypotonia, facial features, congenital heart disease, hand anomalies, dermatoglyphics, and some but not all of the mental retardation of Down syndrome map to this area. Mapping outside this area are the GI abnormalities (such as duodenal atresia), Alzheimer-like changes, immunologic problems, and leukemia found in Down syndrome. Such cryptic rearrangements can be detected by FISH technology using the cosmid DNA probe D21S55 (Fig. 1-10, *I* and *J*). They result from submicroscopic *de novo* or inherited translocations or from unequal crossing over during meiosis involving this small area on the long (q) arm of chromosome 21.

Trisomies 13 and 18

Trisomy 13 and 18 are relatively rare chromosomal abnormalities, the incidence being about 1 in 8000 liveborns for trisomy 18 and 1 in 20,000 for trisomy 13. About 95% of trisomy 18 fetuses and most trisomy 13 fetuses abort spontaneously. The major physical features of each abnormality are listed in Table 1-5 and illustrated in Figs. 1-17 and 1-18. There is often much overlap in physical findings between the two syndromes, making it occasionally difficult to distinguish one from the other solely on the basis of clinical evaluation. Both syndromes result in severe mental retardation and usually lead to death within 1 year. Therefore heroic attempts at medical intervention are not encouraged. Since improved general health care, rare cases of survival for 10 to 30 years have been reported (although with significant developmental delay). Chromosomal mosaicism may allow a somewhat better prognosis, particularly for trisomy 18. A relatively normal albeit mildly retarded 20-year-old woman with diploid/trisomy 18 chromosomal mosaicism has been reported.

As in Down syndrome, meiotic nondisjunction is the mechanism for the chromosome error in most cases of trisomies 13 and 18, with risk increasing with maternal age. Occasionally, cases result from centric fusion translocations (spontaneous or inherited) or postconception mosaicism. The recurrence risk for another chromosomally abnormal liveborn is 1% to 2% at any maternal age (but higher when resulting from an inherited translocation); antenatal diagnosis of fetal chromosomal abnormalities is recommended with subsequent pregnancies.

About 20% of liveborns with the physical features of trisomy 13 are chromosomally normal, probably resulting from single-gene–dominant mutations or less often recessive inheritance. Less commonly, chromosomally normal liveborns have the physical features of trisomy 18.

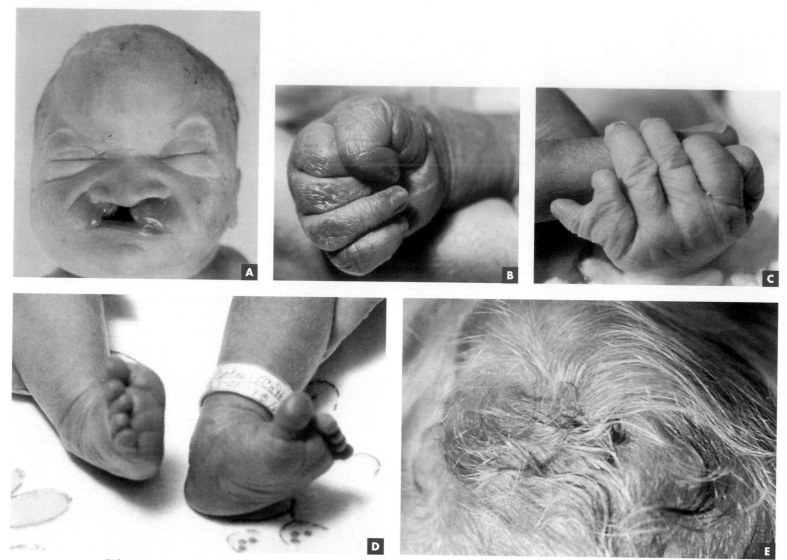

FIG. 1-17 Several physical manifestations of trisomy 13. *A,* Facies showing midline defect. *B,* Clenched hand with overlapping fingers. *C,* Preaxial polydactyly. *D,* Equinovarus deformity. *E,* Typical punched-out posterior scalp lesions. (*A* Courtesy Dr. T. Kelly, University of Virginia Medical Center, Charlottesville; *B* to *E* courtesy Dr. Kenneth Garver, Pittsburgh.)

Such instances may constitute variants of Smith-Lemli-Opitz syndrome, an autosomal recessive trait (see section on Chromosomal-Like Syndromes), or may be the result of maternal ingestion of methotrexate early in pregnancy. The occasional infant who survives methotrexate embryopathy has normal intelligence. However, the prognosis for these other chromosomally normal mimics of trisomy 13 or 18 is not much better than that for the other two. Unfortunately, the negative prognosis is often resisted by parents, physicians, and other health care providers, resulting in fruitless medical-surgical interventions with subsequent frustration and bitterness by all involved. Early frank discus-sions of the realities may be painful but in the long run may be better for all concerned.

Abnormalities of Sex Chromosomes

Turner Syndrome

Turner syndrome is one of the three most common chromosomal ab-normalities found in early spontaneous abortions; only 2% of affected fetuses are born. The phenotype is female. About 1 in 2500 liveborn

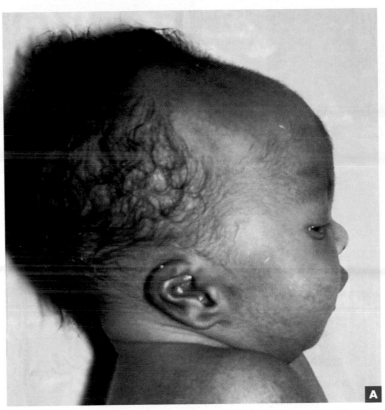

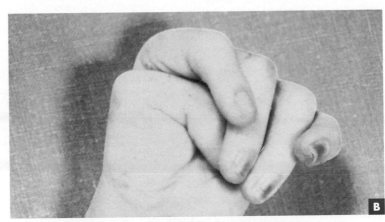

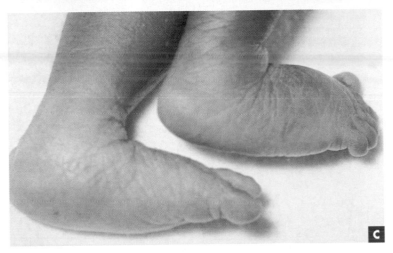

FIG. 1-18 Several physical manifestations of trisomy 18. *A,* Typical profile reveals prominent occiput and low-set, posteriorly rotated malformed auricles. *B,* Clenched hand showing typical pattern of overlapping fingers. *C,* Rocker-bottom feet. (Courtesy Dr. Kenneth Garver, Pittsburgh.)

TABLE 1-5

Physical Abnormalities in Trisomy 13 and 18 Syndromes

Abnormality	Trisomy 13	Trisomy 18
Severe developmental retardation	††††	††††
>90% die within 1st year	††††	††††
Cryptorchidism in males	††††	††††
Low-set, malformed ears	††††	††††
Multiple major congenital anomalies	††††	††††
Prominent occiput	†	††††
Cleft lip and/or palate	†††	†
Micrognathia	††	†††
Microphthalmos	†††	††
Coloboma of iris	†††	†
Short sternum	†	†††
Rocker-bottom feet	††	†††
Congenital heart disease	††	††††
Scalp defects (of skin)	†††	†
Flexion deformities of fingers	††	††††
Polydactyly	†††	†
Hypoplasia of nails	††	†††
Hypertonia in infancy	†	†††
Apneic spells in infancy	†††	†
Midline brain defects	†††	†
Persistence of Hgb F	††††	†
Horseshoe kidneys	†	†††

Relative frequency: ††††, usual; †, rare.

females has Turner syndrome. Primary amenorrhea, sterility, sparse pubic-axillary hair, underdeveloped breasts, and short stature ($4\frac{1}{2}$ to 5 ft) are the usual manifestations. These women have an infantile uterus, and their ovaries consist only of strands of fibrous connective tissue. Other physical features may include webbing of the neck, cubitus valgus, a low hairline, shield chest, renal anomalies, and congenital heart disease, particularly coarctation of the aorta (in 20% of cases) (Fig. 1-19). Newborns often have lymphedema of the feet and/or hands, which can reappear briefly during adolescence. Mental development is usually normal. However, average full-scale IQ is somewhat lower than that of the general population, reflecting a decrease in performance rather than verbal IQ. Schooling and behavioral problems seem to be the same as in age-matched control subjects. Difficulty with spatial orientation, such as map reading, may be a problem. The classic physical findings of Turner syndrome may be absent or so minimal in the newborn that the diagnosis is missed. The first indication may be unexplained short stature in later childhood or failure of the secondary sex characteristics to develop by late adolescence. Thus a chromosome study is indicated as part of the diagnostic workup of adolescent girls with these complaints.

The chromosome error in 60% of individuals with Turner syndrome is 45XO. Most often, the missing sex chromosome is paternally derived, so the risk of Turner syndrome does not increase with parental age. Another 15% of individuals with Turner syndrome are mosaics (XO/XX, XO/XX/XXX, or XO/XY). The physical stigmata may be less marked in mosaics, some of whom may be fertile. If an XY cell line is present, the intraabdominal gonads should be removed because they are prone to malignant change. The remaining cases of Turner syndrome have 46 chromosomes, including one normal plus one structurally abnormal X. The latter may have a short (p) arm deletion or may be an isochrome duplication of the long (q) arm of the X chromosome; usually it is pa-

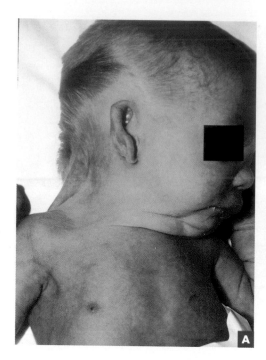
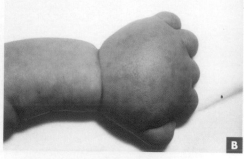
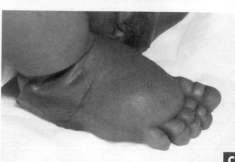

FIG. 1-19 Clinical photographs show several physical manifestations associated with Turner syndrome. *A,* Webbed neck with low hairline, shield chest with widespread nipples, abnormal ears, and micrognathia. *B* and *C,* Lymphedema of hands and feet.

ternally derived. Cases of Turner syndrome with one normal and one abnormal X chromosome are more likely to have other, more serious major anomalies, including mental retardation. A structurally abnormal X chromosome may lead to abnormal X inactivation (Fig. 1-23), resulting in a deleterious dosage effect for X-linked genes. Karyotypes such as 46XYp- or 46Xi(Yq) result in a female with Turner syndrome. Also, recent research suggests that a significant proportion of females with Turner syndrome may have some submicroscopic Y chromosome material in their genome. The clinical significance of this if any is still not clear.

Whereas loss of the short arm of an X chromosome results in full-blown Turner syndrome, deletion of the long arm usually produces only streak (fibrous) gonads with consequent sterility, amenorrhea, and infantile secondary sex characteristics without the other somatic stigmata of Turner syndrome. A buccal smear for sex chromatin is a poor diagnostic test for Turner syndrome because mosaics, partial deletions, and isochromes can be sex-chromatin positive. If the diagnosis is clinically suspected, a G-banded chromosome study should be ordered. Should the affected child be 45XO or a mosaic, the parental risk for recurrence of a chromosomally abnormal liveborn is 1% to 2% but may be higher if a parent carries a structurally abnormal X chromosome.

Antenatal diagnosis of chromosomally abnormal fetuses should be discussed with the parents, and the relatively good prognosis for Turner syndrome liveborns should not be overlooked. Girls with Turner syndrome should receive appropriate hormone therapy during adolescence to develop their secondary sex characteristics and stimulate menses.

Rarely, 45XO women with Turner syndrome have been fertile for a limited number of years. However, infertile women with Turner syndrome can bear children by implantation of an in vitro fertilized donor egg into their hormonally prepared and maintained uterus. Growth hormone therapy has had some limited success with Turner syndrome girls, but its safety and efficacy are still under investigation.

Klinefelter Syndrome

About 20% of aspermic adult men, 1 in 250 men over 6 ft tall, and 1 in 1080 newborn boys have Klinefelter syndrome. The physical stigmata usually are not obvious until puberty, at which time the normal onset of spermatogenesis is blocked by the presence of two X chromosomes. Consequently the germ cells die, the seminiferous tubules become hyalinized and scarred, and the testes become small. Testosterone levels are below the normal adult man's level, though the level varies from case to case (the average is about half as much as normal). This then leads to a wide range of virilization in these cases. At one extreme is the eunuchoid man with a small penis and gynecomastia (Fig. 1-20); at the opposite extreme is the virile mesomorph with a normal penis. Scoliosis may develop during adolescence. Libido may be reduced in adult men, virtually all of whom are sterile. Libido may be improved by testosterone therapy, but whether this reflects a pharmacologic or a psychologic effect is not clear. Homosexuality is not more common with Klinefelter syndrome than in the general population. The average full-scale IQ of men with Klinefelter syndrome is 98, which is about the

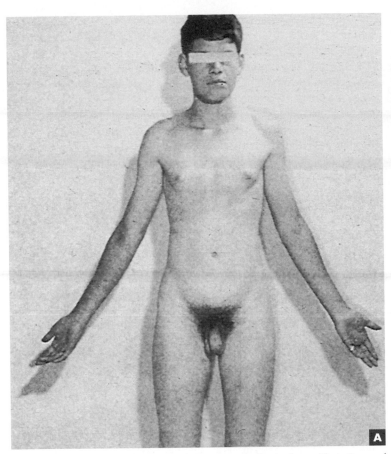

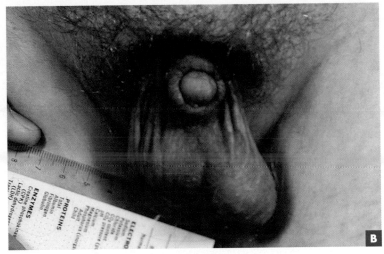

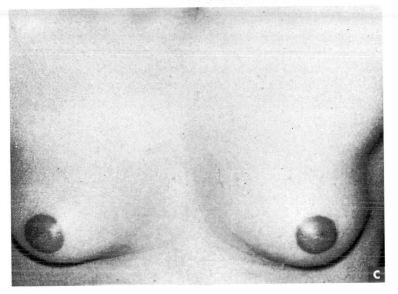

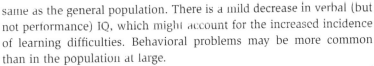

FIG. 1-20 Clinical photographs show several physical manifestations of Klinefelter syndrome. *A*, Eunuchoid body habitus, relatively narrow shoulders, increased carrying angle of arms, female distribution of pubic hair, normal penis, and small scrotum because of small size of testes. *B*, Small testes and penis. *C*, Gynecomastia. (*B* courtesy Dr. Peter Lee, University of Pittsburgh School of Medicine; *C* from Gardner LI, ed: *Endocrine and genetic diseases of childhood*, ed 2, Philadelphia, 1975, WB Saunders.)

same as the general population. There is a mild decrease in verbal (but not performance) IQ, which might account for the increased incidence of learning difficulties. Behavioral problems may be more common than in the population at large.

Testosterone treatment should begin at about 11 or 12 years of age if in vivo levels do not result in virilization. Such treatment also prevents gynecomastia, which occurs in 40% of cases. Once gynecomastia occurs, it can be corrected only by surgery.

The karyotype in Klinefelter syndrome is XXY in 80% of cases and mosaic (XY/XXY) in the other 20%. Rarely the latter type may be fertile. About 60% of cases reflect a chromosome error in oogenesis; 40% an error in spermatogenesis. Risk of having an affected child increases with maternal age. Males with more than two X chromosomes (XXXY, XXXXY) are usually mentally retarded and are more likely to have skeletal and other major congenital anomalies such as cleft palate, congenital heart disease (particularly a patent ductus arteriosus), and microcephaly. The parents' recurrent risk for another chromosomally abnormal liveborn is 1% to 2%; antenatal diagnosis with subsequent pregnancies should be discussed.

XXX and XYY Syndromes

Triple X females have no characteristic physical stigmata. However, intelligence is reduced, and about one fourth are mildly retarded. Educational but not behavioral problems are more common than in age-matched controls. The parental risk for an XXX daughter increases with

maternal age. XXX women are fertile, and their offspring are usually chromosomally normal. About 1 in 1000 liveborn girls is triple X.

About 1 in 350 men over 6 ft tall and 1 in 1000 newborn boys are XYY. Such males have no pathognomonic physical stigmata, and IQ is normal. The prevalence of XYY men in a prison population is severalfold greater than their proportion in the general population. This led to the erroneous conclusion that XYY men must be overly aggressive and antisocial, presumably because of the extra Y chromosome. In fact, XYY males are typically neither. Educational and behavioral problems in XYY young boys are similar to those in age-matched controls. Their disproportionate numbers in prisons—usually for nonaggressive crimes—is for reasons that remain unclear. Since XYY males reflect a chromosomal error in their father's spermatogenesis, the recurrent risk does not increase with parental age. XYY men are fertile, and their offspring are usually chromosomally normal. Because parents of XXX females and XYY males have the usual 1% to 2% recurrent risk for chromosomally abnormal liveborns, antenatal diagnosis should be discussed. It also is advisable for XXX females and XYY males to consider antenatal diagnosis with their own pregnancies.

Sex and Gender

Sex is determined by chromosomes, but gender is a psychosocial definition. The latter is the prime consideration to the medical practitioner. When sex and gender are not compatible, anatomic, physiologic, and psychosocial considerations should determine the final gender assign-

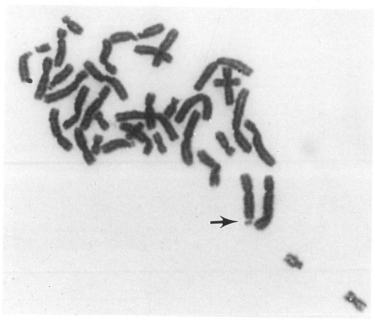

FIG. 1-21 Fragile X chromosome marker in lymphocyte culture. Partial metaphase plate shows the chromosome break at Xq27 (*arrow*) characteristic of fragile X syndrome (solid Giemsa stain).

ment of the individual. Finally, although XO, XXY, XYY, and XXX fetuses can be detected in utero by chorionic villous sampling or amniocentesis and in newborns by routine chromosome screening, the relatively benign clinical course of these conditions should be an important factor in the genetic counseling for these conditions.

Molecular Cytogenetic Syndromes

Advances in molecular genetics during the last 8 to 10 years have provided new insights into the genetic pathogenesis of several syndromes often associated with specific cytogenetic abnormalities.

Fragile X Syndrome

It has been long recognized that there is a significant excess (about 25%) of males in moderately to severely mentally retarded populations. Much of this inordinate male representation is the result of defective recessive X-linked genes. These may represent new mutations or inheritances from normal heterozygous (carrier) mothers. About 1 in 150 individuals, usually male, has some form of X-linked mental retardation—including one fifth with fragile X syndrome.

In 1969, Herbert Lubs noted the in vitro cytogenetic marker now called *fragile X* in short-term lymphocyte cultures. However, its clinical significance was not realized until a 1977 report by G.R. Sutherland in Australia. Under tissue culture conditions that starve the cell of its ability to synthesize thymidilic acid, a chromosome break at Xq27, the distal part of the long arm of the X chromosome (Fig. 1-21), is visible in cells of individuals clinically affected with fragile X syndrome. By pedigree analysis, about 1 in 1100 males has the fragile X gene but only 80% (1 in 1400) show clinical manifestations. About 1 in 750 females has the fragile X gene but only 30% (1 in 2500) are clinically affected (i.e., the fragile X gene is 80% penetrant in males and 30% penetrant in females). Females with the fragile X gene usually are heterozygotes and, when clinically normal, are called *carrier females*. Having only one X chromosome, males with the fragile X gene are of course hemizygous and, when clinically normal, are called *transmitting males*.

Males affected with fragile X syndrome are mentally retarded to borderline IQ; about 90% have an IQ between 20 and 49, and the remainder fall in the 50 to borderline IQ range. The IQ may decline with age. The majority have speech delay, short attention span, hyperactivity, persistence of mouthing objects, and poor motor coordination. Whereas autism is no more frequent than in other mentally retarded children, disciplinary problems, temper tantrums, poor eye contact, perseverative speech, hand flapping, avoidance of socialization, and rocking are common. Physical stigmata may include long, wide, or protruding ears; long face; prominent jaw; flattened nasal bridge; and high arched palate (Fig. 1-22, *A* and *B*). Some have "velvety" skin, hyperextensible joints, and mitral valve prolapse. Relative macrocephaly is more likely than microcephaly. Macroorchidism is found in most adults and 20% of prepubescent boys as a consequence of interstitial testicular edema (Fig. 1-22, *C*), although affected males may still be fertile.

R.J. Hagerman and others have developed a checklist to help diagnose males affected with fragile X syndrome. A total score of 16 or more gives a 50% probability of a correct diagnosis on laboratory testing. The 13 items on the checklist are as follows: mental retardation, hyperactivity, short attention span, tactilely defensive, hand flapping, hand biting, poor eye contact, perseverative speech, hyperextensible metacarpophalangeal joints, large or prominent ears, large testicles, simian crease or Sydney line (a simian crease which is jagged in the middle), and a family history of mental retardation. Each of these items is scored as follows: 0 if not present, 1 if present in the past or borderline, or 2 if present.

Females affected with fragile X syndrome are less severely retarded than males; about 35% fall in the 20-49 IQ range and the remainder fall in the 50 to borderline IQ range. However, learning disabilities; mood disorders, such as unipolar and bipolar diseases; schizoid personality; and significant disturbances in affect, socialization, and communication are common. The physical features often seen in males with fragile X syndrome are less common in females.

In most clinically affected patients, the fragile X chromosome marker can be detected in peripheral blood lymphocytes cultured in special medium, as described previously. Detection is somewhat less feasible using tissue cultures of skin fibroblasts or of fetal aminocytes. The range of expression in cultured lymphocytes is 1% to 50% positive cells (average 25% in affected males, 15% in affected females). Occasionally a normal person expresses the fragile X chromosome marker in no more than 1 in 200 cells. This is of no known significance. Males and females who carry the fragile X gene (by pedigree analysis) but are clinically normal are unlikely to express the fragile X chromosome marker in vitro. Since this test requires special media, the clinician must specify the fragile X test when sending a blood sample to the genetics laboratory for analysis.

Fragile X syndrome is the first example of a trinucleotide repeat disorder. The gene involved, located at Xq27.3, is called *FMR-1* and is active in brain and sperm. At the start of the gene is the DNA trinucleotide CGG, which in the general population is normally linearly repeated about 5 to 50 times (the average being 30). From 52 to 200 linear CGG repeats is considered a fragile X premutation. Individuals with a premutation appear clinically normal. Over 200 linear CGG repeats is considered a full mutation and in males results in fragile X syndrome. In females with over 200 linear CGG repeats, there are clinical effects in 60% and apparently little or no effect in 40%. The reason for this disparity in females most likely is X chromosome inactivation (Fig. 1-23). If the full mutation is on the inactive X chromosome in a female cell, that cell is not harmed by it. Therefore, if by chance the majority of a female's cells have the fragile X mutation on their inactive X chromosome, she is not harmed and vice versa. Premutation and, in females, X inactivation explain lack of penetrance of the fragile X gene discussed earlier.

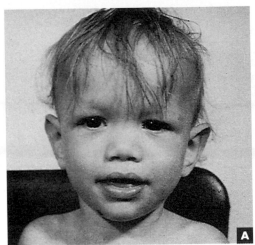 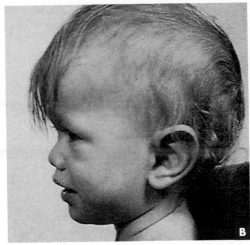 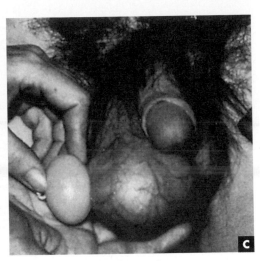

FIG. 1-22 Physical findings in fragile X syndrome. *A* and *B*, Note the long, wide, and protruding ears, elongated face, and flattened nasal bridge. *C*, Macroorchidism in adult man with fragile X syndrome caused by interstitial testicular edema. (*A* and *B* from Simko A, Hornstein L, Soukup S, Bagamery N: Fragile X syndrome: recognition in young children, *Pediatrics* 83(4):547-552, 1989; *C* from Hagerman RJ: Fragile X syndrome. In Lockhart JD, ed: *Current problems in pediatrics,* vol 17, no 2, Chicago, 1987, Year Book Medical Publishers.)

There do not seem to be any new mutations for these FMR-1 gene CGG trinucleotide expansions. That is, all such expansions are inherited from a parent. A man with a premutation passes it on to all of his daughters as a premutation. A man with a full mutation (i.e., affected with fragile X syndrome) also passes on a premutation, not a full mutation, to all of his daughters. The reason for this is as follows: full mutations are unstable in tissues including germ cells so that in some cells full mutations break down into premutations. In cells with a full mutation but not a premutation the FMR-1 gene is inactive because of methylation that turns the gene off. Consequently, only sperm with a premutation and therefore an active FMR-1 gene can fertilize. Men with premutations or full mutations pass neither to their sons because they give their Y chromosome to their sons.

Women heterozygous for either a premutation or full mutation have a 50% chance of passing it on to each child as follows: if she has a full mutation, she passes it on as a full mutation in most instances; if she has a premutation, she passes it on to her child either as a premutation or expanded into a full mutation, depending on the size of her own premutation. A mother with a premutation up to 60 CGG repeats has little chance of an expansion to a full mutation in her child; with 61 to 80 CGG repeats, there is a 30% chance of a full mutation expansion; with 81 to 90 CGG repeats, there is an 80% chance of a full mutation expansion; and if there are over 90 CGG repeats, the chance of expansion to a full mutation in the child is almost 100%.

Laboratory testing for fragile X mutations is done by molecular genetic rather than the cytogenetic techniques described earlier. The standard molecular genetic test is Southern blot analysis of DNA extracted from cells, usually in blood (Fig. 1-24). This requires 5 to 10 ml of blood in a purple top tube. Another molecular genetic technique, polymerase chain reaction (PCR) analysis of DNA, can be done with less blood. These techniques also can be applied to fetal cells for the purpose of antenatal diagnosis. However, if the fetus is a female with a full mutation, it is impossible to predict with certainty whether or not the fetus after birth would be clinically affected with fragile X syndrome because of the influence of X inactivation.

Rarely, an individual may seem to have a mild form of fragile X syndrome but tests negative by these molecular genetic laboratory techniques. In these instances, cytogenetic fragile X testing might be helpful. Apparently, there is another fragile X gene site (FRAXE) distal to the fragile X gene on Xq that is associated with mental retardation and a positive fragile X cytogenetic laboratory test.

The number of known trinucleotide expansion disorders is increasing. Three examples are as follows: Huntington disease, which is caused by a linear CAG trinucleotide expansion in its gene at the end of chromosome 4p; myotonic dystrophy, resulting from a linear CTG expansion in its gene on chromosome 19q; and spinobulbar muscular atrophy because of a linear CAG expansion in its gene on the proximal part of chromosome Xq.

Imprinting Syndromes

Prader-Willi and Angelman Syndromes

Two syndromes associated with chromosomal abnormalities and imprinting are Prader-Willi and Angelman syndromes (Figs. 1-25 and 1-26). Imprinting means that the functioning of a gene is dependent on its parental origin. Newborns affected with Prader-Willi syndrome usually are markedly hypotonic. Decreased fetal movement in utero and a breech fetal position are common. Although birth is usually at term, birth weights tend to be below 3000 g. In neonates, poor sucking and swallowing reflexes predispose to choking episodes that can cause respiratory problems. The cry may be weak. Although Moro and deep tendon reflexes often are decreased, the neurologic evaluation is otherwise unremarkable. Motor development is delayed, and most patients are mildly to moderately mentally retarded (IQ range 35 to 85), with particular delay in speech. Hypotonia abates over the next 2 to 3 years, but patients develop an uncontrollable appetite that rapidly produces marked obesity. The distribution of excess fat is particularly thick over the lower trunk, buttocks, and proximal limbs (Fig. 1-25, *A*). Although the facies are not particularly dysmorphic, they are similar in most Prader-Willi syndrome patients. The eyes often are described as "almond shaped," and strabismus is common. The bifrontal diameter is narrow and the face is "fat" (particularly around the cheeks and chin), the mouth is "fishlike" in shape, and the ears may be slightly dysplas-

X-CHROMOSOME INACTIVATION

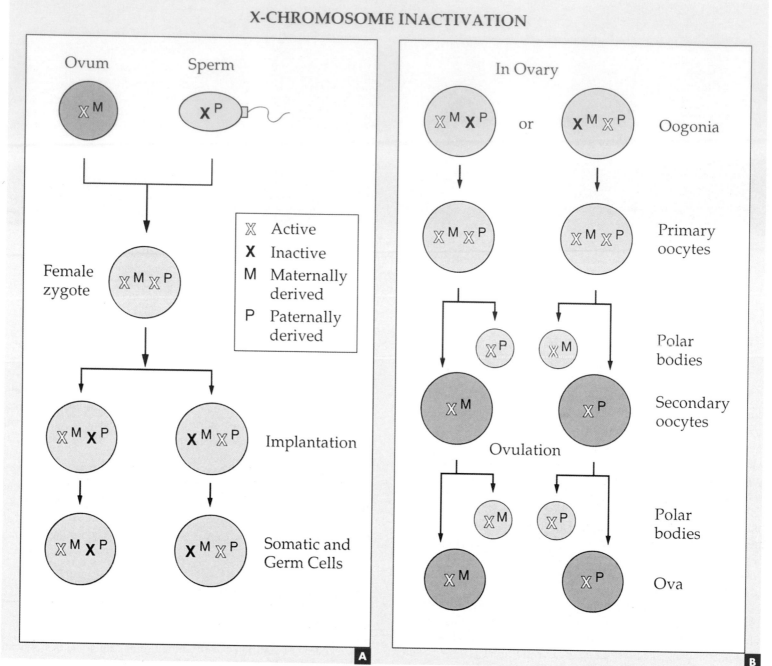

FIG. 1-23 Functional behavior of the X chromosome in XX females. *A,* Somatic and premeiotic germ cells. Implantation occurs 5 days after conception, at which time in each female cell either X^M or X^P is randomly genetically inactivated and remains so in each of the cell's descendants. Because the process is random, by determining the proportion of cells with an inactive X^M or inactive X^P in each of a large population of women, a Gaussian population distribution of women is generated. That is, most women in the population will have an approximate 50/50 mix of cells, in which each cell expresses either X^M or X^P. However, some women will have by chance more cells with an inactive X^M and vice versa. *B,* Meiotic germ cells. When a female germ cell enters in first prophase of meiosis, X inactivation is abolished; both X chromosomes become genetically active through fertilization and continue so until embryonic uterine implantation. Then, as in *A,* random X inactivation in XX females occurs all over again.

tic. Hypopigmentation being common, the patient usually has blonde to light brown hair, blue eyes, and sun-sensitive fair skin. Picking of skin sores can become a problem. Hands and feet are noticeably small from birth (Fig. 1-25, *B*), and the stature of the older child and adult is short. The penis and testes remain small, and the scrotum is atrophic in males with Prader-Willi syndrome (Fig. 1-25, *C*), although the penis can be enlarged by testosterone therapy. If the testes are cryptorchid,

surgical correction should be attempted. Menarche in females is delayed or absent, and menses, when present, are sparse and irregular. The gonadotropic hormone levels are reduced in both sexes. No patient with Prader-Willi syndrome has been known to reproduce.

Of particular concern in older children with Prader-Willi syndrome are the problems of emotional lability and extreme temper tantrums. These conditions and the overeating can often be partly ameliorated by

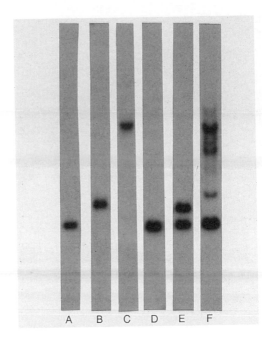

FIG. 1-24 Fragile X Southern blot DNA test. DNA is extracted from cells (usually blood), digested with a restriction enzyme, and then placed in slots at the top of an agarose gel. The smaller the DNA segment, the further down the gel it moves when an electric current is applied to the gel. Next, the electrophoresed DNA is transferred from the gel to a nylon membrane and hybridized with a radioactive labeled DNA probe for part of the FMR-1 gene, which includes the CGG repeat region. Then, x-ray film is applied to the nylon membrane for several days and an autoradiograph results, as above. By comparing the DNA migration to that of a standard, its number of CGG repeats can be calculated. *A,* Normal male; *B,* premutation male; *C,* full mutation male; *D,* normal female; *E,* premutation female showing one normal allele (*bottom*) and one premutation allele (*top*); *F,* full mutation female showing one normal allele (*bottom*) and a full mutation allele (*top*), which has broken down postconception into several alleles of different size. Any one cell, however, would contain only two alleles: the one normal allele and one of the several-sized abnormal alleles. Note that the lower one of the latter here is in the premutation size range. (Courtesy Mr. James H. Cummins, Children's Hospital of Pittsburgh.)

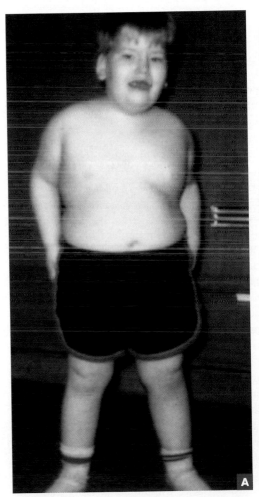

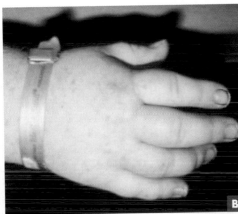

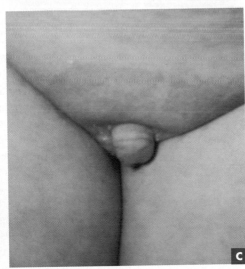

FIG. 1-25 Prader-Willi syndrome. *A,* This patient demonstrates the marked obesity characteristic of Prader-Willi syndrome. Excess fat is distributed over the trunk, buttocks, and proximal extremities. *B* and *C,* Small hands (and feet) and hypoplastic penis and scrotum are other typical features. (*A* courtesy Dr. Jeanne M. Hanchett, The Rehabilitation Institute of Pittsburgh; *B* and *C* courtesy Dr. Holly W. Davis, Children's Hospital of Pittsburgh.)

intensive inpatient behavioral modification programs followed by longitudinal parental support and follow-up in the home. Interestingly, despite a normal basal metabolic rate, weight reduction requires significantly more severe caloric restriction in these patients than in normal persons. Diabetes mellitus can develop in the older child, and its incidence is correlated with the severity of obesity. Although it tends to be insulin resistant, the condition responds well to treatment with oral hy-

poglycemic agents. Life expectancy is shortened by cardiorespiratory complications related to the extreme obesity (pickwickian syndrome).

Angelman syndrome was described about 10 years after Prader-Willi syndrome was first recognized in 1956. Except for the tendency to have hypopigmentation, the clinical phenotypes of the two disorders are quite different. Patients with Angelman syndrome are severely mentally retarded. Speech is impaired or absent, and inappropriate paroxysms of

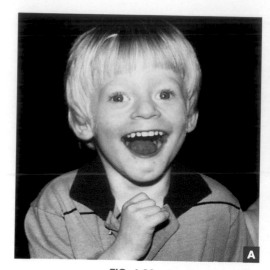
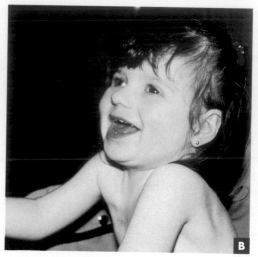
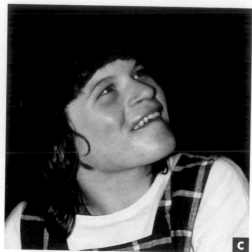

FIG. 1-26   Angelman syndrome. *A* to *C,* Three patients with typical facies. Note the maxillary hypoplasia, large mouth (often with protruding tongue), and prognathism. (Courtesy Drs. C.A. Williams and J. Hendrickson, University of Florida, Gainesville.)

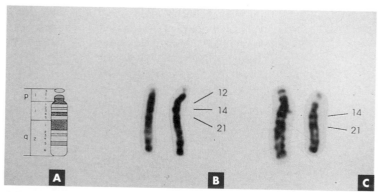

FIG. 1-27   High-resolution banding in Prader-Willi syndrome. The diagram of a high-resolution analysis of chromosome 15 is shown on the left. In pair *B* both chromosomes are normal, whereas in pair *C* the band q12 is deleted from the paternally derived chromosome 15 (*right-most*) in a patient with Prader-Willi syndrome. Note that in higher-resolution chromosome preparations, banding patterns become more and more subdivided. This allows detection of increasingly smaller structural abnormalities. However, as the number of bands increases, cytogenetic analysis becomes progressively more difficult. To avoid error, the clinician should provide sufficient medical information to help the laboratory personnel decide specifically where to look for very small structural abnormalities in the patient's karyotype. Blanket requests for high-resolution chromosome studies should be avoided.

laughter are common. Physical features include microbrachycephaly, maxillary hypoplasia, large mouth with protruding and "flickering" tongue, prognathism, and short stature (in adults) (Fig. 1-26, *A* to *C*). The gait is ataxic, with a tiptoe walk and jerky arm movements resembling those of a marionette, hence its designation as the "happy puppet syndrome." Akinetic or major motor seizures are common. Although survival to adulthood is possible, no patient with Angelman syndrome has been known to reproduce. Prader-Willi and Angelman syndromes are imprinting syndromes; that is, they reflect on the fact that the func-

tion of some genes depends on their parental origin. This seems to be particularly true of some genes located in chromosome area 15q11.2-13. At the more proximal end of this area is a set of genes that normally is turned off on the maternally derived 15 chromosome. In about 70% of Prader-Willi syndrome cases this area is physically deleted on the paternally derived 15 chromosome. Consequently the individual cannot make gene products for this area and has Prader-Willi syndrome. This deletion can be detected most reliably with a FISH SNRPN DNA probe (Fig. 1-10, *C* and *D*). It often can be detected by high-resolution cytogenetic technology (Fig. 1-27). About 28% of Prader-Willi syndrome patients do not have the aforementioned deletion, but rather both of their 15 chromosomes are derived from their mother. This is called *maternal heterodisomy* or *isodisomy*. It results from a trisomy 15 zygote caused by a maternal meiotic error with subsequent early embryonic loss of the paternal 15 chromosome. For deletion and disomy cases, the recurrence risk is less than 1%. A small percentage of Prader-Willi syndrome cases demonstrate neither paternal deletion nor maternal disomy, and in these rare instances there may be a higher recurrence risk.

Angelman syndrome results from the same mechanisms as Prader-Willi syndrome except that the deletion is more distal in the 15q11.2-q13 area and may involve only a single gene normally turned off on the paternally derived 15 chromosome. About 60% of cases demonstrate a deletion here on the maternally derived 15 chromosome using high-resolution cytogenetics (Fig. 1-27) or DNA FISH probe D15S10, which is more accurate. Of Angelman syndrome cases, 2% result from a paternal 15 chromosome disomy and the remaining cases have neither a demonstrable deletion nor disomy. The recurrence risk for the former two is less than 1%, but for those cases without a maternal deletion or paternal disomy, the recurrence risk is 5% to 50% at each conception. Genetic evaluation of the family in this last case might allow for a more precise estimate of recurrence risk.

Chromosomal-Like Syndromes

As already mentioned, some syndromes without a detectable chromosomal abnormality have clinical features that suggest a chromosomal

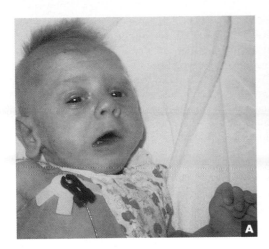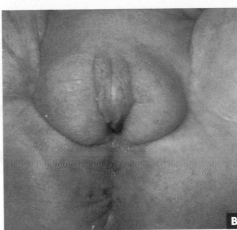

FIG. 1-28 Smith-Lemli-Opitz syndrome. *A,* Note the anteverted nostrils, low-set ears, small chin, and clenched hand. *B,* Hypospadias, cryptorchidism, or ambiguous genitalia as shown here also may be seen. (Courtesy Dr. W. Tunnessen, Children's Hospital of Philadelphia.)

disorder, hence these enter into the differential diagnosis of the latter. Some of the more common syndromes in this class include the CHARGE and VATER associations and the Smith-Lemli-Opitz, Cornelia de Lange, Noonan, and fetal alcohol syndromes.

Smith-Lemli-Opitz Syndrome

Smith-Lemli-Opitz syndrome (SLOS) is an autosomal recessive, simple, mendelian genetic disorder, although it shares many physical features with trisomy 18. Approximately 1 in 20,000 live births is affected. Heretofore there had been no specific laboratory test or treatment for this condition. Recently, however, defective cholesterol biosynthesis has been reported in patients with Smith-Lemli-Opitz syndrome, which might allow a confirmatory laboratory test for the syndrome and perhaps palliative treatment with a high-cholesterol diet and bile acid replacement. Apparently there is a blockage in the final step of cholesterol biosynthesis, resulting in a cholesterol deficiency and an excess of possibly toxic cholesterol precursors, particularly 7-dehydrocholesterol (DHC). The deficiency of cholesterol and the toxicity of DHC are hypothesized to cause the clinical feature of SLOS, particularly deficiency of central nervous system myelination and cataracts. Affected infants tend to be small for gestational age and often are born via breech presentation after a pregnancy noted for decreased fetal movements. Patients have microcephaly with a prominent occiput and narrow frontal area. Facial stigmata include eyelid ptosis, epicanthal folds, strabismus, low-set or posteriorly rotated ears, broad nasal tip with upturned nares, and micrognathia (Fig. 1-28, *A*). Simian crease of the palm and syndactyly of the second and third toes are characteristic; in males, hypospadias with cryptorchidism and even ambiguous genitalia are other usual findings (Fig. 1-28, *B*). Clenched hands, digital abnormalities, cataracts, cleft palate, and bifid uvula also are seen in some cases. Radiographs may reveal stippled epiphyses. Structural abnormalities of the CNS (at times associated with seizures), heart, GI tract, and/or kidneys are common. Initial hypotonia progresses to hypertonia with irritable behavior, shrill screaming, and feeding problems. Affected infants fail to thrive. By age 18 months, 80% of infants with the disorder die, most in the first year. Only a few survive longer than 4 years, and these

are moderately to severely mentally retarded. Cholesterol therapy appears to allow some improvement.

Being an autosomal recessive disorder, the recurrence risk for a couple with an affected child is 25% for each subsequent conception. This risk can be reduced by artificial insemination of the mother; a healthy, unrelated sperm donor should be used. Antenatal diagnosis also may be attempted using high-resolution ultrasound of the fetus to look for intrauterine growth retardation and major organ structural abnormalities and by biochemical analysis of amniotic fluid and cultured amniocytes obtained through amniocentesis.

CHARGE Association

CHARGE is an acronym for a nonrandom association of features including *c*oloboma of the retina or less commonly the iris; *h*eart abnormalities; *a*tresia of the choanae; *r*etarded growth and mental development; *g*enital hypoplasia in males; and *e*ar anomalies that can include deafness. The minimal diagnostic criteria should include abnormalities in four of the six categories—of which at least one must be coloboma or choanal atresia (Fig. 1-29). Cleft lip and/or palate and renal abnormalities sometimes are found, as in the DiGeorge sequence. The syndrome includes congenital heart disease, particularly abnormalities of the aortic arch, right subclavian artery, or ventricular septal defect; agenesis or hypoplasia of the thymus with decreased T-cell production and impaired cell-mediated immunity; partial or less often complete absence of the parathyroid glands, manifested by hypocalcemia and neonatal tetany; and often a facies characterized by wide-spaced, slightly down-slanting eyes, anteverted nares, a short philtrum, and small abnormal ears (see Fig. 4-42). Infants with CHARGE association often die early as a result of their congenital anomalies, but many survive to adulthood. Although there is developmental delay, the IQ range is broad (<30 to 80). Men often have a micropenis that responds to testosterone therapy, whereas women usually have amenorrhea and poor development of secondary sex characteristics.

In the neonate, CHARGE association must be differentiated from chromosomal disorders, such as trisomy 13 or 18, and the more benign nonchromosomal VATER association. Although chromosome studies should be normal in CHARGE association, when the DiGeorge se-

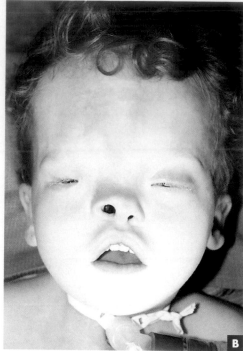

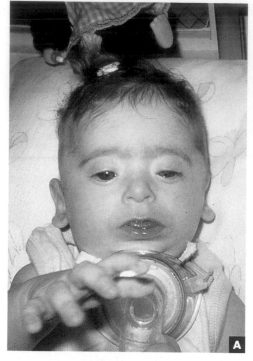

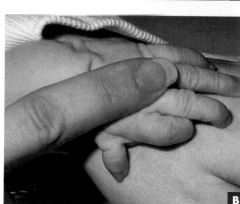

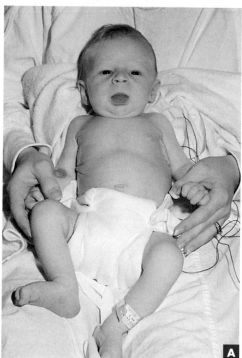

FIG. 1-29 CHARGE association. *A*, Note small left eye with ptosis; low-set, posteriorly rotated, anomalous auricles; and small chin. Choanal atresia necessitated tracheotomy. *B*, Another infant with CHARGE association reveals broad forehead, widespread eyes with narrow palpebral fissures, hypoplastic right nares, low-set ears, and Cupid's bow mouth. (*A* courtesy Dr. W. Tunnessen, Children's Hospital of Philadelphia; *B* courtesy Dr. Timothy McBride, Georgetown University Medical Center.)

FIG. 1-30 Although this child with VATER association has a relatively normal facial appearance, radial dysplasia and an abnormal thumb are present.

quence is present, a small interstitial deletion of chromosome 22 at q11 occasionally is found with high-resolution cytogenetic techniques and FISH DNA probe (Fig. 1-10, *A* and *B*).

The etiology of CHARGE association is unknown, but most likely it is heterogeneous. Although most cases are sporadic, instances of affected siblings and an affected parent and offspring have been reported. The risk of recurrence for a couple with one affected child is about 1% to 4%; however, if there are two affected siblings, this rises to approximately 25% for each subsequent conception. If an affected parent has an affected child, the risk of recurrence is most likely 50%. Antenatal diagnosis may be attempted with high-resolution ultrasound to detect major structural abnormalities in the fetus.

VATER Association

VATER is another acronym for a nonrandom association of *v*ertebral and *a*nal anomalies, *t*racheoesophageal fistula with *e*sophageal atresia, and *r*adial and/or *r*enal abnormalities. Most affected newborns have anomalies in all five categories. The acronym can be expanded to VAC-TERL to include *c*ongenital heart disease (particularly ventricular septal defect, which again is found in a majority of cases) and less often other *l*imb defects (Fig. 1-30). Vertebral anomalies include hemivertebrae and sacral abnormalities. Limb deformities consist of radial aplasia or hypoplasia, abnormal thumbs, polydactyly, and syndactyly. Renal abnormalities include unilateral agenesis and less commonly ectopic or horseshoe kidney. The etiology of VATER association is

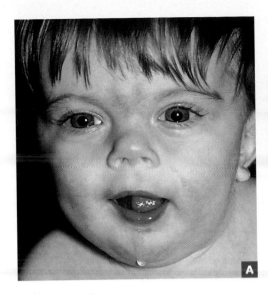
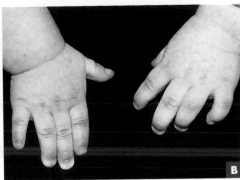

FIG. 1-31 Cornelia de Lange syndrome. *A*, Note heavy eyebrows with developing synophrys, long eyelashes, small upturned nose, long philtrum, and small mouth with thin lips. *B*, Small hands, hypoplastic proximally placed thumb, and small fifth finger with mild clinodactyly. (Courtesy Dr. A.H. Urbach, Children's Hospital of Pittsburgh.)

unknown. Virtually all cases are sporadic, and no chromosomal abnormalities have been detected. The prognosis for growth and development in newborns who survive infancy is good. Most have normal intelligence and eventually achieve normal stature. Consequently, to make optimal management decisions, it is important to distinguish VATER syndrome from more dire chromosomal abnormalities (such as trisomy 18) or nonchromosomal abnormalities (such as CHARGE association).

For the purpose of genetic counseling, VATER association also must be differentiated from Towne syndrome, an autosomal dominant, simple mendelian genetic disorder that shares some features. However, in Towne syndrome there often is a positive family history involving at least two generations; ear abnormalities, including microtia and preauricular and facial skin tags; whereas vertebral anomalies and tracheoesophageal fistula are unusual. The prognosis for growth and development in Towne syndrome patients is good as well. However, the risk for recurrence of Towne syndrome with a positive family history could be 50%, whereas for VATER syndrome the risk should be less than 2%. Antenatal diagnosis for both conditions depends on detecting structural anomalies in the fetus by high-resolution ultrasound.

De Lange or Cornelia de Lange Syndrome

De Lange or Cornelia de Lange syndrome is characterized by intrauterine growth retardation and persistent failure to thrive, severe to moderate mental retardation, and microcephaly with flat occiput and low hairline. Facial features include long, curly eyelashes, bushy eyebrows that by age 16 months meet at the midline (synophrys), small nose with anteverted nostrils, long philtrum, downturned mouth with thin lips (the upper lip may have a midline beak, the lower a corresponding notch), and small chin (Fig.1-31, *A*). Micromelia (small hands and feet) is another characteristic finding (Fig.1-31, *B*). Hirsutism, cutis marmorata, proximally placed thumbs (Fig. 1-31, *B*), flexion contractures of the elbows, aplasia or hypoplasia of limbs, and in males hypospadias with cryptorchidism are common, as are significant abnormalities of various other major organs. Affected adults are short, with average IQ <35 (range 4 to 85). Menses may be normal in older females, who often have a bicornuate uterus.

The incidence of de Lange syndrome is estimated at 1 in 10,000 liveborns. The etiology is unknown but probably is heterogeneous. Although most cases are sporadic, affected siblings are found in 2% to 5% of families with normal parents. A minority of patients with features similar to those of de Lange syndrome have a duplication involving the lower half (q21→qter) of chromosome 3. In effect, these patients have a partial 3q trisomy. This chromosomal abnormality may be a new spontaneous mutation but more often is inherited from a normal parent carrying a balanced chromosomal rearrangement. Various other nonspecific chromosomal abnormalities occasionally are found in individuals with features typical of de Lange syndrome. When there is a chromosomal abnormality, the recurrence risks and antenatal diagnosis are as previously discussed in this chapter. Nevertheless, most patients with de Lange syndrome reveal normal chromosomes even when high resolution techniques are used. It is possible that these cases represent the effect of a new spontaneous dominant gene mutation. In this scenario, instances of affected siblings could suggest gonadal mosaicism for the dominant mutation in one of the normal parents. A more likely etiology for most cases of de Lange syndrome is a submicroscopic chromosome duplication or deletion, possibly in 3q21→qter (i.e., a "contiguous gene syndrome"). The latter implies the duplication or deletion of several unrelated but physically contiguous genes resulting in a syndrome of congenital anomalies. In any event, if a normal couple has a child with de Lange syndrome and the results of chromosome studies for every member are normal by high-resolution cytogenetic techniques, the recurrent risk is 2% to 5%. After the birth of a second affected child the subsequent risk of recurrence approaches 25%. Antenatal diagnosis depends on finding intrauterine growth retardation and/or major structural abnormalities in the fetus by high-resolution ultrasound.

Finally, there have been several case reports of women mildly affected with de Lange syndrome whose offspring were both affected and normal. However, in several of these reports the diagnosis has been questioned. In any event, the recurrence risk in such parent-child cases could be as high as 50% for each conception.

Noonan Syndrome

Noonan syndrome is an autosomal dominant, simple mendelian genetic disorder that shares many clinical features with Turner syndrome. Up to 1 in 1000 individuals may have Noonan syndrome. There is no gender preference. Newborns with Noonan syndrome may have lymphedema of the hands and feet and later in infancy develop a webbed neck. Consequently a chromosome study should be done on such female newborns to distinguish them from newborns with Turner syndrome.

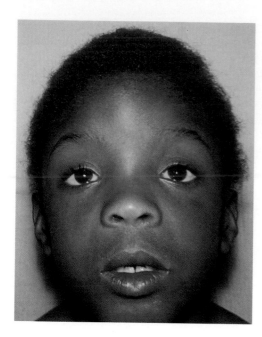

FIG. 1-32 Fetal alcohol syndrome. Note the poorly formed philtrum; slightly narrow and widespread eyes, with inner epicanthal folds and mild ptosis; hirsute forehead; short nose; and relatively thin upper lip.

somy 18, Smith-Lemli-Opitz syndrome, or Noonan syndrome. Although the teratogenic effects were first noted in 1968 in France, they were not widely known until 5 years later through the reports of K.L. Jones working with the late D.W. Smith in the United States. Hallmarks of the syndrome are short palpebral fissures; smooth philtrum; and a thin, smooth upper lip. Other features include mild microcephaly, short nose, and hypoplasia of the nails and distal digits (particularly the fifth toes). Occasionally, affected infants have eyelid ptosis, epicanthal folds, strabismus, small raised hemangiomata, cervical vertebral abnormalities, congenital heart disease, renal anomalies, and hypoplasia of the labia in females (Fig. 1-32).

Newborns with fetal alcohol syndrome tend to be small for gestational age and have poor catch-up growth. They are hypotonic, irritable, and tremulous. Most older children tend to be thin and hyperactive, and more than 80% have some delay in mental development—particularly fine motor function. Their IQs range from 50 to 80. Affected infants with the characteristic dysmorphology have fetal alcohol syndrome, whereas those without the dysmorphology but with the development problems have fetal alcohol effects.

The breakdown products of ethanol (particularly acetaldehyde) ingested by the mother during pregnancy cause fetal alcohol syndrome or effects. Maternal disulfiram (Antabuse) treatment during pregnancy is contraindicated because it also raises serum acetaldehyde levels. Although there may be no absolutely safe level of maternal alcohol consumption throughout pregnancy (particularly in the first trimester), the risk of teratogenesis increases dramatically with increasing degrees of maternal ethanol consumption. Major evidence of fetal alcohol syndrome or effects is observed in 30% to 50% of offspring of mothers who are chronic severe alcoholics (over 7 drinks per day), whereas more subtle effects result from 4 to 6 drinks per day. Prematurity and/or low birth weight for gestational age can result from 2 to 3 drinks per day. It is estimated that some fetal alcohol effects can be seen in 1 of 300 to 1000 liveborns, depending on population drinking norms. The risk to the fetus of occasional maternal alcoholic binges is not clear, but such drinking is best avoided. It is also unclear why some babies are affected and others are not, despite equivalent degrees of maternal alcoholism. This fact may reflect some polygenic maternal or fetal difference in ethanol or acetaldehyde metabolism. Antenatal diagnosis may be attempted with high-resolution ultrasound aimed at detecting intrauterine growth retardation and major structural abnormalities. Also, maternal serum alpha-fetoprotein may be reduced at 16 weeks' gestation if the fetus has fetal alcohol syndrome.

The facies in Noonan syndrome are characterized by a broad forehead and hypertelorism. The eyes tend to slant downward, and there are epicanthi and ptosis, often unilaterally (see Fig. 5-9). Ears are low-set and/or abnormally shaped. Hair tends to be coarse and curly, and there may be excessive keratinization of the hair follicles. The facial features tend to ameliorate with age. Height is less than the 10th percentile in 70% of cases, but head circumference tends to be more in the midrange of normal. Coagulation abnormalities are found in 60% of cases. About 80% of cases have congenital heart disease, pulmonary valvular stenosis being most common. Hypertrophic cardiomyopathy is found in 20% (see Chapter 5). Pectus carinatum or excavatum is common. Most patients with Noonan syndrome have normal intelligence, but learning difficulties and/or mild mental retardation are found in 10%.

Puberty is delayed in individuals with Noonan syndrome, but females are fertile and have normal menses. About 75% of males have undescended testes and 50% are sterile. Most cases of Noonan syndrome result from a new mutation with a parental recurrence risk of about 5% because of gonadal mosaicism for the mutation. It is important, however, to examine the parents carefully for any evidence of Noonan syndrome because an affected individual would have a 50% recurrence risk at each conception for a child with Noonan syndrome. Antenatal diagnosis of an affected fetus might be possible by high-resolution sonography looking for structural abnormalities, such as congenital heart disease.

There is an increased association of the stigmata of both Noonan syndrome and neurofibromatosis I. It is still unclear whether this combination is simply a chance association or a distinct clinical entity in its own right.

Fetal Alcohol Syndrome

The effect of exposure to significant levels of serum alcohol during gestation results in a constellation of clinical features that can resemble tri-

Antenatal Diagnosis

The standard technique for antenatal diagnosis of fetal chromosome abnormalities is by transabdominal amniocentesis at 16 weeks' gestation. This is often performed in the obstetrician's office under local anesthesia. Results are usually available in 21 days or less (minimum 10 days) and should be over 99% reliable. Early antenatal diagnosis of fetal chromosomal abnormalities is possible at $10\frac{1}{2}$ to $12\frac{1}{2}$ weeks' gestation by transcervical or transabdominal chorionic villus sampling (CVS), with results available in 13 days or less. However, CVS is presently limited to highly experienced practitioners in tertiary care medical centers. Although diagnostic accuracy should be over 98%, in about 1% to 2% of cases technical problems or other ambiguities necessitate an amniocentesis at 16 weeks. Both CVS and amniocentesis must be carried out in conjunction with sonography to determine fetal number and viability, gestational age, and placental location. The procedure-related fetal loss (death) rate both for amniocentesis and for CVS is about 0.5% to 1%. There may be some increased risk with CVS for fetal limb reduction defects, but the issue is still controversial. Consequently, when couples are counseled on the need for antenatal diagnosis of fetal chromosomal abnormalities, it must be ensured that they understand their relative risk of having an abnormal liveborn as compared with their risk of losing the pregnancy as a result of the procedure.

Antenatal diagnosis of fetal chromosomal abnormalities should be considered and discussed when a pregnant woman is 35 years of age or older, when a couple has had a previous child with a chromosomal abnormality, or when a parent is known to carry a chromosomal rearrangement. Another indication is an abnormal maternal serum triple-marker screening test at 16 weeks' gestation because this has been associated with increased risk for Down syndrome, trisomy 18, and trisomy 13. Unfortunately, such maternal serum screening for fetal chromosomal abnormalities may not be reliable unless performed in very experienced, high-volume laboratories. This screening method has a relatively low specificity even under the best of circumstances, thereby leading to a need for confirmatory amniocenteses on women, most of whom are carrying normal fetuses.

Because of the potential for loss of a normal fetus associated with invasive procedures such as amniocentesis and CVS, intensive research is underway to attempt cytogenetic analyses of fetal cells that may be present in maternal blood by 9 weeks' gestation. Using FISH Y chromosome DNA probes, the preliminary results indicate that these cells could allow reliable fetal sex determination. Such fetal cells can be nucleated RBCs that, being relatively short lived, are likely to represent the current pregnancy. They can be partially purified from maternal blood by a fluorescent cell sorter. They do not divide, negating the usual metaphase cytogenetic type of analysis. However, they can be analyzed in interphase using FISH DNA probes for specific chromosomes. It is hoped that this noninvasive technique for antenatal fetal cytogenetic analysis will be available within a few years.

An increasingly useful technique for monitoring fetal development in utero is ultrasound scanning (sonography). This technique allows detailed visualization of the fetus by passing high-frequency sound waves through the mother's abdomen and uterus. There is as yet no evidence that this causes structural, physiologic, or genetic damage to the mother or fetus.

Level I ultrasound is used routinely by most obstetricians as an office procedure to monitor pregnancies. Usually this is done between 12 and 20 weeks' gestation, but it can be carried out at any gestational age. Level I ultrasound allows the clinician to confirm gestational age by measuring fetal crown to rump and femoral lengths and biparietal diameter. Serial measurements of the latter compared with abdominal diameter often can detect microcephaly. Fetal viability, cardiac activity, number, position, and growth, as well as placental location, amniotic fluid volume, and pelvic adequacy, can be evaluated by the clinician using level I ultrasound. When initial suspicions of major fetal structural defects, such as anencephaly and spina bifida cystica, arise, further higher-resolution (levels II and III) ultrasound evaluation and/or other antenatal diagnostic procedures are indicated.

High-resolution sonography allows much more detailed evaluation of fetal morphology. Although the equipment used is more sophisticated than that in level I ultrasound, the main difference resides in the expertise of the sonographer. High-resolution ultrasound of the fetus is performed in tertiary care medical centers by radiologists, cardiologists,

and perinatologists specially trained and highly experienced in this technique. Some examples of major fetal structural abnormalities that can be diagnosed by high-resolution ultrasound before 26 weeks' gestation include craniospinal defects such as anencephaly, spina bifida cystica, hydrocephalus, microcephaly, encephalocele, and cysts, all of which can be detected in 95% of instances with over 99% reliability; GI anomalies such as omphalocele, gastroschisis, diaphragmatic hernia, and duodenal atresia (90% detection rate); GU anomalies such as obstructive uropathy, renal agenesis, and infantile polycystic kidneys (95% detection rate); skeletal dysplasia such as osteogenesis imperfecta, abnormal limbs, and achondroplasia (95% detection rate). Detection of fetal cardiac anomalies is best left to specialists in fetal echocardiography (up to 95% detection rate, over 99% reliability). Detection of fetal structural anomalies such as duodenal atresia may be the first indication of a fetal chromosomal abnormality such as Down syndrome. If possible, this should be confirmed by antenatal chromosome studies on the fetus. Finally, in those rare instances when fetal biopsy or fetal blood sampling is diagnostically indicated in the second or third trimester, the procedure is guided by ultrasound.

BIBLIOGRAPHY

Buyse ML, ed: *Birth defects encyclopedia*, Cambridge, Mass, 1990, Blackwell Scientific.

Francke U: Prader-Willi syndrome: chromosomal and gene aberrations, *Growth, Genetics and Hormones* 10:4-7, 1994.

Gorlin RJ, Cohen MM Jr., Levin LS: *Syndromes of the head and neck*, ed 3, New York, 1990, Oxford University Press.

Graham JM Jr.: *Smith's recognizable patterns of human deformation*, ed 2, Philadelphia, 1988, WB Saunders.

Hagerman RJ, Khaled A, Cronister A: Fragile X checklist, *Am J Med Genet* 38:283-287, 1991.

Jones KL: *Smith's recognizable patterns of human malformation*, ed 4, Philadelphia, 1988, WB Saunders.

McKusick VA: *Mendelian inheritance in man*, ed 11, Baltimore, 1994, Johns Hopkins University Press.

Milunsky A, ed. *Genetic disorders and the fetus*, ed 3, Baltimore, 1992, Johns Hopkins University Press.

Patton MA: Noonan syndrome: a review, *Growth, Genetics and Hormones* 10:1-3, 1994.

Rousseau F, Heitz D, Tarleton J, MacPherson J, et al: A multicenter study on genotype-phenotype correlations in the fragile X syndrome, using direct diagnosis with probe StB12.3: the first 2,253 cases, *Am J Hum Genet* 55:225-237, 1994.

Shepard TH: *Catalog of teratogenic agents*, ed 7, Baltimore, 1992, Johns Hopkins University Press.

Spohr H-L, Willms J, Steinhausen H-C: Prenatal alcohol exposure and long-term developmental consequences, *The Lancet* 341:907-910, 1993.

Stevenson RE, Hall JG, Goodman RM, eds: *Human malformations and related anomalies*, New York, 1993, Oxford University Press.

Thompson MW, McInnes RR, Willard HF: *Thompson & Thompson genetics in medicine*, ed 5, Philadelphia, 1991, WB Saunders.

Trask BJ: Fluorescence in situ hybridization, *Trends in Genetics* 7:149-154, 1991.

Wenger SL, Steele MW, Boone LY, Lenkey SG, Cummins JH, Chen X-Q: "Balanced" karyotypes in six abnormal offspring of balanced reciprocal translocation normal carrier parents, *Am J Med Genet* 55:47-52, 1995.

Willard HF, Ferguson-Smith MA, Goodfellow PN, Epstein CJ, Nussbaum RL, Ledbetter DH, Ballabio A: Chromosomes and autosomes. In Scriver CR, Beaudet AL, Sly WS, Valle D, eds: *The metabolic and molecular bases of inherited disease*, New York, 1995, McGraw-Hill.

2

Neonatology

MICHAEL J. BALSAN ❦ IAN R. HOLZMAN

General Techniques of Physical Examination

Assessment of the Newborn

The purposes of the routine newborn assessment are to determine the infant's gestational age, document normal growth and development for a given gestational age, uncover signs of birth-related trauma or congenital anomalies, and evaluate the overall health and condition of the infant. The assessment begins with the establishment of a historical data base. Information may be gleaned from antenatal, labor, delivery, and postpartum records and a brief interview with the parents (Fig. 2-1). The aim of this data gathering is to assess the fetal and neonatal responses to pregnancy, labor, and delivery; estimate the risk for hereditary or congenital diseases; and identify the potential for future difficulties by appraising the family's social history and observing maternal-infant interactions. This background is recorded in the infant's medical record and serves as a guide to the subsequent physical examination (Table 2-1).

Examination requires specialized techniques because of the lack of patient cooperation and the infant's small size and developmental immaturity. If possible, the newborn should be examined in the presence of one or both parents to reassure them about normal variations and to discuss any abnormal findings. The baby should remain at least partially clothed through as much of the examination as possible, although a complete and thorough examination is imperative. The examiner's hands should be warm to minimize the chance that the infant will become uncomfortable because of heat loss.

Observation must be done before the quiet infant is disturbed by the examination. By visual inspection the clinician can assess skin and facies; general tonus and symmetry of movement; respiratory rate, retractions, and color; and abdominal contour. Auscultation of the heart and lungs should be done before more stressful portions of the examination, which are likely to make the infant fussy. Allowing the baby to suck on a pacifier or gloved finger can help quiet him or her. The latter also allows for an assessment of sucking strength, as well as of integrity of the palate. Lifting the infant under the arms (Fig. 2-2) and gently rocking him or her (such that the head swings toward and away from the examiner) is usually calming. This maneuver also induces a reflexive opening of the eyes, which facilitates the ophthalmologic examination. Sucking also induces eye opening. Such maneuvers may be necessary to convince the examiner that the patient does not have a congenital cataract or an intraorbital mass (see Chapter 19) requiring prompt intervention.

When the abdomen is examined, it often helps to gently flex the hip on the side being examined, since this relaxes the abdominal muscles. Most structures in the abdomen are smaller (pyloric olive), softer (liver), more superficial (spleen tip), or deeper (kidneys) than expected. The use of any part of the hand other than the fingertips should be discouraged because maximal sensitivity is essential.

Careful evaluation of the hip joints is a crucial part of every newborn examination because identification and early treatment of congenital dislocation can prevent later disability. Although asymmetry of the buttocks and skin creases or asymmetry of femoral length can be clues to dislocation, the performance of at least one of a number of active motion tests is essential. The Ortolani maneuver involves placing the third or fourth finger over the greater trochanter and the thumb on the medial aspect of the thighs (Fig. 2-3). The thighs are adducted and then abducted with the fingers pushing toward the midline and the thumbs away. A definite "clunk" can be felt and often heard if the femoral head has been dislocated and clunks back into the acetabulum. Often, higher-pitched clicks and snaps that represent nothing more than tendons passing over bone or cartilage can be heard and felt.

Assessment of Gestational Age

One of the unique considerations in the examination of the newborn is the assessment of gestational age. Accurate determination should be the first part of any newborn examination, since this provides the context for the remainder of the evaluation. No differential diagnosis of newborn disease can be made without knowing whether the patient is premature or full-term and whether he or she is small, large, or appropriate for gestational age. Although an accurate menstrual and pregnancy history usually provides firm evidence of gestational age, there are many cases in which data such as the date of the last menses and the date of the onset of fetal movement are unavailable or unreliable.

Many investigators (see Bibliography) have developed examination criteria, both morphologic and neurologic, for the assessment of gestational age. Although these criteria are generally useful because of the ordered patterns of fetal development, the clinician can rely on no single feature or even small group of features to develop at the same rate in all infants. In fact, assessment of paired structures, such as ears, may reveal slightly different degrees of maturation from one side to the other. Thus all of the available methods involve *numerous* physical and neurologic items and at best have a 2-week range of error.

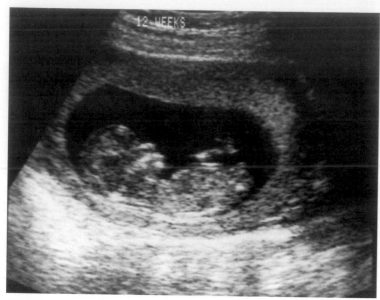

FIG. 2-1 Antenatal assessments. This infant has a normal sonographic appearance at 12 weeks' gestation. Knowledge of the results of in utero evaluations may assist in the provision of appropriate antenatal and postnatal care. (Courtesy Dr. Lyndon Hill, Pittsburgh.)

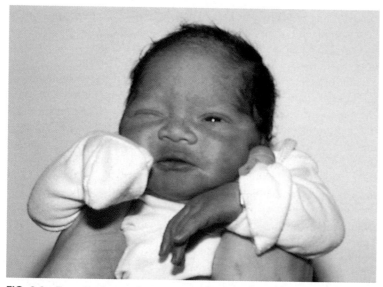

FIG. 2-2 Examination techniques. Holding an infant under the arms and gently rocking calms the infant and reflexively induces eye opening.

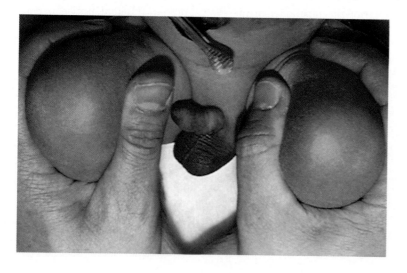

TABLE 2-1

Newborn Historical Data Base

Antenatal Record
- Maternal age
- Maternal medical history
- Obstetric history
  —Number of previous pregnancies
  —Number of term/preterm deliveries
  —Outcomes of previous pregnancies
- Estimations of gestational age
- Antenatal sonogram or fetal surveillance results (if available)
- Complications of pregnancy
- Adequacy of antenatal care

Labor and Delivery Record
- Date and time of delivery
- Duration of labor
- Time of the rupture of membranes
- Complications or abnormalities of labor
- Method of delivery or type of anesthesia
- Placental weight and morphologic condition
- Birth weight
- Need for resuscitation and Apgar scores
- Maternal blood type

Postpartum Record
- Maternal postpartum complications
- Newborn vital sign records
- Nursing documentation of the activity and condition of the infant
  —On admission to the nursery
  —Since admission to the nursery
- Abnormal physical findings noted by the nursing staff
- Feeding, voiding, and stool history
- Observations of maternal–infant interactions

Parental Interview
- Parental perceptions of
  —Pregnancy
  —Labor
  —Delivery
- History of parental and family illnesses
- Health status and growth and development of siblings and other family members
- Degree of education, preparation, and planning for newborn care
- Available social support systems
- Medical follow-up plans

Although morphologic criteria tend to be uninfluenced by events occurring around the time of delivery, neurologic findings may be unreliable in the presence of a number of conditions, including depression secondary to medication, asphyxia, seizures, metabolic diseases, infections, and severe respiratory distress. Even morphologic criteria may be inaccurate if the infant is born with severe edema or growth retardation or suffers effects from maternal drug use. Such factors must be considered in estimating gestational age.

Fig. 2-4 illustrates one of a number of published data tables used in the estimation of the gestational age of newborns. In this version, there

FIG. 2-3 Ortolani maneuver. The proper hand positioning for this maneuver is demonstrated. Abducting the femur produces a palpable clunk in the infant with congenital hip dislocation.

Physical Maturity

	0	1	2	3	4	5
Skin	Gelatinous, red, transparent	Smooth, pink, visible veins	Superficial peeling &/or rash, few veins	Cracking, pale area, rare veins	Parchment, deep cracking, no vessels	Leathery, cracked, wrinkled
Lanugo	None	Abundant	Thinning	Bald areas	Mostly bald	
Plantar creases	No crease	Faint red marks	Anterior transverse crease only	Creases anterior two thirds	Creases cover entire sole	
Breast	Barely perceptible	Flat areola, no bud	Stippled areola, 1-2 mm bud	Raised areola, 3-4 mm bud	Full areola, 5-10 mm bud	
Ear	Pinna flat, stays folded	Slightly curved pinna, soft, slow recoil	Well-curved pinna, soft but ready recoil	Formed & firm with instant recoil	Thick cartilage, ear stiff	
Genitals: male	Scrotum empty, no rugae		Testes descending, few rugae	Testes down, good rugae	Testes pendulous, deep rugae	
Genitals: female	Prominent clitoris & labia minora		Majora & minora equally prominent	Majora large, minora small	Clitoris & minora completely covered	

Maturity Rating

Score	Wks.
5	26
10	28
15	30
20	32
25	34
30	36
35	38
40	40
45	42
50	44

Neuromuscular Maturity

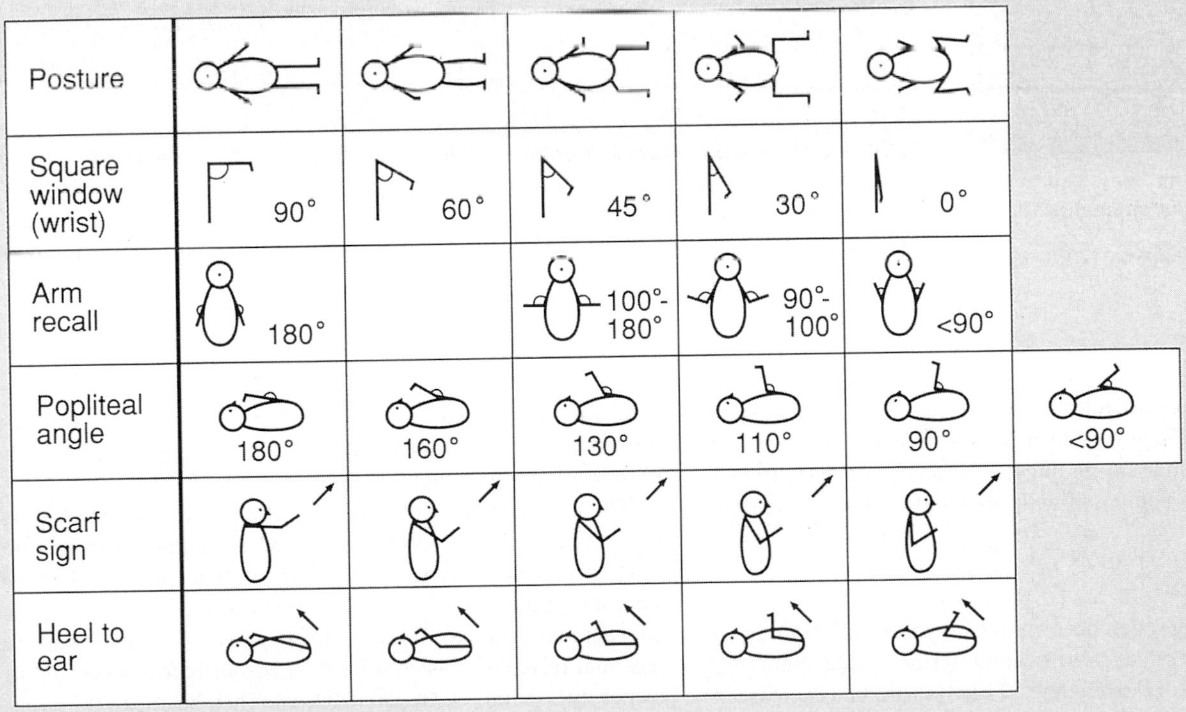

FIG. 2-4 Gestational age assessment. The six morphologic and six neurologic criteria, in aggregate, yield an estimation of gestational age. (From Ballard J, Novak KK, Driver M, et al: A simplified score of assessment of fetal maturation of newly-born infants, *J Pediatr* 95:769-774, 1979.)

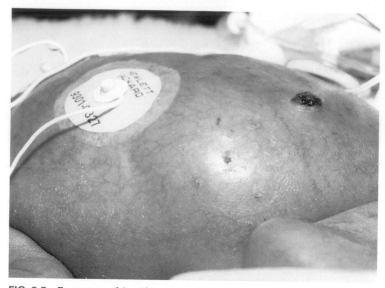

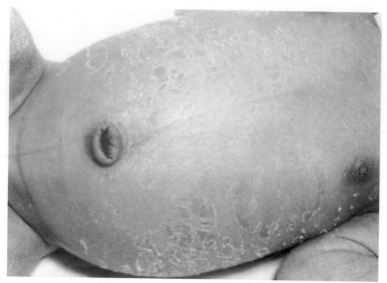

FIG. 2-5 Premature skin. This premature infant demonstrates translucent, paper-thin skin with a prominent venous pattern.

FIG. 2-6 Postterm skin. Peeling and cracking of the skin are characteristics of the infant delivered after 42 weeks' gestation.

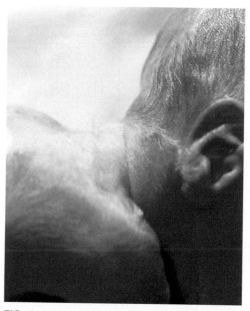

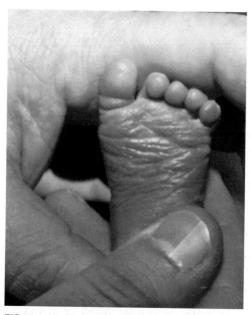

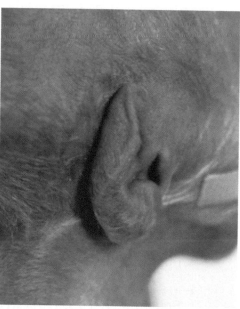

FIG. 2-7 Lanugo. This fine body hair resembling "peach fuzz" is present on infants of 24 to 32 weeks' gestation.

FIG. 2-8 Sole creases. Transverse sole creases cover approximately half the sole in this infant, indicating a gestational age of approximately 34 weeks.

FIG. 2-9 Ear cartilage. The lack of cartilage and the easy foldability (lack of recoil) are evident in the ear of this premature infant at 26 weeks.

are six morphologic and six neurologic criteria that, in aggregate, yield an estimate of gestational age based on an examination performed at 12 to 24 hours of life. Individual findings are scored on a scale from 0 to 5, and the total score is compared with the chart shown on the right of Fig. 2-4.

Physical Maturity

One of the most striking differences among newborns of various gestational ages is the quality of the skin. As intrauterine development proceeds, the chemical nature of skin changes. There is a gradual decrease in water content and a thickening of the keratin layer. Very premature infants (24 to 28 weeks) have nearly translucent, paper-thin skin (Fig. 2-5) that is easily abraded. A diffuse red hue and a prominent venous pattern are characteristic. At term, the skin no longer appears thin, and the general color is a pale pink. Some superficial peeling and cracking around the

ankles and wrists may be visible. Postterm infants (42 to 44 weeks) often have more diffuse peeling and cracking of the skin because the outermost layers are sloughed (Fig. 2-6).

The general quality of scalp hair changes during development from rather fine, thin hair (24 to 28 weeks) to coarser, thicker hair (term). There are, of course, racial differences in hair quality, which can make this change difficult to assess. A second type of hair, known as *lanugo*, appears and disappears during development. Lanugo is very fine body hair that resembles peach fuzz. It is absent before weeks 20 to 22, becomes diffuse until weeks 30 to 32, and then begins to thin. Assessment of the presence and extent of lanugo is best accomplished by observing the back tangentially (Fig. 2-7).

Transverse creases begin to appear on the anterior portion of the soles of the feet at approximately 32 weeks (Fig. 2-8). By 36 weeks, the anterior two thirds of the sole is covered with creases. For adequate assess-

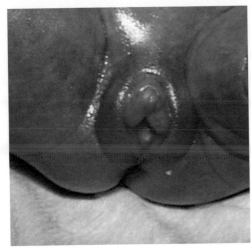

FIG. 2-10 Premature female genitalia. Prominence of the labia minora in a premature female infant at 28 weeks.

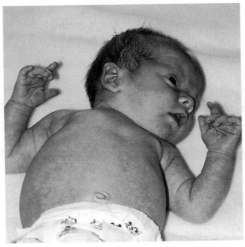

FIG. 2-11 General posture. The typical, marked flexor posture of the term infant.

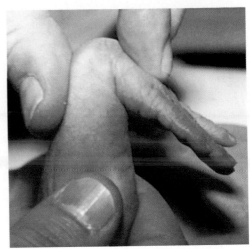

FIG. 2-12 Square-window test. The position for assessing the square window is shown. The 45-degree angle seen between the palm and forearm is consistent with a gestational age of 30 to 32 weeks.

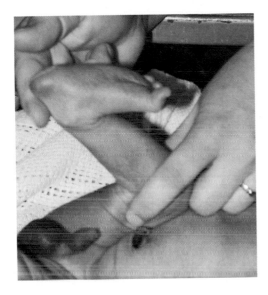

FIG. 2-13 Knee flexion. The position for assessing knee flexion is shown. Note the decreased knee flexibility of this term infant.

ment of this feature, it is necessary to stretch the skin over the sole gently to distinguish wrinkling from true creases. Infants with congenital neurologic dysfunction involving the lower extremities may lack normal creases, as might infants born with severe pedal edema. It is sometimes possible to learn something about gestational age long after birth by reviewing the sole prints made for identification in many hospitals.

Breast tissue, which is responsive to maternal hormonal influences, shows a progressive development as gestational age advances. Infants of gestational ages less than 28 weeks have barely perceptible breast tissue (Fig. 2-5). With advancing age, these tissues show progressive development (Fig. 2-6), and occasionally, a term infant has active glandular secretions termed *witch's milk.*

Cartilaginous development proceeds in an orderly manner during gestation and can be assessed by examination of the external ear. Although the normal incurving of the upper pinnae begins at 33 to 34 weeks and is complete at term, it is more reliable to assess the extent of cartilage in the pinnae by feeling its edge and folding the ear (Fig. 2-9). Until approximately 32 weeks, there is only minimal recoil of a folded ear, but by term, there is instant recoil.

The appearance of the genitalia can be used to assess gestational age. In a boy, the testes descend into the scrotum during the last month of gestation, but they are often palpable in the inguinal canal by 28 to

30 weeks. The appearance of rugae on the scrotum parallels testicular migration. Absence of testicular descent alters the appearance of the scrotum at term. Clearly, congenital cryptorchidism complicates this evaluation. In a girl, the labia majora tend to be overshadowed by the clitoris and labia minora until 34 to 36 weeks (Fig. 2-10). In cases of fetal malnutrition, lack of subcutaneous fat, which should normally be present in the latter part of gestation, can interfere with assessment of the female genitalia.

Neuromuscular Maturity

Numerous neurologic tests and observations can be used to assess gestational age. Most examiners use the tests that seem to best cover the various facets of neurologic function, including range of motion, tone, reflexes, and posture. None is particularly reliable in the presence of illness, and the entire neurologic examination is best done between 12 and 24 hours after birth to allow recovery from the stress of delivery.

The resting supine posture of infants changes with advancing gestational age. The mature infant exhibits a marked flexor posture of the extremities compared with the extensor posture of the premature infant (Fig. 2-11).

Tests for flexion angles assess a combination of muscle tone, ligament and tendon laxity, and flexion-extension development. The inexperienced examiner usually assumes that the very premature infant is the most flexible, but observation of flexion angles demonstrates that this is false. The square-window test of the wrist (Fig. 2-12) is performed by gently flexing the hand on the wrist and assessing the resultant angle. The wrists of babies younger than approximately 32 weeks can be flexed only to 45 to 90 degrees, whereas the wrists of term infants undergo full flexion. Sometime between birth and adulthood this flexion ability is lost. Examination of the flexion of the knees reveals a different pattern of development, with decreasing flexibility as gestational age increases (Fig. 2-13). It is essential to emphasize gentleness in these evaluations because any result can be achieved if the examiner applies undue force.

Active tone and reflex responsiveness may be assessed by examining arm recoil. In this maneuver, the supine infant's forearms are fully flexed for 5 seconds, extended by pulling on the hands, and then released. As gestational age increases, the flexion response is more pronounced.

The resting tone of the upper extremities can be assessed by elicit-

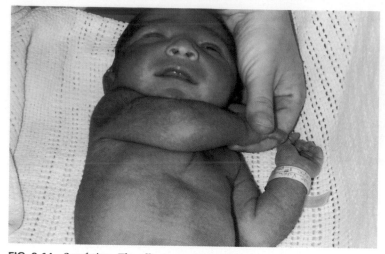

FIG. 2-14 Scarf sign. The elbow cannot be drawn, with gentle traction on the upper extremity, across this term infant's chest. This is in contrast to the marked flexibility of a preterm infant.

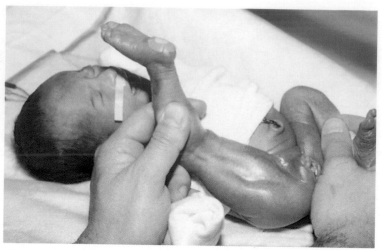

FIG. 2-15 Heel-to-ear maneuver. The position for assessing the heel-to-ear maneuver is demonstrated. The degree of extension seen is consistent with a 28- to 30-week infant.

GESTATIONAL AGE (WEEKS)

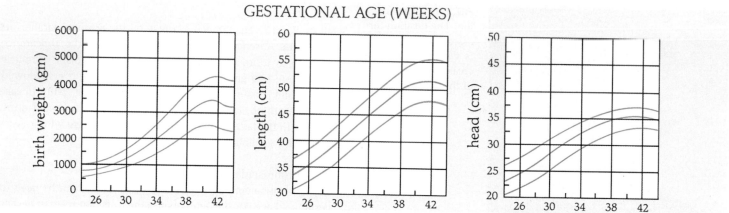

FIG. 2-16 The mean (± 2 standard deviations) weight, length, and head circumference for infants born at various gestational ages. Infants above or below the curves are considered too LGA or too SGA. (From Usher R, McLean F: Intrauterine growth of liveborn Caucasian infant at sea level, *J Pediatr* 74:901-910, 1969.)

ing the scarf sign. Gentle traction of the upper extremities across the chest in a rostral direction ("placing a scarf on the infant") while examining the position of the elbow reveals a decreasing displacement of the elbow as gestational age increases (Fig. 2-14).

In a similar manner, the resting tone of the lower extremities can be assessed by the heel-to-ear maneuver. With the baby on the back, a foot is moved as near to the ipsilateral ear as possible without exerting undue force. The pelvis must be kept flat during the evaluation. Very premature infants can easily touch their heels to their ears (Fig. 2-15). This becomes somewhat more difficult after 30 weeks and impossible by approximately week 34 of gestation.

Abnormalities of Growth

One of the important advances in neonatal medicine has been the realization that the size of a newborn does not necessarily reflect gestational age (Fig. 2-16). The parameter most commonly affected is weight, especially in infants who are small for their gestational age. A number of terms have been applied to small babies, including *small for gestational age (SGA), intrauterine growth retardation (IUGR),* and *fetal malnutrition (FM).* The last is probably most descriptive of newborns whose weight is inappropriately low in relation to length and head circumference. These infants, who appear long and thin, often

have an obvious loss of subcutaneous tissue, which is best seen over the buttocks and within the folds of the neck.

The relationship among weight, length, and head circumference can be useful in understanding the etiology of the small size. Conditions that affect growth during the third trimester of pregnancy, such as preeclampsia, tend to interfere with the normal acquisition of fatty tissue while sparing brain growth (and thus head circumference) and linear growth. These newborns have an asymmetric form of growth retardation. In severe cases, the onset of protein catabolism affects muscle mass. By comparing length or head circumference percentiles with the weight percentile at any given gestational age, the clinician can detect growth retardation even if the actual weight still falls within two standard deviations of normal. Often postmature infants (>42 weeks) have some decrease in weight compared with length or head circumference. Problems beginning earlier than the third trimester tend to produce generalized growth retardation (Fig. 2-17). In very premature infants, such global decreases in growth often complicate assessment of gestational age, since the tools are rather limited in babies born at 24 to 28 weeks' gestation. Two of the most important causes of generalized growth retardation are chromosomal syndromes and congenital infections. A thorough investigation of such problems should be undertaken in any unexplained instance of generalized growth retardation.

bD 5

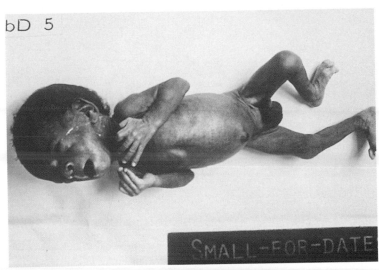

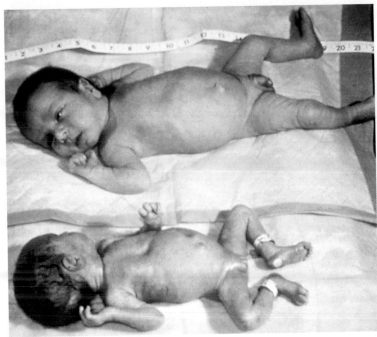

FIG. 2-17 IUGR. This term baby weighed only 1.7 kg. The head appears disproportionately large for the thin, wasted body. This resulted from placental insufficiency late in pregnancy. Hypoglycemia may be a complication. (Courtesy TALC, Institute of Child Health, Bethesda.)

FIG. 2-18 Discordant twins. This is a pair of markedly discordant dizygotic twins. Disturbed placentation accounted for the marked reduction in size of the smaller twin.

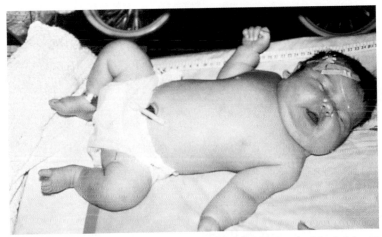

FIG. 2-19 LGA infant. This infant of a diabetic mother weighed 5 kg at birth and exhibits the typical rounded facies.

Multiple-gestation pregnancies often produce newborns who are premature and symmetrically small. Size discordancy (>10% difference in weight) between identical twins occurs because their placentas can share vascular connections, resulting in overperfusion of one twin and underperfusion of the other. This leads to a marked difference in size, with the growth of the underperfused twin being symmetrically retarded. Discordancy may also occur in dizygotic twins (Fig. 2-18) if one has inadequate placentation. Rarely, one twin may be afflicted with a chromosomal abnormality or congenital infection, and the other is normal.

Newborns who are too large for gestational age (LGA) are often the products of pregnancies in diabetic or prediabetic mothers. The effect is usually noted during the third trimester, with infants at term weighing more than 8 pounds. Weight is the most affected parameter, but length and head circumference are often increased as well. Infants of diabetic mothers often are identifiable by macrosomia, round facies (Fig. 2-19), and sometimes plethora and hirsutism (especially of the pinnae). They may also demonstrate visceromegaly, with enlargement particularly of the liver and heart.

Although babies weighing more than 8 pounds are more likely to be from diabetic pregnancies, a significant number of large full-term new-

borns are the product of normal pregnancies. Nevertheless, all LGA infants should be routinely screened for hypoglycemia and their mothers investigated for the possibility of undiagnosed diabetes mellitus. Two fairly unusual syndromes can also cause excessive size: (1) cerebral gigantism, or Soto syndrome, in which macrosomia, macrocephaly, large hands and feet, and ultimately poor coordination and variable mental deficiency occur, and (2) Beckwith-Wiedemann syndrome, whose prominent features include macrosomia, macroglossia, omphalocele, linear ear fissures, and neonatal hypoglycemia (see Chapter 9).

Placenta

Careful examination of the placenta can aid in the diagnosis and treatment of many conditions and diseases. It is unfortunate that the placenta has been relegated to an afterbirth and is often immediately discarded without knowing the condition of the offspring. After the membranes and cord are trimmed, the normal ratio of fetal to placental weight is approximately 4.7 to 1. The configuration, color, condition of the membranes, insertion of the cord, and condition of the fetal and maternal surfaces are all relevant.

The insertion of the umbilical cord into the placenta, which can be central, eccentric, marginal, or velamentous, can be important in understanding unexplained asphyxia or blood loss. In a velamentous insertion (Fig. 2-20), the cord is inserted into the membranes rather than into the disc, leaving the umbilical vessels unprotected for a variable distance. These vessels are more prone to rupture, with resultant fetal hemorrhage (vasa praevia).

At times, placentation itself is abnormal. In a circumvallate placenta (Fig. 2-21), the villous tissue projects beyond the chorionic surface, with a hyalinized fold at the edge of the chorionic plate. This type of placentation may cause antepartum bleeding, premature labor, and increased perinatal mortality.

Premature placental separation (abruptio placentae) can lead to an accumulation of blood behind the placenta (Fig. 2-22). Although the bleeding is usually of maternal origin, fetal blood loss may also occur.

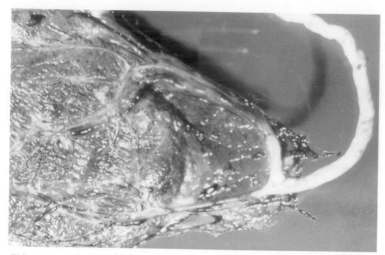

FIG. 2-20 Velamentous cord insertion. The umbilical cord is inserted into the amniotic membranes rather than into the placental disc. This leaves the umbilical vessels relatively unprotected and predisposes them to rupture.

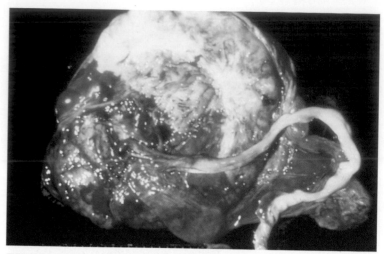

FIG. 2-21 Circumvallate placenta. There is extension of villous tissue beyond the chorionic surface, with a well-defined hyalinized fold at the edge of the chorionic plate.

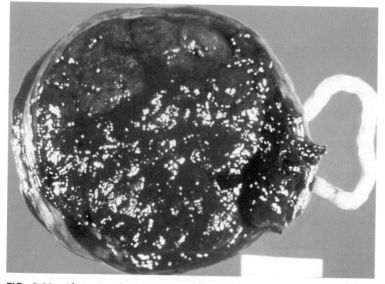

FIG. 2-22 Abruptio placentae. Examination of this placenta reveals a small abruption site, with an adherent blood clot along the margin.

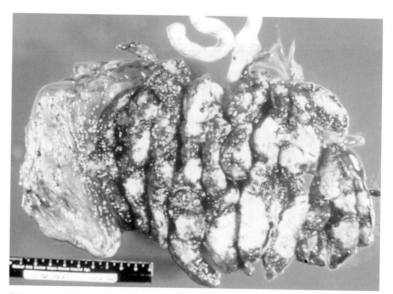

FIG. 2-23 Infarcted placenta. A massive placental infarction comprising the majority of the villous surface is shown. Such an extensive infarction compromises fetal nutrition and oxygenation.

Large abruptions may lead to poor growth, fetal asphyxia, or even death. It is important to distinguish a true abruption, in which an adherent clot compresses the maternal surface, from the nonadherent collection of blood that forms on normal placental separation.

Placental infarctions (Fig. 2-23) are among the more common, easily diagnosed abnormalities. They tend to occur along the margin of the placenta and can vary from red to yellowish-white. When small, they are usually of little significance. However, large (>30% of placental volume) central infarcts can be clinically significant by reducing the placental surface available for fetal oxygenation and nutrition. Infarcts are most common in pregnancies complicated by hypertension.

Chorioamnionitis (Fig. 2-24), inflammation of the fetal membranes, is an immediate clue to potential neonatal infection. On gross examination, the membranes lack their normal sheen and translucency, appearing gray or yellow. Inflammation, confirmable by microscopic examination, can also be found in the fetal vessels of the chorionic plate and umbilical cord.

In pregnancies in which the quantity of amniotic fluid is decreased (oligohydramnios), examination of the amnion may also reveal shiny, gray, flat nodules known as *amnion nodosum* (Fig. 2-25). The presence of these nodules can be an immediate indication of the diagnosis of renal dysfunction or agenesis in the newborn. Because such infants may also

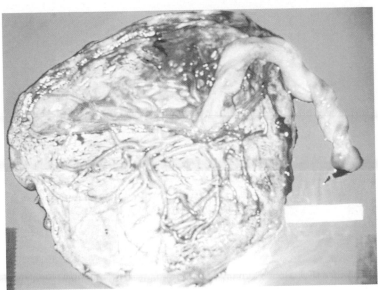

FIG. 2-24 Chorioamnionitis. This is a placental specimen from a pregnancy with documented amniotic fluid infection. The surface of the membranes is opaque and shows yellowish discoloration.

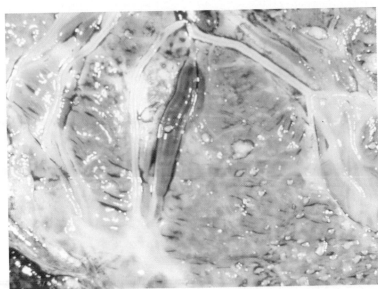

FIG. 2-25 Amnion nodosum. The fetal surface of this placenta from a pregnancy with oligohydramnios demonstrates multiple nodules consistent with amnion nodosum. This finding suggests a strong possibility of renal agenesis or dysgenesis.

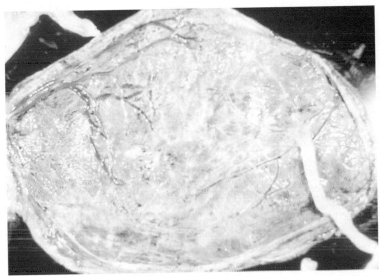

FIG. 2-26 Monochorionic, monoamniotic placenta. Examination of this placenta from monozygotic twins reveals no dividing membranes, thus assuring monozygosity

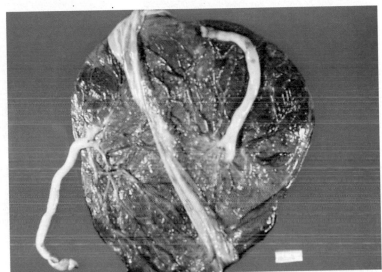

FIG. 2-27 Dichorionic, diamniotic placenta. The presence of two amniotic sacs and separate chorions in this twin placenta precludes determination of zygosity.

have hypoplastic lungs and dysmorphic features (such as occurs in Potter syndrome) early diagnosis can be helpful to the physician and family.

In multiple-gestation deliveries, a careful placental evaluation is crucial. The major distinction to be made is whether there is a single chorion, or outer layer of the fetal membranes. When twins with a single chorion are present in a single amniotic cavity (Fig. 2-26), monozygosity is ensured. For all practical purposes, a single chorion that bridges two amniotic sacs is also evidence of monozygotic twins. In this instance, it is essential to carefully examine the membranes at the site of connection of the two amniotic sacs. When two chorions and two amnions (or a total of four membranes at their interface) are present (Fig. 2-27), twins may be monozygotic or dizygotic. Approximately 36% of monozygotic twins are dichorionic.

Birth Trauma

In the majority of cases, a newborn is relatively unscathed by the birth process. However, sometimes transient and permanent stigmata of birth trauma are evident. Not only is prompt identification of such injuries important for good management, but it can also prevent inappropriate speculation, diagnostic tests, and treatment.

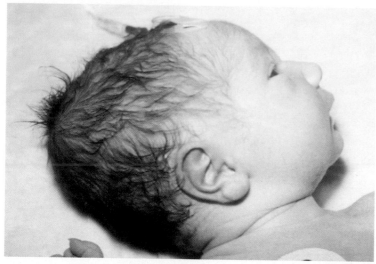

FIG. 2-28 Caput succedaneum. This infant has significant scalp edema as a result of compression during transit through the birth canal. The edema crosses suture lines.

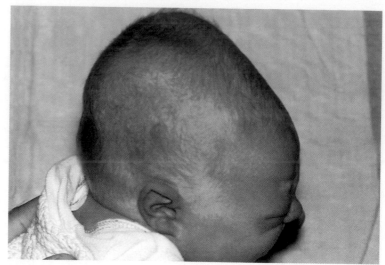

FIG. 2-29 Cephalohematoma. In this infant with bilateral cephalohematomas, the midline sagittal suture remained palpable, confirming the subperiosteal location of the hematomas.

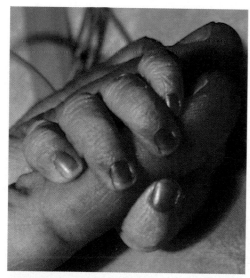

FIG. 2-30 Meconium staining. The marked discoloration of this infant's fingernails resulted from long-standing meconium staining of the amniotic fluid before delivery.

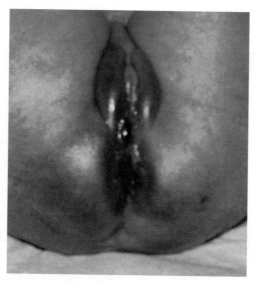

FIG. 2-31 Bruising. This severe bruising of the perineum was the result of a difficult breech labor and delivery.

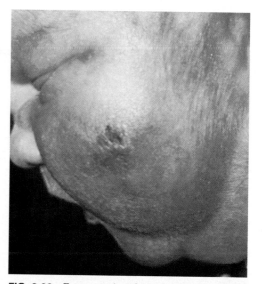

FIG. 2-32 Fat necrosis. This discolored nodular lesion on the cheek is characteristic of subcutaneous necrosis of fat secondary to forceps trauma.

Caput Succedaneum

Normal transit of the fetal head through the birth canal induces molding of the skull and scalp edema, especially if labor is prolonged. The edema, which can be massive, is known as a *caput succedaneum* (Fig. 2-28). Much of this edema is present at birth and tends to overlie the occipital bones and portions of the parietal bones bilaterally. In some cases, bruising of the scalp may also be present (especially if a vacuum extractor was used). The presence of a caput requires no therapy, and spontaneous resolution within a few days is the rule. At times, it can be difficult to distinguish a caput from a rare but serious subgaleal (subaponeurotic) hematoma, which is a collection of blood within scalp tissues extending under the epicranial aponeurosis. Such infants, however, show signs of progressive hypovolemia. Although the exact source and location of bleeding may be unclear initially, awareness of the possibility of massive blood loss extending under a large portion of the scalp as well as prompt replacement can be lifesaving.

Cephalohematoma

Often, confusion arises between the diagnosis of a caput and that of a cephalohematoma. The latter is a localized collection of blood beneath the periosteum of one of the calvarial bones. It is distinguished from a caput by the fact that its borders are limited by suture lines, usually those surrounding the parietal bones. However, diagnosis can be difficult in the immediate newborn period, when there may be overlying scalp edema. Cephalohematoma can be bilateral (Fig. 2-29), but it is more often unilateral. On palpation, the border feels elevated and the center depressed. Most patients have an uncomplicated course of slow resolution over 1 or more months, with possible calcification. Occasionally complications are seen, the most common being jaundice resulting from breakdown and resorption of a large hematoma. Secondary anemia should also be considered when the hematoma is large. Underlying hairline skull fractures occur with some regularity but are rarely of clinical significance. The exception is the uncommon develop-

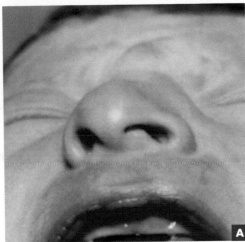 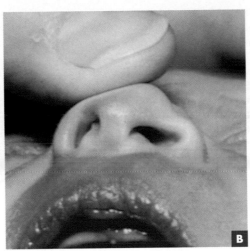 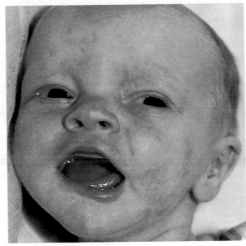

FIG. 2-33 Nasal deformity. This infant incurred dislocation of the triangular cartilage of the nasal septum during delivery. Inspection of the nose reveals deviation of the septum to the right and asymmetry of the nares (A). When the septum is manually moved toward the midline, the asymmetry persists, confirming the dislocation (B).

FIG. 2-34 Facial nerve palsy. This infant incurred injury to the right facial nerve, resulting in loss of the nasolabial fold on the affected side and asymmetric movement of the mouth. The side of the mouth that appears to droop is the normal side.

ment of a leptomeningeal cyst. Radiologic investigation for an underlying depressed fracture is indicated in infants whose histories suggest significant trauma and those having depressed levels of consciousness or neurologic abnormalities on examination. Another potentially serious, though rare, complication is infection, which is more likely when the integrity of the overlying skin is broken. Needle aspiration of a cephalohematoma is contraindicated because of the risk of introducing microorganisms.

Meconium Staining

Meconium is noted in the amniotic fluid in as many as 10% of deliveries. The meconium may have been recently expelled or may have been present in the amniotic fluid for hours or days. Because the timing of the passage of meconium may have significance for the diagnosis of asphyxia, it is useful to examine infants for the presence of meconium staining. Apparently, it takes at least 4 to 6 hours of contact before staining of the umbilicus, skin, and nails occurs (Fig. 2-30). Often, the meconium-stained infant is postmature and has diffuse peeling of the skin and a shriveled, stained umbilical cord.

Bruises and Petechiae

Superficial bruising can occur when delivery is difficult. This is relatively common with breech presentations (Fig. 2-31) and can include swelling and discoloration of the labia or scrotum (to be distinguished from an incarcerated inguinal hernia). When bruises are extensive, significant secondary jaundice may develop as the extravasated blood is broken down and resorbed. In an infant in whom a nuchal cord is found at delivery, the presence of diffuse petechiae around the head and neck is common and does not warrant further investigation. The appearance of new bruises or petechiae after delivery should alert the physician and nurse to the possibility of a bleeding disorder.

Fat Necrosis

Many infants delivered with the aid of forceps show forceps marks after delivery. These marks tend to fade over 24 to 48 hours. Occasionally, a well-circumscribed, firm nodule with purplish discoloration may appear at the site of a forceps mark. This may represent fat necrosis

(Fig. 2-32) and resolves spontaneously over weeks to months. The phenomenon may occur at other sites of trauma.

Nasal Deformities

Abnormalities of the nose are common after delivery, the majority consisting of transient flattening or twisting induced during transit through the birth canal. Less than 1% of nasal deformities are due to actual dislocations of the triangular cartilage of the nasal septum. These can be differentiated from positional deformities by manually moving the septum to the midline and observing the resultant shape of the nares. In a true dislocation, marked asymmetry of the nares persists (Fig. 2-33). Returning the septum to its proper position can be accomplished in the nursery with the guidance of an otolaryngologist. Failure to recognize and treat dislocation may lead to permanent deformity.

Peripheral Nerve Damage

Injury to the peripheral nervous system, especially the facial and brachial nerves, is one of the more common serious occurrences related to birth. Unilateral facial nerve palsy is the most common peripheral nerve injury, with an incidence as high as 1.4 per 1000 live births. Injury can result from direct trauma from forceps or from compression of the nerve against the sacral promontory while the head is in the birth canal. With pronounced nerve injury, there is decreased facial movement and forehead wrinkling on the side of the palsy, eyelid elevation, and flattening of the nasolabial folds and corner of the mouth (Fig. 2-34). Crying accentuates the findings, with the most obvious sign being asymmetric movement of the mouth. The side that appears to droop when crying is the normal side. The differential diagnosis includes Möbius syndrome (usually bilateral) and absence of the depressor anguli oris muscle, which may be associated with cardiac anomalies. The latter condition is distinguishable from facial nerve palsy by the absence of involvement of the forehead, eyelid, or nasolabial area. The prognosis for facial nerve palsies is excellent, and recovery usually occurs within the first month. In the meantime, prevention of corneal drying is essential. Surgery is reserved for cases in which clear-cut severing of the facial nerve has occurred.

The incidence of brachial plexus trauma with current obstetric management is approximately 0.7 per 1000 live births. The mechanism of

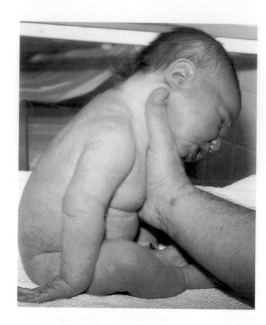

FIG. 2-35 Brachial plexus injury. Traction injury to C5, C6, and C7 spinal cord segments produces this (Erb) palsy. This infant demonstrates the characteristic posture of the limply adducted and internally rotated arm.

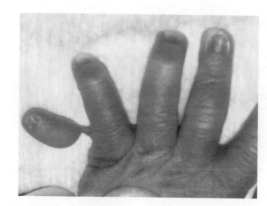

FIG. 2-36 Supernumerary digit. This is the common position for a sixth digit. The thin pedicle distinguishes this anomaly from true polydactyly.

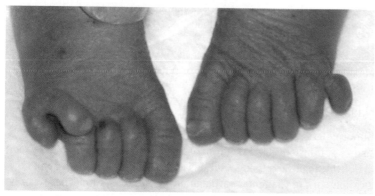

FIG. 2-37 Polydactyly. True bilateral polydactyly of the fifth toe is seen in this infant.

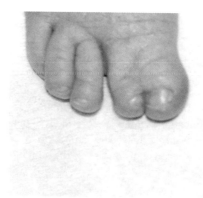
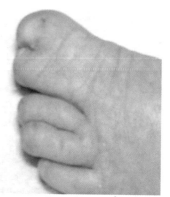

FIG. 2-38 Syndactyly. This child demonstrates bilateral fusion of the soft tissue between the first and second toes.

injury in most instances is traction on the plexus during delivery. Although lesions have classically been divided into those affecting upper spinal segments (Erb palsy) and those affecting lower segments (Klumpke palsy), the distinction may not be clear-cut in some cases. Injury to the C5 and C6 fibers is most often identified by the child's arm hanging limply adducted and internally rotated at the shoulder and extended and pronated at the elbow (Fig. 2-35). Appropriate deep-tendon reflexes are absent. It may be difficult to confirm sensory deficit, and autonomic fibers are often intact. Diagnosis is made clinically, but electromyography may be indicated to assess the severity of the injury and to determine the prognosis in patients not showing improvement after 6 to 8 weeks. Treatment should be deferred for at least 7 to 10 days; then specific physical therapy and splinting should be undertaken. Most infants with brachial plexus palsies demonstrate complete recovery in the first few months of life. The earlier the beginning of recovery, the better is the long-term prognosis.

Congenital Anomalies

Innumerable congenital anomalies, many of a minor nature, can be noted at birth. Although any single minor malformation may be of little medical consequence, the identification of three or more in a single infant may be a clue to more serious errors of morphogenesis. A careful family history, including examination of the parents and siblings, can often place these malformations in proper perspective.

Digits

The majority of minor external anomalies involve the hands, feet, and head. One of the more common abnormalities of digitation, especially in black infants, is the presence of a supernumerary digit (Fig. 2-36), which is most often located lateral to the fifth digit on the hand or foot. This condition is distinguishable from true polydactyly because of the small pedicle that attaches the extra digit to the fifth digit. The supernumerary digit may have a fingernail but often lacks bones. Although usually of no consequence, a supernumerary digit has, on occasion, been associated with major central nervous system (CNS) malformations. Removal may be accomplished by applying a ligature around the pedicle (assuming that it is thin and lacks palpable bony tissue) as close as possible to the surface of the fifth digit and allowing for the extra digit to fall off naturally. This usually takes approximately 1 week. Care should be taken to observe for infection.

True polydactyly (duplication of digits) may also be seen (Fig. 2-37). It is most common on the feet but can also occur on the hands. There may be a family history of this anomaly, or it may occur in association with other, more serious patterns of malformation. Although removal is not required, it may be indicated cosmetically.

Syndactyly, fusion of the soft tissues between digits, is relatively common (Fig. 2-38). Once again, a family history can be helpful.

External Ear

Careful morphologic examination of the external ear may reveal a number of minor anomalies. One of the more common is the presence of

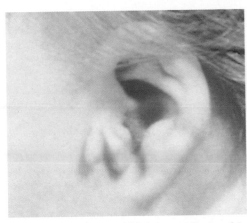

FIG. 2-39 Ear tags. Multiple preauricular skin tags were seen as an isolated finding in this patient.

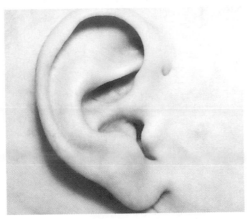

FIG. 2-40 Aural fistula. A pronounced congenital ear pit is seen anterior to the tragus. Its only significance is that it may become infected.

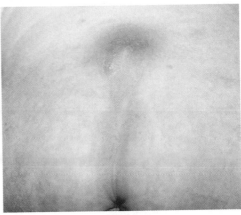

FIG. 2-41 Pilonidal sinus. This midline sinus overlying the sacrum did not extend to the spinal cord.

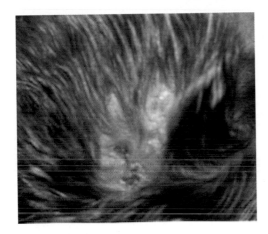

FIG. 2-42 Localized ectodermal dysplasia. An extensive punched-out area lacking all normal dermal elements is seen in the midline of the scalp of this child with trisomy 13.

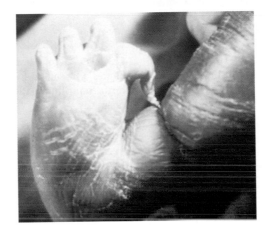

FIG. 2-43 Amniotic bands. A lower extremity amniotic band caused amputation of the toes and constriction around the lower leg.

preauricular skin tags located anterior to the tragus (Fig. 2-39). These tags may be unilateral or bilateral and represent remnants of the first branchial arch. Although often of little consequence, they may be seen in serious malformations of branchial arch development involving multiple structures of the head and neck. Surgical removal may be indicated for cosmetic purposes.

A second, often overlooked malformation is the presence of ear pits or congenital aural fistulae located anterior to the tragus (Fig. 2-40). These may be familial, occur twice as often in girls, and are more common in blacks. They are of little consequence beyond the fact that they may become infected.

Midline Defects

Although major malformations of the spinal column, such as myelomeningocele, are readily identifiable (see Chapter 15), diagnostic differentiation between two other midline defects—pilonidal sinuses and congenital dermal sinuses of the lumbar and sacral spine—can be difficult. A pilonidal sinus tends to be located over the sacrum (Fig. 2-41). The surface opening is usually larger than that of a dermal sinus, but the tract rarely extends into the spinal canal. Therefore although infection can occur, CNS extension is unlikely. A congenital dermal sinus is usually located over the lower lumbar region, with a

sinus tract that can extend farther down the spinal column. The external orifice may be a small dimple or an easily visible opening surrounded by hair. Recognition is important because there may be an underlying spinal dysraphism, and infection of the tract can extend to the CNS. Both types of sinuses may coexist in the same infant. If diagnostic differentiation is difficult, radiographic and neurosurgical evaluations may be indicated.

Another form of midline defect may occur over the posterior parietal scalp and consists of a localized area of ectodermal dysplasia (Fig. 2-42). This lesion appears "punched out" and lacks all normal dermal elements. It may be associated with chromosomal anomalies, especially trisomy 13, but may be present in otherwise normal infants. Similar lesions, often located on the extremities, should be distinguished from those on the scalp, since they often represent a dermatologic defect known as *cutis aplasia*.

Amniotic Bands

A number of serious structural deformations can result from early in utero amniotic rupture and subsequent bandline compression or amputation. The band-induced abnormalities generally affect the limbs, digits, and craniofacial structures (Fig. 2-43). This phenomenon is usually sporadic.

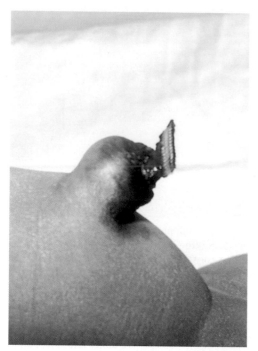

FIG. 2-44 Umbilical hernia. This prominent umbilical hernia was noted at birth in an otherwise normal black infant.

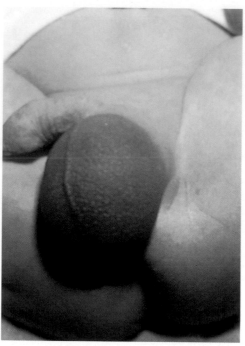

FIG. 2-45 Scrotal swelling. This infant demonstrates a unilateral hydrocele that was noted at birth. Transillumination was consistent with the diagnosis.

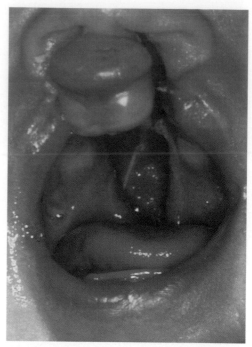

FIG. 2-46 Cleft lip. A prominent bilateral cleft lip with a complete cleft palate is seen in an infant with trisomy 13. The cleft extends from the soft to the hard palate, exposing the nasal cavity.

Umbilical Hernia

An umbilical hernia is a common finding, especially in black infants (Fig. 2-44). The incidence of this defect of the central fascia beneath the umbilicus is also higher in premature infants and those with congenital thyroid deficiency. It is important to distinguish between this relatively benign fascial defect and the more serious defects of the somites that form the peritoneal, muscular, and ectodermal layers of the abdominal wall underlying the umbilicus, resulting in an omphalocele. In the latter condition, a portion of the intestine is located outside the abdominal wall (see Chapter 17). When large, the distinction is obvious, but in its mildest form it resembles a fixed hernia of the umbilicus. True umbilical hernias usually require no therapy because the majority resolve spontaneously in the first few years of life. Those that remain after the age of 3 years can be surgically repaired. Attempts to reduce the hernia with tape or coins are ineffective. Incarceration is rare.

Scrotal Swelling

Swelling of the scrotum in the neonate is relatively common, especially in breech deliveries. Although the differential diagnosis includes hematomas, infections, testicular torsion, and tumors, the majority of cases are attributable to hydroceles or fluid accumulation in the tunica vaginalis. Palpation reveals an extremely smooth, firm, egg-shaped mass that brightly transilluminates (Fig. 2-45). When the hydrocele is noncommunicating, the clinician can often palpate above the mass with the thumb and finger and feel a normal spermatic cord. The testicle may be difficult to palpate but is usually visible on transillumination. With inguinal hernias, the prolapsed intestine may transilluminate as well, but it usually presents visible septa under high-intensity light.

Furthermore, on palpation there is significant thickening of the spermatic cord. Although a hydrocele may persist for months, the majority resolve spontaneously. There is a high association with inguinal hernias, especially in hydroceles that persist. In such cases, the spermatic cord is often noticeably thickened. Given the association with hernias, the possibility of bowel incarceration should be kept in mind. Surgical repair is indicated when a hydrocele persists for more than 6 months or when it is associated with findings suggestive of an inguinal hernia. (See Chapter 17 for a more detailed discussion of inguinal hernias.)

Oral Clefts

Cleft lip and palate are among the most common facial anomalies (Fig. 2-46). These defects represent failure of lip fusion (at 35 days) and, in some cases, subsequent failure of closure of the palatal shelves (at 8 to 9 weeks). Although many cases occur spontaneously, others appear to be inherited, and in a minority of instances the defect is one manifestation of a chromosomal disorder. Adequate assessment necessitates careful examination of all structures of the head and neck and their relationship to each other. For example, cleft palate may be coupled with mandibular hypoplasia (Pierre Robin syndrome), resulting in significant respiratory obstruction. Because of associated eustachian tube dysfunction, otitis media is an almost invariable complication of cleft palate. Specialized feeding techniques are often necessary for these infants. Even in the absence of an overt cleft, palpation and visualization of the palate and uvula should be routine because clefts of the soft palate (associated with a bifid uvula and a midline notch at the posterior border of the hard palate) can lead to later speech problems.

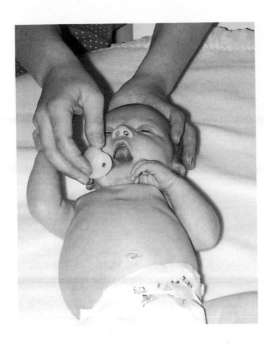

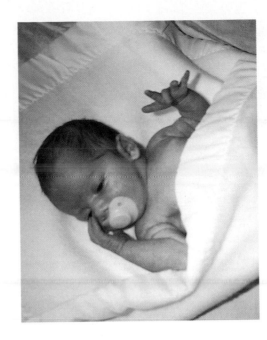

FIG. 2-47 Rooting reflex. The infant opens the mouth and turns the head toward the pacifier stimulating the cheek.

FIG. 2-48 Sucking reflex. Vigorous sucking movements are initiated when an object is placed in the infant's mouth.

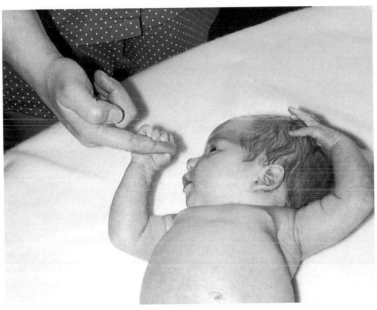

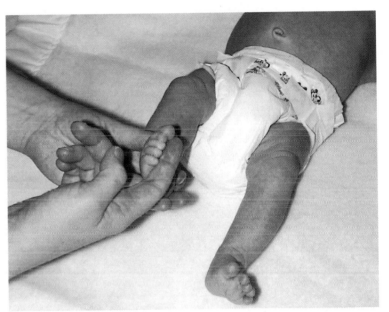

FIG. 2-49 Grasp reflex (palm). Transverse stimulation of the midpalm leads to a grasp by the infant.

FIG. 2-50 Grasp reflex (sole). Transverse stimulation of the midsole triggers a grasp by the infant.

Primitive Reflexes

Normal newborns exhibit a large number of easily elicited primitive reflexes that are often altered or absent in the infant with neurologic impairment. These reflexes may be transiently depressed in the infant who has experienced difficulty in achieving the transition between intrauterine and extrauterine existence. The persistent absence or asymmetry of one or more of these reflexes may be a clue to the potential presence of neuromuscular abnormalities requiring further investigation (see Chapter 3).

The rooting reflex may be elicited by lightly stimulating the infant's cheek and observing the reflexive attempts to bring the stimulating object to the mouth (Fig. 2-47). The sucking reflex is activated by placing an object in the infant's mouth and observing the sucking movements (Fig. 2-48). In the grasp reflex, illustrated in Fig. 2-49 and 2-50, transverse stimulation of the midpalm or midsole leads to flexion of the digits or toes around the examiner's fingers.

The Moro reflex (Fig. 2-51) evaluates vestibular maturation and the relationship between flexor and extensor tone. Elicitation of the reflex involves a short (10-cm), sudden drop of the head when the infant is supine. The full response involves extension of the arms, "fanning" of the fingers, and then upper extremity flexion followed by a cry. An incomplete but identifiable reflex becomes apparent at approximately 32 weeks' gestation, and by 38 weeks it is essentially complete. Very immature infants demonstrate extension of the arms and fingers but no true flexion or sustained cry. Marked asymmetry of response may be associated with focal neurologic impairment.

These reflexes and a host of other less commonly used reflexes are termed *primitive* because they are present at or shortly after birth and normally disappear after the first few months of life. Just as their ab-

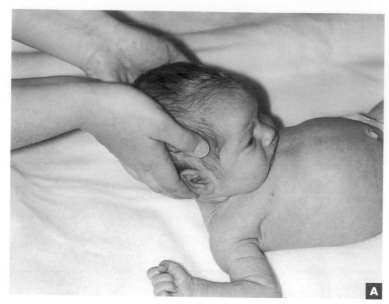

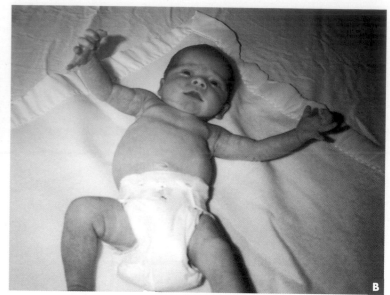

FIG. 2-51   Moro reflex. *A*, To elicit the reflex, the head is supported and allowed to drop to the level of the bed. The initial extension response to vestibular stimulation is shown in *B*. The complete response includes secondary flexion and cry.

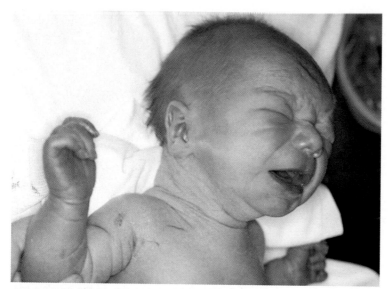

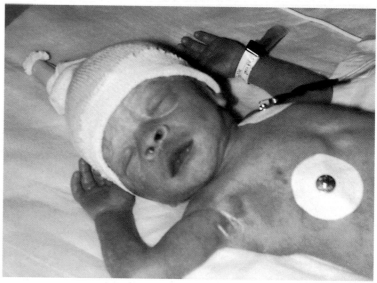

FIG. 2-52   Cyanosis. This critically ill infant exhibits cyanosis and poor skin perfusion.

FIG. 2-53   Flaring. Reflexive widening of the nares may be seen in infants with respiratory distress.

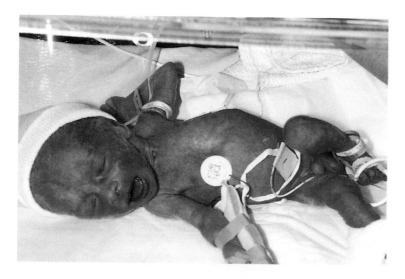

sence may indicate neurologic impairment at birth, their abnormal persistence may also be cause for concern.

Respiratory Distress

The differential diagnosis and the subsequent management of the infant with respiratory distress are the most frequent challenges encountered by the practitioner of newborn medicine. Problems posed by prematurity, the failure of the necessary transition to extrauterine existence, infectious complications, metabolic derangements, and various

FIG. 2-54   Retractions. The inward collapse of the lower anterior chest wall can be seen in this premature infant with RDS.

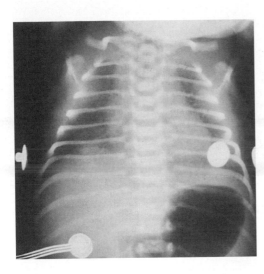

FIG. 2-55 RDS. Note the ground-glass appearance and the presence of air bronchograms.

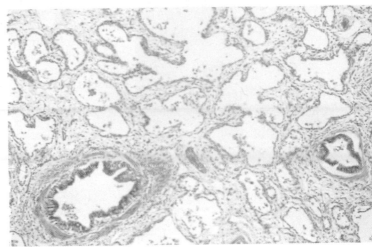

FIG. 2-56 Bronchopulmonary dysplasia. Histologic features include inflammation and fibrosis.

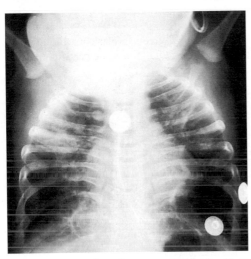

FIG. 2-57 Bronchopulmonary dysplasia. Note the alternating areas of hyperinflation and atelectasis.

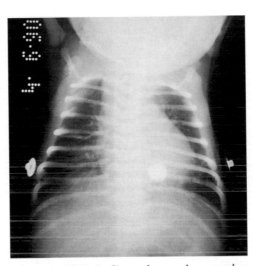

FIG. 2-58 TTN. Radiograph reveals a number of streaky perihilar densities and a visible fluid density in the right major fissure.

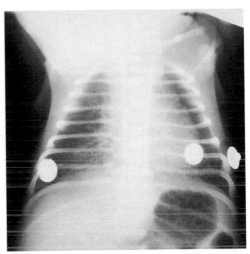

FIG. 2-59 Congenital pneumonia. Cultures from the lungs of this infant were positive for group B streptococci. Note the similarity to previous radiographs.

congenital and acquired abnormalities of the cardiopulmonary system may all lead to a similar presentation in the newborn period.

Infants with respiratory distress may present with tachypnea and/or cyanosis (Fig. 2-52) and varying degrees of a triad of signs termed *grunting, flaring, and retractions (GFR)*. Grunting is a characteristic involuntary guttural expiratory sound made by infants as they exhale against a closed glottis in an attempt to maintain expiratory lung volume. *Flaring* refers to the reflexive opening of the nares during inspiration in such infants (Fig. 2-53). Retractions are the result of increased respiratory effort with high negative intrathoracic pressures leading to an inward collapse of the relatively compliant chest wall of the newborn during inspiration (Fig. 2-54).

Classic respiratory distress syndrome (RDS) is caused by a combination of lung immaturity secondary to preterm delivery and surfactant deficiency. The radiographic findings in such infants consist of a ground-glass appearance (small airway and alveolar atelectasis) and "air bronchograms" (an outline of the large airways superimposed on the relatively airless lung parenchyma) (Fig. 2-55). Infants with RDS usually need supplemental oxygen therapy and often require mechanical ventilatory assistance.

Most infants with RDS recover without sequelae. However, a small proportion develop a chronic lung condition known as *bronchopulmonary dysplasia*. Histologically, this condition is characterized by varying degrees of inflammation and fibrosis (Fig. 2-56). The chest x-ray studies of such infants exhibit areas of hyperinflation alternating with atelectasis (Fig. 2-57).

The most common cause of respiratory distress in term infants is transient tachypnea of the newborn (TTN). Thought to be related to the delayed removal of fetal alveolar fluid, this condition is more common in infants born by cesarean section. Radiographic findings may include streaky perihilar shadows caused by dilated lymphatics and/or visible fluid densities within the intralobar fissures (Fig. 2-58). As its name implies, TTN resolves over time, usually with minimal supportive care.

Unfortunately for the clinician, the early clinical and radiographic findings in infants with potentially life-threatening congenital pneumonias may mimic those seen in RDS or TTN (Fig. 2-59). This diagnostic uncertainty leads to early treatment with antibiotics until bacterial cultures, serial chest radiographs, and clinical improvements reassure the practitioner that the discontinuation of such antibiotics is warranted.

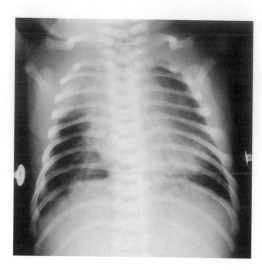

FIG. 2-60 Meconium aspiration. The radiograph reveals irregularly distributed areas of hyperaeration and consolidation.

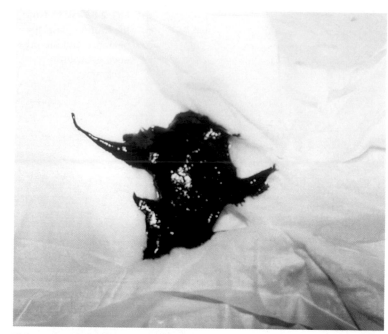

FIG. 2-61 Meconium. A typical, sticky, greenish-black meconium stool consists of accumulated intestinal cells, bile, and proteinaceous material formed during intestinal development.

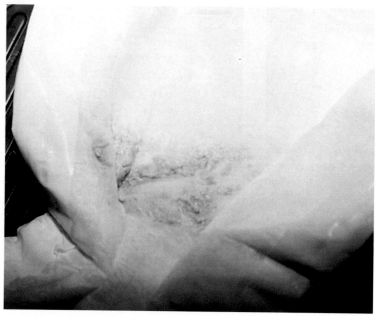

FIG. 2-62 Transitional stool. At 2 to 3 days after delivery, stools become greenish-brown and may contain some milk curds.

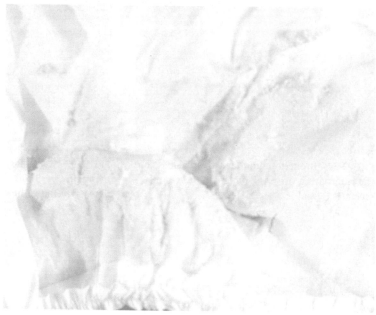

FIG. 2-63 Breast-milk stool. The stools of breast-fed infants are yellow, soft, and mild smelling and typically have the consistency of pea soup.

Meconium aspiration, discussed in the next section, may also manifest with respiratory distress. The radiographic findings consist of irregularly distributed areas of hyperaeration and consolidation throughout the lung parenchyma (Fig. 2-60).

Congenital heart disease (see Chapter 5) and various anomalies of the thoracic cavity or lungs (see Chapter 16) also commonly manifest in the newborn with signs of respiratory distress and should be included in the differential diagnosis when evaluating such infants.

Newborn Stools

An infant's first few bowel movements consist of accumulated intestinal cells, bile, and proteinaceous material formed during intestinal development. The material, termed *meconium* (Fig. 2-61), is a sticky greenish-black product mirroring the shape of the fetal intestine. When passed into the amniotic fluid before delivery, it can, if aspirated into the lung, cause a potentially life-threatening disorder known as *meconium aspiration syndrome.* Such early passage is generally precipitated

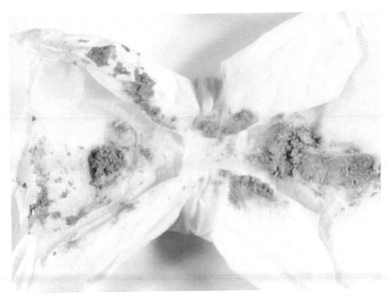

FIG. 2-64 Formula stool. Infants fed commercial formulas typically have darker, firmer stools than breast-fed infants.

After the third to fourth day, the quality and frequency of stool are often functions of the type of milk given. Breast-fed infants have stools that are yellow to golden, mild smelling, and pasty in consistency, resembling pea soup (Fig. 2-63). Although it is commonly thought that the mother's diet directly affects the frequency and consistency of a breast-fed infant's stool, there is little scientific information on this subject. Infants fed cow's milk–based formula have pale yellow to light brown stools that are firm and somewhat more offensive in odor (Fig. 2-64).

There is a wide range of normal stool frequency in neonates. Many infants have a stool after each feeding for the first several weeks, which is due to an active gastrocolic reflex. Other normal infants may have one stool every few days. In general, infants fed cow's milk formula have stools less frequently than those fed breast milk.

A careful history, with emphasis on an infant's stool pattern, feeding history, and any parental attempts (laxatives, rectal manipulation) to induce bowel movements can be extremely important. Normal weight gain in the presence of true diarrhea is unusual. Difficulty passing stools (straining, crying, decreased frequency) may reflect local irritation from anal fissure formation rather than true constipation. The use of a topical lubricant and stool softeners can often overcome constipation. Failure of such measures suggests the possibility of a significant pathologic condition (see Chapter 17 for further discussion).

by fetal distress or asphyxia. Failure to pass meconium in the first 2 days of life may indicate intestinal obstruction resulting from stenosis, atresia, or Hirschsprung disease. The possibility of cystic fibrosis with a meconium ileus should also be considered. In premature infants, failure to pass meconium may reflect meconium plug syndrome (small left colon syndrome), which appears to be a disorder of maturation of intestinal motility. In most cases, a Gastrografin enema leads to prompt passage of meconium without recurrence.

By the third day of life, stools change in character and become known as *transitional stools* (Fig. 2-62). They are greenish brown to yellowish-brown, are less sticky than meconium, and may contain some milk curds. In some infants who are fed generous quantities of milk during the first few days, the stool may have an increased liquid component that contains undigested sugar. This diarrheal stool resolves with moderation in the quantity of feeding, since it is caused by the osmotic effect of undigested lactose.

BIBLIOGRAPHY

Avery GB, ed: *Neonatology: pathophysiology and management of the newborn*, ed 3, Philadelphia, 1987, JB Lippincott.

Ballard JL, Novak KK, Driver M, et al: A simplified score for assessment of fetal maturation of newly-born infants, *J Pediatr* 95:769-774, 1979.

Dubowitz LV, Dubowitz C, Goldberger C: Clinical assessment of gestational age in the newborn infant, *J Pediatr* 77:1-10, 1970.

Fox H: Pathology of the placenta. In *Major problems in pathology*, vol 7, Philadelphia, 1978, WB Saunders.

Jones KL: *Smith's recognizable patterns of human malformation*, ed 4, Philadelphia, 1988, WB Saunders.

Painter MJ, Bergman I: Obstetrical trauma to the neonatal central and peripheral nervous system, *Semin Perinatol* 6(1):89-104, 1982.

Scanlon JW, Nelson T, Grylack LJ, Smith YF: *A system of newborn physical examination*, Baltimore, 1979, University Park Press.

3

Developmental-Behavioral Pediatrics

HEIDI FELDMAN ❦ ROBERTA E. BAUER

Developmental-behavioral pediatrics is the study of the acquisition of functional skills during childhood and variations in sequence or timing that indicate developmental disorders and disabilities. Traditionally, developmental pediatrics concerns itself with cognitive and motor competence and with constitutionally based physical and mental disabilities that limit adaptive functioning. In contrast, behavioral pediatrics emphasizes behavioral and emotional characteristics and the interaction of family and social variables on these characteristics. A union of the terms is preferred. Developmental-behavioral pediatrics thus emphasizes that cognitive and motor skills interact with social and emotional characteristics in normal and disordered development.

The goal of this chapter is to familiarize the reader with developmental-behavioral issues faced in routine pediatric practice. The first half discusses the fundamental principles of development and applies them to each major domain of functioning. Within each domain is a discussion of developmental milestones, methods of assessment, signs of developmental variation, and approaches to children who show developmental delay or deviant patterns. The second half describes several developmental disorders including definitions, diagnostic criteria, the role of physical examination in evaluation, and relevant physical findings.

Principles of Normal Development

For ease of description and investigation, development is commonly discussed in terms of domains of function: gross motor skills refer to the use of the large muscles of the body; fine motor skills to the use of small muscles of the hands; cognition to the use of higher mental processes, including thinking, memory, and learning; language, to the comprehension and production of meaningful symbolic communication; and social and emotional functioning to emotional reactions to events and interactions with others. In fact, these domains are interdependent. Cognitive abilities in infancy cannot readily be distinguished from sensorimotor functioning. Similarly, mature social functioning depends on competent language abilities. Within each domain, develop-

mental change is generally orderly and predictable. Early reflex patterns and congenital sensory and motor capabilities are the building blocks of higher-order skills.

Developmental Assessment

A central component of health maintenance is the assessment of development. The assessment procedure of choice is developmental surveillance, a method in which the physician uses all available clinical tools—history, physical examination, screening tests, and other assessment techniques—to determine a child's developmental status. Observations of the child's accomplishments in each developmental domain can often be ascertained in the course of a complete routine physical examination. Frequent routine assessments promote a longitudinal view of the child and allow parental concerns to be addressed in a timely manner. A formal developmental screening or assessment can be arranged if there are severe or persistent concerns.

Standardized screening methods, such as the Denver Developmental Screening Test, also play an important role in evaluation. Physicians typically use screening tests at selected health maintenance visits, most often at the 9-month visit and again at the 24- or 36-month visit. These tests allow physicians to distinguish normal development from delays and deviations in unselected populations. They are useful adjuncts to history and physical examinations. However, they are inappropriate instruments for populations at risk, who require comprehensive assessment. Screening instruments are more sensitive to severe developmental delays than mild delays; minor developmental problems may be missed. Children who are developing normally may fail a screening test because of shyness, unfamiliarity with the examiner or the materials, or other factors unrelated to developmental competence. When parents have concerns about their child's developmental standing, the screening test can be used to confirm but not describe the nature of the problem. If parental concerns persist despite negative findings, a full evaluation is in order. To ensure that the performance is representative of the child's ability, screening tests should be performed when the child is physically well, familiar with the setting and examiner, and under minimal stress.

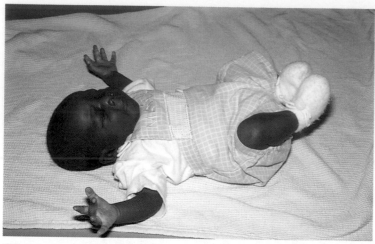

FIG. 3-1 First phase of the Moro response. Symmetric abduction and extension of the extremities follow a loud noise or an abrupt change in the infant's head position.

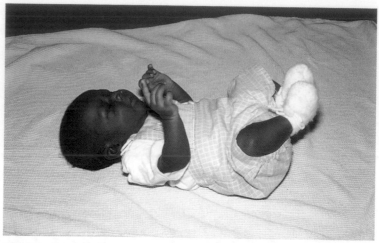

FIG. 3-2 Second phase of the Moro response. Symmetric adduction and flexion of the extremities, accompanied by crying.

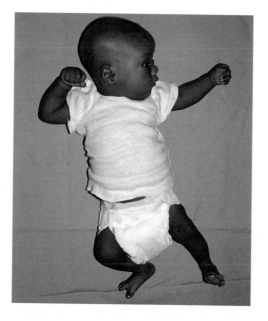

FIG. 3-3 Flexion of the arm and leg on the occipital side and extension on the chin side create the "fencer position."

TABLE 3-1

Primitive Reflexes and Protective Equilibrium Responses

Reflex	Appearance*	Disappearance*
Moro	Birth	4 months
Hand grasp	Birth	3 months
Crossed adductor	Birth	7 months
Toe grasp	Birth	8-15 months
ATNR	2 weeks	6 months
Head righting	4-6 months	Persists voluntarily
Protective equilibrium	4-6 months	Persists voluntarily
Parachute	8-9 months	Persists voluntarily

*Different sources may vary on the precise timing of the appearance and disappearance of these primitive and equilibrium responses.

Gross Motor Development

Early Reflex Patterns

At birth, a neonate's movements consist of alternating flexions and extensions that usually are symmetric and vary in strength with the infant's state of wakefulness. In addition, involuntary reflexes can be elicited; they indicate that the patterns of movement requiring the integrated activity of multiple muscle groups are present even at birth.

Perhaps the best known of these reflex patterns is the Moro response. This reflex can occur spontaneously after a loud noise, but typically, it is elicited during the course of physical examination by an abrupt extension of the infant's neck. The first phase of the response consists of symmetric abduction and extension of the arms with extension of the trunk (Fig. 3-1). The second phase is marked by adduction of the upper extremities, as in an embrace, and frequently is accompanied by crying (Fig. 3-2). The Moro reflex gradually disappears by 4 months of age, secondary to the development of cortical functioning. In children up to 4 months of age, the Moro response can be used to evaluate the integrity of the central nervous system and to detect peripheral

problems such as congenital musculoskeletal abnormalities or neural plexus injuries.

Another early reflex pattern is called the *asymmetric tonic neck reflex (ATNR)* (Fig. 3-3). A newborn's limb motions are strongly influenced by head position. If the head is directed to one side, either by passive turning or by inducing the baby to follow an object to that side, extensor muscle tone increases on that side and in the flexor muscles on the opposite side. This response is not often seen immediately after birth, when the newborn has high flexor tone throughout the body, but it usually appears by 2 to 4 weeks of age. The ATNR allows the baby to sight along the arm to the hand and is considered one of the first steps in the coordination of vision and reaching. This reflex disappears by 6 months of age, secondary to the development of cortical functioning. Other primitive reflexes are listed in Table 3-1.

With the emergence of voluntary control from higher cortical centers, muscular flexion and extension become balanced. Primitive reflexes are replaced by reactions that allow children to maintain a stable posture, even if they are rapidly moved or jolted. A timetable listing the expected emergence and disappearance of some of the protective equilibrium responses is presented in Table 3-1.

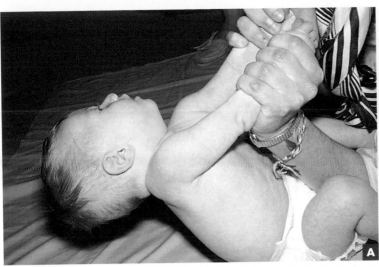
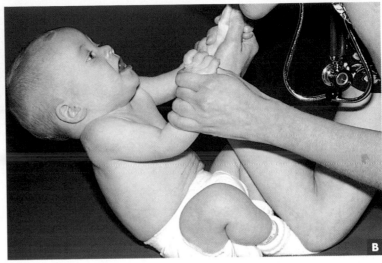

FIG. 3-4 Development of head control on the pull-to-sit maneuver. *A,* At 1 month of age the head lags after the shoulders. *B,* At 5 to 6 months the child anticipates the movement and raises the head before the shoulders.

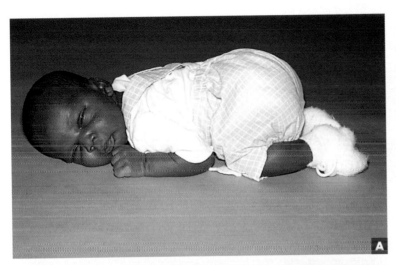
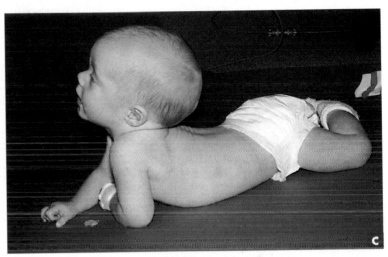
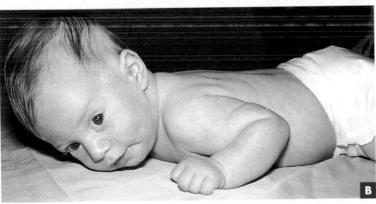

FIG. 3-5 Development of posture in the prone position. *A,* The newborn lies tightly flexed with the pelvis high and the knees under the abdomen. *B,* At 2 months of age, the infant extends the hips and pulls the shoulders slightly. *C,* At 3 to 4 months, the infant keeps the pelvis flat and lifts the head and shoulders.

Antigravity Muscular Control

Head Control

The infant's earliest control task is to maintain a stable posture against the influence of gravity. This control develops in an organized fashion, from head to toe, or in a cephalocaudad progression, paralleling neuronal myelination. For example, neck flexors allow head control against gravity when a child is pulled from the supine to the sitting position. Neonates show minimal control of the neck flexors, holding their heads upright only briefly when supported in a sitting position. When an infant is pulled to a sitting position, the head lags behind the arms and shoulders. At 5 to 6 months of age the infant anticipates the direc-

tion of movement of the pull-to-sit maneuver and flexes the neck before the shoulders begin to lift (Fig. 3-4).

Trunk Control and Sitting

In the prone position a newborn remains in a tightly flexed position and can simply turn the face from side to side along the bedsheets. Progressive control of the shoulders and upper trunk in the first few months of life, plus a decrease in flexor tone, enables the young infant to hold the chest off the bed with the weight supported on the forearms (Fig. 3-5). Evolution of trunk control down the thoracic spine can also be observed with the infant in a sitting position (Fig. 3-6). As control

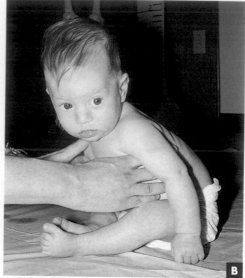
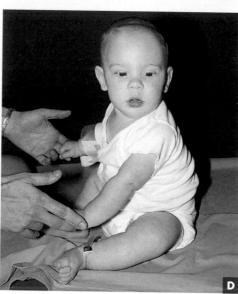
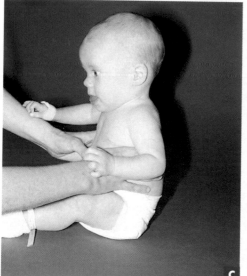
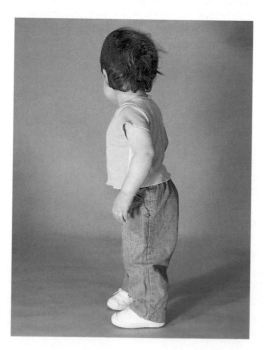

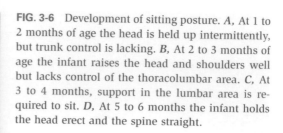

FIG. 3-6 Development of sitting posture. *A,* At 1 to 2 months of age the head is held up intermittently, but trunk control is lacking. *B,* At 2 to 3 months of age the infant raises the head and shoulders well but lacks control of the thoracolumbar area. *C,* At 3 to 4 months, support in the lumbar area is required to sit. *D,* At 5 to 6 months the infant holds the head erect and the spine straight.

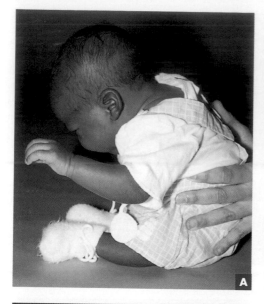

FIG. 3-7 Standing. By 1 year of age, the lordotic curve, exaggerated here by a diaper, is evident.

reaches the lumbar area, the lumbar lordotic curve can be seen when the child is standing (Fig. 3-7).

Head Righting and Parachute Response

Balance and equilibrium reactions also emerge in a cephalocaudal sequence. *Head righting* refers to the infant's ability to keep the head vertical despite a tilt of the body. A 4-month-old infant typically demonstrates this ability in vertical suspension when gently swayed from side to side. As control moves downward, protective equilibrium responses can be elicited in a sitting infant by abruptly but gently pushing the infant's center of gravity past the midline in one of the horizontal planes. This reflex response, which involves increased trunk flexor tone toward the force and an outreached hand and limb away from the force, usually emerges by 6 months of age (Fig. 3-8). At 10 months the child develops the parachute response, an outstretch of both arms and legs when the body is abruptly moved head first in a downward direction (Fig. 3-9). The acquisition of this equilibrium response demonstrates the integrity of the sensations and motor responses of the central nervous system, which allow independent sitting and standing in normal or motor-impaired children.

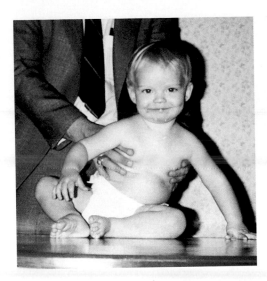

FIG. 3-8 Protective equilibrium response. As the child is pushed laterally by the examiner, he flexes his trunk toward the force to regain his center of gravity while one arm extends to protect against falling (lateral propping).

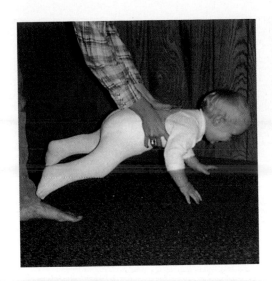

FIG. 3-9 Parachute response. As the examiner allows the child to free fall in ventral suspension, the child's extremities extend symmetrically to distribute his weight over a broader and more stable base on landing.

TABLE 3-2

Early Gross Motor Milestone Normals

Task	Age range*
Sits alone momentarily	4-8 months
Rolls back to stomach	4-10 months
Sits steadily	5-9 months
Gets to sitting	6-11 months
Pulls to standing	6-12 months
Stands alone	9-16 months
Walks three steps alone	9-17 months

From Bayley N: *Bayley scales of infant development*, ed 2, San Antonio, 1993, Psychological Corp, Harcourt Brace.
*Wide ranges in the attainment of these gross motor milestones in healthy children are the rule rather than the exception.

Development of Locomotion

Gross motor milestones can be described in terms of locomotion and antigravity muscular control (Table 3-2). Prone-to-supine rolling usually is accomplished by 3 to 4 months of age, after the child gains sufficient control of shoulder and upper trunk musculature to prop up on the arms. Supine-to-prone rolling requires control of the lumbar spine and hip region, as well as the upper trunk; this is usually present by 5 to 6 months of age. Early commando crawling, accomplished at 5 to 6 months of age (Fig. 3-10, *A*), involves coordinated pulling with upper arms and passive dragging of the legs, akin to a soldier trying to keep the body out of the line of fire. By 6 to 9 months of age, as voluntary control moves to the hips and legs, the child is capable of getting up on the hands and knees, assuming a quadruped position, and creeping (Fig. 3-10, *B*). The next developmental milestone is supported standing. By 9 to 10 months of age, many children like to demonstrate this new skill by holding on to a parent or by walking independently while holding on to furniture. This is called *cruising* (Fig. 3-10, *C*). Increased control to the feet and disappearance of the plantar grasp reflex allow the child to walk independently. Walking three steps alone occurs at a median age of 11.7 months, with a range of 9 to 17 months of age (Fig. 3-10, *D*).

Development of Complex Gross Motor Patterns

Further progress in gross motor skills continues throughout childhood. The developmental sequence beyond walking incorporates improved balance and coordination and progressive narrowing of the base of support. The sequence of milestones is as follows: running, jumping on two feet, balancing on one foot, hopping, and skipping. The child simultaneously learns to use muscle groups in timed sequences. By 13½ months, the child walks well and by 36 months can balance on one foot for 1 second. Most children can hop by age 4. They can throw a ball overhead by 22½ months, but catching develops later, at almost 5 years.

Gross Motor Assessment During Health Maintenance Visits

The evaluation of gross motor skills can often begin when the pediatrician enters the office for a well-child visit. The typical 2-month-old infant is cradled in the parent's arms; the 6-month-old child is sitting with minimal support on the parent's lap or on the examination table next to the parent; the 12-month-old is cruising or toddling through the room. Although there is a wide age range in the onset and duration of each stage, the 6-month-old infant who lacks head control on the pull-to-sit maneuver, who cannot clear the table surface with the chest by supporting weight on the arms when prone, who shows no head righting, or who has persistent primitive reflexes such as a complete Moro response or ATNR is at sufficient variance from peers to warrant evaluation for a possible neuromuscular disorder. When gross motor delays are found in association with verbal and social delays, asymmetric use of one limb or one side of the body, or loss of previously attained milestones, further diagnostic evaluation is indicated.

Evaluation of the older infant or toddler who has mastered walking can occur in the course of the physical and neurologic evaluation. Many children enjoy showing off their abilities to jump, balance on one foot, hop, and skip. Some pediatricians use gross motor testing to establish rapport at the outset of a physical examination. However, since an aroused preschooler may not cooperate with a sedentary evaluation of heart or ears, many pediatricians hold off on motor evaluation until the conclusion of the examination. The Denver Developmental Screening Test includes basic milestones for assessment of children 2 to 6 years of age.

At the discovery of delayed or atypical development, the pediatrician's first task is to develop a differential diagnosis and a plan to establish the specific diagnosis. Potential causes of delayed gross motor development are listed in Table 3-3. Another equally important task is to recommend a treatment program. Physical therapy or infant stimulation programs should be actively considered for children with motor difficulties during infancy through preschool. Adaptive physical educa-

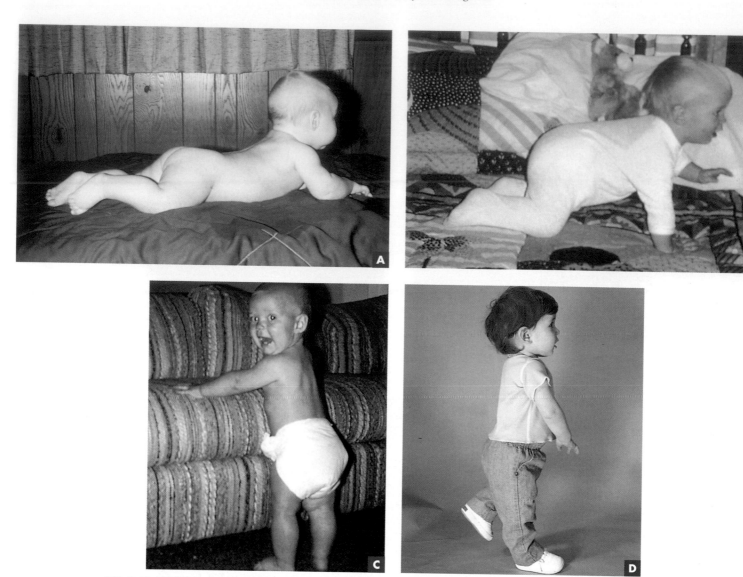

FIG. 3-10 Development of locomotion. *A, Crawling* implies that the belly is still on the floor. *B, Creeping* refers to mobility with the child on the hands and knees (quadruped). *C, Cruising* refers to standing with two-handed support on stationary objects before moving with steps. *D,* Early free walking.

TABLE 3-3

Potential Causes of Delayed Gross Motor Development

Global developmental delay	Motor dysfunction	Motor intact but otherwise restricted
Genetic syndromes and chromosomal abnormalities	Central nervous system damage—kernicterus, birth injury, neonatal stroke, trauma, prolonged seizures, metabolic insult, infection	Congenital malformations—bony or soft tissue defects
Brain morphologic abnormalities		Diminished energy supply—chronic illness, severe malnutrition
Endocrine deficiencies—hypothyroidism, prolonged hypoglycemia	Spinal cord dysfunction—Werdnig-Hoffmann disease, myelomeningocele, polio	Environmental deprivation—casted, non–weight-bearing
Neurodegenerative diseases	Peripheral nerve dysfunction—brachial plexus injury, heritable neuropathies	Familial and genetic endowment—slower myelination
Congenital infections	Motor end-plate dysfunction—myasthenia gravis	Sensory deficits—blindness
Idiopathic mental retardation	Muscular disorders—muscular dystrophies	Temperamental effects—low activity level, slow to try new tasks
	Other—benign congenital hypotonia	Trauma—child abuse

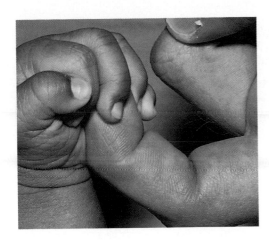

FIG. 3-11 Reflex hand grasp. A newborn reflexively grasps at a finger placed in the palm.

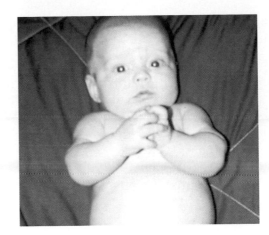

FIG. 3-12 Midline hand play. A 2-month-old infant brings the hands together at the midline.

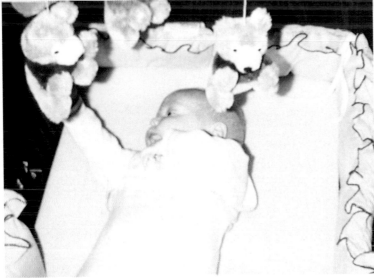

FIG. 3-13 Reaching and swiping. A 3-month-old infant uses his entire upper extremity as a unit in interacting with the toy.

tion programs are available for older children with mild problems that do not seriously impair function.

Fine Motor Development

Involuntary Grasp

At birth, the neonate's fingers and thumb are typically tightly fisted. A newborn grasps reliably and reflexively at any object placed in the palm (Fig. 3-11) and cannot release the grasp. Because of this reflex, the newborn's range of upper extremity motion is functionally limited. Normal development leads to acquisition of a voluntary grasp.

Voluntary Grasp

The reflexive palmar grasp gradually disappears at about 1 month of age. From that point, the infant gains control of fine motor skills in an orderly progression, from the midline to the periphery or from proximal to distal. In the second or third month of life, the infant initially brings both hands together for midline hand play (Fig. 3-12). Shortly after that, the baby begins to swipe at objects held in or near the midline (Fig. 3-13). At this early stage, swiping is in fact a gross motor activity that involves the entire upper extremity as a unit. However, it is

through swiping that the infant increases the exploratory range and fine tunes the small muscles of the wrist, hand, and fingers.

Improvements in fine motor control increase sensory input from the hands and permit greater hand manipulation through space. By 2 to 3 months of age, the hands are no longer tightly fisted, and the infant may begin sucking on a thumb or individual digit rather than the entire fist for self-comfort. A 3-month-old is usually able to hold an object in either hand if it is placed there, although the ability to grasp voluntarily or to release that object is limited. At approximately 4 to 5 months of age, infants begin to use their hands as entire units to draw objects toward them. Neither the hand nor the thumb functions independently at this point, and consequently, the child uses the hand like a rake.

Next, the child develops the ability to bend the fingers against the palm (palmar grasp), to squeeze objects, and to obtain them independently for closer inspection. Differentiation of the parts of the hand develops in association with differentiation of the two hands. Between 5 and 7 months of age, the infant can use hands independently to transfer objects across the midline. Further differentiation of the plane of movement of the thumb allows it to adduct as the fingers squeeze against the palm in a radial-palmar or whole-hand grasp. With time, the thumb moves from adduction to opposition. The site of pressure of the thumb against the fingers moves away from the palm toward the fingertips in what is called an *inferior pincer* or *radial-digital grasp*, seen around 9 months of age (Fig. 3-14). By 10 months of age, differentiated use of the fingers allows the child to explore the details of an object.

Between 9 and 12 months of age, the fine pincer grasp develops, allowing opposition of the tip of the thumb and the index finger (Fig. 3-14). This milestone enables the precise prehension of tiny objects (Fig. 3-15). The infant uses this skill in tasks such as self-feeding and exploration of small objects. By 1 year, the infant can position the hand in space to achieve vertical or horizontal orientation before grasping or releasing an object.

Development of Complex Fine Motor Skills

Early in the second year of life the young child uses the grasp to master tools and to manipulate objects in new ways. Dropping and throwing, stacking, and putting objects in and out of receptacles become favorite pastimes. Mastery of the cup and spoon supplement finger feeding as a more efficient and less messy means of eating (Fig. 3-16).

Advancements in fine motor planning and control can be demonstrated through the child's ability to stack small cubes. After children master stacking, they show consistent patterns of improvement in reproducing structures that they have watched the examiner assemble (Fig. 3-17). The child's ability to copy a variety of drawings also improves during this period.

5 MONTHS RAKE	7 MONTHS RADIAL-PALMAR GRASP	9 MONTHS RADIAL-DIGITAL GRASP	10 MONTHS INFERIOR-PINCER GRASP	12 MONTHS FINE PINCER GRASP
Thumb adducted, proximal thumb joint flexed, distal thumb joint flexed	Raking object into palm with adducted totally flexed thumb and all flexed fingers, OR with two partly extended fingers	Between thumb and side of curled index finger, distal thumb joint slightly flexed, proximal thumb joint extended	Between ventral surfaces of thumb and index finger, distal thumb joint extended, beginning thumb opposition	Between fingertips or fingernails, distal thumb joint flexed
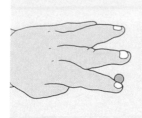	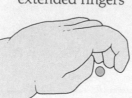	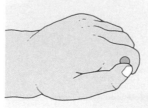	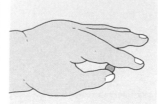	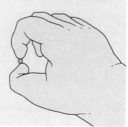

FIG. 3-14 Development of prehension. (Modified from Erhardt RP: *Developmental hand dysfunction: theory, assessment, treatment,* Laurel, Md, 1982, Ramsco.)

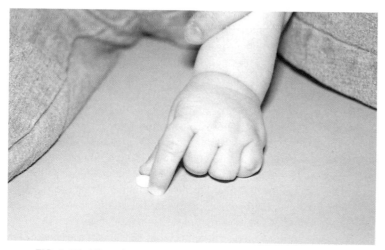

FIG. 3-15 Fine pincer grasp. A 12-month-old child lifts a pill.

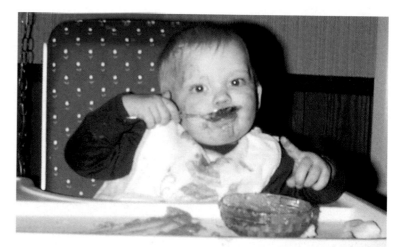

FIG. 3-16 Independent feeding. A 15-month-old child uses fine motor skills to use a spoon independently.

Fine Motor Evaluation and Testing

Fine motor testing can be incorporated readily into a physical examination and may uncover problems with vision, neuromuscular control, or perception, in addition to difficulties with attention or cooperation. The 4-month-old child usually can be encouraged to grasp a tongue depressor. By 6 to 9 months of age, two tongue depressors should be offered, one for each hand, since the child can operate the hands independently. At 9 to 12 months the child spontaneously points with an isolated index finger or picks up small objects with a fine pincer grasp. Children younger than 18 months of age generally use both hands equally well. Therefore the child who develops consistent handedness with neglect of the other limb before that time should have a neurodevelopmental assessment. The child who has not developed use of the thumb and pincer grasp by 1 year of age deserves further evaluation, as does the child who is unable to copy vertical or horizontal lines by age 3 or circles by age 4.

Fine motor activities can be engaging and nonthreatening to the preschool and school-age child; these activities allow the physician to make valuable observations and to establish a rapport. The physician can routinely request that the child use the waiting time or the period of history-taking to draw a self-portrait. These drawings provide a wealth of information not only on the child's capacities for fine motor control, but also on cognitive development and social and emotional functioning. A quick method for analyzing the age level of a drawing is to count the number of features in the drawing. The child receives one point for each of the following features: two eyes, two ears, a nose, a mouth, hair, two arms, two legs, two hands, two feet, a neck, and a trunk. Each point converts to the value of $1/4$ year added to a base age of 3 (Fig. 3-18).

Children with brain damage are at particular risk for problems with perceptual–fine-motor integration, even in the absence of visual problems and with minimal involvement of the upper extremities (Fig. 3-19).

Fine motor skills figure prominently in self-care activities. The child who lacks the dexterity to complete simple daily activities such as zipping, buttoning, or cutting with a knife may lack the self-esteem that accompanies independent self-care. Furthermore, children who contin-

FIG. 3-17 Fine motor tasks.

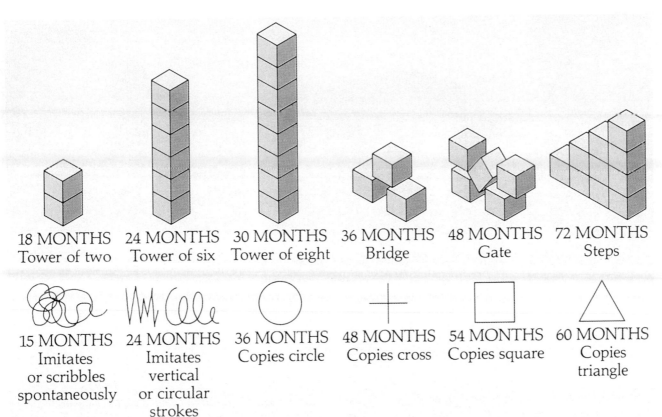

| 18 MONTHS | 24 MONTHS | 30 MONTHS | 36 MONTHS | 48 MONTHS | 72 MONTHS |
| Tower of two | Tower of six | Tower of eight | Bridge | Gate | Steps |

| 15 MONTHS | 24 MONTHS | 36 MONTHS | 48 MONTHS | 54 MONTHS | 60 MONTHS |
| Imitates or scribbles spontaneously | Imitates vertical or circular strokes | Copies circle | Copies cross | Copies square | Copies triangle |

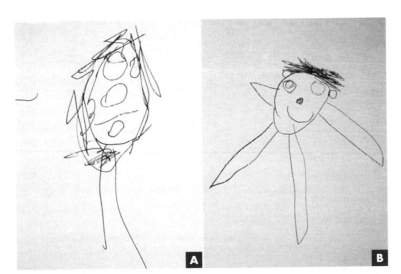

FIG. 3-18 Development of skill at drawing a person. *A,* This drawing by a 4-year-old child includes five features: eyes, nose, mouth, hair, and legs. To calculate an age equivalent, the child earns $1/4$ year for each of the five features, added to a base age of 3 years. This drawing has an age equivalent of $4^1/4$ years. *B,* A drawing by the same child at age 5. Note the inclusion of ears and arms as well as improvements in proportion. This drawing has an age equivalent of $4^3/4$ years.

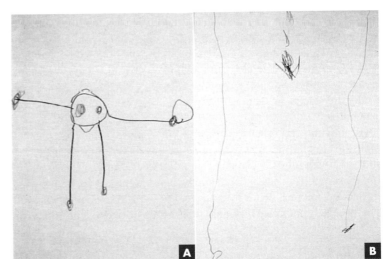

FIG. 3-19 Difficulties with visual–fine motor integration skills in a child with cerebral palsy. *A,* Drawing by a bright 4-year-old who was born prematurely but showed no developmental delays. Note the inclusion of seven features: eyes, hair, mouth, arms, hands, legs, and feet. The age equivalent for this drawing is $4^3/4$ years. *B,* Drawing by a 4-year-old child with spastic diplegia. Difficulties in organization appear related to visuomotor integration skills rather than to problems with fine motor skill.

ually depend on parents or teachers may be viewed by peers, teachers, or perhaps, most damagingly, by themselves as less mature. In the school-age child, inefficient fine motor skills can have a significant impact on the ability to compete with peers in timed tasks, even if the child is possessed of sound academic and conceptual skills. Occupational therapy and special education may enhance fine motor skills and emotional development in these children.

Cognitive Development

Early Sensory Processing

Innate sensory capabilities serve as the building blocks of cognitive development. Even at birth the healthy neonate responds to visual and auditory stimuli. These responses, like the primitive reflexes, take the form of integrated patterns of activity.

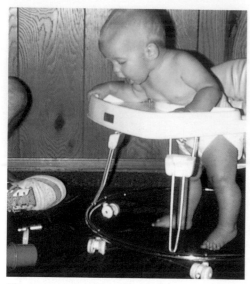

FIG. 3-20   Early object permanence. A 6-month-old infant was able to track his toy through a vertical fall and to search for it on the floor even after his gaze had been interrupted.

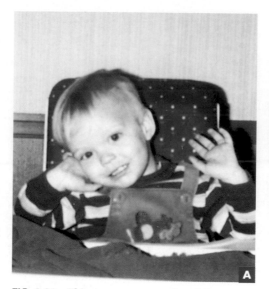
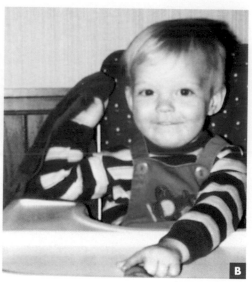

FIG. 3-21   Object permanence. *A* and *B,* An 11-month-old child is able to locate a small, hidden object even if no part of it remains visible. In doing so, he is demonstrating his understanding that objects are permanent.

The visual acuity of the full-term infant is estimated to fall between 20/200 and 20/400 and improves rapidly over the first year of life. Even at birth, it is possible to get the full-term newborn to fix on faces 9 to 12 inches from the face and to track objects horizontally at least 30 degrees. Some neonates, if assessed when calm and fully alert, can track objects 180 degrees across the visual field. Newborns also respond to sound, typically quieting to a human voice or to gentle inanimate sounds such as rattles or music. In the first days of life, many children turn to the source of sound and search for it with their eyes. These maneuvers, found on the Brazelton Neonatal Behavioral Assessment Scale, are useful in demonstrating neurobehavioral characteristics of newborns.

Examination must take place at optimal times, when the infant is alert; if the infant is drowsy or agitated, the ability to track visually or to search for sounds is severely compromised. If, when assessed under optimal circumstances and when fully alert, infants do not demonstrate horizontal tracking of objects, do not look at the toys or people with whom they are involved, or hold their heads in unusual positions, the physician should recommend prompt evaluation for abnormal visual perception or central nervous system development.

Development of Sensorimotor Intelligence

During the first 2 years of life, the sensorimotor period of development, the young child's cognitive abilities can be surmised only through use of the senses and through the physical manipulation of objects. The nature of an infant's thinking is assessed through concrete interaction with the environment. During this period, the child develops an understanding of the concept of object permanence, the ability to recognize that an object exists even when it cannot be seen, heard, or felt. Simultaneously, the child develops an understanding of cause-and-effect relationships. Progress in the child's development of these concepts is an important prerequisite to the development of pure mental activity, reflected in the ability to use symbols and language.

Early progress in the development of object permanence is indicated by the infant's continued though brief gaze at the site where a familiar toy or face has disappeared. At this point, children also repeat actions that they have discovered will produce interesting results. Between 4 and 8 months of age, infants become interested in changes in the position and appearance of toys. They can track an object visually through a vertical fall (Fig. 3-20) and search for a partially hidden toy. They also begin to vary the means of creating interesting effects. In these early months the baby's play consists of exploring toys to gain information about their physical characteristics. Activities such as mouthing, shaking, and banging can provide sensory input about an object beyond its visual features. However, when mouthing of toys persists as the predominant mode of exploration after 12 to 18 months of age, assessment of cognitive function is warranted.

At approximately 9 to 12 months of age, infants are able to locate objects that have been completely hidden (Fig. 3-21). Not surprisingly, peekaboo becomes a favorite pastime at this point. Later, the infant can crawl away from the mother and recall where to return to find her.

As children near 1 year of age, interest in toys extends beyond physical properties (e.g., color, texture). These children may begin to demonstrate their awareness that different objects have different purposes. For example, a child might touch a comb to the hair in a meaningful nonpretend action, typical of the 9- to 12-month age range. Beyond 1 year of age, children begin to vary their behavior to create novel effects. They no longer need to be shown how to work dials or knobs on a busy box, nor do they need to hit something by accident to discover the interesting effect that will result.

By 18 months of age, children can deduce the location of an object even if they have not seen it hidden from view. They can maintain mental images of desired objects and develop plans for obtaining them. The child's understanding of causality also advances; cause-and-effect relationships no longer need to be direct to be appreciated (Fig. 3-22). These developments herald the beginning of a new stage in cognitive development, that of symbolic thinking. They also indicate the need for major changes in the parental approach to discipline.

Development of Symbolic Capabilities

In the second year of life the child demonstrates mental activity independent of sensory processing or motor manipulation. For example, the child observes a television superhero performing a rescue mission and hours later reenacts the scene with careful precision. Clearly, the child has a

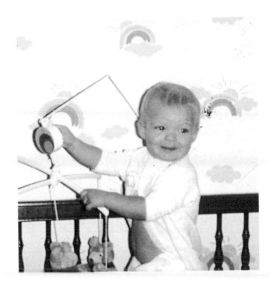

FIG. 3-22 Mature means-end reasoning. A 15-month-old child turns the key of the music box atop the mobile to make it play. The child's understanding has advanced beyond that of direct causality, such as pulling a toy to bring it closer.

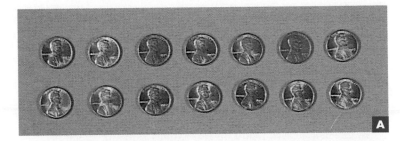
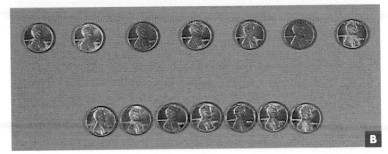

FIG. 3-23 Experimental design to demonstrate preoperational logic. The 3- or 4-year-old child agrees that the two rows in *A* have the same number of pennies. After seeing the pennies moved into the configuration in *B*, the child claims that the top row has more because it is longer.

mental image of the event and uses it to generate the delayed imitation.

As children develop the capacity for pure mental activity, they use objects to represent other objects or ideas. Genuine pretending begins; the child engages in playful representation of commonplace activities, using objects for their actual purpose but accompanied by exaggerated sounds or gestures. Pretend actions are combined into a series of events. For example, the child may hold a phone to the ear and then to a doll's ear or may feed a teddy bear and then put the bear to bed.

The next stage in development allows the child to plan pretend activities in anticipation of the play theme to come, combining many steps into the play. Preparing for play indicates an advance in pretending beyond that of improvising with the objects at hand. For example, the child might be seen preparing the play area or searching for needed objects and announcing what the objects are meant to represent.

Development of Logical Thinking

The preschool child has well-developed capabilities for mental representation and symbolic thinking. However, limited life experience and lack of formal education lead to a unique and charming logic during this period. Preschoolers often assume that all objects are alive like themselves. A car and a tricycle, for example, may be seen as alive, perhaps because they are capable of movement. Similarly, children claim that the moon follows them on an evening walk.

The logic of the preschooler is in large part influenced by the appearance of objects. Since an airplane appears to become smaller as it takes off, the preschooler may assume that all the people on the plane become smaller as well. Piaget demonstrated that preschoolers seem to think that number and quantity vary with appearance (Fig. 3-23). Under certain circumstances a 4-year-old child may show understanding that a quantity remains invariant unless something is added or subtracted. That same child, however, may insist that two rows of pennies are different in number simply because of a compelling visual difference between them.

The idiosyncratic logic of the preschooler is gradually replaced by conventional logic and wisdom. School-age children follow a logic akin to adult reasoning, at least when the stimuli are concrete. Faced with the same question about the pennies, they readily acknowledge that the two rows have the same number regardless of their visual appearance (Fig. 3-23). They also know that the airplane just looks smaller because it has moved farther from the viewer, and they giggle at the suggestion that the people on the plane have shrunk. Their logical limitations become obvious only when they must reason about the hypothetical or the abstract.

Adolescents, at least those with the benefits of formal education, tend to extend logical principles to increasingly diverse problems. They can generate multiple logical possibilities systematically when faced with scientific experiments, and they can also consider hypothetical problems. These principles of reasoning are applied not only to schoolwork but also to social situations. For example, the adolescent may think about who will go with whom to the school prom: "She thinks that I think that she wants to go with him, but I know that she wants to go with me."

Assessing Cognitive Development

Because the observations needed to assess cognitive abilities in the preverbal period are less well known by the general public than the major motor milestones, parents often rely on physicians for guidance. Simple observation of the child's use of toys or objects can help to determine cognitive progress. The pediatrician can induce the infant to look for a hidden toy or to play a game of peekaboo; the infant's anticipation of reappearance indicates the development of the concept of object permanence. Similarly, the toddler's ability to play with a toy telephone indicates the emergence of symbolic thought. Beyond the toddler stage the physician typically relies on conversation and language ability to assess levels of cognitive skill. Children with language delays may need a formal nonverbal assessment of cognitive abilities by a psychologist.

For the parents, a delay in a child's attainment of a well-known milestone may create tremendous fear about ultimate learning potential. In many cases, such parental concerns are put to rest when the physician determines that the child's learning to date is age-appropriate. If a child does show delays in cognitive development, the physician should generate a differential diagnosis (Table 3-4) from knowledge of the child's

T A B L E 3 - 4	

Potentially Remediable Disorders Associated with Developmental Delay

Findings sometimes present on history or examination	Possible disorder
Decreased vision or hearing	Specific sensory deficits
Startling spells, motor automatism	Seizure disorders
Lethargy, ataxia	Overmedication with anticonvulsants
Myxedema, delayed return on DTRs, thick skin and tongue, sparse hair, constipation, increased sleep, coarser voice, short stature, goiter	Hypothyroidism
Irritability, cold sweats, tremor, loss of consciousness	Hypoglycemia
Unexplained bruises in varying stages, failure to thrive	Child abuse and neglect
Short stature, weight below third percentile	Malnutrition or systemic illness producing failure to thrive
Poor purposeful attending in multiple settings	ADHD
No specific findings	Environmental deprivation
Anemia	Iron deficiency or lead exposure
Absent venous pulsations or papilledema on funduscopic examination, morning vomiting, headaches, brisk DTRs in lower extremities	Increased intracranial pressure
Vomiting, irritability and seizures, failure to thrive	Some inborn errors of metabolism (e.g., methylmalonicacidemia)
Hepatomegaly, jaundice, hypotonia, susceptibility to infection, cataracts	Galactosemia
Fair hair, blue eyes, "mousy" odor to urine	Phenylketonuria
Ongoing evidence of active or progressive disease	Chronic infection, inflammatory disease, malignancies

ADHD, Attention-deficit hyperactivity disorder; *DTR*, deep tendon reflex.

level of functioning in multiple domains and aspects of history and physical examination.

Parents should be given information about their child's delay early enough to enable them to make informed decisions about early educational intervention. Pediatricians serve a critical role in referring children to such programs and in monitoring their progress. Active communication between the providers of early intervention and the physician facilitates a comprehensive and cohesive approach.

Physicians frequently need the consultation of colleagues in psychology and education to assess the cognitive abilities of their older preschool and school-age patients. A number of methods have been devised for formal assessment of mental achievement, and almost all parents are familiar with the terms *intelligence quotient* and *IQ*. Although not a means of comprehensively assessing all mental capabilities, normal IQ scores are (albeit imperfect) predictors of which children will have the attention, social skills, motivation, and intelligence to perform well in school. Low IQ scores may reflect a child's poor ability to grasp new concepts, or they may indicate poor purposeful attending behaviors, as seen in depression or in attention-deficit hyperactivity disorder (ADHD). Low scores also may reflect poor social adjustment or limitations in test-taking capabilities, such as sitting in a chair at a table and applying maximal effort to a task requested by an unfamiliar authority figure. Frequently, low scores result from a combination of difficulties in several areas.

If children with sensory or motor impairments are tested with instruments normalized on able-bodied children, they often obtain low scores. Different assessment techniques have been devised to circumvent specific disabilities while obtaining information about a child's cognitive abilities; these are typically administered by psychologists, child development specialists, or special educators (Table 3-5).

Assessment of a child's abilities to learn must go beyond standardized IQ tests. For example, some children who can score in the normal range on IQ tests are unable to learn to read. A diversified and individualized assessment process should precede any educational recom-

mendation. The pediatrician, in the role of advocate, should ensure that assessments include information about the child's strengths and weaknesses, since educational planning should involve attention to all aspects of the child's abilities. Moreover, the pediatrician can encourage families to maintain an active, decision-making role in their children's education.

Language Development

Early Skills in Speech Perception and Production

The use of language—the ability to generate reproducible sounds or gestures that are recognized by others as representative of concepts—begins slowly and subtly in the first year of life. Language skills are subdivided into two realms: receptive skills—the ability to comprehend communication—and expressive skills—the ability to produce communication.

Neonates demonstrate skills that are useful in the eventual development of receptive language abilities. Even before birth, fetuses detect sounds and show preferences for some sounds over others. Pregnant women report that their unborn children may kick after sudden loud noises and that they may kick harder with rock than with classical music. At birth, the newborn is particularly attuned to the human voice and may turn toward a parent who is gently whispering. Children remain interested in sounds as they grow older and turn toward the source of a sound by 3 to 4 months of age (Fig. 3-24).

Children also are able to differentiate speech sounds, even close to birth. Experimental paradigms, using the fact that an infant's heart rate and sucking patterns change when they encounter new environmental stimuli, suggest that infants as young as 1 month of age can differentiate such similar speech sounds as /ba/ and /pa/.

By 2 to 3 months of age, children begin to *coo* or make musical sounds spontaneously. This is the first step toward the development of expressive verbal language.

TABLE 3-5

Tests Used in The Assessment of Cognitive Development

Type of scale	Tests used	Age range
Standard intelligence scales	Stanford-Binet Intelligence Scale —IV	2-adult
	Wechsler Intelligence Scale for Children—III	6-16 years
Nonverbal intelligence scales	Leiter International Performance Scale	2-18 years
Infant development tests	Bayley Scales of Infant Development—II	0-3½ years
	Gesell Developmental Schedules	0-5 years
Developmental scales for the visually impaired	Reynell-Zinkin Scales	0-5 years
	Maxfield-Buchalty Social Maturity for Blind Preschool Children	0-6 years
Screening instruments	Denver Developmental Screening Test (Denver II)	0-5 years
	Draw a Person Test (DAP-Goodenough-Harris Drawing Test)	3-adult

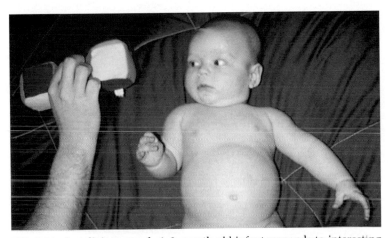

FIG. 3-24 Localizing sound. A 3-month-old infant responds to interesting sounds by looking in the direction of the sound.

By about 6 months of age, children place consonant sounds with vowel sounds, creating what is known as *babble*. In this period the infant says "ma-ma", or "da-da" without necessarily referring to the loving parent. By 9 to 12 months of age, they integrate babble with intonational patterns consistent with the parent's speech. This is called *jargon*.

Later Development

In the second half of the first year the child develops early skills in true receptive language. Milestones are listed in Table 3-6. By 6 months of age, children reliably respond to their names, and at about 9 months, they can follow verbal routines, such as waving bye-bye or showing how big they are. At about the same age, they also learn that pointing shares the focus of attention. The young infant looks at the point, whereas the older infant looks at the object to which the point is directed.

Receptive language can be demonstrated as children follow increasingly complex commands. For example, children will understand one-step commands such as "throw the ball" by approximately 1 year of age. The labeling of commonplace items in pictures is slightly more complex and begins after 1 year of age. The ability to choose between two pictures when asked "show me the..." should be consistent between 18 and 24 months of age.

By 2½ years of age, receptive language skills have advanced beyond the understanding of simple labels. The child is able to identify objects by their use. Continued advances in receptive language occur during the preschool years and are highly susceptible to environmental stimulation or deprivation.

Expressive language skills (Table 3-6) lag behind receptive skills in the first year of life. But even before word production begins, a child's gestures have communicative intent. Many 9- to 10-month-olds are able to communicate that their juice or cereal is "all gone" by placing their hands palms up, at shoulder height. Even older children gesture to make themselves better understood because gross and fine motor skills develop faster than the oropharyngeal musculature used in articulation.

Expressive language at first develops slowly. The child's first meaningful words are produced around the first birthday. Over the next 6 months the child may master only 20 to 50 more words. These early words come and go from the child's vocabulary and tend to be idiosyncratic child-forms. After 18 to 24 months, word usage increases rapidly, standard forms replace baby talk, and word combinations begin.

The child's earliest two-word sentences typically contain important content words but lack prepositions, articles, and verb-tense markings. This two-word phase has been called *telegraphic speech* because, like a telegram, the child leaves out nonessential articles and prepositions. Once the child is capable of three- and four-word utterances, length limitations do not appear to be a significant barrier. By age 3 the child has developed complex language with the use of pronouns and prepositions. The child develops the ability to ask questions, although at age 3 the most frequently posed question is probably "why." The child also can use negation within a sentence. By age 5 the child uses all parts of speech, as well as clauses and complex sentences.

Mastering Intelligibility and Fluency

Sounds required in language are mastered at different rates. Children who are attempting to say words containing sounds they cannot yet produce have a variety of choices on how to proceed: by omission of the difficult sound (*ba* for bottle), by substitution of a different sound (*fum* for thumb), or by distortion (*goyl* for girl). The information presented in Table 3-7 provides an estimate of when mastery of particular sounds, along with estimates of overall intelligibility, might be expected.

TABLE 3-6

Receptive and Expressive Language Milestones

Age range	Receptive response	Expressive response
0-1½ months	Startles or widens eye to sound	Shows variation in crying (hunger, pain)
1½-4 months	Quiets to voice, blinks eyes to sound	Makes musical sounds; coos; participates in recipro-cal exchange
4-9 months	Turns head toward sound; responds with raised arms when parent says "up" and reaches for child; responds appropriately to friendly or angry voices	Babbles; repeats self-initiated sounds
9-12 months	Listens selectively to familiar words; begins to respond to "no"; responds to verbal routine such as wave bye-bye or clap; turns to own name	Uses symbolic gestures and jargon; repeats parent-initiated sounds
12-18 months	Points to 3 body parts (eyes, nose mouth); understands up to 50 words; recognizes common objects by name (dog, cat, bottle, ball, book); follows one-step com-mands accompanied by gestures ("give me the doll," "hug your bear," "open your mouth")	Uses words to express needs; learns 20 to 50 words by 18 months; uses words inconsistently and mixed with jargon, echolalia, or both
18 months-2 years	Points to pictures when asked "show me"; understands *soon, in, on,* and *under;* begins to distinguish *you* from *me;* can formulate negative judgments (a pear is not a cookie)	Uses telegraphic 2-word sentences ("go bye-bye," "up daddy," "want cookie"), 25% intelligibility
30 months	Follows two-step commands; can identify objects by use	Uses jargon and echolalia infrequently; makes aver-age sentence of 2½ words; adjectives and adverbs appear; begins to ask questions, asks adults to re-peat actions ("do it again")
3 years	Knows several colors; knows what we do when we are hungry, thirsty, or sleepy; is aware of past and future; understands *today* and *not today*	Uses pronouns and plurals; can tell stories that begin to be understood; uses negative ("I can't," "I won't"); verbalizes toilet needs; can tell full name, age, and gender; forms sentences of 3 to 4 words, 75% intelligibility
3½ years	Can answer such questions as "do you have a doggie," "which is the boy," and "what toys do you have"; un-derstands *little, funny,* and *secret*	Can relate experiences in sequential order; can say a nursery rhyme; can ask permission
4 years	Understands same versus different; follows three-step commands; completes opposite analogies (a brother is a boy, a sister is a ...); understands why we have houses, stoves, and umbrellas	Tells a story; uses past tense; counts to 3; names pri-mary colors; enjoys rhyming nonsense words, en-joys exaggerations; asks many questions a day
5 years	Understands what we do with eyes and ears; under-stands differences in texture (hard, soft, smooth); un-derstands *if, when,* and *why;* identifies words in terms of use; begins to understand left and right	Indicates "I don't know"; indicates *funny,* and *sur-prise;* can define in terms of use; asks definition of specific words; makes serious inquiries ("how does this work," and "what does it mean"); uses mature sentence structure and form

TABLE 3-7

Phonemes and Intelligibility

Age range*	Sounds mastered	Percent intelligibility (to a stranger)
2 years	—	50
2½ years	—	75
3 years	14 vowels and *p, b, m*	85
4 years	10 vowel blends and *n, ng, w, h, t, d, k, g*	100
5 years	*f, v, y, th, l, wh*	100
6 years	*r, s, z, ch, j, sh, zh,* and consonant blends	100

*The ages presented here are general guidelines, since authorities differ with re-gard to the specific ages associated with articulation and intelligibility.

Assessing Language Development

In the early stages of prelinguistic and linguistic development, direct assessment by the pediatrician may be difficult. Children are likely to remain quiet in new situations, especially in the office where they re-ceived an injection. It is usually easy to engage a normally developing child of age 3 in conversation. Before that age the physician may need to rely on parental report.

The differential diagnosis for delayed expressive language develop-ment includes impaired hearing, global developmental delay or mental retardation, environmental deprivation, autism, and emotional malad-justment. Keeping this in mind, worrisome clinical situations include the 4- to 6-month-old infant who fails to coo responsively, the 9- to 10-month-old child who does not babble or whose cooing and babbling have diminished, and the 18-month-old child whose repertoire of words includes only *mama* or *dada.* Beyond 18 months a convenient rule of thumb is that children 2 years of age should use two-word

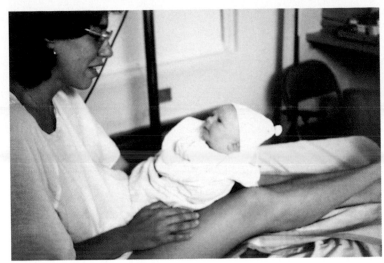

FIG. 3-25 Early social skills. A newborn within an hour of birth fixates on the face of the mother.

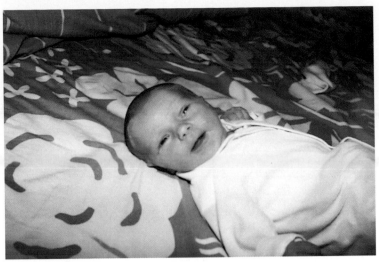

FIG. 3-26 Early smiling. A 19-day-old infant smiles for her parents.

utterances, at least half of which should be intelligible. By 3 years of age, children should use phrases of three or more words, three quarters of which should be intelligible. Children who fail to achieve these developmental milestones should undergo evaluation for hearing loss, as well as for cognitive and emotional impairment.

Families often attribute language delays in their youngster to superficial and easily remediable physiologic or social factors. "Being tongue-tied," for example, is not an explanation for delayed speech. However, it may be the effect rather than the cause, since the frenulum of the tongue may be tight in some children because it has not been sufficiently exercised by early verbal practice. Similarly, children rarely delay language because "they don't need it." Children have tremendous motivation to improve their verbal skills, even if they have older siblings who speak for them. For children who want a particular food, for example, a point toward the cupboard door will not specify precisely what is wanted. The parents must offer the items one at a time and await acceptance or rejection. The use of a verbal label will allow the child to meet needs efficiently.

Delays in the development of intelligibility might include any of the following:

1. Lack of intelligible speech by age 3
2. Frequent omission of initial consonants after age 4
3. Continued substitution of very easy sounds for harder ones after age 5
4. Persistent articulation errors after age 7

If any of these delays persists for 6 months or more, a referral should be initiated.

During the period in which articulation and vocabulary are being mastered, speech dysfluencies are common. Noticeable stuttering or rapid speech beyond age 4 should prompt further attention. The problems of nasality, inaudibility, and unusual pitch sometimes may be helped by a speech pathologist. Furthermore, children of any age who are embarrassed by their speech are appropriate candidates for referral.

Therapy for speech and language disorders helps improve the communication skills of children with language delays and problems of intelligibility. A child whose unusual language pattern is destined to be outgrown will not suffer from monitoring by a communication disorders specialist; the child whose language impairment will not be outgrown has much to lose when help is delayed.

Social Development

Early Capabilities: Social Responsivity

The earliest sociodevelopmental task of newborns is to establish a mutually satisfying relationship with their caregivers. Neonates begin the sociodevelopmental process by fixing visually on faces in preference to other sights, a skill that is evident during the first few days of life (Fig. 3-25). The responsive smile develops soon thereafter (Fig. 3-26). The social smile is another innate behavior, although it may not appear until 4 to 6 weeks of life. Smiling appears in infants from all cultures at about the same time. Infants with visual impairment who cannot appreciate a smile on the faces of their caregivers nonetheless smile at ages comparable with sighted children.

Development of Attachment

During the first 6 months of life, infants are rather indiscriminate in their social behavior, laughing and giggling with anyone willing to play. Evidence of the special relationship between parent and child may be seen when the crying infant can be calmed only by a parent's voice.

Infants develop a sense that their parents exist when out of sight sooner than they learn object permanence. By 6 to 8 months of age, children protest when their parents leave the room. As infants begin to recognize faces of familiar caregivers, they may squirm and cling in the company of unfamiliar people, exhibiting stranger awareness. The severity of the reaction varies with the infant's temperament and with previous experiences. Extreme reactions, known as *stranger anxiety*, are usually characteristic of children who have not had routine care from alternative caregivers. Pediatricians are advised to refrain from holding the 9- to 12-month-old child at the well-child visit. A child who is securely in the parent's arms may remain playful and calm but may fret or cry when wrenched from that security.

By 1 year of age, most children have experienced periods of separation from a parent, whether it be for minutes or hours. Infants who have developed a secure attachment to their parents show signs of recognition and pleasure when they are reunited with them. While progressing in gross motor development, the child initiates separation by walking away independently and exploring at greater distances from parents. Typically, infants return regularly for some verbal encourage-

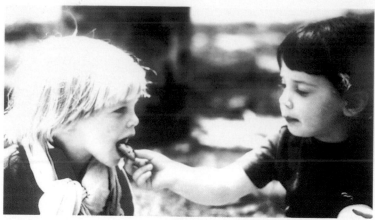

FIG. 3-27 Sharing. Two-year-old children with day-care experience share a special treat.

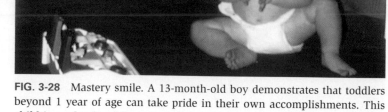

FIG. 3-28 Mastery smile. A 13-month-old boy demonstrates that toddlers beyond 1 year of age can take pride in their own accomplishments. This child is applauding his own success at having made the puppets appear.

ment, eye contact, or hugging and then venture farther. In contrast, infants who have not developed secure attachments may show indifference, ambivalence, or disorganization at reunion with their parents. Their exploration of the environment during the toddler years is limited. These children are at risk for troubled social relationships as they become older.

Development of Social Play

Infants and young toddlers tend to line up and engage in similar activities simultaneously. Play in this age group typically is parallel. Although parents often expect their young toddlers to interact or share with peers, success in this age group is unusual. Sharing for a young toddler involves showing a prized toy to another or handing it to the other child only to take it back within seconds.

By 2 years of age, with the development of symbolic capabilities in cognitive development, children begin to pretend. They will seek to engage their parents in activities that satisfy their growing curiosity. They enjoy reading with caregivers and having their labeling questions answered.

Near 3 years of age, children begin to include one another in their pretending games. At first both children may select the same role (two mothers, for example), whereas later, the roles will become more interactive. The young preschooler is especially interested in imitating the parent of the same gender but shows no preference for same- or opposite-gender playmates.

The child's abilities to share are shaped by social experiences. Children who attend day-care may share successfully at an earlier age than children raised at home (Fig. 3-27). Although it can be achieved through consistent experience, taking turns is also a challenge for the preschooler who possesses a limited concept of time. Impulse control is just developing in the preschool years. Active goals for this age group include learning to gain the cooperation of one's peers, learning to communicate ideas to new friends, and learning to handle conflicts.

By 4 to 5 years of age, peer interactions grow increasingly cooperative and complicated; pretend play involves themes requiring greater feats of imagination and experience, such as trips or parties. Older preschoolers enjoy helping with household tasks and frequently are more interested in participating in gender-specific activities than they were at an earlier age. This interest may relate to cognitive and social development. As children understand that they are in the same category as their same gender parent, they become interested in the implications of category membership. Strict adherence to the rules of cate-

gory membership reflects the concrete and inflexible thinking of the preschooler.

Preschoolers do not often play games with rules. Rules are seen as variable, to be made and broken at the discretion of the players. It is often a challenge to get through a board game with preschoolers who decide not to follow the rules once they discover that the rules are not working in their favor.

Children become capable of playing by rules when they reach school age. With superior logical capabilities, they realize that rules are invariant and must be followed regardless of the personal implications. As they progress through the elementary school years, board games and sports become preferred activities for groups of peers.

Development of Sense of Self

Self-awareness and independence develop gradually throughout life. The earliest indications of an emerging identity occur at 6 to 9 months of age, when infants display interest in their own mirror images. Some 7- to 8-month-olds may prefer to grab the cups and spoons rather than accept passive roles in eating. These infants may resist pressure to do something that they would prefer not to do (e.g., fussing to stand when placed in a sitting position).

Beyond 1 year of age, toddlers rapidly expand their senses of self. They explore their environment with ease, and they are increasingly able to function independently. They can feed themselves and manage a cup and spoon, and they have clear ideas about what they want. Children at 1 to 2 years of age also enjoy their own accomplishments and can clap for their own successes (Fig. 3-28).

An emerging sense of self and the thrust for independence make discipline of the toddler a challenge. Parents may need help in viewing their child's refusals to eat, nap, or be washed as positive steps toward increased independence. They may also need support in setting limits on the child's behaviors.

As the child reaches 2 to 3 years of age, increased independence in verbal abilities, increased awareness of body sensations, and modest skills in donning and doffing clothing combine with the child's desire to imitate adults and to gain parental approval. This allows toilet training to begin. In fact, the developmental milestones mentioned here may be viewed as readiness signs. The pediatrician can review them with families at the 15- or 18-month visit so that parents can time their toilet-training efforts to the child's developmental rate and style. Children differ substantially in their interest in achieving bladder and bowel control, and parents may benefit from counseling to maintain a relaxed approach.

In other areas as well, children need support in their attempts to initiate and control their own activities. Toward this end, parents can be encouraged to allow their child to practice emerging self-care skills, such as zippering or buttoning a coat, even when the practice costs precious time in a rushed schedule. Should the child become frustrated or disappointed, a response of empathy is likely to soothe more effectively than a response of reason, since rational reasoning is limited during this preoperational cognitive period.

By mid to late elementary school, cognitive development has progressed toward abstract and hypothetical thinking such that children are able to reflect self-consciously about themselves and others. First- or second-graders struggle to understand the causes of conflict or their emotional reactions to it. Older elementary-school children and adolescents are able to analyze situations, reasons, and reactions. They begin to understand their own motivations and the environmental triggers of their responses.

Throughout childhood the desire to grow up is in continued conflict with the desire to remain a child. The young preschooler is just beginning to address this issue. Families frequently report that a child's accomplishments in socioemotional functioning backslide when unexpected stresses challenge household equilibrium or when the child becomes ill. As a result, temporary regressions to earlier, safer levels of functioning may occur in some children. It is important that parents learn to view these lapses as expected components of development rather than as intentional lapses on the part of the child. However, if the regression is prolonged and significant, the physician may initiate an evaluation of the child's emotional status.

During elementary-school years, at least in Western cultures, the child's self-image is strongly influenced by success or failure in school. Not only do difficulties with learning put additional pressures on the child, they also may damage the child's sense of self-worth. Parents and teachers of children with learning problems should be especially willing to praise the child for accomplishments and good behavior. Physicians should be particularly sensitive to the higher risk of emotional and behavioral problems in children with learning difficulties so that they can make timely referrals to colleagues in the mental health professions.

Evaluation of Social Development

Subtle indicators of sociodevelopmental status can be gleaned in the course of a routine pediatric visit. The physician has the opportunity to note not only the way the infant behaves but also the style of parental caregiving and the nature of the parent-child relationship. The young infant typically shows social responsiveness to both the parent and the pediatrician, although at 9 months of age, there is a definite preference for the familiar parent. Also at this age, particularly in times of stress, the infant turns to the parent for support and comfort. Children of limited responsiveness, who avoid physical contact, who avert their gaze, or who in other ways fail to contribute to a mutually satisfying reciprocal exchange are of concern. Of equal concern are parents who are harsh, unresponsive, or threatening in response to the infant's needs.

Given the nature of sociodevelopmental change, the assessment of possible problems must rely largely on history. Parents tend to be frank and open about the nature of their relationship with their child if questions are asked in a direct but nonjudgmental way. Difficulties in social development may relate to constitutional and temperamental characteristics of the child, as well as to philosophy and practices of the parent. By remembering the bidirectional nature of causality in social development, the physician can avoid slipping into criticisms or judgments.

The older preschool or school-age child may be able to give, independently, direct information about social development. For example,

the child may be able to name special friends and the activities enjoyed with those friends. Young preschoolers might name both boys and girls and list rough-and-tumble or fantasy play as favorite activities. Older preschoolers might name same-gender friends but similar activities. School-age children might add board games and sports to their list of activities.

Variations in Developmental Patterns

The presence or absence of a single skill at a particular age is rarely sufficient to determine developmental status. Developmental progress is highly dependent on multiple factors: the general health of the child, opportunities for learning, temperamental characteristics, willingness to try new experiences, genetic endowments, coordination and strength, and socioeconomic factors. If delays occur in more than one domain, persist over time, or both, they are considered significant. The challenge for the pediatrician is to differentiate variation from deviation.

Sometimes the parents raise developmental concerns. These concerns must be addressed freely and openly. Parents are rarely comforted by superficial evaluation and pat reassurance, and although prudent waiting may serve some families well, it may arouse anxiety and anger in others. If a comprehensive evaluation of a given problem is beyond the capabilities of the pediatrician, early referral should be considered.

Evaluation of developmental problems proceeds in the same manner as evaluation of other medical concerns: history, physical examination (including neurological and developmental evaluation), and laboratory testing. Important in establishing a diagnosis is consideration of the pattern of development across all domains. For example, findings of hypotonia and selective problems in gross motor skills along with normal development in cognition, language, and social skills suggest a neuromuscular disorder or benign congenital hypotonia. In contrast, hypotonia with global developmental delay suggests a central nervous system problem. It is also important to differentiate delayed behavior from deviant behavior. For example, since even neonates are able to make good eye contact with their caregivers, the toddler who avoids eye contact is showing deviancy rather than delay. The combination of sustained deviant social behavior and delayed language development is suggestive of childhood autism.

Cerebral Palsy

Cerebral palsy is a disorder of movement and posture resulting from injury to the motor areas of the brain. The type of cerebral palsy varies according to the location of the injured area. Injury may occur before birth, during labor and delivery, or after birth, up through the preschool years. The majority of affected patients have a history of perinatal complications. However, in 20% to 30% of cases, no etiology can be established. The key to making the diagnosis is to establish that motor problems are static rather than progressive. Regression of motor skills suggests a different set of diagnostic possibilities, including surgically treatable lesions of the brain or spinal cord, or inherited neurodegenerative diseases.

Physical Examination

A diagnosis of cerebral palsy and a determination of its subtype can be established through physical examination. However, physical findings over the first year of life are highly variable and nonspecific. Early signs may include decreased passive tone in the presence of elicitable, brisk, deep tendon reflexes (DTRs) without concomitant weakness. Early problems with sucking and swallowing may predate evidence of motor delays.

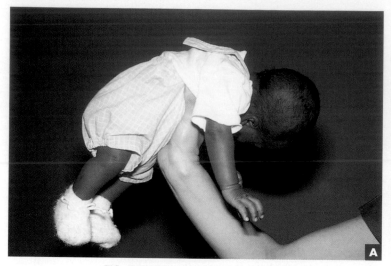
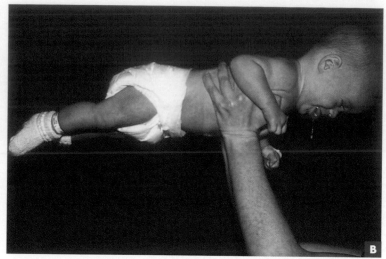

FIG. 3-29 Ventral suspension. *A,* This infant's posture is normal for a 1- to 3-month-old child held in ventral suspension. The head, hips, and knees are flexed. *B,* For a child 4 months of age or older held in ventral suspension with normal posture, the head, hips, and knees may be extended. This finding is abnormal in a child younger than 3 months of age.

TABLE 3-8

The Levine (POSTER) Criteria for Diagnosis of Cerebral Palsy

1. Posturing and abnormal movement patterns—extensor thrusts, blocks
2. Oropharyngeal problems—tongue thrusts, grimacing, swallowing difficulties
3. Strabismus
4. Tone—increased or decreased in muscles
5. Evolutional responses—persistent primitive reflexes or failure to develop equilibrium and protective responses
6. Reflexes—increased deep tendon reflex and extension of the toes during plantar reflexes

---

Because the findings may change, the definitive diagnosis of cerebral palsy should not be made until the child is at least 1 year of age. Beyond that point the diagnosis is based on abnormal findings in four of six major motor areas: posture, oromotor functioning, visuomotor functioning, tone, evolution of primitive reflexes, or muscle-stretch reflexes (Table 3-8).

Abnormalities of Tone. Because damage to the central nervous system prevents the inhibition and balance of the inherent tone of the muscles, abnormalities of tone are particularly significant in the diagnosis of cerebral palsy. After initial hypotonia, a child may develop increased tone between 12 and 18 months of age, showing clearly rigid or spastic hypertonia by age 2.

The child who demonstrates increased extensor tone beginning in early infancy also is at risk for cerebral palsy. Under normal circumstances, infants younger than 3 months of age, when supported ventrally, maintain their heads in slight flexion with the trunks mildly convex (Fig. 3-29, *A*). However, with exaggerated tone in the antigravity muscle group, the infant may elevate the head above the horizontally level trunk (Fig. 3-29, *B*). Similarly, the unknowing parents may be pleased by their child's apparent precocious development of head control when the child is prone or rolls belly-to-back in the first 2 months

of life, when in fact both of these findings suggest excessive extensor posturing.

Further evidence of abnormally increased tone is found when the supine child is pulled to an upright position and extends at the hips and knees, coming to stand on pointed toes rather than ending up in the appropriate sitting posture. This child, when placed in vertical suspension, will not right the head as expected and will later scissor the lower extremities as a result of hypertonia of the leg adductors and internal rotators (Fig. 3-30). Parents may find it difficult to position these infants for diapering and feeding; knowledge of the Marie-Foix maneuver, used to break up excessive extension in the lower extremities (Fig. 3-31), will help them.

Abnormalities in Development of Primitive Reflexes and Equilibrium Responses. Abnormal persistence of primitive reflexes is helpful in making a diagnosis of cerebral palsy. Damage to the central nervous system prevents high levels of control from superseding and inhibiting the influence of the early reflexes. Thus obligate or persistent primitive reflexes are signs of cerebral palsy. For example, in the normal variant of the ATNR, the infant can move out of the posture if the gaze is directed to the other side of the body. In an obligate ATNR, however, the infant remains in the fencer position until the head is passively moved. This finding is not normal in a child of any age and is highly suggestive of the static encephalopathy and motor deficit characterizing cerebral palsy.

Also strongly suggestive of cerebral palsy is the nonobligate ATNR that persists beyond 6 months of age. This is one possible explanation for a consistent preference in a 6- to 12-month-old child to sleep or lie with the head turned in a particular direction. Similarly, persistence of the Moro response beyond 6 months of age is associated with cerebral palsy, as is a lack of development of lateral protective equilibrium reactions by 7 to 8 months or of the parachute reaction by 10 months of age.

Subtypes of Cerebral Palsy

Hemiparesis. Hemiparesis is caused by asymmetric damage to the motor control areas of the central nervous system. In children with hemiparesis, functional discrepancies often predate asymmetric changes in tone or reflexes. The upper extremities may be affected more severely than the lower extremities. Asymmetric use of the upper or lower extremities is rare during the first 4 months of life. When seen in the resting state

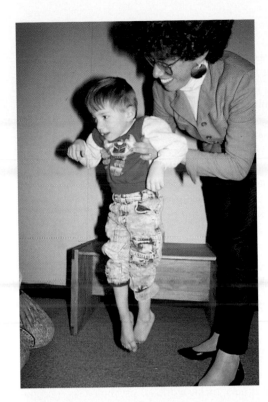

FIG. 3-30 Scissoring. Excessive pull of the hip adductors and internal rotators in this child of 3 years results in his legs crossing in a scissorlike pattern while he is supported in vertical suspension.

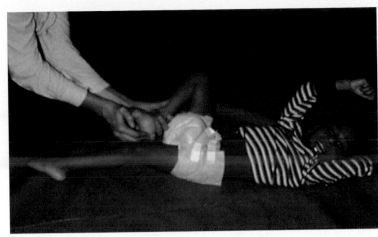

FIG. 3-31 Marie-Foix maneuver. By flexing the child's toes, the therapist can reduce extensor tone enough to obtain abduction of the hip and knee flexion in this child with spastic quadriplegia.

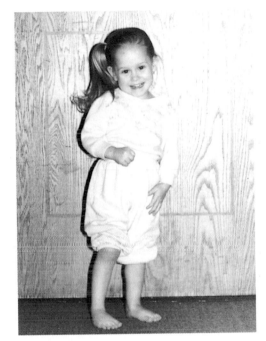

FIG. 3-33 Note the arm held in flexion and internal rotation and the leg circumducted on the involved side in this child with hemiplegic cerebral palsy.

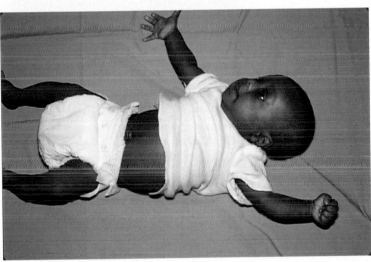

FIG. 3-32 Asymmetric Moro response. Note one hand is fisted and one open. This child warrants a complete neurologic examination and close follow-up.

or when elicited with the ATNR or the Moro response (Fig. 3-32), it is more likely related to lower motor neuron disease than to cerebral injury (see Chapter 2). At 4 to 6 months, during the development of early reaching and grasping, signs of hemiparesis include the presence of one hand that is fisted, the arm getting caught beneath the body when the child tries to prop up on the elbows or hands, and evidence that the arm is not used in simple tasks. Increased resistance to supination at the wrist, limited flopping of one wrist when the upper extremities are gently shaken, or extra beats of unilateral clonus at the ankle are other clues.

Later, during the first year of life, abnormal findings include a failure to develop the protective response of lateral propping or the development of an asymmetric parachute response. In addition, crawling may be uneven, with propulsion coming from one side while the opposite arm and leg are dragged behind.

Children with hemiparesis have sufficient difficulty compensating for their lack of protective responses, their uneven strength, and poor balance. Walking is typically delayed until 2½ to 3 years of age. In mildly affected children, walking may be almost normal, but when asked to run, the child may show posturing of the upper extremity in flexion and internal rotation. Usually, the lower limb rotates internally and the foot may be held in equinus, making it functionally longer on the swing-through part of the gait. To clear the foot from the floor, the child compensates by swinging the leg farther out in abduction or by circumducting the affected side. These patterns, in some cases, also can be observed in standing (Fig. 3-33).

Children with hemiparesis may neglect the visual field on their affected side. Parents should position their infant so that visual stimulation is provided to the intact visual field. Another consideration is that of abnormal bony stresses caused by asymmetric muscle strength. Unequal spinal stresses predispose children with hemiparesis to scoliosis, especially during growth spurts.

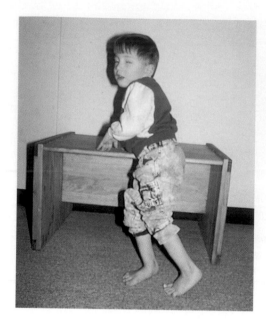

FIG. 3-34 Toe-walking. A 4-year-old child with cerebral palsy cruises on furniture. Notice that the child is crouched because of hamstring tightness and is toe-walking because of gastrocnemius tightness.

phorias and tropias that persist beyond 4 months of age is important to prevent amblyopia.

Hearing loss is also associated with cerebral palsy. Although clinical evaluation may suggest hearing loss, a definitive diagnosis requires an audiologic assessment. Brainstem auditory responses can be obtained to assess hearing capabilities in infants younger than 6 months of age and in older children unable perform in conditioned play audiometry because of motor or intellectual problems.

Approximately 50% of children with cerebral palsy have intellectual limitations or mental retardation. Learning disabilities and attentional weaknesses are more prevalent in this population than in the general population. Furthermore, behavioral problems may develop as a result of the frustration encountered in trying to adjust to motor disabilities.

Prognosis

Overall, the ability of individuals with cerebral palsy to live and work independently depends on the severity of the motor handicap and associated cognitive impairments. If a child is 4 years of age or older and has not achieved sitting balance, independent walking with or without crutches is rarely possible. A child 2 to 4 years of age who cannot sit and has three or more primitive reflexes is also unlikely to walk.

Because cerebral palsy affects multiple systems, children with the disorder are best served by an interdisciplinary team including not only medical professionals, but also social workers, psychologists, occupational and physical therapists, speech and communication therapists, and educational and vocational specialists. In many cases, children require educational support for physical and intellectual problems. They may also require behavioral management training or pharmacologic intervention for attentional weaknesses. Some of the behavioral problems can be prevented by matching developmental expectations to the child's functional capacities. These children and their families benefit enormously from the support of a primary care physician who offers routine health care maintenance, diagnostic and preventative procedures such as referrals to audiology and ophthalmology specialists, and advice and counseling on the interpretation of team evaluations.

Spastic Diplegia and Quadriplegia. Spastic diplegia implies dysfunction of the lower extremities, with normal or limited involvement of the upper extremities. Spastic quadriplegia implies dysfunction of the upper and lower extremities. The child with spasticity may have presenting symptoms that include delayed sitting, crawling, or walking or toe-walking (Fig. 3-34). In the supine position, children with spastic diplegia may keep their lower extremities in the "frog" position, with the hips and knees flexed and the hips externally rotated. In the erect position, the child may internally rotate and adduct the legs, leading to scissoring (Fig. 3-30). The ankles assume the equinus position. The child who toe-walks has brisk DTRs, limited range of ankle motion, Babinski reflexes, and a normally proportioned muscle mass.

The differential diagnosis of toe-walking includes the muscular dystrophies, tethered spinal cords and spinal tumors, peripheral neuropathies, and fixed bony deformities of the feet. Unilateral or asymmetric toe-walking may indicate leg-length discrepancy or a dislocated hip as an isolated finding or in conjunction with spasticity.

Athetoid or Ataxic Cerebral Palsy. In children with athetoid or ataxic cerebral palsy, involuntary movements do not present until after the first year of life. However, affected infants tend to be hypotonic and normoreflexive from the outset, and motor milestones are delayed. Between 1 and 2 years of age, hypotonia is usually replaced by spasticity, and involuntary movements appear. Exaggerated tone and dyskinetic movements reach maximal intensity around age 3. Athetoid cerebral palsy has been associated with bilirubin encephalopathy and damage to the basal ganglia.

Hypotonic Cerebral Palsy. Some hypotonic infants with exaggerated reflexes do not progress to hypertonicity. The putative explanation is cerebellar dysfunction with pyramidal track involvement. The child with hypotonic cerebral palsy usually exhibits severe motor and intellectual disability. The prognosis for independent functioning is quite poor. Hypotonic cerebral palsy must be differentiated from benign congenital hypotonia, an isolated disorder of tone, which spares other developmental areas.

Associated Findings with Cerebral Palsy

As many as 75% of children with diplegia or quadriplegia have strabismus (see Chapter 19). Refractive errors are found in 25% to 50% of children with cerebral palsy. Clumsiness because of motor imbalance of the lower extremities may be exaggerated by altered depth perception resulting from impaired visual function. Ophthalmologic referral for

Mental Retardation

According to the American Association on Mental Deficiency, *mental retardation* refers to substantial limitations in current functioning. It is characterized as "significantly subaverage general intellectual functioning existing concurrently with deficits in adaptive behavior and manifested during the developmental period." *Significantly subaverage functioning* refers to scores obtained on standardized intelligence tests that are about two or more standard deviations below age-group norms; *adaptive behaviors* refers to the broader areas of functioning such as self-care, community survival skills (e.g., using the telephone, making change, and using public transportation), and social interactions; and *developmental period* refers to the period from birth to 18 years of age.

The ability to predict intellectual performance and academic achievement from developmental testing during infancy is quite limited. Only in children falling far behind age expectations should one estimate permanent intellectual disability. Nonetheless, if an infant shows delayed cognitive development, the parents' reasonable concerns can be met with a referral to an early intervention program.

As these children approach school age, particularly if they have had optimal educational support, the ability to predict later difficulties improves. The rate of developmental progress during the preschool years is often a good predictor of later intellectual performance. After initial cognitive developmental delays, if a child is able to achieve 6 months' progress in 6 months, the prognosis for normal intellectual capacity is good. However, if the child achieves, for example, 4 months' progress in 6 months, the rate of development is 67% of the expected rate, and the prognosis for later intellectual functioning is poor. By the time a child is 6 to 7 years of age, limitations as measured on an IQ test typically characterize the individual's abilities throughout life. At that point, the term *mental retardation* is more specific and accurate than *developmental delay.*

Physical Examination

Physical examination can be helpful in determining the cause of mental retardation. Most children classified as mentally retarded function in the mildly retarded range. These children often have a normal physical examination, with no apparent evidence of malformation or deformity. In contrast to children with severe mental retardation, who will be readily identified, children with mild retardation are likely to have normal motor milestones and delays only in adaptive areas such as self-care, language acquisition, or play. The detection of disability in these mildly affected youngsters may not be possible until the child experiences school performance difficulties.

The average IQ of parents of children with mild mental retardation is lower than the population norm. Thus many of these parents also show limitations in intellectual abilities. For this reason the etiology of mild mental retardation is generally felt to be multifactorial, including multiple genetic contributions and limited social enrichment.

The more significant the degree of retardation, the more likely that a specific etiologic factor will be found. Children who score in the moderate, severe, or profound ranges are likely to have congenital malformations of the central nervous system, severe neurologic insults in the prenatal or perinatal period, an inherited disorder, or another specific diagnosis. A systematic approach to the physical examination may reveal clues to the nature of the underlying disorder.

Growth Pattern and Vital Signs. Aberrant growth patterns, which are in and of themselves the cause for assessment, may be associated with developmental delays and mental retardation. Obesity appears as part of a number of syndromes associated with mental deficiency, such as Laurence-Moon syndrome and Prader-Willi syndrome (see Chapter 1). Children who are exceptionally large may have cerebral giantism (Soto syndrome). Small-for-date infants deserve close study for evidence of anomalies or infection; they are also at risk for abnormal development. Extreme to moderate short stature, with or without skeletal dysplasia, is associated with many dysmorphic syndromes that include mental retardation as an associated finding. Growth curves have been prepared for children with various genetic and chromosomal disorders such as Down syndrome, since they tend to be shorter than the general population (Fig. 3-35). However, if children are shorter than expected even for the population of children with the disorder or if children fall off of their own curve after following a percentile, then endocrine-function abnormalities such as hypothyroidism should be investigated.

Skin Findings. Hemangiomas, multiple café au lait spots, and sebaceous adenomas may be evidence of an underlying neurocutaneous abnormality, thereby providing a constitutional basis for a developmental delay. Von Recklinghausen disease and tuberous sclerosis, both examples of neurocutaneous disorders, are inherited as autosomal dominant, although there is a high rate of spontaneous mutation. If these disorders are diagnosed or suspected, examination of the immediate family is warranted (see Chapter 15). Hirsutism occurs in fetal alcohol and fetal hydantoin syndromes (see Chapter 1). Abnormal fingernail formation can signal teratogenic influences or ectodermal dysplasias (see Chapter 8).

Cranial Abnormalities. Head circumference provides an obvious clue to the cause of mental retardation; undergrowth of the cranium may indicate central nervous system damage or dysgenesis; overgrowth may indicate hydrocephalus. Abnormal skull shape may indicate that the underlying nervous system has undergone unusual physical stresses.

Transillumination aids in the diagnosis of porencephalic cysts or of other structural defects in young infants (see Chapter 15). The presence of an intracranial bruit may indicate an arteriovenous malformation, although such bruits are sometimes heard in normal infants. Even in the absence of these signs, children with moderate, severe, and profound mental retardation may warrant an imaging study of the central nervous system because of the high incidence of identifiable abnormalities.

Facial Abnormalities. The presence of certain facial characteristics may suggest a specific etiology of mental retardation. Minor malformations (which include hypotelorism or hypertelorism; epicanthal folds; colobomata; and auricles that are large, abnormally formed, or set low in comparison with the plane of the eyes) are rare in the general population. In isolation, one dysmorphic feature may be insignificant. However, the presence of three or more of these features correlates highly with a major malformation, often of the heart, kidney, or brain. Patterns of dysmorphic features may suggest a specific diagnosis such as a genetic syndrome, chromosomal abnormality, or prenatal exposure. For example, flat facies, upturned palpebral fissures, epicanthal folds, single palmar creases, and clinodactyly are associated with trisomy 21 (Down syndrome) (Fig. 3-36). Likewise, a lengthened philtrum, a thin vermilion border, and microcephaly are clinical features of fetal alcohol syndrome.

Some of these unusual features themselves are clues to the etiology of the intellectual disability or are the result of abnormal functioning, even in prenatal life. For example, aberrant patterning of scalp hair may indicate abnormal cerebral morphology. The pattern of hair growth is affected by pressures from the developing brain on the overlying scalp in early gestation. The absence of a posterior hair whorl or the presence of multiple hair whorls suggests abnormal prenatal brain growth. Small palpebral fissures also result from abnormal brain growth; the eye is an extension of the brain, and small eyes are suggestive of abnormal early brain development. Similarly, a high-arched palate may be secondary to abnormal motor activity of the tongue in utero, suggesting a prenatal origin of motor problems.

Other Physical Abnormalities. Hepatosplenomegaly in the neonatal period may suggest congenital infection or in childhood may indicate a heritable storage disease affecting central nervous system and developmental functioning. Large testes are found in youngsters with fragile X, whereas hypogonadism is a concomitant of the Prader-Willi syndrome. About half of patients with this syndrome have an abnormality on chromosome 15 (see Chapter 1).

Changes in the long bones of the limbs may show evidence of congenital infection; disproportionate bone length may suggest metabolic disorders such as homocystinuria or the osteochondrodysplasias. Errant toe proportions or changed crease patterns on the hands or soles of the feet may suggest early morphogenetic changes associated with certain defined syndromes. Lethargic or pale children may prompt an examination for iron deficiency or lead intoxication, which also may contribute to subnormal intellectual progress.

Prognosis

Some 3% of newborns are classified as mentally retarded at some point in their lives. In a society that prizes intellectual accomplishment, the identification of cognitive delays is upsetting for a family. Findings of unusual features in any aspect of the physical examination may help provide an explanation for abnormal or delayed cognitive development. In evaluating the cause of developmental delay, the greatest need, beyond that of assessing the possibility of remediation, is that of providing the parents with appropriate genetic, behavioral, and educational counseling. Evidence that a child's lack of developmental progress is re-

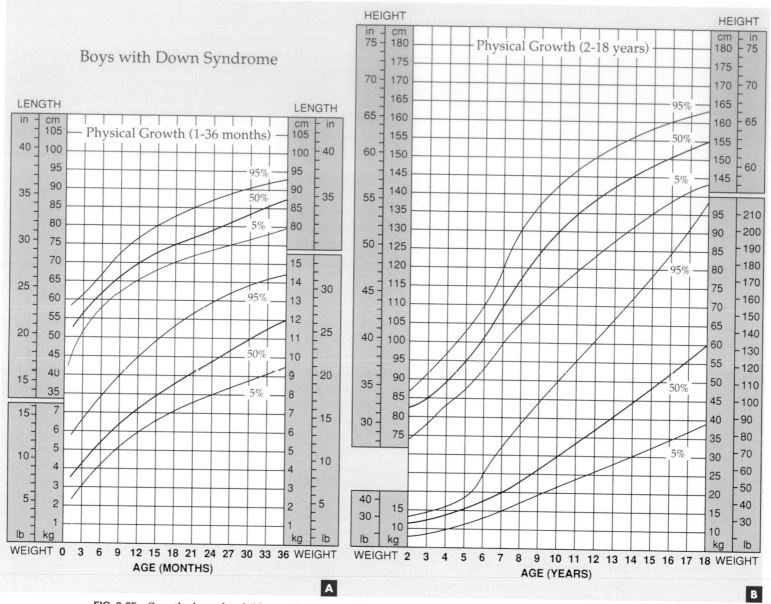

FIG. 3-35 Growth charts for children with Down syndrome. (From Cronk C, Crocker AC, Pueschel SM, et al: Growth charts for children with Down syndrome, *Pediatrics* 81:108, 1988.)

lated to constitutional factors can help relieve parents of guilt feelings.

In the past, physicians have often underestimated the capabilities of children with mild to moderate retardation. Similarly, families often interpret a diagnosis of mental retardation to mean that their child will make no further developmental progress. Estimates of functional abilities for children who are classified as mentally retarded are variable. Children with mild mental retardation (IQ scores two to three standard deviations below the mean [69 to 55]) can be taught to read and write and to do simple mathematics. As adults, they often live independently and hold jobs. The extent of their disability is most prominent during the school years or during times of life crisis beyond school age. Children with moderate mental retardation (IQ scores three to four standard deviations below the mean [54 to 40]) probably will not learn to read and write. Nonetheless, their abilities in language, self-care, and adaptation skills may allow them to live and work in semiindependent supervised settings. Children with severe and profound mental retardation (four to six standard deviations below the mean [39 to 24 and below]) require substantial lifelong support.

The benefits of early intervention are maximized by early identification. Careful documentation of the child's opportunities for interaction with parents, other children, and stimulating environments helps in determining the type and degree of intervention needed. The importance of careful screening of infant and preschool development by informed health professionals and of close collaboration between physicians and early intervention personnel cannot be overemphasized.

Specific Language and Reading Disorders

Delays and disturbances in language development are most frequently associated with mental retardation, hearing impairment, childhood autism, and environmental deprivation. However, language difficulties may occur in an otherwise normal child; in such cases, they are referred to as specific language disabilities, usually of unknown etiology. Some theories stress difficulties with high-level concepts and symbolic capabilities, and others stress auditory perceptual impairments as the root of specific language disorders.

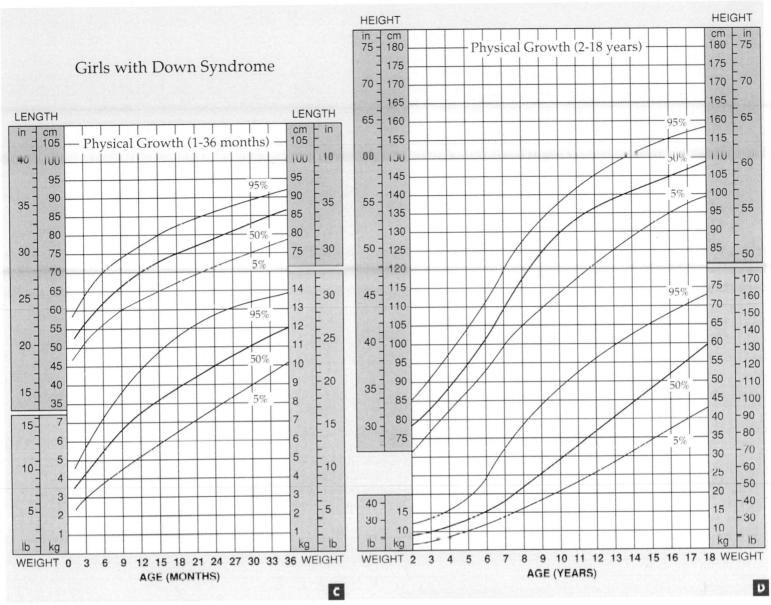

Girls with Down Syndrome

Physical Growth (1-36 months)

Physical Growth (2-18 years)

FIG. 3-35, cont'd For legend see opposite page.

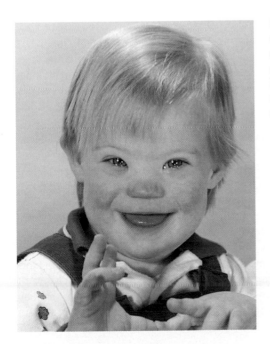

FIG. 3-36 Down syndrome. Note the upslanting palpebral fissures, flat nasal bridge, epicanthal folds, small ears, and small hands.

Physical Examination

There are no specific physical signs associated with specific language disorders. The physician's role is in large part to rule out other disorders with different etiologies and prognoses. Hearing assessment is indicated for any child with delays or deviancies in language development, since hearing loss is treatable. In early infancy, assessment of hearing requires use of brainstem auditory-evoked response, an electrophysiologic measure that records brain waves as a function of sound exposure. In older infants and toddlers, conditioned play techniques are typically used. The child is rewarded for turning toward the source of a sound. In preschoolers, conventional audiometry with the use of headphones allows for evaluation of each ear independently (Fig. 3-37).

Hearing should be assessed in all children with syndromes known to be associated with hearing loss. These include Treacher Collins, Waardenburg, and congenital rubella syndromes and osteogenesis imperfecta. Evaluation should not await delays in language acquisition. Abnormalities of the external ear, including preauricular tags and pits, also may be associated with abnormalities of the ossicular chain and conductive and sensorineural hearing loss. Again, early hearing assess-

AUDIOGRAMS

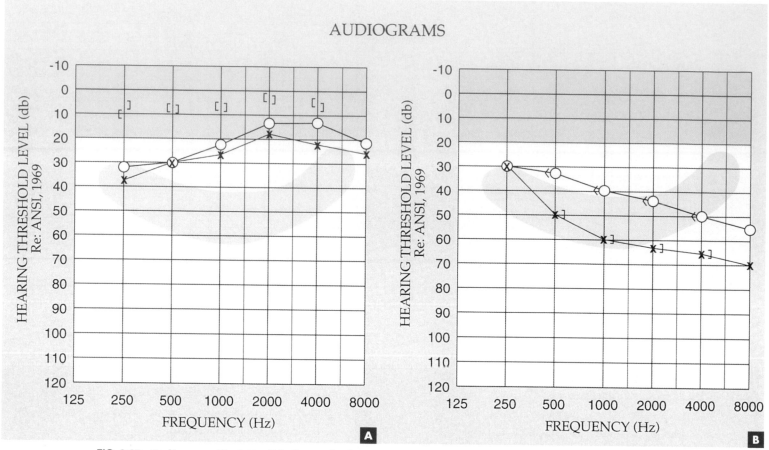

FIG. 3-37 Audiograms. The letter X indicates the threshold for the left ear, and the letter O indicates the threshold for the right ear. Brackets indicate bone conduction. *A,* This audiogram indicates mild conductive hearing loss in both ears. Notice that more energy is required for detection of sound in the low-frequency range. Bone conduction is normal. *B,* This audiogram demonstrates sensorineural hearing loss. The left ear shows a sloping pattern with mild to moderate loss in the low-frequency range and severe loss in the high-frequency range. The right ear shows mild to moderate loss throughout the frequency range.

TABLE 3-9

Conditions Associated with Sensorineural Hearing Loss

Family history of childhood hearing impairment
Congenital perinatal infection (CMV, rubella, herpes, toxoplasmosis, syphilis)
Anatomic malformations of the head or neck
Birth weight less than 1500 grams
Hyperbilirubinemia above levels indicated for exchange transfusion
Bacterial meningitis
Severe asphyxia
Exposure to ototoxic medications

CMV, Cytomegalovirus.

---

ment is advisable for children with abnormalities of the external ear, the palate, or facial structures or for children who are otherwise at risk for hearing impairment (Table 3-9). Conditions associated with varying degrees of hearing loss, their disabling effects, and the interventions required for children with these conditions are listed in Table 3-10.

Some 60% of all cases of sensorineural hearing loss in preverbal children will be of undetermined causes. For these children, an absence of expected hearing behaviors is the best clue to the presence of a hearing problem. Healthy newborns react to sounds with startle responses and with changes in their level of alertness. In the neonatal period, and then again after 3 months of age, the infant should be able to turn toward the source of a sound (Fig. 3-24). Qualitative differences in the early behaviors of children with hearing impairment in comparison with their peers without hearing impairment have been observed in sensorimotor functioning, receptive and expressive language, and social functioning. These abnormalities include indifference to the spoken word, decreased vocalization and sound production, increased visual attentiveness, altered social rapport, and frustrations in communicating.

The relationship between language development and otitis media with effusion is unclear. Chronic otitis media with effusion may be associated with a variable, mild to moderate conductive hearing loss (Table 3-10). Some studies have found an association between frequent bouts of otitis media and delays in speech and language, presumably a consequence of variable hearing loss. However, other studies have found no such relationship. The correlation between the appearance of the tympanic membrane, the results of tympanometry, and the degree of hearing loss in otitis media with effusion is poor. Children who have chronic otitis media with effusion should be assessed through use of audiometry. If hearing loss is documented or if the child shows a delay in language development, aggressive medical or surgical management may be warranted.

TABLE 3-10

Disabling Effects of Hearing Loss

Average hearing 500-2000 Hz (ANSI)	Description	Condition	Sounds heard without amplification	Degree of disability (if not treated in first year of life)	Probable needs
0-15 dB	Normal range	Serous otitis, perforation, monomeric membrane, tympanosclerosis	All speech sounds	None	None
15-25 dB	Slight hearing loss	Serous otitis, perforation, monomeric membrane, sensorineural loss, tympanosclerosis	Vowel sounds heard clearly; may miss unvoiced consonant sounds	Mild auditory dysfunction in language learning	Consideration of need for hearing aid; lipreading; auditory training, speech therapy, preferential seating
25-40 dB	Mild hearing loss	Serous otitis, perforation, tympanosclerosis, monomeric membrane, sensorineural loss	Hears only some louder-voiced speech sounds	Auditory learning dysfunction, mild language retardation, mild speech problems, inattention	Hearing aid, lipreading, auditory training, speech therapy
40-65 dB	Moderate hearing loss	Chronic otitis, middle ear anomaly, sensorineural loss	Misses most speech sounds at normal conversational level	Speech problems, language retardation, learning dysfunction, inattention	All the above; plus consideration of special classroom situation
65-95 dB	Severe hearing loss	Sensorineural or mixed loss from sensorineural loss plus middle ear disease	Hears no speech sounds of normal conversation	Severe speech problems, language retardation, learning dysfunction, inattention	All the above; plus probable assignment to special classes
More than 95 dB	Profound hearing loss	Sensorineural or mixed loss	Hears no speech or other sounds	Severe speech problems, language retardation, learning dysfunction, inattention	All the above; plus probable assignment to special classes

From Stewart JM, Downs MP: Medical management of the hearing-handicapped child. In Northern JL, ed: *Hearing disorders*, ed 2, Boston, 1984, Little, Brown. *ANSI*, American National Standards Institute; *dB*, decibel.

Prognosis

Many toddlers with specific language disorders develop adequate speech, language, and communication skills by the middle of elementary school. There are no variables consistently associated with a good prognosis; however, the prognosis for communication is clearly improved through early communication therapy. Physicians should not hesitate to refer children with speech and language delays for assessment and treatment.

Many toddlers and preschoolers with selective problems in language acquisition develop reading difficulties during the school-age years. Difficulty in a specific aspect of learning that is greater than that expected for the child's overall intellectual functioning qualifies as a learning disability. A reading disorder or dyslexia is a frequent finding in a child with an early history of language delay and a positive family history of reading disability. With increasing age, children with reading difficulties tend to improve. However, in many cases, reading remains an area of relative weakness compared with other cognitive and academic skills.

Children with reading disorders show abnormal or inefficient eye movements in the course of reading. This observation has led to visual training as a treatment strategy. However, the literature supports the notion that in most cases, a reading problem is a high-level language difficulty, not a visual or visuomotor problem.

Attention-Deficit Hyperactivity Disorder

Attention-deficit hyperactivity disorder (ADHD) is a syndrome characterized by persistent inattention, hyperactivity, and impulsivity compared with what is expected for a child at a particular developmental level. Judgments about the degree of deviance in these behaviors are based on the degree of interference they cause in the child's social, academic, or other functioning. The diagnosis of ADHD requires that symptoms have been long-standing, that they be present before at least 7 years of age, and that they occur in multiple settings and not just at either home or school. Multiple genetic, neurologic, toxic, and psychosocial conditions are associated with presence of ADHD. Among children born prematurely and children with mental retardation, ADHD is more prevalent than in the general population.

Though precise diagnostic criteria have changed over the last 2 decades, certain features have recurred in the lists of defining characteristics. Individuals with ADHD have difficulty sustaining attention and persisting to task completion. They become easily distracted. Fre-

TABLE 3-11

Indicators Associated with Neurologic Immaturity

Task	Immature response	Norms
Rapid pronation-supination	Dysdiadochokinesia	Mature by age 7-8 years
Repeated finger-to-thumb apposition	Synkinesis	Markedly decreased after age 9 years
Alternation of squeezing and relaxation of single hand grip	Synkinesis	Markedly decreased after age 9 years
Sensory integration—tactile recognition from visual presentation	Astereognosis	>90% accurate by age 7 years
Indentification of right and left		
On self	Inaccurate	>90% correct by age 7 years
Execution of crossed commands (e.g., touch your left eye with your right hand)	Inaccurate	>90% correct by age 8 years
On examiner	Inaccurate	>70% correct by age 8 years

quently they fail to organize and plan before beginning a task. Because of all these features operating concurrently, these children fail to complete work assignments and eventually may avoid long and demanding tasks. Impulsivity in young children is frequently demonstrated by difficulty waiting for a turn. As children get older, impulsivity is expressed as difficulty delaying responses, blurting out answers, interrupting others, and generally acting before thinking.

The current diagnostic criteria from the *Diagnostic and Statistical Manual of Mental Disorders—IV* identify three different subtypes of ADHD. Most children demonstrate ADHD combined type, a variant that includes symptoms of inattention and hyperactivity-impulsivity. However, ADHD predominantly inattentive type is appropriate for children with symptoms of inattention without hyperactivity or impulsivity. An alternative diagnosis is ADHD predominantly hyperactive-impulsive type, in which inattention may be a feature but less prominent than hyperactivity. The degree of hyperactivity varies in part with the child's age, developmental level, temperament, and style. Young school-age boys with ADHD tend to display excessive fidgetiness and activity, whereas adolescents and girls may be inattentive but not hyperactive.

Most children with ADHD show age-appropriate attention in some highly motivating situations. For example, parents routinely report that their children with ADHD sit for computer games or captivating movies. For this reason, as many as 80% of children whose behavior at home and at school meets diagnostic criteria do not show characteristics of the disorder in the physician's office. Diagnosis rests on historical information from parents and confirmatory reports from teachers. Standardized questionnaires are often used in diagnosis to quantify the degree of behavioral problems.

Children with ADHD can develop secondary maladaptive behavioral problems, including refusal to work, aggression, depression, and social isolation. This fact often makes it difficult to differentiate ADHD from the other externalizing disorders. In conduct disorder, as opposed to ADHD, the child violates the basic rights of others and age-appropriate social norms. In oppositional defiant disorder, the child shows severe and persistent disobedience and hostility directed against authority figures.

Physical Findings

On physical examination, it is important to assess the general characteristics of the child to rule out other similar psychiatric disorders such as autism, depression, anxiety, or oppositional disorder. Physical findings in ADHD may be completely noncontributory. However, findings such as short stature or dysmorphic features may suggest an associated genetic or dysmorphic syndrome such as alcohol-related birth defects. Focal neurologic findings may suggest a static or progressive neurologic cause such as periventricular leukomalacia from prematu-

rity. The presence of motor or vocal tics with ADHD raises the diagnostic possibility of Tourette syndrome.

The physical and neurologic examination of children with suspected ADHD often includes a set of specific maneuvers and tasks referred to as *neurologic soft signs* or *neuromaturational indicators*. Nonnormative performance on these specific motor and sensory tasks can be obtained in children who otherwise show no evidence of a localizing neurologic disorder or pathognomonic patterns indicative of generalized encephalopathy. The soft signs are of clinical interest because they serve as an index for cognitive or behavioral dysfunction.

Table 3-11 includes several tasks for eliciting soft signs, the typical ages of acquisition, and indications of immature or positive findings. On rapid alternating pronation-supination of the hands, developing children typically show resolution of dysdiadochokinesia by age 7 years. On the same task and on repeated finger-to-thumb apposition and alternating squeezing and relaxing of handgrip, children usually show a marked decrease in synkinesis after age 9 years. A single abnormal finding in a series of tasks may be of no significance. Persistence of abnormal findings on several tasks is a nondiagnostic but supporting finding consistent with ADHD. Children with ADHD may show delays in identification of right and left on themselves and the examiner and have difficulty executing crossed commands on themselves beyond 8 years of age. They also may show problems in executing four or more sequential commands from memory. These maneuvers on physical examination may unmask the child's inattention, impulsivity, and disorganization that would otherwise go undetected in the clinical setting. It is clinically worthwhile to include these tasks because parents are often relieved if the physician has the opportunity to observe the traits that have brought the family for evaluation.

Prognosis

Research suggests that ADHD is a lifelong condition. The signs and symptoms of hyperactivity are likely to resolve during adolescence, but relative inattention persists through adulthood. Many individuals with ADHD do better as adolescents and adults than they did as children because they can choose educational programs or occupations that capitalize on their profile. They often prefer vocations that permit frequent shifts in attention and a high energy level and that do not require sustained attention to challenging tasks. Nonetheless, individuals with ADHD have higher rates of automobile accidents, lower job attainment, and greater instability in relationships compared with siblings who do not have the disorder, presumably related to persistent inattention. The prognosis is more favorable in individuals with isolated ADHD, good cognitive skills, no learning disorders, and positive family and peer relationships.

TABLE 3-12

Visually Related Behaviors

Age of infant	Behavior
Term	Focuses on face, briefly tracks vertically and horizontally, turns toward diffuse light source, widens eyes to object or face at 8-12 inches
1 month	Blinks at approaching object, tracks 60 degrees horizontally, 30 degrees vertically
2 months	Tracks across midline, follows movement 6 feet away, smiles to a smiling face, raises head 30 degrees in prone
3 months	Eyes and head track 180 degrees, looks at hands, looks at objects placed in hands
4-5 months	Reaches for object (12-inch cube) 12 inches away, notices raisins 1 foot away, smiles at familiar adult
5-6 months	Smiles in mirror
7-8 months	Rakes at raisin
8-9 months	Notes visual details, pokes at holes in peg board and at elevator buttons
9 months	Neat pincer grasp
12-14 months	Stacks blocks, places peg in round hole

Treatment options for ADHD fall into three categories: behavior management, educational interventions, and psychopharmacology. Combinations of these options often are more effective than a single treatment.

Visual Impairment

Visual experience facilitates the learning of many important concepts of space and form important in the development of motor skills, perception, cognition, and social skills (Table 3-12). Thus in situations of congenital blindness or visual impairment, developmental patterns may be altered and delayed, demonstrating the close interrelationships that exist among developmental domains. Children with visual impairments can learn to increase the use of residual visual functioning and other sensory modalities. The physician's understanding of the impact of visual impairment is important to evaluate whether developmental progress is being achieved as expected in this population and to ensure that unexpected delays and deviancies are appropriately diagnosed and treated.

Gross and Fine Motor Development

Apparently, much of the motivation for the infant with normal vision to raise the head 90 degrees when in the prone position is to increase the visual field. Without the feedback of interesting sights, the infant with severe visual impairment may not attain this milestone until 11 to 12 months of age. In contrast, rolling occurs in infants who are blind at close to the same age as in infants with normal vision. If sitting independently is an active goal, it can occur by 6 to 7 months of age. However, transitional movements from lying to sitting or from sitting to standing occur several months later in infants without sight than in infants able to see.

Protective reactions develop more slowly in infants with severe visual impairment, and these are expected to appear in the 10- to 12-month age range. This delay, as well as the inability to integrate visual cues in attaining balance and equilibrium, and the lack of a visual impetus to explore distant toys may contribute to a typical delay in crawling or walking. Paired auditory-tactile cues presented to children with severe visual impairment may stimulate their interest in objects beyond their reach, thus accelerating gross motor development.

Regarding fine motor development, information gathering by index finger and manual manipulation may be more accurate in the child who is blind than in the child with normal vision. However, the youngster who is blind may experience a delay in the acquisition of precise prehension, which sometimes never develops, with raking favored as a more efficient means of exploration.

Cognitive Development

The development of cognitive skills in the child with visual impairment must of necessity depend on use of the other sensory modalities. For this reason, careful global evaluation of the child with severe visual impairment should be conducted early in infancy to ensure that the other senses are intact.

A child with normal vision develops the understanding that objects are permanent even when they cannot be seen, felt, heard, sniffed, or tasted. For the child with severe visual impairment, the opportunities for object perception are fewer, and thus the understanding of object permanence typically develops later, stimulated by encouragement of the infant to reach for sound cues. Similarly, this child's understanding of conservation of continuous quantity, that a cup of water contains the same volume of liquid in a tall thin container as it does in a short fat one, also develops later than in the child with normal vision.

Haptic perception, the acquisition of information about objects or spaces by exploration with the hands, appears to be more important in the cognitive development of the child with severe visual impairment than in that of the child with normal vision. For this reason, tactile exploration in the child who is blind cannot be promoted at too early an age. In fact, without such encouragement, these children may be fearful and resistant to unfamiliar new feelings.

Language and Intellectual Development

Verbal imitation and receptive language skills may develop normally in healthy children who are blind. As one might expect, these children may have difficulty with words relating to visual concepts, such as *light, dark,* or *color.* They also may have problems with words referring to large things that cannot be touched (*sky* or *stars*), things that change slowly (*age* or *growth*), or the concept "I." However, some children with severe visual impairment show accurate use of all of these concepts and even make the distinction between the words *look* and *see.* In these cases the child probably uses available linguistic information to substitute for visual information.

Although standard IQ tests cannot be used to assess intellectual capabilities of children with severe visual impairment, standardized instruments have been developed to assess their cognitive development. Receptive and expressive language skills figure prominently in these assessments. In addition, interview schedules of adaptive behavior in communication and self-help skills have been normed for children with visual impairment.

Social Development

Infants who are blind lack the opportunity to benefit from face-to-face contact with their caregivers, from the visual reinforcement of smiling, from the use of facial expressions to assist in the interpretation of voices or actions, and from the experience of tracking parents across the room to know that even when they cannot be heard or felt they are still there. These differences in sensory input affect their social and emotional development. Parents of infants with severe visual impairment frequently need to be coached to use touch and sound to reinforce smiling and other desired behaviors in their child.

At about the same time that children with normal vision smile at familiar faces, children who are blind smile in response to familiar touching and kinesthetic handling. Smiling in response to a familiar voice, however, may occur inconsistently up to 1 year of age. The infant who is blind demonstrates attachment by calming to the tactile exploration of the caregiver's familiar face or hands.

Blind children of about 1 year of age may have stranger awareness, although a greater hurdle will be their reaction to separation. Because these children have a limited capacity to track their caregivers, separations from them may induce panic states even among older ones. Similarly, the development of independent caregiving and play may be delayed and may require specific interventions.

Parents should be advised that, without purposeful stimulation, children who are blind may engage in nonpurposeful motor activities such as eye rubbing or rocking and that these stereotypic behaviors, referred to as *blindisms*, are difficult to extinguish. Blindisms can often be channeled to purposeful stimulation by directing the child's hands to exploration of a toy or by distracting the child with conversation or music. These efforts will serve to channel the child's activities in a more socially adaptive direction.

Summary

The tasks of routine developmental surveillance, identification of children with variations, and referral for appropriate developmental services (especially during infancy and in the preschool years) fall largely, and often exclusively, to the primary care clinician. Although we have provided estimates regarding the expected chronology of development, these developmental milestones are guidelines rather than fixed time frames within which behavior acquisition may be judged as normal or abnormal. In evaluating a child, the physician must use these guidelines and clinical judgment, taking into account the child's own personality traits, experiences, and degree of cooperation.

Recommendations for further assessment and treatment should be made in consultation with the family.

BIBLIOGRAPHY

American Academy of Pediatrics Joint Committee on Infant Hearing: Position statement 1982, *Pediatrics* 70:496-497, 1982.

Diagnostic and statistical manual of mental disorders, ed 4, Washington, DC, 1994, American Psychiatric Association.

Dixon SD, Stein MT, eds: *Encounters with children,* St Louis, 1992, Mosby.

Fraiberg S: *Insights from the blind,* New York, 1977, Basic Books.

Illingsworth RS: *The development of the infant and young child abnormal and normal,* ed 7, New York, 1980, Churchill Livingstone.

Knobloch H, Pasamanick B, eds: *Gesell and Amatruda's developmental diagnosis,* ed 3, New York, 1974, Harper & Row.

Levine M, Carey W, Crocker A, Gross R: *Developmental-behavioral pediatrics,* Philadelphia, 1983, WB Saunders.

Louick D, Baland T: Psychological tests: a guide for pediatricians, *Pediatr Ann* 7(12):86-101, 1978.

Northern JL, Downs MP: *Hearing in children,* Baltimore, 1974, Williams & Wilkins.

Opitz JM: Mental retardation: biological aspects of concern to pediatricians, *Pediatr Rev* 2(2):41-40, 1980.

Scheiner AP, Moomaw M: Care of the visually handicapped child, *Pediatr Rev* 4(3):74-81, 1982.

Smith DW, Jones KL: *Recognizable patterns of human malformation,* ed 4, Philadelphia, 1988, WB Saunders.

Smith DW, Simons FER: Rational diagnosis evaluation of the child with mental deficiency, *Am J Dis Child* 129:1285–1290, 1975.

4

Allergy and Immunology

DAVID P. SKONER   ANDREW H. URBACH
PHILIP FIREMAN

isorders of the immune system are diverse and range from mild to severe in their manifestations and impact on normal function. This chapter emphasizes physical findings and characteristic symptoms of children with disorders of hypersensitivity and immunodeficiency, as well as diagnostic techniques and radiographic findings. Topics have been chosen on the basis of their prevalence and importance in the pediatric population and their association with characteristic physical findings.

Immunologic Hypersensitivity Disorders

Hypersensitivity disorders of the human immune system have been classified by Gell and Coombs into four groups (Table 4-1) based on the different mechanisms by which immune reactions may initiate tissue inflammation. Type I reactions occur promptly after the sensitized individual is exposed to an antigen and are mediated by a specific immunoglobulin E (IgE) antibody. This mechanism is responsible for the common disorders of immediate hypersensitivity, such as allergic rhinitis and urticaria. Type II reactions involve antibodies directed against antigenic components of peripheral blood or tissue cells, resulting in cell destruction. Examples of this type include autoimmune hemolytic anemia and Rh and ABO hemolytic disease of the newborn, which is discussed in Chapter 11. In type III reactions, antigen-antibody complexes are deposited in or near blood vessels, stimulating tissue inflammation mediated by complement or toxic leukocyte products. Examples of this type of reaction are hypersensitivity pneumonitis, serum sickness, and the immune-complex–mediated renal diseases. Type IV reactions occur 24 to 48 hours after antigen exposure and involve cell-mediated (T-lymphocyte–mediated) tissue inflammation. Examples of this type are tuberculin and fungal delayed cutaneous hypersensitivity reactions and contact dermatitis (see Chapter 8).

Type I Disorders

The development of type I, or immediate, hypersensitivity depends on hereditary predisposition, sensitization, and subsequent reexposure to specific antigens known as *allergens*. The mechanism of antigen-induced mediator release in type I hypersensitivity reactions is shown in Fig. 4-1. Type I reactions may occur in one or more target organs, including the upper and lower respiratory tracts, skin, conjunctivae, and

gastrointestinal tract. Manifestations depend on the systems involved, as shown in Fig. 4-2. The acuteness or chronicity of target organ manifestations depends on the particular allergens to which the individual is sensitized. Inhalation of pollens produces seasonal symptoms, and inhalation of indoor molds, house dust, mite fragments, or animal danders produces year-round or perennial symptoms. Foods, insect venoms, and drugs produce intermittent symptoms depending on time of exposure.

Allergic Rhinitis

Allergic rhinitis, characterized by inflammation, edema, and weeping of the nasal mucosa, is the most common allergic disorder and occurs in 10% to 20% of the population. Diagnosis is based on characteristic history, physical findings, and laboratory (skin test) results. Common presenting symptoms include nasal congestion and pruritus, clear rhinorrhea, and paroxysms of sneezing. Congestion may be bilateral or unilateral or may alternate from side to side. It is generally more pronounced at night. Whereas older children blow their noses frequently, younger children do not. Instead, they sniff, snort, and repetitively clear their throats. Nasal pruritus stimulates grimacing and twitching (Fig. 4-3) and picking or rubbing the nose (allergic salute). Picking and repetitive sneezing and blowing may produce enough irritation to cause epistaxis. In the case of allergy to seasonal pollens, the symptoms may be acute, have an explosive onset, and be confined to the period during which the particular airborne pollen is detectable. Trees and grass typically pollinate in the spring, whereas ragweed (classic "hay fever") pollinates in the fall. In contrast, symptoms may be chronic and more indolent in the case of allergy to perennial allergens, including molds, dust mites, and animal danders.

Many patients have prominent itching and watering of the eyes with nasal symptoms, and some experience pruritus of the throat or ears. Associated symptoms include (1) disturbed sleep and snoring; (2) morning dryness and irritation of the throat as a result of mouth breathing; (3) lassitude, fatigue, and irritability from sleep interruption; (4) early nighttime cough; and (5) if the maxillary, frontal, and ethmoidal sinuses are affected, a sensation of pressure over the cheeks, forehead, and bridge of the nose.

Many children with long-standing allergic rhinitis can be recognized by their facial characteristics. Ocular manifestations of the allergic disposition include cobblestoned conjunctivae (Fig. 4-23), the allergic shiner, and the Dennie sign. Allergic shiners, bluish discolorations or

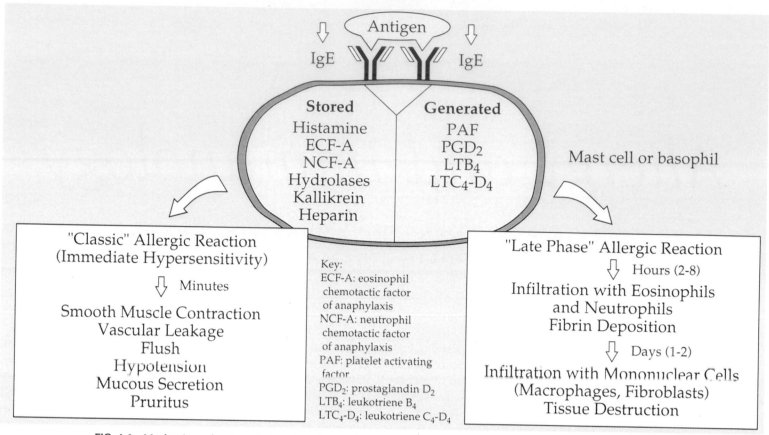

FIG. 4-1 Mechanism of antigen-induced mediator release in type I hypersensitivity. Note that an early (classic) and late phase reaction can follow antigen exposure. Cytokines are also produced and can play a role in these reactions.

T A B L E   4 - 1

Classification of Hypersensitivity Disorders

		Interval between exposure and reaction	Effector cell or antibody	Target or antigen	Examples of mediators	Examples
Type I	Anaphylactic		IgE	Pollens, foods, drugs, insect venoms		Anaphylaxis
	a. Immediate	<30 minutes			a. Histamine	Allergic rhinitis
	b. Late phase	2-12 hours			b. Leukotrienes	Allergic asthma
						Urticaria
Type II	Cytotoxic	Variable (minutes to hours)	IgG, IgM	Red blood cells, lung tissue	Complement	Immune hemolytic anemia
						Rh hemolytic disease
						Goodpasture syndrome
Type III	Immune complexes	4-8 hours	Antigen with antibody	Vascular endothelium	Complement Anaphylatoxin	Serum sickness
						Poststreptococcal glomerulonephritis
Type IV	Delayed type	24-48 hours	Lymphocytes	*Mycobacterium tuberculosis,* chemicals	Lymphokines	Contact dermatitis
						Tuberculin skin test reactions

From Gell PGH, Coombs RRA: *Clinical aspects of immunology,* ed 2, Philadelphia, 1968, FA Davis.

dark circles beneath the eyes, are commonly observed in patients with allergic rhinitis (Fig. 4-4). This finding may represent chronic venous congestion and/or chronic melanocyte stimulation related to repeated rubbing in response to itching. The Dennie sign is prominent folds or creases on the lower eyelid (Fig. 4-5) running parallel to the lower lid margin. Although these lines were originally thought to indicate a predisposition to allergy, data suggest that they may be present in any condition associated with periocular pruritus and scratching and/or chronic nasal congestion. Frequent upward rubbing of the nose with the palm of the hand to alleviate itching (the allergic salute [Fig. 4-6]) promotes development of a transverse nasal crease across the lower third of the nose (Fig. 4-7). Chronic obstruction produced by nasal mucosal edema may result in the typical open-mouthed, adenoid-type facies (Fig. 4-8).

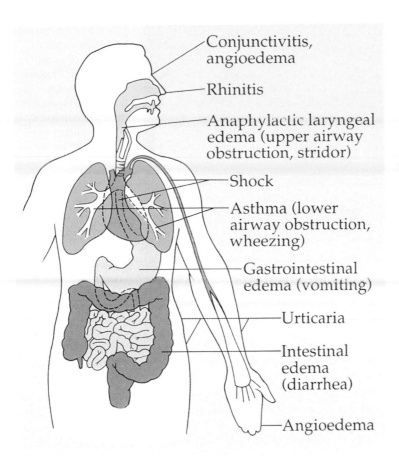

Conjunctivitis, angioedema

Rhinitis

Anaphylactic laryngeal edema (upper airway obstruction, stridor)

Shock

Asthma (lower airway obstruction, wheezing)

Gastrointestinal edema (vomiting)

Urticaria

Intestinal edema (diarrhea)

Angioedema

FIG. **4-2** Systemic manifestations of type I hypersensitivity disorders. Note the characteristic physical findings of each affected organ system.

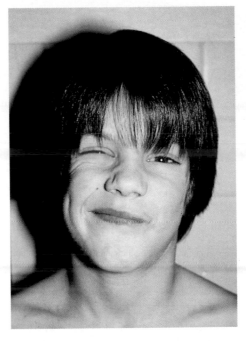

FIG. **4-3** Facial grimacing and twitching caused by nasal itching in patient with allergic rhinitis. These are frequently repeated and easily noted during patient evaluation.

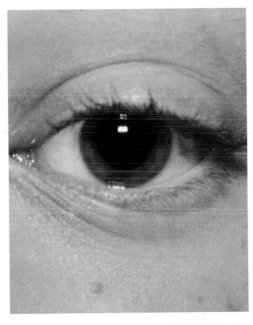

FIG. **4-5** Dennie sign originates in the inner canthus and traverses one half to two thirds the length of the lower lid margin in an arc nearly parallel to it.

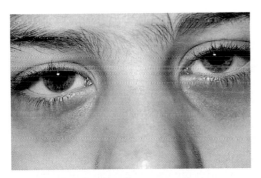

FIG. **4-4** Allergic shiners, or dark circles beneath the eyes, in patient with allergic rhinitis.

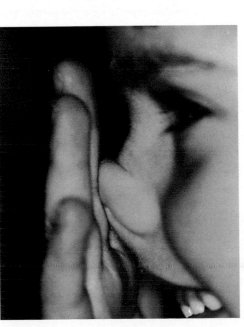

FIG. **4-6** The allergic salute is characteristic of children with allergic rhinitis and nasal itching and is usually noticed by parents.

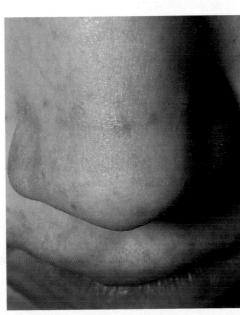

FIG. **4-7** The nasal crease across the lower third of the nose results from chronic upward rubbing of the nose with the hand (allergic salute). (Courtesy Dr. Meyer B. Marks.)

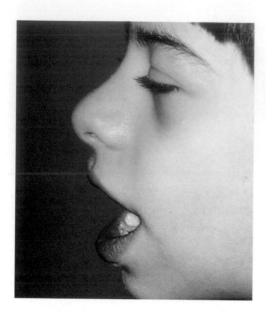

FIG. 4-8 Characteristic adenoid-type facies in a patient with long-standing allergic rhinitis. Note the open mouth and gaping habitus.

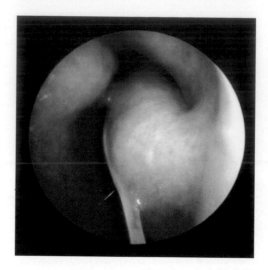

FIG. 4-9 Pale, edematous inferior nasal turbinate of patient with allergic rhinitis, as seen through a fiberoptic rhinoscope. Even though this tool is not routinely used in evaluations, the physical findings are well illustrated, including watery nasal secretions.

On rhinoscopy, attention should be focused on the position of the nasal septum; nasal patency; mucosal appearance; and presence and character of secretions, polyps, or foreign bodies (see Chapter 22). Use of a vasoconstrictor spray may be necessary to decrease edema and improve the examiner's view. The typical rhinoscopic findings in allergic rhinitis include a marked decrease in nasal patency resulting from swollen inferior turbinates, which appear wet and bluish-gray (Fig. 4-9). The degree of nasal obstruction may be estimated by digitally occluding one nostril and maintaining normal breathing through the other with the mouth closed. It is roughly proportional to the intensity of inspiratory nasal sounds, except when there is complete occlusion (no sounds). The mucosa appears edematous, and secretions are clear and watery or white. Examination of a Wright-stained smear of this discharge typically reveals eosinophils (Fig. 4-63).

Depending on the specific allergies, allergic rhinitis may be acute, recurrent, or chronic and must be distinguished from a number of non-allergic conditions. This necessitates a thorough medical and family history and careful examination. In some instances, response to a trial of medication and/or observations over time may be necessary to confirm the diagnosis. When symptoms are seasonal or regularly associated with exposure to specific allergens, the distinction is generally clear. In evaluating patients with perennial or recurrent but nonseasonal symptoms, allergy, recurrent infection, eosinophilic nonallergic rhinitis, and vasomotor rhinitis must be considered.

Children with frequent upper respiratory infections and/or persistent nasal congestion can present a major diagnostic challenge. In some cases the phenomenon is due to frequent or heavy exposure to pathogens. This is particularly true of children in their first year of day-care or nursery school. In other patients, tonsillar and adenoidal hypertrophy provides favorable conditions for recurrent infections (see Chapter 22). Atopic (allergic) children may have increased risk of infection because of impaired flow of secretions from mucosal edema, and infectious symptoms may be more protracted. They often have a history of frequent colds (more than the average of six to eight per year), which are unusually prolonged, lasting 1 to 2 weeks rather than the typical 3 to 5 days. During the course of infections, nasal eosinophilia disappears, and the character of the nasal discharge often changes. With viral infections, nasal discharge tends to be clear or white, but with bacterial infection it is often cloudy and yellow or green. Diagnosis of underlying atopy in these children is facilitated by a thorough past medical and family history with questions specifically directed at possible allergic symptoms and environmental allergens. Having the parents keep a symptom record

with the patient on and off antihistamine therapy and reexamination at a time when the child is not acutely infected can be valuable as well.

Other forms of rhinitis that must be distinguished from allergic rhinitis are enumerated in Table 4-2. Although characterized by eosinophilia, eosinophilic nonallergic rhinitis does not produce nasal pruritus, and patients lack specific IgE antibodies as measured by skin testing or serum radioallergosorbent testing (RAST). Patients with vasomotor rhinitis do not complain of pruritus, have a clear discharge without eosinophils, and also lack specific IgE antibodies. Vasomotor rhinitis is thus considered a form of noninflammatory rhinitis, the etiology of which is unknown. The condition is diagnosed most frequently in adults but may affect children. A vasocongestive form, characterized by marked nasal congestion but not secretion, and a vasosecretory form, characterized by a chronic, profuse, clear rhinorrhea but minimal congestion, have been identified. Nonspecific precipitants of symptoms, such as sudden changes in environmental temperature and humidity, should be avoided, because pharmacologic management frequently is unsuccessful. Rhinitis medicamentosa is a condition seen in patients who have been using alpha-adrenergic vasoconstrictor nose drops as decongestants for more than a few days. The disorder is characterized by rebound vasodilation that produces an erythematous, edematous mucosa in association with profuse clear nasal discharge.

Some children with perennial allergic rhinitis have congestion that is so constant and severe that it produces signs of chronic nasal obstruction. This must be distinguished from other acquired and congenital causes (see Chapter 22). Again history, physical findings, and results of nasal smears and therapeutic trials of antihistamines are major clues to the diagnosis, which may then be confirmed by IgE testing.

The majority of patients with allergic rhinitis have mild symptoms that are easily controlled by intermittent antihistamine administration and/or environmental control. In many of these the pattern of symptoms suggests the probable responsible allergens, obviating the need for specific IgE testing. Those with severe symptoms only partially alleviated by antihistamines, topical antiinflammatory agents, and environmental control and those with perennial symptoms who require daily therapy should be referred for specific IgE testing and possible desensitization therapy.

Respiratory Distress

Respiratory distress in children (tachypnea with or without grunting, flaring, retractions, and cyanosis) of any etiology (allergic, infectious, anatomic) must be promptly evaluated and treated, since failure

TABLE 4-2

Comparison of Allergic and Nonallergic Rhinitis

	Allergic	Nonallergic ENR	Nonallergic Vasomotor
Usual onset	Childhood	Childhood	Adulthood
Family history of allergy	Usual	Coincidental	Coincidental
Collateral allergy	Common	Unusual	Unusual
Symptoms			
Sneezing	Frequent	Occasional	Occasional
Itching	Common	Unusual	Unusual
Rhinorrhea	Profuse	Profuse	Profuse
Congestion	Moderate	Moderate to marked	Moderate to marked
Physical examination			
Edema	Moderate to marked	Moderate	Moderate
Secretions	Watery	Watery	Mucoid to watery
Nasal eosinophilia	Common	Common	Occasional
Allergic evaluation			
Skin tests	Positive	Coincidental	Coincidental
IgE antibodies	Positive	Coincidental	Coincidental
Therapeutic response			
Antihistamines	Good	Fair	Poor to fair
Decongestants	Fair	Fair	Poor to fair
Corticosteroids	Good	Good	Poor
Cromolyn	Fair	Unknown	Poor
Immunotherapy	Good	None	None

From Fagin J, Friedman R, Fireman P: Allergic rhinitis, *Pediatr Clin North Am* 28:(4):797–806, 1981.
ENR, Eosinophilic nonallergic rhinitis.

to do so may result in progression to respiratory failure, apnea, coma, and death. The first step in approaching respiratory distress is to differentiate upper from lower airway disorders. Once the level of involvement has been established, the cause can be promptly assigned on the basis of specific symptoms and signs. Appropriate therapy must be initiated without delay and is based on the severity of distress and the type of disorder. At times, various degrees of upper and lower airway obstruction may coexist, as in laryngotracheobronchitis.

An algorithm for determining the etiology of respiratory distress in children (Fig. 4-10) demonstrates differences in physical findings between upper and lower airway obstructive disorders. Upper airway obstruction causes difficulty moving air into the chest, whereas lower airway obstruction causes difficulty moving air out of the chest. This difference results in the characteristic physical findings in each type. In general, lower airway obstruction produces prolongation of the expiratory phase of respiration and typical expiratory wheezing, whereas upper airway obstruction prolongs the inspiratory phase. *Wheezing* is defined as musical or whistling auscultatory sounds heard more often on expiration than on inspiration. Inspiratory stridor, seen with upper airway obstruction, can mimic wheezing. Both can be detected concomitantly, but their differentiation is seldom confusing to the experienced observer. *Stridor* is defined as a crowing sound usually heard during the inspiratory phase of respiration. It tends to be loud when the obstruction is subglottic and quiet when obstruction is supraglottic.

All forms of acute upper airway obstruction present with suprasternal, supraclavicular, and subcostal retractions, which increase as the obstruction progresses. Mild to moderate increases in respiratory and heart rates are common. In lower airway disorders such as pneumonitis and asthma, retractions are primarily intercostal and when present usually indicate a significant degree of obstruction. Respiratory and

heart rates are often markedly increased. Retractions are usually generalized in severe airway obstruction of any etiology.

This chapter concentrates on disorders in which respiratory distress stems from hypersensitivity. These include anaphylactic laryngeal edema, in which upper airway obstruction is the result of an acute allergic reaction, and three lower airway disorders: asthma, hypersensitivity pneumonitis, and allergic bronchopulmonary aspergillosis. Infectious causes of acute upper airway obstruction and foreign body aspiration are discussed in Chapter 22.

Anaphylactic Laryngeal Edema. Anaphylactic (type I hypersensitivity) laryngeal edema typically presents with symptoms and signs of subglottic obstruction such as tightness or pressure in the upper chest, stridor, dyspnea, and retractions. Onset is immediate and explosive after bee stings, drug administration, or food ingestion. Asphyxiation may result from delays in diagnosis or treatment. Frequently, other organ systems are also involved. Facial angioedema is common, and many patients have associated urticaria. Wheezing reflecting pulmonary involvement and vomiting resulting from gastrointestinal reaction may also be seen. In severe cases there is massive third spacing of fluid, resulting in cardiovascular shock with an initial phase of flushing and warm extremities resulting from vasodilation. This phase is superseded by pallor and cold related to vasoconstriction. Therapy depends on severity and ranges from the administration of antihistamines to the use of epinephrine, steroids, volume expansion, and pressor agents.

Acute and Chronic Asthma. Type I hypersensitivity reactions can occur in the large and small airways of the lungs and result in the disorder termed *asthma.* The most widely accepted definition of *asthma* includes the following characteristics: (1) lower airway obstruction that is partially or fully reversible either spontaneously or with bronchodilator or antiinflammatory treatments, (2) the presence of airway

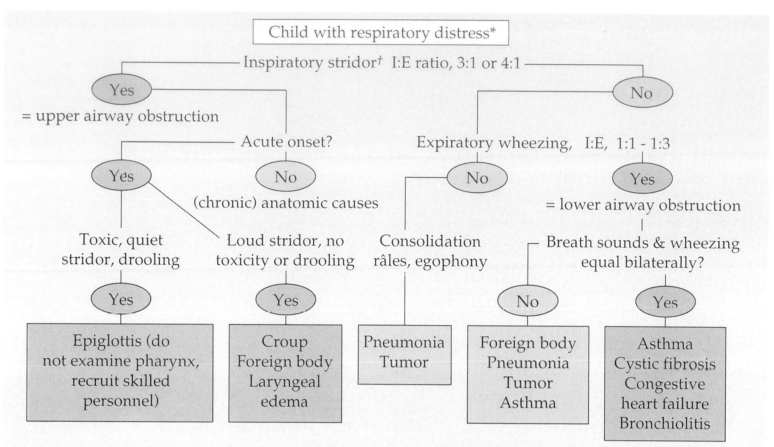

FIG. 4-10 Algorithm to determine the etiology of respiratory distress in children.

Tachypnea, with or without accessory muscle use, cyanosis, flaring or retractions. (Flaring and retractions are seen predominately in upper airway obstruction, also in advanced lower airway obstruction.)

†*Supraglottic-quiet stridor (may be audible only with stethoscope over mouth). Subglottic-loud stridor (may be audible across the room).*

inflammation, and (3) increased lower airway responsiveness (hyperreactivity). The last is characterized by inherent hyperreactivity of the airways to one or more of several stimuli, including allergens, infections, exercise, chemical agents such as methacholine, cold or dry air, emotions, and weather changes. Hence in some cases asthma has an atopic basis, and in others it does not. Specific allergens implicated in atopic patients are pollens, molds, house dust mites, animal danders, drugs, food, and insect venoms. On exposure, these allergens, via type I hypersensitivity, produce the characteristic features of asthma: mucosal edema, increased mucus production, and smooth muscle contraction that results in airway inflammation, airway hyperreactivity, and bronchoconstriction. These responses combine to produce obstruction of the large and small airways, which if recurrent and reversible with bronchodilator and/or antiinflammatory drugs, is the hallmark of asthma.

Any child undergoing an evaluation for asthma should also be evaluated for possible allergic rhinitis and atopic dermatitis, which are frequent concomitant disorders. This evaluation should include a close inspection of the skin and nasal mucosa and possibly allergy skin testing to identify offending allergens (see other sections). Affected individuals are usually aware of the specific stimuli that trigger their asthma. Viruses are the most common precipitants of acute asthma in children, especially respiratory syncytial virus, parainfluenza viruses, and rhinoviruses. These infections usually affect the upper and lower airways, producing rhinorrhea, nasal congestion, and fever in addition to

wheezing, which tends to develop insidiously. In contrast, allergy-triggered episodes typically lack fever and have a more explosive onset of wheezing.

Asthma is one of the leading causes of pediatric morbidity. Indeed, approximately 5% to 10% of children in the United States show signs and symptoms compatible with asthma at some time during childhood. Peak incidence of onset is before the age of 5 years. In childhood, boys are affected 30% more often than girls and tend to have more severe disease. Beyond puberty, the gender distribution is equal. Asthmatic children with respiratory allergy and eczema usually have more severe courses than those who wheeze only with upper respiratory infections.

Recently, an unexplained, worldwide increase in asthma-related morbidity and mortality rates has been noted. Indeed, deaths resulting from asthma have now exceeded 5000 per year in the United States. In an effort to reverse this trend, a national (National Institutes of Health [NIH]) educational program has resulted in the publication of suggested guidelines on the diagnosis and management of asthma (see references).

Emergency department visits, hospitalizations, and intensive care unit admissions for asthma usually peak in the late fall or early winter months and, to a lesser extent, in the spring (Fig. 4-11). These seasonal patterns may be related to environmental temperature and humidity changes, allergen exposure, or respiratory infections.

The diagnosis of asthma is frequently based on historical findings alone, indicating the importance of taking a thorough history. Recently published NIH guidelines have stressed the importance of comple-

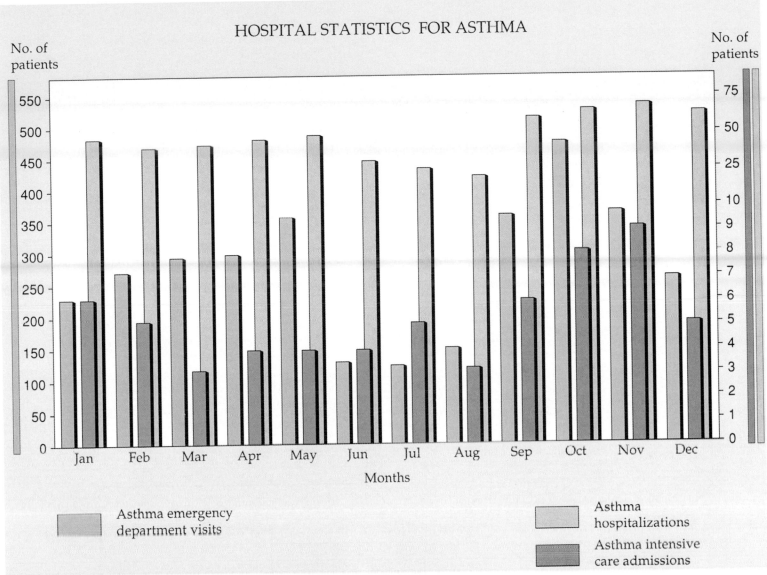

HOSPITAL STATISTICS FOR ASTHMA

No. of patients

No. of patients

Asthma emergency department visits

Asthma hospitalizations

Asthma intensive care admissions

Months

FIG. 4-11 Number of emergency department visits for wheezing (1986-1987) and number of asthma admissions (1982-1985) to Children's Hospital of Pittsburgh and number of asthma intensive care unit admissions to Children's Hospital of Los Angeles (1969-1977) by month of year. (Data from Friday GA, Fireman P: Morbidity and mortality of asthma, *Pediatr Clin North Am* 35(5):1153, 1988; Richards W, Lew C, Carney J, et al: Review of intensive care unit admissions for asthma, *Clin Pediatr* 18(6):346, 1979; and Fireman P, Slavin RG: *Atlas of allergies*, New York, 1990, Gower.)

menting good history taking with the use of objective measurements of lung function (Fig. 4-12). This can include in-office pulmonary function testing and home monitoring of peak expiratory flow rates in children 6 years of age and older. Peak expiratory flow rates, which must be referenced by percentage to the patient's personal best value or to predicted values (Table 4-3), can be used to diagnose and treat asthma. These values allow the establishment of well-defined zones to guide management (Fig. 4-13). Green zones (80% to 100% of predicted or personal best) indicate normal values. Yellow zones (50% to 80%) signal caution and a possible need for a temporary and/or long-term increase in medication. Finally, a red zone (<50%) indicates a medical emergency, whereby an inhaled bronchodilator should be used immediately and the clinician should be notified if the values do not improve and stay in the yellow or green zones. Transport to an emergency facility may be indicated if the response is inadequate. This also signals the need for an initiation or increase in corticosteroid medication.

Even though asthma is a familial disorder, its clinical expression requires not only a hereditary predisposition, but also specific environmental factors. Family history often reveals affected siblings, parents, or first-degree relatives. An environmental survey can determine possible provocative factors, especially allergens, infections, occupational exposures, smoking, exercise, stress, climate, and medication use (aspirin, propranolol). The history should emphasize the frequency, duration, and intensity of suspected episodes. A description of symptoms between acute episodes aids in the determination of chronicity (night cough, exercise intolerance, fatigue, school absenteeism, social function). Individuals with asthma commonly present with recurrent episodes of wheezing that, depending on the severity, may require emergency treatment. Episodes may be infrequent and/or seasonal but may occur as frequently as every day. The spectrum of presenting complaints, however, is broad, and affected individuals may complain only of mild, occasional wheezing or shortness of breath with exercise

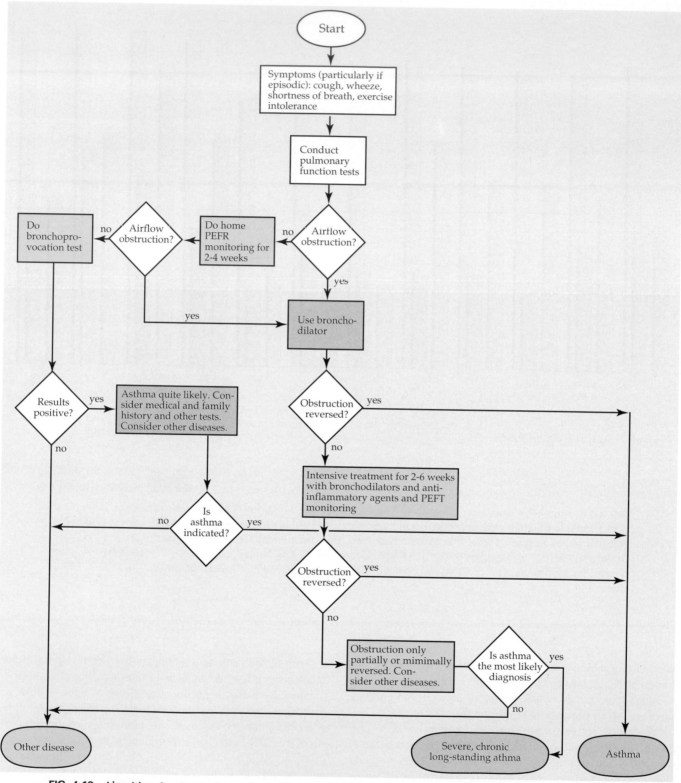

FIG. 4-12 Algorithm for diagnosing asthma. (From National Asthma Education Program: *Guidelines for the diagnosis and management of asthma*, Pub No 91-3042, Bethesda, Md, 1991, National Heart, Lung, and Blood Institute, National Institutes of Health.)

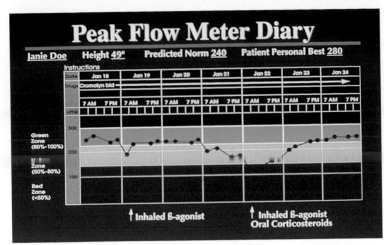

FIG. 4-13 Example of a peak flow meter diary and ways that the values can be used to guide the use of various forms of therapy.

	TABLE 4-3		

Predicted Average Peak Expiratory Flow for Normal Children and Adolescents*

Height (Inches)	Boys and girls	Height (inches)	Boys and girls
43	147	56	320
44	160	57	334
45	173	58	347
46	187	59	360
47	200	60	373
48	214	61	387
49	227	62	400
50	240	63	413
51	254	64	427
52	267	65	440
53	280	66	454
54	293	67	467
55	307		

Modified from Polger G, Promedhat V: *Pulmonary function testing in children: techniques and standards*, Philadelphia, 1971, WB Saunders. As appears in National asthma education program: *Guidelines for the diagnosis and management of asthma*, Pub No 91-3042, Bethesda, Md, 1991, National Heart, Lung, and Blood Institute, National Institutes of Health.
*In liters per minute.

and/or colds or a persistent dry, hacking cough. The diagnosis of asthma is usually considered established after three or more episodes have been successfully treated with bronchodilators. The frequency and severity of acute asthma episodes and the level of symptoms between episodes can be used to grade asthma severity and guide therapy (Table 4-4).

The early stages of an asthma exacerbation in children are characterized by the onset of cough, rhinorrhea, and chest tightness, as well as chest retractions or audible wheezing. The parents should be educated to critically and accurately observe their child for the warning signs and, in collaboration with the managing physician, identify the onset of asthmatic exacerbation at home. As previously mentioned, peak flow assessment may be useful under these circumstances. The institution of appropriate therapy can halt the progression of airway obstruction and reduce the number of visits to the emergency department.

Asthma should be considered part of the differential diagnosis in any child with recurrent or chronic lower respiratory symptoms or signs. Even though a high index of suspicion must be maintained, excessive or erroneous diagnoses may result if they are made hastily without appropriate supportive evidence; normal children or those with potentially more severe disorders may be mistakenly labeled with the stigma of asthma and inappropriately treated. Parents must be instructed that physician assessment is essential during suspected episodes of asthma so that wheezing or other signs of lower airway obstruction and reversibility may be documented. If the diagnosis is unclear on clinical grounds, then specific laboratory studies must be performed to document asthma and rule out disorders that mimic asthma. Pulmonary function tests in asthmatic children older than 5 years show airway obstruction at baseline or after appropriate challenge with methacholine, exercise, or cold air and document reversibility after administration of an aerosolized bronchodilator (Fig. 4-14). In children younger than 5 years or those in whom testing is unreliable, the diagnosis must be made on the basis of historical and physical findings and

clinical response to bronchodilator or antiinflammatory medication. Lack of an immediate response to a bronchodilator does not eliminate asthma as a diagnostic consideration, however.

A thorough physical examination provides valuable information regarding the diagnosis of asthma and its severity and chronicity. The physical findings in asthma vary with the chronicity and state of activity of the disease process at the time of examination. The findings of acute asthma are markedly different from those of chronic and latent or quiescent asthma. Between episodes, the examination usually is entirely normal. Often, however, gentle compression of the anterior chest with the hand, at the end of the expiratory phase, elicits auscultatory wheezing over the posterior chest. If a patient with prolonged obstruction has not received appropriate therapy, signs of chronic lung disease may be present. These include a paucity of subcutaneous fatty tissue and a barrel-chest configuration (Fig. 4-15). Rales, wheezing, rhonchi, and decreased intensity and duration of the inspiratory phase of respiration are commonly noted on auscultation. Clubbing as a sign of chronic asthma is rare and if present in a wheezing child suggests another chronic pulmonary disease.

During acute asthma, the following historical features should be noted: time of onset, possible triggers, present medications, comparison with previous episodes, and presence of complicating factors (e.g., vomiting, fever, chest pain). Examination should document the presence and degree of the following:

1. Dyspnea (the patient's own assessment of breathlessness); wheezing; accessory muscle use (visible contractions of the scalene and/or sternocleidomastoid muscles); and suprasternal, intercostal, or substernal retractions (visible depression in the chest wall during inspiration), all of which are graded as absent, mild, moderate, or severe

2. Cyanosis (central, involving the lips, and/or peripheral, involving the nail beds)

3. Inspiratory breath sounds (normal or decreased)

TABLE 4-4

Guidelines for Defining Asthma Severity

Characteristics	Mild	Moderate	Severe
Pretreatment			
Frequency of exacerbations	Exacerbations of cough and wheezing no more often than 1-2 times/week.	Exacerbation of cough and wheezing on a more frequent basis than 1-2 times/week. Could have history of severe exacerbations, but infrequent. Urgent care treatment in hospital emergency department or doctor's office <3 times/year.	Virtually daily wheezing. Exacerbations frequent, often severe. Tendency to have sudden severe exacerbations. Urgent visits to hospital emergency departments or doctor's office >3 times/year. Hospitalization >2 times/year, perhaps with respiratory insufficiency or, rarely, respiratory failure and history of intubation. May have had cough syncope or hypoxic seizures.
Frequency of symptoms	Few clinical signs or symptoms of asthma between exacerbations.	Cough and low-grade wheezing between acute exacerbations often present.	Continuous albeit low-grade cough and wheezing almost always present.
Degree of exercise tolerance	Good exercise tolerance but may not tolerate vigorous exercise, especially prolonged running.	Exercise tolerance diminished.	Very poor exercise tolerance with marked limitation of activity.
Frequency of nocturnal asthma	Symptoms of nocturnal asthma occur no more often than 1-2 times/month.	Symptoms of nocturnal asthma present 2-3 times/week.	Considerable, almost nightly, sleep interruption due to asthma. Chest tight in early morning.
School or work attendance	Good school or work attendance.	School or work attendance may be affected.	Poor school or work attendance.
Pulmonary function			
Peak expiratory flow rate (PEFR)	PEFR >80% predicted. Variability* <20%.	PEFR 60%-80% predicted. Variability 20%-30%.	PEFR <60% predicted. Variability >30%.
Spirometry	Minimal or no evidence of airway obstruction on spirometry. Normal expiratory flow volume curve; lung volumes not increased. Usually a >15% response to acute aerosol bronchodilator administration, even though baseline near normal.	Signs of airway obstruction on spirometry are evident. Flow volume curve shows reduced expiratory flow at low lung volumes. Lung volumes often increased. Usually a >15% response to acute aerosol bronchodilator administration.	Substantial degree of airway obstruction on spirometry. Flow volume curve shows marked concavity. Spirometry may not be normalized even with high-dose steroids. May have substantial increase in lung volumes and marked unevenness of ventilation. Incomplete reversibility to acute aerosol bronchodilator administration.
Methacholine sensitivity	Methacholine PC_{20} >20 mg/ml.†	Methacholine PC_{20} between 2 and 20 mg/ml.	Methacholine PC_{20} <2mg/ml.
After optimal treatment is established			
Response to and duration of therapy	Exacerbations respond to bronchodilators without the use of systemic corticosteroids in 12-24 hours. Regular drug therapy not usually required except for short periods of time.	Periodic use of bronchodilators required during exacerbations for a week or more. Systemic steroids also usually required for exacerbations. Continuous around-the-clock drug therapy required. Regular use of antiinflammatory agents may be required for prolonged periods of time.	Requires continuous, multiple, around-the-clock drug therapy including daily corticosteroids, either aerosol or systemic, often in high doses.

From National Asthma Education Program: *Guidelines for the diagnosis and management of asthma,* Pub No 91-3042, Bethesda, Md, 1991, National Heart, Lung, and Blood Institute, National Institutes of Health.
Variability means the difference either between a morning and evening measure or among morning peak flow measurements each day for a week.
†While the degree of methacholine/histamine sensitivity generally correlates with severity of symptoms and medication requirements, there are exceptions.
PC_{20}, Provocative concentration of methacholine causing a 20% fall in forced expiratory volume in 1 second.

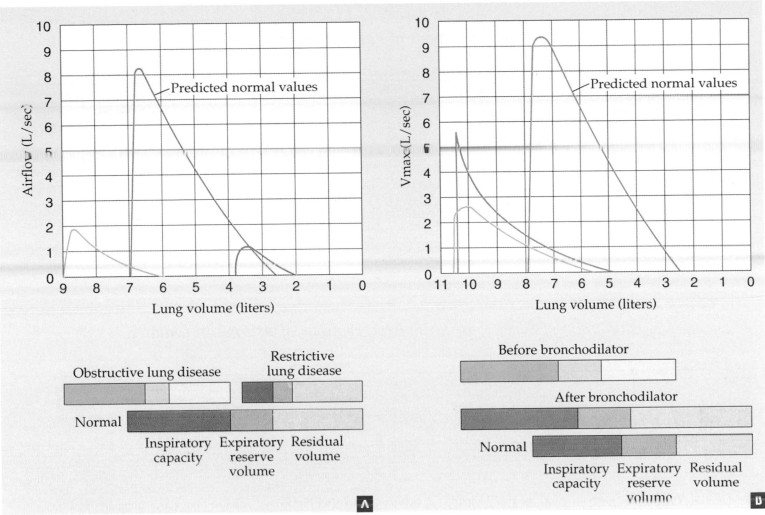

FIG. 4-14 *A,* Maximum expiratory flow rates are reduced in obstructive lung diseases such as asthma and restrictive lung disease. However, in asthma, the airflow is limited at high lung volumes, in contrast with restrictive lung disease, in which airflow is limited because lung volume is decreased. *B,* Bronchoconstriction characteristic of hyperreactive airways is generally reversible. Indices of expiratory airflow in asthmatic patients thus improve after inhalation of a nebulized bronchodilator (e.g., a beta-adrenergic agonist). (From Cherniack RM: Continuity of care in asthma management, *Hosp Pract* 22(9):119-143, 1987.)

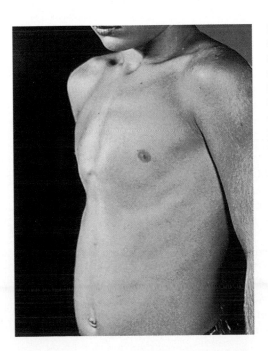

FIG. 4-15 The barrel-chest configuration of chronic asthma. Physical findings include an increased anteroposterior diameter of the chest and decreased respiratory excursion of the chest wall. (Courtesy Dr. Meyer B. Marks.)

4. Air exchange (normal, decreased, or absent)

5. Abnormalities of the inspiration:expiration ratio

In addition, rales are often heard, and pulse, respiratory rate, and blood pressure are frequently elevated. Pulsus paradoxus, an exaggerated decrease in systolic blood pressure during inspiration (Table 4-5), correlates highly with the degree of airway obstruction and can serve as an indicator of severity and a guide to therapy. This phenomenon may result from physical forces on the pericardium that impede venous return and reduce cardiac output during forced inspiration. Normally, the inspiratory decrease in systolic blood pressure is less than 10 mm Hg and is not discernible during routine sphygmomanometry. In acute asthma, it is usually greater than 10 mm Hg (up to 30 and 40 mm Hg) and is easily detectable. The presence of pulsus paradoxus is generally correlated with a forced expiratory volume in 1 second of less than 20% predicted.

Individuals with asthma may be distinguished by their characteristic symptoms and signs during acute episodes, which typically change as the degree of airway obstruction increases. Symptoms usually consist of progressively increasing shortness of breath and difficulty breathing with or without rhinorrhea, low-grade fever, and vomiting.

TABLE 4-5

Measurement of Pulsus Paradoxus

	Blood pressure in relation to time and respiratory phase (mm Hg)				
	Expiration	Inspiration	Expiration	Inspiration	Expiration
Normal (no airway obstruction)	125/70	120/70	125/70	120/70	125/70
Asthma (airway obstruction)	125/70	100/70	125/70	100/70	125/70

Method

1. Pump sphygmomanometer cuff to occlude the peripheral pulse.
2. As the cuff pressure falls, listen carefully for the onset of the first Korotkoff sound.
3. Note the pressure at which the first Korotkoff sound is detected. This should be heard only during expiration. (In above example, 125 = normal and asthma.)
4. Continue to slowly decrease the cuff pressure until the first sound is detected during inspiration and expiration. Note this pressure. (In above example, 120 = normal; 100 = asthma.)
5. When the difference between the two pressures is greater than or equal to 10, pulsus paradoxus is present. (In above example, 5 = normal, no pulsus paradoxus, and 25 = asthma, pulsus paradoxus.)

TABLE 4-6

Estimation of Severity of Acute Exacerbations of Asthma in Children

Sign or symptom	Mild	Moderate	Severe
PEFR*	70%-90% predicted or personal best	50%-70% predicted or personal best	<50% predicted or personal best
Respiratory rate, resting or sleeping	Normal to 30% increase above the mean	30%-50% increase above the mean	Increase over 50% above the mean
Alertness	Normal	Normal	May be decreased
Dyspnea†	Absent or mild; speaks in complete sentences	Moderate; speaks in phrases or partial sentences; infant's cry softer and shorter, infant has difficulty suckling and feeding	Severe; speaks only in single words or short phrases; infant's cry softer and shorter, infant stops suckling and feeding
Pulsus paradoxus‡	<10 mm Hg	10-20 mm Hg	20-40 mm Hg
Accessory muscle use	No intercostal to mild retractions	Moderate intercostal retraction with tracheosternal retractions; use of sternocleidomastoid muscles; chest hyperinflation	Severe intercostal retractions, tracheosternal retractions with nasal flaring during inspiration; chest hyperinflation
Color	Good	Pale	Possibly cyanotic
Auscultation	End expiratory wheeze only	Wheeze during entire expiration and inspiration	Breath sounds becoming inaudible
Oxygen saturation	>95%	90%-95%	<90%
P_{CO_2}	<35	<40	>40

From National Asthma Education Program: *Guidelines for the diagnosis and management of asthma*, Pub No 91-3042, Bethesda, Md: 1991, National Heart, Lung, and Blood Institute, National Institutes of Health.
NOTE: Within each category, the presence of several parameters, but not necessarily all, indicates the general classification of the exacerbation.
*For children 5 years of age or older.
†Parents' or physicians' impression of degree of child's breathlessness.
‡Pulsus paradoxus does not correlate with phase of respiration in small children.

On examination, expiratory wheezing or a prolonged expiratory phase may be the only manifestation of mild asthma. However, as the obstructive process progresses, the expiratory phase becomes longer and the wheezing louder. Eventually, airways collapse, and signs of hyperinflation develop (low diaphragms, decreased lateral excursions of the chest wall with breathing, and hyperresonance to percussion). There are visible sternocleidomastoid contractions; increased anteroposterior chest diameter; circumoral cyanosis; and suprasternal, intercostal, and substernal retractions. Subjectively, the patient experiences chest tightness and anxiety and works harder to breathe. Accessory muscle use and retractions develop with or without a marked degree of wheezing on auscultation. To maximize air exchange, the child assumes a characteristic sitting posture, bending slightly forward. Frequent examinations are warranted, and any change in sensorium requires prompt evaluation. As respiratory muscles tire, the patient becomes lethargic and cyanotic, even with supplemental oxygen. Maximal effort to breathe produces feeble air exchange manifested by decreased intensity and duration or lack of inspiratory breath sounds. This is due to the decrease in audible sounds associated with respiration as air exchange decreases. Consequently, a patient with severe obstruction and impending respiratory failure may not be wheezing because he or she is moving too little air to do so. With extreme fatigue, respiratory muscles fail, retractions decrease, and respiratory failure is imminent unless appropriate therapy is promptly initiated. After initial examination, serial assessment of the degree of respiratory distress using the parameters outlined in Table 4-6 facilitates determination of the response to therapy.

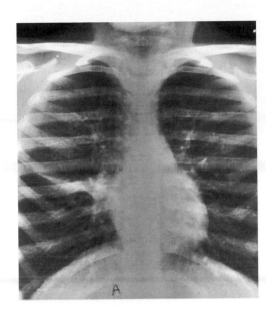

FIG. 4-16 Anteroposterior chest radiograph of child with acute asthma. Note the flattened diaphragm, hyperinflation, peribronchial thickening, and right middle lobe atelectasis.

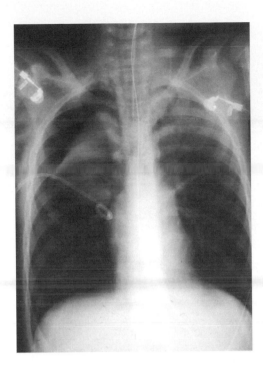

FIG. 4-17 Chest radiograph showing right-sided pneumothorax in an intubated patient with acute asthma and respiratory failure. Clinical manifestations include pleutitic chest paint, dyspnea, cyanosis, tachypnea, and cough. Also, note the marked hyperinflation of the lungs, which can result in cardiac compression (narrow cardiac shadow) and compromise of cardiac venous return, as well as extensive right-sided subcutaneous emphysema. (Courtesy Dr. Beverly Newman, Pittsburgh.)

TABLE 4-7

Respiratory Rates of Normal Children, Sleeping and Awake

Age	Sleeping			Awake			Mean difference between sleeping and awake
	No.	Mean	Range	No.	Mean	Range	
6-12 months	6	27	22-31	3	64	58-75	37
1-2 years	6	19	17-23	4	35	30-40	16
2-4 years	16	19	16-25	15	31	23-42	12
4-6 years	23	18	14-23	22	26	19-36	8
6-8 years	27	17	13-23	28	23	15-30	6

From Waring WW: The history and physical exam. In Kendig E, Chernick V, eds: *Disorders of the respiratory tract in children*, Philadelphia, 1983, WB Saunders. As appears in National Asthma Education Program: *Guidelines for the diagnosis and management of asthma*, Pub No 91-3042, Bethesda, Md: 1991, National Heart, Lung, and Blood Institute, National Institutes of Health.
*In breaths per minute.

A particularly useful aspect of the physical examination is the respiratory rate, which increases as the degree of airway obstruction progresses. Respiratory rates of normal children are shown in Table 4-7.

Histopathologic features of acute asthma include airway infiltration with inflammatory cells, increased intraluminal mucus with plugging of small airways, edema, bronchoconstriction, and smooth muscle hypertrophy. Because asthma has bronchoconstrictive and inflammatory components, the ideal therapeutic regimen should incorporate a combination of bronchodilator and antiinflammatory agents. Education is a key component of asthma therapy, incorporating information about disease pathogenesis; use of peak flow meters; avoidance of environmental triggers (including second-hand tobacco smoke exposure); benefits and risks of medications; and a written, individualized therapeutic plan for chronic and acute management.

The radiographic features of the hyperinflation, peribronchial cuffing, and atelectasis, which are characteristic of uncomplicated acute asthma, are illustrated in Fig. 4-16. Complications are generally diagnosed radiographically (Fig. 4-17) but may be suggested by symptoms and signs. Pneumothorax should be suspected in any asthmatic person who develops pleuritic chest pain associated with dyspnea, cyanosis,

tachypnea, and occasionally cough. Examination reveals respiratory distress, marked hyperinflation and decreased chest wall excursion, and decreased or absent breath sounds on the affected side. With tension pneumothorax, the trachea, mediastinum, and cardiac landmarks may be shifted to the opposite side. Pneumomediastinum and subcutaneous emphysema (Fig. 4-18), usually involving the neck and supraclavicular areas, are more common than pneumothorax. When mild, they may be asymptomatic and may be detected incidentally on chest or neck radiograph. With more extensive air dissection the patient may complain of neck and chest pain, and the subcutaneous emphysema may be visibly evident as a soft tissue swelling of the neck and chest that is crepitant (has a crunching sensation) on palpation. Pneumothorax and pneumomediastinum can produce characteristic auscultatory findings, including a crackling "mediastinal crunch" at the base of the heart and a systolic crunch or knock. The latter sound has been referred to as *noisy pneumothorax* and frequently is audible to the patient and physician without the aid of a stethoscope.

Other complications diagnosable on physical examination include those induced by chronic systemic steroid use, such as weight gain, "moon-type" facies, hirsutism, polycythemia (red, ruddy complexion)

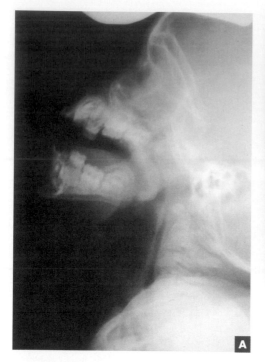

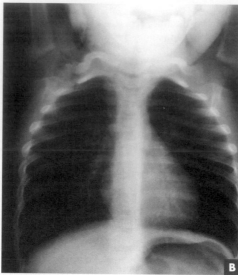

FIG. 4-18 Pneumomediastinum in a 16-month-old child with asthma. Note the dissection of air in the soft tissues just anterior to the vertebrae (A) and in the mediastinum and subcutaneous tissues of the right arm (B). This highlights the often subtle findings of pneumomediastinum in the chest and the more striking findings in the neck. Also note the hyperinflation (B). (Courtesy Dr. Beverly Newman, Pittsburgh.)

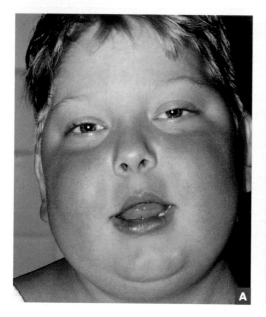

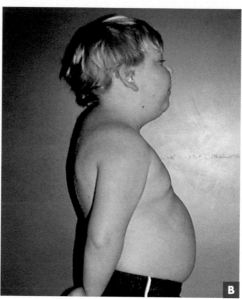

FIG. 4-19 Complications of corticosteroid therapy for chronic asthma. Moon-type facies (A) and buffalo hump (B), both resulting from abnormal fat distribution.

(Fig. 4-19), and short stature (see Chapter 9). Such side effects of excessive oral or parenteral steroid therapy for chronic asthma should be avoidable and are generally not associated with inhaled steroid therapy at the manufacturer's recommended doses.

In children with recent onsets of wheezing, asthma must be differentiated from other disorders associated with wheezing. In infants, this differentiation includes bronchiolitis, the features of which are listed in Table 4-8 (see Chapter 16). Many asthmatic exacerbations are triggered by infection; 30% to 50% of children with recurrent bronchiolitis are later diagnosed with asthma. Even though these two entities may be different manifestations of the same or a similar disease, the distinction remains a clinically useful one for the following reasons: (1) the children with bronchiolitis who do not develop asthma may be inappropriately labeled with the stigma of asthma and (2) children younger than 2 years of age frequently may not respond to inhaled or injected bronchodilators. Depending on the response to a trial dose, the ongoing bronchodilator therapy characteristic of asthma management may be indicated in children with bronchiolitis. Although children with pneumonia (particularly of viral origin) may wheeze, they are more likely to have rales or normal findings on auscultation, with the diagnosis suggested by tachypnea in association with retractions, nasal flaring, or expiratory grunting. Other causes of wheezing are listed in Table 4-9. Airway compression by anomalous vessels (see Chapter 5) or mass lesions is often distinguishable from bronchiolitis by virtue of absence of signs of infection and from asthma by failure to respond to bronchodilators. The history and presence of infiltrates help in the diagnosis of aspiration, which can mimic asthma closely, often responding to bronchodilator therapy. Radiographic studies such as barium swallow with fluoroscopy can be very helpful in distinguishing among these entities (Fig. 4-20). pH-Probe testing may be required to identify gastroesophageal reflux (see Chapter 10).

In older children who have sudden onsets of wheezing and respiratory distress, the differential diagnosis includes respiratory infections, left ventricular failure, and aspiration. Respiratory infections such as

Differentiating Features of Asthma and Bronchiolitis in Children

	Asthma	Bronchiolitis
Primary etiologies	Viruses, allergens, exercise, and so on	Respiratory syncytial virus, other viruses
Age of onset	50% by 2 years of age 80% by 5 years of age	<24 months
Recurrent wheezing	Yes (characteristic)	70% (≤2 episodes) 30% progress to asthma (≥3 episodes)
Onset of wheezing	Acute if allergic or exercise-induced	Insidious
Concomitant symptoms of upper respiratory infection	Yes, if infectious	Yes
Family history of allergy and asthma	Frequent	Infrequent in children with ≤2 episodes
Nasal eosinophilia	With allergic rhinitis	Absent
Chest auscultation	If viral, as in bronchiolitis Nonviral: high-pitched expiratory wheezes	Fine, sibilant rales, and coarse inspiratory and expiratory wheezes
Concomitant allergic manifestations	If allergic asthma	Usually absent
IgE level	Elevated (if allergic)	Normal
Response to bronchodilator	Yes (characteristic)	Unresponsive or partially responsive

Associated Symptoms and Signs in the Wheezing Child that are Helpful in Differential Diagnosis

Symptoms and signs	Diseases associated with wheezing	
	In infants	In older children
Positional changes	Anomalies of great vessels, gastroesophageal reflux	Gastroesophageal reflux
Failure to thrive	Cystic fibrosis, tracheoesophageal fistula, bronchopulmonary dysplasia	Cystic fibrosis, chronic hypersensitivity pneumonitis, alpha₁-antitrypsin deficiency, bronchiectasis
Factors associated with feeding	Tracheoesophageal fistula, gastroesophageal reflux	Gastroesophageal reflux
Environmental triggers	Allergic asthma	Allergic asthma, allergic bronchopulmonary aspergillosis, acute hypersensitivity pneumonitis
Sudden onset	Allergic asthma, croup	Allergic asthma, foreign body aspiration, croup, acute hypersensitivity pneumonitis
Fever	Bronchiolitis, pneumonitis	Infectious asthma, acute hypersensitivity pneumonitis, croup
Rhinorrhea	Bronchiolitis, pneumonitis	Infectious or allergic asthma, croup
Concomitant stridor	Tracheal or bronchial stenosis, anomalies of the great vessels, croup	Foreign body aspiration, croup
Clubbing	—	Cystic fibrosis, bronchiectasis, bronchopulmonary dysplasia

croup may be distinguished by their characteristic histories and tendencies to involve the upper airways (see Chapter 22). Lower respiratory infections (pneumonia) generally produce fever and more localized findings of rales, decrease the number of and change the quality of breath sounds, and produce egophony. Left ventricular failure, especially with pulmonary edema, may present with acute respiratory distress and wheezing. A history of cardiac disease, diffuse crackles or basilar rales, and a third heart sound on auscultation help distinguish this condition from asthma. Aspiration of a foreign body with lodgment in the stem bronchus may produce wheezing (Fig. 4-21). A history of a choking episode and physical findings of unilateral wheezing and hyperresonance aid in distinguishing aspiration from asthma but do not confirm the diagnosis. It is important to remember that wheezing resulting from foreign body aspiration may respond at least in part to bronchodilator therapy.

In the older child with mild, infrequent episodes of wheezing that respond to bronchodilator therapy, asthma is readily diagnosed. However, with daily wheezing, frequent exacerbations, lack of response to bronchodilators, or poor growth, other diagnoses must be considered, including chronic obstructive pulmonary disease, cystic fibrosis, alpha₁-antitrypsin deficiency, carcinoid syndrome, and associated immunologic deficiency. Chronic obstructive pulmonary diseases, which include chronic bronchitis, emphysema, bronchiectasis, and bronchopulmonary dysplasia, are distinguished by their lack of significant reversibility with bronchodilator therapy. Cystic fibrosis may present with chronic cough, wheezing, and recurrent infections. In addition, malabsorption with bulky, foul-smelling stools; failure to thrive; and clubbing of the nail beds are common. Alpha₁-antitrypsin deficiency, an inherited autosomal recessive disorder, is characterized by the onset of progressive emphysema in a young adult, and is one cause of neonatal hepatitis.

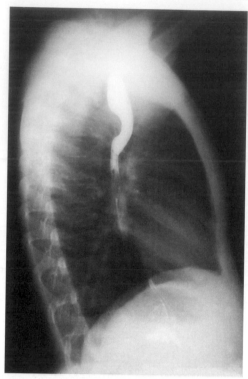

FIG. 4-20 Barium swallow (lateral chest radiograph) shows upper airway compression by a right-sided aortic arch with aberrant left subclavian and diverticulum at the left subclavian origin. Note the round indentation on the posterior wall of the esophagus and the anterior displacement and compression of the trachea, which can cause wheezing and mimic asthma. (Courtesy Beverly Newman, Pittsburgh. From Fireman P, Slavin RG: *Atlas of allergies,* New York, 1990, Gower.)

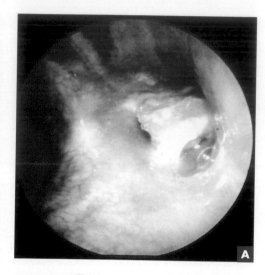

FIG. 4-21 Piece of carrot lodged in the right stem bronchus just below the carina, as visualized during bronchoscopy. Foreign bodies such as this can cause airway obstruction that is partially responsive to bronchodilator therapy. (Courtesy Dr. Sylvan Stool, Pittsburgh. From Fireman P, Slavin RG: *Atlas of allergies,* New York, 1990, Gower.)

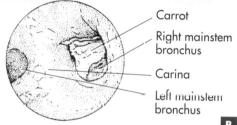

Carrot

Right mainstem bronchus

Carina

Left mainstem bronchus

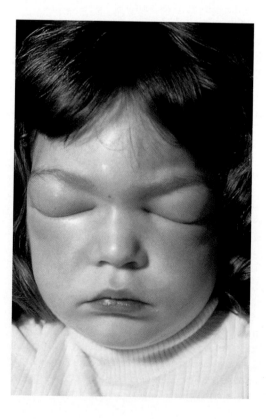

FIG. 4-22 Eyelid angioedema in child with a venom allergy. The onset was explosive after exposure to the bee sting. (From Fireman P, Slavin RG: *Atlas of allergies,* New York, 1990, Gower.)

Ocular Allergy

Ocular allergic reactions may involve the eyelid and/or conjunctiva. The eyelids have a rich blood supply and loose connective tissue. This facilitates edema collection in response to inflammation generated by histamine release in allergic conditions or by trauma. Immediate hypersensitivity reactions that produce eyelid angioedema may be triggered by a vast number of stimuli, including pollens, dusts, insect stings or bites, foods, or drugs. These reactions are characterized by a sudden onset of periorbital edema, pruritus, and erythema after exposure to an allergen (Fig. 4-22). The disorder is distinguished from cellulitis by lack of induration, absence of tenderness and fever, and the fact that involvement is usually bilateral (see Chapter 22).

Allergic conjunctivitis may be acute or chronic and seasonal or perennial, depending on the allergens to which the individual is sensitized. Commonly implicated allergens include weed, tree, and grass pollens; molds; dust; and animal dander. In the acute seasonal form, onset may be explosive and may coincide with the beginning of ragweed pollination. This condition frequently accompanies seasonal allergic rhinitis and commonly is due to ragweed and grass pollen. Itching and excessive tearing are the most prominent symptoms. Pruritus often interferes with sleep, and vision may be impaired by excessive discharge.

Physical findings depend on the degree of chronicity. In the acute form, these findings consist of diffuse bilateral conjunctival edema and

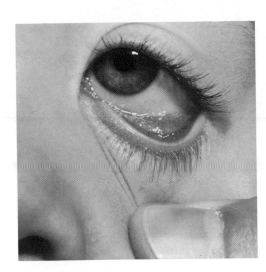

FIG. 4-23 Allergic cobblestoning of the conjunctiva in chronic allergic conjunctivitis. This granular appearance is due to edema and hyperplasia of the papillae.

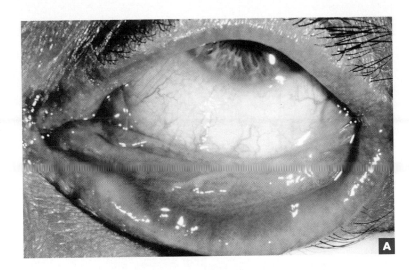

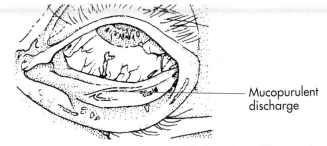

FIG. 4-24 Atopic keratoconjunctivitis with chronic papillary conjunctivitis. Note the stringy mucopurulent discharge often seen in this disorder. (From Fireman P, Slavin RG: *Atlas of allergies,* New York, 1990, Gower.)

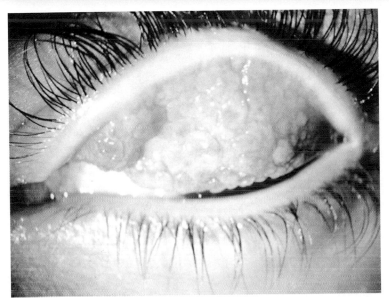

FIG. 4-25 Vernal conjunctivitis, palpebral form. The giant papillary elevations are easily seen without magnification. (From Fireman P, Slavin RG: *Atlas of allergies,* New York, 1990, Gower.)

hyperemia. Photophobia, profuse tearing, and mild lid swelling are commonly associated. In the chronic form, the conjunctivae appear pale, with mild edema and hyperplasia of the papillae. This may result in a fine, granular appearance of the conjunctivae, which is termed *allergic cobblestoning* (Fig. 4-23). Prominent cobblestoning is seen in vernal conjunctivitis. The clinical diagnosis may be confirmed by finding eosinophilia on a smear of conjunctival secretions and skin testing for the suspected allergens.

The differential diagnosis of allergic conjunctivitis includes atopic conjunctivitis, atopic keratoconjunctivitis, and vernal conjunctivitis. Individuals with atopic conjunctivitis have a history of asthma, allergic conjunctivitis, or infantile eczema. Serum IgE levels are elevated during the active phase of the disease, but there is no seasonal variation in severity. The disease usually begins in the late teens, and many patients experience a remission during adulthood. The eyelids manifest a thickened, lichenified, red, exudative or dry rash.

Atopic keratoconjunctivitis occurs in patients with atopic dermatitis and is characterized by erythema and thickening of the conjunctivae (Fig. 4-24). This may progress to scarring and vascularization of the cornea in severe cases. Ocular disease activity parallels that of cutaneous disease.

Vernal conjunctivitis is uncommon and chronic in nature. Its typical occurrence during the spring and summer is suggestive of an allergic etiology, but this is unproved. Young, atopic boys are affected most frequently. Symptoms include severe itching, photophobia, blurring of vision, and lacrimation. Physical examination reveals white, ropy secretions containing many eosinophils. A palpebral form manifests hypertrophic nodular papillae that resemble cobblestones on the upper eyelids (Fig. 4-25). The papillae consist of dense fibrous tissue with eosinophilic infiltrates. In the bulbar form, nodules appear as gelatinous masses called *Trantas dots,* usually found at the corneoscleral junction (Fig. 4-26). This disease usually remits with maturity and is rarely seen in adults. Giant papillary conjunctivitis, which appears clinically and histologically to be a mild form of vernal conjunctivitis, is associated with the use of hard and soft contact lenses (Fig. 4-27). The stimulus is believed to be foreign material that accumulates on the surface of the contact lenses. Whether this material is antigenic and the condition an immune-mediated disease is not known.

Urticaria and Angioedema

Hypersensitivity reactions in which the skin is the major target organ are manifested clinically as diffuse erythema, urticaria, or an-

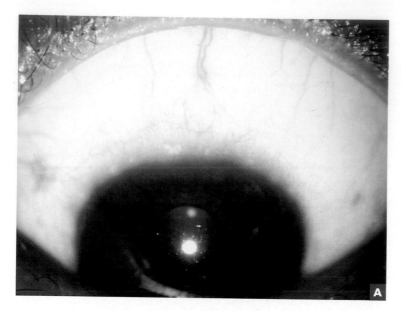

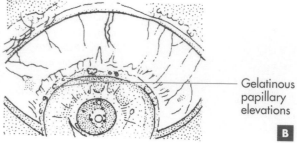

FIG. 4-26   Vernal conjunctivitis, limbal form. Note the gelatinous papillary elevations of the limbal tissue. (From Fireman P, Slavin RG: *Atlas of allergies,* New York, 1990, Gower.)

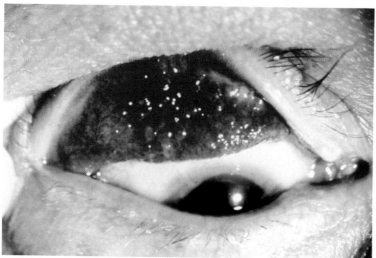

FIG. 4-27   Characteristic lesions of giant papillary conjunctivitis. These hobnail-like elevations of the upper tarsal conjunctiva, evident on eversion of the upper eyelid, occur when the upper lid meets a foreign body such as a contact lens, prosthesis, or exposed suture. (From Fireman P, Slavin RG: *Atlas of allergies,* New York, 1990, Gower.)

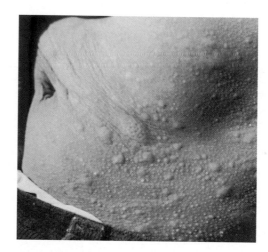

FIG. 4-28   Urticarial lesions. Note the well-demarcated borders, redness, elevation, and occasional confluence of the palpable lesions. (Courtesy Dr. Michael Sherlock.)

gioedema. Type I hypersensitivity to inhalants, foods, insect venoms, and drugs is the most common mechanism, but urticaria and angioedema may also accompany type II (transfusion reaction) or type III reactions (cutaneous vasculitis, serum sickness). These disorders result from increased vascular permeability. The resultant edema collects in the dermis in urticaria and primarily in the subcutaneous tissues in angioedema. Although frequently seen in combination, urticaria and angioedema may also appear individually. Urticaria is most frequently an acute disorder that resolves spontaneously. When the duration of recurrences exceeds 6 weeks, the condition is arbitrarily termed *chronic urticaria.* In contrast to acute urticaria, extensive evaluations frequently do not reveal the causes of chronic urticaria.

Urticarial lesions are well-circumscribed, raised, palpable wheals that blanch with applied pressure (Fig. 4-28). They are usually erythematous but may be pale or white with red halos. Typically, the lesions are intensely pruritic; however, in some instances the pruritus is mild. Angioedema is characterized by diffuse subcutaneous tissue swelling with

normal or erythematous overlying skin. Itching is usually intense. The face, hands, feet, and perineum are most commonly involved (Fig. 4-29).

Skin involvement may be generalized or localized to body parts exposed to a provoking stimulus. Careful history taking concerning recent exposures and medications is often rewarding. In cases with associated fever and respiratory and/or gastrointestinal symptoms, infectious diseases resulting from viruses (including enterovirus, hepatitis B virus, and Epstein-Barr virus), group A beta-hemolytic streptococcus, and helminth infestation should be considered. Generalized urticaria with or without angioedema may also be the initial manifestation of erythema multiforme or Henoch-Schönlein purpura. Thus in cases in which a specific etiology is unclear, parents should be informed of the possible evolution and instructed regarding observation of signs and symptoms.

Urticaria associated with serum sickness is due to a necrotizing vasculitis involving small venules. Histamine release associated with IgE-dependent reactions and complement activation may contribute to the

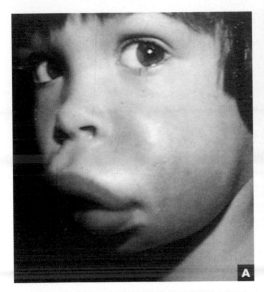
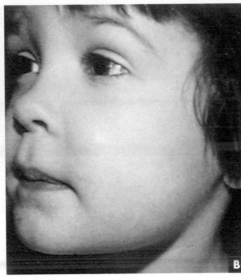

FIG. 4-29 Angioedema involving the lips. *A,* Onset was sudden. *B,* Resolution was complete within 24 hours.

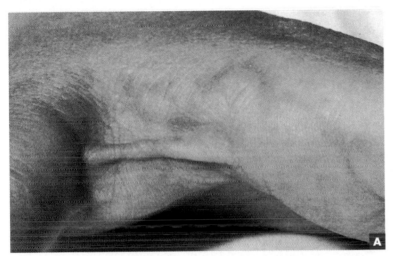
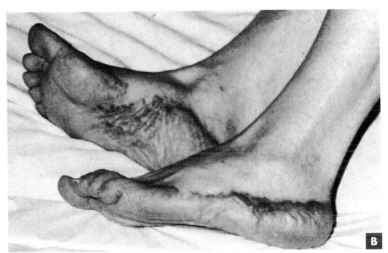

FIG. 4-30 Cutaneous eruptions on the sides of the hands and feet of patients with serum sickness. *A,* The finger web of a patient is shown in the early stages of serum sickness; a scalloped band of erythema can be seen on the side of the finger at the margin of palmar skin. *B,* The feet of a thrombocytopenic patient are shown at the clinical peak of serum sickness. At the margin of plantar skin is a band of purpura. The purpura was preceded by a band of erythema. (From Lawley TJ, Bielory L, Gascon P, et al: Prospective clinical and immunologic analysis of patients with serum sickness, *N Engl J Med* 311:1407–1413, 1984.)

pathophysiologic manifestations of this form of urticaria. Typically, type I hypersensitivity produces intense pruritus, whereas type II and III hypersensitivity reactions may be associated with a burning sensation. In addition to urticarial lesions, patients with serum sickness may present with fever, malaise, arthralgias, gastrointestinal disturbances, and lymphadenopathy. These patients also may have characteristic serpiginous erythematous and purpuric eruptions on the hands and feet at the junction of the palmar and plantar skin (Fig. 4-30), which is considered a cutaneous marker for the disease. The most common cause of serum sickness is a hypersensitivity reaction to drugs. Erythema multiforme, a cutaneous hypersensitivity disorder, also can be caused by drugs and involves the surfaces of the palms and soles and at times the mucosal surfaces (Stevens-Johnson syndrome). The cutaneous lesions associated with erythema multiforme can be distinguished from those related to serum sickness by their symmetric distribution and by the characteristic appearance of the initial lesion. This lesion is a dusky red macule or erythematous wheal that evolves into an iris or target lesion, which is the hallmark of erythema multiforme (see Chapter 8).

A subgroup of urticarial disorders results from hypersensitivity to

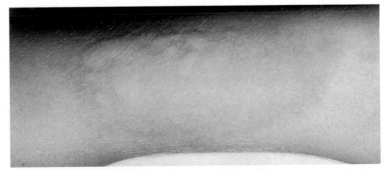

FIG. 4-31 Positive ice-cube test in child with cold urticaria. An ice cube placed on the arm for 10 minutes results in urticaria of the exposed skin. Onset is usually immediate but may be delayed for up to 4 hours after cold exposure.

physical and mechanical factors. These include cold urticaria, pressure-induced urticaria and angioedema, aquagenic and solar urticaria, and exercise-induced urticaria. The history and distribution of lesions often help in identifying the source, which can then be confirmed by challenge (Fig. 4-31).

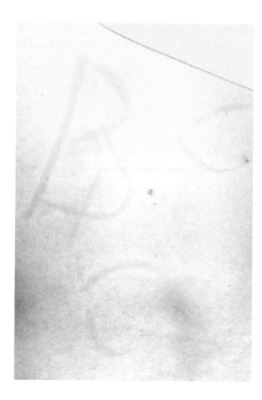

FIG. 4-32 Dermographism or writing on the skin is the most common type of urticaria induced by physical or mechanical factors. Firm stroking of the skin with a fingernail or tongue blade results in urticaria of the traumatized skin.

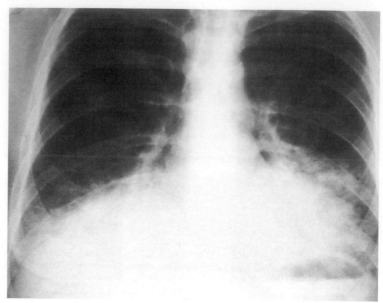

FIG. 4-33 Chest radiograph of patient with acute hypersensitivity pneumonitis. Note the soft, patchy coalescent infiltrates in both lower lung fields.

Dermographism, translated literally as the "ability to write on the skin" (Fig. 4-32), is a form of trauma-induced pressure urticaria. It is elicited by stroking the skin with a fingernail or tongue blade. The initial white line secondary to reflex vasoconstriction is supplanted by pruritic, erythematous linear swelling, as seen in a classic wheal and flare reaction. The condition is chronic and the etiology unclear. Patients with dermographism suspected of having an atopic disorder cannot be skin tested for specific IgE antibody because all tests appear positive.

Type III Disorders

Hypersensitivity Pneumonitis

Although IgE-mediated allergic respiratory diseases (allergic rhinitis, asthma) are the most common manifestations of inhalant sensitivities in humans, other immunologic respiratory diseases, involving non-IgE immune mechanisms, may result from the inhalation of antigens from the susceptible individual's environment. A wide variety of inhaled biologic dusts may induce an inflammatory lung disease involving the interstitium, alveoli, and airways. The most common form of hypersensitivity pneumonitis is caused by inhalation of thermophilic actinomycetes (*Micropolyspora faeni),* antigens present in moldy vegetable compost, and is termed *farmer's lung.* Other forms (and their causative dusts and antigens) include malt-worker's lung (moldy malt, *Aspergillus* species) and bird-breeder's lung (avian dust, avian proteins). The disorder is termed *hypersensitivity pneumonitis* or *extrinsic allergic alveolitis* and appears to be immune-complex mediated.

Hypersensitivity pneumonitis is a syndrome with a broad spectrum of presenting symptoms and signs. The clinical features depend on the following factors: (1) the nature of the inhaled dust, (2) the intensity and frequency of inhalation exposure, and (3) the immunologic responsiveness of the exposed individual. A concomitant upper respiratory infection or another pulmonary insult may be an important factor in induction. Development of sensitization to the inhaled organic dust requires several months to years.

In the acute form, systemic and respiratory symptoms usually develop explosively within 4 to 6 hours of exposure. These consist of cough, dyspnea, fever as high as 104° F, chills, myalgia, and malaise.

Symptoms may persist up to 18 hours, subside spontaneously, and recur with each subsequent exposure. During such attacks, the patient appears acutely ill and dyspneic on physical examination. On chest auscultation, bibasilar end-inspiratory rales may be noted, and these may persist for weeks after the episode subsides. Chronic disease results from mild, continuous exposure. Progressive dyspnea, decreased exercise tolerance, productive cough, anorexia, and weight loss develop insidiously. Episodes of chills and fever are less common than in the acute form. Physical findings in these patients include wheezing, cyanosis, and clubbing. Evidence of cor pulmonale develops as pulmonary inflammation and fibrosis progress.

Chest radiographs may show normal structures if attacks are widely spaced but more commonly show the characteristic findings of fine, sharp nodulations; reticulation; and coarsening of bronchovascular markings. During an attack, soft, patchy, ill-defined parenchymal densities that tend to coalesce may be seen bilaterally (Fig. 4-33). Diffuse fibrosis with parenchymal contraction or honeycombing is a sign of end-stage disease. Pulmonary function tests reveal restrictive lung disease, especially in the chronic form, and challenge with the offending antigen may result in an immediate and a delayed response.

The differential diagnosis of hypersensitivity pneumonitis should include other conditions that cause interstitial lung disease and intermittent, explosive, and progressive pulmonary and systemic symptoms (drug-induced lung disease, recurrent pneumonias, allergic bronchopulmonary aspergillosis, sarcoidosis, collagen vascular diseases). Environmental and immunologic studies, along with close observation of the patient during periods of exposure and avoidance, are useful in diagnosing this disorder. Environmental studies can include a history and collection of antigenic materials, and immunologic studies include tests for serum IgG precipitins to thermophilic actinomycetes, *Aspergillus* species, or avian protein.

Allergic Bronchopulmonary Aspergillosis

Aspergillus species, in addition to being one cause of hypersensitivity pneumonitis and allergic asthma, cause a disorder termed *allergic bronchopulmonary aspergillosis.* This entity is characterized by migrating pulmonary infiltrates and peripheral blood and sputum eosinophilia.

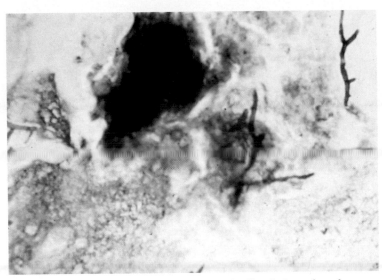

FIG. 4-34 Sputum smear from patient with allergic bronchopulmonary aspergillosis. Note the fungal mycelia characteristic of this disorder. (From Slavin RG, Laird TS, Cherry JD: Allergic bronchopulmonary aspergillosis in a child, *J Pediatr* 76:416-421, 1970.)

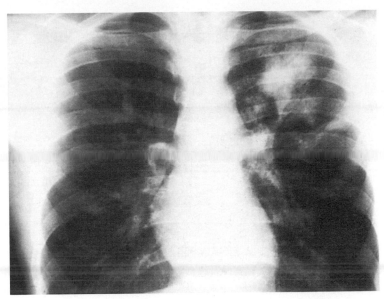

FIG. 4-35 Chest radiograph of patient with allergic bronchopulmonary aspergillosis. These patients are frequently asymptomatic despite extensive areas of consolidation. (Courtesy Dr. Raymond G. Slavin, St Louis.)

Type I and type III hypersensitivity are thought to be involved in the pathogenesis. Affected individuals are usually atopic and have a history of asthma. They present with anorexia, headache, generalized myalgias, loss of energy, temperature elevation, and acute episodes of wheezing and dyspnea. Sputum production is prominent, and parents often report that their child's cough is productive of solid mucoid lumps of different sizes, shapes, and colors, ranging from dirty green to brown or beige. Physical findings include the general signs of lower airway obstruction (see section on asthma). On auscultation, crepitant rales are frequently heard over areas of pulmonary consolidation.

Laboratory studies that assist in diagnosis include the following:

1. Direct examination of sputum plugs reveals fungal mycelia (Fig. 4-34) and large numbers of eosinophils in most patients. Cultures are not considered diagnostic because they may be negative during episodes of pulmonary consolidation and positive at other times.
2. Peripheral blood examination reveals eosinophilia (generally greater than 1000/mm³).
3. The serum IgE level (*A. fumigatus* specific and nonspecific) is markedly elevated and may be as high as 78,000 ng/ml.
4. Even though a positive immediate wheal and flare reaction to *A. fumigatus* is not considered diagnostic of allergic bronchopulmonary aspergillosis, a negative reaction during skin testing makes the diagnosis unlikely. Most patients also experience a secondary skin reaction (Arthus-type) at the injection site, first noted at 3 to 4 hours. This reaction consists of erythema and poorly defined edema, reaching a peak at 8 hours and resolving by 24 hours.
5. The serum precipitating antibody (IgG) to *A. fumigatus* is found in most patients, but the titer has a poor correlation with disease activity and intensity of the clinical picture.
6. Chest radiography commonly shows a massive homogeneous consolidation without fissure displacement. The upper lobes are commonly involved, and infiltrates characteristically shift rapidly from one site to the other. Remarkably, radiographic findings do not correlate well with clinical severity, and patients with extensive consolidation may be asymptomatic (Fig. 4-35).

7. Bronchography reveals the distinctive findings in allergic bronchopulmonary aspergillosis. These include saccular bronchiectasis of the proximal bronchi with normal filling of distal ones, in distinct contrast to usual forms of bronchiectasis.

Allergic bronchopulmonary aspergillosis is being recognized with greater frequency as awareness increases. The diagnosis requires a high index of suspicion and should be considered in any asthmatic person who has pulmonary infiltrates or suddenly uncontrollable disease. Allergic bronchopulmonary aspergillosis and hypersensitivity pneumonitis are frequently confused. Early diagnosis and corticosteroid treatment are necessary to prevent progression to severe, irreversible, end-stage lung disease.

Immunologic Deficiency Disorders

Normal Development of the Immune System

The integrity of the immune system is essential to maintaining appropriate host defense mechanisms, which consist of humoral antibody, cell-mediated immunity, phagocytic, and complement systems. Defects of one or more of these host defense mechanisms result in immunodeficiency disorders, many of which are familial with a potential molecular genetic defect. In addition, skin and mucosal surface abnormalities may result in the breakdown of the physical barriers that ordinarily prevent the invasion of microorganisms.

Cellular and humoral immunity depends on the maturation of two distinct lymphoid cell lines, the T- and B-lymphocytes, both originating from a common bone marrow stem cell. T- and B-lymphocytes undergo a complex series of maturational changes before arriving at a stage at which they are capable of antigen-stimulated differentiation (Fig. 4-36). The thymus-dependent T-lymphocytes are responsible for cell-mediated immune responses directed against viruses, fungi, or less common pathogens, such as *Pneumocystis carinii*. Other functions of T-lymphocytes include graft rejection and tumor cytotoxicity. Subpopulations of T lymphocytes also collaborate in immunoregulation by the expression of helper and suppressor functional activities. On the other hand, the thymus-independent B-lymphocytes are precursors of plasma cells. Plasma cells

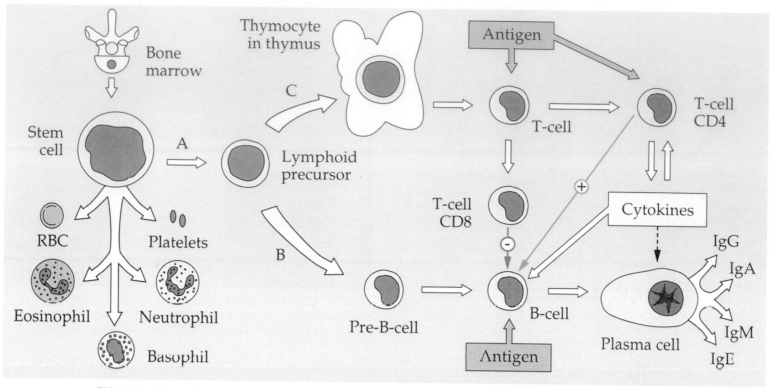

FIG. 4-36   Schematic representation of T- and B-lymphocyte ontogeny. Defects along pathway A result in combined immunodeficiencies. Pathway B is responsible for normal antibody production, whereas normal cell-mediated immunity requires the integrity of pathway C. Cytokines are soluble products of activated lymphocytes and include interleukins and interferons.

TABLE 4-10	
Indications for Immunodeficiency Evaluation	
Family history	Positive for early unexplained death, sepsis, recurrent infections, or specific immunodeficiency diagnosis
Frequency of infection	Elevated (>8 upper respiratory infections per year, >2 episodes of pneumonia per year)
Chronicity of infection	Persistent sinusitis and otitis media, bronchiectasis, recurrent abcesses
Severity of infection	Severe systemic sepsis or meningitis
Complication of infection	Present (e.g., mastoiditis complicating otitis media)
Site of infection	Multiple, not single, sites
Infecting organism	Opportunistic or recurrent
Response to therapy	Poor or recurring after antimicrobial discontinuation
Other signs	Failure to thrive, dermatitis, recurrent diarrhea

produce the various classes of immunoglobulins that serve as functional antibodies for antigen recognition. Deficiencies of one or more of the immunoglobulin classes (IgG, IgA, IgM) constitute humoral or serum antibody immunodeficiency. Despite having normal numbers of B-lymphocytes and plasma cells and normal serum immunoglobulin levels, some patients are nonetheless immunodeficient because they lack functional antibodies. Many of the immunodeficiency disorders described in later sections result from an arrest in cell maturation or a defect in the im-

munoregulatory cell interactions necessary for antigen recognition. Abnormalities in the maturation of T- or B-lymphocytes result in humoral or cellular immunodeficiency, respectively. Abnormalities in the maturation of both cell lines result in combined immunodeficiency.

Abnormal Function of the Immune System: Suspicion and Evaluation

Deficiencies of the immune system can involve lymphocytes (humoral and/or cellular immunodeficiency), phagocytes (chronic granulomatous disease), the complement system (hereditary angioedema), and the mucosal barrier (immotile cilia syndrome). Humoral (antibody) deficiency disorders are characterized by recurrent infections with high-grade extracellular encapsulated bacterial pathogens and chronic sinopulmonary infections. In contrast, cellular deficiencies are manifested by recurrent infections with low-grade or opportunistic infectious agents such as fungi, viruses, or *P. carinii* and are associated with growth retardation, wasting, and diarrhea. These patients are susceptible to graft-versus-host disease if given fresh blood and can have fatal reactions from live virus vaccination.

Other immune deficiencies, such as mucosal barrier defects, may present in a more subtle fashion, with few life-threatening infections and normal growth. Thus the clinician frequently is confronted with the question of whether a patient should be evaluated for immunodeficiency. In general, children with infections that are frequent, are recurrent or chronic, and are caused by unusual organisms or respond poorly to therapy should be evaluated for immunodeficiency. Moreover, growth retardation or a family history of early death should raise the clinician's level of suspicion (Table 4-10). In the screening for immunodeficiency, quantitative and functional aspects of the components of

TABLE 4-11

Suggested Laboratory Screening Tests for Children With Suspected Immunodeficiency

Immune system component	Example of immunodeficiency	Screening tests
B-lymphocyte	Bruton agamma-globulinemia	Quantitative immunoglobulin serum levels (IgG, IgA, IgM) Serum antibodies to tetanus, polio, *Haemophilus influenzae* B, other vaccine antigens
T-lymphocyte	DiGeorge syndrome	Total lymphocyte count Delayed hypersensitivity skin tests (*Candida*, tetanus, mumps)
Phagocyte	Chronic granulomatous disease	Total neutrophil count NBT reduction test
Complement	C3 deficiency	C3 and C4 complement serum levels CH_{50} (hemolytic complement)

TABLE 4-12

Chromosomal Map Locations of Primary Immunodeficiency Disorders

	Chromosome	Locus
X-linked SCID	X	q13.1-13.3
X-linked agammaglobulinemia	X	q21.3-22
Immunodeficiency with hyper-IgM	X	q24-27
Wiscott-Aldrich syndrome	X	p11.22-11.3
ADA deficiency	20	q13.11
PNP deficiency	14	q13.1
DiGeorge syndrome	22	q11.2(10p)
Ataxia-telangiectasia	11	22-23
Leukocyte adhesion deficiency	21	q22.3

From Fireman P, ed: *Atlas of allergies,* ed 2, London, 1996, Times-Mirror.

the immune system are considered. A simple office evaluation for immunodeficiency should include quantitation of serum IgG, IgA, and IgM and specific functional antibody titers to tetanus (or other antigens) for the evaluation of humoral immunity; delayed hypersensitivity skin testing for cellular immunity; a nitroblue tetrazolium (NBT) test for phagocyte function; and levels of C3, C4, and total hemolytic complement for evaluation of complement component quantity and function. These screening tests can be performed in most laboratories and can identify severe immunodeficiency disorders (Table 4-11).

Pathogenesis

The immunodeficiency diseases make up a group of illnesses that are heterogeneous not only in their clinical and immune expression but also in their basic pathophysiologic mechanisms. The faulty genes in some of the inherited immunodeficiencies have been localized to specific sites on the X chromosome. These include X-linked hypogammaglobulinemia (Bruton agammaglobulinemia), X-linked immunodeficiency with hyper-IgM, Wiskott-Aldrich syndrome, X-linked severe combined immunodeficiency disease (SCID), X-linked lymphoproliferative syndrome (Duncan syndrome), properdin deficiency, and chronic granulomatous disease. The abnormal gene in DiGeorge syndrome has been localized to chromosome 22, the faulty gene for adenosine deaminase (ADA) deficiency SCID to chromosome 20, the gene for purine-nucleoside phosphorylase (PNP) deficiency to chromosome 14, the gene for ataxia-telangiectasia to chromosome 11, and that for leukocyte adhesion deficiency to chromosome 21 (Table 4-12).

Recent advances in molecular biology have helped identify the primary biologic defect in a small but growing number of these inherited deficiencies, which can be designated as inborn errors of the immune system. In X-linked hypogammaglobulinemia, there is an intrinsic defect of pre–B-lymphocyte to B-lymphocyte differentiation because of a defect of B-lymphocyte–specific tyrosine kinase (btk). In X-linked SCID a point mutation of the alpha subunit of the interleukin-2 receptor leads to defective development of T- and B-lymphocytes. Defective synthesis of the CD40 ligand required for the immunoglobulin isotype switch from IgM to IgG synthesis has been found in patients with X-linked immunodeficiency with hyper-IgM. In leukocyte adhesion deficiency, there is an abnormal beta chain subunit of CD18, which results in deficiency of the adhesion protein leukocyte function–associated antigen and several complement receptors (CR3).

In patients with ADA deficiency and SCID, the T- and B-lymphocyte deficiency is due to the toxic metabolites that build up from the interruption of purine catabolism because of the enzyme deficiency. ADA catalyzes the conversion of adenosine to inosine and deoxyadenosine to deoxyinosine, and in its absence, there is excessive deoxyadenosine, which inhibits synthesis of deoxyribonucleic acid (DNA). A similar situation exists in patients with PNP deficiency. PNP catalyzes the conversion of inosine to hypoxanthine and of deoxyguanosine to guanine, the step in purine metabolism beyond that catalyzed by ADA. The excessive deoxyguanosine also inhibits DNA synthesis. It has been postulated that there is greater T- and B-lymphocyte immunodeficiency with ADA deficiency than PNP deficiency because resting T-lymphocytes are destroyed by deoxyadenosine, whereas only dividing T-lymphocytes are killed by deoxyguanosine. It is anticipated that additional biologic defects in the other immune deficiencies will be identified as the tools of molecular biology are further refined.

Humoral Immunodeficiency (B-Lymphocyte)

Congenital Hypogammaglobulinemia

Congenital hypogammaglobulinemia may be X-linked (Bruton) or autosomal-recessive. Affected infants are clinically well for the first few months of life because of placentally acquired maternal antibodies but

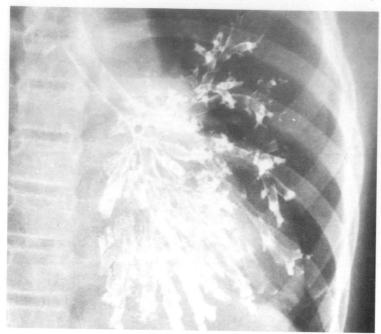

FIG. 4-37 Bronchogram reveals bronchiectasis of the left lower lobe in an older child with hypogammaglobulinemia. Symptoms consisted of chronic cough and sputum production.

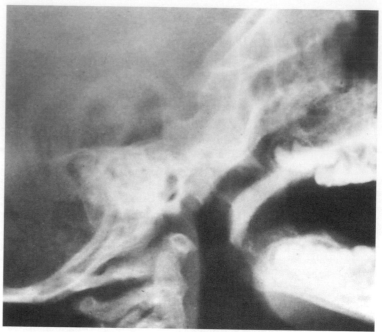

FIG. 4-38 Lateral neck radiograph shows absent adenoids in patient with congenital hypogammaglobulinemia.

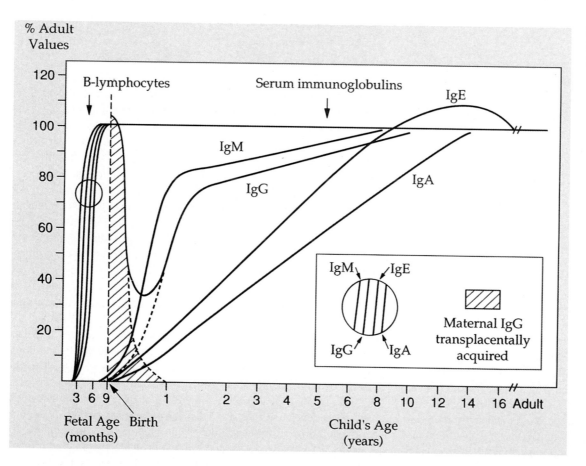

FIG. 4-39 Ontogeny of serum immunoglobulin levels before and after birth.

subsequently develop recurrent or chronic infections with virulent bacterial pathogens such as gram-positive cocci and *H. influenzae.* The infections may localize in the upper and lower respiratory tracts, resulting in sinusitis, otitis media, and pneumonia. Sepsis, meningitis, and skin infections are also common. One of the complications of the chronic lower respiratory infections to which they are predisposed is bronchiectasis. This is characterized clinically by chronic cough with increased sputum production and by abnormal chest radiographs (Fig. 4-37). In the absence of chronic lung disease, growth is usually unimpaired, and survival to adulthood is common with appropriate gammaglobulin and antibiotic therapy.

The physical findings are those of localized infection, with specific signs depending on the particular structures infected. In addition, these children frequently manifest a paucity of adenoidal, tonsillar, and other

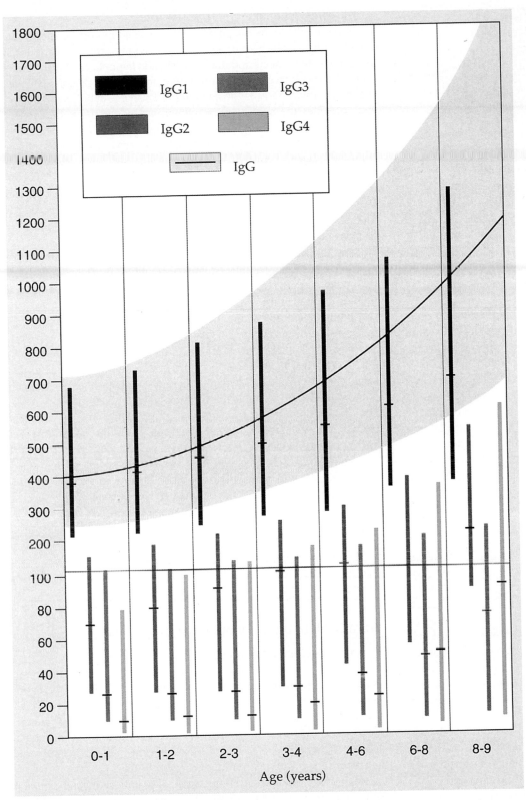

FIG. 4-40 Age-related normal values for serum IgG and IgG subclasses. (From Smith TF: Immunodeficiency in chronic pediatric respiratory illness, *Hosp Pract* 21(8):145, 1986.)

lymphoid tissues (Fig. 4-38). The diagnosis of hypogammaglobulinemia should be considered in any child who has recurrent infections with virulent bacterial pathogens and is confirmed by finding markedly decreased levels of the immunoglobulin classes (IgG, IgA, IgM) in the serum.

Transient Hypogammaglobulinemia of Infancy

As shown in Fig. 4-39, term infants are born with high levels of serum IgG because of active placental transport of maternal IgG. The serum IgG level normally declines during the first 7 months of life while the infant progressively attains the ability to actively synthesize IgG. The diagnosis of transient hypogammaglobulinemia is applied to in-

fants in whom the low serum IgG concentration observed during the first 7 months of life is prolonged. Serum IgG levels in these infants usually attain age-appropriate values by 18 to 24 months. Despite the low levels of serum IgG, these infants can synthesize specific antibodies to tetanus and other antigens. Gamma-globulin replacement therapy is generally not indicated for this condition.

IgG Subclass Deficiency

Serum IgG immunoglobulin comprises four subclasses termed IgG1, IgG2, IgG3, and IgG4. Normal serum values for each are age related (Fig. 4-40). IgG1 is the most plentiful of the subclasses and is considered the subclass that responds immunologically to foreign protein anti-

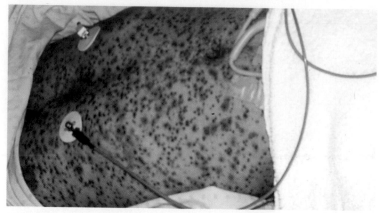

FIG. 4-41 Adolescent with abnormal T-lymphocyte function and disseminated varicella, in whom pneumonia resulted in respiratory failure.

gens such as tetanus toxoid. Conversely, polysaccharide antigens of the encapsulated *H. influenzae* or pneumococcus are considered to stimulate antibody synthesis predominantly in the IgG2 subclass. The specific antibody functions of IgG3 and IgG4 are not well defined.

Some clinical immunologists have defined a role for quantitation of IgG subclasses in the evaluation of immunodeficiency. IgG subclass deficiency is defined by a low IgG subclass concentration but must be combined with a deficient functional antibody response of that subclass. These patients usually present with a history of chronic sinopulmonary infections but have a normal growth pattern. Gamma-globulin replacement therapy along with appropriate antibiotics is indicated in this condition.

Selective IgA Deficiency

Selective IgA deficiency, which affects 1:500 to 1:700 of the population, is the most common humoral antibody deficiency. Even though these patients are deficient in mucosal secretory IgA, only half of affected individuals manifest symptoms. Synthesis of IgG and IgM is usually normal. Most cases are sporadic, but siblings with IgA or other immunodeficiencies have been frequently reported.

IgA deficiency has been associated with a variety of clinical syndromes. Chronic infections of the sinuses and middle ear are common, but severe or recurrent lower respiratory disease is unusual unless another form of immunodeficiency coexists with the IgA deficiency. Individuals with selective IgA deficiency may have severe malabsorption manifesting as chronic diarrhea and have an increased incidence of autoimmune syndromes (collagen vascular disease) and of atopy. Therefore the patient with a history of recurrent upper respiratory or sinopulmonary infections, malabsorption, or arthritis should be investigated for serum IgA deficiency. There is no replacement IgA therapy.

Cellular (T-Lymphocyte) Immunodeficiency

Isolated defects of T-lymphocyte, or cell-mediated, immunity are rare. Since normal T-lymphocyte function is necessary for regulation of antibody production, many cellular immunodeficiencies are also associated with humoral immunodeficiencies. Patients with T-lymphocyte deficiencies experience an increased frequency of severe infections with viral agents such as herpes simplex and cytomegalovirus, certain fungi, intracellular parasites, and other organisms of relatively low virulence. PNP deficiency is a rare syndrome associated with defective T-lymphocyte function. Fig. 4-41 demonstrates a severe disseminated varicella infection in a child with congenital cellular immunodeficiency.

DiGeorge Syndrome

DiGeorge syndrome is a pure T-lymphocyte immunodeficiency disorder characterized by absent T-lymphocytes with normal or near-normal B-lymphocyte numbers and function. Thymic hypoplasia, which results from abnormal development of the third and fourth branchial pouches during embryogenesis, is the hallmark of DiGeorge syndrome. The thymus provides the necessary microenvironment for the maturation of lymphoid precursors into functioning T-lymphocytes. When the thymus is absent, this normal maturation does not proceed, resulting in cellular immunodeficiency. Since major cardiovascular structures and the parathyroid glands are derived from the same branchial pouches, affected children frequently present with signs of congenital heart disease and hypocalcemic tetany or seizures within the first few days of life. Associated abnormalities include unusual facies (Fig. 4-42), esophageal atresia, and hypothyroidism.

Even though the T-lymphocyte defect may be transient and resolve spontaneously, many of these infants succumb to overwhelming infections with bacteria, viruses, and fungi unless reconstituted with fetal thymus or bone marrow transplantation.

Chronic mucocutaneous candidiasis is a T-lymphocyte disorder typified by superficial candidal infections of the mucous membranes, skin, and nails. This illness may be sporadic or familial. The disorder is often associated with an endocrinopathic condition, and variants of this syndrome may include hypoparathyroidism, hyperthyroidism, and polyendocrinopathy. Candidal infections typically begin in early childhood but may be delayed for up to 20 years. Other manifestations of chronic mucocutaneous candidiasis result from the associated endocrinopathic conditions, of which hypoparathyroidism is the most common. Abnormalities of the immune system include absent cutaneous delayed hypersensitivity to *Candida* organisms and lack of lymphokine production by *Candida*-stimulated lymphocytes. Other mechanisms of host defense, including immunoglobulins, are normal. Treatment of chronic mucocutaneous candidiasis involves long-term antifungal therapy. Local application of nystatin and clotrimazole may prevent progression but is rarely curative. Ketaconazole given orally has resulted in dramatic clinical improvement and decreased morbidity in affected patients.

Combined T- and B-Lymphocyte Disorders

Severe Combined Immunodeficiency Disorders

SCID is a heterogeneous group of disorders with varying etiologies. The consequent defects in stem cell maturation ultimately result in abnormalities of humoral and cellular immunity (Fig. 4-36). Inherited deficiency of the enzyme ADA is also associated with combined immunodeficiency. The mechanism involves the accumulation of metabolic substrates that are toxic to T- and B-lymphocytes. ADA deficiency may be responsible for up to 25% of all cases of SCID.

Having deficiencies of cell-mediated (T-lymphocyte) and humoral (B-lymphocyte) immunity, these infants have recurrent severe bacterial, viral, fungal, and protozoal infections. Manifestations typically appear in the first few months of life and are often associated with failure to thrive, diarrhea, and candidiasis (Fig. 4-43). Affected infants may be distinguished from normal babies by the frequency and severity of infections and their recalcitrance to appropriate antimicrobial therapy. Presenting symptoms usually involve the respiratory tract, since pneumonia resulting from *P. carinii* or virulent bacterial pathogens is common. In addition to the clinical findings of infection, examination discloses hypoplastic or absent tonsils and lymph nodes. Laboratory abnormalities include peripheral blood lymphopenia; decreased serum IgG, IgA, and IgM levels; and defective lymphocyte responses to mitogens such as phytohemagglutinin. Histologic examination of tonsillar,

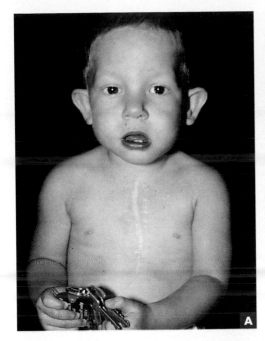

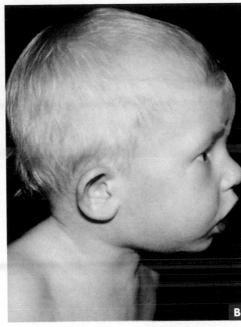

FIG. 4-42 Characteristic facial features of a child with DiGeorge syndrome, frontal *(A)* and lateral *(B)* views. Note the micrognathia; hypertelorism; low-set, malformed ears; and midline sternotomy scar after repair of a congenital heart defect.

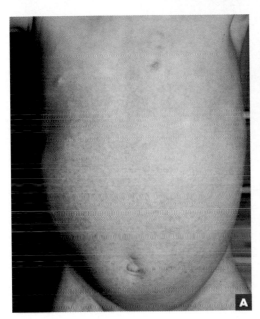

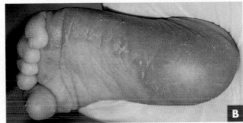

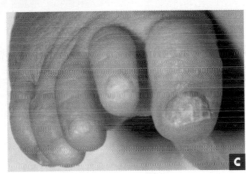

FIG. 4-43 Widespread fungal dermatitis with *C. albicans* over the trunk *(A)* and foot *(B)* of child with SCID. Note the dystrophic changes of the nails secondary to chronic infection *(C)*. Normal immune surveillance usually prevents persistent infection with this ubiquitous organism.

adenoidal, and lymph node remnants reveals immature lymphoid tissue. The thymus is typically dysplastic histologically and radiographically (Fig. 4-44); normal lobulation and corticomedullary differentiation are lacking, and the number of lymphocytes is decreased.

Once the diagnosis of SCID is considered, the child must be placed in protective isolation and given appropriate supportive therapy, including intravenous gamma-globulin. All administered blood products must be irradiated to prevent the potential development of severe graft-versus-host disease. These patients can be successfully immunologically reconstituted with bone marrow transplants. SCID patients with ADA deficiency have been the initial recipients of gene therapy, and the long-term results are eagerly awaited.

Partial Combined Immunodeficiency Disorders

Congenital Disorders. Wiskott-Aldrich syndrome is an X-linked recessive disorder characterized by eczema, thrombocytopenia with cutaneous petechiae, and recurrent infections that begin in infancy (Fig. 4-45). The immunodeficiency may result in infectious complications later in life. Inability to form antibody to bacterial capsular polysaccharide antigens is the most commonly reported immunologic defect, but some patients also manifest a partial defect in T-lymphocyte responses.

Ataxia telangiectasia is a complex and intriguing immunodeficiency disorder with autosomal-recessive inheritance. The pathogenesis is unclear, since no theory has been developed to explain the hallmark multisystem involvement characteristic of this disorder: telangiectasia, pro-

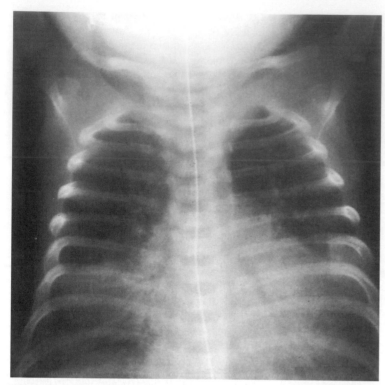

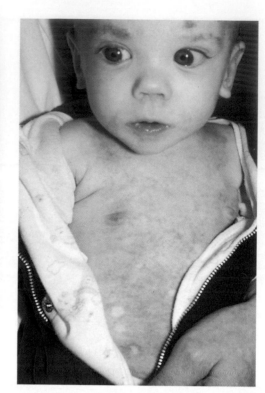

FIG. 4-45 Child with Wiskott-Aldrich syndrome. The skin eruptions on the trunk and face are eczematoid and pruritic but not always similar to atopic dermatitis in flexural distribution. Many of these patients have thrombocytopenia that results in petechiae of varying distribution and intensity. (From Fireman P, Slavin RG: *Atlas of allergies,* New York, 1990, Gower.)

FIG. 4-44 Chest radiograph of infant with SCID. Note the absent thymic shadow and bilateral pulmonary infiltrates.

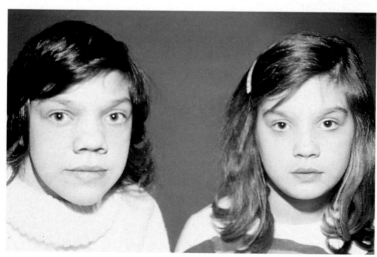

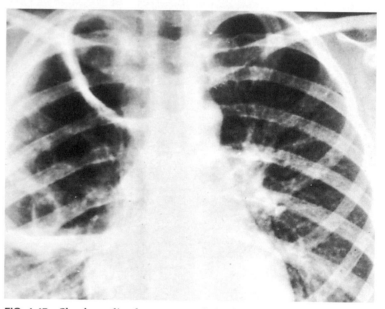

FIG. 4-46 Coarse facial features of female with hyper-IgE syndrome *(left).* Her sister *(right)* has IgA deficiency. Although distinct in etiology, these girls illustrate the frequency with which immune deficiencies are observed in family members of IgA-deficient individuals.

FIG. 4-47 Clearly outlined pneumatocele in the right lung of patient with hyper-IgE syndrome. This encapsulated lesion frequently complicates *Staphylococcus aureus* pneumonia.

gressive ataxia, and variable immunodeficiency. Most patients develop ocular telangiectasia and ataxia during the first 6 years of life (see Fig. 15-23). The ataxia is cerebellar in nature and characteristically progressive. Neurologic involvement may be extensive, including abnormalities of speech, movement, and gait and mental retardation. The progressive, variable immunodeficiency commonly consists of selective IgA deficiency and depressed T-lymphocyte function. Selective IgG subtype and IgG deficiencies have also been reported. Recurrent sinus and pulmonary infections, which may lead to bronchiectasis, are common and may be responsible for early death. These patients, in addition to those with other forms of immunodeficiency, have a higher incidence of neoplasia.

The hyper-IgE syndrome is a disorder of autosomal-recessive inheritance characterized by marked elevation of serum IgE. Clinical features include recurrent staphylococcal infections, a pruritic eczematoid dermatitis, and coarse facial features (Fig. 4-46). Recurrent staphylococcal skin infections, including impetigo and furuncles, are especially common and typically resistant to therapy. Staphylococcal pneumonia complicated by pneumatocele formation (Fig. 4-47) and lung abscesses is frequent. Other organisms of relatively low virulence, including *Candida albicans,* may cause infection. Immunologic findings include markedly elevated IgE levels (often greater than 10,000 IU/ml), eosinophilia, abnormal cell-mediated immunity, and in certain patients, abnormal polymorphonuclear leukocyte chemotaxis.

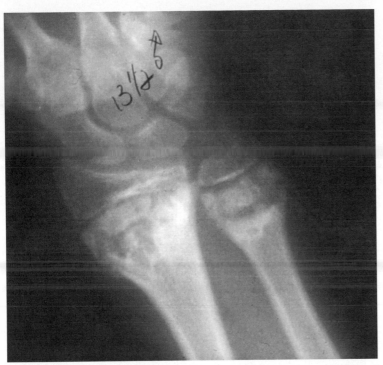

FIG. 4-48 Wrist radiograph of a 13½-year-old boy with short-limbed dwarfism and metaphyseal dysplasia. Note the normal epiphysis. (Courtesy Drs. Beverly Newman and Jocyline Medina, Pittsburgh.)

Short-limbed dwarfism is an autosomal-recessive disorder associated with metaphyseal or spondyloepiphyseal dysplasia and immunodeficiency usually involving T-lymphocyte function. Since the immunodeficiency is variable, many affected children have no increase in the frequency or severity of infections, whereas others develop fatal, overwhelming infections. At birth, the head size is normal, the hands and limbs are short, and elbow extension is limited. Radiographic abnormalities include flaring of the ribs, sclerosis, and cystic changes of the widened metaphyses (Fig. 4-48). A variant consists of short-limbed dwarfism and cartilage-hair hypoplasia, in which fine sparse hair is characteristic.

Acquired Disorders. Acquired immunodeficiency syndrome (AIDS) represents the most severe form of infection by human immunodeficiency virus (HIV). Over 6000 children (younger than 13 years of age) in the United States have been reported to the Centers for Disease Control and Prevention (CDC) with AIDS. Estimates suggest that 1 million children worldwide have been infected with the virus. By the year 2000, 4 times that number will have been infected. Of these children, the majority acquire the virus perinatally from their HIV-infected mothers. Studies indicate a 20% to 30% risk of an HIV-positive mother transmitting the virus to her offspring. Antepartum and intrapartum treatment with zidovudine (ZDV) of some groups of HIV-infected women (and their offspring for the first 6 weeks of life) appears to decrease the risk of vertical transmission by two thirds. Nevertheless, worldwide estimates suggest that 35 million women (mostly of childbearing age) are currently infected, and 3000 new infections occur daily. These staggering figures, along with the problem of accessing these individuals for antenatal therapy, suggest a sobering projection for the future.

In addition to perinatal transmission, breast-feeding and sexual abuse can result in HIV transmission to young children. The blood bank screening procedures introduced in 1985 have greatly reduced the risk of transmission from exposure to HIV-infected blood products. Like adults, adolescents acquire HIV through high-risk behaviors such as unprotected sexual activity and needle sharing during intravenous drug use. Adolescents account for less than 1% of cases of AIDS reported to the CDC. Given the average incubation period of 10 years associated with adult AIDS, it is clear that much adult AIDS is ascribable to HIV infection acquired during the teenage years. Transmission by casual contact with an HIV-infected individual in normal living conditions and school settings has not been reported to date. Under very unusual circumstances, contact between HIV-infected blood and open skin lesions or mucous membranes of an unifected individual can result in virus transmission.

HIV-1 is a retrovirus and is the major etiologic agent of AIDS throughout the world. A second virus, HIV-2, is endemic in West Africa and accounts for the remainder of AIDS cases. HIV is a ribonucleic acid virus that is trophic for CD4$^+$ (helper) T-lymphocytes as well as some monocytes, macrophages, and microglial cells of the central nervous system that bear CD4$^+$ surface markers. The virus becomes integrated into the host genome and hence persists in the infected individual for life.

The timing of symptom development in HIV-infected children varies. Some infants present in the first months or year of life with one or more of the characteristic AIDS-indicator conditions, suggesting intrauterine infection.

HIV-infected infants often present with failure to thrive (Fig. 4-49), developmental delay or loss of developmental milestones, hepatosplenomegaly, lymphadenopathy, candidal skin or mucosal infections (Fig. 4-50), diarrhea, chronic pneumonitis (lymphoid interstitial pneumonitis), and recurrent or particularly severe bacterial infections. The last include meningitis, sepsis, pneumonia, abscess, cellulitis, otitis media, and sinusitis. Common pathogens are *Streptococcus pneumoniae*, *H. influenzae*, *Salmonella*, *S. aureus*, and gram-negative organisms. The repeated bacterial infections that characterize perinatally acquired HIV usually develop during the first 2 to 5 months of age but are seen throughout the first few years.

Other infants, perhaps those who acquire the infection very late in pregnancy or during delivery, will have more indolent courses, manifesting features of immunodeficiency only after the first year of life and in some cases not until after a decade or more. HIV infection is often suspected because of a history of maternal high-risk behaviors or because of a child's clinical presentation. A broad range of clinical manifestations have been described in children infected with HIV. Because many of these presenting symptoms are nonspecific, a high index of suspicion is necessary. Because most children are infected perinatally, HIV tends to be an illness that is diagnosed early in childhood. Approximately 50% present with the infection by the age of 1 year and 82% by 3 years.

Although bacterial infections are often seen in HIV-infected infants, opportunistic infections related to defects in cell-mediated immunity also occur. One of the most common of these is *P. carinii* pneumonia (Fig. 4-51), which occurs in more than one third of symptomatic HIV-infected children. Other opportunistic infections include *Mycobacterium avium* complex, candidal esophagitis, cytomegalovirus infection, cryptosporidiosis, infection from herpes simplex virus, cryptococcosis, toxoplasmosis, and infection from a variety of other organisms

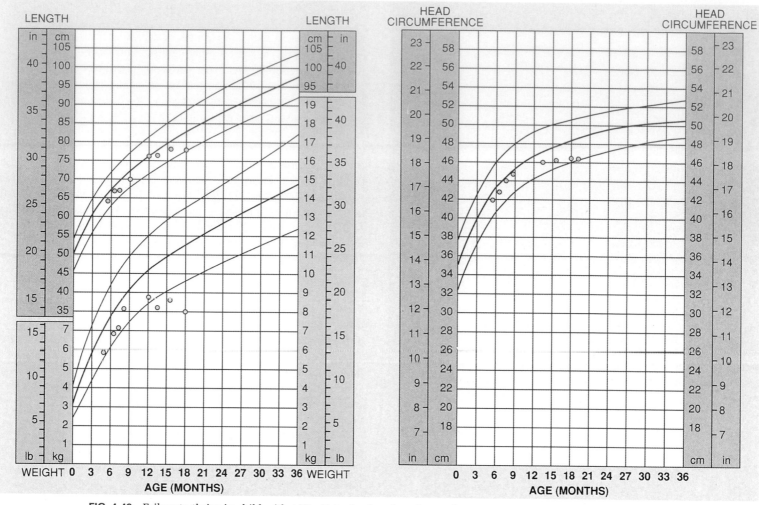

LENGTH
LENGTH
HEAD
CIRCUMFERENCE
HEAD
CIRCUMFERENCE

FIG. 4-49   Failure to thrive in child with AIDs. Note deceleration of growth parameters for length, weight, and head circumference.

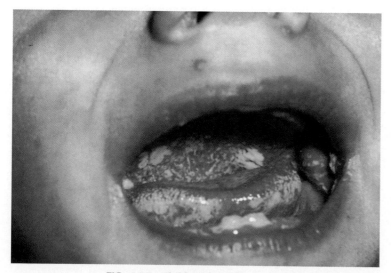

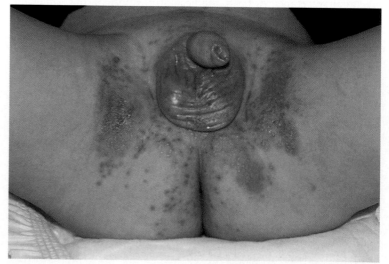

FIG. 4-50   Child with AIDS. *A*, Oral thrush. *B*, Candidal diaper dermatitis. (*A* courtesy Drs. G.B. Scott and M.T. Mastrucci, Miami.)

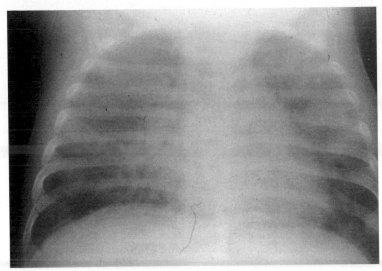

FIG. 4-51 *Pneumocystis carinii* pneumonia in a child with AIDS. Note diffuse bilateral haziness. (Courtesy Drs. G.B. Scott and M.T. Mastrucci, Miami.)

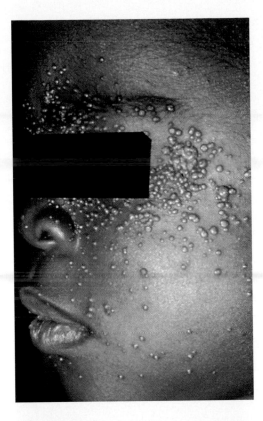

FIG. 4-52 Severe molluscum contagiosum in a patient with AIDS. (Courtesy of Drs. G. B. Scott and M. T. Mastrucci, Miami.)

(Fig. 4-52). Of particular note is *M. avium* complex, which may cause fever, weight loss, diarrhea, and abdominal pain.

An especially devastating feature of HIV infection is the encephalopathic condition that leads to developmental delay, loss of developmental milestones, and behavioral alterations. Also seen are pyramidal tract signs, paresis, ataxia, pseudobulbar palsy, and decreased tone. Computed tomographic scans and magnetic resonance imaging studies often show severe brain atrophy with increased ventricular size and calcifications in the basal ganglia and frontal lobes (Fig. 4-53). The course of HIV related neurologic disease is variable and may be intermittent, static, or relentlessly progressive.

Lymphoid interstitial pneumonitis, leading to chronic interstitial pneumonitis, occurs commonly in AIDS patients (Fig. 4-54). This form of chronic lung disease presents insidiously over the course of several years with cough, wheezing, clubbing of the fingers (Fig. 4-55), hypoxemia, radiologic features of a diffuse reticulonodular infiltrate, and at times, hilar and mediastinal adenopathy. Children with this condition often have lymphadenopathy, hepatosplenomegaly, parotid gland enlargement, and a longer survival than children who have opportunistic infections.

As with many immunodeficiencies, malignancies also occur in children with AIDS, although at rates significantly lower than in adults. Kaposi sarcoma (Fig. 4-56) and lymphoma have been reported in affected children.

Other clinical manifestations of HIV include diarrhea, hepatitis, pancreatitis, cardiomyopathy (Fig. 4-57), eczema, nephrotic syndrome, and pancytopenia. HIV infection therefore presents with a multitude of clinical patterns. The clinical pattern of disease reflects direct HIV infection as well as immune system dysregulation, including evidence of immunodeficiency and autoimmune disease. A variety of immunologic abnormalities occur with HIV infection (Table 4-13).

Diagnosis of HIV infection in children older than 18 months of age is reliably established by detecting serum IgG antibodies to a number of specific HIV antigens using two assays. The enzyme-linked immunosorbent assay (ELISA) is used as a highly sensitive screening test. Sera reported as positive by ELISA assay need to be confirmed by the

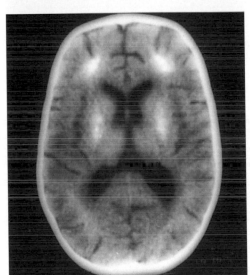

FIG. 4-53 CT scan in infant with AIDS. Note the frontal lobe and basal ganglia calcification and increased ventricular size secondary to cerebral parenchymal volume loss.

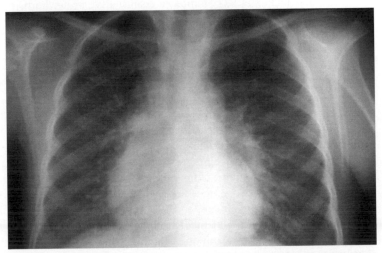

FIG. 4-54 Lymphoid interstitial pneumonitis in a child with AIDS. Note the diffuse bilateral reticulonodular infiltrates.

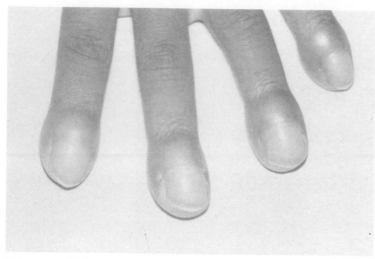

FIG. 4-55 Clubbing in patient with lymphoid interstitial pneumonitis and AIDS. (Courtesy Drs. G.B. Scott and M.T. Mastrucci, Miami.)

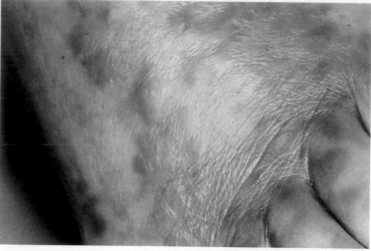

FIG. 4-56 Cutaneous manifestations of Kaposi sarcoma. The purplish hyperpigmented plaques and nodules are characteristic.

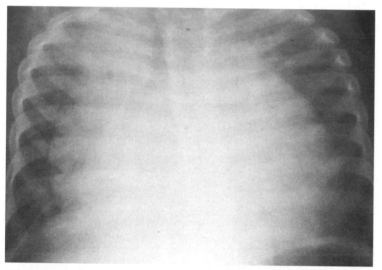

FIG. 4-57 Cardiomyopathy in a patient with AIDS. Note the massively increased heart size. (Courtesy Drs. G.B. Scott and M.T. Mastrucci, Miami.)

TABLE 4-13

Selected Abnormalities of the Immune System in AIDS

Lymphopenia (more common in adults)
Decreased helper T-lymphocytes (T4)
Decreased helper:suppressor ratio (T4:T8 ratio)
Decreased T- and B-lymphocyte mitogen responses (pokeweed, phytohemagglutinin, concanavalin A)
Decreased specific antibody response to antigen
Increased immunoglobulin levels (IgG, IgD, IgA, IgM, IgG subclasses)
Deficient serum isohemagglutinin levels
Positive test for antinuclear antibodies
Positive Coombs test
Positive circulating immune complex levels

Western blot assay, which, to be considered positive, must indicate the presence of antibodies against a requisite number of HIV-specific antigens. Because of the ubiquitous presence of passively acquired maternal antibodies (including IgG antibodies against HIV) in newborns of HIV-infected mothers, conventional ELISA and Western blot serologic assays are not helpful in establishing a diagnosis of HIV infection in children younger than 18 months. Detection of anti-HIV IgA antibodies (which do not cross the placenta) has proved to be a diagnostic tool for establishing HIV infection within the first 3 months of life with sensitivity that has varied in the hands of different investigators.

HIV culture and the detection of proviral DNA using the polymerase chain reaction (PCR) amplification technique have proved to be powerful tools in establishing the diagnosis of HIV infection in infants. In the first month of life, both techniques, which are available at medical centers or selected laboratories, have a sensitivity of approximately 50%; by 3 to 6 months of age, they are capable of detecting more than 90% of cases of vertically transmitted HIV infection. A diagnosis of HIV infection established by one of these techniques should be confirmed by the other method or by repetition of the test using a second sample. Conventional p24 antigen detection is not sufficiently sensitive to make it a useful technique in diagnosing HIV infection in infants. However,

when HIV antibodies are separated from antigens using acid hydrolysis (the immune-complex–dissociated p24 antigen [ICDp24] assay), high degrees of sensitivity and specificity have been reported among HIV-infected infants in the first 3 months of life. This assay, which is technically simpler and cheaper than PCR and HIV culture, may become an increasingly important diagnostic tool.

Therapy includes trimethoprim-sulfamethoxazole prophylaxis for *P. carinii* pneumonia, intravenous gamma-globulin infusions, and ZDV for selected patients. Prognosis remains poor, but with new therapies for HIV itself and its related complications, the importance of early diagnosis and aggressive management is heightened.

Phagocytic Disorders

Polymorphonuclear leukocytes and mononuclear cells play vital roles in the defense against acute infections. Normal neutrophil numbers, intact neutrophil chemotaxis, phagocytosis, and killing are necessary for the rapid elimination of microorganisms that invade the skin or mucous membranes. Patients with neutropenia are vulnerable to bacterial infections, as are patients with disorders of phagocyte function. The neutropenias and Chédiak-Higashi syndrome are discussed in Chapter 11.

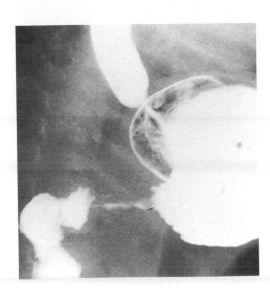

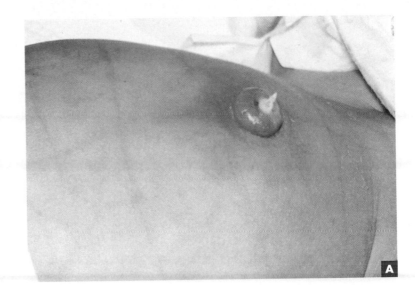

FIG. 4-58 Barium contrast radiogram demonstrating the "string sign," a thin line of barium that represents narrowing of the gastric antrum secondary to granuloma formation. This child had persistent vomiting but none of the usual stigmata of chronic granulomatous disease.

Chronic granulomatous disease of childhood is one example of neutrophil dysfunction. Neutrophil chemotaxis and phagocytosis are intact, but killing of ingested microorganisms is defective. The responsible biochemical defect results in abnormal leukocyte oxidative metabolism and inability to kill microorganisms. Intracellular survival of ingested bacteria, even those not typically associated with granuloma formation, can lead to development of granulomatous lesions. An NBT test is used to diagnose this disorder (see section on diagnostic techniques). Because of its X-linked recessive inheritance, the disorder predominantly affects boys; girls are affected less frequently. Clinically, children with chronic granulomatous disease become symptomatic early in life. The most common presenting problems are severe, recurrent infections of the skin and lymph nodes with *S. aureus*. The skin infections often become chronic and heal slowly. Suppurative lymphadenitis often requires surgical drainage. Pneumonitis may progress to produce pneumatoceles (Fig. 4-47). Osteomyelitis of the small bones of the hand and foot is common. Hepatosplenomegaly is a constant physical finding and presumably represents involvement of the reticuloendothelial system. Granulomas may also develop in other organ systems and may not be palpable on examination. In the patient whose radiograph is seen in Fig. 4-58, the diagnosis of chronic granulomatous disease was suggested by the finding of antral narrowing secondary to granulomatous involvement of the gastric antrum. Cytokine therapy with gamma-interferon is an important adjunct to antibiotic therapy with trimethoprim-sulfamethoxazole.

Intercellular adhesion molecule (ICAM) deficiency, also called *leukocyte adhesion factor deficiency*, is a recently defined, rare syndrome resulting from deficiency of one or more of a group of cell-membrane glycoproteins termed *intercellular adhesion molecules* and normally used by phagocytes to move and adhere to surfaces. The patients have a variety of symptoms and signs, all of which are related to the inability of phagocytes to adhere and move toward a chemoattractant. These include delayed umbilical cord severance (Fig. 4-59, *A*), persistent peripheral blood granulocytosis (lack of vascular margination), recurrent soft tissue infections, and impaired wound healing. Since these patients do not mobilize neutrophils in response to infection, many aspects of the normal inflammatory response are lacking, including the formation of pus (Fig. 4-59, *B*). This may confound the diagnosis when infection is suspected. ICAM deficiency should be suspected in any infant with periumbilical problems and persistent peripheral blood leukocytosis (frequently > 50,000 cells/mm³).

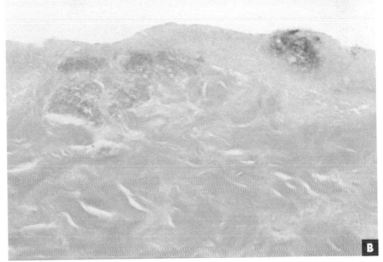

FIG. 4-59 Infants with ICAM deficiency. *A*, Infection involving and surrounding the umbilical cord. *B*, Histopathologic appearance of a scalp abscess. Note the presence of bacterial colonies (purple staining) and distinct lack of host cellular inflammatory response. (A courtesy Dr. Kenneth Schuit, Pittsburgh; B courtesy Dr. Kenneth Schuit and William Robichaux, Pittsburgh.)

Complement System Disorders

The complement system is a complex system of nine distinct serum proteins, designated C1 through C9, that require serial activation through the classical or alternative complement pathways. Complement mediates and amplifies many of the biologic functions of the immune system. These functions include (1) enhancement of phagocytosis (opsonization) and viral neutralization, (2) mediation of inflammation via chemotaxis and alteration of vascular permeability, (3) cell lysis, and (4) modulation of the immune response. Defects of the complement system result from decreased levels of or absence of components or from production of components that function abnormally. Although rare, inherited deficiencies of most complement components have been reported. Clinical presentation varies, depending on the specific complement protein involved. Frequent modes of presentation for complement component deficiencies are collagen vascular diseases for C1 through C4, disseminated infections with pyogenic bacteria for C3, and disseminated neisserial infections for C5 through C8.

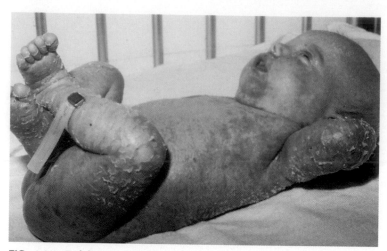

FIG. 4-60 Exfoliative dermatitis characteristic of severe seborrhea in an infant with Leiner disease.

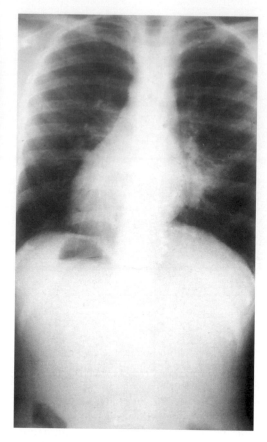

FIG. 4-61 Dextrocardia and situs inversus of abdominal organs in a patient with Kartagener syndrome. Abnormal ciliary motion is thought to result in malrotation during embryogenesis.

Leiner Disease

Shortly after the turn of the century, Leiner described an infantile syndrome characterized by recurrent infections, severe seborrheic dermatitis, intractable diarrhea, and failure to thrive (Fig. 4-60). These children were subsequently observed to have a functional abnormality of C5 and an inability to opsonize yeast particles. Yeast opsonization has been used to identify individuals with Leiner disease, since other functional and antigenic assays of C5 are normal in these patients. Mothers of these children lack functional C5 in their breast milk; therefore this disease occurs almost exclusively in breast-fed babies and not those fed cow milk–based formulas, which do contain functional C5. The disorder is self-limited, tending to resolve by age 2 months, coincident with the appearance of endogenous functional C5.

Hereditary Angioedema

Hereditary angioedema is an autosomal-dominant disorder characterized by the absence or abnormal function of a protein in the complement cascade known as *C1 esterase inhibitor.* Inhibitors of the complement system are naturally occurring and are capable of blocking activated complement components. C1 esterase inhibitor binds to activated C1 and thereby prevents further activation of the classical pathway. In the absence of C1 inhibitor, complement activation proceeds unchecked. This results in increased vascular permeability and the observed clinical features of angioedema. Many clinicians do not consider hereditary angioedema an immunodeficiency disorder because these patients do not have recurrent infections. Nevertheless, a defect in the complement system is responsible for the clinical manifestations. This disorder is characterized by recurrent bouts of swelling that involve any part of the body but that typically involve the face, extremities, and respiratory and gastrointestinal tracts. The swelling is generally self-limited and episodic. Laryngeal edema is a frightening, life-threatening complication that may result in asphyxia. Involve-

ment of the gastrointestinal tract is characterized by severe abdominal pain, bloating, vomiting, and rarely intestinal obstruction resulting from intussusception.

Mucosal Barrier Disorders

Intact mucosal barriers are of crucial importance in preventing the entrance of ubiquitous microorganisms into the host. The respiratory and gastrointestinal mucosa aid in host defense by secreting antibodies (predominantly IgA) into their lumina. Also, physical factors such as saliva flow in the oral cavity, intestinal peristalsis, and the coughing reflex are important in the "washing out" effect on potential pathogens.

Immotile cilia syndrome is characterized by a defect in mucociliary transport, another component of the mucosal barrier. This disorder was first described as Kartagener syndrome, which consists of a triad of situs inversus viscerum (Fig. 4-61), chronic sinusitis, and bronchiectasis. These patients were also noted to be infertile, because their spermatozoa were poorly motile as a result of lack of dynein arms in the ultrastructure of their tails. Studies revealed similar defects in mucosal cilia and led to recognition of the fact that the phenomenon could exist in the absence of situs inversus viscerum. The resultant ciliary dysfunction impedes mucus clearance and produces a combination of the following signs and symptoms: (1) early onset of chronic rhinorrhea (2) chronic otitis media, (3) chronic sinusitis with opaque sinuses on radiography, (4) chronic productive cough, (5) bronchiectasis, (6) digital clubbing, and (7) nasal polyps. The disorder should be suspected in any child with chronic or recurrent upper or lower respiratory tract infections. When situs inversus viscerum is not present, the diagnosis of immotile cilia syndrome requires confirmation by electron microscopic analysis of cilia obtained from a biopsy of the nasal or tracheobronchial mucosa (Fig. 4-62).

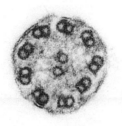
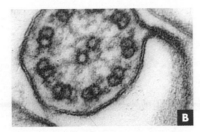

FIG. 4-62 *A,* Electron micrograph of cilia from a patient with immotile cilia syndrome. Note the absence of dynein arms from the outer doublets. *B,* Normal cilia with dynein arms. (From Bluestone C, Stool S: Pediatric *otolaryngology,* vol 1, Philadelphia, 1983, WB Saunders.)

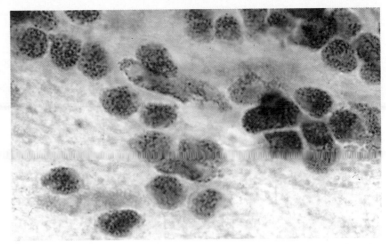

FIG. 4-63 Eosinophilia on nasal smear from a patient with allergic rhinitis.

Diagnostic Techniques in Allergy and Immunology

Skin Testing: Immediate Hypersensitivity

For over 100 years, hypersensitivity skin tests have been used to confirm the diagnosis of allergy. This in vivo method detects the presence of IgE antibody specific to the test antigen. The prick skin test is the safest and most specific test and correlates best with symptoms. It involves placing a drop of antigen solution on cleansed skin. A blunt needle is passed through the drop, punctures the skin, and is rapidly withdrawn without scratching the skin. The test site is "read" in 15 to 20 minutes by recording the presence or absence of a wheal and surrounding flare (erythema) and their sizes. A typical scoring system is listed below.

Although the prick skin test is very specific, it is less sensitive than intradermal skin tests. If prick tests are negative, intradermal tests should be performed. This test involves injecting 0.02 ml of antigen solution intradermally and is also read in 20 minutes. The scoring system used for interpretation follows:

Grade 0(-)	Wheal <3 mm, erythema 0-5 mm
Grade 1+	Wheal 3-5 mm, erythema 0-10 mm
Grade 2+	Wheal 5-10 mm, erythema 5-10 mm
Grade 3+	Wheal 10-15 mm, erythema >10 mm
Grade 4+	Wheal >15 mm or with pseudopods, erythema >20 mm

Although intradermal tests are more sensitive, their results do not correlate as well with symptoms as do those of prick tests. Appropriate antigen solutions must be used to ensure reliability, and results must be correlated with clinical symptoms. In addition, drugs that inhibit or suppress histamine action or release, such as antihistamines and cromolyn, must be discontinued 24 to 48 hours before skin testing. In vitro correlates of skin testing are the serum RAST or ELISA tests, which correlate well with history but are less sensitive and more expensive than skin testing.

Nasal Smear

The nasal smear is another helpful tool in diagnosing allergic and nonallergic nasal disease. Mucus is obtained by having the patient sneeze into wax paper or by swabbing the posterior nares. The secretions are then applied in a thin layer onto a microscope slide. The slide is stained with Wright or Hansel stain, and the percentage of eosinophils is noted (Fig. 4-63). The presence of eosinophilia (> 25%), along with positive skin tests, is very suggestive of allergic disease. When skin tests are negative, the presence of nasal eosinophilia can differentiate eosinophilic nonallergic rhinitis from vasomotor rhinitis. This distinction has important therapeutic implications.

Skin Testing: Delayed Hypersensitivity

Traditionally, cell-mediated immunity has been assessed by the delayed hypersensitivity skin test. Intradermal injection of 0.1 ml of antigen solution in a sensitized individual is followed by the development of an indurated erythematous reaction over several hours. This reaction peaks at 24 to 48 hours and is recorded at 48 hours. A positive test occurs when 10 mm or more of induration and erythema are present. Using an antigen such as *C. albicans,* the majority of children with intact cellular immunity have positive tests after 12 months of age. Other antigens such as diphtheria and tetanus, if tested within 6 to 12 months of booster immunization, frequently show delayed hypersensitivity. Purified protein derivative (PPD) is used to document exposure and sensi-

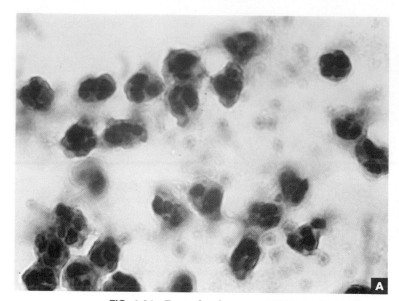 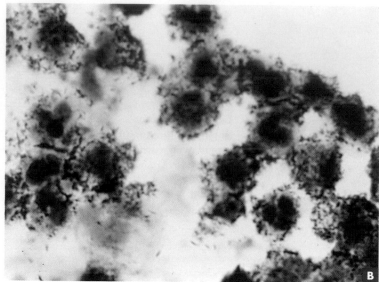

FIG. 4-64 Example of a normal NBT test (×1000). Neutrophils in the unstimulated state display virtually no dye reduction *(A)*, but nearly all of the neutrophils display the purple color after incubation with phorbol myristate acetate for 15 minutes at 37°C *(B)*. In normal patients, more than 99% of stimulated neutrophils display the color, whereas patients with chronic granulomatous disease have less than 1% NBT-positive granulocytes. (Courtesy Dr. Sandra Kaplan.)

tization to the tubercle bacillus. If delayed hypersensitivity skin tests are negative in a child with suspected immunodeficiency, a thorough evaluation of the T-lymphocyte system is indicated. For the diagnosis of patients with contact dermatitis, delayed hypersensitivity skin testing is performed by the patch test technique (see Chapter 8).

Nitroblue Tetrazolium

Chronic granulomatous disease (CGD) is diagnosed by an abnormal NBT test. This test is based on the increased metabolic activity of normal granulocytes after phagocytosis and the absence of such an increase in CGD. The respiratory burst that the stimulated neutrophils normally undergo results in a reduction of the colorless dye NBT to purple formazan, which is easily visible in the responsive cells microscopically (Fig. 4-64). A typical phagocytic stimulus used in this test is latex particles. The leukocytes of patients with CGD cannot reduce NBT in the normal fashion, and this defect is correlated with their inability to generate superoxide and hydrogen peroxide and to kill certain microorganisms.

BIBLIOGRAPHY

Annunziato PW, Frenkel LM: The epidemiology of pediatric HIV-1 infection, *Pediatr Ann* 22:401-405, 1993.

Buckley RH: Immunodeficiency, *J Allergy Clin Immunol* 72:627-644, 1983.

Burrows B, Martinez FD, Halonen M, et al: Association of asthma with serum IgE levels and skin-test reactivity to allergens, *N Engl J Med* 320:271-277, 1989.

Church JA: Clinical aspects of HIV infection in children, *Pediatr Ann* 22:417-427, 1993.

Djukanovic R, Roche WR, Wilson JW, et al: Mucosal inflammation in asthma, *Am Rev Respir Dis* 142:434-457, 1990.

Falloon J, Eddy J, Wiener L: Human immunodeficiency virus infection in children, *J Pediatr* 114:1-30, 1989.

Frenkel LD, Gaur S: Perinatal HIV infection and AIDS, *Clin Perinatol* 21:95-107, 1994.

Henderson FW, Clyde WA, Collier AM, et al: The etiologic and epidemiologic spectrum of bronchiolitis in pediatric practice, *J Pediatr* 95:183-190, 1979.

International Consensus Report on Diagnosis and Management of Asthma, Washington, DC, 1992, US Department of Health and Human Services, Public Health Service, National Institutes of Health.

International consensus report on the diagnosis and management of rhinitis: International Rhinitis Management Working Group, *Allergy (Euro J Allergy Clin Immunol)* 49(19):1-34, 1994.

Kline MW: Introduction, *Semin Pediatr Infectious Dis* 5:251, 1994.

Laitinen LA, Laitinen A, Haahtela T: Airway mucosal inflammation even in patients with newly diagnosed asthma, *Am Rev Respir Dis* 147:796-704, 1993.

Lawley TJ, Bielory L, Gascon P, et al: A prospective clinical and immunologic analysis of patients with serum sickness, *N Engl J Med* 311:1407-1413, 1984.

Middleton E Jr, Reed CE, Ellis EF, et al, eds: *Allergy: principles and practice,* ed 4, St Louis, 1993, Mosby.

Mofenson LM: Epidemiology and determinants of vertical HIV transmission, 5:252-265, 1994.

National Asthma Education Program: *Guidelines for the diagnosis and management of asthma,* Pub No 91-3042, Bethesda, Md: 1991, National Heart, Lung, and Blood Institute, National Institutes of Health.

Peter G, ed: *Report of the Committee on Infectious Diseases ("The Red Book"),* ed 23, Elk Grove, Ill, 1994, American Academy of Pediatrics.

Primer on allergic and immunologic diseases, *JAMA* 268(20):2790-2992, 1992.

1994 revised classification system for human immunodeficiency virus infection in children less than 13 years of age, *MMWR* 43(RR12): 1994.

Rosen FS, Cooper MD, Wedgewood RJ: The primary immunodeficiencies. I. *N Engl J Med* 311:300-310, 1984.

Rubinstein A: Pediatric AIDS, *Curr Probl Pediatr* 16:362-409, 1986.

Schnittman SM, Fauci AS: Human immunodeficiency virus and acquired immunodeficiency syndrome: an update, *Adv Intern Med* 39:305-355, 1994.

Steihm ER, Fulginiti VA, eds: *Immunologic disorders in infants and children,* ed 3, Philadelphia, 1989, WB Saunders.

5

Cardiology

LEE B. BEERMAN   ❦   F. JAY FRICKER
SANG C. PARK   ❦   CORA C. LENOX

The practice of cardiology as a pediatric subspecialty continues to evolve with new imaging technology. Complex structural congenital anomalies previously delineated only at autopsy can now be defined in great detail by a combination of techniques that include echocardiography, angiography, and nuclear magnetic resonance imaging. The medical cost associated with these new technologies is significant, and a proper initial assessment of the child with suspected congenital heart disease helps to avoid the expense of unnecessary testing. The emphases of this chapter remain the physical examination, chest x-ray examination, and electrocardiogram. In addition, we cover two-dimensional echocardiography and color flow Doppler imaging of common congenital heart lesions to reflect their important contribution to the practice of pediatric cardiology.

The three prerequisites to a good cardiovascular examination are a proper environment, a cooperative child, and the conviction on the part of the physician that the examination is important. The heart murmur is not the only part and often is not even the most important part of the cardiac physical examination. Blood pressure determination, character of the pulse and precordial activity, observation of cyanosis, clubbing of the nail beds of the fingers or toes, and dysmorphic facial or other physical features may provide clues to the diagnosis and nature of congenital heart lesions before auscultation is even performed.

Physical Diagnosis of Congenital Heart Disease

Cyanosis and Clubbing

Even before mild desaturation is detectable, early clubbing and cyanosis may be seen (Figs. 5-1 and 5-2). The base of the nail, especially the thumbnail, may show loss of angle as early as 3 months of age (see Chapter 16). Elevated hemoglobin and hematocrit and loss of nail angle indicate hypoxemia and the presence of a right-to-left intracardiac shunt (Fig. 5-3).

Observation of the lips and mucous membranes for the presence of cyanosis is best done in good daylight, since fluorescent light may produce a false cyanotic tinge. In the presence of polycythemia with hemoglobin in the 18- to 20-g range and hematocrit over 60%, the conjunctival vessels become engorged and plethoric (Fig. 5-2). Differential cyanosis between the upper and lower extremities is an unusual clinical finding. If the patient has pulmonary vascular disease, reverse flow through a patent ductus arteriosus, and no right-to-left intracardiac

shunting, cyanosis and clubbing should be found in the lower extremities but not in the hands (Fig. 5-4).

Blood Pressure and Pulse

Blood pressure determination in infants and children is an integral part of the cardiac physical examination. Attention to proper cuff size prevents the misdiagnosis of systolic hypertension from an undersized cuff. In general, it is better to use an oversized cuff because overestimation in systolic blood pressure can be avoided. Blood pressure can be tracked in children over time, and tables depicting normal blood pressure range for age have been published. Blood pressure determination in both arms and a lower extremity will detect coarctation of the aorta, lend support for the diagnosis of supravalvular aortic stenosis (blood pressure higher in the right arm than in the left arm), and help to assess the severity of aortic valve disease—including aortic valve stenosis (narrow pulse pressure) and aortic regurgitation (wide pulse pressure).

Heart Murmur Evaluation

In the newborn, a common innocent heart murmur originates from the branch pulmonary arteries because of their relatively small size compared with the main pulmonary artery resulting from the normal fetal flow pattern, which delivers very limited flow to the right and left pulmonary arteries. Characteristically, this murmur is early systolic and loudest over both axillae and the back. The murmur of branch pulmonary artery stenosis has the same distribution as the structural lesions that cause increased pulmonary blood flow. Transient systolic murmur at the middle-low left sternal border in the newborn can be due to tricuspid regurgitation, and a soft systolic ejection murmur at the upper left sternal border may arise from a closing patent ductus arteriosus. A large ventricular septal defect will not produce a murmur in the newborn period because the initially high pulmonary vascular resistance results in minimal shunting across the defect. On the other hand, pathologic systolic murmurs in the newborn are caused by restrictive ventricular septal defects and lesions producing left and right ventricular outflow tract obstruction (i.e., tetralogy of Fallot and valvular aortic or pulmonary stenosis). In the newborn, it can be difficult to distinguish the murmur of a small restrictive ventricular septal defect from that of a severe right ventricular outflow tract obstruction in tetral-

111

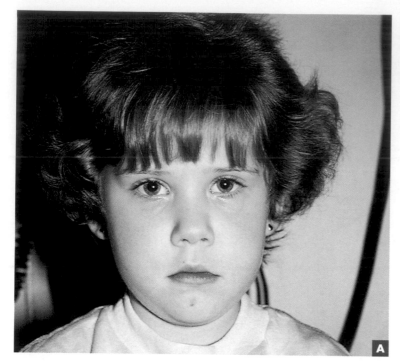
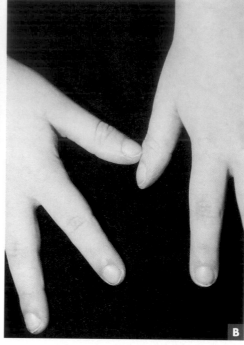

FIG. 5-1   *A,* This child shows no obvious cyanosis of the face and lips, although the photograph in *B* demonstrates clubbing: loss of nail angle and curvature of nails, especially of the thumb.

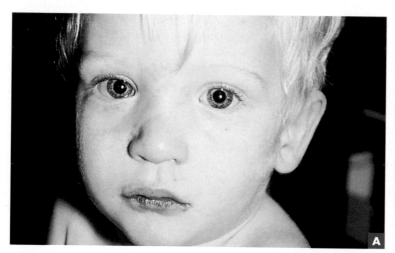
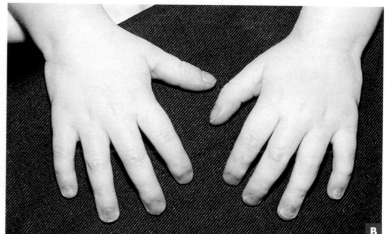

FIG. 5-2   This child demonstrates moderate cyanosis of the lips *(A)* and nails *(B).* Note also the reddish discoloration of the eyes resulting from conjunctival suffusion.

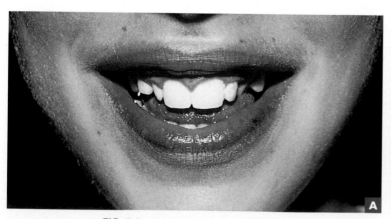
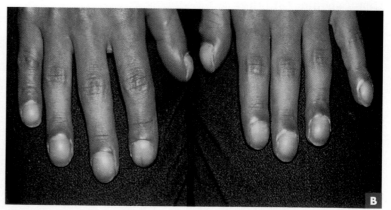

FIG. 5-3   Severe cyanosis of the lips, tongue, and mucous membranes can be noted in *A,* associated with marked clubbing and cyanosis of the nails in *B.*

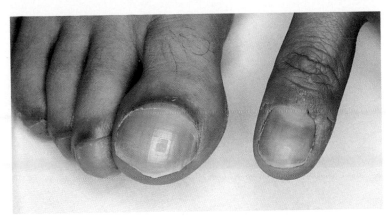

FIG. 5-4 Differential cyanosis and clubbing resulting from reverse shunting through a patent ductus arteriosus in a patient with pulmonary vascular disease. Note marked cyanosis and clubbing of the toes, although the finger appears to be normal. (Courtesy Dr. J.R. Zuberbuhler, Pittsburgh.)

TABLE 5-1

Innocent Murmurs Mimicking Congenital Heart Disease

Innocent heart murmur	Structural congenital heart disease
Systolic Ejection Murmur at the Base of the Heart	
High left sternal border	Pulmonary valve stenosis
	*Ejection click
	*Transmission to back
	Atrial septal defect
	*Parasternal lift
	*S2 wide split
	*Diastolic murmur of tricuspid flow
High right sternal border	Aortic valve stenosis
	*Ejection click
	*Radiation to neck
Still Murmur	
Vibratory quality	Ventricular septal defect
Location: left midsternal border	*Character of murmur
	Discrete subaortic stenosis
	*Radiation to aortic area
	Subpulmonic stenosis
	*Radiation to pulmonic area
	*Soft P2
Venous Hum	
Continuous	Patent ductus arteriosus
Location: neck and under clavicles	*Location under left clavicle
	*No change with position
Usually loudest when sitting, disappears in supine posture	Coronary AV malformation
	*Accentuated in diastole
Carotid and Cranial Bruits	
Murmur over carotids and head	Aortic stenosis
	AV malformation
	*Continuous murmur would support AV malformation

*Distinguishing features
AV, Atrioventricular.

TABLE 5-2

Syndromes and Trisomies, With Associated Cardiovascular Abnormalities

Syndrome	Common cardiac defect
Ellis–van Creveld	Atrial septal defect or single atrium
Fetal alcohol	Ventricular septal defect
Holt-Oram	Atrial and ventricular septal defects, arrhythmias
Marfan	Dilation of ascending aorta/aortic sinus, aortic and mitral insufficiency
Noonan	Dysplastic pulmonic valve, atrial septal defect
Turner	Coarctation of the aorta, bicuspid aortic valve
Williams	Supravalvular aortic stenosis, pulmonary artery stenosis
Trisomy	
13	Patent ductus, septal defects, pulmonic and aortic stenosis (atresia)
18	Ventricular septal defect, polyvalvular disease, coronary abnormalities
21 (Down)	Atrioventricular septal defects, ventricular septal defect, patent ductus, anomalous subclavian artery

ogy of Fallot or left ventricular outflow obstruction. The implications of this differential diagnosis are such that an echocardiogram is recommended for infants with this clinical presentation.

Contrary to popular belief, the presence of a continuous murmur from a patent ductus arteriosus is extremely rare in a full-term newborn. If a continuous murmur is heard in the newborn, patent ductus–dependent pulmonary blood flow or systemic to pulmonary collateral in association with pulmonary atresia complex should be considered.

It is common for preschoolers and school age children to be referred for evaluation of a heart murmur. Innocent murmurs of childhood fall into four major categories: systolic ejection murmurs at the base; vibratory, or Still, murmurs; venous hums; and carotid and cranial bruits. In most instances there are associated clinical and laboratory studies that can distinguish the innocent from the pathologic murmur. Table 5-1 summarizes the distinguishing features and differential diagnosis. Fig. 5-5 illustrates the sites where murmurs resulting from various cardiovascular lesions are best heard.

Syndrome-Associated Physical Findings

Dysmorphology of the face and habitus suggests certain syndromes associated with congenital heart disease (Table 5-2).

The typical features in Down syndrome (trisomy 21) are demonstrated in Chapter 1. About 40% of children with this syndrome have structural lesions such as atrioventricular septal defects, isolated ventricular septal defects, patent ductus arteriosus, or anomalous origin of the subclavian arteries.

Although many infants with Down syndrome have chronic congestive heart failure and growth failure, there is a subset that grows and develops appropriately. Pulmonary vascular resistance does not decrease in the usual fashion in this group, and these children develop early pulmonary vascular disease. Because this presentation may be silent, it is important that all children with Down syndrome be thor-

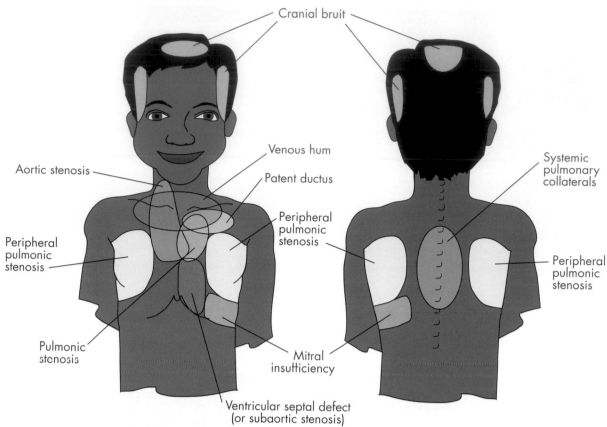

FIG. 5-5   Sites where murmurs resulting from various cardiovascular lesions are best heard.

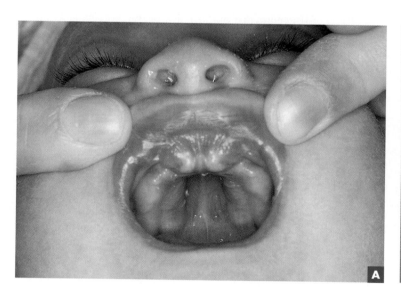

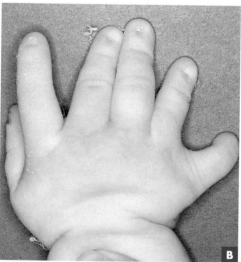

FIG. 5-6   This infant with Ellis–van Creveld syndrome demonstrates characteristic facial features *(A)* and multiple digits (polydactyly) *(B)*.

oughly evaluated during early infancy. The evaluation should include an echocardiogram to rule out congenital heart disease.

Ellis–van Creveld syndrome is an autosomal recessive disorder characterized by multiple gingival frenula, natal teeth, and polydactyly (Fig. 5-6). The patient with this syndrome frequently has an atrial septal defect or a common atrium.

Holt-Oram syndrome, an autosomal-dominant disorder, is associated with upper limb deformities consisting of narrow shoulders, hypoplasia of the radius, and phocomelia (Fig. 5-7). Absence of both radius and thumb or proximal displacement of the thumb is the most frequent

finding. Commonly associated cardiovascular abnormalities include an atrial septal defect, ventricular septal defect, and dysrhythmias (atrial and ventricular ectopy, and atrioventricular block).

Marfan syndrome also has an autosomal-dominant inheritance; it manifests as a connective tissue disorder in which the elastic fibers are disrupted, causing cystic medial necrosis of the aorta, as well as joint laxity and subluxation of the ocular lens. Affected patients are tall, with increased limb length compared with the trunk. Their arm span exceeds their height. The cardiovascular abnormalities consist of aneurysmal dilation of the aorta, aortic sinuses, and mi-

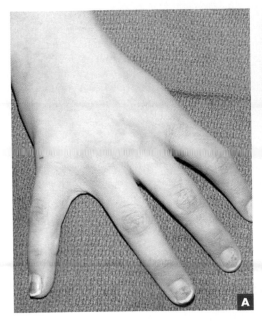

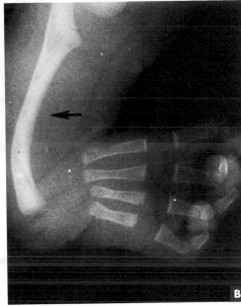

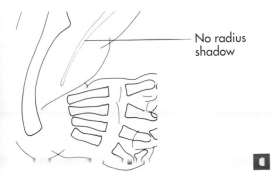

FIG. 5-7 Clinical photograph (*A*) reveals the absence of the radius and thumb in a patient with Holt-Oram syndrome. The associated cardiovascular abnormality is an atrial septal defect. Radiographic examination (*B* and *C*) demonstrates the absence of a radius shadow; the missing thumb is apparent.

No radius shadow

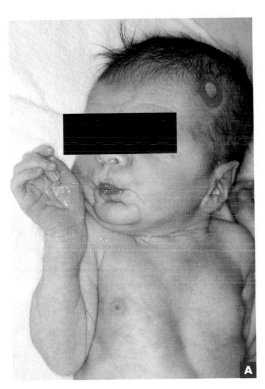

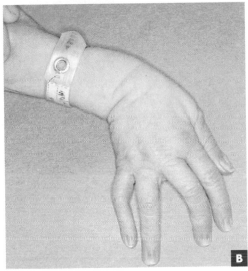

FIG. 5-8 Infant with Marfan syndrome. *A*, Note the narrow elongated face, pectus excavatum, laxity, and long arms and fingers. *B*, A close-up view of the infant's hand.

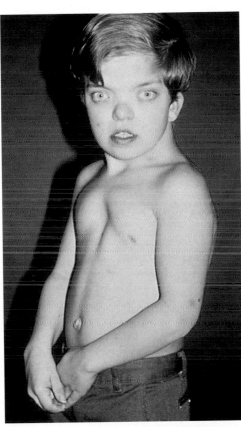

FIG. 5-9 This child displays characteristic features of Noonan syndrome: widely spaced eyes, low-set ears, webbing of the neck, shield chest, pectus, and increased carrying angle of the arms.

tral valve prolapse. Associated aortic and mitral valve regurgitations are common (Fig. 5-8).

Patients with Noonan syndrome have features characteristic of Turner syndrome but possess normal chromosomes. Clinically, these children have phenotypic findings of Turner, including webbing of the neck, pectus, shield chest with widely spaced nipples, short stature, epicanthal folds, low-set ears, and increased carrying angle of the arms (Fig. 5-9). Common cardiovascular defects include pulmonary stenosis in association with a dysplastic pulmonary valve and an atrial septal

defect. Occasionally, there may be dysplasia of all cardiac valves and later development of myocardial hypertrophy. The syndrome appears as an autosomal-dominant disorder; multiple members of a family often are affected.

The most common cardiac defects in Turner syndrome are coarctation of the aorta and a bicuspid aortic valve. (See Chapters 1 and 9 for a detailed discussion of Turner syndrome.)

Patients with Williams syndrome characteristically have "elfin" facies: a broad maxilla, a small mandible with full mouth and large up-

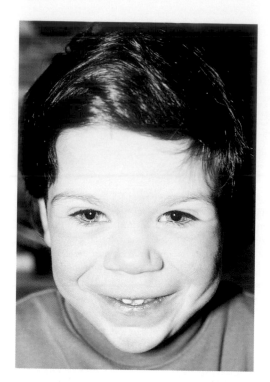

FIG. 5-10 A child with elfin facies (Williams syndrome). Note the wide-set eyes, upturned nose, large maxilla, prominent philtrum, and pointed chin. (Courtesy Dr. R.A. Mathews, Philadelphia.)

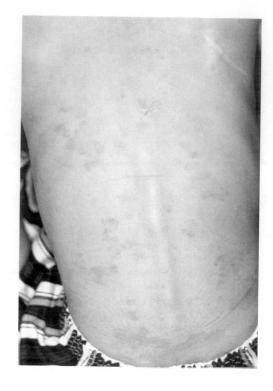

FIG. 5-11 Erythema marginatum rash in a child with acute rheumatic fever. Note the wavy margins in the distribution on the trunk.

TABLE 5-3

Genetic Syndromes and Inborn Errors of Metabolism, With Associated Cardiovascular Findings

Genetically determined diseases	Cardiac findings
Metabolic	
Pompe disease (glycogen storage)	Cardiomyopathy (storage of glycogen in myocardium)
MPS	Storage of MPS in arteries, coronaries, and valves with insufficiency and stenosis Hurler (MPS I H), Hunter (MPS II), Scheie (I S, I H/S), Morquio (MPS IV)
Hyperlipoproteinemia, familial type II	Premature atherosclerosis of arteries, including coronaries
Neurologic	
Friedreich ataxia	Cardiomyopathy (congestive or hypertrophic)
Muscular dystrophies	Myocardial degeneration and fibrosis

Inborn error of metabolism (no proven genetic basis)	Cardiac findings
Progeria	Hypercholesterolemia, atherosclerotic changes in arteries, including coronaries

MPS, Mucopolysaccharidosis.

per lip (philtrum), upturned nose, and a full forehead (Fig. 5-10). This syndrome has been associated with hypercalcemia in infants and may have a genetic but undefined hereditary basis. Supravalvular aortic stenosis and pulmonary artery branch stenosis are common cardiovascular abnormalities.

In addition, there are many genetically determined diseases and inborn errors of metabolism with cardiac involvement, the most common of which are listed in Table 5-3.

Visible Clues in Acute Rheumatic Fever

Examination of the skin in a patient with acute rheumatic fever may reveal the typical rash of erythema marginatum, although this rash is not specific for rheumatic fever. It is nonpruritic, has sharp serpiginous margins, and is found on the inner aspects of the upper arms and thighs and on the trunk (Fig. 5-11). The differential diagnosis includes: (1) drug rash, which is papular and pruritic; (2) rash of glomerulonephritis, which is macular and has no sharp margins; (3) rash of juvenile rheumatoid arthritis, which is pink, macular, and lacks wavy margins, and which may be transient; and (4) the cutaneous findings of Kawasaki syndrome (see Chapter 7).

Subcutaneous nodules are rare in chronic rheumatic heart disease, but if found, they are almost always associated with severe carditis. These movable, nontender, cartilage-like swellings vary in size from 2 mm to 1 cm and are never transient. They are seen over the bony prominences of the large joints and external surfaces of the elbows and knuckles of the hands, knees, and ankles. They also may be felt along the spine and over the skull. Although difficult to photograph, they are easily palpated (Fig. 5-12).

Signs of Bacterial Endocarditis

Although the clinical presentation of bacterial endocarditis varies according to the infecting organism, it should be suspected in any patient

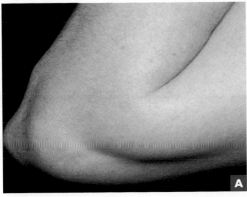
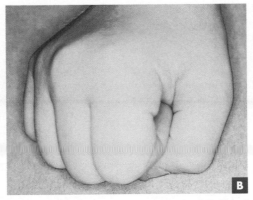
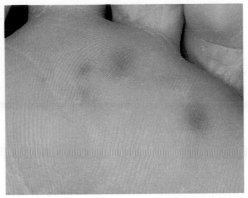

FIG. 5-12 Subcutaneous nodules over bony prominences of the elbow *(A)* and knuckles of the hand *(B)* in a patient with chronic rheumatic heart disease.

FIG. 5-13 Janeway lesions, small painless nodules on the sole of a patient with bacterial endocarditis.

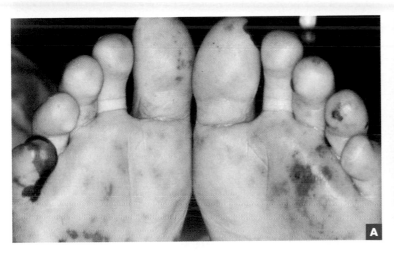
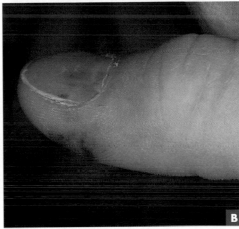

FIG. 5-14 *A*, Hemorrhagic lesions in a patient with acute bacterial endocarditis. *B*, Subungual splinter hemorrhages. (*A* courtesy Dr. W.H. Neches.)

with congenital or acquired heart disease who has prolonged fever without apparent cause. The classic skin lesions include petechiae, splinter hemorrhages of the nails, conjunctival hemorrhages, and Janeway lesions (Fig. 5-13), all of which are manifestations of vasculitis. Vegetations occasionally dislodge and embolize in an end artery, which results in hemorrhagic or gangrenous lesions (Fig. 5-14). Osler nodes, which present as small tender erythematous nodules, are found in the intradermal pads of the fingers and toes or in the thenar or hypothenar eminences (Fig. 5-15). All the aforementioned findings are often associated with a new heart murmur, splenomegaly, spiking fever, and positive blood culture. Clubbing of the fingers may occur in chronic cases.

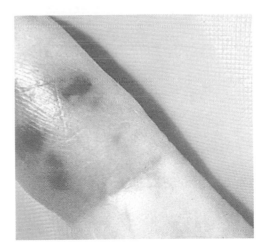

FIG. 5-15 Osler nodes, painful erythematous nodular lesions resulting from infective endocarditis. (Courtesy Dr. J.F. John, Jr.)

Laboratory Aids in the Diagnosis of Congenital Heart Disease

In addition to a comprehensive physical examination, the chest roentgenogram, electrocardiogram, and, particularly, cross-sectional echocardiograic images have provided valuable information concerning specific congenital heart lesions and have allowed therapeutic decisions to be made without cardiac catheterization.

Chest Roentgenography

The chest x-ray examination is useful to screen patients with suspected congenital heart disease. It will exclude apparent pulmonary problems such as pneumothorax, pneumomediastinum, or parenchymal lung disease mimicking cyanotic congenital heart disease. The review of any chest roentgenogram requires a systematic approach.

Cardiac Apex and Visceral Situs

The location of the cardiac apex and visceral situs provides important diagnostic clues. Discordance of the situs and cardiac apex (i.e., apex to

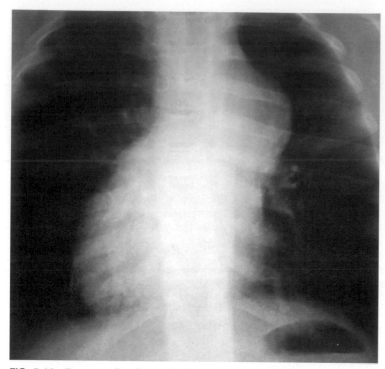

FIG. 5-16 Dextrocardia (heart in the right side of the chest) associated with situs solitus. This pattern is commonly associated with ventricular inversion (corrected transposition of the great arteries). The prominent vascular shadow noted along the left-sided cardiac border is the aorta.

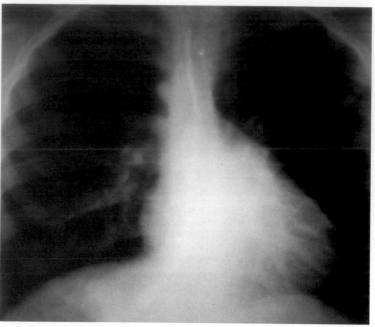

FIG. 5-17 Levocardia with situs inversus. Discordance of the apex of the heart and visceral situs often is associated with structural congenital heart defects. The hepatic portion of the inferior vena cava is absent in this patient, and there is azygos vein continuation. Note the prominence of the shadow at the high right-sided cardiac border.

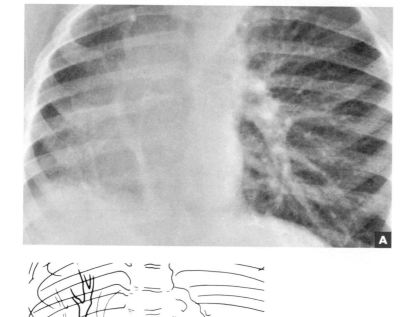

Scimitar shadow

Systemic artery

FIG. 5-18 *A,* Radiographic appearance of scimitar syndrome with a hypoplastic right lung. The scimitar-shaped shadow is formed by pulmonary veins draining the sequestered segment and connecting to the inferior vena cava. *B,* Note also the systemic artery coursing diagonally upward from the abdominal aorta to the sequestered lobe.

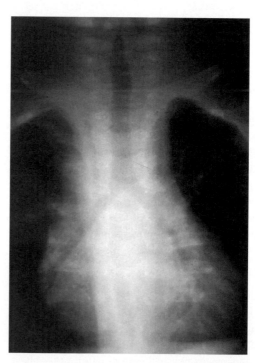

FIG. 5-19 Atrial isomerism should be suspected when the heart is midline on the chest x-ray and with situs ambiguus. The best radiographic sign of right or left atrial isomerism pertains to the symmetry of bronchial anatomy, with right atrial isomerism being related to bilateral right bronchi and left atrial isomerism to bilateral left bronchi.

the right with situs solitus or apex to the left with situs inversus) often is associated with structural congenital heart disease (Figs. 5-16 and 5-17). Dextrocardia (apex to the right) with situs solitus is a frequent presentation of ventricular inversion or corrected transposition of the great arteries (Fig. 5-16). Dextrocardia also can be seen with primary pulmonary problems. Scimitar syndrome comprises dextrocardia with hypoplasia of the right lung (Fig. 5-18). In this case a major portion of the right lung (usually the right lower lobe) has its arterial supply by way of

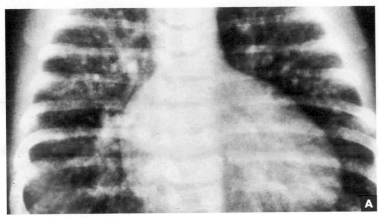

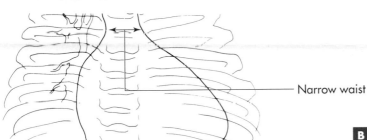

FIG. 5-20 "Egg on a string" heart shadow resulting from transposition of the great arteries. The main pulmonary artery is posterior and slightly to the left of the aorta, contributing to the narrow waist (the "string").

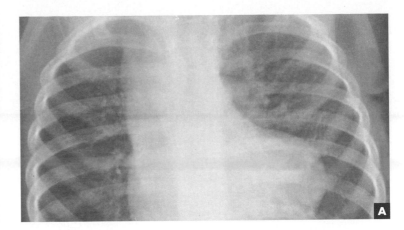

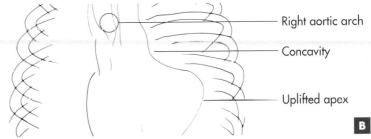

FIG. 5-21 Tetralogy of Fallot with pulmonic stenosis produces this "boot-shaped" heart. Because of right ventricular hypertrophy, the apex is tilted upward, and the small right ventricular infundibulum and small main pulmonary artery cause the concavity in the left upper border of the heart. Right aortic arch is present.

a systemic artery from the descending aorta, and the pulmonary venous return from that lung drains abnormally into the inferior vena cava, forming a scimitar (Fig. 5-18). Patients with levocardia (apex to the left) with either situs inversus or situs ambiguus frequently have complex congenital heart diseases such as transposition of the great arteries, pulmonary atresia, and atrioventricular septal defects. Atrial isomerism can be recognized as bilateral symmetric short or long bronchi. This is best demonstrated with a magnified penetrated chest x-ray examination focusing on bronchial anatomy (Fig. 5-19). Almost all patients with this anomaly have complex congenital heart disease.

Shape and Size

Cardiac size is important, but the shape of the cardiac image may provide a clue as to which heart chambers are enlarged and the likely structural diagnosis. In the cyanotic newborn with transposition of the great arteries, the cardiac image appears as an "egg on a string" (Fig. 5-20). If the thymic shadow does not obscure it, the mediastinal shadow shows a narrow waist resulting from the posteromedial position of the main pulmonary artery. This produces the "string." Pulmonary vascular markings usually are increased, although vascularity may be normal in the immediate newborn period.

In tetralogy of Fallot with pulmonic stenosis, the heart appears "boot-shaped" because right ventricular hypertrophy causes the apex (toe of the boot) to turn upward (Fig. 5-21). The concavity of the left upper cardiac border is due to the small right ventricular outflow tract and pulmonary artery segment.

In tetralogy of Fallot with pulmonary atresia, the heart is shaped like an "egg on its side" (Fig. 5-22). The pulmonary blood flow to the lungs

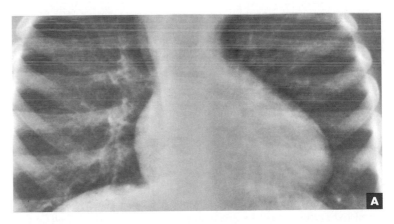

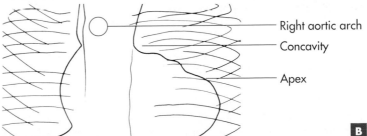

FIG. 5-22 Tetralogy of Fallot with pulmonary atresia produces this "egg on its side" appearance. Note the uplifted apex resulting from the right ventricular hypertrophy. There is concavity because of the absence of right ventricular outflow and small main pulmonary artery segment. Note also the right aortic arch.

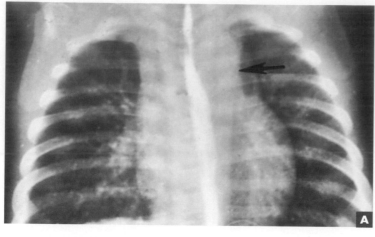

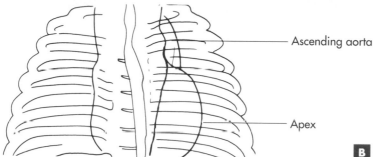

FIG. 5-23   Radiograph shows the "valentine-shaped" heart characteristically found in transposition of the great arteries. Note the ascending aorta on the left side.

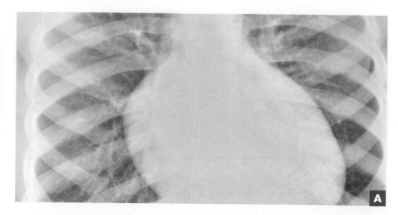

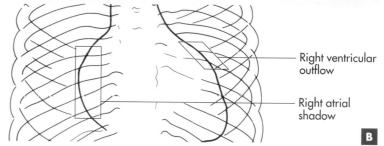

FIG. 5-24   Radiograph demonstrates the "box-shaped" heart associated with Ebstein anomaly of the tricuspid valve. Note the enlarged right atrium and right ventricular outflow tract.

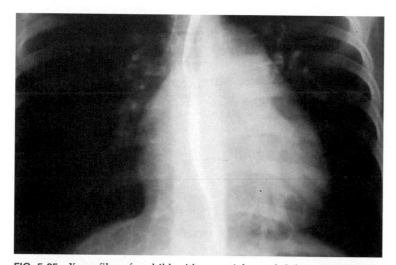

FIG. 5-25   X-ray film of a child with an atrial septal defect. Note the enlarged right atrium, right ventricle, and pulmonary artery, as well as the increased pulmonary vascular markings.

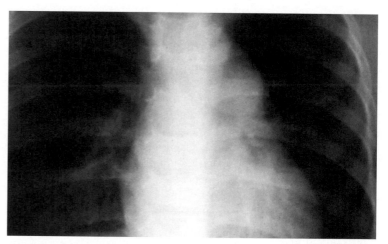

FIG. 5-26   Prominence of the main and left pulmonary arteries is the only radiographic abnormality in this child with pulmonic valve stenosis.

may be supplied by either a patent ductus arteriosus or systemic arterial collateral vessels. The pulmonary vascular markings are decreased if pulmonary blood flow is patent ductus–dependent and increased if large systemic collaterals supply pulmonary blood flow.

In corrected transposition of the great arteries, the heart has a "valentine" or "heart" shape with the apex pointing downward just to the left of the midline, as shown in Fig. 5-23. The fullness in the left upper border is due to the ascending aorta.

Massive cardiac enlargement is typical in patients with Ebstein anomaly, or malformation of the tricuspid valve. In this anomaly there is displacement of the inferior and septal leaflets of the tricuspid valve

into the ventricle, causing severe tricuspid valve regurgitation or stenosis. As a result the right atrium becomes markedly enlarged and, along with the right ventricle, contributes significantly to a cardiac image of a box-shaped heart (Fig. 5-24).

Left-to-right shunt lesions from atrial septal defects, ventricular septal defects, or a patent ductus arteriosus demonstrate specific chamber enlargement and increased pulmonary vascular markings. A significant atrial defect will show enlargement of all right-sided cardiac chambers, including right atrium, right ventricle, and pulmonary artery (Fig. 5-25). A patent ductus arteriosus shows enlargement of all left-sided cardiac chambers, including the aorta. In patients with a ven-

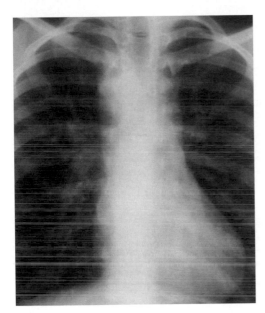

FIG. 5-27 The only radiographic sign of aortic valve stenosis in children is dilation of the ascending aorta.

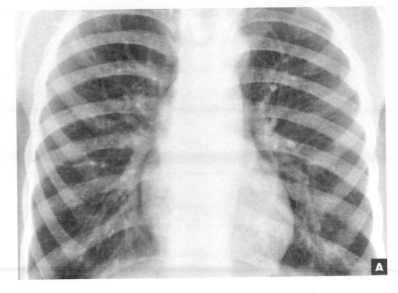

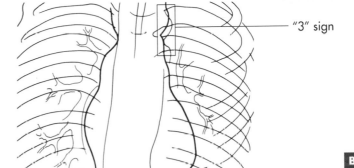

FIG. 5-28 Radiograph of a 5-year-old child reveals the characteristic signs of coarctation of the aorta. The site of the stenosis can be observed at the center of the "3" sign with pre- and poststenotic dilation of the aorta.

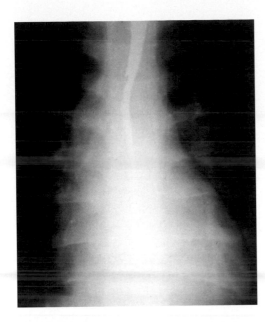

FIG. 5-29 Right aortic arch in a child with truncus arteriosus is demonstrated by deviation of the tracheal air column to the left.

tricular septal defect, the right atrium is the only heart chamber that is not enlarged.

Great Vessels

The radiographic appearance of the great arteries also may suggest a specific structural congenital heart defect. The main and left branch pulmonary arteries usually are enlarged in patients with pulmonary valve stenosis (Fig. 5-26). The characteristic radiographic finding of congenital aortic valve stenosis is dilation of the ascending aorta, best seen as an overlapping shadow with the superior vena cava along the right upper cardiac border (Fig. 5-27). Coarctation of the aorta not di-

agnosed in a timely fashion may show the distinct radiographic finding of a reversed E or 3 sign caused by poststenotic dilation of the descending aorta (Fig. 5-28).

The normal left aortic arch causes a shift of the tracheal air column to the right, whereas a right arch causes a similar deviation to the left (Fig. 5-29). A right aortic arch has been associated with tetralogy of Fallot or truncus arteriosus in about 30% of patients with those lesions.

The addition of a barium swallow to the chest x-ray examination is an important diagnostic tool in the assessment of patients with upper airway obstruction from vascular rings. If a bilateral indentation is noted on the barium esophagram, a double aortic arch should be sus-

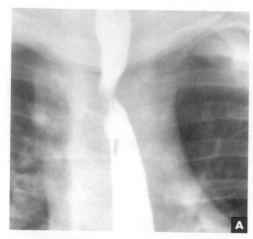

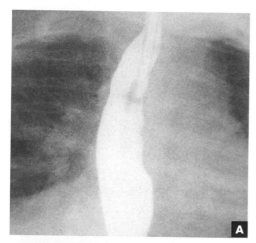

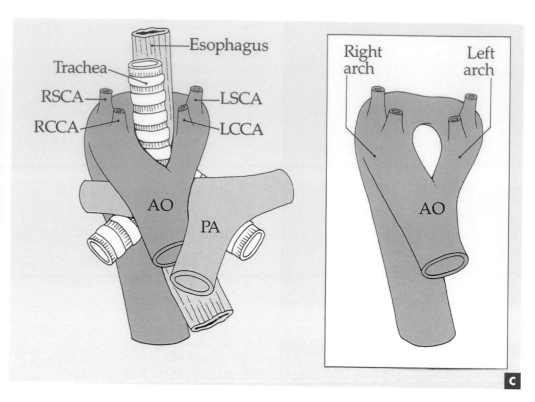

FIG. 5-30 A barium esophagram is essential when infants with stridor are evaluated. In this child the bilateral compressions and marked retroesophageal indentation are caused by a double aortic arch.

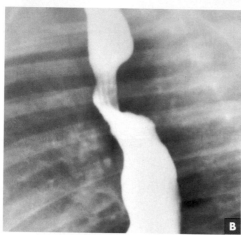

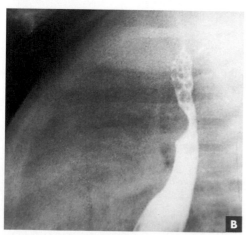

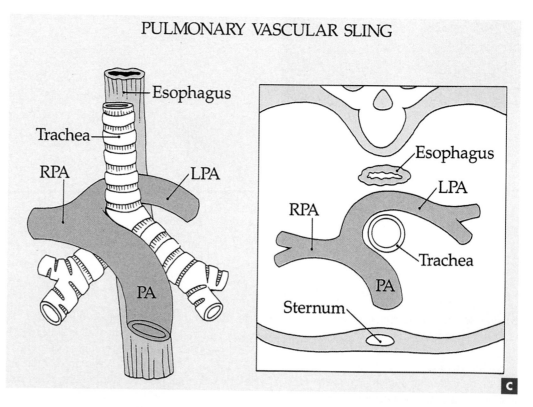

PULMONARY VASCULAR SLING

FIG. 5-31 Anomalous left pulmonary artery (the pulmonary artery sling) can be observed as a rounded indentation between the barium-filled esophagus posteriorly and the air-filled trachea anteriorly.

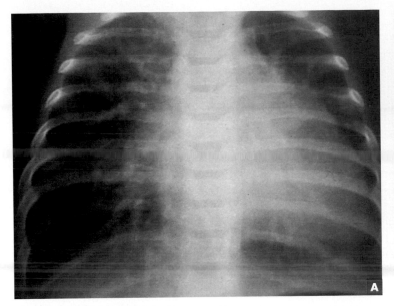

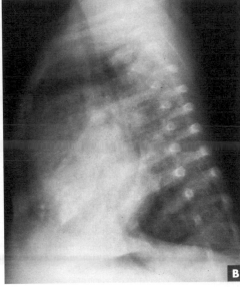

FIG. 5-32 Postero-anterior *(A)* and lateral *(B)* radiographs from a 2-month-old infant with a large left-to-right shunt from a ventricular septal defect. The lung hyperinflation with flattened hemidiaphragms is clearly seen on the lateral projection. This finding is predictive of associated pulmonary hypertension.

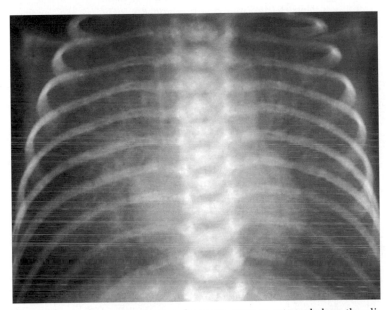

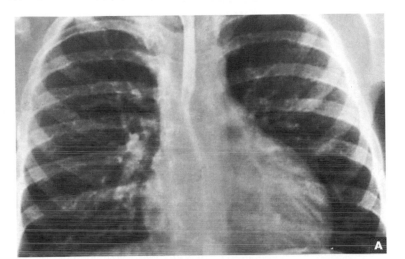

FIG. 5-33 A total anomalous pulmonary venous return below the diaphragm leads to a radiographic finding of severe pulmonary venous obstruction and pulmonary edema, mimicking a respiratory distress syndrome.

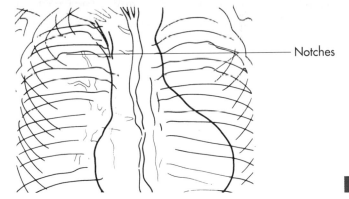

— Notches

FIG. 5-34 Rib notching can be observed here, resulting from coarctation of the aorta in the older child.

pected (Fig. 5-30). A right aortic arch with distal origin of the left subclavian or a left aortic arch with distal origin of the right subclavian also produces posterior indentation on the barium esophagram, but usually it is not associated with airway compromise. An anterior esophageal indentation is almost always caused by distal origin of the pulmonary artery coursing between the trachea and esophagus and causing a pulmonary sling (Fig. 5-31).

Pulmonary Vascularity

Left-to-right shunt lesions are associated with increased pulmonary blood flow that causes primarily arterial or a combination of arterial and venous markings on the chest radiograph. Hyperinflation seen on the chest x-ray film is a characteristic finding in infants with a large left-to-right shunt associated with pulmonary hypertension (Fig. 5-32). Patients with pulmonary venous obstruction, such as infradiaphragmatic total anomalous pulmonary venous return, show a fine reticular pattern of pulmonary venous obstruction, which may mimic respiratory distress syndrome in the neonate (Fig. 5-33). It should be cautioned that the in-

terpretation of pulmonary vascularity can be quite difficult and should always be interpreted within the context of other clinical findings.

Skeletal Abnormalities

Attention also should be given to the thoracic cage, including the spine and ribs. Although abnormal fusions of ribs and hemivertebrae are not pathognomonic for specific congenital heart lesions, there is a higher incidence when these findings are present. Rib notching is a distinct radiographic finding in patients with coarctation of the aorta (Fig. 5-34).

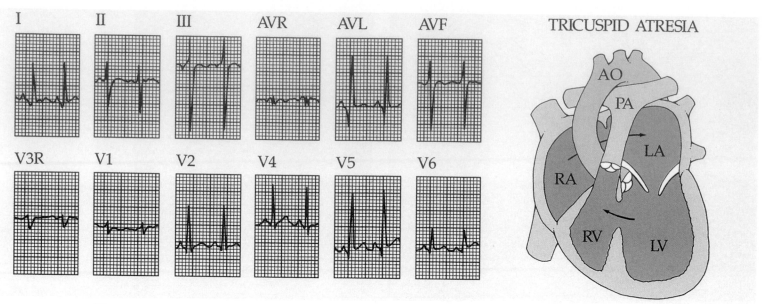

FIG. 5-35 Electrocardiogram of a child with tricuspid atresia. Note the left axis deviation, left atrial enlargement, and left ventricular hypertrophy. *AO*, Aorta; *LA*, left atrium; *LV*, left ventricle; *PA*, pulmonary artery; *RA*, right atrium; *RV*, right ventricle.

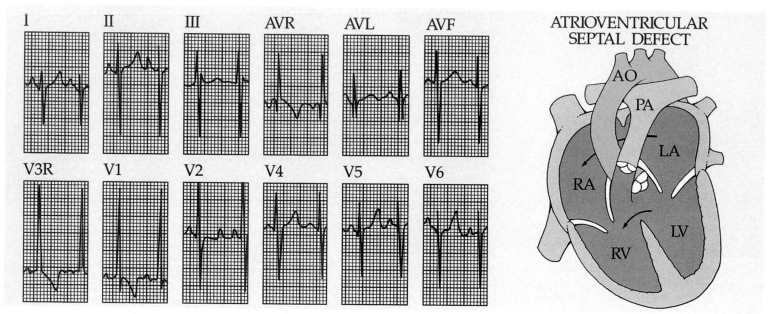

FIG. 5-36 Typical electrocardiogram of a child with an atrioventricular septal defect. Note the superior (northwest) axis deviation and right ventricular hypertrophy.

Scoliosis is a common finding in teenage patients with cyanotic congenital heart disease. Pectus excavatum may cause a false impression of cardiac enlargement because of a "pancaking" effect on the heart from a narrow anteroposterior thoracic diameter.

Electrocardiography and Dysrhythmias

Electrocardiography

It is impractical and unnecessary for pediatricians to have a thorough knowledge of detailed electrocardiogram interpretation; however, it is valuable to be able to recognize certain typical electrocardiographic patterns that yield important diagnostic information. For instance, it is common for children to have a frontal plane axis that is either normal (0 to 90 degrees) or in the right axis deviation range from 90 to 120 degrees. A superior axis suggests specific defects. A left axis deviation that includes the range 0 to −90 degrees and is associated with a QR pattern in leads I and AVL is frequently seen in the following situations:

a cyanotic newborn with tricuspid atresia (Fig. 5-35), an atrioventricular septal defect with or without Down syndrome (Fig. 5-36), Noonan syndrome, or some of the varieties of single ventricle. When the frontal plane axis falls between 180 and 270 degrees, it is usually referred to as a *northwest axis* and is frequently found in atrioventricular septal defects or other lesions that lead to severe right ventricular hypertrophy.

It is difficult to be certain about hypertrophy in the pediatric age group because of the wide range of normal values that vary with age. This is particularly true of right ventricular hypertrophy, which can be a physiologic finding in the first several years of life. On the other hand, left ventricular predominance in the newborn is almost always a pathologic finding and usually indicates one of the hypoplastic right heart syndromes, such as tricuspid atresia or pulmonary atresia with an intact septum.

Conduction abnormalities, such as Wolff-Parkinson-White syndrome, prolonged corrected Q-T interval, and atrioventricular block are readily apparent on the 12-lead electrocardiogram and are discussed further in the following section on dysrhythmias.

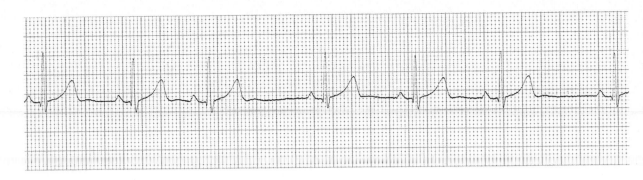

FIG. 5-37 Sinus arrhythmia. Note variable QRS cycle lengths without change in the P wave–QRS relationship.

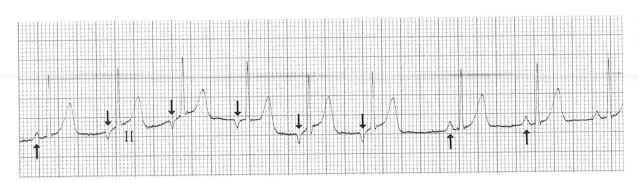

FIG. 5-38 Wandering atrial pacemaker. The morphology of the P wave varies, indicating origin from either the sinus node *(upward arrows)* or an ectopic atrial site *(downward arrows)*.

TABLE 5-4

Pediatric Dysrhythmias

Treatment not required	Treatment required
Sinus arrhythmia	Supraventricular tachycardia
Wandering (ectopic) atrial pacemaker	Ventricular tachycardia
Isolated premature atrial contractions	Third-degree atrioventricular block with symptoms
Isolated premature ventricular contractions	
First-degree atrioventricular block	

Dysrhythmias

Disorders of heart rate or rhythm are not nearly as common in childhood as they are in adulthood, but it is vital that pediatricians are familiar with dysrhythmias that may occur in otherwise healthy children. An outline of these disorders based on the need for treatment is presented in Table 5-4. For the numerous rhythm disorders not listed, management must be individualized, taking into account the presence or absence of associated heart disease.

Transient dysrhythmias may present in the following manner: an asymptomatic child with an irregular heartbeat noted on examination, palpitations, chest pain (a common complaint among children less than 10 years of age when they sense a tachycardia), dizziness or presyncope, or actual syncope with or without seizure activity. More sustained dysrhythmias may lead to congestive heart failure, cardiogenic shock, or even death. The most common irregularity of heart rhythm seen in children is a sinus arrhythmia. This is a normal variant that reflects a healthy interaction between autonomic respiratory and cardiac control activity in the central nervous system. Typically the heart rate increases during inspiration and decreases during expiration and may sound wildly irregular on auscultation unless careful attention is paid to the relationship between the heart rate and respirations (Fig. 5-37). Another normal variant occurs when the atrial pacemaker transiently shifts from the sinus node to another atrial site with only minimal variation in the heart rate. This is often referred to as a *wandering atrial pacemaker* (Fig. 5-38). Premature atrial contractions are generally benign when they occur in the absence of underlying heart disease. They are particularly common during the newborn period, when they are often associated with aberrant conduction (Fig. 5-39) or apparent pauses (Fig. 5-40) resulting from failure of conduction to the ventricle of the premature atrial impulse. *Isolated premature ventricular* beats are not common but may be seen with an incidence of 0.3% to 2.2% and rarely require treatment as long as there is no associated heart disease. This form of ectopy is rec-

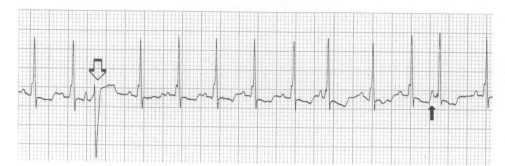

FIG. 5-39 Premature atrial contractions. These premature complexes may be associated with aberrant conduction of the QRS *(open arrow)* or normal conduction *(solid arrow).*

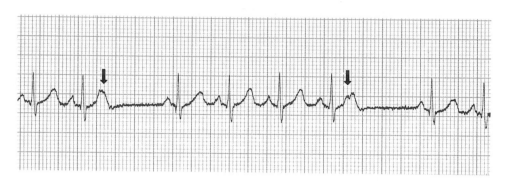

FIG. 5-40 Nonconducted premature atrial contractions. Arrows indicate premature atrial beats that are not conducted, resulting in apparent pauses.

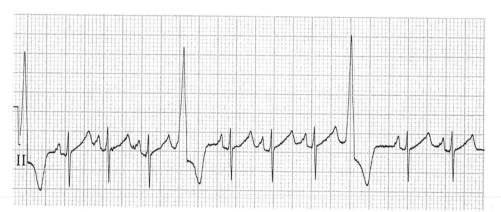

FIG. 5-41 Premature ventricular contractions. The obvious wide QRS premature complexes demonstrate an abnormal T wave, fully compensatory pause, and absence of a preceding P wave.

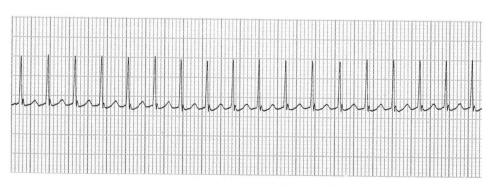

FIG. 5-42 Supraventricular tachycardia. This is a normal QRS complex tachycardia at a rate of 214 beats per minute. Note lack of visible P waves.

ognizable by a wide QRS, a T wave opposite in direction to the QRS in any given lead, dissocation from the P wave, and usually a full compensatory pause (Fig. 5-41). For the abovementioned abnormality, an appropriate initial workup includes a 12-lead electrocardiogram and rhythm strip and brief exercise in the office to see if the ectopy is suppressed or becomes more frequent as the heart rate increases. An exacerbation of the dysrhythmia with this maneuver would warrant further cardiologic investigation.

By far the most common dysrhythmia requiring treatment in the pediatric population is supraventricular tachycardia (SVT). The most frequent age of presentation is in the first 3 months of life, with secondary peaks occurring at 8 to 10 years and again during adolescence. This rhythm disorder is characterized by a regular, narrow complex tachycardia with rates that vary with the patient's age. The overall average rate for SVT at all ages is 235 beats per minute; however, in the first 9 months the average is 270 beats per minute compared with 210 beats per minute in older children (Fig. 5-42). Discrete P waves are usually difficult to define, but if present, there is always a one-to-one relationship to the QRS. There may be dramatic ST segment changes during tachycardia that resolve shortly after conversion to sinus rhythm.

Two important points with regard to SVT include differentiating sinus tachycardia in an infant and the value of the 12-lead electrocardio-

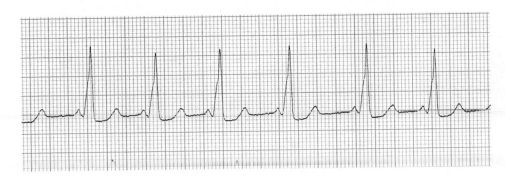

FIG. 5-43 Wolff-Parkinson-White syndrome. Characteristic findings include short P-R interval, slurred upstroke of QRS (delta wave), and prolongation of the QRS interval.

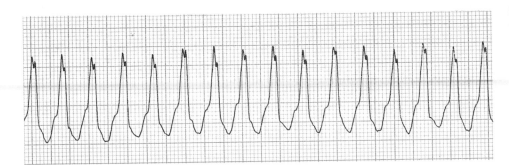

FIG. 5-44 Ventricular tachycardia. Wide QRS complex tachycardia at a rate of 188 beats per minute.

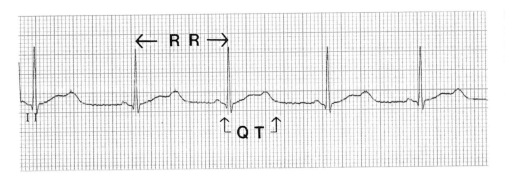

FIG. 5-45 Prolonged Q-T syndrome. The corrected Q-T interval is prolonged at 0.57 second (upper limit of normal is 0.44 second). The Q-T interval must be corrected for heart rate by using the formula: measured Q-T interval (0.56 second) divided by the square root of the preceding RR interval (0.96 second).

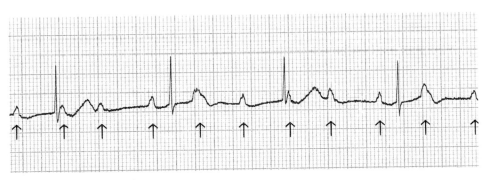

FIG. 5-46 Complete heart block. Tracing demonstrates atrial activity *(arrows)* independent of a slower ventricular rhythm.

gram after conversion to sinus rhythm. In a child less than 1 year of age, during periods of severe stress such as sepsis or high fever, the sinus rate may reach 220 to 250 beats per minute. At this rate the P wave will be lost in the T wave. Facial ice water immersion or intravenous adenosine may be invaluable in differentiating this form of rapid sinus tachycardia from SVT: in the latter case the intervention will terminate the tachycardia abruptly, whereas in the former it will produce only transient slowing and the P waves will become evident on the downstroke of the T wave. With regard to the postconversion 12-lead electrocardiogram, it is important to recognize the presence of Wolff-Parkinson-White syndrome, which occurs in 25% of patients with SVT. This syndrome is characterized by a short PR interval, a delta-wave, and prolongation of the QRS complex (Fig. 5-43) and will not be evident when the tachycardia is present.

Sustained ventricular tachycardia is distinctly uncommon in childhood, and the patient must be thoroughly investigated for underlying heart disease. This dysrhythmia is usually associated with hemodynamic compromise and is characterized by a regular wide-complex tachycardia usually with atrioventricular dissociation if P waves are visible (Fig. 5-44). This life-threatening disorder most commonly occurs in children who have had open-heart surgical repair for tetralogy of Fallot or other complex anomalies or who have a cardiomyopathy, myocarditis, or myocardial tumor. It is also important to look for a prolonged corrected Q-T interval because this abnormality of repolarization may lead to recurrent syncope and sudden death secondary to ventricular tachycardia or fibrillation (Fig. 5-45). Symptomatic bradycardia is rarely encountered in the pediatric age group. One condition that needs to be recognized is congenital third-degree atrioventricular block (Fig. 5-46).

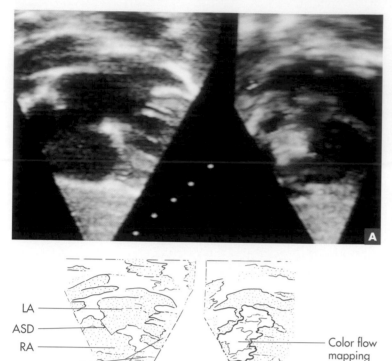

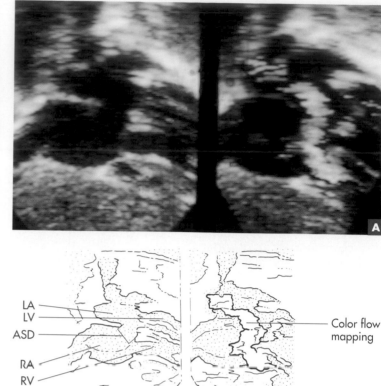

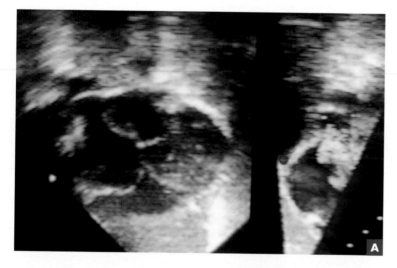

LA
ASD
RA
RV

Color flow
mapping

B

FIG. 5-47 A large secundum atrial septal defect *(left)* is seen in the fossa ovale area on the subcostal view *(arrow)*. Color flow mapping *(right)* confirms marked left-to-right shunt *(dotted)*.

LA
LV
ASD
RA
RV

Color flow
mapping

B

FIG. 5-48 A partial form of an atrioventricular septal defect *(left)* is seen in the inferior portion of the atrial septum *(arrow)*. Significant left-to-right shunt is shown on color flow mapping *(right)*.

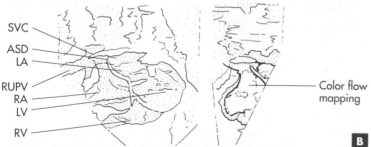

SVC
ASD
LA
RUPV
RA
LV
RV

Color flow
mapping

B

FIG. 5-49 Sinus venosus defect *(left)* appears in the posterosuperior portion of the atrial septum, where the right upper pulmonary vein (RUPV, *arrow*) opens directly into the superior vena cava (SVC, *arrow*). Shunts from the anomalous drainage from the right upper pulmonary vein and from the left atrium are seen on color flow mapping *(right)*.

This may occur with associated structural heart disease but more frequently with an otherwise normal heart. The presence of maternal connective tissue disease or antinuclear antibodies should always be sought as a possible cause when a newborn with congenital atrioventricular block is detected.

When a patient is evaluated for a history of syncope or new onset seizures, it is highly recommended that the physican obtain an electrocardiogram to look for "footprints" of a possible dysrhythmic cause. The possibilities include: Wolff-Parkinson-White syndrome (providing a substrate for rapid supraventricular tachycardia), prolonged corrected Q-T interval (predisposing to severe ventricular dysrhythmias), or atrioventricular block (leading to Stokes-Adams attacks).

Echocardiography

Cross-sectional echocardiography was the most important advance in the investigation of congenital heart defects in the early 1980s. The echocardiographic image in various cross-sectional views can accurately identify common and complex structural congenital heart defects. The addition of Doppler and color flow mapping provides another dimension to the accuracy of anatomic diagnosis and noninvasive hemodynamic assessment. Thus cross-sectional echocardiography and Doppler technique have provided invaluable assistance to the management of patients with congenital heart disease and represent complementary tools to cardiac catheterization and angiography.

All types of septal defects can be readily visualized by cross-sectional echocardiography. The atrial septal defects are reliably demonstrated by the subcostal approach. The most common type is the secundum defect, which involves the middle portion of the atrial septum (Fig. 5-47). An ostium primum defect known as *a partial form of an atrioventricular septal defect* is seen in Fig. 5-48. The sinus venosus

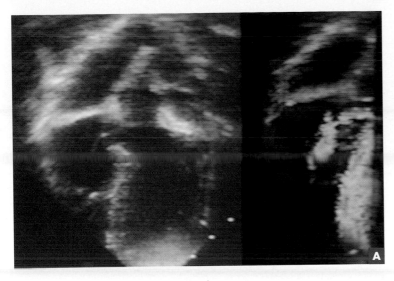

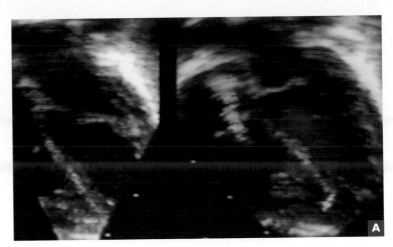

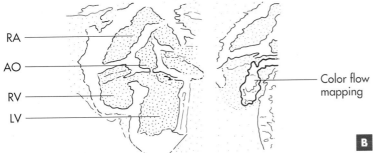

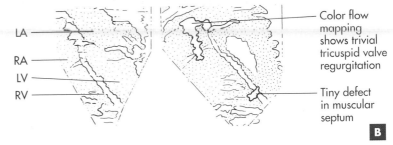

FIG. 5-50 On apical four-chamber views, a perimembranous ventricular septal defect *(left)* is seen in the ventricular septum *(arrow)*. Significant left-to-right shunt through the defect is confirmed by color flow mapping *(right)*.

FIG. 5-51 Muscular ventricular septal defect. No apparent defect in the ventricular septum could be visualized on 2-dimensional imaging *(left)*. However, color flow mapping *(right)* confirmed a tiny defect in the muscular septum near the apex by showing a jet *(yellowish-red jet)*. In addition, a trivial tricuspid valve regurgitation is noted *(blue jet)*.

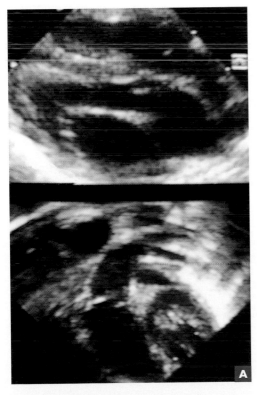

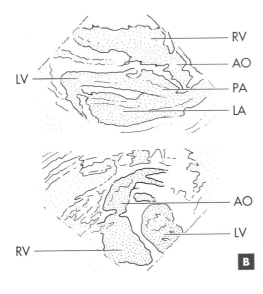

FIG. 5-52 Transposition of the great arteries. *A* and *B* The parasternal long axial view shows a parallel arrangement of the great vessels *(top)*. Origination of the aorta from the right ventricle is confirmed in the apical four-chamber view *(bottom)*.
Continued

type of atrial septal defect is located in the posterosuperior portion of the atrial septum at the opening of the superior vena cava and is associated with partial anomalous pulmonary venous return of the right upper pulmonary vein (Fig. 5-49).

Similarly a ventricular septal defect can be accurately diagnosed by using the apical four-chamber view, as shown in Fig. 5-50. The most common defect is in the perimembranous septum located in the subaortic area bordered by the atrioventricular valves. However, a defect located in the muscular septum can be difficult to image, particularly if it is located near the apical trabecular area of the ventricle. However, color flow mapping techniques facilitate the detection of even the smallest defect when imaging of the defect is not possible (Fig. 5-51).

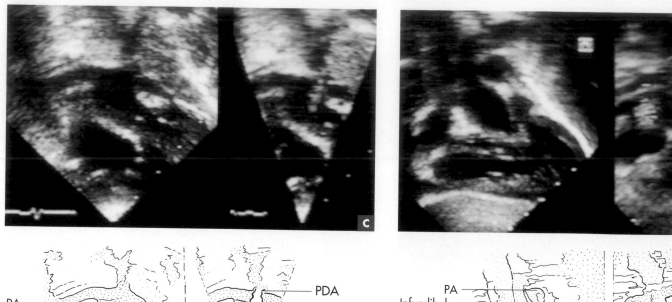

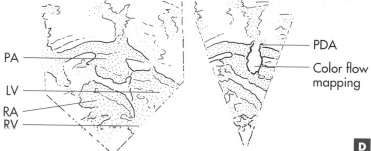

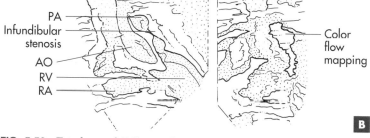

FIG. 5-52, cont'd *C* and *D,* Connection of the pulmonary artery with the left ventricle *(left)* confirms the diagnosis. The color flow map *(right)* shows left-to-right shunt through a small patent duct (PDA) appearing as a yellowish-red jet.

FIG. 5-53 Tetralogy of Fallot. Subcostal view shows both valvular pulmonic and infundibular stenotic components *(left).* Color flow map *(right)* confirms formation of turbulence *(mosaic color)* across the stenotic area.

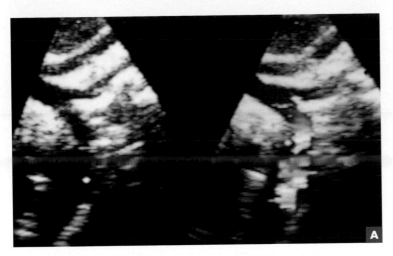

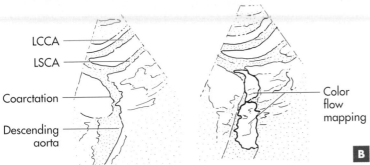

FIG. 5-54 Coarctation of the aorta. Suprasternal view *(left)* demonstrates a discrete narrowing *(arrow)* in the proximal portion of the descending aorta. Color flow map *(right)* confirms the turbulent flow pattern *(aliasing)* across the coarctation. LCCA, left common carotid artery; LSCA, left subclavian artery.

Accurate diagnosis of most structural congenital heart diseases, whether simple or complex, can be made by echocardiography. A systematic approach to define major intracardiac connections is a useful starting point: (1) venoatrial connection (systemic or pulmonary venous return to the right or left atrium), (2) atrioventricular, and (3) ventriculoarterial connection (ventricle to the great vessels).

If the pulmonary veins are not communicated with the left atrium, total anomalous pulmonary venous return should be suspected. Corrected transposition is the most likely diagnosis when the atrioventricular connection is not concordant, whereas transposition of the great arteries is suspected when the ventriculoarterial connection is discordant. The rather characteristic finding of parallel takeoff of the great vessels from both ventricles is seen in transposition of the great arteries, with the aorta arising anteriorly from the right ventricle and the pulmonary artery originating posteriorly from the left ventricle (Fig. 5-52).

Typical findings in another common cyanotic heart lesion, tetralogy of Fallot, are a dilated aortic root that overrides the ventricular septum, a large perimembranous ventricular septal defect, and right ventricular outflow obstruction (Fig. 5-53). The aortic arch is best visualized by a suprasternal approach, and the diagnosis of interrupted aortic arch or coarctation of the aorta can be readily diagnosed in most cases (Fig. 5-54).

BIBLIOGRAPHY

French JW, Guntheroth WG: An explanation of asymmetric upper extremity blood pressures in supravalvular aortic stenosis: the Coanda effect, *Circulation* 42:31-36, 1970.

Greenwood RD: Cardiovascular malformations associated with extracardiac anomalies and malformation syndromes, *Clin Pediatr* 23(3):145-151, 1984.

National Heart, Lung, and Blood Institute Task Force on Blood Pressure Control in Children: Report, *Pediatrics* 59(suppl):797-820, 1977.

Spicer RL: Cardiovascular disease in Down syndrome, *Pediatr Clin North Am* 31(6):1331-1343, 1984.

Zuberbuhler JR: *Clinical diagnosis in pediatric cardiology*, Edinburgh, 1981, Churchill Livingstone.

6

Child Abuse and Neglect

HOLLY W. DAVIS ❧ MARY M. CARRASCO

Child abuse and neglect constitute a pediatric public health problem of enormous magnitude. Their relative contribution to morbidity and mortality in children is especially prominent in developed nations, where sanitation, immunization, and high standards of medical care have substantially reduced the sequelae of infectious diseases.

Although the incidence of abuse and neglect appears to have increased within the past century, improved reporting must also be considered. Caffey in the late 1940s and then Kempe and coworkers in the early 1960s fostered a marked increase in the recognition of the physical manifestations of abuse and of the real needs and problems of child abuse victims. Subsequent passage of legislation mandating that suspected cases be reported to the proper authorities has further improved the incidence of reporting. Thus, while some of the increasing incidence is real, much is probably the result of these developments. Additionally, societal standards have changed, for much of what is currently regarded as abuse was once sanctioned as discipline.

Four major forms of abuse have been delineated: physical abuse, sexual abuse, physical neglect, and emotional abuse. Not infrequently, an individual child is found to be the victim of more than one form. For purposes of reporting under abuse laws, the abuse or neglect generally must result from the acts or omissions of a parent, guardian, custodian, or other caretaker of the child.

Statistics (National Center on Child Abuse and Neglect, U.S. Dept. of Health and Human Services) for the United States in 1995 underline the extent of the problem: 3.1 million cases were reported, representing an increase of 24% over 6 years. Thirty-two percent of these reports were substantiated by child protection authorities. Of these, 53% involved neglect, 26% physical abuse, 10% sexual abuse, and 3% emotional maltreatment. An average of 1100 fatalities (most occurring in children less than 1 year of age) resulting from abuse were recognized during the 6 years from 1989 to 1995. These figures may significantly underestimate the actual number: it is estimated that for every case reported, two go unreported. Furthermore, findings from recent investigations indicate that many fatal cases of abuse are listed as resulting from natural causes or accidents, because many coroners and pathologists have not received thorough training in the manifestations of abuse and neglect. Obtaining full skeletal surveys on all unexplained infant death victims could uncover a significant percentage who were victims of abuse.

Epidemiology

The incidence of child abuse per capita is greatest in lower socioeconomic groups, probably stemming in part from the chronic stresses of living in poverty and problems of socialization. Nevertheless, abuse is a phenomenon found in all socioeconomic, cultural, racial, and religious subsets of society although children of lower socioeconomic status are more likely to be reported.

Parental Risk Factors

1. **Past history of being an abused child.** NOTE: Not all abused children grow up to become abusive adults. Those who do not have been found to have had a strong long-standing and supportive relationship with a nonabusive adult. This appears to have enabled them to develop better social support systems. They are also more able to recall their childhood and express their feelings about it and are less ambivalent about having and raising children.
2. **Poor socialization and lack of trust in others.** Such people have difficulty with relationships, and thus they are inadequately nurtured as adults and socially isolated because they are poorly equipped to develop and utilize support systems. They also tend to have little understanding of child development and therefore of reasonable expectations and children's emotional needs. A common pattern involves an unmarried mother, living with a series of paramours, each of whom stays for a short period and then leaves to be replaced by another. These men have no investment in the woman's children and tend to have little patience with them.
3. **Limited ability to cope with stress, anger, and frustration and a tendency to lash out violently, either verbally or physically, in response to negative feelings.**
4. **Alcoholism, addiction, or psychosis.** The recent increase in crack addiction has had a particular impact, resulting in a disturbing rise in cases of gross neglect and unusually brutal physical abuse.
5. **Membership in certain fringe group cults or sects.**

Child Risk Factors

1. **Age less than 3 years.** Young children are unable to escape attack, are incapable developmentally of meeting many expectations, and frequently are negativistic and stubborn.
2. **Infants separated from their mothers at birth because of illness or prematurity** (perhaps resulting in part from impaired bonding by a high-risk mother).

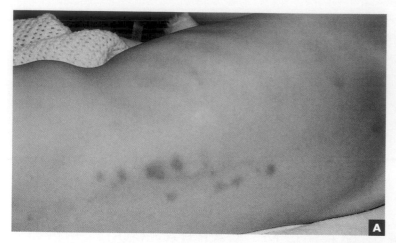
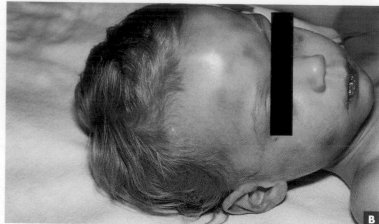
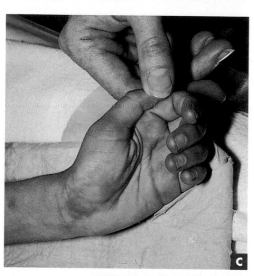
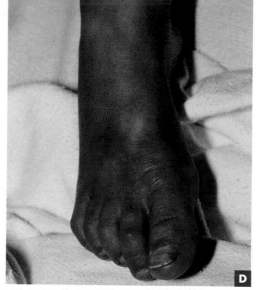
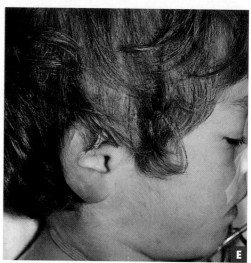

FIG. 6-1 Inflicted bruises found in unusual locations. *A,* Multiple ecchymoses are evident over the back and upper chest of this child who presented in a poorly nourished condition but whose coagulation study findings were normal. *B,* The same patient with multiple bruises of the face and forehead. *C* and *D,* This child had severe contusions over the hands and feet, which were inflicted with a ruler. *E,* The same child also had a markedly swollen and contused ear.

3. **Infants born with congenital anomalies and children with chronic illness** (possibly resulting from parental grieving and guilt compounded by the chronic stress of caring for a handicapped child).
4. **Children who are seen as difficult or different.**
5. **Foster children and, less commonly, adopted children.**

A common thread connecting all of these risk factors appears to be one of unmet expectations, either unrealistic parental expectations of the child or the child's inability to meet realistic expectations as the result of developmental delay, hyperactivity, or inconsistent disciplining.

With the preceding as background, the approach to diagnosis of the major forms of abuse can now be addressed more specifically. Checklists for use in evaluation of patients with suspected physical and sexual abuse are presented in Appendices A and B.

Physical Abuse

Physical abuse is defined as the infliction of injury that causes significant pain, leaves physical evidence, impairs physical functioning, or significantly jeopardizes the child's safety. It is usually repetitive and, as already noted, tends to escalate in severity over time. Given this, early recognition, reporting, and intervention are essential to prevent-

ing future, more severe injuries. The increasing incidence of severe and fatal cases had led to an effort to detect identifiable risk factors that might be predictive of fatal outcome. The majority of perpetrators of such abuse who have been studied have been found to have been severely abused themselves as children. Poverty, unemployment, a long history of family violence, drug and alcohol abuse, and adolescent parenthood are common threads. Fathers and paramours are by far the most common perpetrators, responsible for up to 58% of the cases. Babysitters have been identified as abusers in up to 21% of severe cases and mothers in up to 13%. Overall, male caretakers are responsible for nearly 70% of severe cases of physical abuse. Crying and toilet training accidents are the most common triggering events. Victims frequently have histories or evidence of prior suspicious injuries, and often of a series of injuries of increasing severity, before the final beating.

The diagnosis of inflicted injury is established on the basis of a constellation of factors, including historical, physical, and behavioral observations. Radiographs and laboratory studies are often useful in confirming injuries and in ruling out other differential diagnostic possibilities.

Historical Factors
In many instances, one or more of the following historical red flags provides the first clue to abuse:

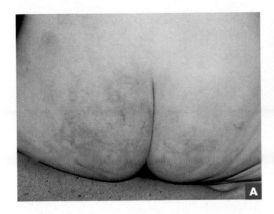
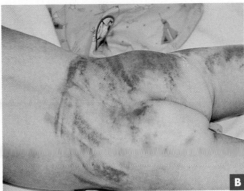
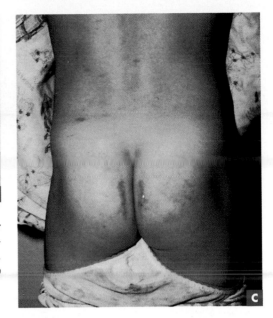

FIG. 6-2 Buttock bruises. *A,* At first glance this toddler appeared to have a diaper rash, but on closer inspection the lesions were found to be petechiae produced by a severe spanking. *B,* The severe contusions of the buttocks and lower back seen in this child were inflicted by hand, hairbrush, and belt. *C,* A linear pattern of petechial hemorrhages is seen on either side of the gluteal cleft in this boy who was subjected to repeated rapid-fire blows across the gluteal crease.

1. **The history is incompatible with the type or degree of injury;** for example, the distribution of lesions or type of injury does not fit the mechanism reported, or the history is suggestive of a minor injury but major trauma is found.
2. **The history of the way in which the injury occurred is vague,** or the parent has no idea of how it happened.
3. **The history changes** each time it is told to a different health care worker.
4. **The parents, when interviewed separately, give contradictory histories.**
5. **The history is not credible.** The child may be said to have done something developmentally impossible; for example, having climbed and fallen when yet unable to sit.

Behavioral Factors

1. **There is often a significant delay between the time of injury and the time of presentation.**
2. **The parent may not show the degree of concern appropriate** to the severity of the child's injury.
3. **A pathologic parent-child interaction may be observed** if it is the abusive parent who brings the child for care. Here unrealistic expectations, inappropriate demands, or angry impulsive behavior are expressed by the parent toward the child. Such parents are often unaware of their child's needs and insensitive to behavioral cues.

Miscellaneous Observational Red Flags

1. **History or evidence of repeated visits** necessitated by "accidents" or injuries.
2. **History or evidence of repeated fractures or old scars suggestive of prior inflicted injury.**
3. **History of evidence of repeated ingestions.**

Although some victims of physical abuse are brought in with a chief complaint of abuse, many (if not most) are not. The latter may come with a chief complaint of an accidental injury or may have an unrelated or somewhat peripheral chief complaint. Whenever the physician's suspicion is aroused by historical or observational findings, he or she should seek more detailed information concerning the family's current living situation, stresses, and emotional support systems. Particular attention should be paid to personal (ill health, job loss, separation) and environmental (pending eviction, heat or utilities discontinued) crises, degree of isolation (no family or social supports, no phone), and prior problems with family violence, alcohol, or drugs. Answers to questions about methods of discipline and parental reactions to common triggering events such as stubborn behavior, pro-

longed crying, and toilet training accidents can be most illuminating. This and the medical history should be obtained in a supportive, nonjudgmental manner, because interrogation will only serve to alienate the parent, limiting the value of the data obtained. Bear in mind that the person who has brought the child in for care may not be the abuser, and that many parents of abused children truly want help. Typically they feel very alone, guilt-ridden, and inadequate as persons and parents, their own abusive behavior or their inability to protect their child from abuse by others often evoking painful memories of having been abused themselves.

In approaching the child, one must recognize that his parents are the only ones he knows, that he loves them and usually his other caretakers, and that he may feel in some way deserving of abuse. Young children rarely acknowledge that a parent or other caretaker has injured them, especially when questioned directly, and may have been sworn to secrecy. If they can be interviewed alone (when old enough to give a history) in pleasant, nonthreatening surroundings, helpful historical information can often be obtained by means of nonleading questions and through drawings or play.

Physical Findings and Patterns of Injury

Surface Marks

The most obvious manifestations of physical abuse are those visible on the surface of the skin. They include bruises, welts, scars, tourniquet and bite marks, and burns. Despite differing opinions on the appropriateness or inappropriateness of physical methods of discipline, there is a good rule of thumb in distinguishing the boundary between discipline and abuse: Discipline does *not* inflict pain and does *not* cause physical injury.

All external signs of trauma should be carefully documented in writing, on body diagrams, and in photographs, preferably with a ruler and color wheel in the frame.

Bruises, Welts, and Scars

Inflicted bruises and welts are often found in places that are unusual sites for accidental injury. These include the back, buttocks, upper arms, thighs, chest, abdomen, face (other than the chin or forehead), ears, hands, and feet (Figs. 6-1 to 6-4). This is in contrast to the "usual" small bruises seen over bony prominences in normally active children

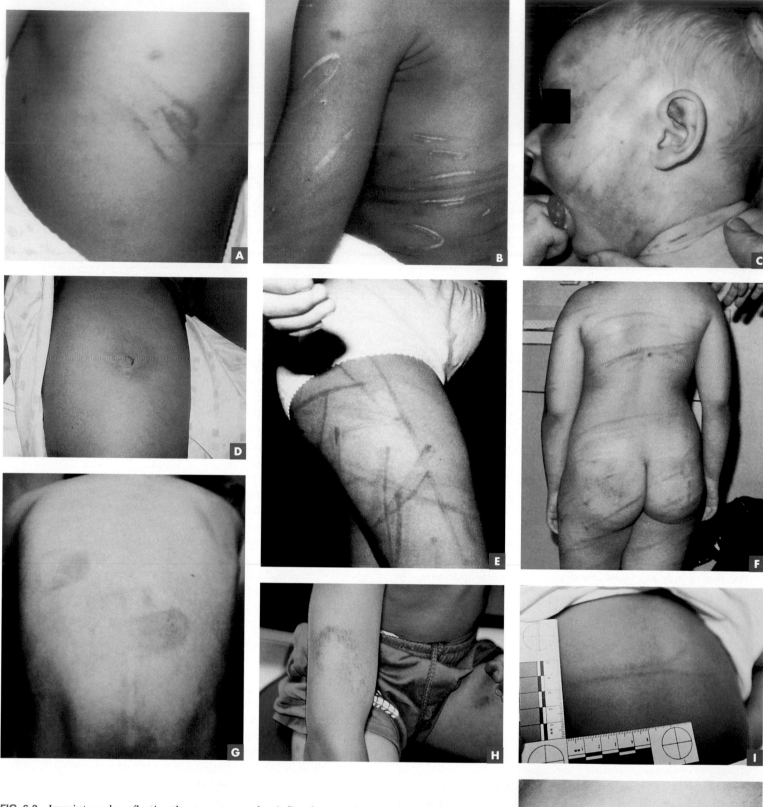

FIG. 6-3 Imprint marks reflecting the weapons used to inflict them. *A,* Fresh looped-cord marks and, *B,* hypopigmented and hyperpigmented scars that were the result of beatings with a looped electrical cord. *C,* The characteristic pattern of parallel lines that results from blows with a belt. *D,* This contusion in the configuration of a closed horseshoe with a central linear abrasion was inflicted with a belt buckle. *E,* The red linear contusions on this child's thigh were the result of repeated blows with a switch. *F,* These acute linear contusions over the back and buttocks were inflicted with a belt and a switch. *G,* This boy was hit with a slipper with such force that the imprint of the heel is evident. *H,* The heel prints of a running shoe left on this boy's arm and thigh were distinct enough to enable identification of his abuser. *I,* This girl was hit forcefully with a spatula. *J,* This boy was struck with a chain, leaving a clear imprint of the links.

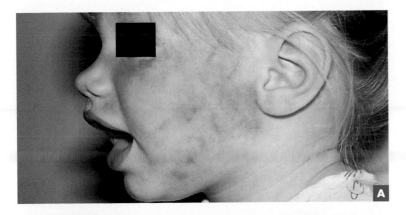

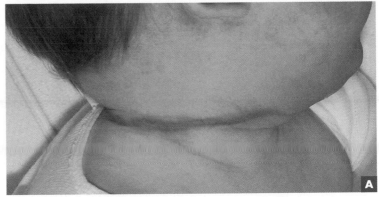

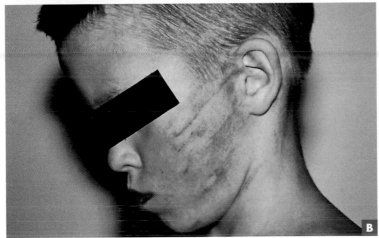

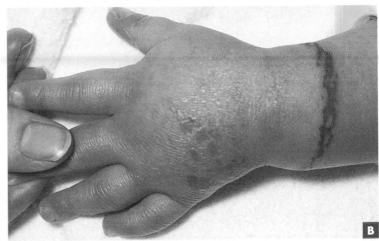

FIG. 6-4 Hand prints. *A* and *B*, These children were slapped so forcefully that the outlines of their abuser's fingers are clearly evident.

FIG. 6-5 Strangulation and restraint marks. *A*, This circumferential cord burn was the result of an attempted strangulation. *B*, A deep, circumferential rope burn of the wrist with considerable edema and early skin breakdown of the hand is seen in this infant who was tied to the siderails of her crib.

after they have begun to walk (see the section Differential Diagnosis and Fig. 6-26). Although bruises resulting from severe spankings are often seen over the curvature of the buttocks and lower back (Fig. 6-2, *A* and *B*), another pattern of linear bruising over the gluteal crease has also been noted (Fig. 6-2, *C*). This is due to rapid-fire blows delivered across the gluteal crease, which maximally distort capillaries and cause petechial hemorrhages on each side of the cleft.

In many instances the surface marks are recognizable imprints of the weapon used to inflict the injury. Those most commonly seen are looped-cord marks, caused by whipping the child with a looped electrical cord (Fig. 6-3, *A* and *B*), belt and belt-buckle marks (Fig. 6-3, *C, D,* and *F,* and Fig. 6-2, *B*), and switch marks (Fig. 6-3, *E* and *F*); but almost any implement can be used, including hairbrushes (Fig. 6-2, *B*), shoes (Fig. 6-3, *G* and *H*), kitchen utensils (Fig. 6-3, *I*), and chains (Fig. 6-3, *J*). Marks left by forceful slaps can be identified because they leave a petechial outline of the fingers where maximal capillary distortion occurs on impact (Fig. 6-4). Impressions of fingers are sometimes left at sites, such as the upper arms, trunk, or thighs, where the patient has been held tightly while being shaken or forcibly restrained. If such bruises are found over the medial thighs, the child should also be examined carefully for signs of concurrent sexual abuse. These finger-shaped bruises can at times lead to identification of the perpetrator if carefully photographed under ultraviolet light, thereby allowing the print to be lifted.

The initial appearance of bruises and the time it takes for them to resolve vary widely, depending on the degree of force used, their depth, their location on the body, and the patient's complexion. Bruises may be difficult to detect in patients with dark skin. Superficial bruises appear almost immediately and resolve more quickly than deeper contusions, which may not discolor the overlying skin for days and may take up to

2 weeks to resolve. Bruises of the face and perineum, where the skin is more loosely attached to underlying soft tissues, also appear early. Furthermore, the evolution of bruises in terms of color change is also quite variable. Although red, blue, and black are more typical colors of fresh bruises, these colors can persist in some cases until resolution. Yellow, green, and brown are more characteristic of older bruises but can be seen relatively early in superficial bruises. Hence, it is difficult to determine precisely the ages of ecchymotic lesions and to be certain that bruises of differing colors are truly of different ages. One can only say that they appear fresh or old and clearly document the size, color, and configuration. This is best done with photographs that have a standard color wheel in the frame, thereby ensuring that the lesion's true color can be determined even if there are problems with exposure or photographic technique. Despite the difficulties in determining the ages of bruises, finding old scars that reflect prior use of a weapon in a child with acute injuries can be helpful in identifying abuse or confirming prior abuse (Fig. 6-3, *B*).

To avoid errors in diagnosis, children who present with multiple bruises in unusual locations that do not reflect use of a weapon should be thoroughly examined to check for evidence of an underlying coagulopathy, and screening coagulation studies should be performed before arriving at a final diagnosis.

Strangulation, Restraint, and Tourniquet Injuries

Strangulation and restraint marks result from attempts to hang, choke, or, in some instances, tie the child to a crib, bed, or chair (Fig. 6-5). On rare occasions, bizarre tourniquet injuries are encountered (Fig. 6-6). These are more likely to be found in the children of psychotic or addicted parents and can result in severe ischemia and necrosis.

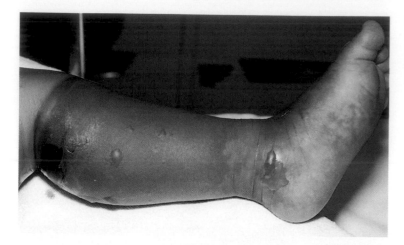

FIG. 6-6 Tourniquet injury. This toddler was brought in with severe skin, soft tissue, and muscle necrosis of his entire lower leg. His mother reported finding a strap wrapped tightly around the leg below the knee on checking him in the morning. She did not know how it had gotten there and denied hearing his cries of pain, which surely lasted for hours.

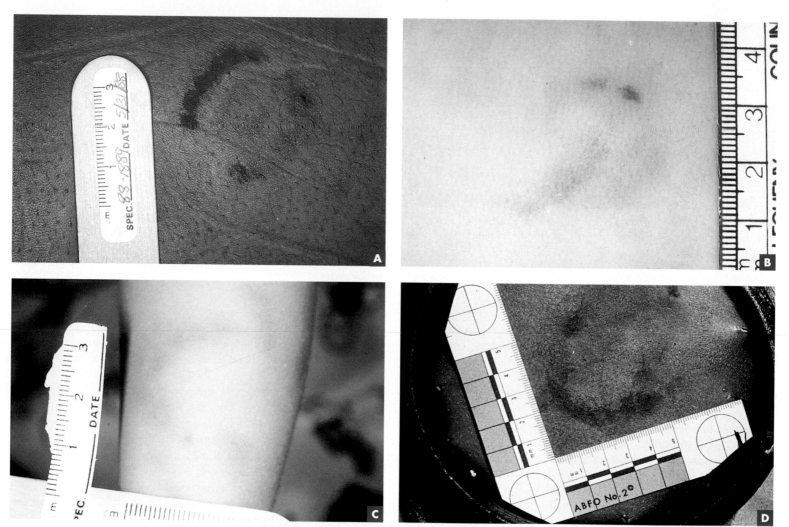

FIG. 6-7 Bite marks. *A,* This adolescent was bitten by another teenager. Deep abrasions, left especially by the upper arch, clearly reflect the imprint of the incisors. *B,* In this bite mark inflicted on a toddler by a 6-year-old child, the configuration of the upper central incisors is clearly seen (note the diastema). The lower arch has left indistinct abrasions and contusions. *C,* At first glance this fading bite mark could be mistaken for a bruise; however, on close inspection, the outline of the dental arch becomes evident. The size of the arch is clearly that of an adult or adolescent. *D,* Viewed under ultraviolet light, bite marks that are weeks to months old can still be identified, even though the skin overlying the site has returned to normal. (*A, B,* and *C* courtesy Dr. Michael N. Sobel, Pittsburgh; *D* courtesy Dr. Thomas J. David, Atlanta.)

Bite Marks

Bite marks can be yet another manifestation of physical abuse. In children in whom the resulting imprint is distinct, it is as identifiable as a fingerprint and its size enables the examiner to clearly distinguish between the bite of another child and that of an adult (Fig. 6-7, *A* to *C*).

Each bite mark should be carefully photographed in its entirety, and then photos should be taken perpendicular to the plane of the imprint of each arch, with a ruler or measuring tape in each photo. Such evidence can enable a forensic dentist to make a model of the perpetrator's dentition, which can specifically reveal his or her identity. Ultra-

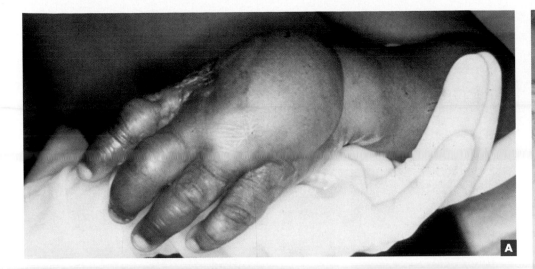

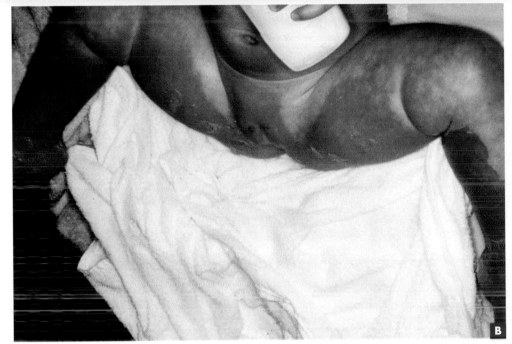

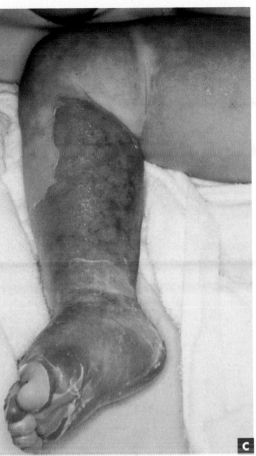

FIG. 6-8 Inflicted scalds. *A,* This child suffered severe second-degree dip burns on both hands and wrists. *B,* Patient seen 2 days after receiving dip burns to the lower extremities and perineum. *C,* Close-up of severe second-degree burns of the foot and lower leg. (Courtesy Dr. Thomas Layton, Mercy Hospital, Pittsburgh.)

violet photography can disclose a clear image of bite marks weeks or months after all surface marks have disappeared (Fig. 6-7, *D*). This has proved highly useful in identifying abusers of children with a past history of being bitten, but who have no acute lesions. Finally, if the patient has not bathed or washed the bite wound since it was inflicted, swabbing the area with a saline-soaked cotton-tipped applicator is indicated, to obtain a sample of the perpetrator's saliva. Crime laboratory analysis of this material can positively identify the perpetrator.

Burns

Although burns are generally accidental, they are also a fairly common mode of abusive injury. Here, too, inconsistency of history, the pattern of injury, and the delay in seeking medical attention are valuable clues.

Immersion scalds are among the most common forms of inflicted burns. Typical patterns include symmetrical burns of both hands or both feet in a stocking-glove distribution, with a sharp line of demar-

cation at the level of the water line (Fig. 6-8, *A*); circumferential burns of the feet and lower legs along with burns of the perineum and flexor surfaces of the thighs are seen in children who are held under the axillae and knees and have their legs dipped in scalding water (Fig. 6-8, *B* and *C*). If the child is forcibly held down in a sink or tub as it fills with scalding water, partial sparing of the palms, soles, and buttocks may be noted because they were pressed against the cooler sink or tub surface.

Despite claims to the contrary, immersion burns are rarely accidental. Table 6-1 shows the time required to produce a full-thickness burn in adult skin at different water temperatures. Although the time may be slightly shorter for a child, normal children would, if they accidentally put a hand or foot into water over 120°F, withdraw it in a fraction of a second, after the tips of their fingers or toes made contact with the water, leaving them with only superficial burns of the tips of their fingers or toes.

Branding injuries show the imprint of the instruments used to inflict them. For example, one may see the full-thickness imprint of a hot iron

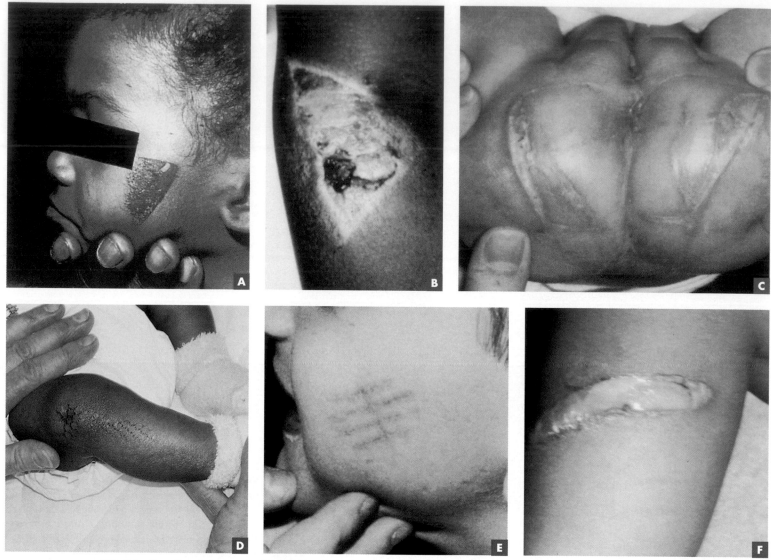

FIG. 6-9 Branding injuries. *A*, This child, who was acting out while his mother ironed, was punished by having her hold the tip of the iron against his cheek. *B*, A healing full-thickness burn in the shape of an iron was found when this boy's shirt was removed prior to his being given an immunization injection. *C*, These linear full-thickness burns were incurred when this infant was forced to sit on the hot grille of a space heater. *D*, This infant presented with a history of irritability and a rash. The "rash" has a honeycomb configuration that matched that of a radiator cover in her home. She also had multiple fractures. *E*, These facial burns are the result of being branded with the grille of a hair dryer. *F*, The hot wand of a curling iron leaves a cigar-shaped, partial- to full-thickness burn.

or of the grill of a space heater or radiator cover (Fig. 6-9, *A* to *D*). No child with normal sensation would remain in contact with these objects long enough to incur such a burn. Burns caused by holding a hot hair dryer next to the skin leave an imprint of the screen that covers the heating element (Fig. 6-9, *E*), and those inflicted with a curling iron produce cigar-shaped second-degree or full-thickness imprints (Fig. 6-9, *F*). Most of these burns are found in unusual locations such as the extensor surfaces of the arms or legs, the back, chest, abdomen, or buttocks, where they are less likely to be noticed by the public.

Inflicted cigarette burns leave sharply circumscribed, full-thickness imprints approximately 7 to 8 mm in diameter (5 mm if a slim cigarette is used), over which a thick, black eschar soon forms (Fig. 6-10, *A*). If this eschar is removed, one sees full-thickness skin loss. Subacutely,

TABLE 6-1

Duration of Exposure Required to Produce Full-Thickness Burn in Water at Various Temperatures

Water temperature	Duration of exposure
120°F	10 minutes
130°F	30 seconds
140°F	5 seconds
150°F	2 seconds
158°F	1 second

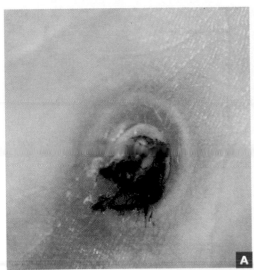
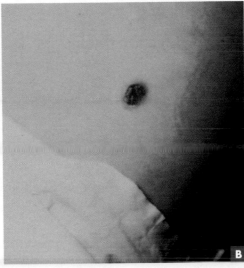
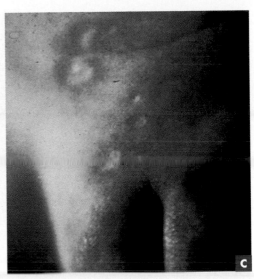

FIG. 6-10 Cigarette burns. *A,* This sharply circumscribed burn was inflicted through the child's sock. The burn is perfectly circular with a blistered rim and a full-thickness punched-out center to which charred fabric adheres. The configuration did not fit the history that he had accidentally stepped on a cigarette. *B,* This older burn has begun to granulate in. *C,* Full-thickness, punched-out scars are characteristic of healed cigarette burns. (*A* courtesy Dr. David Evanko, Butler, Pa.; *C* courtesy Dr. Marc Rowe, Children's Hospital of Pittsburgh.)

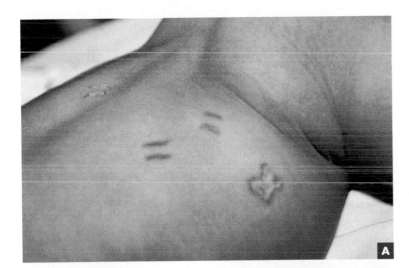

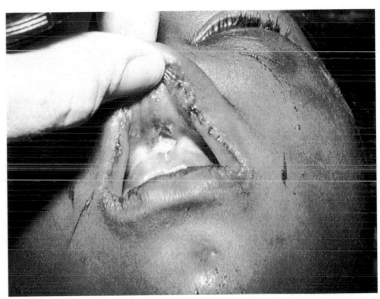

FIG. 6-12 Frenulum tear. This badly beaten boy incurred a torn frenulum when his abuser tried to muffle his cries by forcibly holding his hand over the child's mouth. Note the facial bruises. (Courtesy Dr. Robert Hickey, Children's Hospital of Pittsburgh.)

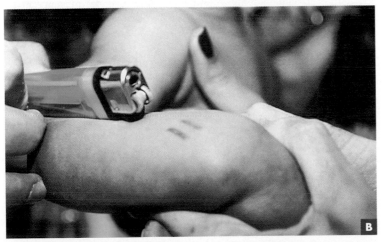

FIG. 6-11 Cigarette lighter burns. *A,* Two pairs of lesions with the appearance of parallel serrated lines and a deep burn in the shape of a butterfly were found on examining this infant who was brought to the emergency department for treatment of a rash. *B,* Clever deduction on the part of a case worker led to the discovery that a heated cigarette lighter wheel had been used to inflict the burns.

these lesions fill in with granulation tissue (Fig. 6-10, *B*), and on completion of healing, the child is left with a deep, punched-out scar (Fig. 6-10, *C*). An unusual pattern of serrated first- and second-degree burns in parallel lines is made when a butane lighter is lit, the flame is tilted so that it heats the wheel that strikes the flint, and then the hot wheel is pressed or run over the child's skin (Fig. 6-11).

Oral Injuries

Occasionally, child abuse results in oral bruises and lacerations. One of the most typical patterns is bruising of the mucosa of the upper lip or the maxillary gingiva associated with tearing of the frenulum (Fig. 6-12). This can be produced when the perpetrator holds a hand

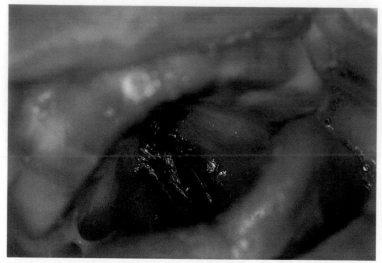

FIG. 6-13   Inflicted palatal lacerations. This infant's soft palate was shredded by repeated stabs with a sharp object. He presented with a complaint of spitting up blood and no history of trauma.

tightly over the child's mouth to silence screaming or tries to force a bottle or pacifier into a crying infant's mouth. Gag marks at the corners of the mouth can be mistaken for cheilosis or for impetiginous or candidal lesions. On rare occasions, bizarre intraoral lacerations are found (Fig. 6-13). Their usual mode of presentation is a complaint of spitting or vomiting blood.

Skeletal Injuries

Depending on the series reported, between 5% and 18% of abused children have fractures. The incidence is especially high in younger children, with more than 80% of cases of inflicted skeletal trauma seen in infants and children under 18 months of age. Children with abuse-related skeletal injuries may have a history of minor injury or a reported mechanism of injury that does not fit the fracture pattern. Frequently the chief complaint is one of unexplained irritability; sometimes it is totally unrelated (e.g., a rash, vomiting, or upper respiratory tract infection) with no history of injury given. Since presentation is often delayed, fractures identified on radiographs commonly show signs of healing, for example, callus or subperiosteal new-bone formation. The degree of callus formation and the extent of periosteal new-bone formation and remodeling are clues to the ages of the various fractures. The periosteum in infants and very young children resists tearing and has great osteogenic potential; consequently, many nondisplaced fractures are no longer tender or only subtly tender at the time of examination.

Two radiographic fracture patterns are pathognomonic for abuse. The first is multiple, unexplained fractures (often symmetrical) of varying ages involving the long bones and ribs of an infant or young child who has otherwise normal bones (Fig. 6-14). Often these fractures are transverse, resulting from a blow delivered perpendicularly to the long axis of the bony shaft, or oblique, resulting from twisting. Rib fractures (Fig. 6-15) are most common over the posterior portion of the ribs near the costovertebral articulations. They result from violent shaking of the baby while holding him or her by the chest, during which the posterior portions of the ribs are bent against the fulcrum of the vertebrae, producing the fractures. Rib fractures can also occur anterolaterally as a result of direct blows delivered to the anterior chest and sternum.

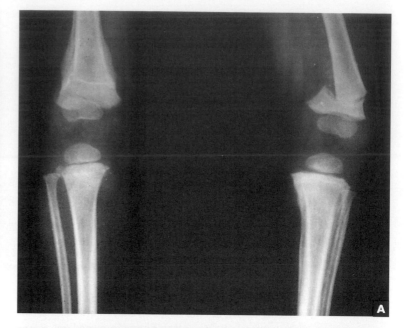

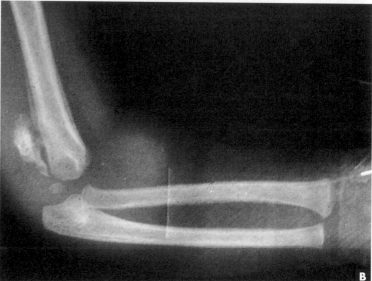

FIG. 6-14   Multiple fractures of varying ages. This child was seen because of a chief complaint of refusing to bear weight. On examination, he was found to have marked swelling, tenderness, and crepitance over the distal left femur. *A,* Radiographic examination confirmed the presence of an acute transverse fracture and also revealed multiple additional fractures in various stages of healing. These include old fractures of the distal right femur with callus and subperiosteal new-bone formation, relatively new metaphyseal chip fractures seen in the right proximal tibia, and vigorous subperiosteal new-bone formation encompassing the left tibia. *B,* On skeletal survey, he was also found to have a healing fracture of the distal humerus with vigorous callus formation, subperiosteal new-bone formation, and considerable soft tissue swelling. Note that the cortices of his long bones are of normal thickness. (Courtesy the Department of Radiology, Children's Hospital of Pittsburgh.)

The second type of pathognomonic fracture is sometimes termed a *metaphyseal chip* or *corner fracture.* Perhaps it is more appropriately described as a *bucket-handle fracture,* because the fracture line actually traverses the primary spongiosa of the entire metaphysis, just beneath its junction with the epiphysis. The fracture then crosses the outer aspects of the metaphysis. In many cases the central portion of the fracture is radiographically invisible and only the metaphyseal chips on the medial and lateral aspects of the involved long bone are seen on standard A-P x-ray views (Fig. 6-16, *A*; see Fig. 6-14, *A*). In some cases a thin meta-

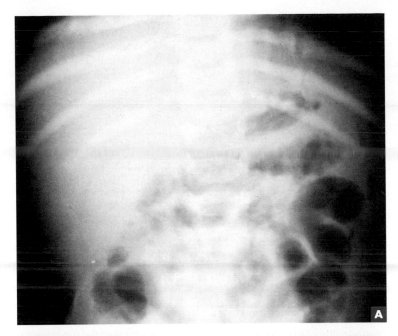

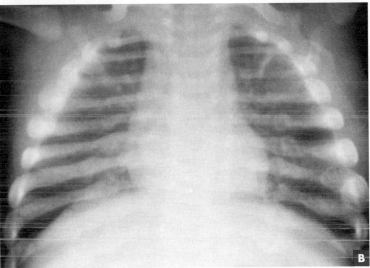

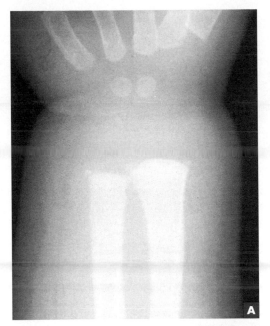

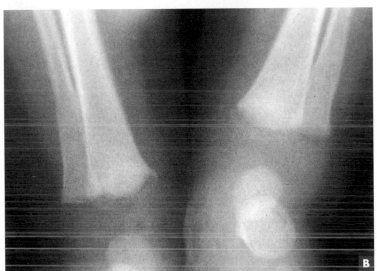

FIG. 6-15 Rib fractures. *A,* This infant was seen because of a history of vomiting and irritability. An abdominal film obtained to rule out intestinal obstruction showed a normal bowel gas pattern but revealed multiple posterior rib fractures in various stages of healing, which were missed. *B,* When the infant was finally tracked down 2 months later, her chest x-ray showed in excess of 20 healing rib fractures, some posterior and others anterolateral. (Courtesy the Department of Radiology, Children's Hospital of Pittsburgh.)

FIG. 6-16 What appear as metaphyseal chip fractures on this AP view of the distal radius and ulna *(A)* are actually bucket-handle fractures as shown in this oblique view of both distal tibias *(B).* The fracture lines traverse the entire width of the distal metaphyses and are the result of violent shaking. (*A* courtesy the Department of Radiology, Children's Hospital of Pittsburgh; *B* courtesy Dr. Bruce Rosenthal, Mercy Hospital, Pittsburgh.)

physeal lucency may be evident, although often special oblique views are necessary to reveal this (Fig. 6-16, *B*). This type of fracture is usually caused by rapid acceleration and deceleration forces produced by violent shaking while holding the child by the trunk, the hands, or the feet. They can also be caused by violent yanking of the end of the extremity.

Long-bone fractures, particularly transverse and oblique fractures of the humerus and femur in the absence of a clear history of a consistent major mechanism of injury, are highly suspect, as are any rib fractures in infants or toddlers. In fact, the ribs of children under 5 years of age are so flexible that accidental fractures are rarely found, even after major motor vehicle accidents and falls.

The frequency of skeletal injury in young abused children necessitates that examination of the suspected abuse victim include careful palpation of *all* bones for evidence of tenderness, crepitus, or callus formation. Because of the greater probability of multiple occult fractures in the infant and toddler, a skeletal survey is advisable in children less than 2 years of age. In older children, careful physical examination should reveal areas requiring radiographic evaluation.

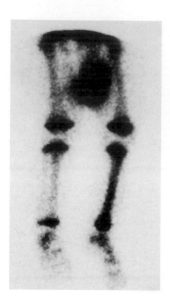

FIG. 6-17 Bone scan of a child abuse victim. This 14-month-old child was seen because of low-grade fever and refusal to walk. Radiographs were normal. The scan, obtained because of suspicion of infection, revealed increased uptake throughout the entire left tibia. Findings from a workup for infection were normal, and repeat radiographs obtained 2 weeks later revealed healing fractures and extensive subperiosteal new-bone formation.

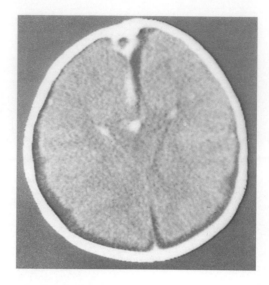

FIG. 6-18 Subdural hematomas in the shaken-baby syndrome. This CT scan reveals subdural hematomas along the falx and over the cerebral convexities. These are seen as a dark rim along the falx and between the bony calvarium and the brain substance. (Courtesy the Division of Neuroradiology, University Health Center of Pittsburgh.)

Bone scans can reveal occult (radiographically invisible) fractures within hours of injury (Fig. 6-17), and they can be particularly helpful in detecting acute posterior rib fractures in infants. However, although more sensitive than standard radiographs, they are less specific. Radiographs have to be taken of sites detected by scan to help distinguish fractures from other lesions and help determine the mechanism of injury. Bone scans are also less available and more time-consuming and expensive, the children usually need to be sedated, they involve more radiation, and their accuracy is highly dependent on the technician and interpreter. This imaging method is thus best reserved for patients whose standard radiographs show normal findings, yet the index of suspicion of fracture remains high.

Central Nervous System Injuries and the Shaken-Baby Syndrome

Head injuries are the major source of morbidity and mortality in child abuse victims. Findings reported in the recent literature reveal that approximately 65% of all head injuries and 95% of serious intracranial injuries in infants under a year of age are inflicted and that 80% of the deaths resulting from head injury in children less than 2 years of age are caused by abuse. Studies of the victims of falls witnessed by people other than caretakers and of children who fell from beds and examining tables in hospitals have shown that falls from less than 10 feet (3 meters), even onto hard surfaces, do not cause serious, let alone life-threatening, head injuries. These findings have led to the recognition that study populations described in earlier literature on pediatric head trauma included many unrecognized cases of abuse, and to a refutation of the conclusions of the investigators that short falls and relatively minor mechanisms of injury could result in serious head trauma.

An infant's head is uniquely vulnerable to injury, whether from impact or from shaking, for several reasons:

1. It is relatively large, accounting for up to 10% of body weight, as opposed to 2% in the adult. This weight adds to the momentum of acceleration and deceleration forces with shaking and accounts for the fact that infants who are dropped or thrown (whether bodily or ejected from motor vehicles) tend to land on their heads.
2. Highly elastic, underdeveloped cervical ligaments; relatively weak neck muscles; shallow, horizontally oriented cervical facet joints; and incompletely ossified and anteriorly wedged cervical vertebrae hinder an infant's ability to protect against whiplash forces. Together they make the infant susceptible to extreme hyperflexion and hyperextension of the neck.

3. The soft calvarium, which elongates with acceleration and deceleration, and the relatively large subarachnoid space make the bridging veins between the dura mater and cerebral cortex more vulnerable to tearing. In addition, with impact the pliable skull tends to transfer the force to the underlying brain rather than fracturing and absorbing some of the force along the fracture line. Fractures that do occur tend to be large, diastatic burst fractures.
4. The increased plasticity and thin axons of the unmyelinated brain make it more vulnerable to shearing injuries, especially at the gray-white matter interface.

The first type of inflicted head injury recognized was that seen in the *shaken-baby syndrome*, a constellation of findings that included subdural hematomas (Fig. 6-18), retinal hemorrhages (Fig. 6-19), and metaphyseal chip fractures (Figs. 6-14, *A*, and 6-16) attributed to shaking. Most victims of suspected shaking are less than 1 year of age, frequently under 6 months, and most have no external signs of injury (although careful inspection may reveal faint finger impression bruises). On the basis of confessions and videotapes obtained with hidden cameras, it is known that the infant may be held by the trunk, the upper arms and shoulders, or the hands or feet and is subjected to repetitive, violent shakes. Studies using monkeys, conducted in the late 1960s, showed that violent shaking generates rapid acceleration and deceleration forces, which have both linear and rotational components, and that either the rotational forces or the combination of forces was necessary for producing the subdural, subarachnoid, and retinal hemorrhages seen in the animals.

Advances in neuroimaging and forensic examination, together with improvements in the identification of inflicted head trauma, have expanded our knowledge of the spectrum of central nervous system (CNS) injuries seen in the shaken-baby syndrome. In addition to subdural hematomas (seen particularly in the interhemispheric fissure along the falx as well as over the cerebral convexities), subarachnoid hemorrhages, cerebral contusions, diffuse axonal injury with shearing at the gray-white matter interface, and white matter tears have been reported. Epidural and subdural hematomas at the cervicomedullary junction in association with ventral cord contusions at high cervical levels have also been linked to shaking.

In the past decade, however, the role of shaking in producing these injuries has been called into question by a group of investigators who developed an infant model using a doll with a weighted head. They concluded that shaking alone failed to generate sufficient G forces to cause the CNS injuries attributed to shaking in human infants and noted on close examination that many of their victims showed signs of

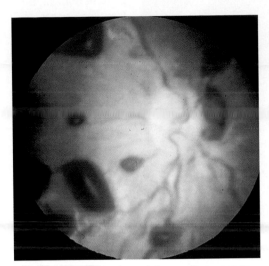

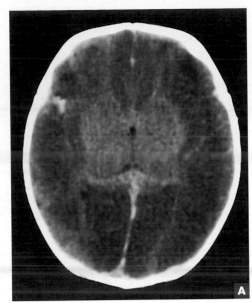

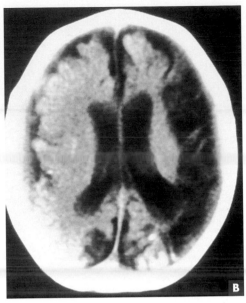

FIG. 6-19 Multiple retinal hemorrhages are seen on funduscopic examination of this infant who was a victim of the shaken-baby syndrome. Subdural hematoma and multiple metaphyseal "shake" fractures are typical associated findings. (Courtesy Dr. Stephen Ludwig, Children's Hospital of Philadelphia.)

FIG. 6-20 Hypoxic injury. *A,* This infant, who was found unresponsive in his crib, has a pattern of diffuse cortical hypodensity on CT scan indicative of extensive cerebral infarction caused by hypoxia. *B,* Three months later, the patient remained significantly impaired neurologically and repeat CT scan showed severe cerebral atrophy.

impact injury. They then postulated that some form of impact was necessary for these injuries to occur. They further suggested that the impact in patients with no evidence of impact injury may have been on a soft surface such as a mattress. Subsequent investigators have found that although many shaken infants do indeed have evidence of an associated impact injury, a significant percentage (11% to 50%, depending on the series), especially of very young infants, do not; further, on the basis of confessions, it does appear that severe CNS injury can result from violent shaking alone. The validity of the model has also been questioned, because the doll's neck is capable of less hyperflexion than an infant's. Thus, some victims' injuries appear to be due solely to shaking, others result from a combination of shaking and impact trauma, and still others from impact alone.

The metaphyseal fractures described earlier, posterior rib fractures, and retinal hemorrhages appear to be nearly pathognomonic for shaking. Retinal hemorrhages are found in 75% to 90% of infants and children with inflicted head injury and in nearly 100% of those who suffer serious sequelae and death. Although the uniqueness of the association of retinal hemorrhages with shaking has also been the subject of some controversy, studies of infants and children whose accidental severe head trauma was witnessed have shown that the incidence of retinal hemorrhages is vanishingly small and that this injury is largely limited to children who have incurred severe crush injuries to the head or chest, or both, or who suffered high-velocity, lateral-impact rotational injuries. Similarly, research on children who have undergone cardiopulmonary resuscitation has revealed a very low incidence of retinal hemorrhages, and the children so affected were abuse victims or suffering from malignant hypertension, coagulopathy, or septic shock.

Many episodes of severe shaking or impact result in loss of consciousness, frightening the perpetrator who then leaves the baby to rest, hoping that he or she will revive. (Studies have shown that the person alone with the child at the time symptoms are first "noted" is often the perpetrator.) During the ensuing interval, intracranial pressure may increase and seizures may occur, resulting in hypoventilation or respiratory arrest, adding hypoxic injury to the physical trauma

(Fig. 6-20). Most fatalities result from a combination of hypoxia and uncontrollable cerebral edema.

Modes of presentation vary depending on the severity of the CNS injury and include unrelated chief complaints, a history of a minor fall, lethargy, irritability, seizures, respiratory distress, choking, apnea and being found unresponsive. Unless the infant is thrown down on a hard object or against a wall after the shaking, there is little or no evidence of external injury.

Physical findings may include lethargy, increased or decreased tone, rhythmic eye opening, bicycling movements of the extremities, and sometimes posturing. Decreased ability to follow the examiner's face, decreased responsiveness to pain, and poor suck and grasp are important findings. The fontanelle is usually full but may or may not be tense. Because retinal hemorrhages (Fig. 6-19) are found in 75% to 90% of shaken babies, dilated ophthalmoscopy should be performed in all infants who are suspected to be victims of abuse and in all infants seen because of the sudden onset of an altered level of consciousness. These infants should also undergo meticulous inspection of the skin, looking for evidence of fingerprint marks.

Inflicted impact injuries or blunt head trauma are seen in infants and children who have been thrown to the floor, against a wall, or into other objects, or who have received direct blows to the head with a fist or other blunt object. Injuries range from surface hematomas and linear fractures to complex skull fractures, subdural and epidural hematomas, diffuse cerebral swelling, and cerebral contusions with attendant cerebral edema (Figs. 6-21 to 6-23).

Children with moderate and severe degrees of blunt head injury tend to present acutely, with one or more of the following complaints: bump on the head, vomiting and irritability, altered level of consciousness, seizures, or abnormal posturing. On occasion, infants may be in shock resulting from massive subgaleal or intracranial hemorrhage or a history of respiratory arrest is given. A history of trauma may be vague or nonexistent. The reported mechanism of injury may be inconsistent with the type or severity of injuries found. Patients who have incurred milder trauma tend to be seen subacutely with one or more of the fol-

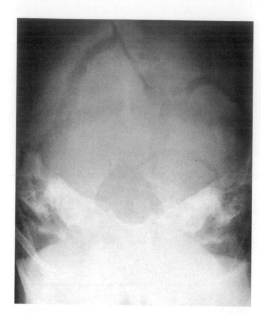

FIG. 6-21 Multiple occipital fractures are seen in a child who presented with a history of a minor fall and scalp swelling. It was later acknowledged that he had been thrown against a brick wall. (Courtesy the Department of Radiology, Children's Hospital of Pittsburgh.)

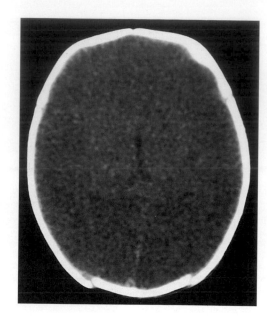

FIG. 6-22 Massive cerebral edema. This CT scan from an infant who presented with altered level of consciousness and seizures reveals occipital fractures and diffuse cerebral swelling causing ventricular compression. Note the loss of gray-white matter differentiation. (Courtesy the Division of Neuroradiology, University Health Center of Pittsburgh.)

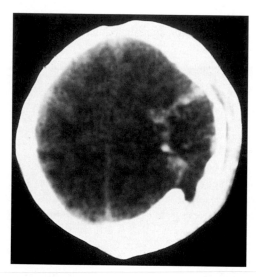

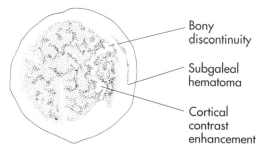

FIG. 6-23 Cerebral contusion. CT scan from a 4-week-old infant, who allegedly rolled out of his crib while the siderails were up, shows a large subgaleal hematoma obscuring an underlying fracture, severe cerebral swelling with a shift of the midline, and cortical contrast enhancement indicative of a cerebral contusion. (Courtesy the Division of Neuroradiology, University Health Center of Pittsburgh.)

lowing: intermittent vomiting and irritability, rapidly increasing head circumference with split sutures and a full fontanelle, failure to thrive, and developmental delay typically affecting social more than motor development.

Careful external, general, neurologic, and funduscopic examinations are warranted in evaluating these patients. Neurologic examination may reveal an altered level of consciousness, signs of increased intracranial pressure, alterations in tone, or, on occasion, focal abnormalities.

Neuroimaging

Computed tomography (CT) has proved valuable in the acute assessment of CNS injuries. Although routine skull radiographs may be better for detecting most skull fractures, especially in patients with completely normal neurologic findings, CT is indicated whenever there is any suspicion of intracranial injury. It clearly delineates most intracranial hemorrhages and cerebral edema as well as subdural hematomas and many fractures. It is especially good at revealing interhemispheric subdural hematomas along the falx in the parietooccipital area seen in the victims of shaking (Fig. 6-18). These may be accompanied by a midline shift caused by extracerebral blood collec-

tion or concomitant cerebral contusion or edema, as well as by subdural blood over the convexities (Fig. 6-18). In more severe cases, one may see an infarct pattern consisting of hypodensities of the cortex and underlying white matter or even a loss of gray and white matter differentiation (Figs. 6-20, *A*, and 6-22). These changes result in part from hypoventilation and hypoxia, which in turn are caused by increased intracranial pressure. Diffuse axonal injury is characterized by low-density changes, often seen in association with hemorrhages at the gray-white matter junction. Both sets of findings indicate a poor prognosis for recovery (Fig. 6-20, *B*).

CT does have limitations, however; it may not reveal the full extent of injuries and may fail to reveal small subdural hemorrhages and subtle cerebral contusions or hemorrhages. Studies in which magnetic resonance imaging (MRI) was used have shown that it is up to 50% more sensitive in detecting small subdural hematomas over the convexities (Fig. 6-24, *A* and *B*). MRI can also detect subdural hemorrhages of differing ages, because the imaging intensity changes as blood begins to break down (Fig. 6-24, *C*). Subdural hematomas of varying ages may result from repetitive injury or from spontaneous rebleeding. MRI is far superior to CT in detecting subtle contusions and small parenchymal hemorrhages, in identifying diffuse axonal injury, and in detecting abnormalities of posterior fossa structures and the cervical cord.

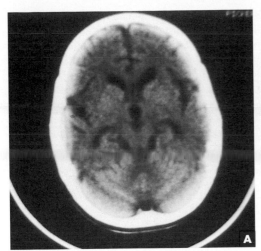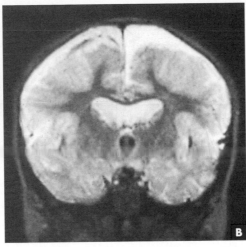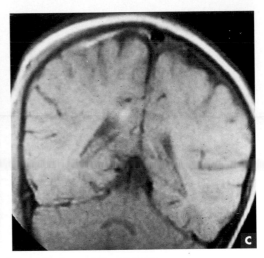

FIG. 6-24 *A* and *B,* This 3-year-old abuse victim presented with lethargy, vomiting, hyporeflexia, and the acute on-set of blindness. The CT scan reveals ventricular enlargement and cortical atrophy, which were the result of severe shaking 1 year earlier, but no hemorrhage. The MRI shows small, bilateral subdural hemorrhages that were missed on CT. *C,* This 5-month-old infant with head and facial bruises, bilateral retinal hemorrhages, and multiple rib frac-tures was found to have subdural hemorrhages of differing ages on MRI. The white subdural hematoma is between 0 and 14 days old, and the gray subdural hematoma is more than 14 days old. (Courtesy Dr. Randall Alexander, Uni-versity of Iowa.)

Abdominal and Chest Injuries

Although less common than surface injuries and skeletal and head trauma, abdominal and chest injuries have been found in up to 2% of victims of physical abuse and can be quite severe, with a mortality of up to 50%. Young children are more vulnerable to internal abdominal injury with blunt trauma than adolescents or adults, for three major reasons: (1) their abdominal muscles are relatively weak, (2) the distance between the abdominal wall and the vertebral column is relatively short, and (3) their costal margins are more horizontally oriented, affording less protection to underlying viscera. Midabdominal structures that are fixed in place by pedicles of overlying ligaments (small intestines, liver, and pancreas) are particularly vulnerable to injury. Typically these injuries result from being punched or kicked forcefully or from being thrown to the floor or against a wall or piece of furniture. External findings are often minimal or absent; trauma often goes unreported or is ascribed to a minor mechanism. Presentation often is delayed but may be prompt if signs and symptoms are severe.

The major types of abdominal pathology seen are duodenal hema-tomas, small intestinal or mesenteric tears, pancreatic and renal contusions, and contusions or lacerations of the liver or spleen. Patients with duodenal hematoma typically show signs of intestinal obstruction (e.g., vomiting and abdominal pain). Plain radiographs may reveal an air-fluid level in a dilated duodenal loop proximal to the hematoma, and upper gastrointestinal series and ultrasound studies reveal narrowing of the lumen and thickening of the duodenal wall respectively (Fig. 6-25). Children with small intestinal or mesenteric tears generally complain of diffuse abdominal pain and have signs of diffuse tenderness, distension, and peritoneal irritation. Children with splenic and hepatic lacerations may show similar findings or may have signs of hypovolemia, shock, or even sudden collapse that is often unexplained by history. In most instances of inflicted abdominal trauma, abuse is not confirmed until special radiographic studies including sonography and CT scans have been obtained or surgery has been performed.

Findings from a recent study indicate that the true incidence of intra-abdominal injury in abuse victims may have been significantly underestimated. Using transaminase levels as screening tests, the investigators found evidence of hepatic injury, including three liver lacerations involving the left lobe as detected by CT, in four of 49 patients being evaluated for possible physical abuse. Although some patients had clinical evidence of head injury and some had facial or thoracic bruises, none had any external evidence of abdominal trauma or any abdominal tenderness. All were under 5 years of age. This indicates that serum transaminase levels should be checked in suspected victims of physical abuse who are under 5 years of age, much as a skeletal survey is recommended for those under 2 years.

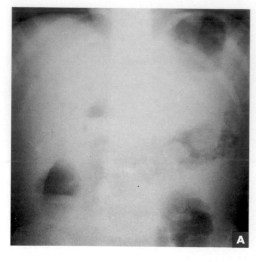 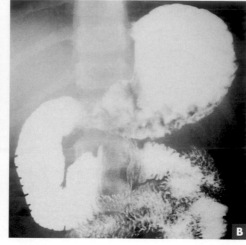

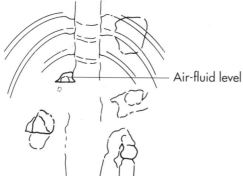 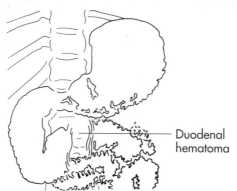

Air-fluid level

Duodenal hematoma

FIG. 6-25 Duodenal hematoma. *A,* Abdominal film reveals an air-fluid level in a dilated duodenal loop proximal to the duodenal hematoma. *B,* This upper gastrointestinal series shows narrowing of the duodenal lumen and widening of the duodenal wall at the site of a hematoma. The obstruction is partial, because some barium has passed through the narrowed segment. (Courtesy the Department of Radiology, Children's Hospital of Pittsburgh.)

Inflicted thoracic injuries include pulmonary and myocardial contusions, pulmonary lacerations, and thymic or subpleural hemorrhages. Rarely a severe blow causes myocardial or aortic rupture and the child is dead on arrival after sudden collapse. The chief complaint on presentation may be respiratory distress, chest pain, or sudden collapse. Typically there is no history of injury or a report of only minor trauma.

Differential Diagnosis of Inflicted Injuries Versus Findings Due to Accident or Illness

Although it is highly important to detect injuries resulting from abuse in order to protect children from future and potentially more serious trauma, it is also most important to avoid erroneously diagnosing abuse, because this subjects innocent families to the ordeal of a child protective services investigation, causing tremendous emotional stress. Accurate diagnosis requires clear knowledge not only of patterns of injury seen following abuse, but also of mechanisms of injury and their resulting findings, the types of accidental injuries commonly seen at various ages, and the diseases and congenital disorders that predispose to bleeding or increased bony fragility. If doubt exists, the services of experienced clinicians with expertise in the fields of child abuse, orthopedics, pediatric surgery, and neurosurgery should be sought.

Differential Diagnosis of Surface Bruises

Accidental Bruises

Ordinary, play-related bruises can be distinguished from those resulting from abuse by virtue of the fact that they tend to be small and nonspecific in configuration. They are typically located over the bony prominences of the shins, knees, elbows, extensor forearms, chin, or forehead (Fig. 6-26, *A*). Larger bruises, and even those with configurations suggesting they were inflicted by an object, can also be accidental or the result of an altercation with another child. In such cases, however, presentation for care is prompt, the mechanism of injury is consistent with the findings, and in most instances, the incident was witnessed.

Black eyes following forehead contusions may be mistaken for inflicted bruises. If the initial injury produces a large forehead hematoma, subsequent tracking of blood through the facial soft tissues is likely to occur over the ensuing 24 to 72 hours, producing ecchymotic discoloration along the sides of the nose and under the lower eyelids (Fig. 6-26, *B*). This gives the illusion of an injury resulting from direct periorbital trauma. The history, presence of residual forehead contusion, and absence of tenderness in the periorbital area help confirm the true origin of these findings.

Bruises Due to Subcultural Healing Practices

The influx of immigrants from Southeast Asia to the United States and Canada since the late 1970s has made it important to be aware of

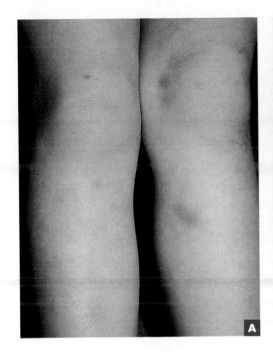
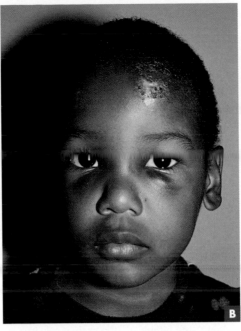

FIG. 6-26 Normal bruises. *A,* Numerous small, nonspecific bruises are present over the knees and shins of this active youngster. *B,* Black eyes occurring after a forehead contusion. This boy had fallen from a slide 3 days before. Blood from his forehead hematoma had tracked down through the facial soft tissues, creating these shiners, which were nontender.

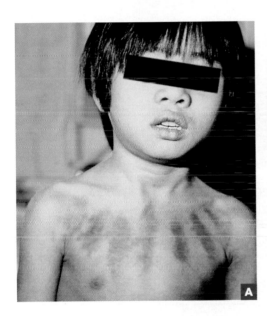
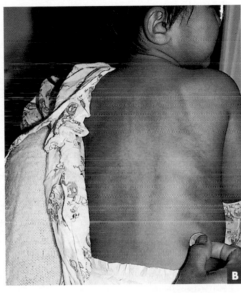

FIG. 6-27 Coin rubbing. *A,* Vigorous stroking of the skin of a febrile child with a coin produces a peculiar bruising pattern. *B,* Here the father of another child demonstrates the technique. (*A* courtesy Dr. Thomas Daley, Bronx-Lebanon Hospital.)

nonabusive healing practices which produce unusual bruising patterns. The most common of these is coin rubbing in which the skin of the trunk and back are rubbed vigorously with the edge of a coin as a means of treating fever. This leaves a pattern of bruises resembling the branches of a fir tree (Fig. 6-27). In another practice termed *cupping,* a candle is lit and placed under a small cup. The cup is then applied to the forehead or trunk. As oxygen is consumed by the flame, a vacuum is created and the cup adheres to the skin. On removal, a round imprint is left on the skin. As the indentation resolves, a characteristic circular ecchymosis remains that encircles central petechiae (Fig. 6-28).

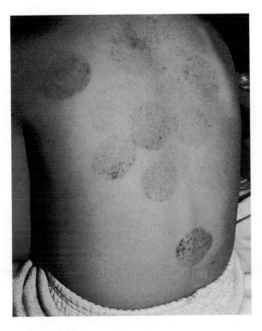

FIG. 6-28 Cupping. These circular bruises with central petechiae are the sequelae of the Southeast Asian practice of cupping. (Courtesy Dr. Robert Hickey, Children's Hospital of Pittsburgh.)

Purpura Due to Bleeding Disorders or Vasculitis

Purpuric lesions associated with coagulopathies and acute vasculitic disorders must also be recognized and distinguished from inflicted bruises.

Thrombocytopenia

Patients with acute idiopathic thrombocytopenic purpura (ITP) and acute leukemia can have purpuric lesions located anywhere on the

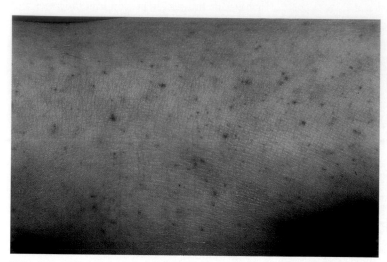

FIG. 6-29 Idiopathic thrombocytopenic purpura. This school-age child was seen with a chief complaint of a rash after a viral upper respiratory tract infection. Examination revealed diffuse petechiae, shown here over her ankle, and scattered purpuric lesions. Her hemoglobin and white blood cell count and differential were normal, but her platelet count was markedly reduced.

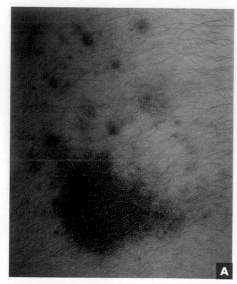 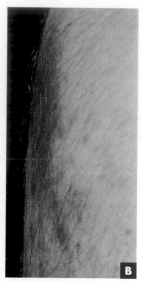

FIG. 6-30 *A,* Dramatic bruises with thick round centers can be seen in children with aplastic anemia or with clotting factor deficiencies. *B,* This view from the side shows the elevation of the indurated central portion of the ecchymosis in a patient with chronic aplastic anemia.

body. Because they are caused by thrombocytopenia, they are usually associated with petechiae (Fig. 6-29). Children with ITP commonly have a history of an antecedent viral illness, and those with leukemia may have a history of fatigue and weight loss and usually have adenopathy and splenomegaly. Patients with aplastic anemia can have bruises with round, thick, indurated centers similar to those seen in children with clotting factor deficiencies (Fig. 6-30). These hematologic abnormalities usually are readily detected by a complete blood count with differential and platelet count.

Clotting Factor Deficiencies

Children with clotting factor deficiencies—the hemophilias and von Willebrand's disease—tend to bruise easily, and their bruises are often much more impressive than one would ordinarily expect from the reported mechanism of injury. Although severe hemophilia in most males is diagnosed in early infancy (frequently following circumcision), those with mild disease may not be identified until they start crawling and show prominent ecchymoses over their knees, along with other evidence of easy bruising. Children with von Willebrand's disease, which occurs in both males and females and is characterized by partial factor VIII deficiency and platelet dysfunction, may escape detection for years, and this can be a source of confusion. Von Willebrand's disease is diagnosed in some patients when they suffer unexpectedly severe bleeding after surgery; the disease in many girls is identified when they suffer menorrhagia during adolescence or have severe bleeding following childbirth. Clues to an underlying factor deficiency include (1) bruises with round, thick, indurated centers (Fig. 6-30); (2) a clear mechanism of injury consistent with the configuration but not the severity of the bruise; (3) a family and child who seem well adjusted and interact appropriately. There also may be a positive family history for bleeding problems, especially after surgery or the birth of a baby. Whenever any question exists about a possible factor deficiency, a full coagulation profile is recommended, as many patients with von Willebrand's disease will have a normal prothrombin time and partial thromboplastin time.

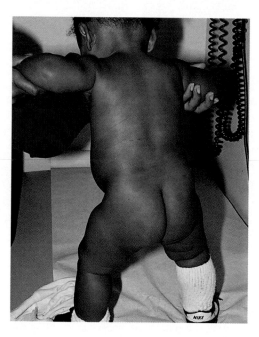

FIG. 6-31 This toddler, referred from a day care center because of "multiple bruises," actually had an unusual number of hyperpigmented mongolian spots.

Vasculitis

Patients with vasculitic disorders may develop diffuse purpuric lesions that can be mistaken for inflicted bruises. In the pediatric population, Henoch-Schönlein purpura is by far the most common of these. Knowledge of the pattern and course of evolution of its exanthem can help prevent misdiagnosis. Affected children often have a history of antecedent viral or streptococcal infection, followed by the appearance of the exanthem. In many, the initial lesions are urticarial, although pruritus is mild or absent. The purpuric lesions appear in crops, with the first located below the waist. Subsequent crops tend to involve the extensor forearms, cheeks, and ears. Periarticular swelling and stocking-glove angioedema, which wax and wane, are common, as is crampy or colicky abdominal pain (see Chapters 7 and 8).

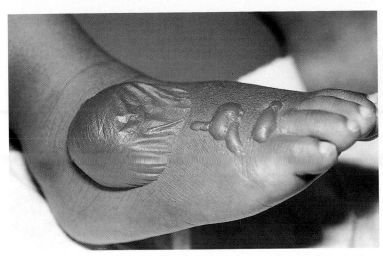

FIG. 6-32 Accidental scald. The splash-and-droplet pattern of an accidental scald is evident on the foot of a toddler who grabbed a hot cup of tea
from the table while sitting on his grandmother's lap.

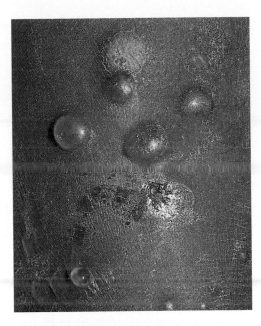

FIG. 6-33 Vesicula-
tion due to mite bites.
These pruritic vesicles
are relatively thick
walled and almost
perfectly round and
show no evidence of
splash.

Mongolian Spots

Most dark-skinned infants have patchy areas of hyperpigmentation
("mongolian spots") in which the epithelial cells contain increased
amounts of melanin. These are most commonly located over the
sacrum and buttocks, although they may be found elsewhere on the
trunk and extremities. These areas are flat, nontender, and typically a
bit more blue or green than true acute ecchymotic lesions (Fig. 6-31; see
also Chapter 8).

Differential Diagnosis of Accidental
Versus Inflicted Burns

All children incur accidental burns in the course of growing up, and it
is important to be able to distinguish these from inflicted burns. Many
are so small and minor that no medical care is sought. Children with
accidental burns usually present soon after the incident, and the history is consistent with the physical findings. Presentation may be delayed, however, if a minor burn being treated at home becomes secondarily infected.

Accidental Scalds

Accidental scalds typically occur when a hot liquid is spilled, producing a splash and droplet pattern (Fig. 6-32). The child usually has
grabbed a cup of hot coffee, tea, or cocoa, or the handle of a pot on the
stove. In some instances, a parent or older sibling has stumbled while
carrying a pan of hot liquid or food. Such burns commonly involve the
chest, a hand, a foot, or occasionally the head.

Vesicular Reactions to Insect Bites

Some mites inject a blistering agent that causes vesiculation. Such
vesicles and blisters have been mistakenly attributed to sprinkling the
child with scalding water. On close inspection, however, the lesions
(which are pruritic rather than painful) are found to be almost perfectly
round with no evidence of splash and the roof of each blister or vesicle is noted to have a thicker wall than that of the blister of a second-
degree burn (Fig. 6-33).

Accidental Iron Burns

Pulling an iron down from the ironing board by yanking on its cord
is the classic scenario for an accidental iron burn in a young child. The
iron being heavier at one end falls end over end, producing a configuration of two or three linear or patchy first- or second-degree burns sep-

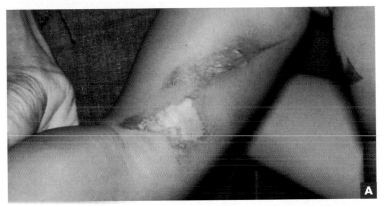

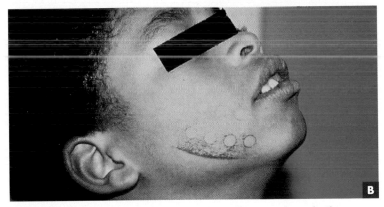

FIG. 6-34 Accidental iron burns. *A,* These linear and patchy burns are
characteristic of an accidental iron burn. In this case the patient's brother
pulled the iron down while she had her back turned. *B,* This hyperactive
boy decided to test the iron on his cheek while his mother went to answer
the phone. Though the imprint of the iron is clear, the superficial degree
of the burn is more consistent with an accidental than with an inflicted
burn.

arated by gaps (Fig. 6-34, *A*). In older children and adolescents, burns
are more often acquired in the course of ironing and usually consist of
small, superficial, linear burns of the hand or fingers. Occasionally, impulsive behavior results in self-inflicted burns, which also tend to be
superficial (Fig. 6-34, *B*).

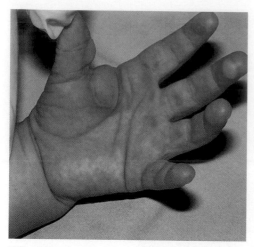

FIG. 6-35 Accidental curling iron burn. Second-degree burns are seen over the palm and flexor surfaces of the fingers of this toddler who grabbed her mother's curling iron.

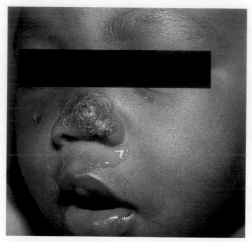

FIG. 6-36 Impetigo. This infant was initially suspected of having a cigar burn, but close inspection revealed a new peripheral bullous rim. This and the presence of another early impetiginous lesion on the cheek enabled the correct diagnosis to be made.

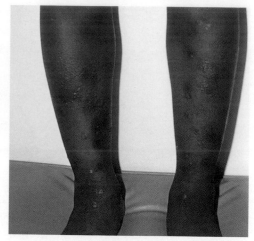

FIG. 6-37 Postinflammatory hyperpigmentation after insect bites. When this child was seen at a follow-up visit for the treatment of flea bites, he was found to have a multitude of round, hyperpigmented spots at the sites of the original bites. Their macular appearance and their distribution distinguish them from cigarette burn scars. (Courtesy Dr. Michael Sherlock.)

Accidental Curling Iron Burns

Accidental curling iron injuries occur most commonly when an older infant, toddler, or preschool-age child grabs the hot wand of a curling iron that has been left unattended by a parent or older sibling. The resulting first- and second-degree burns thus involve the palm and flexor surfaces of the fingers of one hand (Fig. 6-35). Preadolescent and adolescent girls may incur superficial burns on the ears or nape of the neck if they are not careful when curling their hair.

Accidental Space Heater Burns

During winter months, accidental burns can be incurred as a result of brushing up against the grid of a space heater while walking or running by it or when engaging in wrestling or horseplay near it. The lesions produced tend to be superficial and tangential and usually involve the dorsum of a hand or occasionally the lateral aspect of the lower leg or forearm. Less commonly, crawling infants and toddlers engaged in exploration may grab the grid, incurring palmar burns, or may fall against it.

Accidental Cigarette Burns

Unintentional cigarette burns usually occur when a child accidentally brushes against the lit end of an adult's cigarette. They tend to be single superficial, tangential burns and usually involve one hand, a forearm, or the cheek.

Lesions Often Mistaken for Cigarette Burns

On occasion, impetiginous lesions have been mistaken for cigarette or cigar burns. This is often the case with bullous impetigo, in which the initial central bulla has ruptured and crusted over. On careful inspection, one can detect the formation of a bullous rim around the more central crusts and other lesions usually can be found nearby (Fig. 6-36). Removal of the crust will reveal that the lesion is very superficial, in contrast to the full-thickness depression seen upon removal of the eschar from an inflicted cigarette or cigar burn.

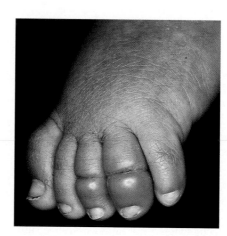

FIG. 6-38 Hair tourniquet. The mild erythema and edema of the third and fourth toes are the result of constriction by hairs that accidentally became wrapped around them. (Courtesy Dr. Thomas J. Daley, Bronx-Lebanon Hospital, New York.)

After resolution of the acute inflammatory phase of insect bites, children are often left with round, hyperpigmented or hypopigmented areas that have been mistaken for healed cigarette burns (Fig. 6-37). However, their usual distribution is over the lower legs above the sock line. The fact that these are macular and not punched-out scars should enable the clinician to distinguish between these and the scars left by cigarette burns.

Accidental Tourniquet Injuries

Perhaps the most common form of accidental tourniquet injury is that caused by a hair that becomes tightly wrapped around the toe of an infant (Fig. 6-38). The constriction causes pain and irritability, which prompts the parent to seek the cause. Hence, such patients are brought in promptly before circulatory compromise occurs. If they are not, neglect should be suspected. We have also seen young children with mild hand edema as a result of putting colored rubber bands around their wrists for bracelets.

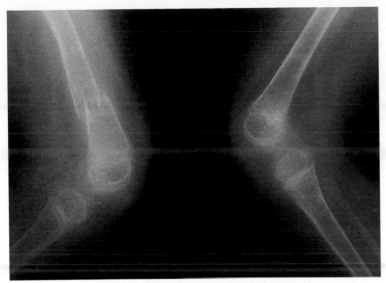

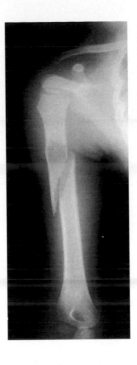

FIG. 6-40 Fracture through a unicameral bone cyst. This boy was seen because of intense pain and swelling of his upper arm after a relatively minor fall. The radiograph reveals a pathologic fracture through a unicameral bone cyst, which has caused considerable cortical thinning. (Courtesy the Department of Radiology, Children's Hospital of Pittsburgh.)

FIG. 6-39 Demineralization from disuse. Severe osteopenia and a femur fracture incurred during physical therapy are evident in this child who was left quadriplegic as the result of an earlier injury. Courtesy the Department of Radiology, Children's Hospital of Pittsburgh.)

Differentiation of Accidental and Pathologic Fractures from Inflicted Fractures

Accidental Fractures

In most instances, it is relatively easy to recognize a truly accidental fracture: the incident is usually witnessed, and the mechanism of injury is clearly reported. Care is typically sought promptly, although occasional exceptions occur, especially if the patient is a stoic athlete with a minor fracture who avoids complaining in order not to miss an important game. Accidental fractures are usually single or isolated or involve both bones of the forearm or lower leg.

Knowledge of the types of fractures produced by various mechanisms of injury facilitates accurate diagnosis. Some of the most common fractures and their mechanisms include:

Buckle (torus) and greenstick fractures of the radius and ulna (see Figs. 21-25 and 21-26)	Fall forward on an outstretched arm
Distal or midclavicular fracture (see Fig. 21-19)	Direct blow to clavicle, fall sideways onto outstretched arm
Supracondylar humerus fracture (see Fig. 21-33)	Fall backward onto hyperextended outstretched arm
Toddler's fracture, spiral fracture of distal to mid tibia (see Fig. 21-42)	Fall with a twist, while trying to extricate a caught foot, following a sudden turn while running, or on landing from a jump

One type of accidental humerus fracture, only recently described, can be easily mistaken for an inflicted injury. This spiral fracture of the humeral shaft can occur unintentionally when someone turns an infant from prone to supine without completely lifting his trunk from the surface on which he is lying. This occurs if the infant, while lying prone, has one arm extended out from his body, palm down, and while held by the opposite axilla, is rolled over to the supine position. Being unable to adduct the extended arm as he is turned, his upper arm is then subjected to a twisting force that produces the fracture.

Conditions Associated With Pathologic Fractures

Three relatively unusual conditions account for most pathologic fractures seen in the pediatric population: osteogenesis imperfecta, demineralization from disuse, and bone cysts.

Osteogenesis Imperfecta. The term *osteogenesis imperfecta* (OI) refers to a group of heritable conditions in which abnormal collagen formation results in osteoporosis and increased susceptibility to fractures (see Chapter 21). Children with OI types II (10% of cases) and III (18% of cases) are born with multiple fractures and deformities and have blue sclerae and extreme osteoporosis, making the diagnosis evident at the time of delivery (see Figs. 21-108 and 21-109). Patients with OI types I (66% of cases) and IV (6% of cases) have less severe bony fragility. Most patients with OI type I have blue sclerae and lax ligaments, and many have a family history of hearing impairment. They also tend to have mild short stature, with lower extremity bowing, and dentinogenesis imperfecta (see Chapter 20); all have wormian bones seen on skull x-ray studies (see Fig. 21-107). When these children do incur fractures, they present early, as do normal children with accidental fractures, and the mechanism of injury fits the fracture pattern described, although the force of impact may be less than that ordinarily required to produce a fracture. Their injuries usually involve the shafts of the long bones of the forearms or legs, and they tend to have clear radiographic evidence of cortical thinning (see Fig. 21-107).

The greatest difficulty in differential diagnosis may occur in an infant or young child with OI type IV, at which time osteopenia may not be apparent. These patients do not have blue sclerae and may not have abnormal teeth. In these cases a skull x-ray study can be of great help, as wormian bones usually will be present in this form of the disorder as well. Family history may also be helpful. The incidence of OI type IV in the population is extremely low, being 1 in 1 to 3 million.

Demineralization from Disuse. Children with severe cerebral palsy, advanced neuromuscular diseases, paraplegia, or quadriplegia that essentially leaves them confined to bed or a wheelchair develop muscular atrophy and bony demineralization as the result of disuse. Cortical thinning is marked (Fig. 6-39) and makes the patient vulnerable to frac-

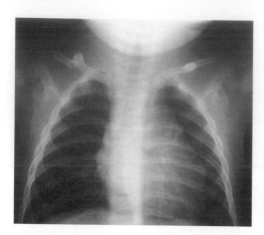

FIG. 6-41 Congenital pseudarthrosis of the clavicle. The overlapping ends of bone near the midpoint of this infant's clavicle are smooth, rounded, and well corticated, distinguishing this congenital anomaly from a fracture.

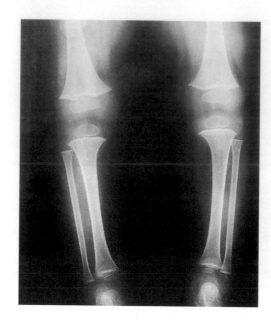

FIG. 6-42 Scurvy. Note the increased density of the zones of provisional calcification and the lucency of the underlying spongiosa. The metaphyses are also widened, and early spur formation is seen. (Courtesy the Department of Radiology, Children's Hospital of Pittsburgh.)

tures after the application of even minor forces, whether in minor falls or in the process of manipulation during physical therapy.

Bone Cysts. Benign bone cysts in pediatric patients are usually seen near the metaphyseal ends of long bones. As they enlarge, they cause cortical thinning, leaving the bone vulnerable to fracture (Fig. 6-40). Similar pathologic fractures may occur at sites of osteomyelitis or in portions of bone replaced by tumor.

Conditions Associated With or Mimicking Fractures

Congenital Pseudarthrosis of the Clavicle. Congenital pseudarthrosis of the clavicle is a rare congenital anomaly that usually involves the right clavicle and probably results from failed maturation of an ossification center. The clavicle appears foreshortened and has a visible bulbous deformity near its midportion (see Fig. 21-78). Hypermobility and crepitance are felt on palpation over the bump. This is distinguishable from a fracture because the site is nontender and the patient has full range of motion of the shoulder without pain. On radiography the two ends of the clavicle at the point of deformity are seen to be smooth and rounded and covered with a well-formed bony cortex (Fig. 6-41).

Rickets. Radiographic changes seen in rickets include metaphyseal irregularities, periosteal reaction, and fractures. The obvious cupping and fraying of the metaphyses and cortical thinning make it easy to distinguish these findings from fracture healing in an infant with a normal skeleton. Clinically, widened metaphyses and costochondral beading also help to establish the diagnosis (see Chapter 10).

Premature infants who, because of severe illness or lung disease, have prolonged nutritional problems necessitating total parenteral nutrition (TPN) are particularly vulnerable to rickets with attendant bony fragility. Because these infants often require chest physiotherapy, they may incur multiple rib fractures. When these are detected on chest x-ray studies obtained during evaluation of a respiratory illness following discharge from the nursery, abuse is often suspected. Given a history of prematurity and prolonged hospitalization, it is wise to contact the hospital where the child was cared for and review prior films before diagnosing abuse. Careful inspection of the current films often shows residual metaphyseal and costal changes characteristic of rickets.

Copper Deficiency. Copper deficiency is an exceptionally rare phenomenon that should be readily distinguishable from abuse. It occurs in nutritional and inherited forms. Prematurity; a change in early infancy to whole, powdered, or evaporated milk; severe malabsorption

syndromes; and prolonged TPN without copper supplementation are the major predisposing factors. Clinically, affected infants have pale skin, hypopigmented hair, edema, enlarged scalp veins, and seborrhea, with or without failure to thrive or developmental delay. All have neutropenia and a hypochromic microcytic anemia that is resistant to iron therapy; radiographically their bones are found to be grossly abnormal. Findings include overt osteoporosis, cupped metaphyses, metaphyseal spurs, widened anterior ribs, periosteal reaction, and at times, soft tissue calcification (see Chapter 10).

Menkes' kinky hair syndrome is the inherited form and results from an X-linked recessive defect in copper absorption. These children are markedly pale and have a characteristic facies with pudgy cheeks; horizontal, twisted eyebrows; and little facial expression. Their hair is dull or lusterless, sparse, and kinky with pili torti (see Chapter 8). Affected infants are also grossly abnormal neurologically, with hypertonia, decreased movement, lethargy, myoclonic seizures, and difficulty maintaining normothermia being major findings.

Scurvy. Although children with vitamin C deficiency (now exceedingly rare) tend to bruise easily because of vascular fragility, the disorder should be readily distinguishable from abuse on the basis of radiographic findings. Although a periosteal reaction resulting from subperiosteal hemorrhage is seen and there may be fractures through the zone of provisional calcification and through metaphyseal spurs, their cortices are thin and the ends of the long bones show characteristic changes consisting of increased density of the zone of provisional calcification and increased lucency of the underlying spongiosa (Fig. 6-42). These infants are irritable, tend to move little because of bone pain, and often have gingival bleeding.

Hypervitaminosis A. Chronic vitamin A intoxication produces a thick, wavy periosteal reaction, which most commonly involves the ulnas and metatarsals, although other long bones can be affected. Hard, tender swellings may be evident on palpation. Absence of fractures and metaphyseal abnormalities should help distinguish this from abuse. The history and findings of papilledema or split sutures on skull x-ray studies resulting from concomitant pseudotumor cerebri also aid in differentiation.

Leukemia. Children with acute leukemia may develop diffuse demineralization, periosteal reactions, and osteolytic lesions. Lucent metaphyseal bands, termed *leukemic lines,* are also seen (Fig. 6-43). The relative osteopenia and typical absence of fractures, combined with the antecedent history, often of fatigue, anorexia, and weight loss;

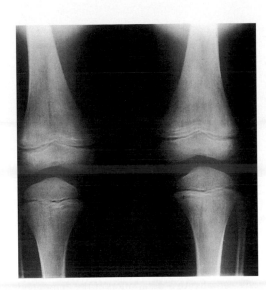

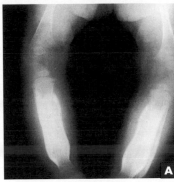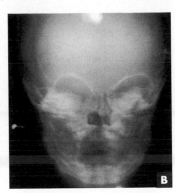

FIG. 6-43 Leukemic lines. These lucent metaphyseal bands can be seen in some children with acute leukemia or other severe systemic illnesses. However, they are rarely associated with fractures. (Courtesy the Department of Radiology, Children's Hospital of Pittsburgh.)

FIG. 6-44 Caffey's disease. *A,* Intense periosteal reaction and cortical thickening are seen in the lower extremities. *B,* Mandibular involvement has resulted in dramatic thickening. These findings, associated symptoms, and absence of fractures distinguish this condition from the skeletal changes characteristic of abuse. (Courtesy the Department of Radiology, Children's Hospital of Pittsburgh.)

physical findings which may include adenopathy, visceromegaly, and sternal tenderness; and the results of hematologic tests should distinguish these findings from those of abuse.

Caffey's Disease. A rare disorder of unknown etiology, Caffey's disease is characterized by cortical thickening and a painful periosteal reaction (Fig. 6-44). Bones are otherwise normally mineralized, and fractures are not seen. Involvement of the mandible, seen in 75% of affected patients, results in dramatic thickening. The clavicle and ulna are other common sites, although other bones can be involved. Most patients are under 6 months of age, and all have fever, anorexia, and marked irritability. The skin overlying affected sites is neither warm nor discolored. There is no soft tissue swelling, and palpation reveals bony-hard thickening below the subcutaneous tissues, which are adherent to the underlying bone.

Differential Diagnosis of Accidental Versus Inflicted Head Injuries

Accidental head injuries are common in childhood as a result of falls and other accidents, and the vast majority are minor. Presentation is usually prompt because a head injury, no matter how minor, tends to provoke considerable parental anxiety. Again, the history is usually clear and the mechanism is consistent with the physical findings. Mild forehead and scalp contusions with or without small lacerations or abrasions are by far the most common injuries seen. Linear skull fractures can result from relatively mild falls onto hard surfaces, but these do not tend to be associated with significant changes in level of consciousness or with intracranial injury. More severe injuries are incurred as a result of more serious mechanisms, including major falls, bicycle and sports accidents, and motor vehicle accidents.

Differentiation of Accidental from Inflicted Oral Injuries

Falls and sporting and bicycle accidents are the usual sources of accidental oral injuries. These include lip and chin lacerations; loosened or avulsed teeth; and gingival, palatal, or retropharyngeal lacerations, the last resulting from falls with an object in the mouth (see Chapters 20 and 22). These injuries, like head injuries, provoke considerable parental anxiety and result in prompt presentation for care, with a clear history and consistent mechanism of injury.

Differential Diagnosis of Accidental Versus Inflicted Chest and Abdominal Injuries

Accidental chest and abdominal injuries in children are predominantly the result of major blunt force trauma and are similar in nature to those caused by abuse. However, victims of accidental injuries have a clear history of a major mechanism of injury that was often witnessed. Immediate care is sought, and findings are consistent with the history.

Sexual Abuse

In sexual abuse the perpetrator misuses his or her power over a child, involving her or him in sexual activities that may or may not involve physical contact. The best available data indicate that the rising number of reports of sexual abuse stem from increased public and professional awareness and an increased willingness of victims to disclose abuse, rather than from a true rise in incidence. Despite this, sexual abuse continues to be underreported. Data from 1993 indicate that approximately 150,000 cases of sexual abuse were substantiated by child protection agencies. Given the fact that 20% of adult women and 5% to 10% of adult men report having been sexually abused before 18 years of age, it is estimated that substantiated cases constitute less than a third of all cases of sexual abuse.

Extrapolating current prevalence data to a pediatric practice of 1500 children, it is likely that 12 of them will be abused each year, eight of whom will disclose their abuse to a professional. Child protective services will be able to substantiate only half of the cases disclosed. It is also of concern that only 40% of cases disclosed to professionals are reported to authorities, despite mandatory reporting laws.

Sexual abuse may involve visual exposure to exhibitionistic, masturbatory, or copulatory behavior; fondling, masturbation, and digital manipulation; oral/genital contact; and direct genital contact, including penetration or attempted penetration of the vagina or anus. Twenty to twenty-five percent of cases reported retrospectively by women involve vaginal or orogenital penetration. Data regarding perpetrators indicate that approximately 40% are parents or stepparents and 25% are other relatives. Strangers probably constitute no more than 10% of the perpetrators. The rest are people who are known by but unrelated to the victim. The vast majority of perpetrators are male, but adult females are responsible for 20% of abusive sexual contact with prepubescent boys and 5% of such contact with prepubescent girls.

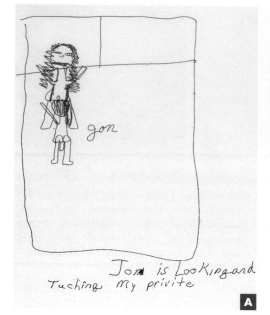

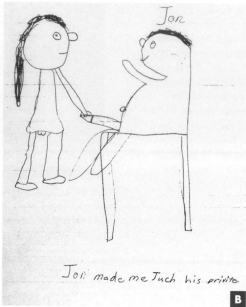

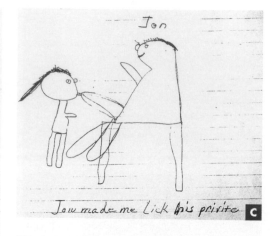

Jon is Looking and Tuching my privite **A**

Jon made me Tuch his privite **B**

Jon made me Lick his privite **C**

FIG. 6-45 *A, B,* and *C,* Drawings of a school-age sexual abuse victim. Though the child had difficulty verbalizing a description of the abuse, she was able to clearly depict the acts in her drawings.

If the perpetrator is a family member or acquaintance, the encounter is more likely to be physically nonviolent, with persuasion, bribery, or threats used to enlist the victim's cooperation. Not infrequently, these experiences are repetitive and occur over long periods. There is also a well-described pattern of escalating levels of involvement, with initial fondling and digital manipulation progressing to actual penetration over time. The victim's silence is ensured by various means, including bribes, gifts, praise, threats of dire consequences if the child discloses it, and fear of the perpetrator's power. Thus, the victim bears both the guilt of engaging in unwanted sexual activity and the pressure of keeping it a secret. Absence of physical violence or injury does not imply consent, as the offender is usually in a position of power over the victim, making it difficult for the child to refuse to engage in the activity and to disclose it. Episodes involving strangers are more likely to be isolated incidents and more frequently involve physical violence, often adding the emotional stress of being in a potentially life-threatening situation.

Forensic requirements for a detailed history, physical examination, and often multiple laboratory specimens (all carefully documented) necessitate a lengthy evaluation, which, if not sensitively handled, can compound the existing emotional trauma. This can be minimized if the physician approaches the patient and family with patience, gentleness, and tact. If the disclosed sexual abuse does not involve allegations that necessitate collection of evidence of ejaculate, the physical examination may be postponed, conducted in stages, or if necessary, performed under anesthesia or conscious sedation.

Because physical findings are usually normal and, if present, are frequently nonspecific, the history is usually the key aspect of the evaluation. Hence, it is essential that historical information be documented meticulously (and, if possible, verbatim), since many of these cases have the potential for legal prosecution (usually months later). It is also important to avoid asking leading questions, although in certain situations, after all other avenues have been exhausted, they may be necessary in order to elicit enough information to ensure protection of the child. The parent or persons accompanying the child should be interviewed first, if possible, apart from each other and separately from the child. During this interview one can obtain information about the child's emotional status and recent behavior; present and past history; family psychosocial situation; household members or other persons caring for the child, or people who live in or visit the home who might

have unwitnessed access to the child; the events that appear to have led to the disclosure; and terms used by the child for body parts. When the chief complaint is not sexual abuse, but findings on examination point to molestation, this information should be sought in a further interview with the parent, or parents, after the examination, with the child out of the room.

In approaching the child, it is essential for the clinician to show kindness, empathy, and gentleness. If the child is willing and able to give a history, it, as well as the exact phrasing of the questions asked, should be documented verbatim. In the initial portion of the interview, talking about favorite subjects such as friends, favorite toys, games, and activities helps to reduce the child's anxiety and establish rapport between the child and clinician. Thereafter, it is best to ask general questions, reserving more specific questions for situations in which the child is unable to disclose and there is a very strong suspicion of sexual abuse. If the child is unwilling to discuss the episode or episodes and there is a strong suspicion of sexual abuse, a return visit or referral for a play therapy session with a trained clinician is recommended. In such interviews a variety of alternative techniques can be used if the child still has difficulty disclosing verbally. These include having the child try to draw what happened (Fig. 6-45), demonstrate what happened with anatomically correct dolls, or write about the incidents.

Documentation of the manner in which disclosure occurs is also important. When children give spontaneous detailed descriptions of sexual experiences in language appropriate to their developmental level, these are usually accurate and not imagined. Asking nondirective questions to ascertain the site where the activity occurred and the number of times it happened, and questions related to such things as clothing worn, can be useful in documenting the child's credibility. It is also important to determine the patient's understanding of the need for accuracy in relating the history and of the difference between telling the truth and telling a lie. This helps in determining the child's ability to testify. Recent recognition of the problem of false accusations of sexual abuse made in the heat of child custody battles has raised questions regarding the veracity of many such claims. Findings from ongoing research suggest that if the child's disclosure is made without benefit of leading questions and is reported with feeling and often some hesitancy and in age-appropriate terms, the report is more likely to be accurate. In contrast, children coached to make false claims tend to relate a history in a rote manner and often use adult-oriented words.

TABLE 6-2

Most Common Substitute Complaints in Sexual Abuse Cases*

Any age	Preschool age	School age	Adolescence
Abdominal pain	Excessive clinging	Decreased school performance	Same as school age plus:
Anorexia	Thumbsucking	Truancy	Runaway behavior
Vomiting	Speech disorder	Lying, stealing	Suicide attempts
Constipation	Encopresis/enuresis	Tics	Commission of sexual offenses†
Sleep disorders	Excessive masturbation†	Anxiety reaction	
Dysuria		Phobic and obsessional states	
Vaginal discharge‡		Depression	
Vaginal bleeding‡		Conversion reaction	
Rectal bleeding		Encopresis/enuresis	

*Most of these complaints are also symptomatic of disorders more prevalent than sexual abuse.
†Symptoms highly suggestive of sexual abuse.
‡Symptoms somewhat suggestive of sexual abuse.

Yet another problem has arisen stemming from the child being required to repeat the history to multiple authorities—family, physician, social worker, psychologist, attorney, and the like. Many such victims begin to sound robotic in their reporting (raising questions regarding their truthfulness), and many others become so traumatized by the repetition and the impact on their family that they recant their story to avoid further painful questioning.

A thorough and complete physical examination is warranted for all patients suspected of having been sexually abused, with examination of the genitalia and rectum deferred until last. Each part of the examination should be explained as the examiner proceeds. If possible, and if the child so chooses, a parent or supportive adult should be present. Because the parents are usually anxious, it is important that details of the examination be described to them before it is begun. In cases of elective referrals this should be done before the appointment, because many mothers erroneously assume there will be a speculum examination of the prepubertal child, which they often associate with discomfort themselves and understandably feel will be traumatic for their child. If an attempt to inspect the perineum provokes anxiety which cannot be allayed, the procedure should be deferred, unless there is gross bleeding, pain and discharge, or evidence of venereal disease. Under these circumstances, the patient should be admitted, and the examination and specimen collection should be performed with the patient under general anesthesia or conscious sedation. If the patient is asymptomatic and there is no evidence of trauma, bleeding, discomfort, or discharge, the procedure can be deferred and performed at a follow-up visit. It is most important that the child not feel that he or she is being assaulted yet again during the examination and interview process.

In our experience with prepubescent patients, external inspection of the genitalia suffices in the vast majority of cases and the insertion of a speculum is rarely indicated. Speculum use can be painful, provides little in the way of useful information, and usually provokes much parental anxiety. In the few instances in which internal examination is required in the prepubescent patient, it should be performed with the patient under general anesthesia.

Modes of Presentation

Because the vast majority of cases of sexual abuse do not involve physical violence, most patients have no signs of injury, and in most in-stances, physical findings are completely normal. In cases of sexual assault involving violence and resulting in injury, a significant proportion of victims seek medical care promptly, most acknowledge the nature of the problem at the time of presentation, and physical findings are more often positive.

Although there has been a significant increase in the percentage of patients who have disclosed inappropriate touching prior to presentation, it continues to be true that many victims of long-term sexual abuse present with vulvovaginitis with vaginal discharge caused by a sexually transmitted pathogen or with substitute complaints generated by physical or emotional sequelae (Table 6-2). There is a myriad of such complaints, which are somewhat age dependent and each of which has many potential causes other than sexual abuse. While there is a wide range of differential diagnostic possibilities in patients presenting with these problems, sexual abuse should be considered and addressed among the diagnostic considerations. When sexual abuse is the underlying source of the problem, diagnosis can be difficult if, as is usual, physical findings are normal. It is appropriate to ask questions of parent and child separately about the possibility of inappropriate touching, and if there is any suspicion of this, a more detailed psychological assessment performed by a specially trained clinician is warranted. It is of note that a significant proportion of sexual abuse victims who have substitute chief complaints do not disclose immediately. This, in our experience, seems to be particularly true of children seen because of a sexually transmitted disease. However, after repeated visits with a single clinician during a stepwise evaluation for the underlying cause of their problem, many may develop enough trust to be able to disclose sexual abuse or another source of their stress.

Examination Techniques

Perineal Examination

Several techniques may be used for examination of the genital and perianal areas in different age groups. In the postpubescent age group, a standard gynecologic examination usually can be performed with the patient in the lithotomy position (see Chapter 18). In cases of acute injury, consideration must be given to the severity and extent of the injuries before proceeding. If examination and specimen collection are likely to cause extreme physical pain or emotional distress, or if internal injuries are likely, consideration should be given to examination under anesthesia (EUA).

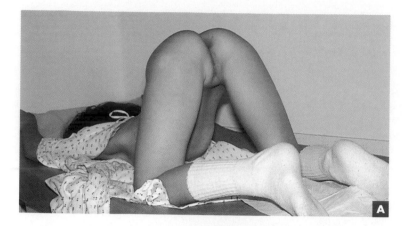

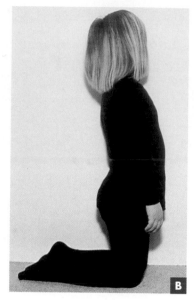

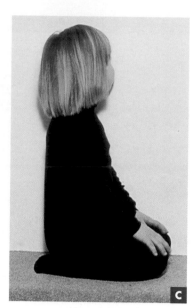

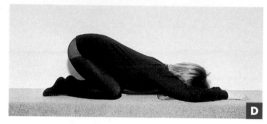

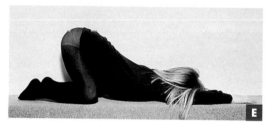

FIG. 6-46 Knee-chest position. *A,* The sway-back position with knees widely separated facilitates examination and provides the best visualization of anatomic structures and abnormalities. *B* to *E,* After looking at enlargements of this series of photographs, we have the patient practice getting into position while still fully clothed. The steps are *(B)* kneel, *(C)* sit back, *(D)* stretch arms out and place arms and chest on table, and *(E)* scoot forward. This helps children become more comfortable with being examined from behind.

The purposes of the perineal examination in the prepubescent child are: (1) to obtain full visualization of the patient's perineal and perianal anatomy; (2) to detect any evidence of acute injury, infection, distortion of anatomy, or scarring indicative of prior injury; (3) to assess the amount and appearance of hymenal tissue and determine the size and configuration of the hymenal orifice; and (4) to collect specimens as indicated. As noted earlier, internal speculum examination is not necessary unless there is evidence of internal extension of injury and, in such cases, the examination, specimen collection, and repair should be done in the operating room under general anesthesia.

In examining prepubescent patients, a number of positions may be used to achieve visualization of the genital area. The one most commonly used is the **supine frog-leg position** with the patient lying supine on the examining table. This position can also be achieved with the child semireclining on the parent's lap—**semisupine frog-leg position.** We have also had good success with the **semisupine lithotomy position** (see Fig. 18-5, *A* and *B*). The latter is accomplished by having the parent sit on the examining table and lean back against the wall. The child sits on her lap, with the buttocks resting just above the parent's knees, and leans back. The parent then places her hands under the patient's knees, flexing them and abducting the hips. The **knee-chest position** (Fig. 6-46, *A*) provides the best exposure of perineal structures and generally a clearer picture of anatomic features and abnormalities (Figs. 6-47 and 6-53). It is therefore preferred by experts in sexual abuse evaluation. In using this, it is important that the child's shoulders and chest touch the table, achieving a

sway-back posture. The knee-chest position is difficult to use in children under 2 years of age, however, and some older children object to it. Nevertheless, most children can be made comfortable with the knee-chest position and helped to relax by engaging them in an ongoing conversation about an unrelated subject, having the child count as high as she can, or using a variety of visually interesting toys (e.g., kaleidoscopes, oil-based timers) held by an assistant at eye level. We also have the child practice the position before the examination while fully clothed (Fig. 6-46, *B* to *E*).

To facilitate visualization of the introitus in the supine or semisupine frog-leg or lithotomy positions, the labia must be manually separated. In the **labial separation** method, the examiner places the index fingers over the lower portion of the labia majora and gently presses downward and laterally. In the **labial traction** technique, the labia majora are grasped between the thumbs and index fingers and gently pulled toward the examiner. The latter usually achieves better visualization of the hymen and its orifice and the greatest hymenal opening. It is also generally possible to see the posterior aspect of the lower third of the vagina using this technique (see Fig. 18-6).

In the **knee-chest position,** exposure of the introitus is facilitated by placing the thumbs over the edge of the gluteus muscles at the level of the introitus, lifting them upward. Because decrease in hymenal tissue can be an important finding in some sexual abuse victims, it should be assessed. Transverse diameter does vary with position and degree of relaxation; hence, it is important to document not only the diameter, but also the position of the patient in which the measurement was obtained

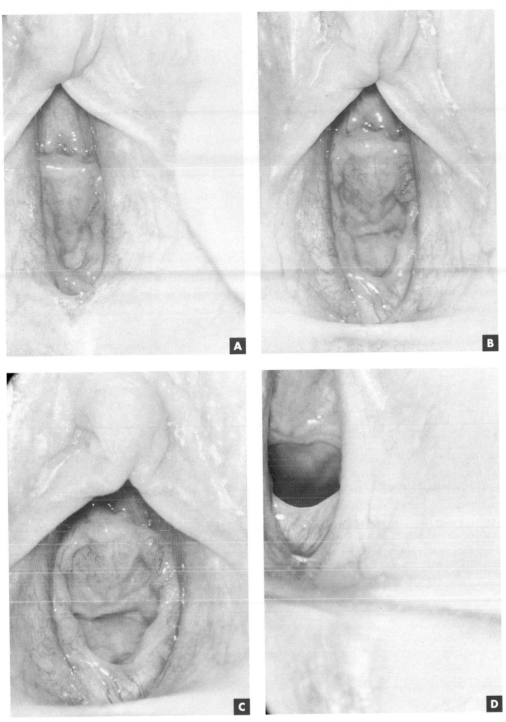

FIG. 6-47 Variation in the transverse or horizontal hymenal diameter with position and technique. *A,* Supine with labial separation. *B,* Supine with labial traction. *C,* Lithotomy with more labial traction. *D,* Knee-chest position. Note that the hymenal orifice is widest with good traction and that the hymen appears wrinkled and thickened in *B* and *C.* This is due to a mild redundancy seen in the knee-chest position, in which the hymen is seen to be thin with smooth, sharp edges when fully stretched out.

(see Figs. 6-47 and 18-6). It is now recognized that measurements of the hymenal orifice are less useful than are assessment of the appearance of the hymen and surrounding tissues.

Good lighting and magnification are also important. Use of a colposcope is ideal, but this device is not readily available to most practitioners. Alternatively, a magnifying halogen lamp or an otoscope may be used. The latter is the device most readily available, but the child must be reassured that this is only being used to get a good view with the light and that no speculum will be used as it is for ear examinations.

It is very important that a complete description of the appearance of the genitalia be documented on the chart (Fig. 6-48), and if possible,

magnified photographs of the genital area should be taken. These obviate the need for reexamination if a second opinion is requested.

Documentation should include: (1) Tanner staging; (2) the presence or absence of erythema or discharge; (3) the presence or absence and location of bruises, abrasions, or lacerations of the labia majora and perineum; (4) the appearance of the vestibule and (5) of the labia minora; (6) the presence and extent of labial adhesions; (7) the appearance of the posterior fourchette and presence or absence of scarring; and (8) the configuration of the hymen (annular, crescentic, redundant), the transverse diameter of its orifice (the position in which it was measured), and the appearance of its edges (e.g., thin and sharp, thickened or rolled, notched). Such documentation requires

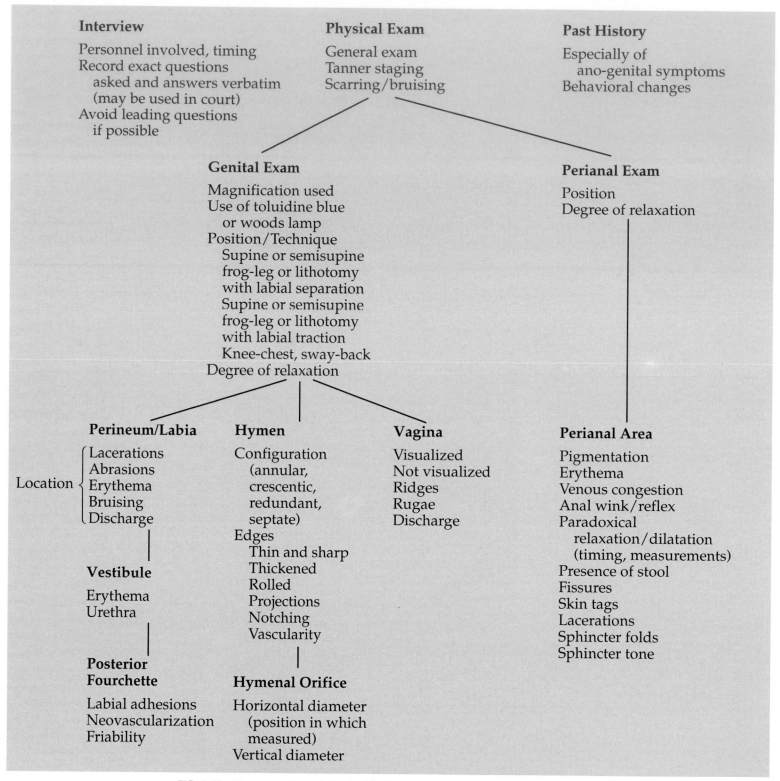

Interview

Personnel involved, timing
Record exact questions
   asked and answers verbatim
   (may be used in court)
Avoid leading questions
   if possible

Physical Exam

General exam
Tanner staging
Scarring/bruising

Past History

Especially of
   ano-genital symptoms
Behavioral changes

Genital Exam

Magnification used
Use of toluidine blue
   or woods lamp
Position/Technique
   Supine or semisupine
   frog-leg or lithotomy
   with labial separation
   Supine or semisupine
   frog-leg or lithotomy
   with labial traction
   Knee-chest, sway-back
Degree of relaxation

Perianal Exam

Position
Degree of relaxation

Perineum/Labia

Location { Lacerations
Abrasions
Erythema
Bruising
Discharge

Vestibule

Erythema
Urethra

Posterior Fourchette

Labial adhesions
Neovascularization
Friability

Hymen

Configuration
(annular,
crescentic,
redundant,
septate)
Edges
   Thin and sharp
   Thickened
   Rolled
   Projections
   Notching
   Vascularity

Hymenal Orifice

Horizontal diameter
(position in which
measured)
Vertical diameter

Vagina

Visualized
Not visualized
Ridges
Rugae
Discharge

Perianal Area

Pigmentation
Erythema
Venous congestion
Anal wink/reflex
Paradoxical
   relaxation/dilatation
   (timing, measurements)
Presence of stool
Fissures
Skin tags
Lacerations
Sphincter folds
Sphincter tone

FIG. 6-48 Documentation of physical findings required in sexual abuse evaluation.

knowledge of basic gynecologic anatomy and terminology, which are shown in Fig. 6-49 and given in Table 6-3 (see also the section Differential Diagnosis of Sexual Abuse that follows and the section Normal Developmental Changes in Chapter 18).

If external contusions or tears are seen, internal injury must be suspected. The prepubescent girl is particularly vulnerable to severe internal trauma as a result of forceful penetration of either the vagina or the rectum (Fig. 6-51). This stems from the fact that the structures are relatively small and the tissues more delicate and rigid. Young children with mild external injuries may in fact have major internal tears, including perforation of the peritoneum and damage to pelvic vessels, mesentery, and intestine (see Figs. 18-16 to 18-19). Signs of internal pathology may be subtle, but such patients will have evidence of vaginal bleeding or vaginal hematoma,

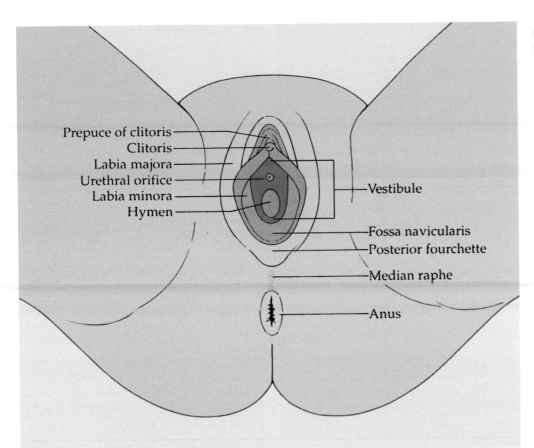

FIG. 6-49 Normal anatomy. Location of the genital structures of the prepubescent female.

TABLE 6-3

Gynecologic Anatomic Terminology

Anal verge	The tissue overlying the subcutaneous external anal sphincter at the most distal portion of the anal canal, extending exteriorly to the margin of the anal skin.
Anterior commissure	The union of the two labia minora anteriorly.
Clitoris	A cylindrical, erectile body situated at the superior portion of the vulva, covered by a sheath of skin called the *clitoral hood*.
Fossa navicularis/ Posterior fossa	Concavity of the lower part of the vestibule situated inferiorly to the vaginal orifice and extending to the posterior fourchette (posterior commissure).
Hymen	A thin membrane located at the junction of the vestibular floor and the vaginal canal which partially covers the vaginal orifice.
Labia majora	Rounded folds of skin forming the lateral boundaries of the vulva.
Labia minora	Thin longitudinal folds of tissue enclosed within the labia majora, which in the child extend from the clitoral hood to the midpoint of the lateral wall of the vestibule. After puberty, they lengthen and join to form the posterior commissure.
Median raphe	Ridge or furrow that marks the line of union of the two halves of the perineum.
Mons pubis	Rounded, fleshy prominence, created by the underlying fat pad which overlies the symphysis pubis.
Perianal folds	Wrinkles or folds of the skin of the anal verge which radiate out from the anus.
Perineal body	The central tendon of the perineum located between the vulva and the anus in the female and between the scrotum and anus in the male.
Perineum	The pelvic floor and associated structures bounded anteriorly by the symphysis pubis, laterally by the ischial tuberosities, and posteriorly by the coccyx.
Posterior commissure	The union of the two labia minora posteriorly, seen after puberty.
Posterior fourchette	The junction of the two labia minora inferiorly. This area is referred to as a *posterior commissure* in the prepubescent child, because the labia minora are not completely developed to connect inferiorly until puberty, when it is referred to as the *fourchette*.
Vagina	The uterovaginal canal extending from the inner aspect of the hymen to the uterine cervix.
Vaginal vestibule	Anatomic cavity containing the opening of the vagina, the urethra, and the ducts of Bartholin's glands; bordered by the clitoris superiorly, the labia laterally, and the posterior commissure (fourchette) inferiorly, and encompassing the fossa navicularis immediately inferior to the vaginal introitus.
Vulva	The external genitalia or pudendum of the female; includes the clitoris, labia majora, labia minora, vaginal vestibule, urethral orifice, vaginal orifice, hymen, and posterior fourchette (or commissure).

Courtesy the American Professional Society on the Abuse of Children.

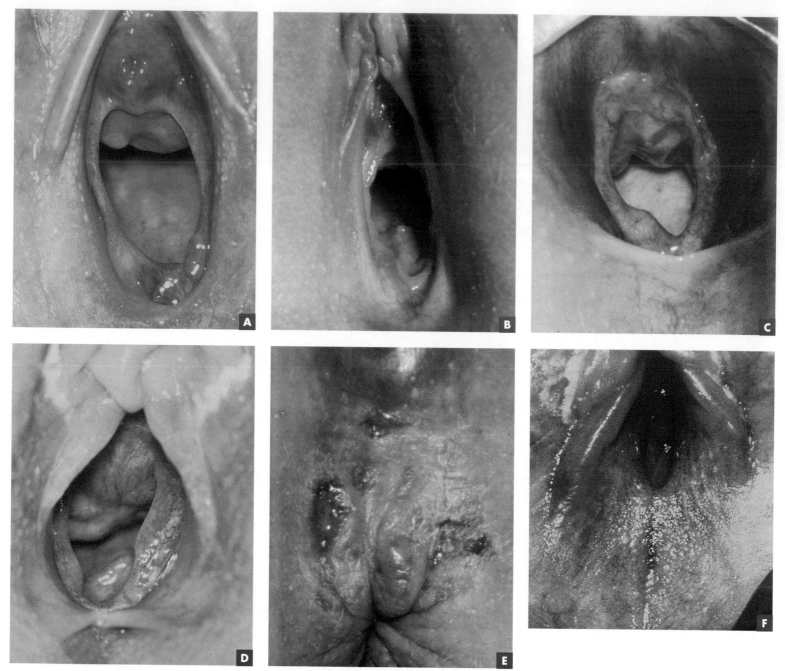

FIG. 6-50 Abnormal findings as a result of chronic sexual abuse. *A,* This child has a wide hymenal orifice with little remaining hymenal tissue. The latter is not thickened, however. *B,* The hymen is almost completely absent and that remaining has slightly thickened, rolled margins. There is a subtle bump at 7 o'clock and a notch at 5 o'clock. *C,* The hymenal rim is markedly thickened in this child and has rolled margins and a bump at 7 o'clock. *D,* This hymen has a deep posterior notch. *E,* Scarring, edema, and fresh excoriations of the perineal body extending to the anterior anal rim are seen in this repetitively abused child. *F,* The adhesed labia minora in this child are markedly thickened secondary to chronic frictional trauma incurred during sexual abuse. (*C* and *E* courtesy Dr. Pat Bruno, Sunbury, Pa.; *F* courtesy Dr. John McCann, University of California at Davis.)

and often have lower abdominal tenderness or evidence of occult blood loss. Therefore, when such findings are present, EUA is indicated. The postpubescent female can usually be adequately assessed by careful pelvic examination, unless, despite good emotional support, reassurance, and careful preparation, she is emotionally unable to tolerate the procedure, in which case an EUA would also be advisable.

Rectal examination is necessary in acute cases for assessment of internal rectal tears, pelvic tenderness, and sphincter tone, and for bimanual palpation.

Perianal Examination

Sodomy is a common form of sexual abuse in both boys and girls. To achieve optimal visualization, the perianal examination should be conducted in the knee-chest position. Care should be taken to look for evidence of abrasions, tears, fissures, or other lesions, and for evidence of rapid dilation of the external sphincter in the absence of stool in the rectum. The absence of physical findings is the norm and does not make the history any less credible. After specimen collection, a digital rectal examination should be performed to assess sphincter tone in patients with acute trauma.

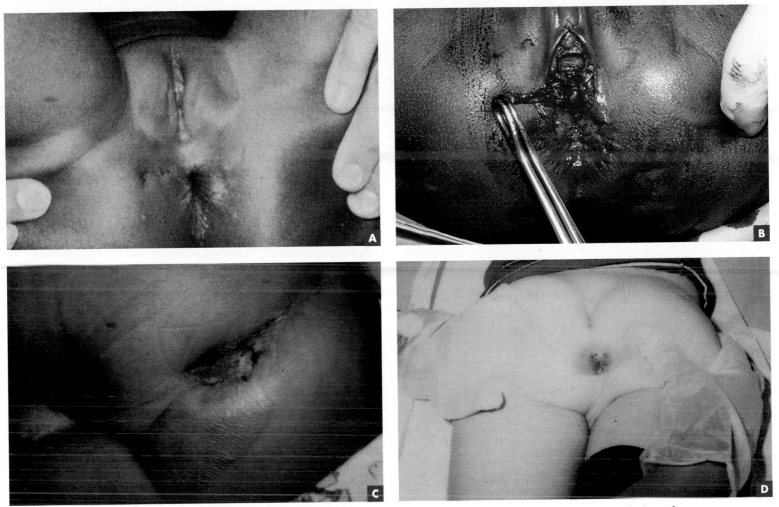

FIG. 6-51 Acute traumatic findings seen in victims of sexual abuse and assault. *A,* Abrasions, contusions, and punctate tears of the perineum and perianal areas can be seen in this prepubescent girl. *B,* Severe genital trauma in a prepubescent girl after rape. Inspection reveals a hymenal tear at 6 o'clock, extending posteriorly through the perineal body to the rectum. With the patient under anesthesia, a 1-inch (2.5-cm) long vaginal tear was discovered, along with a rectal tear and complete disruption of the external anal sphincter. *C,* Perianal lacerations, abrasions, and burns are apparent in this prepubescent boy. It is suspected that the burns were inflicted to obscure the evidence of sodomy. *D,* Prominent, perianal ecchymoses were found in this 3-year-old boy who had been sodomized. (*B* courtesy Dr. Kamthorn Sukarochana, Children's Hospital of Pittsburgh.)

Physical Findings

The changes in appearance of the female genitalia with age are described in Chapter 18. It is most important for practitioners to be familiar with the normal anatomy at different ages and with normal variations. Only recently has an extensive, carefully done study documented in detail the many normal variants, some of which have been mistaken for abnormal findings in the past (see the section Differential Diagnosis of Sexual Abuse).

Abnormal and Suspicious Findings in Cases of Sexual Abuse

Perineal Abnormalities. As noted earlier, findings on examination in victims of molestation or incest are totally normal in up to 80% of cases. In the remaining 20%, abnormal or suspicious findings can be detected with careful examination. There is, however, considerable controversy over the significance of some findings. One of these is enlargement of the hymenal orifice. Hence, mild widening in the absence of other abnormal findings should not be used in isolation as evidence for sexual abuse. For unknown reasons, obese children may have an increased hymenal diameter, but the significance of this is unclear. Marked enlargement is highly suspicious, however (Fig. 6-50, *A* to *C*). Other physical findings associated with chronic sexual abuse include a thickened, rolled hymenal rim with little remaining hymenal tissue (Figs. 6-50, *C,* and 6-53, *C*) and notching of the rim, especially between 3 and 9 o'clock (Fig. 6-50, *C* and *D*). Presence of bumps along the rim between 3 and 5 o'clock and 7 and 9 o'clock in patients with loss of hymenal tissue (Fig. 6-50, *B* and *C*); the presence of abnormal blood vessels over the posterior portion of the hymenal membrane; and excoriations and scarring of the perineal body (Fig. 6-50, *E*) are also abnormal findings seen as a result of sexual abuse. We have also seen lichenification due to chronic abrasive action (Fig. 6-50, *F;* see Fig. 18-23). Erythema is a common but totally nonspecific finding.

Acute Traumatic Findings of Sexual Assault and Sexual Abuse

Victims of sexual assault often show evidence of physical trauma other than genital injuries. Bruises and abrasions of the head, face, neck, chest, forearms, knees, and thighs are common. Occasionally, even more severe nongenital injuries are encountered.

Genital and rectal examination may reveal contusions, erythema, abrasions, or lacerations (Fig. 6-51; see Figs. 18-14 to 18-19). Perineal lesions tend to be located in the posterior portion of the introitus, as opposed to lesions caused by straddle injury, which are usually more anterior or located over the labia majora and inner thighs (see Figs. 6-62 and 18-16). These are usually unilateral and rarely involve the hymen in isolation. It is also important to note that perineal injuries often heal very quickly and completely, with no residual scarring. At times, evidence of seminal products in the form of a vaginal discharge are observed if the patient is seen within 24 to 72 hours of the latest incident and has not bathed (Fig. 6-52). Seminal fluid has been reported to fluoresce under Wood's lamp, but in our tests, we have found only weak fluorescence when it has been wet and none when dry. Under normal light, the seminal products are practically invisible after drying. If a history of ejaculation is obtained and the area has not been washed, swabbing the perineum and inner thighs with saline-moistened cotton swabs may yield a sample of dried seminal fluid which can be identified by the crime laboratory. Swabs should be air-dried after the collection process.

In some cases, when labial separation or traction is performed with the victim in the supine or semisupine frog-leg or lithotomy position, findings can be obscured by redundant hymenal tissue. If this occurs in suspected abuse victims, examination with the child in the knee-chest position, with its superior visualization, is important to avoid missing abnormal findings (Fig. 6-53, *A* to *C*).

Male victims may have evidence of urethral discharge and mild abrasions and contusions of the penis, scrotum, or median raphe.

Oral Abnormalities. Forceful orogenital contact may result in perioral and intraoral injuries. These may include fissuring or tears at the corner of the mouth and gingival and palatal contusions. Such oral lesions are unusual, however. In contrast, asymptomatic gonococcal infection of the pharynx is relatively common.

Anal and Perianal Abnormalities. Patients who have been repetitively sodomized may manifest paradoxical anal sphincter relaxation in response to gluteal stroking to assess for an anal wink reflex, or they may exhibit immediate dilation of the anal sphincter to greater than 2 cm when placed in the knee-chest position. If the latter phenomenon is seen in the absence of stool in the rectal vault, the findings are highly suspicious. Repeated sodomy also is said to result in funneling "of the perianal area." This rare finding occurs as a result of a loss of fatty tissue. The presence of tears in the perianal area and fissures is suspicious, although the latter are not specific to sexual abuse, being seen frequently in children with chronic or recurrent constipation. Tears that extend beyond the hair follicle–bearing areas are thought to be more characteristic of abuse. Evidence of perianal bruises or burns (Fig. 6-51, *C* and *D*) is strongly suggestive of abuse, and burns may be inflicted in an attempt to obscure injuries resulting from sodomy.

Evidence of Sexually Transmitted Disease. The presence of sexually transmitted diseases in the prepubescent child is strongly suggestive of sexual abuse, except in occasional instances in which other modes of transmission can be documented. In fact, many victims are identified upon presenting with a vaginal or urethral discharge that is positive for a venereal pathogen. In females, this usually is manifested by vulvovaginitis with a vaginal discharge, with *Neisseria gonorrhoeae* and *Chlamydia trachomatis* the most commonly identified pathogens (see Chapter 18). Asymptomatic vulvovaginal infection does occur but is unusual, in contrast to oral and rectal gonococcal infections, which typically are subclinical. Males may have overt urethritis or asymptomatic urethral infection.

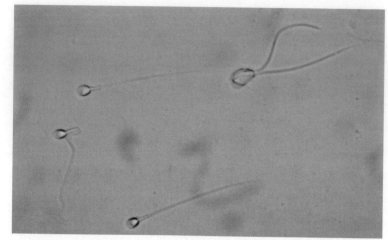

FIG. 6-52 Microscopic appearance of seminal fluid removed from a young rape victim. If a vaginal discharge is found in a patient presenting within 72 hours of sexual abuse, a wet mount may reveal sperm. A portion of the discharge should also be collected for acid phosphatase, blood grouping, and enzyme studies.

Vulvovaginal, urethral, oral, and rectal infections with gonococcus are almost always acquired through sexual contact, as is vulvovaginal *Chlamydia* infection in the child over 2 to 3 years old (see later discussion) and *Trichomonas* infection in the peripubescent child. Development of *Condylomata acuminata* after infancy is highly suspicious, though not diagnostic for abuse (Fig. 6-54). In the very young child, genital herpes infections may be acquired through sexual contact but are probably more often the result of spread from oral or hand lesions from the patient or a parent as a result of poor attention to hand-washing (see Fig. 18-33, *A*). In the latency age child, sexual contact is the more likely source. Nonspecific vaginal discharges, especially if chronic or recurrent, are also suspect. All should be tested for the presence of sperm.

Nonsexual transmission of gonococcus, *Chlamydia*, *Trichomonas*, and human papillomavirus occurs primarily during vaginal delivery. Gonococcal infections tend to produce symptoms early in the neonatal period. Perinatally acquired *Trichomonas* infection causes a copious vaginal discharge in the neonate, which abates even without treatment, although the organism can persist for months. In contrast, *Chlamydia* infection acquired neonatally may persist for 18 months to 3 years. Hence, finding this organism in the very young child cannot be considered diagnostic of sexual abuse. Because of its prolonged incubation period, the human papillomavirus may not produce lesions until several months after delivery, despite being transmitted at birth.

Finally, it must be noted that in some instances children acquire sexually transmitted diseases as the result of sexual contact with other infected children. In such cases, aggressive case finding can result in identification of the index child who is an abuse victim.

Specimen Collection

Laboratory studies are designed to augment the physical assessment of injury, identify sexually transmitted pathogens, and document the presence or absence of seminal fluid. The likelihood of finding the latter is so small after 72 hours that these studies can be omitted if the patient seeks attention 3 or more days after the last incident. Cultures should be obtained regardless of time of presentation or absence of symptoms, as infections may be asymptomatic. Although asymptomatic vaginal infection in prepubescent girls is rare, oral and rectal gonorrhea infections are typically asymptomatic.

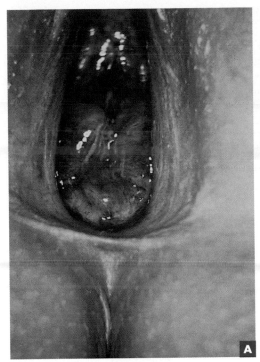
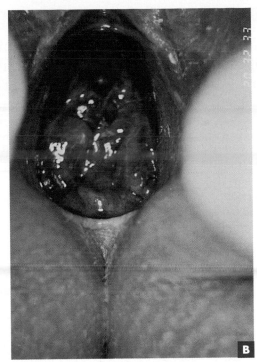
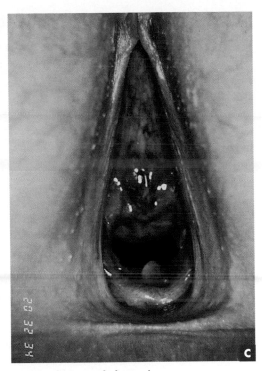

FIG. 6-53 The superiority of visualization using the knee-chest position is demonstrated in this sexual abuse victim whose redundant tissues made it difficult to see the true configuration of her hymen when she was supine with *(A)* labial separation or *(B)* labial traction. *C,* In the knee-chest position the hymenal rim can be seen to be obviously narrowed and thickened. (Courtesy Dr. John McCann, University of California at Davis.)

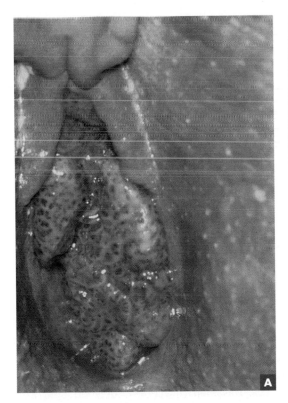
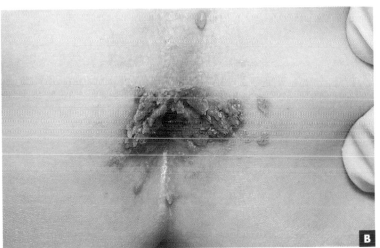

FIG. 6-54 Condylomata acuminata. *A,* When condylomata are restricted to the hymen, as seen in this child, sexual abuse is the likely source. This child also reported that the perpetrator had visible genital warts. *B,* Coalescent and discrete condylomata are seen in the perianal area of this 4-year-old boy with a history of being sodomized.

In the prepubescent child with vaginal discharge, all cultures may be obtained from the discharge on the perineum, except for *Chlamydia* cultures, which necessitate swabbing the vaginal wall. (Note: The ELISA or Chlamydiazyme test is not indicated in prepubescent patients, because it is inaccurate in this age group and because in court the result does not constitute adequate legal evidence of infection.) In the absence of discharge, vaginal specimens are needed. It is important to note that the hymen is extremely sensitive and that touching it with a swab will induce a significant amount of pain in most patients. Application of topical lidocaine ointment to the hymenal area prior to collection of specimens can help to reduce discomfort and is probably a wise measure for girls with small hymenal openings or redundant hymenal tissue. Saline-moistened calcium alginate swabs on thin metal wires are the easiest to insert atraumatically. Instillation of saline via an 18- or 19-gauge soft-rubber catheter is an alternative method sometimes useful for patients with very small hymenal orifices. The saline is instilled with the child

TABLE 6-4

Documentation Required in Sexual Abuse Evaluation: Guidelines for Specimen Collection in Sexual Abuse Examination at Children's Hospital, Pittsburgh

Orogenital contact	Genital contact		Anal contact
	No evidence of penetration	**Evidence consistent with vaginal penetration**	

1. Swabs: use two at a time†
    a. For wet mount for sperm‡
    b. For two air-dried slides‡
    c. For GC culture
    d. Consider *Chlamydia* culture if patient older than 3 years
 2. Consider baseline RPR (repeat in 4-6 weeks if initial result is negative)
 3. Consider HIV testing with repeat test in 3-6 months
	1. Urinalysis for occult blood
	 2. Vaginal swabs or aspirate*†
	    a. For wet mount for sperm‡, *Trichomonas* and *Candida*
	    b. For two air-dried slides‡
	    c. For GC and routine culture*
	    d. For *Chlamydia* culture if patient older than 3 years*
	    e. For Gram's stain if vaginal discharge is present*
	 3. Consider baseline RPR (repeat in 4-6 weeks if initial result is negative)
	 4. Consider HIV testing with repeat test in 3-6 months
		1. Urinalysis for occult blood
		 2. If external tears seen:
		    a. Consult surgeon for possible EUA
		    b. If EUA done, collect specimens then
		 3. Vaginal swabs or aspirate*†
		    a. For wet mount for sperm*‡, *Trichomonas* and *Candida*
		    b. For two air-dried slides‡
		    c. For GC and routine cultures*
		    d. For *Chlamydia* culture if patient older than 3 years*
		    e. For Gram's stain if vaginal discharge present*
		 4. Consider RPR (repeat in 4-6 weeks if initial result is negative)
		 5. Consider HIV testing with repeat test in 3-6 months
			1. If external tears seen:
			    a. Consult general surgeon for possible EUA
			    b. If EUA done, collect specimens then
			 2. Swabs: use two at a time and insert no more than 1 cm† (must be done before rectal examination)
			    a. For wet mount for sperm‡
			    b. For two air-dried slides‡
			    c. For GC and routine cultures
			    d. For *Chlamydia* culture if patient older than 3 years
			 3. If no tears:
			    a. Rectal exam
			    b. Stool guaiac: if positive, consult general surgeon
			 4. Consider baseline RPR (repeat in 4-6 weeks if initial result is negative)
			 5. Consider HIV testing with repeat test in 3-6 months

*In postpubescent patients, cervical swabs must be obtained for GC and *Chlamydia* cultures and for Gram's stain.

†Two of the swabs used to obtain specimens should be air-dried and placed in a sterile test tube for acid phosphatase, blood group, and enzyme studies. When specimens are obtained by vaginal aspirate, a small amount of aspirate should be applied to two swabs, which should then be processed in the same manner.

‡Omit if seen >72 hours after the last incident, except in patients with vaginal discharge.

NOTE: Follow-up in 2-4 weeks is recommended, with additional specimen collection as needed.

GC, Gonococcal; *RPR*, rapid plasma reagin (test); *EUA*, examination under anesthesia.

in the semisupine lithotomy position and allowed to remain for 20 to 30 seconds. It then can be aspirated back as the mother lowers the child's legs and the saline bubbles out. As the knee-chest position produces maximal hymenal opening, this is the optimal position for vaginal specimen collection if the child will tolerate it.

In the postmenarchal patient, cervical cultures for gonorrhea and *Chlamydia* infection in addition to cultures of the vaginal pool are indicated. The possibility of pregnancy must also be considered in all such patients.

In obtaining rectal specimens for gonorrhea and *Chlamydia* cultures, the swab should be inserted no more than 1 to 2 cm to avoid fecal contamination, which interferes with culture results.

Patients with evidence of trauma need urinalysis and rectal examination to check for evidence of bleeding, and may require sonography or CT if physical findings are suggestive of internal extension of injury. Prepubescent girls with evidence of vaginal bleeding or a vaginal hematoma must have an internal examination performed under anesthesia. In such instances, specimen collection is deferred until that time.

Table 6-4 presents guidelines for specimen collection in sexual abuse cases, and Table 6-5 enumerates the additional specimens required by law enforcement authorities in rape cases. Because the examination is for the purpose of gathering forensic evidence in addition to assessing the patient's physical status, procedure must be meticulous. Each specimen for the crime laboratory should be packaged and labeled immediately after collection. All evidence should then be kept together and must remain under the direct supervision of the physician or nurse who was present at the time of collection until it is signed over to hospital

TABLE 6-5

Additional Specimens Needed in Rape Cases (Seen Within 72 Hours)

Specimens may be obtained by the physician or nurse. All containers used in evidence collection
should be paper and must be labeled with:

Patient's name	Body site	Initials of collector
Type of specimen	Date and time	

Clothing	If the patient is wearing the same clothes, they should be collected along with debris, as this may provide valuable clues regarding the assailant. The patient should disrobe while standing on a towel or sheet. Each article, including the towel or sheet, should then be placed in a separate paper bag. Avoid shaking the articles. Each bag is then labeled and sealed.
Fingernail scrapings*	These may provide bits of skin, fiber, and debris from the assailant. Scraping from beneath the nails or nail clippings should be obtained. Specimens from each hand should be collected over separate sheets of paper, and placed in separate paper envelopes, sealed, and labeled.
Hair samples*	Any loose or suspected foreign hairs should be collected, placed in an envelope, and labeled. If patient is post-pubescent, comb pubic hairs onto a sheet of clean paper, fold, place in an envelope with the comb, label "combed pubic hair," and seal. Then, gently pull a small clump of the patient's pubic hair (12 hairs are needed), place on clean paper, fold, put in envelope, label "standard pubic hair," and seal. Then, comb and obtain head hairs in this same manner.
Blood sample	5 ml of blood should be drawn for blood grouping and enzyme typing, and placed in a purple-top tube.
Saliva sample	This enables testing of the patient's secretory status. The specimen should be obtained either by wiping the patient's oral mucosa with a gauze pad or by having the patient expectorate onto a gauze pad. The pad is then placed in an envelope, sealed, and labeled.

Destination of Specimens

The following specimens are handled by the hospital laboratories or performed in the ER:

Urinalysis	Gram's stains	RPR
Wet preps	Stool guaiac	Cultures

All other specimens are to be signed over to police custody for transport to the crime laboratory.

Maintaining an Unbroken Chain of Evidence

Evidence should be packaged and labeled upon collection. All evidence should be kept together and must remain under the direct supervision of the physician, the nurse, or a hospital security guard until signed over to the police. Receipt for release of evidence to police should be signed before evidence is given over to the police.

*Omit if patient has already bathed and shampooed.

security or law enforcement. Finally, police should sign a receipt for release of evidence upon accepting the specimens. Commercially available rape assessment kits greatly facilitate this process. Failure to adhere to these procedures breaks the chain of evidence and invalidates its use in legal proceedings. If the rape has been perpetrated by a stranger (e.g., not a caretaker), the patient or parent usually must sign a consent form before collection of evidence.

Differential Diagnosis of Sexual Abuse

Not only is there a wide range of nonabusive causes of the physical and behavioral symptoms which serve as presenting complaints of many sexual abuse victims, but in addition, physical findings, when present, are variable and often nonspecific, and many have a variety of other causes. Furthermore, as the result of McCann's pioneering work, the wide variation in normal findings is only beginning to be appreciated. Erythema of the vaginal vestibule is seen commonly in asymptomatic nonabused prepubescent girls. It can also be seen in abuse victims and in children with irritant and other forms of vulvovaginitis (see Fig. 18-33).

There is a wide variation in normal hymenal configuration and shape of orifice (see Figs. 18-3 and 18-6) and some degree of variation in diameter that must be appreciated by the examining physician (Fig. 6-55; see Fig. 18-3). Several normal anatomic variants are now recognized as well. **Septal remnants** (Fig. 6-56), seen as tags near the midline on either the anterior or posterior portion of the hymenal membrane (see Chapter 18) and even anterolateral **hymenal flaps** (Fig. 6-57) are normal findings, as are periurethral bands. These and **in-**

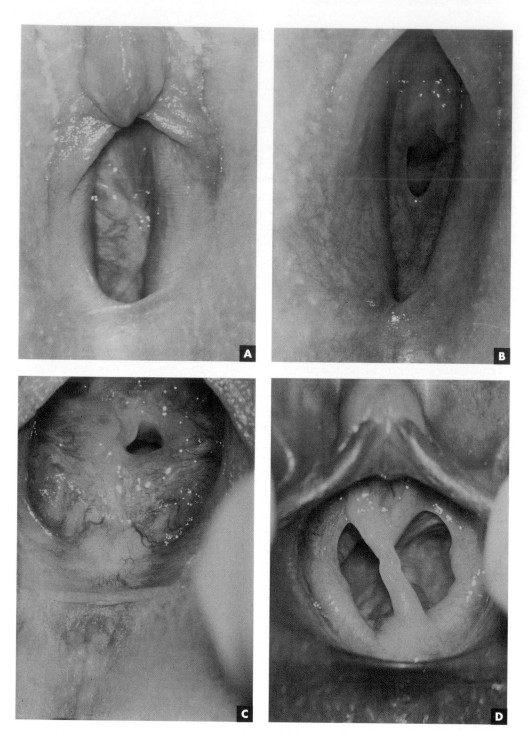

FIG. 6-55 Variations in normal hymenal configuration. *A,* A redundant hymen. *B,* A crescentic hymen with thin smooth edges. *C,* A somewhat redundant hymen with an annular orifice. *D,* A septate hymen resulting from failure of lysis of the embryonic hymenal septum.

travaginal ridges (Fig. 6-58) were once erroneously thought to be the result of scarring. Thin **labial adhesions** are a common finding in normal children, as well (Fig. 6-59).

Vulvovaginitis has a wide variety of causes, many of which are noninfectious, including chemical irritation, poor perineal hygiene or aeration, nonabusive frictional trauma, and contact dermatitis (see Chapter 18). Many infectious cases are caused by respiratory or gastrointestinal pathogens or are seen concurrently with urinary tract infections (see Chapter 18). Thus, vulvovaginitis resulting from sexually transmitted disease probably constitutes a minority of vulvovaginal complaints in prepubescent children. To avoid misdiagnosis of abuse, it is wise to defer diagnosis until definitive culture results are obtained.

The clinical findings of **urethral prolapse** (Fig. 6-60) have been mistakenly attributed to sexual abuse because the purplish-red, prolapsed mucosal tissue that protrudes between the labia minora bleeds easily and often overlies the vaginal orifice, simulating edematous, trauma-

tized, redundant hymenal folds. The condition is often first discovered when blood or serosanguineous discharge is found on the diaper or underwear, as dysuria is unusual and urination is not impeded. With magnification, the urethral orifice can be seen at the center of the mass, which is soft and markedly tender to touch. After application of topical Xylocaine, the prolapse can be lifted, revealing the hymen underneath. The condition is unusual, and tends to occur only in children under 12 years of age; two thirds of affected girls are black. The cause is unknown.

Lichen sclerosus et atrophicus has often been mistakenly attributed to sexual abuse. The involved perineal skin is paper thin and hypopigmented and often has areas of superficial ulceration that bleed easily (Fig. 6-61). Its etiology remains unknown.

As noted earlier, trauma inflicted in the course of attempted or actual sexual penetration generally results in contusions and tears of the posterior portion of the hymen and introitus. In contrast, **straddle in-**

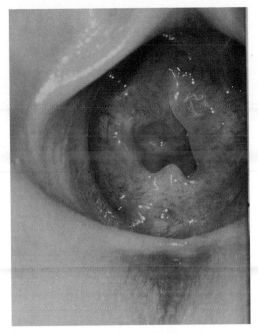

FIG. 6-56 Septal remnant. This skin tag at 6 o'clock is a remnant of a vaginal septum present earlier in fetal development and is a normal finding seen in about 5% of girls.

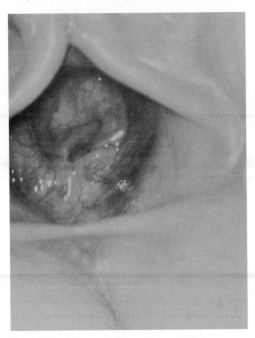

FIG. 6-57 Hymenal flap. This child has a redundant hymen with an everted anterolateral flap, another normal variant.

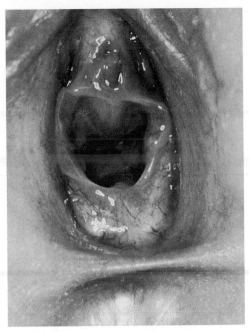

FIG. 6-58 Intravaginal ridges. The bands of tissue along the vaginal walls that here appear to extend medially and downward from the 11 and 2 o'clock positions are normal features of the vaginal walls, which in the past were erroneously thought to be the result of scarring. (Courtesy Dr. John McCann, University of California at Davis.)

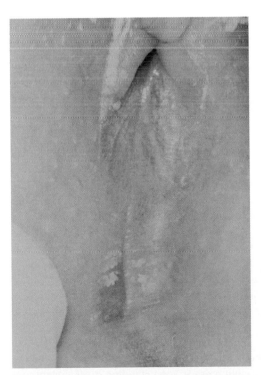

FIG. 6-59 Labial adhesions. The labia minora are fused in the midline as a consequence of prior inflammation. They are separated by a thin lucent line, and the epithelium of the labia is normal.

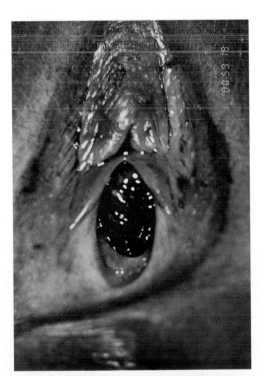

FIG. 6-60 Urethral prolapse. This child was referred for evaluation for possible sexual abuse when blood was noted on her underwear and "traumatized tissue" was seen on examination. On close inspection this was found to be edematous, friable prolapsed urethral mucosa.

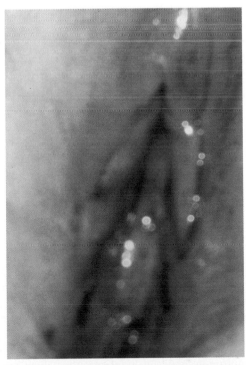

FIG. 6-61 Lichen sclerosus et atrophicus. Multiple small points of bleeding dot the atrophic mucosa in this child.

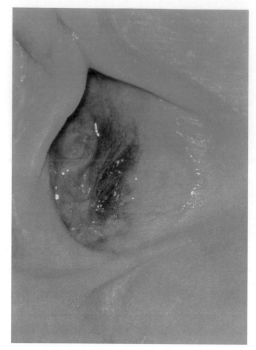

FIG. 6-62 Accidental trauma caused by a straddle injury. This child complained of dysuria and was noted to have a small amount of blood on her underwear after a straddle injury. This superficial laceration between the hymen and labia minora was barely visible in regular light but was brought out by viewing it through a green filter.

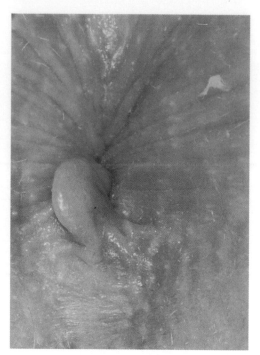

FIG. 6-63 Perianal skin tag. This is a common finding, particularly in children with a history of constipation and prior problems with anal fissures.

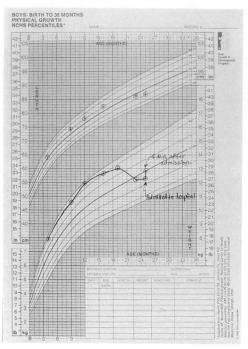

FIG. 6-64 Growth chart of a child with psychosocial failure to thrive. This boy's growth was normal until he was 15 months of age, when his mother became addicted to crack. His weight gain slowed between 15 and 19 months, after which he showed a precipitous weight loss and slowing of height growth. He showed rapid catch-up growth within a week of removal from the home.

juries produce lesions of the anterior and anterolateral portions, as these are tissues most likely to be crushed between the pubic ramus and the object on which the child falls. Findings include contusions, abrasions, and superficial lacerations, the latter being frequently found at the junction of the labia majora and minora (Fig. 6-62).

Finally, **anal fissures** and **perianal skin tags** (Fig. 6-63) are most commonly sequelae of constipation. The fissures do not extend beyond the perianal skin bearing hair follicles, whereas tears produced by sodomy usually exceed this limit. Spontaneous sphincter relaxation occurring 30 seconds to 3 or 4 minutes after adopting the knee-chest position is also normal, while immediate relaxation in the absence of stool is suspicious. Perianal erythema, hyperpigmentation, and venous engorgement also are common findings in normal children.

Passive Abuse or Neglect

Passive abuse or neglect is by far the most commonly reported type of abuse, accounting for over 50% of cases each year (53% in 1995). In its mildest form, this may be seen as a lack of vigilance and safeguarding of the young child, who is thereby at greater risk for accidents and ingestions. In its more severe form the patient presents with failure to thrive and developmental delay as a result of inadequate or ineffective nurturing. Typically, in infancy, the patient has been fed irregularly and inadequately, given little interactional attention, and received minimal basic care. In some cases it appears that the infant may have picked up on maternal anxiety and depression and developed secondary anorexia and autonomic disturbances of intestinal motility. Some of these infants actually begin to resist contact and become difficult to feed.

Risk factors are similar to those seen in cases of active physical abuse, with a few additions. More of these infants were unplanned and unwanted, and often little or no prenatal care was sought. In numerous cases there is a history of the father leaving the mother upon learning of the pregnancy. Mothers of such infants are more likely to be frankly depressed or mentally dull and to have difficulty caring for the children they already have. The incidence of maternal drug abuse as a predisposing factor has increased substantially over the past decade.

Frequently the parent appears relatively unconcerned about the child's failure to thrive, having brought the child for treatment of a minor unrelated problem, such as a cold, rash, vomiting, or constipation. Some present with a history of colic, crying "all the time," or a feeding problem. There are often glaring inconsistencies in the feeding history (e.g., "he takes 6 ounces every 4 hours" yet "he takes 16 ounces in 24 hours"). Many mothers readily acknowledge that they often do not hold the baby for feedings but instead prop the bottle on a towel or against the side of the crib. When they do hold the infant during a feeding, they often do not make good eye contact and tend to put him or her down immediately afterward. A high percentage of these infants have received little or no professional well-child care and are behind on their immunizations.

On examination, the child is usually found to be significantly undergrown. Weight may be below the 3rd percentile, or there may be evidence of plateauing of weight gain. In long-standing cases, height and head circumference are abnormally low as well. Comparison with birth parameters and measurements made at prior visits (if any) reveal that the child has "fallen off the curve" (Fig. 6-64). In the more severe case, the child presents with decreased subcutaneous tissue (most notable over the buttocks, thighs and upper arms), a pinched face, and sunken prominent eyes. In some there are frank physical findings of multiple vitamin deficiencies, which include a nonspecific or seborrhea-like dermatitis that can progress to skin breakdown, cheilosis, glossitis and stomatitis, and erythema and thinning of the skin over the palms and soles (Fig. 6-65, *A* to *E*).

These children tend to look serious, smile infrequently, appear apathetic and withdrawn when left alone, and often lie on their backs with their arms up beside their heads. They show more interest in inanimate objects than in people, and although they appear vigilant toward people at a distance, they tend to become upset when someone approaches and avoid making eye contact. They often object to being touched, held, or cuddled. When health care personnel persist in trying to get them to interact, they find they must work hard to get them to calm down and sit in their lap; and when put back in the crib, the child cries only briefly, if at all. Vocalization is sparse, and development is delayed and uneven, with social milestones being farther behind than motor development. We have even seen some who have had abnormal tone, scissoring, and posturing suggestive of a neurologic problem, which promptly abated within a few days of hospitalization. Poor hygiene, dirty clothes, and badly neglected diaper rashes are common additional findings suggestive of neglect (Fig. 6-66).

The easiest, least traumatic way to confirm the diagnosis of psychosocial failure to thrive is to remove the infant from his or her home environment and observe his or her growth in a nurturing situation. Children with milder cases will gain weight promptly, while marasmic infants may take 1 to 2 weeks before resuming growth (see Fig. 6-65, *F*).

Although pure psychosocial failure to thrive is the most common form of growth failure in infancy, accounting for over 40% to 50% of cases, up to 25% of cases are of purely organic origin; in another 25%, growth failure is due to a combination of organic and psychosocial factors. In the latter instances, affected infants often have suffered prenatal or perinatal insults that have resulted in growth retardation and/or physical conditions that make them difficult to feed and care for.

CNS, cardiac, genetic, pulmonary, renal, and endocrine disorders account for organically based growth failure, in descending order of frequency. The vast majority of such disorders are recognized during physical examination because of the obvious abnormalities seen. The rest tend to be revealed by history or are readily diagnosed on the basis of a few simple screening laboratory tests.

Severe cerebral palsy, neuromuscular disorders, encephalopathies, and neurodegenerative diseases are the major CNS problems associated with failure to thrive. Poor suck; problems coordinating sucking and swallowing; and lethargy, irritability, and altered level of consciousness are the more common factors that impede adequate intake in these infants. Some also have excess losses as the result of vomiting. Neurologic dysfunction may also impair an infant's ability to provide interactive feedback to his or her mother.

A wide variety of gastrointestinal problems cause growth failure, and numerous mechanisms are responsible. Oral malformations, including cleft lip and palate, severe micrognathia, and macroglossia, interfere with sucking and swallowing. Many of these are also associated with chronic or recurrent ear and nasopharyngeal infections. Esophageal and gastric disorders can interfere with growth by causing pain on swallowing, resulting in decreased intake, or repetitive vomiting (abnormal losses), with or without aspiration. These include esophageal stricture, stenosis, or atresia; external esophageal compression by abnormal vessels, an enlarged heart, or mass lesions; and chalasia, achalasia, or severe gastroesophageal reflux.

Malabsorption is the major mechanism of growth failure in patients with small or large intestinal and pancreatic disease. Pain associated with eating caused by gas, hyperperistalsis, or inflammation may cause

anorexia. Such patients have a history of excessive stool losses, and stool examination often reveals the underlying cause. Carbohydrate malabsorption is characterized by large, watery stools, which are positive for reducing substances, have a low pH, and are accompanied by considerable gas. Fat malabsorption results in large, bulky, greasy stools, and protein malabsorption in foul-smelling stools. Infants with blind-loop syndromes resulting from webs, bands, or stenoses have large, watery stools as a result of bacterial overgrowth in the gut lumen proximal to the site of partial obstruction. Short-gut syndrome following surgical resection and parasitic infections with *Giardia* or *Strongyloides* organisms are other causes of malabsorption. It must also be remembered that malnutrition itself causes malabsorption. Impaired bile acid metabolism results in fat malabsorption in infants with severe liver disease. Associated anorexia, malaise, and fatigue impede intake in these children, and vomiting contributes to caloric losses.

Severe cardiac disorders, including those characterized by chronic congestive heart failure, large shunts, or pulmonary hypertension, appear to result in growth failure primarily as a result of dyspnea with feeding and secondarily decreased intake. The role of hypoxia and malabsorption (resulting from impaired intestinal lymphatic drainage in children with congestive heart failure) remains unclear. Many of these patients also have recurrent pulmonary infections, and in some, intrauterine growth retardation, congenital infections, and genetic disorders play a role.

The genetic disorders associated with impaired growth include chromosomal disorders, storage diseases, skeletal disorders and dysplasias, inborn errors of metabolism, idiopathic hypercalcemia, and heritable CNS defects. All are characterized by obvious physical stigmata.

Of the pulmonary disorders associated with failure to thrive, bronchopulmonary dysplasia and persistent viral infections are the two main sources. Dyspnea with feeding and secondarily decreased intake appear to be the major underlying mechanisms, often compounded by recurrent infection. Cystic fibrosis can be put in this category, but it is malabsorption more than pulmonary dysfunction that appears to affect the growth of these patients.

Renal diseases that involve the interstitium and tubular structures are the major nephric causes of growth failure. These include dysplasia, multicystic or polycystic kidney disease, severe hydronephrosis with azotemia, chronic obstructive uropathy, renal tubular acidosis, nephrogenic diabetes insipidus, chronic or recurrent urinary tract infections with severe reflux or other anatomic abnormalities, and chronic renal failure. Inability to concentrate the urine, abnormalities of urinary sediment, or abnormal serum chemistry values are found on screening tests in these patients. Inadequate intake stemming from anorexia and protein restriction; malabsorption; abnormal vitamin D absorption and secondary hyperparathyroidism with renal osteodystrophy; decreased somatomedin levels; and abnormal peripheral utilization and degradation of insulin may all contribute to growth failure in these children.

Among the endocrine disorders, diabetes mellitus and pituitary, thyroid, and adrenal disorders can all be associated with growth impairment. Urinary losses of glucose, dehydration, and excessive protein catabolism result in weight loss in children with diabetes mellitus. A history of polyuria, polydipsia, and polyphagia and tests for serum and urine glucose readily enable diagnosis. The growth curves of children with isolated growth hormone deficiency and panhypopituitarism level off between 9 and 12 months of age, with height affected more than weight. Such patients appear well nourished for height but often have an elfin physiognomy. Congenital hypothyroidism is characterized by an open posterior fontanelle, umbilical hernia, macroglossia, mottled skin, prolonged physiologic jaundice, and constipation. Although height is short and bone age markedly delayed, weight is normal or in-

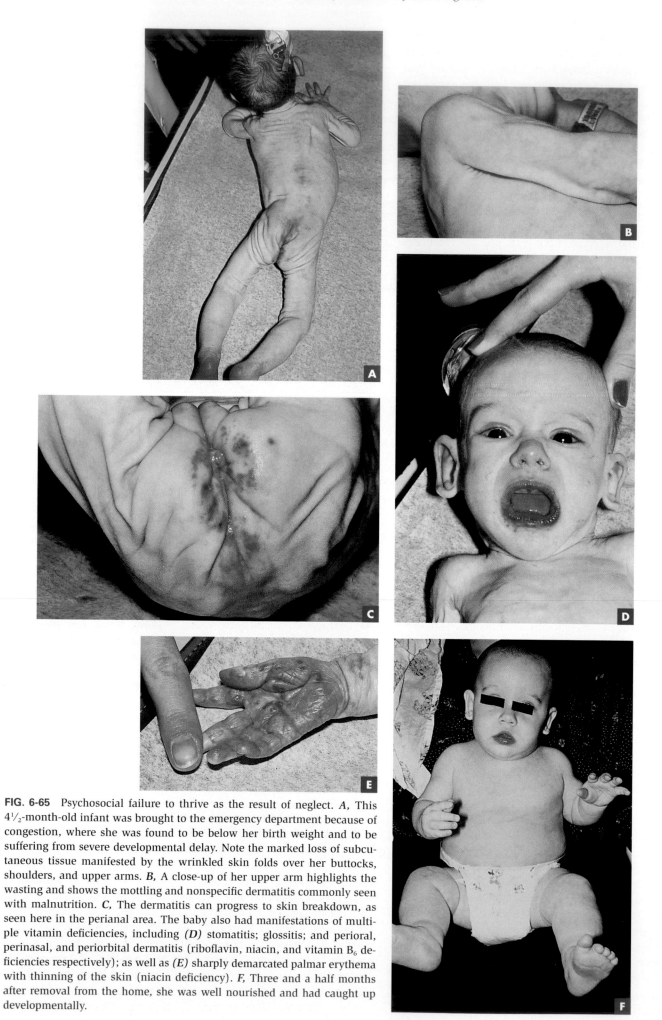

FIG. 6-65 Psychosocial failure to thrive as the result of neglect. *A,* This 4½-month-old infant was brought to the emergency department because of congestion, where she was found to be below her birth weight and to be suffering from severe developmental delay. Note the marked loss of subcutaneous tissue manifested by the wrinkled skin folds over her buttocks, shoulders, and upper arms. *B,* A close-up of her upper arm highlights the wasting and shows the mottling and nonspecific dermatitis commonly seen with malnutrition. *C,* The dermatitis can progress to skin breakdown, as seen here in the perianal area. The baby also had manifestations of multiple vitamin deficiencies, including *(D)* stomatitis; glossitis; and perioral, perinasal, and periorbital dermatitis (riboflavin, niacin, and vitamin B₆ deficiencies respectively); as well as *(E)* sharply demarcated palmar erythema with thinning of the skin (niacin deficiency). *F,* Three and a half months after removal from the home, she was well nourished and had caught up developmentally.

TABLE 6-6

Findings in Failure to Thrive in Infancy

Cause	Approximate percentage of all cases	History	System-specific physical findings	System-specific laboratory studies
Psychosocial	50% or more	Vague, inconsistent feeding history, history of bottle propping	None. May have soft neurologic signs	None
Central nervous system	13%	Poor feeding, gross developmental delay, vomiting	Grossly abnormal neurologic findings	Frequent gross abnormalities on EEG and CT scan or grossly abnormal neuromuscular function
Gastrointestinal	10%	Chronic vomiting and/or diarrhea, abnormal stools	Often negative, may have abdominal distension	Abnormal barium or endoscopic study, abnormal stool findings (pH-reducing substances, fat stain, Wright's stain)
Cardiac	9%	Slow feeding, dyspnea and diaphoresis with feeding, restlessness and diaphoresis during sleep	Often cyanotic or have signs of congestive heart failure	Abnormal echocardiogram, ECG, catheterization findings
Genetic	8%	May have positive family history or developmental delay	Often have facies typical of a syndrome, skeletal abnormalities, or neurologic abnormalities, visceromegaly	May have typical radiographic findings, chromosomal abnormalities, abnormal metabolic screens
Pulmonary	3.5%	Chronic or recurrent dyspnea with feeding, tachypnea	Grossly abnormal chest examination findings	Abnormal chest radiographs
Renal	3.5%	May be negative or may have history of polyuria	Often negative, may have flank masses	Abnormal urinalysis, frequently elevated BUN and creatinine, signs of renal osteodystrophy on x-rays
Endocrine	3.5%	With hypothyroidism, constipation and decreased activity level; with diabetes, polyuria, polydipsia	With hypothyroidism, no wasting but mottling, umbilical hernia, often open posterior fontanelle. With diabetes, often without specific abnormality, but may have signs of dehydration, ketotic breath, and hyperpnea. With hypopituitarism and isolated growth hormone deficiency, growth normal until 9 months or later, then plateaus, but normal weight for height; delayed tooth eruption	Decreased T4, increased TSH; glucosuria and hyperglycemia; abnormal pituitary function study results

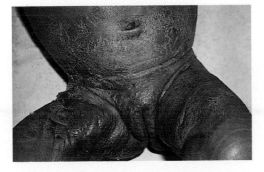

FIG. 6-66 Neglect. Another infant with severe failure to thrive has a badly neglected case of irritant diaper dermatitis.

creased for height. Characteristic physical stigmata facilitate diagnosis. Congenital hyperthyroidism results in failure to thrive because of poor feeding and frequent loose stools. Affected infants are irritable and hyperactive and have tachypnea, tachycardia, and diaphoresis. The presence of goiter makes this condition obvious. Patients with adrenocortical insufficiency grow poorly because of anorexia, vomiting, and diarrhea, which also predisposes them to dehydration. Basic serum chemistry tests reveal hyponatremia and hyperkalemia.

Given the frequency of psychosocial failure to thrive and combined psychosocial and organic failure to thrive, and given the stresses of caring for infants with severe organic disorders, it is essential in evaluating the infant with poor growth to obtain a thorough psychosocial and family history as well as a detailed medical history. The latter should include information regarding duration of the problem, mode of onset, and pattern of growth. It is also helpful to ask the parents how easy or difficult it is to take care of this child. A complete review of systems—gastrointestinal, cardiorespiratory, neurologic, genitourinary, and endocrine—emphasizing intake and output is often helpful. A thorough general physical examination will reveal gross abnormalities in patients with underlying CNS, cardiopulmonary, or genetic problems.

A few basic screening tests (complete blood count and differential; urinalysis and culture; sedimentation rate; stool pH, reducing substance, and fat stain; and urea nitrogen, electrolytes, and creatinine) can serve to rule out most other organic causes of failure to thrive. Table 6-6 summarizes the most common causes of infantile growth failure and their major findings on evaluation.

Emotional Abuse

Emotional abuse accompanies all of the other forms of abuse described previously but can also occur in isolation. It can range from inattentiveness to frank rejection, scapegoating, or even terrorization. Because emotional abuse is very difficult to document since it leaves no visible stigmata, it accounts for the smallest proportion of reported cases (3% in 1995). Victims may present with chronic severe anxiety, agitation, hyperactivity, depression, or frank psychotic reactions. Many are socially withdrawn, have trouble relating to peers, and generally perform poorly in school. Low self-esteem is the rule. If it is suspected, psychological testing and psychiatric examination may prove helpful in confirming its existence.

Reporting

Each state has regulations requiring health care providers, hospitals, and professionals involved in child care to report suspected cases of abuse and neglect to child protective service agencies. Although these regulations are similar, they vary from state to state and clinicians should become familiar with the regulations in their respective states. The suspected abuse or neglect must result from the acts or omissions of a parent, stepparent, or other person in a caretaking role. For abuse to be reported, reasonable grounds for suspicion are required, not clinical certainty. There is no penalty for reporting in good faith, but there can be severe penalties for failure to report.

In many states, cases involving severe abuse (potentially life-threatening or threatening a vital sense organ or limb) as well as sexual abuse cases must be reported to the police, as well. This can be done by the clinician evaluating the patient or by child protective services, but the latter often do not notify police promptly. Cases of stranger rape, physical assault, or abuse perpetrated by a person in a noncaretaking role must be reported to law enforcement.

Conclusion

Although treatment and follow-up are beyond the scope of an atlas of physical diagnosis, a few additional points bear emphasis. Use of a team approach, including physicians, nurses, and social workers or psychologists, greatly facilitates evaluation of victims of abuse and their families and reduces the burden on any one health care worker. Reporting requirements necessitate only *reasonable* grounds for suspicion and place the onus of full investigation on state agencies. Close follow-up, though highly important, is often neglected, especially when patients get caught up in large bureaucratic systems. Having improved our performance on identification and documentation of cases, we must increasingly apply ourselves to facilitating better long-term outcome.

BIBLIOGRAPHY

Ablin DS, Greenspan A, Reinhart M, Grix A: Differentiation of child abuse from osteogenesis imperfecta, *Am J Radiol* 154:1035-1046, 1990.

Alexander R, Sato Y, Smith W, Bennett T: Incidence of impact trauma with cranial injuries ascribed to shaking, *Am J Dis Child* 144:724-726, 1990.

Alexander RC, Schor DP, Smith WL: Magnetic resonance imaging of intracranial injuries for child abuse, *J Pediatr* 109:975-979, 1986.

Bauer CH, ed: Failure to thrive, *Pediatr Ann* 7(11):737-795, 1978.

Bays J: Substance abuse and child abuse: impact of addiction on the child, *Pediatr Clin North Am* 37:881-904, 1990.

Bays J, Chewning M, Keltner L, Sewell R, Steinberg, M, Thomas P: Changes in hymenal anatomy during examination of prepubertal girls for possible sexual abuse, *Adolesc Pediatr Gynecol* 3:42-46, 1990.

Bruce DA, Zimmerman RA: Shaken impact syndrome, *Pediatr Ann* 18(8):482-494, 1989.

Caffey's pediatric x-ray diagnosis, ed 7, Chicago, 1978, Year Book.

Chadwick DL, Berkowitz CD, Kerns DL, McCann J, Reinhart MA, Strickland SL: *Color atlas of child sexual abuse*, Chicago, 1989, Year Book.

Chadwick DL, Chin S, Salerno C, Landsverk J, Kitchen L: Deaths from falls in children: how far is fatal, *J Trauma* 31:1353-1355, 1991.

Coant PN, Kornberg AE, Brody AS, Edwards-Holmes K: Markers for occult liver injury in cases of physical abuse in children, *Pediatrics* 89:274-278, 1992.

Duhaime AC, Gennarelli TA, Thibault LE, Bruce DA, Margulies SS, Wiser R: The shaken baby syndrome: a clinical, pathological and biomechanical study, *J Neurosurg* 66:409-415, 1987.

Feldman KW: Patterned abusive bruises of the buttocks and pinnae, *Pediatrics* 90:633-636, 1992.

Finkelhor D: Current information on the scope and nature of child sexual abuse, *Future Child* 4(2), Summer/Fall 1994.

Gilliand MGF, Folberg R: Shaken babies—some have no impact injuries, *J Forens Sci* 41:114-116, 1996.

Green FC, ed: Incest and sexual abuse, *Pediatr Ann* 8(5):1-103, 1979.

Hadley MN, Sonntag VKH, Rekate HL, Murphy A: The infant whiplash-shake injury syndrome: a clinical and pathological study, *Neurosurgery* 24:536-540, 1989.

Hammerschlag MR, Rettig PJ, Shields ME: False positive results with the use of chlamydial antigen detection tests in the evaluation of suspected sexual abuse in children, *Pediatr Infect Dis J* 7:11, 1988.

Helfer RE: The neglect of our children, *Pediatr Clin North Am* 37:923-942, 1990.

Helfer RE, Kempe HC, eds: *The battered child,* ed 3, Chicago, 1980, University of Chicago Press.

Helfer RE, Kempe HC, eds: *Child abuse and neglect: the family and the community,* Cambridge, MA, 1976, Ballinger.

Homer MD, Ludwig S: Categorization of etiology of failure to thrive, *Am J Dis Child* 135:848-851, 1981.

Huffman JW: *Gynecology of childhood and adolescence,* ed 2, Philadelphia, 1981, WB Saunders.

Hymel KP, Jenny C: Abusive spiral fractures of the humerus: a videotaped exception, *Arch Pediatr Adolesc Med* 150:226-227, 1996.

Johnson CF: Inflicted injury versus accidental injury, *Pediatr Clin North Am* 37:791-814, 1990.

Kleinman PK: *Diagnostic imaging of child abuse,* Baltimore, 1987, Williams & Wilkins.

Kleinman PK, Blackbourne BD, Marks SC, Karellas M, Belanger PL: Radiologic contributions to the investigation and prosecution of cases of fatal infant abuse, *N Engl J Med* 320:507-511, 1989.

Kleinman PK, Marks SC, Blackbourne B: The metaphyseal lesion in abused infants: a radiologic-histopathologic study, *Am J Radiol* 146:895-905, 1986.

Krugman RD: Recognition of sexual abuse in children, *Pediatr Rev* 8:25, 1986.

Lavy U, Bauer CH: Pathophysiology of failure to thrive and gastrointestinal disorders, *Pediatr Ann* 7(11):10-33, 1978.

Levin AV, Magnusson MR, Rafto SE, Zimmerman RA: Shaken baby syndrome diagnosed by magnetic resonance imaging, *Pediatr Emerg Care* 5:181-186, 1989.

McCann J: Use of the colposcope in childhood sexual abuse examinations, *Pediatr Clin North Am* 37:863-880, 1990.

McCann J, Voris J, Simon M, Wells R: Perianal findings in prepubertal children selected for non-abuse: a descriptive study, *Child Abuse Negl* 13:179-193, 1989.

McCann J, Voris J, Simon M, Wells R: Comparison of genital examination techniques in prepubertal girls, *Pediatrics* 85:182-187, 1990.

Merten DF, Carpenter BLM: Radiologic imaging of inflicted injury in the child abuse syndrome, *Pediatr Clin North Am* 37:815-838, 1990.

Munger CE, Peiffer RL, Bouldin TW, Kylstra JA, Thompson RL: Ocular and associated neuropathologic observations in suspected whiplash-shaken infant syndrome: a retrospective study of 12 cases, *Am J Forens Med Pathol* 14:193-200, 1993.

Muram D: Child sexual abuse: genital tract findings in prepubertal girls. I. The unaided medical examination, *Am J Obstet Gynecol* 160:328-332, 1989.

Neinstein LS, Goldenring J, Carpenter S: Non-sexual transmission of sexually transmitted diseases: an infrequent occurrence, *Pediatrics* 74:67-76, 1984.

Newberger EH: Pediatric interview assessment of child abuse: challenges and opportunities, *Pediatr Clin North Am* 37:943-954, 1990.

Paradise JE: The medical evaluation of the sexually abused child, *Pediatr Clin North Am* 37:839-862, 1990.

Reece RM: Unusual manifestations of child abuse, *Pediatr Clin North Am* 37:905-922, 1990.

Reiber GD: Fatal falls in childhood: how far must children fall to sustain fatal head injury? Report of cases and review of the literature, *Am J Forens Med Pathol* 14:201-207, 1993.

Rosenn DW, Loeb LS, Jura MB: Differentiation of organic from nonorganic failure to thrive syndrome in infancy, *Pediatrics* 66:698-704, 1980.

Sills RH: Failure to thrive, *Am J Dis Child* 132:967-969, 1978.

Starling SP, Holden JR, Jenny C: Abusive head trauma: the relationship of perpetrators to their victims, *Pediatrics* 95:259-262, 1995.

Thoennes N, Tjaden PG: The extent, nature and validity of sexual abuse allegations in custody/visitation disputes, *Child Abuse Negl* 14:151-163, 1990.

West MH, Billings JD, Frair J: Ultraviolet photography: bite marks on human skin and suggested technique for exposure and development of reflective ultraviolet photography, *J Forensic Sci* 32:1204-1213, 1987.

Williams JJ: Child abuse. In Reisdorff EJ, Roberts MR, Wiegenstein JG, eds: *Pediatric emergency medicine,* Philadelphia, 1993, WB Saunders.

Williams JJ: The cycle of abuse. In Monteleone JA, Brodeur AE, eds. *Child maltreatment: a clinical guide and reference,* St. Louis, 1994, Mosby–Year Book.

Woodlong BA, Kossosis PD: Sexual misuse, *Pediatr Clin North Am* 28:481-499, 1981.

Physical Abuse Checklist

Suspect Physical Abuse When

History

Incompatible with degree and/or extent of injury
Vague explanation
Parents reluctant to impart information
Contradictory histories from the accompanying adults
Different histories to different personnel
Impossible story
Repeated visits for unexplained or poorly explained injuries
Repeated ingestion
ER care at multiple places
Several failed routine appointments

Psychosocial Factors

Delay in seeking care
Inappropriate affect in relation to severity of injury
Poor parent-child interaction

Physical

Bruises in unusual locations
Bruises of different ages
Injuries in form of handprint or foreign object (e.g., looped cords, belts)
Bite marks attributable to adult dentition

Burns with the imprint of object
Immersion burns (clear line of demarcation)
Flame burns (deep in small prescribed spot)
Cigarette burns

Multiple fractures of different ages and locations
Metaphyseal chip fractures
Spiral fractures in the preambulatory child

Retinal hemorrhages
Unexplained visceral injury
Factitious disease (Munchausen syndrome by proxy)
Failure to thrive

What to Ask

Who brought the child in and why? Why now? (Get name, address, and phone number)

What happened? Get separate histories from the child and each of the accompanying adults. Quote verbatim where possible. Record the alleged time, manner, and mechanism of the injury.

What is the past history? Ask about well child care, illnesses, injuries, surgeries, or ingestion; note where the child was seen in each instance.

Where does the child live? Who lives in the home? (names, ages, relationships)

Who cares for the child during a typical day? (name, relationship, address, phone, location of care) Who else has access to the child?

How are things going in the family? (recent stresses) Family support systems?

What has the child been like? (personality, behavior, "difficulty")

What to Look For

Observe the child's behavior and interaction with the parent and document pertinent findings.

Developmental level and growth.

Examine the entire surface of the skin (including scalp) for bruises, ecchymoses, imprints of objects, lacerations, and scars. Describe any findings clearly with measurements in inches and indications of how painful they are. Note the color and shape. Draw the location of injuries on a body chart and take photographs of all external findings plus two of patient's face.

Palpate all bones for signs of recent or old fractures.

Palpate abdomen and regional lymph nodes.

What Tests to Consider

If bruises do not follow pattern of injury, or if petechiae present, get CBC, differential, platelets, PT, and PTT. If history indicates possibility of von Willebrand's disease or bruising seems excessive, get full coagulation profile.

If child is less than 2 years old and has external injuries or failure to thrive, obtain a skeletal survey, with focal films as indicated by exam.

Consider a CT or MRI if shaken-baby syndrome is a possibility.

APPENDIX 6-B

Sexual Abuse Checklist

When to Suspect Sexual Abuse

- recurrent urinary tract infections
- erythema of genital area; vaginal, vulval, or urethral discharge
- genital bleeding
- vaginal or anal laceration
- enuresis or encopresis
- excessive or compulsive masturbation
- fear of dark or sleep disturbance
- withdrawn or regressive behavior
- excessive sexual play
- school phobia
- anorexia, eating disorders
- grief, guilt, anger
- adolescent delinquency, promiscuity

What to Ask

Who brought the child? (Name address, phone number, relationship, how long in current custody), Why? Why now?

Who lives or works in the home?

Where has the child been? (e.g., baby sitter's, nursery school)

What happened? Get separate histories from adult(s) accompanying child and the child. Document verbatim as much as possible.

Talk with the child alone and use simple clear language that the child can understand. A good rule of thumb is that a question should contain only one more word than the child's age in years. Do not ask leading questions.

Sample questions: Could you tell me what happened? Did anything else happen? Would you tell me more about it? Where were you? Where was Mommy? Daddy? Grandma? etc. How many times did it happen? What do you call this part of your body? Has anyone touched you there? Does anyone wash you there? Does anyone put medication on you there? Does anyone else ever touch you there? *(Leventhal)*

What was the alleged perpetrator's private access to the child? How were their activities presented?

Was there progression in intensity and frequency over time? Was there use of rewards, threats, bribes, or coercion? How did the child experience the activities? (Don't make assumptions, and try not to convey shock or disgust to the child.) *(From SGROI)*

Ask if there is a history of: excessive masturbation, genital injury, bleeding, surgery, infection or discharge, UTI, enuresis, dysuria, constipation, encopresis, rectal bleeding or pain, warts, or menses.

What to Look For

Look for general scarring or bruising; note Tanner stage.

Examine the genitals in the lithotomy, frog-leg, or knee-chest position.

On the perineum, look for erythema or bruising of the labia or discharge. In the vestibule, look for erythema or synechiae, or abnormalities of the urethra. Look for condlylomata acuminata. In the posterior fourchette, check for labial adhesions, scars, neovascularity, avascular areas, or friability.

Describe the hymen in detail; note whether it is crescentic, annular, septate, septal remnant, cribriform, or imperforate. Are the edges: thin or thick, rolled or sharp, smooth, even or notched? Record the location of any apparent abnormalities.

In the perianal exam, look for diliatation, presence or absence of stool in the anal vault, venous congestion, pigmentation. Are the sphincter folds even or irregular? If there are tears or fissures, how far do they extend?

What Specimens to Get

If it is less than 72 hours since the alleged abuse, use a rape kit and follow instructions.

Do wet mount for *Trichomonas* and *Gardnerella*. Routine vaginal culture if discharge.

Gonococcal and *Chlamydia* cultures of pharynx, rectum, vagina and cervix (postmenarchal), or urethra. (*Chlamydia* antigen detection tests are not legally acceptable.)

Obtain serology if there is evidence of any other STD; herpes simplex cultures if inflamed areas. Test for HIV if history of multiple or high-risk perpetrators, stranger rape, or anal penetration.

When Is the Assessment of Sexual Abuse Emergent?

Most sexual abuse is chronic rather than acute. The most important thing is to determine whether the child is still exposed to the alleged perpetrator. If the child may still be exposed to the perpetrator, the interview should be performed as soon as possible but the **physical may be scheduled, if the child does not have bleeding, discharge, or discomfort, or if the alleged assault took place more than 72 hours ago.** If less than 72 hours has elapsed since the time of the alleged abuse, a rape kit should be used and the instructions followed in obtaining specimens.

7

Rheumatology

ANDREW H. URBACH ❦ ALDO VINCENT LONDINO, JR.

The rheumatic diseases of childhood are a heterogeneous group of disorders usually manifest by signs and symptoms of inflammation. Although significant progress has been made in the understanding of the pathophysiology of these disorders, their etiologies remain largely unknown. Despite advances in the laboratory diagnosis of these entities, especially with respect to specific antibodies defining disease subsets, the cornerstones of diagnosis remain the history and physical examination. Knowledge of the natural history of these disorders is also key to correct diagnosis and management.

The majority of the common rheumatic diseases that occur during childhood are classified as inflammatory arthritis or enthesitis syndromes, connective tissue disorders, and vasculitides, although overlap does occur. This chapter illustrates the more distinctive clinical features of these unique disorders.

Musculoskeletal History

A meticulous rheumatologic history is the foundation of accurate diagnosis (Table 7-1). The exact location that the patient complains about should be given careful attention. Muscle, bone, and tendon or ligament insertion pain (enthesitis) may be interpreted as joint pain unless the clinician quite specifically describes the symptomatology. As a result, a vastly different differential diagnosis may be pursued in error. The patient's age and gender serve as initial guides to a possible etiology. For instance, an 18-month-old child with fever and arthritis probably does not have acute rheumatic fever, but systemic onset juvenile rheumatoid arthritis (JRA) is possible. By similar reasoning, an adolescent girl is much less likely to have ankylosing spondylitis than a boy of the same age.

A history of prior illnesses, immunizations, trauma, bites, and the acuteness of symptoms can be a clue to diagnosis. Objective joint symptoms such as swelling, redness, warmth, and decreased range of motion (arthritis) carry a different meaning than simple joint pain (arthralgia). The duration and the persistent or fleeting occurrence of these findings in a particular joint also may be helpful. The child with acute rheumatic fever (ARF) tends to have acute migratory symptoms, whereas JRA generally causes more indolent and persistent joint changes. Morning stiffness or gel phenomenon can be an important clue in the diagnosis of a rheumatologic disease. This sense of impaired movement through a joint's range of motion can occur after napping, sleeping, or any inactivity. If this symptom occurs regularly over time

and is severe, the suspicion of rheumatic disease is enhanced. As the day progresses, the child with JRA may become more limber and may even appear normal. Persistent joint symptoms and signs that develop gradually and occur daily typify JRA. More acute and fleeting findings support other diagnoses, such as trauma, Henoch-Schönlein purpura, and ARF.

Differences in presentation also exist among the various rheumatoid diseases themselves. Joint movements of the patient with systemic lupus may be more painful than with JRA but also may be intermittent in nature even when the symptoms span a period of months. The joint swelling of lupus is often minimal compared with the pain, whereas the JRA joint is often less painful than it is swollen. The complaint of aching "everywhere" is typical of lupus, and the patient may be unable to localize a site of the symptoms. The joints of ARF also can be distinguished from those of JRA by the presence of exquisite pain that is out of proportion to physical findings. Migratory arthritis and rapidly additive arthritis (sequential joint involvement) are common with ARF and can assist in differentiation of these two entities. A rapid response to nonsteroidal antiinflammatory drugs further supports a diagnosis of ARF.

A careful family history incorporates information about similar or related symptoms in family members. Arthritis, back pain, iritis, head pain, ileitis, psoriasis, or prostatis add to the clinician's suspicion of a rheumatic illness.

Although the depth and subtlety of pediatric history taking is vast, the aforementioned approach serves as a primer on how to begin diagnosis of a child with joint symptoms and signs.

Physical Examination of the Musculoskeletal System

The only way to confirm the diagnosis of JRA is to demonstrate arthritis by physical examination of the joints. The elucidation of joint inflammation and synovitis by examination may be the only indication of any rheumatic disease. Since most joints are near the surface of the body, the examiner has an excellent opportunity to obtain significant information about many diseases. A rheumatological diagnosis requires a thorough joint examination and meticulous general physical examination with special attention to the skin and muscles.

The physical examination begins with observation of the child and parents walking from the waiting area to the examination room. The physician notes the general appearance of the patient and interactions

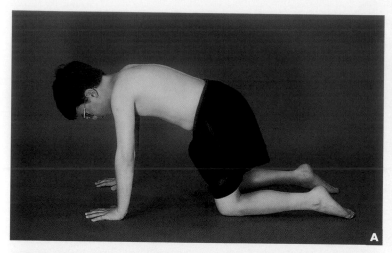
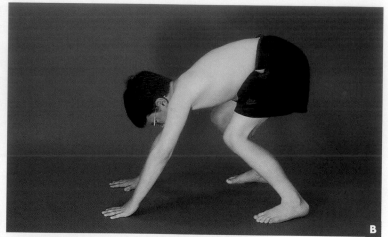
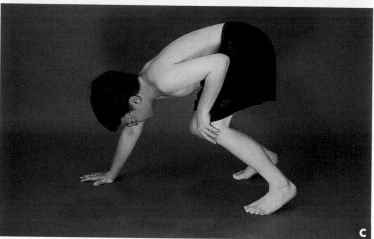
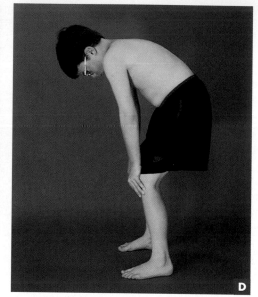

FIG. 7-1   Gower sign. The child begins in a supine position and is asked to stand. The child is unable to rise without rolling over and progressively pushing to the knees and using hands to push up to a standing position.

TABLE 7-1

Important Factors in the Rheumatologic History

1. Age and gender
2. Chief complaint
3. Location of musculoskeletal discomfort
4. Onset characteristics
5. Duration of symptomatology
6. Swelling
7. Morning stiffness
8. Aggravating factors
9. Course, frequency of complaints
10. Severity
11. Associated symptoms
12. Psychosocial history
13. Family history

Modified from Rennebohm RM: Rheumatic diseases of childhood, *Pediatr Rev* 10(6):183-190, 1988.

between family members. Nutritional status and an incremental graph of height and weight must be carefully documented. Certain skin and mucous membrane changes provide valuable information (Table 7-2). Muscle strength must be evaluated first by attempting to elicit a Gower sign (Fig. 7-1) and then by testing resistance capacity of individual muscle groups and grading them on a standard scale (Table 7-3).

The hallmark of a good physical examination of the musculoskeletal system is a careful examination of the joints, consisting of inspection, palpation, and measurement of each individual joint's range of motion. The examiner should develop a standard order for examining joints and follow the same pattern so no joints are missed. Effusions are easily felt and often ballottable; synovial hypertrophy may be more subtle and has a doughy, spongy, boggy feel. Synovial outpouchings are common in children with arthritis and can resemble "ganglion cysts," especially in the wrists and ankles. A ganglion cyst does not cause pain. In children with arthritis the findings may be subtle and often appreciated only because of pain or decreased range of motion.

Temporomandibular Joint

The temporomandibular joint (TMJ) permits three types of motion: (1) opening and closing of the jaw, (2) anterior and posterior motion,

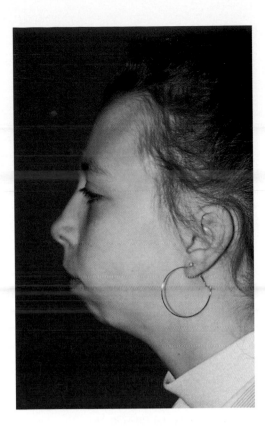

FIG. 7-2 Micrognathia. Note the underdevelopment of the jaw and retracted chin. This occurs in patients with JRA.

TABLE 7-2

Skin, Nail, and Mucous Membrane Changes that Suggest Rheumatic Disease

1. Malar rash
2. Discoid rash—rare in childhood; often heals with atrophy and scarring
3. Periungual erythema
4. Telangiectasias
5. Raynaud phenomenon—triphasic color change in response to cold (white to blue to red)
6. Fingertip ulcers
7. Alopecia and fracturing of frontal hair
8. Heliotrope violaceous eyelid edema
9. Gottron papules—scaly, symmetric, erythematous papules over MCPs and PIPs
10. Sicca (dry eyes); xerostomia (dry mouth)
11. Skin thickening, contractures, calcinosis
12. Palpable purpura
13. Livido reticularis—lacey, fishnet appearance of skin
14. Evanescent salmon-pink rash
15. Erythema nodosum—panniculitis with septal inflammation
16. Rheumatoid extensor nodules
17. Psoriasis
18. Onycholysis (lifting up of the distal portion of the nail), nail pits
19. Mouth and genital ulcers
20. Balanitis circinata—small, shallow, painless ulcers of the glans penis and urethral meatus
21. Keratodermia blennorrhagicum—clear vesicles on erythematous bases that progress to macules, papules, and keratototic nodules

TABLE 7-3

Standard Muscle Strength Grading

Muscle grade	Description
5	Complete range of motion against gravity with full resistance
4	Complete range of motion against gravity with some resistance
3	Complete range of motion against gravity
2	Complete range of motion with gravity eliminated
1	Evidence of slight contractility; no joint motion
0	No evidence of contractility

and (3) lateral or side-to-side motion; each type should be carefully measured. Careful observation of the TMJ may reveal micrognathia, a clue to the diagnosis of JRA (Fig. 7-2).

Cricoarytenoid Joint

The cricoarytenoid joint is rarely involved in JRA but can present a life-threatening complication if edema and scarring interfere with respira-

tion. An early symptom is hoarseness because arytenoid movement is important to phonation.

Acromioclavicular Joint

The acromioclavicular (AC) joint is formed by the lateral end of the clavicle and the medial margin of the acromial process of the scapula; it allows for "shrugging" of the shoulders.

Sternoclavicular Joint

The two sternoclavicular (SC) joints are the only points of articulation between the shoulder girdle and trunk; they move with any motion of the shoulders. The SC joints can be involved in the spondyloarthropathies and rarely in JRA, where they become ankylosed (fused).

Shoulder

The shoulder is usually involved only in severe polyarticular JRA. It is an extremely complicated joint, but range of active motion can be conveniently tested by having the child perform three simple maneuvers (Fig. 7-3). These maneuvers require 180 degrees of abduction, 45 de-

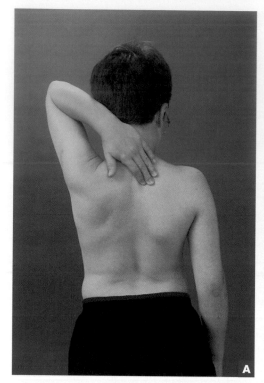 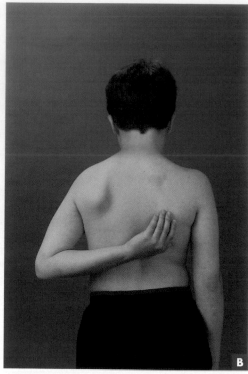 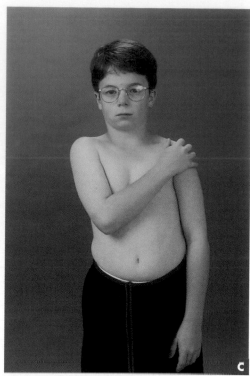

FIG. 7-3 *A,* Place hand behind head on opposite shoulder (external rotation and abduction). *B,* Place back of hand behind the back and touch opposite scapula. *C,* Place hand on opposite shoulder. (*B* and *C* test internal rotation and adduction).

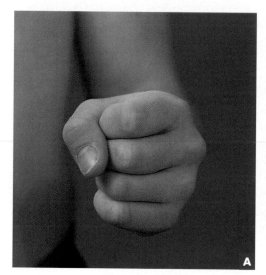 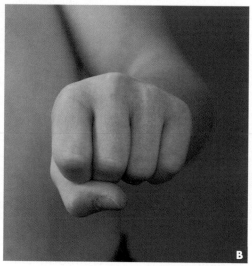 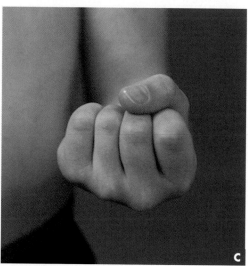

FIG. 7-4 Supination and pronation of the elbow. The elbow should be held flexed at 90 degrees and against the body. The fist in a neutral vertical position *(A),* then rotated 90 degrees in pronation *(B),* and 90 degrees in supination *(C).*

grees of adduction, 90 degrees of flexion, and 45 degrees of external rotation of the glenohumeral joint and related articulations.

Elbow

The examiner must distinguish swelling in the olecranon bursa from involvement of the true elbow joint. The elbow is frequently affected in all forms of JRA and is the most common upper extremity joint affected in spondyloarthropathy. Range of motion of the elbow is easily tested (Figs. 7-4 and 7-5).

Wrist and Hand

Children do not require much extension to perform most activities of daily living and thus can lose strength and mobility in the wrist, which may go unnoticed. The wrist is frequently affected in childhood arthritis, and thus a careful range of motion examination is essential. Normal is 70 degrees of extension, 80 degrees of flexion (Fig. 7-6), 20 degrees radially, and 30 degrees to the ulnar side.

Metacarpophalangeal joints (MCPs) extend 30 degrees and flex 90 degrees. Normal range of motion for the proximal interphalangeal joints (PIPs) is illustrated in Fig. 7-7.

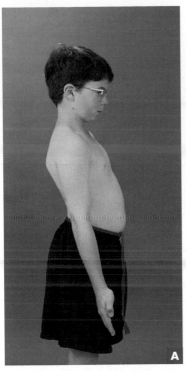
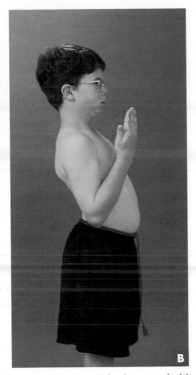

FIG. 7-5 The elbow should extend from 0 degrees with the arm held down *(A)* to 150 degrees in flexion *(B)*.

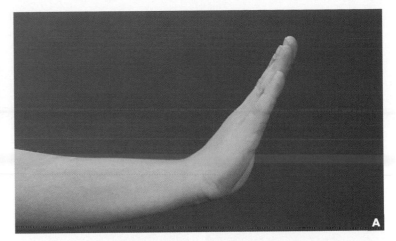

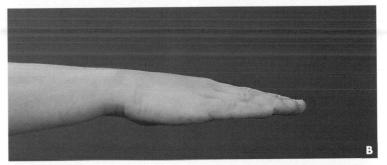

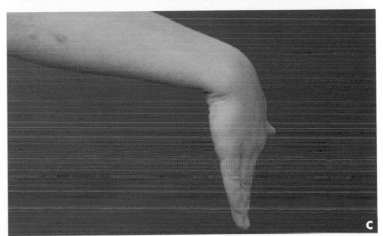

FIG. 7-6 The wrist should extend to 70 degrees *(A)* from neutral position *(B)* and flex to 80 degrees *(C)*.

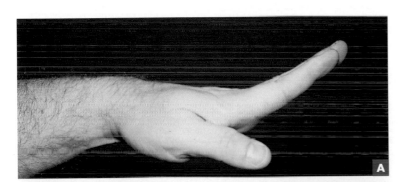

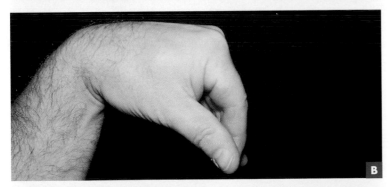

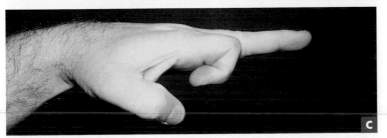

FIG. 7-7 The MCP joints can extend 30 degrees *(A)* and flex 90 degrees *(B)*. Note the normal range of motion for the PIP joints *(C)*.

Spinal Column

In children the neck can be extended so that the head can touch the back and flexed so that the chin touches the chest; 90 degree rotation and 45 degree lateral bending in each direction is also normal (Fig. 7-8).

The entire spine including all spinous processes should be carefully palpated to elicit pain. Flexion, extension, and lateral motion of the spine should be measured using S1 as the focal point. Thirty degrees of extension and 50 degrees of lateral motion are normal. Careful examination of the sacroiliac joints (Fig. 7-9) may be an important clue to the diagnosis of a spondyloarthropathy in an adolescent. Chest expansion,

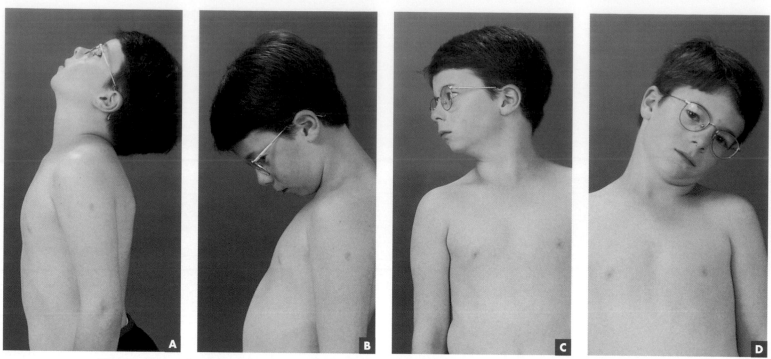

FIG. 7-8   The neck normally can be extended so the head touches the back *(A)*, flexed so the chin touches the chest *(B)*, rotated 90 degrees *(C)*, and tilted laterally 45 degrees *(D)*.

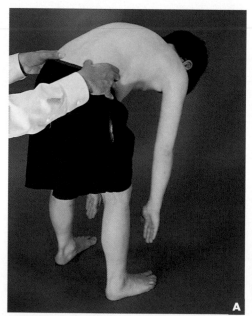

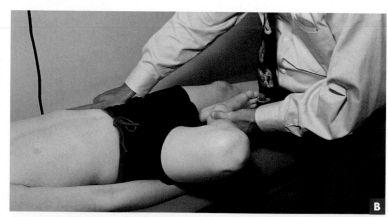

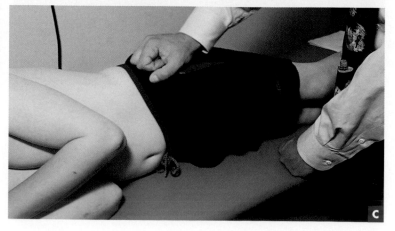

FIG. 7-9   Clinical tests for sacroiliitis. *A,* Application of direct pressure by thumbs over the sacroiliac joints to elicit tenderness. *B,* With knee flexed and hip flexed, abducted, and externally rotated, downward pressure applied on the flexed knee and the contralateral anterosuperior iliac spine. *C,* Compression of the pelvis with patient lying on side. *D,* Patient lying supine, with flexed knee pushed maximally toward the opposite shoulder. *E,* Anterosuperior iliac spines forced laterally apart.

Continued

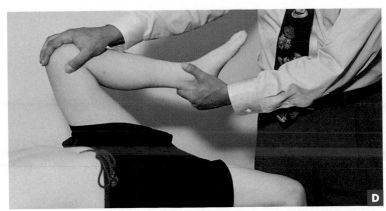

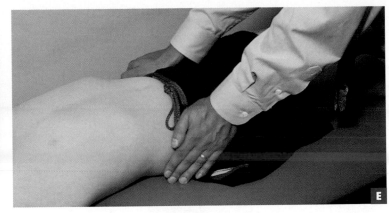

FIG. 7-9, cont'd For legend see opposite page.

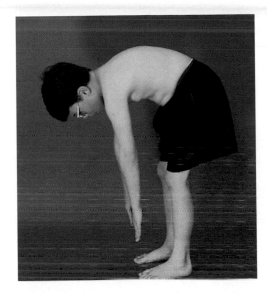

FIG. 7-10 With feet together, the child bends forward. The measurement from floor to fingertip is recorded and compared with subsequent examination.

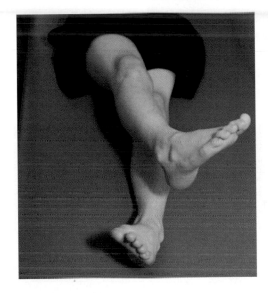

FIG. 7-11 The normal hip can be adducted 20 degrees.

occiput to wall, and finger to floor measurements (Fig. 7-10) are useful in following patients with inflammatory back disease. To detect limitation of forward flexion of the lumbar spine, the Schober test is quite useful. The patient is asked to stand erect and the skin overlying the spinous process of the fifth lumbar vertebra (usually at the level of the "dimples of Venus") and another point 10 cm above in the midline is marked. The patient is asked to maximally bend the spine forward without bending the knees. If the lumbar spine is mobile, the distance between the two points increases by 5 cm or more; that is, the distance between the two points becomes equal to or greater than 15 cm. An increase of 4 cm or less indicates decreased mobility of the lumbar spine.

Hip

The normal hip examination consists of 45 degrees of abduction and 10 degrees of adduction (Fig. 7-11) with the knee bent 20 degrees. The hip can extend 30 degrees, externally rotate to 45 degrees, and internally rotate to 35 degrees. An increase in lumbar lordosis may be the first sign of decreased hip flexion. Normally, hip flexion reaches to about 135 degrees (Fig. 7-12).

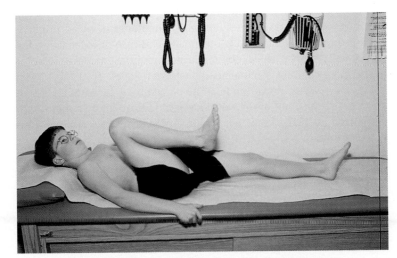

FIG. 7-12 The normal hip can be flexed 135 degrees.

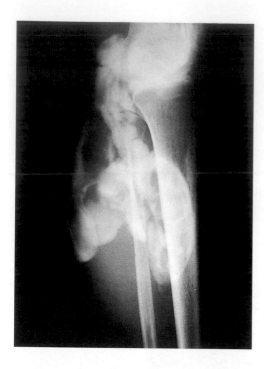

FIG. 7-13 Arthrogram demonstrates communication of Baker cyst with synovial cavity of knee joint.

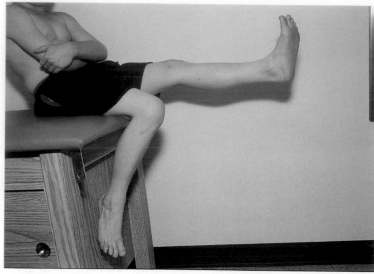

FIG. 7-14 Normal knee range of motion extends from 10 degrees hyperextension (*left knee*) to 130 degrees of flexion (*right knee*).

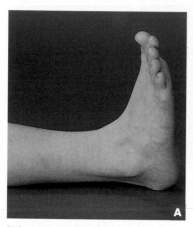
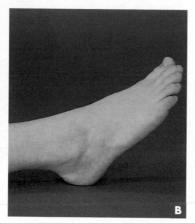
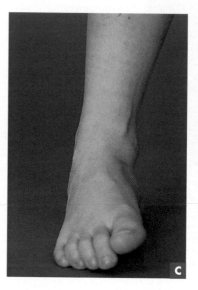
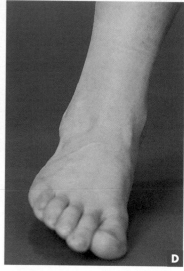

FIG. 7-15 The ankle normally can flex to 20 degrees *(A)* and extend to 45 degrees *(B)*. Inversion occurs to 30 degrees *(C)* and eversion to 20 degrees *(D)*.

Knee

The knee bends and straightens more than 600 times a minute during vigorous walking and is the joint most commonly involved in childhood arthritis. Swelling of the knee may be diffuse or localized to the suprapatellar bursa, which communicates with the true knee joint, or to the gastrocnemius-semimembranous bursa (Baker cyst) (Fig. 7-13), which may dissect down the leg. The patella must be carefully evaluated for "roughening of the undersurface" indicative of chondromalacia patella, which is not uncommon in teenage girls. Normal knee range of motion is illustrated in Fig. 7-14.

Foot and Ankle

The foot and ankle can offer valuable clues to the diagnosis of arthritis in childhood. Evidence of Achilles tendinitis or plantar fasciitis suggests a spondyloarthropathy. First metatarsalphalangeal (MTP) joint involvement is also a strong clue to the diagnosis of a spondyloarthropathy. Normal ranges of motion of the true ankle joint and subtalar joint are

illustrated in Fig. 7-15, and decreased range of motion is common in early onset (type 1) and late onset (type 2) pauciarticular JRA.

Careful flexion and extension of all interphalangeal joints of the feet must be evaluated, especially the first MTP (80 degrees extension to 35 degrees of flexion). The MTPs should be squeezed enough to wrinkle the skin; pain suggests MTP involvement with arthritis.

Leg Length

Leg length discrepancy (Fig. 7-16) is common in JRA because of hyperemia of an affected joint and subsequent overgrowth. Compensatory scoliosis also may develop.

Juvenile Rheumatoid Arthritis

JRA is the most common rheumatic disease in children. The American College of Rheumatology criteria for the diagnosis of JRA are

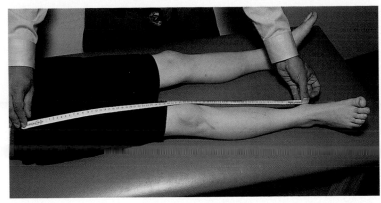

FIG. 7-16 Leg length is measured from the anterosuperior iliac spine to the medial malleolus.

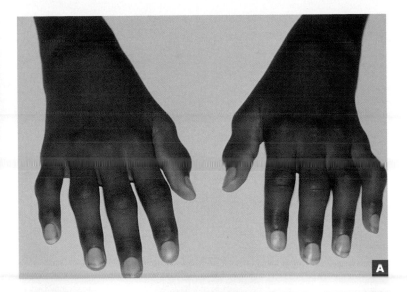

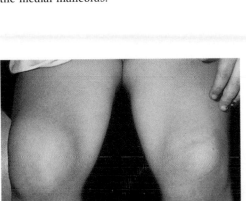

FIG. 7-18 The toddler with pauciarticular JRA has unilateral knee swelling with slight erythema. The right knee demonstrates loss of the normal anatomic landmarks.

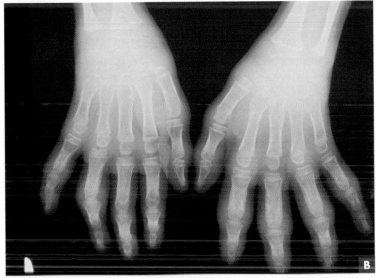

FIG. 7-17 Swelling and inflammation of the small joints of the hands in a patient with polyarticular JRA. *A,* Note the inability to fully extend the fingers. *B,* On x-ray examination, fusiform swelling of the PIP joints with demineralization and diffuse soft-tissue swelling are seen.

the most frequently used in North America (Table 7-4).

The true incidence of JRA is not known. However, recent data from the Mayo Clinic provide an incidence of 13.9 cases per 100,000 children per year, with 95% confidence limits of 9.9 to 18.7. The prevalence of JRA in the Mayo Clinic survey was 113.4 per 100,000 children, with 95% confidence limits of 69.1 to 196.3. Some estimate the prevalence of JRA in the United States to be approximately 250,000 affected persons; however, these figures undoubtedly are conservative.

The first clear description of these entities was presented by George Still in 1897. He postulated multiple etiologies for JRA, and this concept is still supported today. JRA can be a systemic, polyarticular, or pauciarticular disease, all having inflammation of the synovial tissue as one of their cardinal features. Synovium is usually hypertrophied, and joint effusions may occur. On physical examination, joint swelling (Fig. 7-17), loss of normal anatomic landmarks, tenderness, decreased joint mobility, warmth, erythema, and joint deformity (Fig. 7-18) may be noted. It is typical for the child with JRA to have constant and daily pain. Symptoms often develop gradually over a period of weeks or months before

TABLE 7-4

Criteria for the Diagnosis of JRA

1. Age at onset less than 16 years
2. Arthritis (swelling, effusion, or presence of two or more of the following signs: limited range of motion, tenderness or pain on motion, and increased heat) in one or more joints
3. Duration of disease 6 weeks or longer
4. Onset type defined by type of disease in first 6 months:
   (a) Polyarthritis: 5 or more inflamed joints
   (b) Oligoarthritis: <5 inflamed joints
   (c) Systemic: arthritis with characteristic fever
5. Exclusion of other forms of juvenile arthritis

Modified from Cassidy JT, Levinson JE, Bass JC, et al: A study of classification for a diagnosis of juvenile rheumatoid arthritis, *Arthritis Rheum* 29:274-281, 1986.

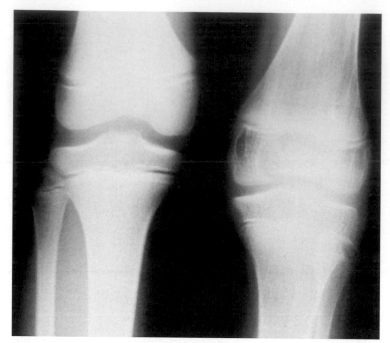

FIG. 7-19 Demineralization of the left femur and tibia with soft-tissue swelling and hypertrophy of the epiphyses secondary to hyperemia.

FIG. 7-20 Rash of systemic onset JRA is erythematous, macular, and often evanescent. It can be more prominent during periods of fever. The rash was pruritic in this patient.

TABLE 7-5

Classification of JRA

Type	Percent	Characteristics	Gender ratio	Rheumatoid factor/ANA	Iridocyclitis	Severe arthritis
Systemic	15	Systemic symptoms; L and S*	M > F	−/−	−	25%
Polyarticular						
RF−	30	Early or late onset of symptoms; L and S	F > M	−/25%	15%	10%-15%
RF+	5	Late onset of symptoms; L and S Rheumatoid nodules	F > M	+/50%-75%	−	Majority
Pauciarticular						
Early onset	35	Few joints; hips and SI joints not involved	F > M	−/60%	50%	Not usually severe
Late onset	15	Few joints; SI, hips involved, HLA B27 75%	M > F	−/−	Occasional	Ankylosing spondylitis sometimes present

Modified from Schaller JG: Juvenile rheumatoid arthritis, *Pediatr Rev* 2(6):163-174, 1980.
*L, Large joints affected; S, small joints affected; M, male; F, female.

evaluation. Morning stiffness is often reported and must last longer than 1 hour in the morning to indicate inflammatory arthritis. The duration of morning stiffness also correlates well with the degree of disease activity in children with JRA. Similar symptoms such as napping and prolonged sitting may occur after inactivity; this is referred to as the *gel phenomenon*. Weather changes may exacerbate symptoms, though they have no impact on the underlying pathology of the disease. Although arthralgia alone can be the initial presentation of JRA without actual joint swelling, the diagnosis cannot be confirmed without the presence of true arthritis. An extremely painful, hot joint with intense erythema (especially if it is monoarticular) suggests the diagnosis of septic arthritis rather than JRA. The child with acute rheumatic fever often has exquisitely tender joints in a migratory pattern, however, with a very acute onset. Again this presentation directs the clinician away from the diag-

nosis of JRA. Despite objective arthritis, the JRA patient may not experience pain. When inflammation persists for a long enough period of time, destruction of the articular surface and bony structures may occur (Fig. 7-19). Because of the poor regenerative properties of articular cartilage, these deformities are usually permanent. Fortunately, most cases of JRA are not associated with permanent joint deformity.

The group of diseases placed under the JRA rubric combines diverse entities, generally divided into three categories: (1) systemic onset disease, (2) polyarticular disease (rheumatoid factor negative or rheumatoid factor positive), and (3) pauciarticular disease (early childhood onset [EOPA, or type 1] and late onset pauciarticular [LOPA, or type 2]). The classification of the disease is based on its presentation during the first 6 months of illness (Table 7-5). On occasion the presenting subtype of JRA is not the child's ultimate disease course. For example, 5% of

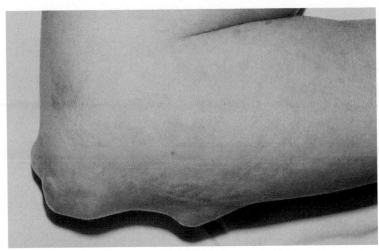

FIG. 7-21 Subcutaneous nodules over the pressure points of the elbow.

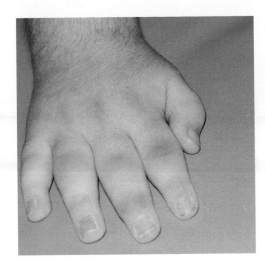

FIG. 7-22 Swelling of the PIP and MCP joints in this patient with polyarticular JRA produces spindle-shaped fingers.

pauciarticular JRA type 1 evolves into a polyarticular course with a much worse prognosis. This subtype has also been referred to in the literature as *extended oligoarticular arthritis.*

Systemic Onset

Systemic onset JRA (Still disease) accounts for anywhere from 10% to 20% of all children with JRA. Fever, rash, irritability, arthritis, and visceral involvement dominate the clinical presentation. The patient's temperature usually rises to greater than 39°C and often occurs twice daily in a double "quotidian" pattern. Chills are associated with fever, but rigors rarely occur. Though the late afternoon is a typical time for a temperature rise, many other patterns may occur. Other manifestations of systemic onset JRA, such as rash and joint symptoms, may wax and wane during febrile periods. One helpful clinical feature during the febrile phase is one subnormal temperature during every 24-hour period, which suggests JRA.

The rash of JRA is macular, 2 to 6 mm in diameter, evanescent, salmon or red in color, with slightly irregular margins (Fig. 7-20). There is often an area of central clearing. The rash usually occurs on the trunk and proximal extremities but also may be distal in distribution, with palms and soles affected. Although the rash generally does not produce discomfort, some older patients report pruritus. Superficial mild trauma to the skin or exposure to warmth and stress may precipitate the rash. Whereas the rash is seen with polyarticular JRA, it does not occur with pauciarticular disease. Arthritis may not occur invariably at the onset of systemic onset JRA, and thus the diagnosis may not be readily apparent. When fever of unknown origin is the sole initial presentation of systemic onset JRA, it must remain a diagnosis of exclusion until the clinician observes true inflammatory arthritis. Arthralgia and myalgia can be prominent early, as can hepatosplenomegaly and lymphadenopathy. Serositis, pleuritis, pericarditis, hyperbilirubinemia, liver enzyme elevation, leukocytosis, and anemia also have been seen with this illness. Although only about 25% of systemic onset JRA progresses to chronic inflammatory arthritis, this is a poor prognostic sign and usually warrants aggressive treatment.

Polyarticular Onset

Polyarticular onset of disease accounts for approximately 35% of all children with JRA. To make the diagnosis, five or more joints must be involved in the absence of prominent systemic signs and symptoms.

There appear to be two subgroups within this category—rheumatoid factor negative and rheumatoid factor positive. The seropositive group is believed to be nearly identical to the adult entity of rheumatoid arthritis (RA). Although onset can occur as early as 8 years of age, it usually occurs in the early teens and girls predominate, as they do in the seronegative form of the disease. Whereas 80% of all adult patients are seropositive, only 5% of children have a positive rheumatoid factor.

In addition to the joint findings of warmth, swelling, erythema, and tenderness seen in both subgroups, seropositive disease provides some additional clues to diagnosis. The subcutaneous nodules that occur in seropositive disease are firm, nontender nodules on the skin surface with a predilection for pressure points or extensor areas (Fig. 7-21). The most common location is the elbow, but the nodules also occur on the heels, hands, knees, ears, scapula, sacrum, and buttocks. Other features of seropositive disease may include cutaneous vasculitis, Felty syndrome (leukopenia and splenomegaly), and Sjögren syndrome (keratoconjunctivitis sicca and xerostomia with or without parotid swelling).

The onset of polyarthritis may be insidious or acute. Whereas the seropositive subgroup progresses to destructive synovitis and a prolonged chronic course in more than half of the patients, children with seronegative disease generally have a better prognosis but approximately 5% to 10% of these children also progress to severe joint destruction and severe flexion contractures and have a long, protracted duration of symptoms. Any synovial joint may be involved in the inflammatory process, including the knees, wrists, elbows, ankles, small joints of the feet, and the PIP and the MCP joints (Fig. 7-22). The lumbosacral spine is usually spared.

Pauciarticular Onset

Pauciarticular onset JRA is strictly defined as onset of disease in fewer than five joints, though clearly children with additional joints may informally belong to this category. The large joints (knees, ankles, and elbows) are often asymmetrically involved. Two subgroups exist under this heading—early and late onset. In early onset pauciarticular (EOPA) disease there is female predominance, the ANA is positive in 25%, and onset is usually before the fifth birthday. As with polyarticular disease, systemic symptoms do not dominate the clinical picture. If the disease does not progress to polyarticular involvement within the first 6 to 12 months of illness, the patient often maintains the pauciarticular pattern. Although joint disease may be visible, pain is rarely severe. This disease entity is particularly unique because of its 50% association

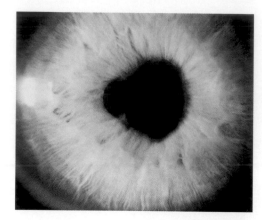

FIG. 7-23 Iridocyclitis with an irregular pupil in a patient with pauciarticular JRA. Note synechiae projecting posteriorly toward the lens.

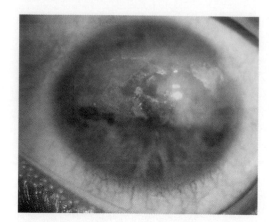

FIG. 7-24 Band keratopathy in a patient with JRA. Note the calcium deposits in Bowman layer.

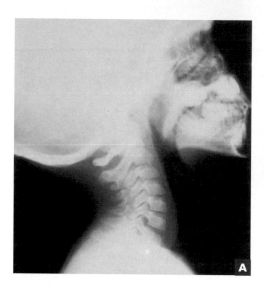

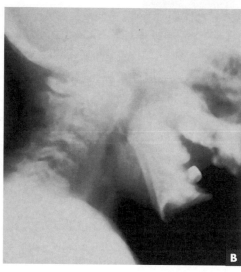

FIG. 7-25 Ankylosing spondylitis with fusion of C2, C3, C4 occurring during an 18-month period between *A* and *B*.

with chronic asymptomatic iridocyclitis. In the disease's earliest stages, diagnosis often depends on slit-lamp examination, though photophobia, eye pain, and erythema can occur. Guidelines for ophthalmologic examination of children with JRA were recently outlined by the American Academy of Pediatrics Section on Rheumatology and Section on Ophthalmology. The guidelines are referenced in Table 7-6. The first clinical sign of uveitis is cellular exudate in the anterior chamber. If the uveitis is left untreated, synechiae (adhesions) between the iris and lens may develop, leading to an irregular and poorly functioning pupil (Fig. 7-23). Further along in the clinical course, band keratopathy (calcium deposits in the cornea) (Fig. 7-24) may occur, as well as cataracts or glaucoma. For these reasons, strict adherence to the recommendations for eye examination outlined in Table 7-6 is necessary to help prevent visual handicap in these children. Ophthalmologic complications do not parallel the activity of the arthritis.

Although fulfilling the criteria of JRA, late onset pauciarticular disease may be more logically placed among the seronegative spondyloarthropathies (Fig. 7-25). Affected patients are generally boys, older than 8 years, with involvement of hips, knees, ankles, and foot joints (especially with acute Achilles tendinitis) or other areas of enthesitis. Onset can be acute and of a more prolonged nature in children with a family history of spondyloarthropathies or associated conditions such as psoriasis. In the child who progresses to lumbar and sacral joint disease, the designation juvenile ankylosing spondylitis is appropriate. Other children manifest findings of Reiter syndrome (a seronegative asymmetric arthropathy associated with urethritis, cervicitis, dysentery, inflammatory acute uveitis, or other mucocutaneous disease), and some develop limitation of spine flexion. Still others never progress to

TABLE 7-6

*Frequency of Ophthalmologic Visits for Children With JRA and Without Known Iridocyclitis**

	Age at onset	
JRA subtype at onset	<7 years†	>7 years‡
Pauciarticular		
+ANA	H§	M
−ANA	M	M
Polyarticular		
+ANA	H§	M
−ANA	M	M
Systemic	L	L

Modified from Guidelines for ophthalmologic examinations in children with JRA, *Pediatrics* 92(2)295-296, 1993.

*High risk (H) indicates ophthalmologic examinations every 3 to 4 months. Medium risk (M) indicates ophthalmologic examinations every 6 months. Low risk (L) indicates ophthalmologic examinations every 12 months. ANA indicates antinuclear antibody test.

†All patients are considered at low risk 7 years after the onset of their arthritis and should have yearly ophthalmologic examinations indefinitely.

‡All patients are considered at low risk 4 years after the onset of their arthritis and should have yearly ophthalmologic examinations indefinitely.

§All high risk patients are considered at medium risk 4 years after the onset of their arthritis, hence 6-month interval examinations are needed.

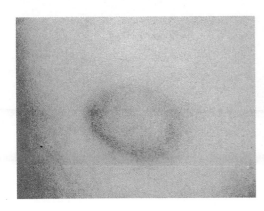

FIG. 7-26 Erythema chronicum migrans in a patient with Lyme arthritis. The lesion may be a large erythematous macule with central clearing, occurring singly or multiply.

TABLE 7-7

Extraarticular Manifestations of JRA

	Poly-articular (%)	Pauci-articular (%)	Systemic disease (%)
Fever	30	0	100
Rheumatoid rash	10	0	95
Rheumatoid nodules	10	0	5
Hepatosplenomegaly	10	0	85
Lymphadenopathy	5	0	70
Chronic uveitis	5	20	0
Pericarditis	5	0	35
Pleuritis	1	0	20
Abdominal pain	1	0	10

Modified from Cassidy JT: *Textbooks of pediatric rheumatology,* New York, 1982, John Wiley.

TABLE 7-8

Differential Diagnosis of JRA

Systemic Onset
Systemic lupus erythematosus
Kawasaki syndrome
Acute rheumatic fever
Henoch-Schönlein purpura
Polyarteritis nodosa
Dermatomyositis
Systemic sclerosis
Inflammatory bowel disease
Malignancy (leukemia, neuroblastoma)
Lyme disease
Viral syndrome
Familial Mediterranean fever

Polyarticular Onset
Systemic lupus erythematosus
Psoriatic arthritis
Hypermobility syndrome
Enthesitis syndrome
Reactive arthritis

Pauciarticular Onset
Septic joint (monarthritis)
Reiter syndrome
Juvenile ankylosing spondylitis
Pigmented villonodular synovitis
Psoriatic arthritis
Lyme disease

a spondyloarthropathy, and hence the designation of JRA continues to be most appropriate.

Extraarticular Manifestations

Many extraarticular features of JRA have been reported. The more common ones are listed in Table 7-7. Linear growth retardation is common in the child with active JRA, especially with systemic onset JRA or polyarticular disease. The degree of retardation and the ultimate prognosis for reaching adult height are related to the severity and duration of inflammation and the use of corticosteroids. Pauciarticular or oligoarticular arthritis, however, can present with bizarre growth abnormalities usually confined to leg length discrepancy or an enlarged hand or foot related to refractory ankle or wrist involvement. Leg length measurements must be recorded on a regular basis to avoid a compensatory scoliosis in these children. During early illness, bony development may be advanced; later in the course of the illness the opposite may be true. Premature epiphyseal fusion may occur. In addition, corticosteroids themselves may inhibit linear growth. Careful use of standardized growth curves assists in the early detection of growth failure. This may in turn guide the long-term therapeutic approach. Rarely, failure to grow may be the only early clinical manifestation of JRA.

Cardiac involvement occurs in more than one third of systemic onset JRA patients. Pericarditis, myocarditis, and endocarditis occur, with pericarditis being the most common. Chest pain, a friction rub, tachycardia, dyspnea, and supportive x-ray findings may occur. These episodes may last for weeks to months and are usually associated with a generalized flare of disease.

A variety of other extraarticular manifestations, including hepatosplenomegaly and lymphadenopathy, are particularly common in systemic onset JRA. Patients can also experience double vision related to a tenosynovitis of the extraocular muscles.

Differential Diagnosis

Because JRA is largely a clinical diagnosis, very strict clinical criteria have been established to make the diagnosis of JRA. Most authors suggest the presence of objective joint findings (arthritis) for a minimum of 6 consecutive weeks coupled with the exclusion of other causes of arthritis in children (Table 7-8). The extraarticular features of JRA, as discussed earlier, may solidify the diagnosis purely because of their distinctiveness (i.e., uveitis, rheumatoid nodules and evanescent rash).

Because of its destructive nature, pyogenic arthritis (staphylococci, streptococci, *Haemophilus influenzae*, etc.) must be ruled out in any child with active joint disease, especially monoarthritis. The intensely red and tender joint, well beyond the degree usually seen with JRA, should raise suspicions of a bacterial pathogen. This combined with systemic symptoms of infection (fever, chills, malaise, rigors) should prompt the clinician to perform an arthrocentesis early in the course of the illness. If the joint in question is the hip, suspicion should be even higher because of the rarity with which the hip is the first affected joint in JRA. Other infectious etiologies include Lyme arthritis. This spirochetal form of arthritis is tick-borne and usually affects the knee, elbow, or wrist in a monoarthritic pattern with spontaneous exacerbations and remissions. Malaise, fever, myalgia, lymphadenopathy, headache, meningismus, and weakness also may occur in the first phase of the illness. The distinctive rash, known as

TABLE 7-9

*Criteria for the Classification of Systemic Lupus Erythematosus**

Malar (butterfly) rash
Discoid-lupus rash
Photosensitivity
Oral or nasal mucocutaneous ulcerations
Nonerosive arthritis
Nephritis†
   Proteinuria >0.5 g/d
   Cellular casts
Encephalopathy†
   Seizures
   Psychosis
Pleuritis or pericarditis
Cytopenia
Positive immunoserology†
   Antibodies to nDNA (*n*ative or *d*ouble-stranded DNA)
   Positive LE-cell preparation
   Biologic false-positive test for syphilis
Positive antinuclear antibody test

Modified from Tan EM, Cohen AS, Fries JF, et al: The 1982 revised criteria for the classification of systemic lupus erythematosus, *Arthritis Rheum* 25:1271-1277, 1982.
*Four of 11 criteria provide a sensitivity of 96% and a specificity of 96%.
†Any one item satisfies this criterion.

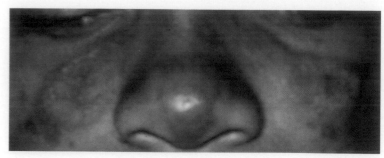

FIG. 7-27 Typical malar rash of SLE. Erythema, erosion, and atrophy are present. Note sparing of nasolabial folds.

erythema chronicum migrans (Fig. 7-26), begins as an erythematous macule or papule. After this clears, the borders of the lesion expand to form an erythematous circular lesion that can be as large as 30 cm in diameter. These lesions can initially occur singularly but can progress to multiple lesions over the legs, arms, and trunk. Other manifestations of Lyme disease include neurologic complications such as seventh nerve palsy, meningitis, radiculoneuritis, and the cardiac manifestations of heart block and myopericarditis. Bilateral Bell palsy or seventh nerve paralysis even more strongly suggests the diagnosis of Lyme disease. *Salmonella, Shigella, Yersinia,* and *Campylobacter* organisms should also be considered. A multitude of viruses cause arthritis. These include rubella; hepatitis B; adenovirus; and herpesviruses, including Epstein-Barr virus, cytomegalovirus, varicella zoster, and herpes simplex. Parvoviruses, mumps, and enteroviruses, including echovirus and coxsackievirus, are associated with acute polyarthritis and occasionally have been recovered from joints. Other viruses result in reactive arthritis and may not infect the joint directly.

Malignancies such as neuroblastoma and leukemia may appear to present with joint disease. More careful evaluation generally reveals bone pain. Sickle cell disease, particularly in the form of dactylitis, can have prominent digital involvement. Inflammatory bowel disease, acute rheumatic fever, hemophilia, trauma, hypermobility syndrome, psoriasis, and Henoch-Schönlein purpura also must be considered in the patient with arthritis. All of the connective tissue diseases can have significant joint disease; however, their clinical features and laboratory tests usually distinguish them from JRA. Differential diagnoses of JRA are proposed in Table 7-8 with respect to disease onset as outlined in Table 7-5.

Systemic Lupus Erythematosus

Systemic lupus erythematosus (SLE) is a complex autoimmune disease with a myriad of clinical presentations. SLE is a syndrome composed of multiple disease subsets, which may be identified by particular antibodies that may define particular disease types. SLE may present in an insidious fashion and hence escape early diagnosis, or it may present acutely and progress rapidly, leading to the patient's demise. As with other collagen vascular diseases, the etiology of SLE is unknown. The disease may involve just one organ system, or more commonly it may be a multisystem disease. Because of the large number of serologic markers known to occur in SLE, it is considered by many to be the prototype of autoimmune diseases. To increase diagnostic accuracy, the American College of Rheumatology revised its classification criteria of lupus (Table 7-9). This classification is highly sensitive and specific for the diagnosis of this disease; however, the criteria are not meant for the clinical application of diagnosis and, although 4 of the 11 criteria must be present to make the diagnosis, they should be used as a study guide rather than applied to the clinical arena.

The word *lupus,* which means wolf, alludes to the erosive nature of the rash of SLE ("wolf bite") (Fig. 7-27). This feature of the disease was critical to the diagnosis of SLE until the discovery of the lupus erythematosus (LE) cell in 1948. The LE cell represents a healthy neutrophil, which has phagocytized the nuclear debris of a nonliving cell that has been coated with antibody. The antibody is directed against deoxyribonucleoprotein (DNP), which is made up of both DNA and histones. The presence of this serologic marker for lupus greatly expanded the recognized clinical entity of SLE. Although the LE prep has proved to be of historic interest, time has shown that it is a nonspecific immunologic phenomenon and has no specificity with respect to the diagnosis of SLE.

Although SLE accounts for 10% of patients with rheumatic diseases, its incidence and prevalence are largely unknown. The incidence among children younger than 15 years of age is estimated at 0.53 to 0.6 per 100,000, although no recent data are available. There are no accurate prevalence data, although it has been inferred that there are between 5,000 and 10,000 children with SLE in the United States. The disease is much more common in teenage girls. Girls are affected five times more than boys, and black patients are more commonly affected than white patients. The disease is rare in children under the age of 5, and before menarche the boy/girl ratio is equal. The incidence of other connective tissue diseases is higher among family members of patients with SLE. Hematologic malignancies and immunodeficiencies are also

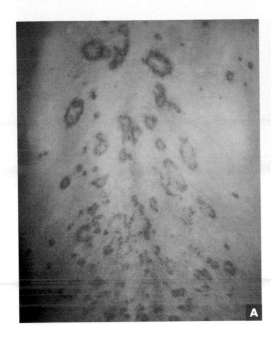

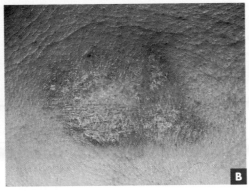

FIG. 7-28 *A,* The localized erythematous rash of SLE in a nonmalar distribution. *B,* The rash of SLE often has a slight white scale.

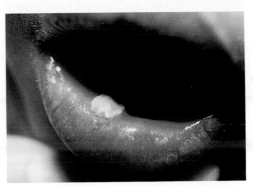

FIG. 7-29 Mucosal ulceration of the lip as evidence of vasculitis in SLE.

reported in increased frequency among SLE relatives. These well-described phenomena may reflect a genetic alteration of immunity or, as some researchers suggest, the effects of a transmissible agent. Drugs induce a lupuslike reaction, and their withdrawal leads to a resolution of this syndrome usually within 6 months. Many patients on certain drugs such as hydralazine, procainamide, isoniazid (INH), chlorpromazine, or certain anticonvulsants develop a positive ANA without developing a lupus syndrome, and this is not an absolute reason to discontinue the medication. Oral contraceptives also have been shown in some studies to be associated with a lupuslike syndrome. The high incidence of disease in girls, SLE's common exacerbation during pregnancy, and the induction of disease by birth control pills support the role of hormonal factors as contributing or modulating agents to the pathogenesis of SLE. Other investigators suggest the influence of viruses, sunlight, and emotional stress on those developing lupus.

Although immunologic markers have made the diagnosis of SLE considerably easier, a high index of suspicion is still necessary to obtain these studies. The early symptoms are often nonspecific and sometimes go unrecognized as harbingers of serious disease. Fever, fatigue, malaise, anorexia, and weight loss may be the only symptoms. In the adolescent population these symptoms may be all the more difficult to interpret. Conversely this multisystem disease may present with a plethora of physical findings, and the presentation may be so dramatic that the diagnosis is readily apparent. Among the more commonly involved areas are the skin, joints, muscles, liver, spleen, lymph nodes, kidneys, heart, and lungs.

Cutaneous manifestations of SLE occur at some time during the course of the disease in 80% of affected individuals. The classic butterfly rash in the malar distribution is seen in about one third of cases (Fig. 7-27). In contrast to patients with dermatomyositis (Fig. 7-46), the nasolabial fold of patients with SLE is spared. The rash of lupus is often reddish-purple and raised with a whitish scale (Fig. 7-28). When the scale is removed, the underlying skin often shows "carpet-tack–like" fingers on the unexposed side of the scale itself. Carpet tacking is caused by the contouring of the scale into the skin follicles. These fingerlike projections on a scale strongly suggest the diagnosis of lupus. Purplish-red urticarial lesions also occur, but these do not produce scales and do not cause atrophy as other lupus lesions do. If the skin manifestations are left untreated, the patient's appearance will be

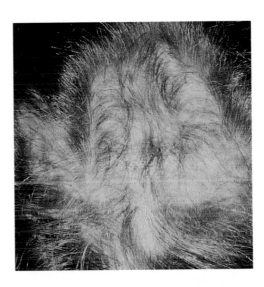

FIG. 7-30 Scarring alopecia seen in SLE.

marred by hypopigmentation and hyperpigmentation. Mucosal erosions and ulcers of the oral cavity and nasal mucosa are part of lupus as well (Fig. 7-29). Alopecia (Fig. 7-30) occurs in 20% of patients and may present as broken hair shafts or patchy, red, scaling areas on the scalp, which may eventually scar and cause permanent hair loss. Other reported mucocutaneous findings are livedo reticularis (lacey, fishnet appearance of the skin), urticaria, atrophy, and telangiectasia. The presence of livedo reticularis may be the clinician's only clue to an associated hypercoagulable state manifest by antiphospholipid antibodies. This tendency can be diagnosed by obtaining an RPR, PTT, and anticardiolipin antibodies of the IgG and IgM classes. Although the antiphospholipid antibody syndrome can occur as an entity alone, it is commonly associated with SLE, a hypercoagulable state, and a tendency toward venous and arterial thrombosis. Though rare in children, discoid lupus refers to the absence of systemic disease in the presence of typical lupus dermatologic pathology. Another entity, referred to as *subacute cutaneous lupus,* in which the traditional ANA is sometimes negative but the SS-A (Sjögren syndrome A, or anti-Ro) is positive recently has been described. This syndrome can occur in an annular pattern or psoriaform pattern and often progresses to full-blown SLE.

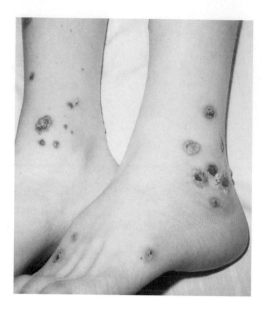

FIG. 7-31 Cutaneous vasculitis in SLE. Purpuric, ulcerative, and necrotic skin lesions of active disease.

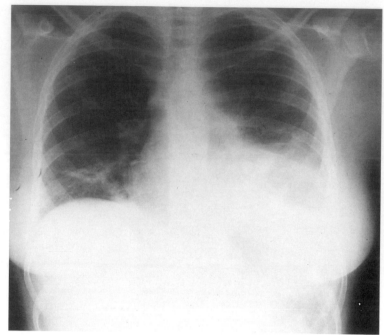

FIG. 7-32 Atelectasis, pleural effusions, and pulmonary infiltrates in a teenage girl with SLE.

The vasculitis of lupus, a small-vessel vasculitis, is responsible for a number of easily recognizable clinical findings. The skin may be purpuric, or in more severe instances necrotic lesions may result (Fig. 7-31). The vasculitic component of lupus also may present with full-blown Raynaud phenomenon. With repeated tissue injury, glossy, atrophic, ulcerated skin and distorted nail architecture may be present.

The heart is often significantly involved in patients with lupus. Although the pericardium is involved most commonly, the myocardium and the endocardium also may be of clinical importance. Pericarditis can be painless and may present only as cardiomegaly on a chest radiograph or as pericardial effusion on an echocardiogram. However, chest pain may be noted or a friction rub auscultated. Although pericarditis is usually mild, it can progress to life-threatening cardiac tamponade. If the myocardium is affected, life-threatening complications, including dysrhythmia, heart failure, and infarction can result. *Libman-Sacks endocarditis* is the term given to the verrucous projections of fibrinoid necrosis in the endocardium. These lesions rarely cause clinical symptoms, though the presence of a murmur raises suspicion of endocardial disease. The mitral valve is most commonly involved, although aortic and tricuspid valves may be similarly infected. The presence of Libman-Sacks endocarditis should also alert the clinician to the possibility of an underlying antiphospholipid antibody syndrome.

Pulmonary manifestations of lupus are particularly difficult to diagnose noninvasively. Migrating pneumonitis, particularly involving the lung bases, suggests "lupus lung," however, distinguishing these entities from infection may be impossible without invasive procedures. Typically, patients have atelectasis, pleural effusions, interstitial pneumonitis, or hemorrhage (Fig. 7-32). These sequelae may present as cyanosis, dyspnea, or almost any other form of respiratory distress. Patients with SLE can also develop a "shrinking lung" syndrome. This is manifest by diaphragmatic involvement and progressively smaller lung volumes recorded by pulmonary function testing. Also, the clinician should always be suspicious of the diagnosis of SLE in the setting of hematuria and hemoptysis and must rule out other entities such as

Wegener granulomatosis, hemolytic uremic syndrome, Goodpasture syndrome, and infective endocarditis.

Unlike the destructive arthritis of JRA, lupus arthritis is more transient and episodic and rarely results in loss of function. "Jaccoud" arthropathy, which is a nondeforming, easily reversible, soft-tissue arthritis that can mimic the boutonniere (flexion of PIP, hyperextension of DIP) and swan-neck (hyperextension of PIP and flexion of DIP) deformities associated with JRA, is strongly associated with the diagnosis of SLE. The fact that arthralgia is more predominant than arthritis has been noted consistently. Any joint may be involved, but the fingers are particularly susceptible. Myalgia and weakness also occur as features of lupus but do not dominate the clinical picture as they do in dermatomyositis.

Central nervous system (CNS) signs and symptoms of lupus are a great challenge to physicians. A wide range of neurologic and psychiatric manifestations of the disease have been described. Further complicating the spectrum of CNS lupus is the difficulty in distinguishing the disease itself from side effects of therapy such as corticosteroid psychosis, emotional response to disease, and a non-CNS etiology of CNS pathology such as hypertensive encephalopathy. Chorea is a common neurologic manifestation of lupus and must be distinguished from the chorea of rheumatic fever. Focal neurologic defects occurring in lupus also suggest the possibility of cerebral vascular accident and again alert the clinician to look for the antiphospholipid antibody syndrome. It is estimated that approximately one quarter of all lupus patients have some form of CNS disease. The findings range from mononeuritis multiplex (inflammatory lesions of multiple nerves located in anatomically unrelated parts of the body) to ataxia, peripheral neuropathy, seizures, headaches, psychosis, pseudotumor cerebri, and intellectual impairment. The thorough investigation of a large number of neurologic signs and symptoms mandates screening serologies for lupus. As a direct extension of the brain, the retina not surprisingly may also show evidence of disease. The best known ocular manifestation is the cotton-wool spot, an exudative, whitish lesion of the retina. Hemorrhage and pap-

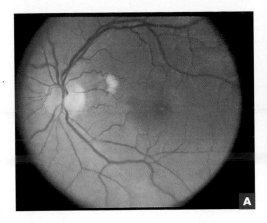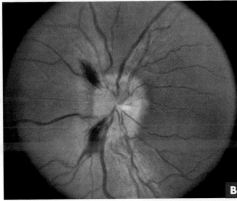

FIG. 7-33 *A,* A white exudate (cotton-wool spot) between the disk and macula. *B,* Papilledema with flame hemorrhages.

TABLE 7-10

World Health Organization Classification of Lupus Nephritis

Class	Characteristic
I	Normal
II	Mesangial
IIA	Minimal alteration
IIB	Mesangial glomerulitis
III	Focal and segmental proliferative glomerulonephritis
IV	Diffuse proliferative glomerulonephritis
V	Membranous glomerulonephritis
VI	Glomerular sclerosis

Modifed from Cassidy JT, Petty RE: *Textbook of pediatric rheumatology,* Philadelphia, 1995, WB Saunders.

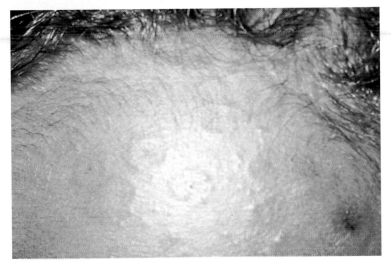

FIG. 7-34 The rash of neonatal SLE.

illedema also are seen (Fig. 7-33). As might be expected, the CNS effects of lupus are responsible for much morbidity and mortality.

At least as important as CNS disease in determining ultimate prognosis is the degree of renal involvement. Approximately 75% of all children with SLE have some degree of clinically apparent renal disease. This often manifests itself in the first 2 years of illness but can also appear many years after the initial diagnosis. The type of pathology largely relates to the nature of immune complex deposition at various sites in the kidney, that is, size and electrical charge of the immune complexes. At a histologic level, renal involvement is classified using the World Health Organization classification of lupus nephritis (Table 7-10). A pathologic diagnosis must be made in children with rapidly progressive renal problems or change in their renal disease to rule out diffuse proliferative glomerulonephritis with the presence of subendothelial deposits on electron microscopy. Other than the glomeruli, the tubules, interstitium, and blood vessels can be involved. From the clinician's point of view, these lesions are difficult to distinguish. More importantly, renal involvement must be monitored at frequent intervals because of the possible development of diffuse proliferative glomerulonephritis. This is best accomplished by urinalysis for protein, hematuria, red cell casts, and abnormalities in the specific gravity patterns over time. The clinician also must obtain BUN and creatinine levels, 24-hour urine for creatinine clearance, and protein levels at periodic intervals. Hypertension also may direct the clinician to the presence of renal disease, and control of hypertension is as important as any other therapeutic maneuver in delaying the progression to renal failure. To complicate the clinical

picture, histologic evidence of renal pathology may be present even when all of the clinical parameters are normal. The timing of renal biopsy in a patient with SLE is extremely controversial in the rheumatologic and renal literature. There is no substitute, however, for careful serologic and clinical monitoring of these patients, and biopsies should be obtained as soon as a change occurs in the clinical picture.

Additional clinical findings in SLE include lymphadenopathy with or without hepatosplenomegaly, hepatitis, anemia, leukopenia, thrombocytopenia, disorders of esophageal motility, pancreatitis, malabsorption, diarrhea, and abdominal pain. Lupus also occurs in infants whose mothers have the disease. SS-A antibody of the IgG class is passed via the placenta to the fetus, leading to positive serologies and the diagnosis of neonatal lupus. The presence of rash (Fig. 7-34), thrombocytopenia, Coombs-positive hemolytic anemia, liver function abnormalities, and congenital heart block should suggest the diagnosis of neonatal lupus. The majority of infants with congenital heart block and neonatal lupus have entirely asymptomatic mothers, although a percentage of these women develop Sjögren syndrome rather than SLE. Fortunately, neonatal lupus is transient, lasting only a few months until the disappearance of passively transferred maternal antibody; however, the congenital heart block is permanent.

Perhaps more than any other rheumatic disease, the clinical diagnosis of lupus can be confirmed serologically. The antinuclear antibodies (ANAs) represent a group of antibodies found in serum and are directed against antigens within the cellular nuclei of lupus patients. ANAs usually are reported with a titer and a pattern. The patterns are

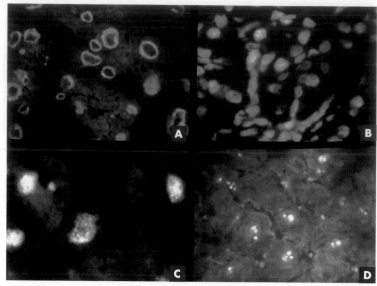

FIG. 7-35　*A,* Peripheral. Correlates with anti-dsDNA double-stranded—active renal disease. *B,* Homogeneous. Nonspecific, SLE. *C,* Speckled. Seen with SLE, MCTD. To further delineate a diagnosis, anti-RNP is present in MCTD and Smith (Sm) antibody is present in SLE. *D,* Nucleolar. Suggests scleroderma.

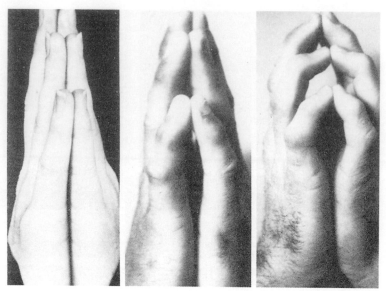

FIG. 7-36　Cheiroarthropathy, or arthropathy of the hand, as seen in diabetes mellitus. Note the progressive deformity over time with flexion contractures of the finger joints.

TABLE 7-11

Antibodies Found in SLE Patients

Antibody	Patients (%)
Native DNA (double-stranded)	50 to 60
DNP (DNA and histone protein)	Up to 70 (usually high titer)
RNP (RNA and non-histone protein)	30 to 40
Histones	
All SLE patients	60
Drug-induced lupus patients	95
SS-A (Ro)	30 to 40
SS-B (La)	15
Sm	30

Modifed from Tan EM: Antinuclear antibodies in diagnosis and management, *Hosp Pract* 18:74-79, 1983.

either peripheral, homogenous, speckled, or nucleolar (Fig. 7-35).

Other antibodies found in SLE patients are listed in Table 7-11. Antinative DNA antibodies are detected in 50% to 60% of lupus patients and are specific for the diagnosis of SLE. It also should be noted that antidouble stranded DNA or native DNA antibodies correlate well with disease activity, especially renal and CNS disease. Antibodies to single-stranded DNA are also present in SLE; however, their presence in many entities limits their clinical utility, and they are of no value in following disease activity. Ribonucleoprotein (RNP), though better known for its presence in high titers in mixed connective tissue disease, is also seen in low titers in 30% to 40% of lupus patients. Other SLE antibodies include SS-A and SS-B also known as anti-Ro and anti-La, respectively. As previously noted, anti-Ro or SS-A antibodies are associated with the neonatal lupus syndrome and congenital heart block in infants. Lastly, the clinician finds antibodies to Smith antigen (Sm), a nonhistone antigen that also appears to be very specific for the diagnosis of lupus.

In summary, SLE is a chronic disease with a variable course and with periods of varying activity. Although the mortality and morbidity remain high, marked improvement in prognosis has occurred in recent years.

Scleroderma

Scleroderma, or "tight skin," remains an enigmatic entity with no known etiology and no consistently effective therapy. The estimated annual incidence of scleroderma is from 4.5 to 12 per million, but childhood onset is extremely rare. In children, the localized forms of scleroderma are much more common than systemic sclerosis (SSc), although the exact numbers are unknown. Systemic sclerosis occurs with equal frequency in boys and girls under the age of 8, whereas girls outnumber boys 3:1 when disease onset is after the eighth birthday.

Scleroderma can be a primary idiopathic disease or a secondary phenomenon (Table 7-12 and Fig. 7-36). The classification of idiopathic scleroderma consists of (1) systemic disease—diffuse or limited, the former known as *progressive systemic sclerosis* (PSS) and the latter

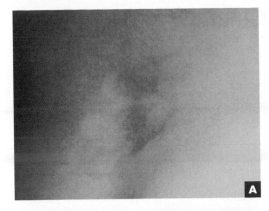

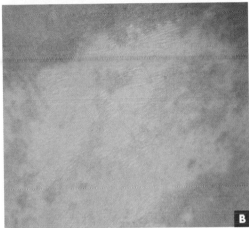

FIG. 7-37 Forms of morphea. *A,* Hypopigmented plaque of scleroderma with skin atrophy. *B,* "Salt-and-pepper" appearance of a plaque in a patient with scleroderma. Note the hyperpigmentation within the hypopigmented lesion.

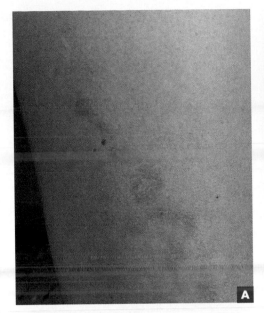

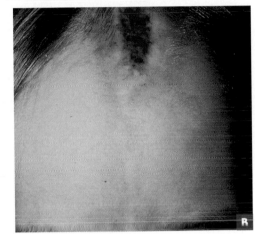

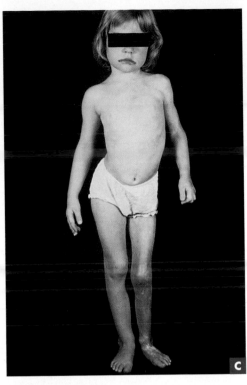

FIG. 7-38 *A,* Linear scleroderma. Localized involvement of a dermatome with hyperpigmentation. *B,* An unusual form of local scleroderma affecting the scalp, termed *en coup de sabre* (stroke of the saber). *C,* Linear scleroderma affecting the left side of the body.

referred to as the *CREST syndrome* (Fig. 7-39) and (2) local disease—morphea, linear scleroderma, or *en coup de sabre* (stroke of the sabre).

Local scleroderma is a group of disorders in which fibrosis is confined to skin, subcutaneous tissue, or muscle. Early active lesions are characterized by a violaceous inflammatory border. Morphea may present in the form of plaques or drops (the "guttate" variety) or with diffuse cutaneous involvement (Fig. 7-37). Linear scleroderma affects a single dermatome and can cause severe deformity and growth arrest in an affected limb. When this lesion occurs on the face or scalp, it is referred to as *scleroderma "en coup de sabre"* because of its resemblance to a scar from a dueling sword (Fig. 7-38). Parry-Romberg syndrome is a rare congenital dysplasia of subcutaneous tissue, muscle, bone, and neurologic disease, consisting of headache, seizure, and transient ischemic attacks that may represent a form of linear scleroderma. Sedimentation rate, total eosinophil count, serum immunoglobulin levels, and single-stranded DNA titers may be useful markers of disease activity in local scleroderma.

The ultimate prognosis of children with systemic sclerosis depends on the nature and extent of visceral involvement. In 1980 the American College of Rheumatology developed criteria for the clinical diagnosis of scleroderma. The single major criteria is the presence of proximal scleroderma or the typical cutaneous manifestations of the disease proximal to the wrist. The three minor criteria are sclerodactyly (Fig. 7-39, *C*), digital pitting ulcers (Fig. 7-40), and lastly bilateral basilar pulmonary fibrosis (Fig. 7-41). Children with systemic sclerosis almost always have

TABLE 7-12

Classification of Scleroderma and Related Disorders

Primary

Systemic sclerosis
Diffuse (PSS)
Limited (CREST syndrome)

Local scleroderma
Morphea
Linear and "en coup de sabre"

Eosinophilic fasciitis

Secondary
Graft-versus-host disease
Drug or chemical induced
  Vinyl-chloride
  Bleomycin
  Pentazocine
  Tryptophan
  Silicone
  Toxic-oil syndrome

Scleroderma-like illnesses
Phenylketonuria
Progeria
Werner syndrome
Scleredema
Porphyria cutanea tarda
Diabetic cheiroarthropathy*

*Arthropathy of the hand (Fig. 7-36).

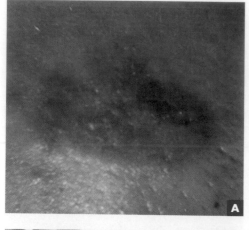

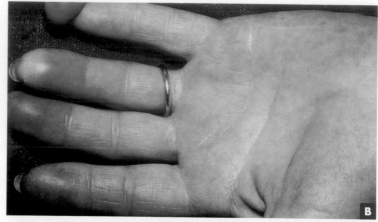

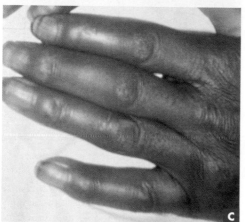

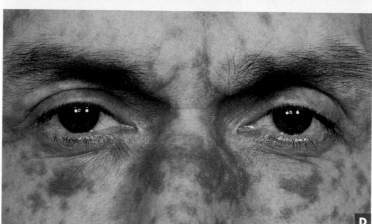

FIG. 7-39 CREST syndrome. *A,* Cutaneous calcinosis. *B,* Raynaud phenomenon (note cyanosis and pallor of the finger-tips). *C,* Sclerodactyly. *D,* Telangiectasia. Esophageal dysmotility may also occur.

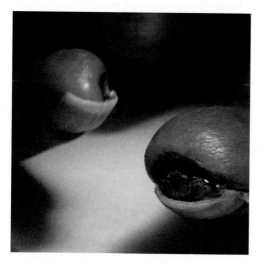

FIG. 7-40 Digital pitting ulcers. One of the three minor diagnostic criteria for scleroderma.

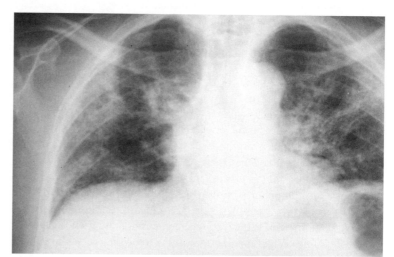

FIG. 7-41 Bilateral pulmonary fibrosis in a patient with scleroderma.

Raynaud phenomenon (Fig. 7-39, *B*), which is a triphasic color change of the hands (first white because of vasoconstriction, then blue secondary to cyanosis, and finally red because of reperfusion with subsequent swelling and pain). This phenomenon can occur in response to cold or stressful stimuli. In its most severe form, fixed vasospasm can lead to gangrene and autoamputation.

The presence of Raynaud phenomenon can be helpful in distinguishing local forms of scleroderma such as morphea or even eosinophilic fasciitis from systemic disease, the former not being associated with Raynaud phenomenon. Raynaud phenomenon can also occur as a "disease" not associated with any particular underlying connective tissue disease.

Systemic sclerosis is divided into two major subtypes: (1) diffuse disease and (2) limited disease or "CREST" syndrome. CREST syndrome is an acronym for *C*alcinosis cutis, *R*aynaud phenomenon, *E*sophageal abnormalities, *S*clerodactyly, and *T*elangiectasias (Fig. 7-39). CREST syndrome also is characterized by a distinct pulmonary lesion indistinguishable from primary pulmonary hypertension as opposed to systemic

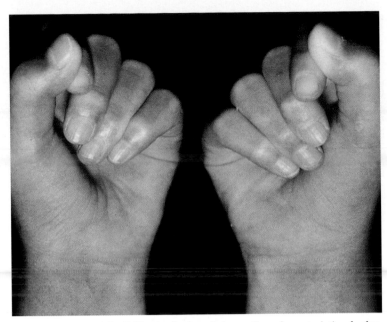

FIG. 7-42 Lack of flexibility in the hands is another characteristic of scleroderma.

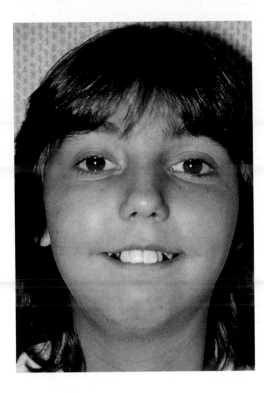

FIG. 7-43 Facial features of scleroderma. The skin appears tight and drawn, without evidence of wrinkles. (Courtesy Dr. J. Jeffrey Malatack, Philadelphia.)

TABLE 7-13

Clinical and Laboratory Characteristics of Patients With Systemic Sclerosis According to Serum Autoantibody Type

Autoantibody	Pattern	Clinical association
Centromere	Centromere	Limited
Th	Nucleolar	—
U1RNP	Speckled	Overlap
PM-Scl	Nucleolar	Overlap with myositis
U3RNP	Nucleolar	Pulmonary hypertension
RNA polymerase I, III	Speckled/nucleolar	Diffuse
Scl-70	Speckled/nucleolar	Diffuse

ACA, Anticentromere antibody; *RNP,* ribonucleoprotein; *PM-Scl,* polymyositis-scleroderma; *Scl,* scleroderma; *Scl-70,* antitopoisomerase.

sclerosis that is characterized by pulmonary fibrosis and secondary pulmonary hypertension. The antibody picture is also helpful in defining subsets of systemic sclerosis (Table 7-13).

Many organ systems can be involved in the child afflicted with scleroderma. Cutaneous manifestations frequently bring children to medical attention, but because of the insidious and subtle onset of skin lesions, there is often a delay in diagnosis. Early in the clinical course, the skin is edematous with particular predilection for the distal extremities; rarely, more proximal limb, face, and trunk involvement is present. The induration phase, for which scleroderma is named, is characterized by loss of the natural pliability of the skin and the presence of a palpable skin thickness. The skin takes on a shiny, tense appearance, with distal tapering of the fingers (Fig. 7-39, *C*). The visual impression that movement might be impaired is supported by the lack of flexibility in the hands (Fig. 7-42). The typical scleroderma facies of tight skin and skin atrophy produce the appearance of a fixed stare, pinched nose, thin pursed lips, small mouth, prominent teeth, and characteristic grimace (Fig. 7-43).

Subcutaneous calcium deposits (calcinosis cutis) may occur at pressure points and may occasionally extrude through the skin in a fashion similar to dermatomyositis (Fig. 7-44). These lesions may be painful and may ulcerate. Often, generalized hyperpigmentation occurs with punctuated areas of hypopigmentation or vitiligo (complete depigmentation) (Figs. 7-37 and 7-38). Telangiectasias of three varieties are known to occur (1) linear telangiectasis of the cuticles, (2) well-defined macules of various sizes and shapes, and (3) the reddish-purple papules typical of Osler-Weber-Rendu disease (tiny circular lesions positioned eccentrically from their telangiectatic spokes) (Fig. 7-39, *D*).

Gastrointestinal symptoms occur in approximately half of the children. More detailed investigation often indicates the presence of abnormalities in a larger percentage. Esophageal dysmotility associated with gastroesophageal reflux often leads to dysphagia and symptoms of esophagitis. In some affected individuals, aspiration or cough may occur and esophageal strictures can develop if the process of reflux is chronic. If the small bowel is involved, cramps, diarrhea, and constipation may result from peristaltic dysfunction. Bacterial overgrowth,

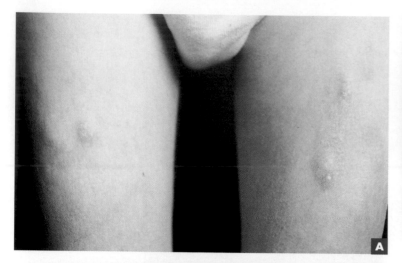

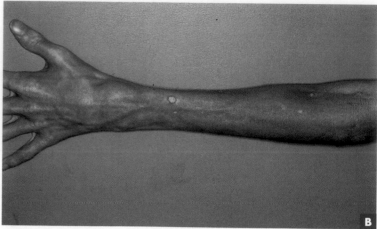

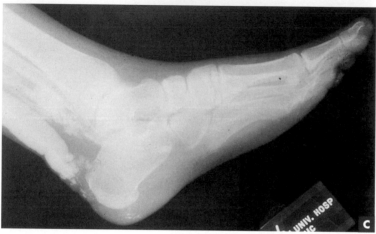

FIG. 7-44 *A,* Nodular calcific densities in thighs of patients with dermatomyositis (DM). *B,* Atrophy, hyperpigmentation, and subcutaneous calcium deposits in the arm of a patient with "burned-out" DM. *C,* Radiologic evidence of soft-tissue calcification in a patient with DM.

TABLE 7-14

Clinical Characteristics of Children With MCTD

Characteristic	Patients (%)
Arthritis	93
Raynaud phenomenon	85
Scleroderma skin	49
Rash of SLE	33
Rash of DM	33
Fever	56
Abnormal esophageal motility	41
Cardiac	30
Pericarditis	27
Myositis	61
CNS disease	23
Pulmonary	43
Renal	26

children with scleroderma usually die a cardiopulmonary death. Cardiac involvement includes heart block, congestive heart failure, ECG changes, and pericardial effusion, rarely including cardiac tamponade. These abnormalities appear to be a result of myocardial fibrosis, vascular insufficiency, and inflammation.

Mixed Connective Tissue Disease

A syndrome characterized by features of rheumatoid arthritis, systemic sclerosis, SLE, and dermatomyositis and associated with high titer anti-RNP antibodies was first described in 1972 and termed *mixed connective tissue disease* (MCTD). Clinical characteristics of MCTD in children are summarized in Table 7-14.

Cardiopulmonary disease and esophageal dysmotility are common in MCTD; nephritis occurs but is less common and usually less severe than in SLE. Anti-RNP antibodies are strongly associated with the diagnosis of MCTD. Rheumatoid factor (RF) is common, but other autoantibodies are unusual.

The outcome and course of children with MCTD is variable. Of the children who die, the majority die a cardiopulmonary death similar to systemic sclerosis. Some children die from renal failure similar to SLE.

Dermatomyositis

Dermatomyositis (DM) is a rare but distinctive disease that accounts for approximately 5% of all rheumatic disease in childhood. Though it was first described in 1887, its etiology remains largely unknown. The hall-

steatorrhea, weight loss, volvulus, and even perforation can occur. Colonic disease occurs in the form of wide-mouth diverticula and a loss of the normal colonic architecture.

Whereas morbidity and mortality in adults with systemic sclerosis is usually related to hypertension and renal failure caused by scleroderma renal crisis with involvement at the level of the arcuate renal arteries,

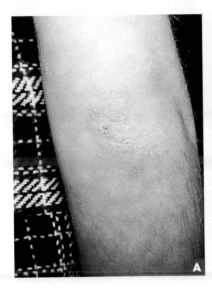

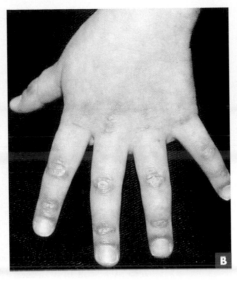

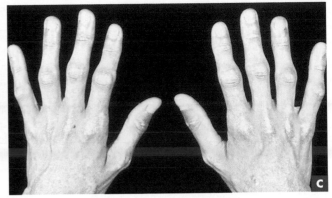

FIG. 7-45 Typical rash of DM, as seen on the elbow *(A)* and the hands *(B* and *C)*, showing erythema and pale, atrophic skin changes (Gottron papules).

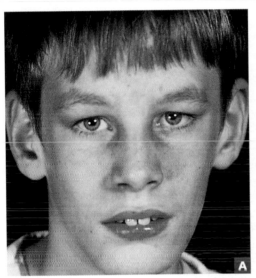

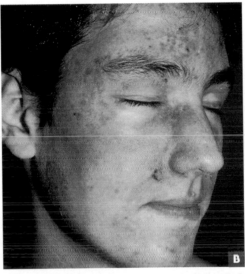

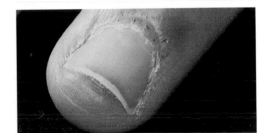

FIG. 7-47 Nail bed telangiectasia. Erythema can be seen around the nail edge. The pinpoint telangiectasia may require a magnifying lens to identify.

FIG. 7-46 *A,* Facial rash of DM with a violaceous color around the eyes and malar region. *B,* More severe, erythematous, scaly rash involving almost the entire face. Note involvement of nasolabial folds.

marks of this entity are various skin manifestations coupled with non-suppurative inflammation of muscle. DM affecting the adult generally carries a worse prognosis than that encountered in the pediatric age group. There is no association with malignancy in pediatric DM patients, though it does appear to be a paraneoplastic syndrome in certain adult populations. Nevertheless, vasculitis of varying severity is often seen earlier in the course of the illness in children, and there is a relatively high incidence of calcinosis (nodular calcium deposits) in nonvisceral tissues such as muscle and subcutaneous tissue (Fig. 7-44). Pressure points and severely affected soft tissue are particularly susceptible.

Though the age range for DM is broad, the 5- to 14-year-old child is particularly at risk. Girls predominate by a 2:1 ratio. There is no racial bias nor is there any evidence of a familial predisposition.

Clinically, patients usually have fatigue and symmetrical, proximal muscle weakness, particularly affecting the hip girdle and legs. Although weakness is the hallmark of the disease, muscle pain can exist. Though shoulders and arms are often involved, this may not be detected as easily in the child. The first complaints are often inability to climb stairs and disturbances of gait. Dysphagia, dysphonia, and dysp-

nea may occur if the respective muscles for these functions are affected. The involved muscles may be tender and indurated, with a superficially edematous appearance. A pathognomonic rash found in three quarters of DM patients can confirm the diagnosis. Even in the absence of this distinctive rash, all patients have some degree of cutaneous disease. The rash is symmetric and erythematous, with atrophic changes located over the extensor surfaces of the knees and elbows. Such changes over the PIP and MCP joints are called *Gottron papules* (Fig. 7-45). DM of childhood can exist with skin involvement only, and skin involvement can antedate muscle involvement for months to years. Other features of the rash include a violaceous discoloration of the eyelids, eyelid edema, a scaly red rash in a malar distribution, telangiectasia (Fig. 7-46), and the characteristic dystrophic skin changes. As opposed to SLE, which also has a malar rash, the nasolabial folds are not spared in DM. Nail bed telangiectasia (Fig. 7-47), digital ulceration, and hyperpigmentation or hypopigmentation of the skin also occur. The rash of DM, similar to that of SLE, may be extremely photosensitive. However, because of the pathognomonic features of the rash, the diagnosis of DM often can be suspected before overt symptoms occur. Constitutional symptoms such as anorexia, malaise, weight loss, and fever may

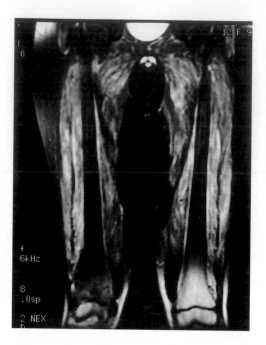

FIG. 7-48 MRI of the thigh (T2 fat-suppressed image) illustrates marked diffuse muscle edema and inflammation caused by dermatomyositis. Note patchy white area in muscle similar in appearance to fluid in bladder.

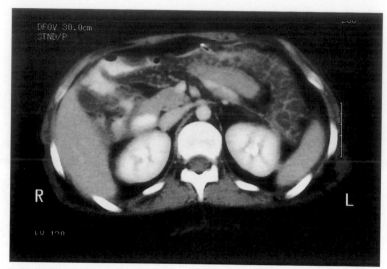

FIG. 7-49 CT scan of abdomen in patient with dermatomyositis demonstrates bowel wall thickening and edema in the transverse colon. Patient eventually perforated bowel because of active vasculitis.

TABLE 7-15

Characteristics of the Most Common Myositis-Specific Autoantibodies

Autoantibodies	Clinical manifestations
Antisynthetases	Arthritis, ILD*, fevers, Raynaud phenomenon
Antisignal recognition particle (anti-SRP)	Cardiac involvement with palpitations, myalgias
Anti-Mi-2	Classic dermatomyositis with rash, cuticular overgrowth

*ILD, Interstitial lung disease.

be present. The illness may progress at variable rates in different patients; however, the majority of patients have a more insidious rather than acute course. Unfortunately, long delays in diagnosis can occur, particularly in the insidious group. Other more uncommon findings are mouth ulcers, retinitis, hepatosplenomegaly, pulmonary infiltrates, myocarditis, and pericarditis. Although calcinosis occurs in 40% of children with DM, it does not occur during the acute phase of the illness. On the other hand, in chronic indolent disease it may be the presenting complaint and often may be the most difficult feature of the disease to control, causing significant morbidity.

About 20% to 30% of patients with DM have a positive antibody, usually to cytoplasmic antigens. In the majority of children with DM the specific antigen of the autoantibody is unknown, although recently antibodies to synthetases and antibodies to signal recognition particle have been described (Table 7-15).

The clinical diagnosis of DM can be supported by an abnormal electromyography. Muscle biopsy and an abnormal magnetic resonance image (T-2 weighted image with fat suppression) can show edema and active inflammation in the case of myositis (Fig. 7-48). Elevated muscle enzymes may be the first clue to the diagnosis of inflammatory muscle disease, the CK, SGOT (AST), SGPT (ALT), aldolase, and LDH should be checked serially because they can be useful in following disease activity. Only one or even none of the aforementioned muscle enzymes may be elevated in the setting of floridly active myositis. The erythrocyte sedimentation rate has little role in the diagnosis or monitoring of myositis disease activity. Corticosteroids are the mainstay of therapy, and their early use often preserves muscle function and minimizes the potentially destructive nature of this disease, and they may prevent the development of calcinosis universalis (Fig. 7-44). One of the most dreaded and potentially lethal complications of DM in childhood is perforation of the intestines secondary to active vasculitis. The clinician must maintain a high index of suspicion because many of the classic signs of an acute condition in the abdomen may not be present in the setting of high-dose corticosteroid therapy. This complication of dermatomyositis may be an indication for cytotoxic therapy (Fig. 7-49).

Systemic Vasculitides

The vasculitides are a broad group of disorders with a common pathology characterized by blood vessel inflammation. The type of inflammation, organ system affected, and size of the vessels vary with each disease entity. Any attempt at classification of the vasculitides has been unsatisfactory, but most have attempted to group these disorders according to the size of the blood vessel involved. A useful classification of the systemic vasculitides is noted in Table 7-16. Kawasaki syndrome is a common form of vasculitis affecting children and is discussed further later in this chapter. Polyarteritis nodosa (PAN) is the prototype of

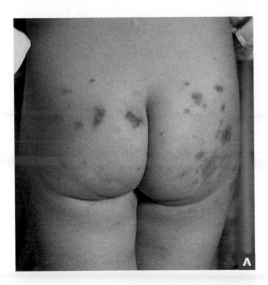

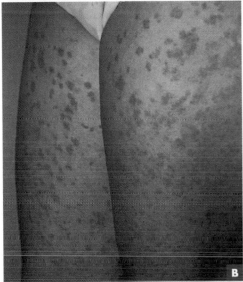

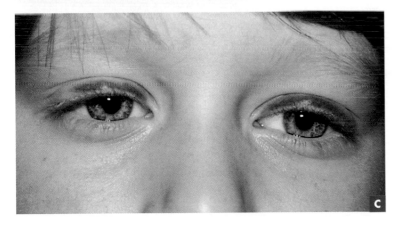

FIG. 7-50 The distinctive rash of HSP. *A* and *B*, It characteristically involves the buttocks and lower extremities, with purpuric coalescent lesions. Note the striking waist-down distribution. *C*, Eye-lid involvement has been reported.

A Classification of Primary Systemic Vasculitis in Children

Large Vessel Vasculitis	**Small Vessel Vasculitis**
Kawasaki syndrome	Henoch-Schönlein purpura
Takayasu arteritis	Hypersensitivity angiitis
Giant cell arteritis	Hypocomplementemic urticarial vasculitis
Medium Vessel Vasculitis	Mixed cryoglobulinemia
Nongranulomatosis	
Polyarteritis nodosa (PAN)	**Other Vasculitides**
Cutaneous polyarteritis	Behçet's syndrome
Microscopic polyarteritis	Mucha-Habermann disease
Cogan syndrome	Köhlmeir-Degos syndrome
Granulomatosis	
Allergic granulomatosis	
Wegener granulomatosis	
Lymphomatoid granulomatosis	
Primary angiitis of the central nervous system	

clastic, vasculitis is characterized by inflammation of small vessels such as arterioles, capillaries, and venules. The venule is the most common vessel involved in producing a venulitis. Henoch-Schonlein purpura is the prototype of these illnesses and is discussed at length in the following section.

Henoch-Schönlein Purpura

Henoch-Schönlein syndrome (HSP), or anaphylactoid purpura, consists of nonthrombocytopenic purpura, arthritis and arthralgia, gastrointestinal symptomatology, and a variety of renal findings. Of cases 75% occur in children less than 10 years of age with the median age being 5 years. Children less than 2 years of age will generally develop milder disease with less frequent gastrointestinal and renal involvement. Most authors report that this syndrome occurs after an upper respiratory infection or other viral illness, though HSP has also been reported after bacterial infections, insect bites, dietary allergens, immunizations, and use of numerous drugs. There does not appear to be a familial predilection, and all races have been affected. Seasonal peaks occur, but a definite etiology remains elusive.

The clinical picture of HSP is that of a previously well child who acutely develops a distinctive skin rash, arthritis, and abdominal pain. The skin rash allows for definitive diagnosis, and hence it is said to occur in all patients with HSP. Of patients 50% present with rash, which usually involves the buttocks, lower extremities, and the hands (waist-down distribution) with the trunk and face generally being spared (Fig. 7-50). The lesions begin as petechial or approximately 0.5-cm purpuric areas that coalesce and become confluent with nearby lesions. They begin as red macules or papules and progress with time to purplish and then brownish areas. Early in the course of the disease the rash may blanch with pressure, but with time this feature disappears. Typically, varying stages of eruption are simultaneously present. On occasion, ulceration and vesicles occur. Some patients have lesions that mimic urticaria, pruritus can be a feature of the rash, and about 25% have subcutaneous edema (Fig. 7-51). The edema is nonpitting, painless, evanescent, and most commonly affects the hands (Fig. 7-51, *B*) and feet.

the medium-sized vessel vasculitis, can occur in older children, and is occasionally noted in the setting of poststreptococcal infection. The major clues to the diagnosis of PAN are hematuria, hypertension, abdominal pain, arthritis, and fever. Wegener granulomatosis and Churg-Strauss vasculitis are systemic necrotizing vasculitides with a granulomatous component. They frequently present with pulmonary and upper respiratory manifestations, can also have neurologic involvement in the form of a mononeuritis multiplex, and are extremely unusual in childhood. The most common forms of vasculitis are the hypersensitivity, or leukocytoclastic, vasculitides. Hypersensitivity, or leucocyto-

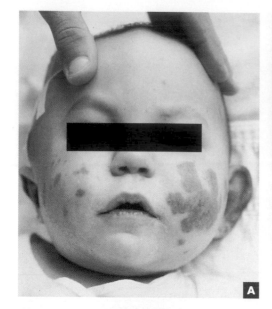

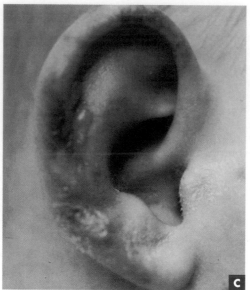

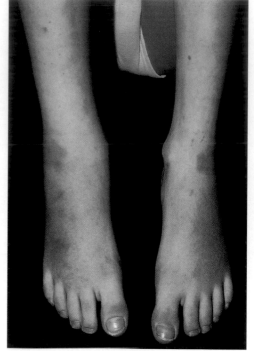

FIG. 7-51   An infant with HSP. *A,* The rash may occur on the face along with edema. *B,* Rash and edema may be present in the extremities. *C,* Ulceration and vesicles are an unusual manifestation of HSP.

FIG. 7-52   The arthritis of HSP. Note the swelling of the right ankle in addition to the purpuric rash.

The child less than 2 years of age is most likely to have edema as a feature of this illness. The younger child is also more likely to display facial involvement (Fig. 7-51, *A, C*).

Approximately 85% of patients display some form of gastrointestinal symptomatology. Simple colicky abdominal pain can be the only symptom, but its severity can raise physician concerns about more threatening abdominal complications. Massive gastrointestinal hemorrhage or intussusception is seen in 5% of patients, and complete perforation rarely occurs. Melanotic stools, vomiting, ileus, and hematemesis may be present as well. In rare circumstances abdominal pain can precede the other features of HSP, making diagnosis difficult until the characteristic rash appears.

The periarticular swelling that occurs presents as arthritis or arthralgia and is a part of HSP in three quarters of reported cases. Knees and ankles are the most common sites of involvement (Fig. 7-52). Warmth and erythema are not usually associated with the pain and swelling that occur. The joints are never affected permanently, and this feature of HSP generally resolves in several days. As with the gastrointestinal symptoms, arthritis can precede the rash. For this reason, HSP should be considered in the child with acute onset of arthritis.

Although renal involvement is detected in only half of HSP patients, it is important because the degree of renal pathology generally affects the patient's ultimate prognosis. Renal manifestations can be as mild as hematuria or proteinuria, but they may be as severe as nephrotic syndrome, nephritis, and, in about 1% of patients, end-stage renal disease. Patients usually declare themselves within several months, but cases of renal failure and hypertension have occurred many years after the initial illness. Berger disease (IgA glomerulonephritis) is believed by many to be HSP without rash and hence an alternative manifestation of the same pathologic process.

Other features of HSP include low-grade fever, malaise, scrotal swelling with pain, headache, cerebral vasculitis, CNS bleeding, seizures, nosebleeds, parotitis, pancreatitis, hydrops of the gallbladder, and cardiopulmonary disease.

The course of the illness varies with age. The majority of patients are over their initial illness in 4 weeks; however, 50% have at least one recurrence. Recurrences generally are limited to cutaneous and mild abdominal symptomatology.

Clotting functions are generally normal but can be abnormal, and platelet counts in these patients are normal or elevated. The presence of IgA complexes in the glomeruli, skin, and serum of affected individuals may be a clue to diagnosis. Elevated serum IgA levels are found in about half of HSP patients. Since there are no diagnostic laboratory examinations for this syndrome, the history and physical examination provide clues to the successful recognition of HSP.

Kawasaki Syndrome

Although the exact etiology of Kawasaki syndrome has eluded investigators, the clinical features and natural history of this distinctive vasculitic entity are very well described. The need to rapidly recognize the presentation of this disease is heightened by its potentially devastating cardiac sequelae. New developments in treatment alter the incidence of these sequelae; therefore the early recognition of Kawasaki syndrome favorably impacts on morbidity and mortality.

Kawasaki syndrome, first described in 1967 in Japan by Tomisaku Kawasaki, consists of a unique constellation of clinical findings initially labeled as mucocutaneous lymph node syndrome. This multisystem syndrome was independently described by Melish in 1976 in Hawaii. Since that time the syndrome has been recognized in all racial groups

8

Dermatology

BERNARD A. COHEN ❦ HOLLY W. DAVIS
SUSAN B. MALLORY ❦ JOHN A. ZITELLI

M̲ost of us think of our skin as a simple durable covering for our skeleton, muscles, and internal organs. However, the skin is a complex organ, consisting of many parts and appendages (Fig. 8-1). The outermost layer, the stratum corneum, is an effective barrier to irritants, toxins, and organisms, as well as a membrane that holds in body fluids. The remainder of the epidermis manufactures this protective layer. Melanocytes within the epidermis help protect us from the harmful effects of ultraviolet light, and Langerhans cells are one of the body's first lines of immunologic defense.

The dermis, consisting largely of fibroblasts and collagen, is a tough, leathery, mechanical barrier against cuts, bites, and bruises. Its collagenous matrix also provides structural support for a number of cutaneous appendages. Hair, which grows from follicles deep within the dermis, is important for cosmesis and protection from sunlight and particulate matter. Sebaceous glands are outgrowths of the hair follicles. Oil produced by these glands helps to lubricate the skin and contributes to the protective epidermal barrier. The nails are specialized organs of manipulation that also protect the sensitive digits. Thermoregulation of the skin is accomplished by eccrine sweat glands and changes in cutaneous blood flow, which is regulated by glomus cells. The skin also contains specialized receptors for heat, pain, touch, and pressure. Sensory input from these structures helps to protect the skin surface against environmental trauma. Beneath the dermis, in the subcutaneous tissue, fat acts as stored energy and as a soft, protective cushion.

Defects or alterations in any component of the skin may result in serious systemic disease or death. Each and every part of the skin can be affected by congenital, inflammatory, infectious, and degenerative disorders and tumors. For example, an altered stratum corneum is seen in ichthyosis, melanocytes are selectively destroyed in vitiligo, the epidermis proliferates in psoriasis, excess collagen is produced in the connective tissue nevus of tuberous sclerosis, hair is preferentially infested by certain fungi, and so on. In addition the skin is affected by many systemic diseases and thus may provide visible markers for internal disorders. A skin examination may demonstrate lesions of vasculitis, explaining a child's hematuria. The white macules of tuberous sclerosis may give insight into the cause of seizures.

Examination and Assessment of the Skin

The skin is the largest, most accessible, and most easily examined organ of the body and is the organ of most frequent concern to the patient. Therefore physicians should be able to recognize basic skin diseases and dermatologic clues to systemic disease.

Optimal examination of the skin is performed in a well-lit room. The physician should inspect the entire skin surface including hair, nails, scalp, and mucous membranes. This may be particularly problematic with infants and teenagers, since it may be necessary to examine the skin in small segments to prevent cooling or embarrassment. Although no special equipment is required, a hand lens and side lighting aid in the assessment of skin texture and small discrete lesions.

Despite the myriad conditions affecting the skin, a systematic approach to the evaluation of a rash or exanthem facilitates and simplifies the process of developing a manageable differential diagnosis. After assessing the patient's general health, the practitioner should obtain a detailed history of the skin symptoms, including the date of onset, inciting factors, evolution of lesions, and presence or absence of pruritus. Recent immunizations, infections, drugs, and allergies may be directly related to new rashes. The family history may suggest a hereditary or contagious process, and the clinician may need to examine other members of the family. Review of nursery records and photographs helps to document the presence of congenital lesions. Attention should then turn to the distribution and pattern of the rash. The term *distribution* refers to the location of the skin findings, whereas the term *pattern* defines a specific anatomic or physiologic arrangement. For example, the distribution of a rash may include the extremities, face, or trunk, and the pattern could be flexural or intertriginous. Identification of a pattern can assist in the development of a differential diagnosis before the detailed morphology of the skin lesions is studied. Other common patterns include sun-exposed sites, acrodermatitis (involvement primarily of the distal extremities), pityriasis rosea, clothing-covered sites, acneiform rashes, and dermatomal configurations (Fig. 8-2).

Next, the clinician should consider the local organization of the lesions, defining the relationship of primary and secondary lesions to one another in a given location. Are the lesions scattered or clustered (herpetiform)? Are they linear, serpiginous, confluent, or discrete?

Finally, the practitioner should identify the morphology of the cutaneous lesions. Primary lesions (macules, papules, wheals, plaques, vesicles, bullae, nodules, and tumors) arise *de novo* in the skin. Secondary lesions (pustules, erosions, ulcers, crusts, excoriations, fissures, lichenification, atrophy, and scars) evolve from primary lesions or result from the patient's manipulation (e.g., scratching, picking, or popping) of primary lesions. Delineation of the primary and secondary lesions allows the clinician to develop a differential diagnosis based on

211

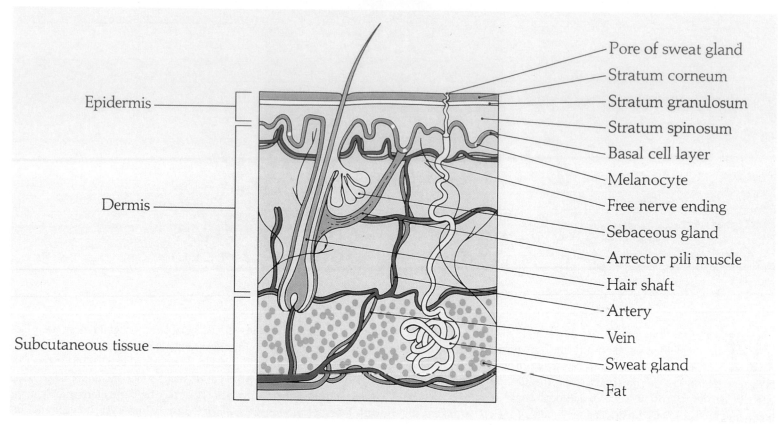

Epidermis

Dermis

Subcutaneous tissue

Pore of sweat gland
Stratum corneum
Stratum granulosum
Stratum spinosum
Basal cell layer
Melanocyte
Free nerve ending
Sebaceous gland
Arrector pili muscle
Hair shaft
Artery
Vein
Sweat gland
Fat

FIG. 8-1 Schematic diagram of normal skin anatomy.

the anatomic level of the skin lesions. Disorders restricted to the epidermis may be associated with macular pigmentary changes, such as in vascular telangiectasias, freckles, and vitiligo. In epidermal disorders, surface markings are commonly altered by scales, vesicles, pustules, crusts, and erosions. Bullous impetigo, atopic dermatitis, and ichthyosis are primarily epidermal disorders. When the dermis is also involved, lesions usually display distinct borders because of dermal inflammation and edema. Disorders with both epidermal and dermal changes include psoriasis, lichen planus, and erythema multiforme. Inflammatory disorders or tumors restricted to the dermis do not usually alter the surface markings. Lesional borders are distinct, and color changes and edema may be present. Examples of dermal disorders include granuloma annulare, intradermal nevi, urticaria, and hemangiomas. The diagnosis of subcutaneous disorders is made by careful palpation. The surface markings are normal, and the color of the skin may be normal or red. There is altered skin firmness, and tenderness may be present. Subcutaneous lesions include lipomas, hemangiomas, hematomas, subcutaneous fat necrosis, and erythema nodosum.

Because an outline of specific pediatric dermatoses defies any one scheme of organization, this text follows a clinically practical format. First, this chapter covers common papulosquamous and vesiculopustular eruptions, which account for a majority of rashes seen in children. This is followed by sections covering reactive erythemas, insect bites and infestations, tumors and infiltrations of the skin, neonatal dermatology, vascular lesions, congenital and acquired nevi, and disorders of

pigmentation. The chapter concludes with a discussion of disorders of the hair and nails and complications of topical therapy.

Papulosquamous Disorders

Papulosquamous eruptions share the morphologic features of papules and scales. However, the clinician must understand that the diverse papulosquamous disorders are produced by a variety of different mechanisms. In psoriasis, increased production of keratinocytes by the basal cell layer results in a markedly thickened epidermis and stratum corneum (scaly surface layer). In dermatitic processes such as atopic dermatitis, contact dermatitis, seborrheic dermatitis, pityriasis rosea, and fungal infections, inflammation results in increased production and abnormal maturation of epidermal cells, with subsequent scale production. Increased adherence of cells in the stratum corneum may result in the retention hyperkeratosis characteristic of ichthyosis vulgaris, which is frequently found in association with atopic dermatitis.

Psoriasis

Psoriasis is a common disorder characterized by red, well-demarcated plaques with dry, thick, silvery scales. These tend to be located on the extensor surfaces of the extremities, the scalp, and the buttocks (Fig. 8-3, *A* and *B*). In some patients the distribution consists of large lesions over the

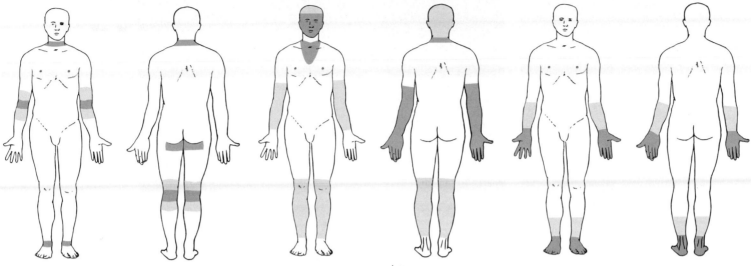

Flexural Rashes

Atopic dermatitis (childhood)
Infantile seborrheic dermatitis
Intertrigo
Candidiasis
Tinea cruris
Epidermolytic hyperkeratosis (ichthyosis)
Inverse psoriasis

A

Sun-Exposed Sites

Phototoxic reaction (sunburn)
Photocontact dermatitis
Lupus erythematosus
Polymorphous light eruption
Viral exanthem
Porphyria
Xeroderma pigmentosum

B

Acrodermatitis

Papular acrodermatitis (viral exanthem)
Acrodermatitis enteropathica
Atopic dermatitis (infantile)
Tinea pedis with "id" reaction
Dyshidrotic eczema
Poststreptococcal desquamation

C

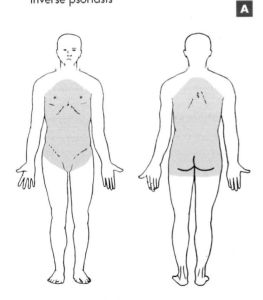

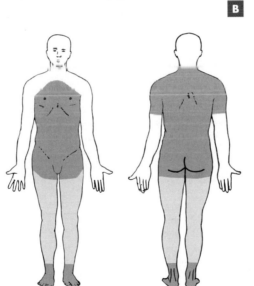

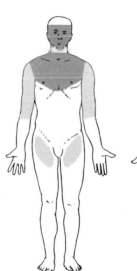

Pityriasis Rosea

Pityriasis rosea
Secondary syphilis
Drug reaction (e.g., gold salts)
Guttate psoriasis
Atopic dermatitis

D

Clothing-Covered Sites

Contact dermatitis
Miliaria
Psoriasis (in summer)

E

Acneiform Rashes

Acne vulgaris
Drug-induced acne (e.g., prednisone,
   lithium, isoniazid)
Cushing syndrome (endogenous steroids)
Chloracne

F

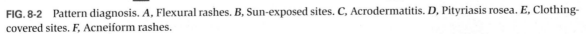

FIG. 8-2 Pattern diagnosis. *A,* Flexural rashes. *B,* Sun-exposed sites. *C,* Acrodermatitis. *D,* Pityriasis rosea. *E,* Clothing-covered sites. *F,* Acneiform rashes.

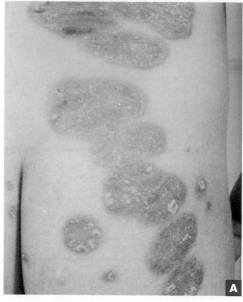

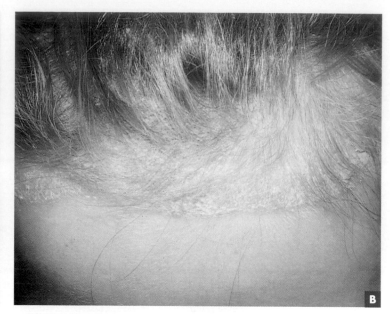

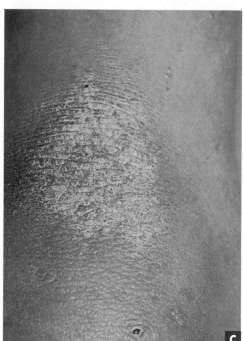

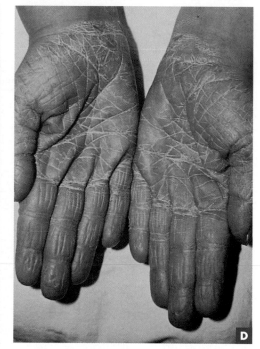

FIG. 8-3 Psoriasis. *A,* Typical erythematous plaques are topped by a silver scale. *B,* Thick tenacious scale on a red base extends from the forehead to the scalp of this 10-year-old girl. *C,* This large plaque is located over the pressure point of the knee. *D,* The skin of the palms is markedly thickened, with silvery fissuring of the palmar creases. (*C* and *D* courtesy Dr. Michael Sherlock.).

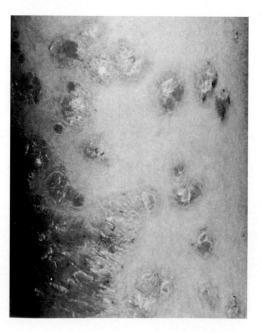

FIG. 8-4 Guttate psoriasis. Small plaques with typical scales quickly developed in a generalized distribution after a streptococcal pharyngitis.

knees and elbows (Fig. 8-3, *C*). Thickening and fissuring of the skin of the palms also may be seen (Fig. 8-3, *D*). In other children, many droplike (guttate) lesions are scattered over the body (Fig. 8-4). In infants, psoriasis may present as a persistent diaper dermatitis (Fig. 8-43). Lesions of psoriasis are often induced in areas of local injury, such as scratches, surgical scars, or sunburn, a response termed the *Koebner phenomenon* (Fig. 8-5). Nail changes include reddish-brown psoriatic plaques in the nail bed (oil-drop changes), surface pitting, and distal hyperkeratosis (Fig. 8-124).

The factors initiating the rapid turnover in epidermal cells that produce the psoriatic plaques are unknown, although an inherited predisposition is suspected and upper respiratory tract and streptococcal infections precipitate lesions, especially in cases of guttate psoriasis. Though the increased epidermal growth causes a thickening of the skin in the psoriatic plaque, there are also areas between the epidermal ridges where the skin is very thin and the scale is close to the subepidermal vessels. Thus when the scale is removed, small bleeding points are often seen. This is called the *Auspitz sign,* and it is the hallmark of psoriasis (Fig. 8-6).

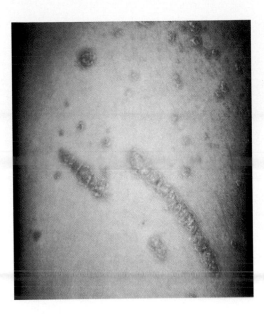

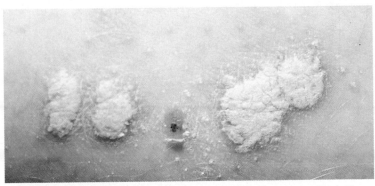

FIG. 8-5 Koebner phenomenon in psoriasis. Lesions are often induced in areas of local trauma such as these scratches.

FIG. 8-6 Auspitz sign. Removal of the thick scale from a psoriatic plaque produces small points of bleeding from tortuous capillaries.

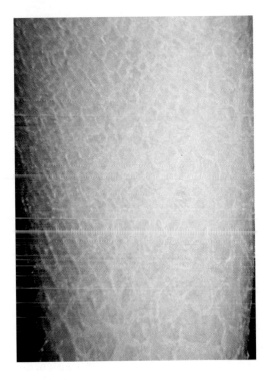

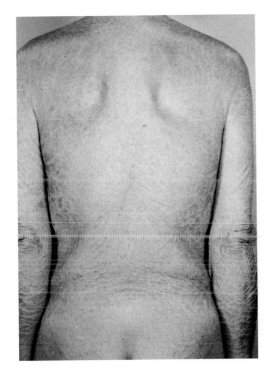

FIG. 8-7 Ichthosis vulgaris. The typical fish-scale appearance is seen in this close-up of a fair-skinned patient's shin.

FIG. 8-8 Sex-linked ichthyosis. "Dirty" brown scales persist on the flanks, elbows, and shoulders despite the use of topical lubricants.

The course of psoriasis is chronic and unpredictable, marked by remissions and exacerbations. Although psoriasis is thought to be rare in childhood, 37% of adults with the disorder first develop lesions before the age of 20.

The Ichthyoses

Ichthyosis refers to a group of inherited dermatoses characterized by dry, scaly skin. Various types have been identified according to clinical course, histopathology, and biochemical markers.

Ichthyosis Vulgaris

Ichthyosis vulgaris is transmitted as an autosomal dominant trait and affects about 0.5% of the population. Although the rash is not present at birth, by 3 months of age, thick, fishlike scales may be apparent on the shins and extensor surfaces of the arms (Fig. 8-7). Occasionally scales become more generalized, involving the trunk, but the flexures are usually spared. Lesions tend to flare during the winter (because of the drying effect of central heating) and improve during the summer, particu-

larly with increasing age. Biopsy of involved skin shows retention hyperkeratosis and a thinned granular layer in the epidermis. Topical emollients usually keep pruritus and scaling under control.

Sex-Linked Ichthyosis

Sex-linked ichthyosis occurs in 1 in 6000 males, although findings are occasionally present in hemizygous female carriers. Affected newborns may have a collodion membrane (Fig. 8-86) that peels during the first several weeks of life and is followed by the development of generalized "dirty" brown scales, particularly on the abdomen, back, and anterior legs and feet (Fig. 8-8). The central face and flexures are spared. Skin biopsy demonstrates an increased granular layer and stratum corneum, and biochemical studies demonstrate decreased or absent steroid sulfatase in the serum and skin.

Lamellar Ichthyosis

Lamellar ichthyosis is a rare autosomal dominant disorder occurring in less than 1 in 250,000 births. Infants are usually born with a collodion membrane (Fig. 8-86). During the first month of life, thick, brownish-

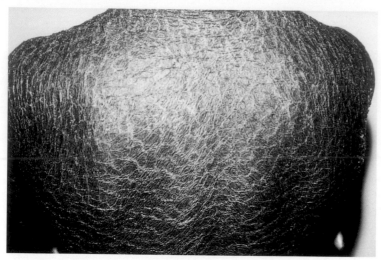

FIG. 8-9 Lamellar ichthyosis. Note the thick, brown scales covering the entire skin surface.

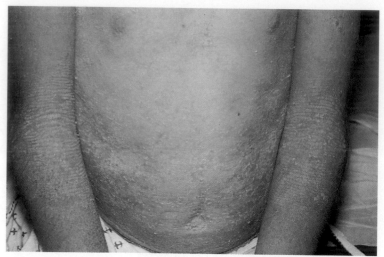

FIG. 8-10 Epidermolytic hyperkeratosis is characterized by thick, warty scales and intermittent blistering. The flexural creases are particular sites of involvement.

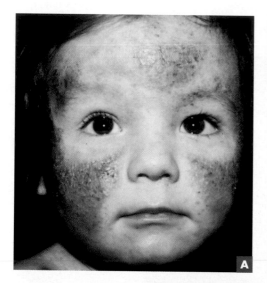

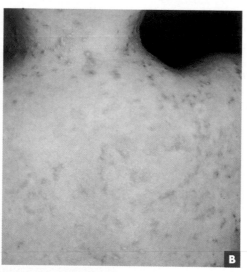

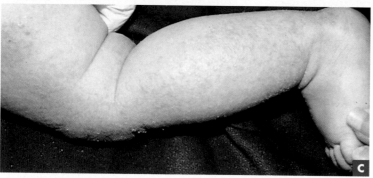

FIG. 8-11 Infantile atopic dermatitis or eczema. *A,* This infant has an acute, weeping dermatitis on the cheeks and forehead. *B* and *C,* Involvement of the trunk and the extremities, with erythema, scaling, and crusting, are evident. Usually the diaper area is the only portion of the skin surface that is spared. (*B* and *C* from Fireman P, Slavin RG: *Atlas of allergies,* New York, 1991, Gower.)

gray, sheetlike scales with raised edges appear. Scaling is prominent over the face, trunk, and extremities (Fig. 8-9). In contrast to ichthyosis vulgaris, the flexural areas are involved in the lamellar form. Eversion and fissuring of the eyelid margins (ectropian) and lips (eclabium) are common complications. The palms and soles show thick keratoderma with fissuring. Some improvement of the scaling occurs with age, and topical keratolytics such as lactic acid and salicylic acid may provide some benefit. Severe cases may respond to oral administration of retinoids such as 13-*cis*-retinoic acid.

Epidermolytic Hyperkeratosis

Epidermolytic hyperkeratosis is a rare autosomal dominant form of ichthyosis characterized by the development of generalized, thick, warty scales and intermittent blistering with severe involvement of the flexures (Fig. 8-10). In newborns blisters may be widespread, suggesting a diagnosis of herpes simplex or epidermolysis bullosa. Histologically, massive hyperkeratosis is associated with ballooning of squamous cells and formation of microvesicles. Epidermal turnover is also markedly increased. The mainstay of treatment includes use of kera-

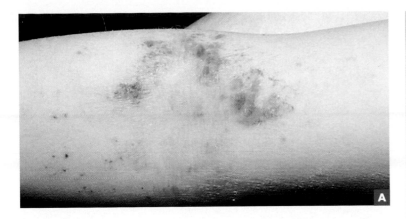

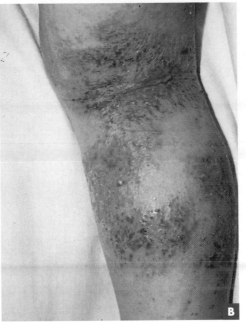

FIG. 8-12 Childhood atopic dermatitis with lesions on the arms *(A)* and the legs *(B)*. In childhood, eczema involves the flexural surfaces of the upper and lower extremities. The neck, ankles, wrists, and posterior thighs also may be severely affected. (*A* from Fireman P, Slavin RC: *Atlas of allergies,* New York, 1991, Gower; *B* courtesy Dr. Michael Sherlock.)

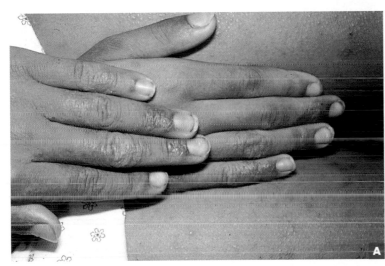

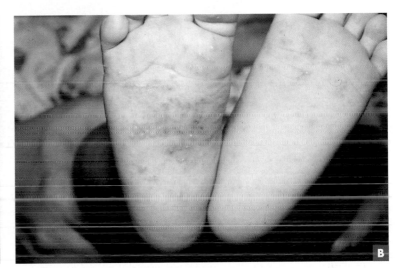

FIG. 8-13 Involvement of the hands and feet in eczema. *A,* A 10-year-old atopic child has ichenification of the skin over the dorsum of his fingers and "buff" nails from chronic rubbing. *B,* This infant has numerous red excoriated lesions over the soles of his feet.

tolytics, lubricants, and antibiotics for secondary infection, which is common and usually caused by *Staphylococcus aureus.* Oral retinoids also may significantly decrease scaling.

The Dermatitides

Depending on duration of involvement, the dermatitides are characterized clinically by acute changes (including redness, edema, and vesiculation) and/or chronic changes (such as scaling, lichenification, increased and decreased pigmentation) in the skin. Microscopically these disorders are characterized by infiltration of the dermis with inflammatory cells, variable thickening of the epidermis, and scaling.

Atopic Dermatitis (Eczema)

Atopic dermatitis, or eczema, is one of the most common and annoying skin disorders in children. This entity is divided into three phases based on the age of the patient, each having a different distribution.

The *infantile phase* of atopic dermatitis begins between 1 and 6 months of age and lasts about 2 or 3 years. Characteristically the rash is manifest by red, itchy papules and plaques that ooze and crust. Lesions are distributed over the cheeks, forehead, scalp, trunk, and extensor surfaces of the extremities, and patches are often symmetrical (Fig. 8-11).

The *childhood phase* of atopic dermatitis occurs between ages 4 and 10 years. The dermatitis is typically dry, papular, and intensely pruritic. Circumscribed scaly patches are distributed on the wrists, ankles, and antecubital and popliteal fossae (Fig. 8-12); these patches frequently become secondarily infected, probably as a result of organisms introduced by intense scratching. Cracking, dryness, and scaling of the palmar and plantar surfaces of the hands and feet are also common (Fig. 8-13). Remission may occur at any time, or the disorder may evolve into a more chronic type of adult dermatitis. Of children with atopic dermatitis, 75% improve between the ages of 10 and 14; the remaining children may go on to develop chronic dermatitis.

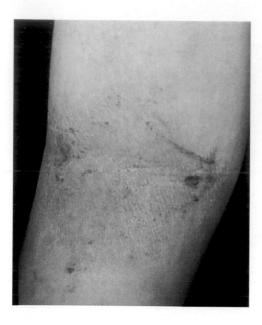

FIG. 8-14 Adult atopic dermatitis. Erythematous excoriated plaques with indistinct borders are seen in the antecubital areas. Note the dried blood from recent excoriation.

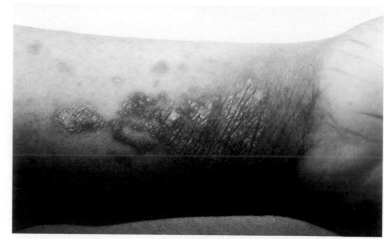

FIG. 8-15 Lichenification. Marked thickening of the skin in an area of chronic scratching. In addition, this patient shows postinflammatory hyperpigmentation.

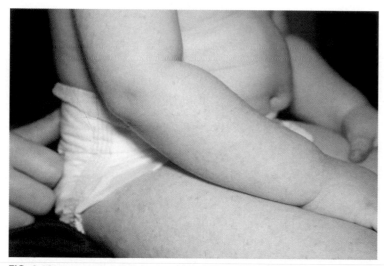

FIG. 8-16 Keratosis pilaris. Fine follicular papules are symmetrically distributed over the extensor surfaces of the arms and legs of this toddler.

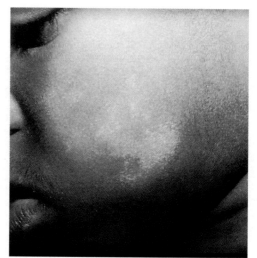

FIG. 8-17 Pityriasis alba. In some atopic individuals, subtle inflammation may result in development of poorly demarcated, hypopigmented patches that are covered by a fine superficial scale.

The *adult phase* of atopic dermatitis begins around age 12 and continues indefinitely. Major areas of involvement include the flexural areas of the arms, neck, and legs (Fig. 8-14). Eruptions are sometimes seen on the dorsal surfaces of the hands and feet and between the fingers and toes. Lichenification may be marked (Fig. 8-15).

Other associated findings include xerosis (dryness); ichthyosis vulgaris (Fig. 8-7); *keratosis pilaris* (keratin plugging of hair follicles and formation of perifollicular scales over the extensor surfaces of the extremities) (Fig. 8-16); hyperlinearity of the palms; Dennie-Morgan folds (double skin creases under the lower eyelid [see Chapter 4]); hyperpigmentation and hypopigmentation, which may be marked and at times may be the predominant findings (Figs. 8-106 and 8-107); and altered cellular immunity, which is manifest by an unusual susceptibility to certain cutaneous infections such as warts, herpes simplex, and molluscum contagiosum. Patients with eczema should be warned to avoid people with cold sores because they are at great risk for developing generalized eczema herpeticum. Parents of children with eczema who themselves have recurrent herpes simplex lesions should be taught hygienic techniques that reduce the risk of transmitting the virus to their children.

In the rash of *pityriasis alba*, which is common in patients with atopic dermatitis, inflammatory changes are minimal. Poorly defined, hypopigmented, scaly patches measuring 2 to 4 cm in diameter are noted most commonly on the face and extremities (Fig. 8-17), although they may involve the trunk as well.

The cause of atopic dermatitis remains elusive. An immunologic etiology is suggested by the chronic elevation of immunoglobulin E (IgE) seen in a majority of patients. Some investigators propose an aberrant cutaneous response to histamine and other mediators of inflammation as a primary mechanism. However, laboratory findings vary from patient to patient and in the same patient at different times in the course of their disease. Atopic dermatitis seems to occur in families and in association with other atopic conditions, including asthma, allergic rhinitis, and food allergies, suggesting some degree of genetic predisposition. Pathophysiologically, a number of external factors, including dry skin, soaps, wool fabrics, foods, infectious agents, and environmental antigens, may act in concert to produce pruritus, which is universal in atopics. The resultant scratching leads to the acute and chronic changes typical of atopic dermatitis. On occasion, patients with scabies develop

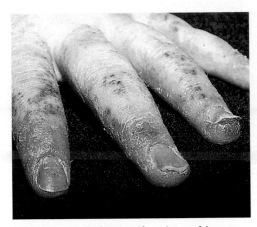

FIG. 8-18 Dyshidrosis. Chronic cracking, oozing, and scaling develop after the tiny pruritic vesicles have been scratched.

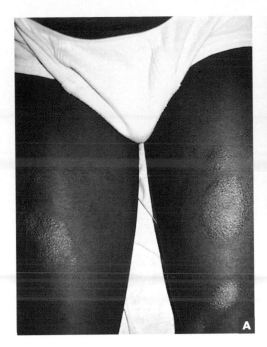

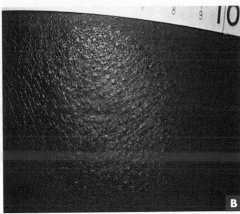

FIG. 8-19 Nummular excema. *A,* These round-to oval-shaped lesions are typically located over the extensor thighs or abdomen. *B,* On close inspection, they are seen to be studded with tiny vesicles. These lesions do not show central clearing. (Courtesy Dr. Michael Sherlock.)

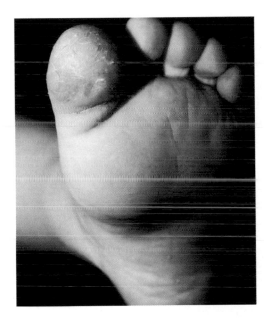

FIG. 8-20 Juvenile plantar dermatosis. This variant of atopic dermatitis is localized to the plantar surfaces of the toes and feet. Note the erythema, scaling, and cracking.

classic eczema as a result of intense scratching, though on close inspection the primary lesions usually can be identified.

The differential diagnosis of atopic dermatitis includes seborrhea, contact dermatitis, pityriasis rosea, psoriasis, fungal infections, histiocytosis X, and acrodermatitis enteropathica. It can be distinguished from seborrhea based on distribution of lesions; atopic dermatitis spares moist, intertriginous areas, such as the axillae and perineum, where seborrhea is prominent. Exposure history and distribution help distinguish contact dermatitis, and discreteness of lesions and distribution distinguish pityriasis. The thick, silvery scale and Koebner phenomenon help distinguish psoriasis, and central clearing with an active microvesicular border helps differentiate tinea corporis. The rash of histiocytosis is greasier and more generalized. It is associated with petechiae and often accompanied by chronically draining ears and hepatosplenomegaly (Fig. 8-78; see Chapter 11). The acral distribution of lesions and gastrointestinal symptoms help in distinguishing acrodermatitis (see Chapter 10).

The mainstays of atopic dermatitis treatment are elimination or avoidance of predisposing factors, hydration and lubrication of dry skin, use of antipruritic agents to relieve itching and break the itch–scratch cycle, application of keratolytic agents for keratosis pilaris, and topical steroids. Because secondary infection is common, it should be looked for carefully and treated promptly with systemic antibiotics.

Dyshidrotic eczema, nummular eczema, juvenile plantar dermatosis, and lip-licking and thumb-sucking eczema often occur in association with atopic dermatitis. However, they may present as independent entities.

Dyshidrotic Eczema

Dyshidrosis is a severely pruritic, chronic, recurrent, vesicular eruption affecting the palms, soles, and lateral aspects of the fingers and toes. Characteristically the vesicles are symmetrical, multilocular, and 1 to 3 mm in diameter. These lesions rupture, leaving scales and crust on an erythematous base (Fig. 8-18). Pathologically this eruption demonstrates spongiotic vesicles and normal eccrine sweat glands. The cause is unknown; however, frequent exposure to water, wet or sweat-soaked shoes, or chemicals (on the hands) may trigger or exacerbate the condition. Treatment is similar to that for acute atopic dermatitis. Use of charcoal-impregnated foam insoles can significantly improve conditions affecting the foot.

Nummular Eczema

Nummular eczema is an acute papulovesicular eruption named for its coin-shaped configuration. Lesions are intensely pruritic, well circumscribed, round to oval, red, scaly patches studded with 1 to 3 mm vesicles (Fig. 8-19). They are usually located on the extensor thighs or abdomen of children who also may have atopic dermatitis and/or keratosis pilaris and dry skin. Lack of central clearing helps distinguish these lesions from tinea corporis (Fig. 8-33). Although the rash is often resistant to therapy, it may respond to the treatment for acute dermatitis outlined previously. Application of occlusive dressings may be useful in recalcitrant cases.

Juvenile Plantar Dermatosis

Juvenile plantar dermatosis ("sweaty sock syndrome") is common in toddlers and school-age children. Chronic, red, scaly patches with cracking and fissuring typically begin in the fall or winter on the anterior plantar surfaces of the feet and big toes (Fig. 8-20). Although the

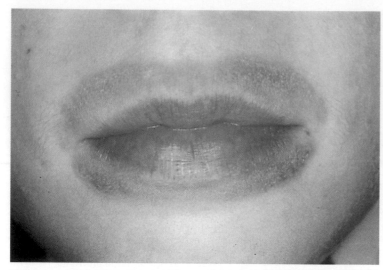

FIG. 8-21   Lip-licking eczema. The perioral skin is inflamed, scaly, and thickened as a result of repetitive licking of the lips. (Courtesy Dr. Douglas W. Kress, Children's Hospital of Pittsburgh.)

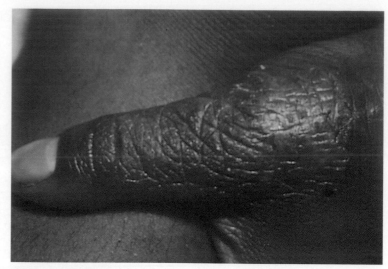

FIG. 8-22   Thumb-sucking eczema. Repeated wetting and drying from persistent thumb-sucking result in eczematoid changes with cracking, fissuring, and lichenification. (Courtesy Dr. Michael Sherlock.)

cause is unknown, the condition is triggered by excessive sweating and/or repeated wetting of the skin inside the child's shoes (especially those made of synthetic materials that do not breathe), followed by drying of the skin at night. Consequently the mainstay of treatment consists of lubricating and covering the feet at night. Topical steroids may be necessary in severe cases. The eruption tends to subside in the summer, and resolution in adolescence is common. Use of charcoal-impregnated foam insoles is also helpful.

Lip-Licking and Thumb-Sucking Eczema

The repeated wetting and drying from persistent lip licking (especially in winter) or thumb sucking can produce eczematoid changes of the perioral skin (Fig. 8-21) or the skin of the involved thumb (Fig. 8-22).

Seborrhea

Seborrheic dermatitis is characterized by a red, scaling eruption that occurs predominantly on hair-bearing and intertriginous areas, such as the scalp, eyebrows, eyelashes, perinasal, presternal, and postauricular areas and the neck, axillae, and groin (Fig. 8-23). In affected infants,

scalp lesions consist of a greasy, salmon-colored, scaly dermatitis called *cradle cap* (Fig. 8-24). A severe type may be more generalized. In adolescents the dermatitis may manifest as dandruff or flaking of the eyebrows, postauricular areas, or flexural areas.

Although the pathogenesis of seborrheic dermatitis is unknown, *Pityrosporum* and *Candida* species have been implicated as causative agents. A role for neurologic dysfunction is suggested by the increased incidence and severity in neurologically impaired individuals.

The dermatitis of seborrhea is usually nonpruritic and mild in nature. Most cases respond to topical steroids and many clear spontaneously. Antiseborrheic shampoos also may be helpful for patients with scalp involvement. In infants and young children, atopic dermatitis can have a greasy, scaly appearance and may be confused with seborrhea. However, infantile atopic dermatitis produces intense pruritus and invariably spares moist sites such as the diaper area and axillae. The differential diagnosis of seborrhea also includes histiocytosis X (in which the rash is generalized, in part petechial, and usually associated with chronic draining of the ears and hepatosplenomegaly) and tinea corporis (in which lesions usually are more circumscribed, with an active

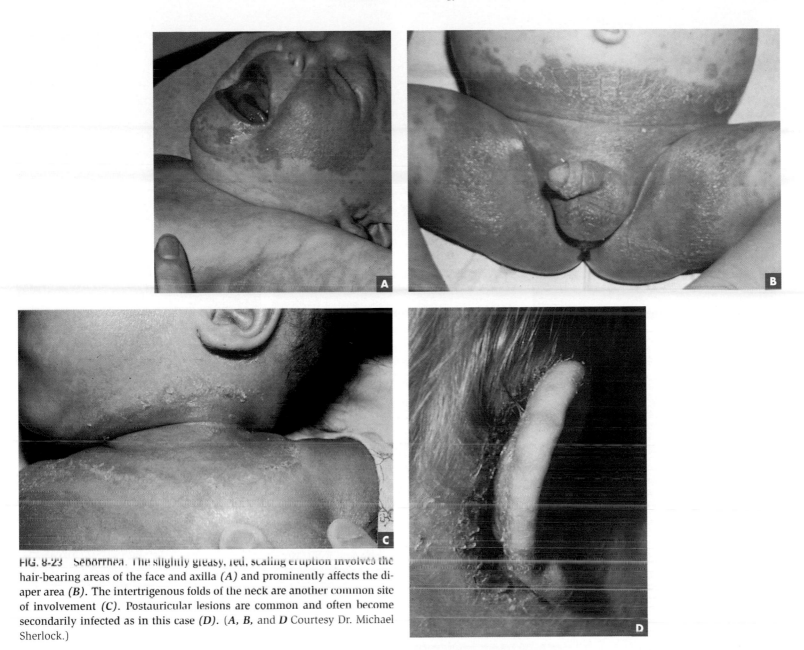

FIG. 8-23 Seborrhea. The slightly greasy, red, scaling eruption involves the hair-bearing areas of the face and axilla *(A)* and prominently affects the diaper area *(B)*. The intertrigenous folds of the neck are another common site of involvement *(C)*. Postauricular lesions are common and often become secondarily infected as in this case *(D)*. *(A, B,* and *D* Courtesy Dr. Michael Sherlock.)

border and central clearing). Scalp lesions may be difficult to differentiate from psoriasis.

Pityriasis Rosea

Pityriasis rosea is a benign, self-limited disorder that can occur at any age but is more common in adolescents and young adults. A prodrome of malaise, headache, and mild constitutional symptoms occasionally precedes the rash. The typical eruption begins with the appearance of a "herald patch" (Fig. 8-25, *A*), which is a large, isolated, oval lesion, usually pink in color and slightly scaly; it may occur anywhere on the body. Occasionally it clears centrally, simulating tinea corporis. From 5 to 10 days later, other smaller lesions appear on the body, frequently concentrated on the trunk but also seen on the extremities, especially the thighs. These begin as small, round papules that enlarge to ovals up to 1 to 2 cm in size, with a scaly surface. They are usually somewhat raised but can be macular as well. The long axes of the ovals often run parallel to the lines of the cleavage of the skin, creating a "Christmas tree" pattern over the thorax (Fig. 8-25, *C*). The rash reaches its peak in several weeks, and then slowly fades over 4 to

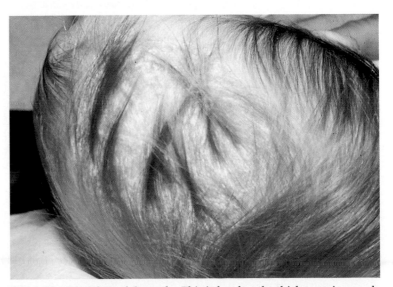

FIG. 8-24 Seborrhea of the scalp. This infant has the thick tenacious scale typical of cradle cap.

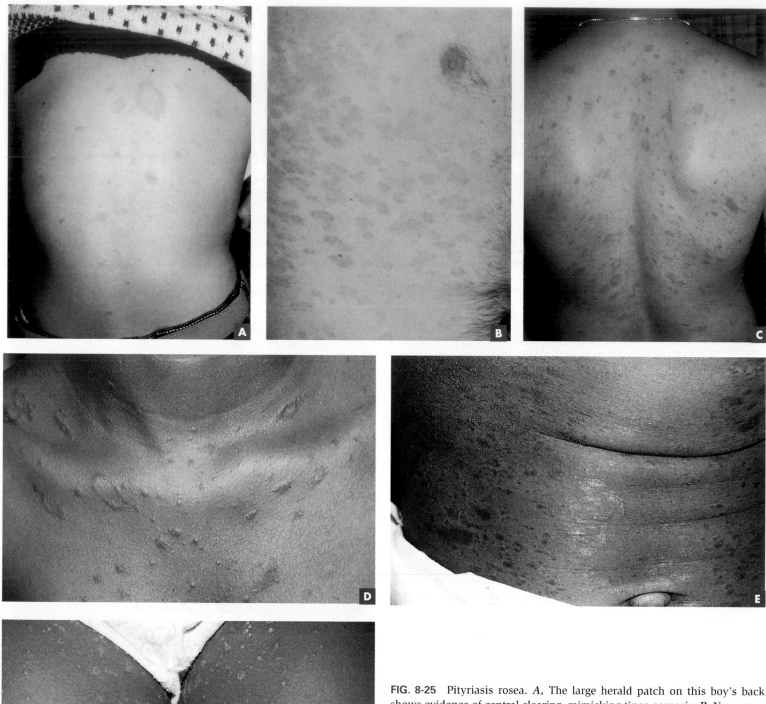

FIG. 8-25 Pityriasis rosea. *A*, The large herald patch on this boy's back shows evidence of central clearing, mimicking tinea corporis. *B*, Numerous oval lesions are seen on this patient's trunk with their long axes oriented along lines of cleavage. *C*, This feature creates the appearance of a fir tree distribution on the back. *D* to *F*, Lesions can be raised, macular, or scaly. (*A* to *C* Courtesy Dr. Douglas W. Kress, Children's Hospital of Pittsburgh; *D* and *E* Courtesy Dr. Michael Sherlock.)

6 weeks. The average total duration is 2 to 3 months. Ultraviolet light may hasten the disappearance of the eruption. Although the cause is unknown, the peak incidence in late winter and the low recurrence rate favor an infectious, probably viral, etiology.

Other eruptions that can resemble pityriasis rosea include guttate psoriasis, viral exanthems, measlelike (morbilliform) drug eruptions, and secondary syphilis. As noted, earlier, the appearance of the herald patch may simulate tinea corporis, but a KOH prep will be negative.

Contact Dermatitis

Contact dermatitis refers to a group of conditions in which a dermatitic or inflammatory reaction in the skin is triggered by direct con-

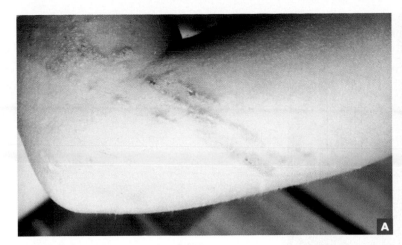

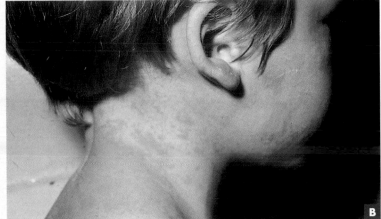

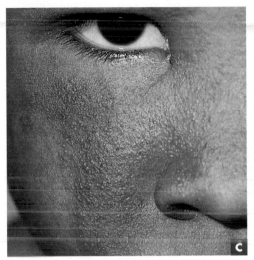

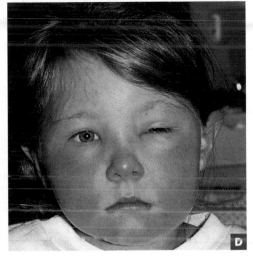

FIG. 8-26   Poison ivy, or rhus dermatitis. *A,* Linear streaks of pruritic vesicles are typical of contact dermatitis to a plant. *B* and *C,* With heavier exposure, however, the eruption can develop in relatively large patches. Also note the microvesicular appearance of the facial lesion in the child shown in *C. D,* Reactions involving the face and genitalia can provoke impressive swelling.

tact with environmental agents. In the most common form, *irritant contact dermatitis,* changes in the skin are induced by caustic agents such as acids and alkalis, hydrocarbons, and other primary irritants. Anyone exposed to these agents in a high enough concentration for a long enough period of time develops a contact dermatitis. The rash is usually acute, with well-demarcated erythema, crusting, and/or blister formation.

In contrast, allergic contact dermatitis is a T-lymphocyte–mediated immune reaction to an antigen coming into contact with the skin. Although it frequently presents with acute onset of erythema, vesiculation, and pruritus, the rash may become chronic with scaling, lichenification, and pigmentary changes. Often, the allergen is obvious, as is the case with poison ivy or nickel jewelry. However, in other cases careful questioning may be required to detect the inciting agent.

The initial reaction occurs after a 7- to 14-day period of sensitization in susceptible individuals. Once sensitization has occurred, reexposure to the allergen provokes a more rapid reaction, sometimes within hours. This is a classic example of type IV (delayed) hypersensitivity (see Chapter 4).

Rhus Dermatitis (Poison Ivy)

The most common allergic contact dermatitis in the United States is poison ivy or rhus dermatitis. This typically appears as linear streaks of erythematous papules and vesicles (Fig. 8-26, *A*); however, with heavy exposure, the rash may appear in relatively large patches (Fig. 8-26, *B* and *C*). When lesions involve the skin of the face or genitalia, impressive swelling can occur (Fig. 8-26, *D*).

Direct contact with the sap of poison ivy, poison oak, or poison sumac, whether from leaves, stems, or roots (whether the plant is alive or dead), produces the dermatitis (Fig. 8-27). Contact with clothing that has brushed against the plant, with logs or railroad ties on which the vine has been growing, or with smoke from a fire in which the plant is being burned are other means of exposure. Areas of skin exposed to the

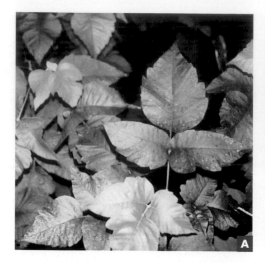

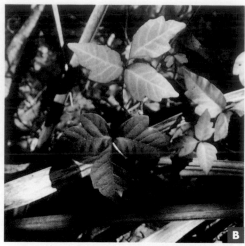

FIG. 8-27 *A,* Poison ivy. The plant has characteristic shiny leaves in groups of three. It may resemble a vine or a low shrub or bush. *B,* Poison oak. This also has leaves in groups of three, although the edges tend to be more scalloped than those of poison ivy. (*B* Courtesy Dr. Mary Jelks.)

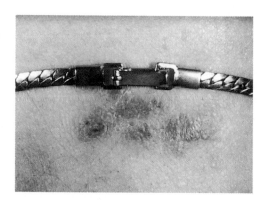

FIG. 8-28 Nickel contact dermatitis. The location of the rash is helpful in determining the cause of a contact dermatitis.

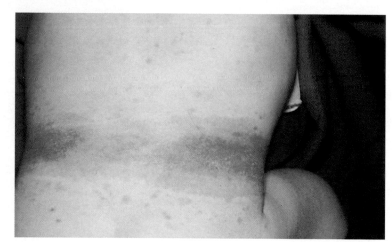

FIG. 8-29 Rubber contact dermatitis. This child had become sensitized to the elasticized waist bands of his underpants.

highest concentration of plant oil develop changes first. Other sites that received lower doses then vesiculate in succession, giving an illusion of spreading. However, within about 20 minutes after contact, the rhus oil becomes tissue fixed to the epithelial cells and cannot be spread further. Thorough washing within minutes of exposure can prevent the eruption.

Other common offending agents are nickel (Fig. 8-28), rubber (Fig. 8-29), glues and/or dyes in shoes (Fig. 8-30), ethylenediamine in topical lotions, neomycin, and topical anesthetics (Fig. 8-31).

Photocontact Dermatitis

Some allergens, known as *photosensitizers,* require sunlight to become activated. Photocontact dermatitis caused by drugs (e.g., tetracyclines, sulfonylureas, and thiazides) characteristically erupts in a sym-

metric distribution on the face, the V of the neck, and the arms distal to the end of the shirt sleeves. Topical photosensitizers (dyes, coal tar, furocoumarins, and halogenated salicylanilides) produce localized patches of dermatitis when applied to sun-exposed sites (Fig. 8-32). These allergens are found in cosmetics, sunscreens, dermatologic products, and germicidal soaps.

"Id" Reaction

Occasionally the local reaction in a contact dermatitis is so severe that the patient develops a widespread secondary eczematous dermatitis. When the dermatitis appears at sites that have not been in contact with the offending agent, the reaction is referred to as *autoeczematization* or an *"id" reaction.*

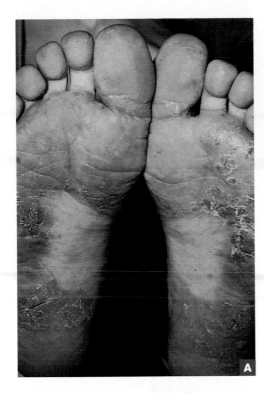

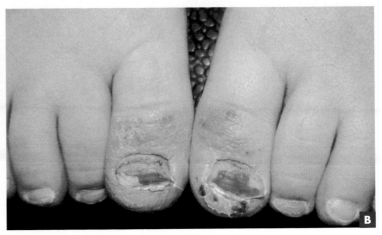

FIG. 8-30 Contact dermatitis of the foot. *A,* This adolescent became sensitized to the glue under the insoles of his shoes. Note the sparing of the instep. *B,* This child had a similar problem with the toe reinforcers in his shoes. Note that the web spaces are spared. (*A* Courtesy Dr. Michael Sherlock; *B* Courtesy Dr. Douglas W. Kress, Children's Hospital of Pittsburgh.)

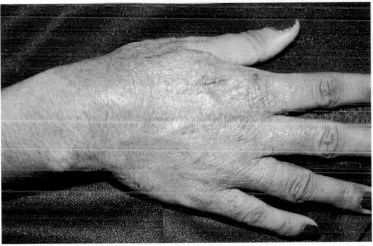

FIG. 8-31 Contact dermatitis. This adolescent became sensitized to the Lanacaine in a moisturizing cream that she applied to her hands daily. Note the line of demarcation at the wrist.

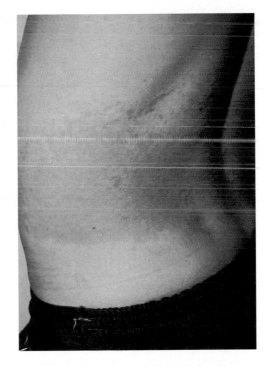

FIG. 8-32 Photocontact dermatitis. This boy developed contact dermatitis after sun exposure while swimming. The offending agent was found to be in his soap. (Courtesy Dr. Michael Sherlock.)

Basic Principles of Management

Although localized patches of contact dermatitis are best treated topically, widespread reactions require a 2-week tapering course of systemic corticosteroids beginning at 0.5 to 1.0 mg per kg per day. Patients may experience rebound of the rash if treated with a shorter course. Response usually occurs within 48 hours. Oral steroids also may be indicated in localized reactions involving the eyelids, extensive areas of the face, genitals, and/or hands, where swelling and pruritus may become incapacitating.

Prevention requires identification of the offending agent and then its avoidance. Children with rhus dermatitis should be shown pictures of the causative plants and taught where they are commonly found. Pa-

tients sensitive to nickel must ensure that jewelry, particularly earring posts, are made of gold or silver with no nickel. However, painting watchband buckles with clear nail polish every several weeks can obviate the difficult task of trying to find watchbands with pure gold or silver buckles.

Fungal Infections

Two types of fungal organisms produce clinical cutaneous disease: dermatophytes and yeasts. Dermatophytes include the tinea or ringworm fungi, and yeasts include *Candida* species, which are associated with diaper dermatitis, and *Pityrosporum* species, which cause tinea versicolor.

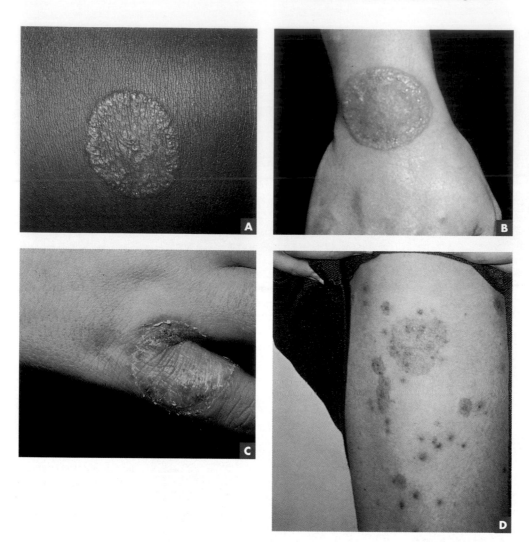

FIG. 8-33 Tinea corporis. The characteristic annular lesions show many variations in appearance. *A*, This lesion has a very raised, active border and shows central clearing. *B*, In this case the inflammatory response is very intense and only partial central clearing is seen. *C*, The sharply circumscribed lesion shown here is macular and is more prominently erythematous and scaly. *D*, The evolution of lesions from papules and pustules into larger papulosquamous patches is seen on this girl's leg. (*B* Courtesy Dr. Douglas W. Kress, Children's Hospital of Pittsburgh; *C* and *D* Courtesy Dr. Michael Sherlock.)

Tinea Corporis

Tinea corporis is a superficial fungal infection of the nonhairy or glabrous skin. It has been labeled "ringworm" because of its characteristic configuration consisting of pruritic, annular lesions with central clearing and an active vesicular border made up of microvesicles that rupture and then scale (Fig. 8-33, *A* to *C*). Lesions, which may be single or multiple, typically begin as red papules or pustules that rupture and evolve to form papulosquamous lesions. These lesions then spread out from the periphery as new vesicles form and begin to clear centrally (Fig. 8-33, *D*). Over a period of several weeks, the patches may expand up to 5 cm in diameter. Tinea corporis can be found in any age group, and it is usually acquired from an infected domestic animal *(Microsporum canis)* or through direct human contact *(Trichophyton tonsurans)*.

Clinically, tinea may be differentiated from atopic dermatitis by the propensity for autoinoculation from the primary patch to other sites on the patient's skin, by the spread to close contacts, and by the central clearing noted in many lesions. Moreover, the rash of atopic dermatitis tends to be symmetric, chronic, and recurrent in a flexural distribution. Unlike tinea, patches of nummular eczema are self-limited and do not clear centrally. The herald patch of pityriasis rosea is often mistaken for tinea. However, it is KOH-negative, and the subsequent development of the generalized rash with its characteristic truncal distribution is distinctive (Fig. 8-25). The clinical pattern, findings, and chronic nature of psoriasis and seborrhea help differentiate them from tinea. Though granuloma annulare produces a characteristic ringed eruption, on palpation the lesions are firm and they usually do not show epidermal changes (scales, vesicles, pustules) unless scratching has been intense. Lesions of granuloma annulare usually are only slightly pruritic or asymptomatic (Fig. 8-79).

The diagnosis of tinea corporis is confirmed by potassium hydroxide examination of the skin. The first step is to obtain material by scraping the loose scales at the margin of a lesion (Fig. 8-34, *A*). These should be mounted onto the center of the slide, with one or two drops of 20% KOH added. Next, a glass coverslip is applied and gently pressed down with the eraser end of a pencil to crush the scales (Fig. 8-34, *B*). The clinician then heats the slide, taking care not to boil the KOH solution, and again the coverslip is pressed down. When viewing the slide under the microscope, the clinician sets the condenser and light source at low levels to maximize contrast, with the objective at ×10. On focusing up and down, true hyphae are seen as long, branching, often septate rods of uniform width that cross the borders of epidermal cells (Fig. 8-35). Cotton fibers, cell borders, or other artifacts may be falsely interpreted as positive findings.

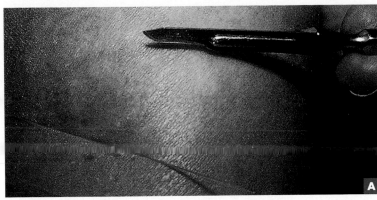
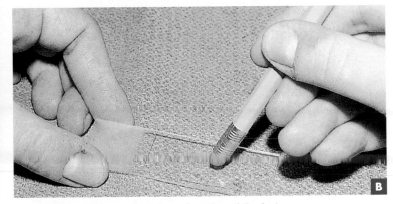

FIG. 8-34 Potassium hydroxide (KOH) preparation. *A,* Small scales should be scraped from the edge of the lesion onto a microscope slide. *B,* To more easily visualize the fungus, the scales should be crushed, making a thin layer of cells.

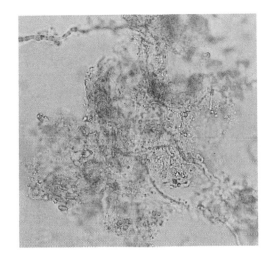

FIG. 8-35 Positive KOH preparation of skin scrapings. Fungal hyphae are seen as long septate branching rods at the margins and center of the scales.

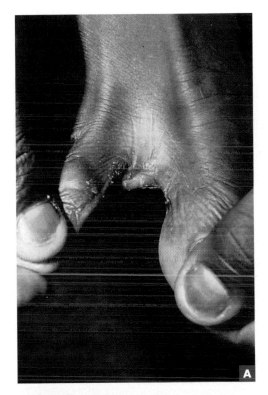

Tinea infections on glabrous skin readily respond to topical antifungal creams (e.g., imidazoles such as miconazole, clotrimazole, econazole, naftifine, ketoconazole, and tolnaftate). When lesions are multiple and widespread, oral therapy with griseofulvin is indicated.

Tinea Pedis

Commonly referred to as *athlete's foot,* tinea pedis is a fungal infection of the feet with a predilection for the web spaces between the toes. It is quite common in adolescence, somewhat less so in prepubertal children. The infecting organisms are acquired from contaminated shower, bathroom, locker room, and gym floors, and their growth is fostered by the warm, moist environment of shoes.

In some cases scaling and fissuring predominate; in others vesiculopustular lesions and maceration are found. The infection begins between and along the sides of the toes, where it may remain (Fig. 8-36, *A*). However, lesions can extend over the dorsum of the foot (Fig. 8-36, *B*) and may involve the plantar surface as well, particularly the instep and the ball of the foot. Patients complain of a combination of burning and itching, which is frequently intense.

This diagnosis often can be made on clinical grounds and is confirmed by KOH preparation of skin scrapings. The mainstays of treatment are topical antifungal creams or powders and adopting measures

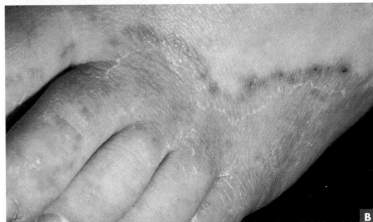

FIG. 8-36 Tinea pedis. *A,* Cracking and scaling are seen in the web space. *B,* In this patient the lesions extend from the web spaces onto the dorsum of the foot. Note the active border. (*B* Courtesy Dr. Douglas W. Kress, Children's Hospital of Pittsburgh.)

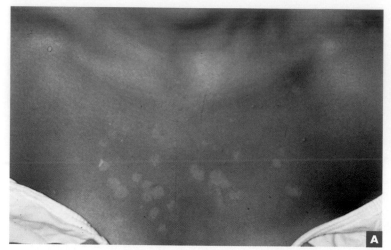

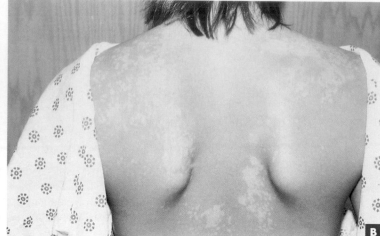

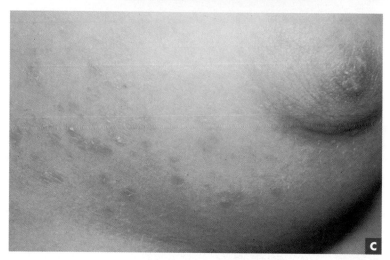

FIG. 8-37 Tinea versicolor. *A* and *B*, Multiple oval patches are seen in a guttate or raindrop pattern over the upper chest and back of two patients. *C*, In areas not exposed to sunlight, lesions are darker than surrounding skin, whereas in *A* and *B* sun-exposed lesions fail to tan, remaining lighter than surrounding skin. (Courtesy Dr. Michael Sherlock.)

designed to reduce foot moisture. The latter include careful drying of the feet after bathing, wearing cotton rather than synthetic socks, and wearing shoes that do not promote sweating or better still sandals. In patients with severe inflammatory lesions, oral antifungal agents may be required. Secondary bacterial infection (particularly with gram-negative organisms) may be a problem.

Tinea pedis is distinguished from contact dermatitis of the feet by virtue of the fact that the latter spares the interdigital web spaces. Dyshidrosis can have a similar distribution, but KOH preparation is negative.

Tinea Versicolor

Tinea versicolor is a common dermatosis characterized by multiple small, oval, scaly patches measuring 1 to 3 cm in diameter, usually located in a guttate or raindrop pattern on the upper chest, back, and proximal portions of the upper extremities of adolescents and young adults (Fig. 8-37, *A* and *B*). However, all ages may be affected, including infants. Facial involvement occurs occasionally. The eruption is caused by a dimorphous form of *Pityrosporum* organism. Warm, moist climates, pregnancy, immunodeficiency, and genetic factors predispose people to the development of infection.

The rash is usually asymptomatic, although some patients complain of mild pruritus. Typically patients go to the physician because they are bothered by the cosmetic appearance of the lesions. Lesions may be light tan, reddish, or white in color, giving rise to the term *versicolor*. They are darker than surrounding skin in non–sun-exposed areas (Fig. 8-37, *C*), and lighter in areas that have tanned on exposure to sunlight (Fig. 8-37, *A* and *B*).

The diagnosis of tinea versicolor can generally be made on the basis of the clinical appearance of lesions and their distribution. It can be confirmed by examining the lesions under a Wood lamp, which reveals a characteristic tan to salmonish-pink glow. A KOH preparation of the surface scale demonstrates short hyphal and yeast forms that resemble spaghetti and meatballs (Fig. 8-38). Although pathogenesis of the color change under a Wood lamp is not fully understood, the fungus is known to produce a substance that interferes with tyrosinase activity and subsequent melanin synthesis.

The differential diagnosis of tinea versicolor includes postinflammatory hypopigmentation and vitiligo. The history and distribution help to distinguish tinea versicolor from postinflammatory hypopigmentation; the presence of fine superficial scaling and some residual pigmentation (even in hypopigmented areas) help rule out vitiligo.

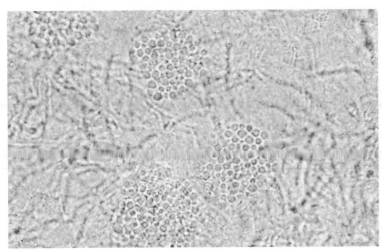

FIG. 8-38 Positive KOH preparation for tinea versicolor. The combination of hyphal and yeast forms of the fungus simulates the appearance of spaghetti and meatballs.

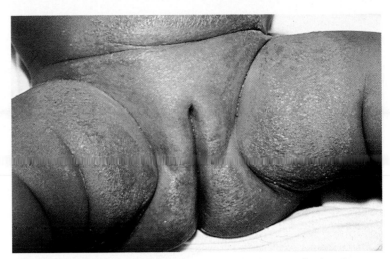

FIG. 8-39 Irritant or ammoniacal diaper dermatitis. Note the involvement of the convex surfaces and the sparing of the intertrigenous creases.

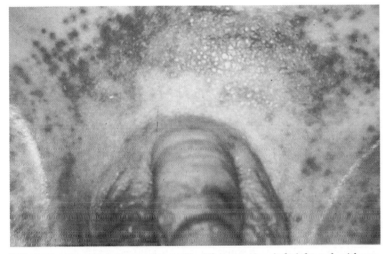

FIG. 8-40 Candidal diaper dermatitis. The eruption is bright red with numerous pinpoint satellite papules and pustules. Intertrigenous areas are prominently involved.

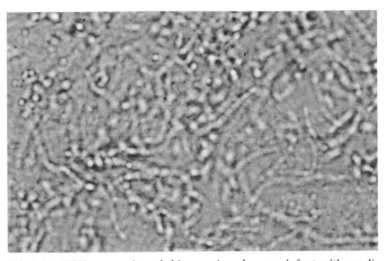

FIG. 8-41 KOH preparation of skin scrapings from an infant with candidal diaper dermatitis demonstrating pseudohyphae and spores.

Topical desquamating agents such as selenium sulfide and propylene glycol produce rapid clearing of the superficial lesions. Localized eruptions may be treated with topical antifungal creams such as miconazole, and recalcitrant cases respond to oral ketoconazole. Patients must be counseled about the high risk of recurrence and reminded that pigmentary changes may take months to clear, even after eradication of the fungus.

Diaper Dermatitis

Because the diaper area is warm, often moist, and frequently contaminated by feces laden with organisms, diaper dermatitis is one of the most common skin disorders of infancy and early childhood.

Irritant Diaper Dermatitis

The diaper area is a prime target for irritant dermatitis because it is bathed in urine and feces and occluded by plastic diaper covers. Failure to change diapers frequently is a major predisposing factor because it provides time for fecal bacteria to form ammonia by splitting the urea in urine. Harsh soaps, irritant chemicals, and detergents contribute to the process. Irritant diaper dermatitis is usually confined to the convex surfaces of the perineum, lower abdomen, buttocks, and proximal thighs, sparing intertriginous areas (Fig. 8-39). When neglected, this may progress with further skin breakdown and ulceration. Frequent diaper changes, gentle, thorough cleansing of the area, and application of lubricants and barrier pastes usually result in clearing of the dermatitis. A short course of low-potency steroids may hasten resolution.

Persistent diaper dermatitis that does not resolve with conservative therapy may be due to other disorders such as candidiasis, seborrheic dermatitis, and psoriasis. These should be suspected particularly when intertriginous areas are involved.

Candidal Diaper Dermatitis

Candidal diaper dermatitis appears as a bright red eruption, with sharp borders and pinpoint satellite papules and pustules (Fig. 8-40). Examination of pustule contents by KOH preparation reveals the typical budding yeasts and pseudohyphae of *Candida* organisms (Fig. 8-41). Candidal diaper dermatitis is occasionally associated with oral thrush, and it is a common sequela of oral or parenteral antibiotic therapy. One should suspect a secondary invasion by *C. albicans* whenever intertriginous areas are involved or a diaper rash fails to respond to symptomatic treatment. Most cases respond well to topical antifungal therapy.

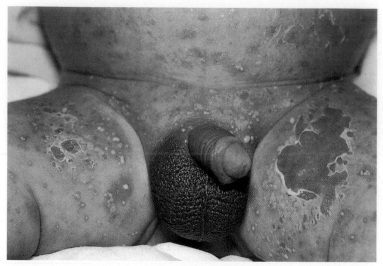

FIG. 8-42 Staphylococcal diaper dermatitis. There are numerous thin-walled pustules surrounded by erythematous halos, as well as multiple areas in which pustules have ruptured, leaving a collarette of scale around a denuded erythematous base.

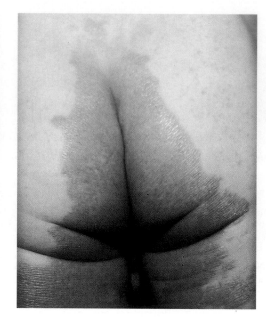

FIG. 8-43 Psoriatic diaper dermatitis. This child had a persistent diaper rash that did not respond to routine therapy. Note that scaling is not as intense as in psoriatic lesions seen elsewhere on the body.

Staphylococcal Diaper Dermatitis

Irritant diaper dermatitis is frequently complicated by secondary staphylococcal infection, or pustules may appear as primary lesions, especially in the first few weeks of life. The presence of thin-walled pustules on an erythematous base (larger than those seen with candidiasis) alert the clinician to the diagnosis. Typically these rupture rapidly and dry, producing a collarette of scaling around the denuded red base (Fig. 8-42). A Gram stain of pustule contents demonstrates neutrophils and clusters of gram-positive cocci. Bacterial cultures are confirmatory but are rarely necessary. Early diagnosis and treatment with oral and topical antibiotics result in rapid resolution.

Seborrheic Diaper Dermatitis

Seborrheic diaper dermatitis is characterized by salmon-colored, greasy lesions with a yellowish scale. The rash is particularly prominent in the intertriginous areas (Fig. 8-23, *B*). Unless secondarily infected with *Candida* organisms (which is common), satellite lesions are not seen. Typically, seborrheic dermatitis of the scalp, face, and postauricular areas is seen in association with this form of diaper dermatitis.

Psoriatic Diaper Dermatitis

Psoriasis occasionally begins as an erythematous, scaling eruption in the diaper area (Fig. 8-43). Although lesions may develop subsequently on the trunk and extremities, the rash may persist for months in the diaper area alone. Failure of a diaper rash to respond to empiric therapy over several weeks should raise psoriasis as a diagnostic possibility. Skin biopsy is the only way to confirm the diagnosis.

Vesiculopustular Disorders

Vesiculopustular eruptions range from benign, self-limited conditions to life-threatening diseases. Early diagnosis, especially in the young child, is mandatory. Systematic evaluation of the clinical findings and a few rapid diagnostic techniques allow these various disorders to be readily differentiated from one another.

Viral Infections

Viral infections, including herpes simplex and varicella-zoster, produce characteristic vesiculopustular exanthems, which are discussed in Chapter 12. However, the technique of confirming the suspicion of an herpetic lesion by preparing a Tzanck test is discussed here.

The Tzanck smear is obtained by removing the roof of the blister with a scalpel or scissors and scraping its base to obtain the moist, cloudy debris. This is then spread onto a glass slide with the scalpel blade, air dried, and stained with Giemsa or Wright stain. The diagnostic finding in viral blisters is the multinucleated giant cell (Fig. 8-44). This is a syncytium of epidermal cells with multiple, overlapping nuclei; hence, it is much larger than other inflammatory cells. Unfortunately, a positive Tzanck test cannot be used to differentiate one blistering viral exanthem from another, and a viral culture should be obtained when the clinical situation dictates.

Bacterial Infections

Several common cutaneous bacterial infections present with vesiculopustular reactions as well. In impetigo the eruption tends to be discrete and localized, whereas in staphylococcal scalded skin syndrome (SSSS) it tends to be associated with a diffuse erythroderma. Gram staining of material aspirated from bullae or removed from the base of an impetigenous lesion is positive for organisms. However, in patients with SSSS, the organism must be sought from noncutaneous sources (nasopharynx, conjunctivae, sinuses, lungs, bone, etc.) because the diffuse cutaneous blistering is due to elaboration of epidermolysin by the infecting organism and not to the organism's direct action within individual lesions (see Chapter 12).

Toxic Epidermal Necrolysis

Toxic epidermal necrolysis (TEN) is a serious vesiculopustular disorder in which generalized erythroderma is followed by widespread necrosis and sloughing of the epidermis. Although the cause may be unclear, hypersensitivity reactions to medications, antecedent viral infections, con-

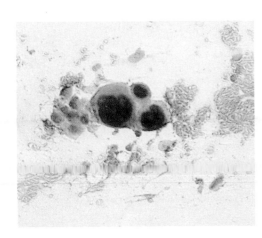

FIG. 8-44 Tzanck preparation. Note the multinucleated giant cell characteristic of viral infection with herpes simplex and varicella-zoster.

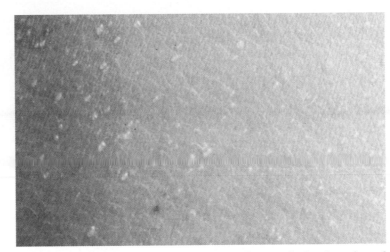

FIG. 8-45 Miliaria crystallina. Found primarily over the head, neck, and upper trunk, these tiny thin walled sweat-retention vesicles rupture readily, then quickly desquamate.

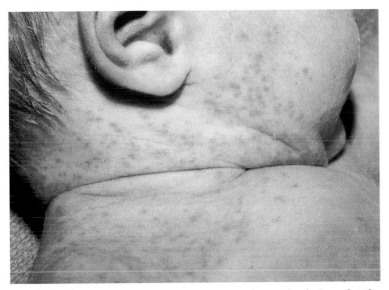

FIG. 8-46 Miliaria rubra. Numerous tiny papulopustular lesions dot the skin around the folds of this infant's neck.

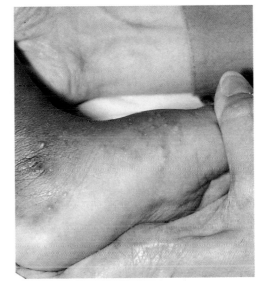

FIG. 8-47 Infantile acropustulosis. Intensely pruritic papulopustular lesions are seen over the foot and ankle of this infant. He had had multiple episodes, and had been treated repeatedly for scabies. (Courtesy Dr. Sylvia Suarez, Children's Hospital of Pittsburgh.)

nective tissue disorders, and malignancy have been implicated. A prodrome of fever, malaise, and sore throat usually precedes the appearance of the erythroderma, which is then superceded in 24 to 48 hours by diffuse cleavage at the dermal-epidermal junction (in contrast to SSSS, in which the plane of cleavage is high in the epidermis). The Nikolsky sign is present as in SSSS. TEN is also characterized by diffuse mucous membrane involvement, including the oral mucosa, conjunctivae, airway, urethra, vagina, and anus. Erythema, hemorrhage, and crust formation are marked, and healing may be associated with the development of ectropion and formation of scars. This also helps distinguish TEN from SSSS, in which the nose and conjunctivae tend to be the only mucous membranes involved and in which Gram stain and culture of the exudates from these sites are usually positive for the offending organism.

Because the line of cleavage is so deep in TEN, fluid and electrolyte losses are proportionately greater, and recovery takes considerably longer (up to 1 month). Intensive supportive therapy is required to prevent complications from these losses and secondary bacterial infection, which is an ever-present danger.

Although the initial target lesions are characteristic, bullous erythema multiforme or Stevens-Johnson syndrome may progress to a clinical picture indistinguishable from TEN. Triggering factors and course are also similar (see section on Reactive Erythemas).

Miliaria

Miliaria Crystallina

Miliaria crystallina is a condition in which obstruction of the eccrine sweat ducts in the outer layer of the epidermis results in the formation of multiple 2 to 3 mm sweat-retention vesicles. Being thin-walled, these vesicles are readily ruptured (Fig. 8-45). In infants, lesions form over the head, neck, and upper trunk. In older children, they more commonly occur in areas of desquamating sunburn.

Miliaria Rubra

Sweat duct obstruction deeper in the epidermal or dermal layers produces an erythematous papulopustular eruption known as *miliaria rubra* (prickly heat) (Fig. 8-46). This rash is common in infants and

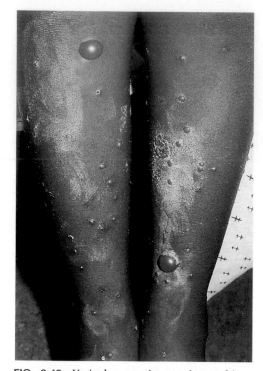

FIG. 8-48 Vesicular reaction to insect bites. This child's lower legs are studded with numerous thick-walled vesicles and bullae that have formed in response to mite bites.

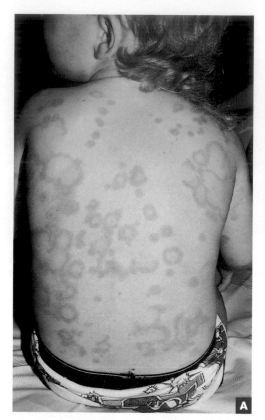

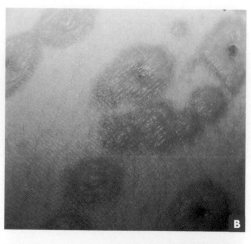

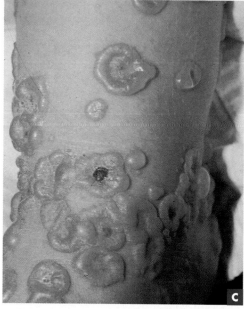

FIG. 8-49 Erythema multiforme. *A,* The characteristic target lesions are symmetrically distributed. *B,* In these typical target lesions with central dusky areas, the peripheral rims are beginning to vesiculate. *C,* In this case the peripheral rims have become frankly bullous. (*C* Courtesy Dr. Michael Sherlock.)

children, especially over the face, upper trunk, and the intertriginous area of the neck, as a result of tight-fitting clothing or use of occlusive lubricants, particularly during hot, humid weather. Wearing lightweight, loose-fitting clothing, eliminating greasy topical agents, and using corn starch or powder facilitates clearing of the rash.

Infantile Acropustulosis

This remitting and exacerbating disorder of unknown etiology occurs primarily in African American boys less than 2 to 3 years of age. Lesions begin as pinpoint erythematous papules, which evolve to form papulopustules or vesiculopustules (Fig. 8-47) that are highly pruritic. They appear in crops over the hands and feet, at times extending onto the wrists and ankles. After 10 to 21 days they resolve, only to recur within a few weeks. Ultimately the disorder resolves by 2 to 3 years of age. Differential diagnostic considerations include scabies, dyshidrosis, erythema toxicum, and transient neonatal pustular melanosis. Steroids are ineffective, and only very high doses of antihistamine relieve the itching. Treatment with erythromycin may be helpful.

Vesiculation Following Insect Bites

Inflammatory reactions to insect bites, though often beginning as edematous papules, may evolve into pruritic vesicles and bullae on red bases (Fig. 8-48). This is particularly true of the bites of grass and sand mites. The eruption is frequently misdiagnosed as chickenpox or bul-

lous impetigo. The lack of systemic complaints, localization to exposed areas (especially the lower legs), and seasonal occurrence point to the correct diagnosis. Furthermore, the vesicles have thicker walls than those of bullous impetigo, and they do not rapidly umbilicate and crust as is true of varicella lesions. Tzanck tests and Gram stains also are negative in bullous insect bite reactions (see section on Bites, Stings, and Infestations).

Reactive Erythemas

The term *reactive erythema* refers to a group of disorders characterized by erythematous patches, plaques, and nodules that vary in size, shape, and distribution. Unlike other specific dermatoses, they represent cutaneous reaction patterns triggered by a variety of endogenous and environmental agents. In children the most common reactive erythemas include erythema multiforme, erythema nodosum, urticaria, vasculitis, and drug eruptions.

Erythema Multiforme

Erythema multiforme (EM) is a distinctive, acute hypersensitivity syndrome that may be caused by many different types of agents, including drugs, viruses, bacteria, foods, and immunizations. It may also arise in association with connective tissue disorders. Infectious diseases and medications are the most common causes in children.

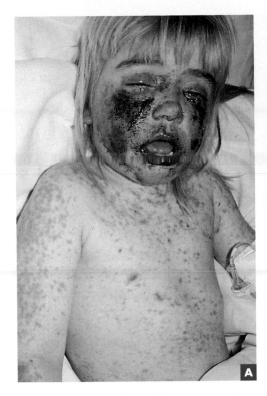

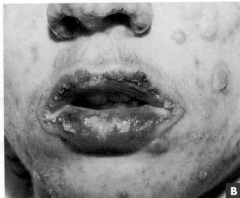

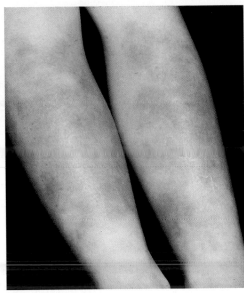

FIG. 8-51 Erythema nodosum. Note the typical, red, raised, tender nodules overlying the pretibial surfaces of the legs.

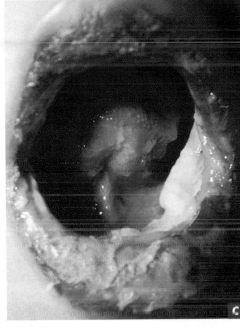

FIG. 8-50 Stevens-Johnson syndrome. *A*, Severe bullous and erosive lesions cover the face, neck, and extremities. *B*, Typical bullae, target lesions, and erosions of the lips are seen in this boy. *C*, This child has numerous vesicles and bullae of the oral mucosa along with formation of a shaggy white membrane consisting of sloughed debris. (*C*, Courtesy Dr. Michael Sherlock.)

The classic eruption is symmetrical and may occur on any part of the body, although it typically appears on the dorsum of the hands and feet and the extensor surfaces of the arms and legs. Involvement of the palms and soles is typical. The initial lesions are dusky, red macules or erythematous wheals that evolve into iris- or target-shaped lesions, the hallmark of EM (Fig. 8-49, *A* and *B*). In many instances the initial crop of lesions closely simulates diffuse urticaria, although EM lesions are typically much less pruritic. The target configuration is due to formation of a central depression that may be blue, violaceous, or white, whereas the elevated periphery tends to remain erythematous. In some cases vesicles or bullae develop centrally, and in others the peripheral rings may vesiculate or become bullous (Fig. 8-49, *C*). The eruption continues in crops that last from 1 to 3 weeks. In most patients the disease is self-limited, and systemic manifestations are limited to low-grade fever, malaise, and myalgia.

Stevens-Johnson Syndrome (Bullous Erythema Multiforme)

Rarely, erythema multiforme progresses to become Stevens-Johnson syndrome, with large areas of epidermal and mucous membrane necrosis and shedding. Hence, Stevens-Johnson syndrome is thought to represent the most severe end of the spectrum of erythema multiforme. In this disorder, constitutional symptoms are prominent, including high fever, cough, sore throat, vomiting, diarrhea, chest pain, and arthralgias. Vesiculation occurs early and is often hemorrhagic and extensive (Fig. 8-50, *A* and *B*). Mucous membrane involvement, particularly of the oral, conjunctival, and urethral mucous membranes, is routine and

often severe. It consists of formation of fragile, thin-walled bullae that rupture early, leaving shallow ulcerations that are rapidly covered by a gray, yellow, or white membrane (Fig. 8-50, *C*). Conjunctival involvement can progress to involve the cornea, resulting in scarring unless aggressive ophthalmologic treatment is instituted early on. Fluid and electrolyte imbalances caused by losses from ruptured bullae and secondary infection are major risks in this disorder, which has a mortality rate ranging between 5% and 25%.

Erythema Nodosum

Erythema nodosum is characterized by symmetrical, red, tender nodules, 1 to 5 cm in diameter, which are usually located over the pretibial surfaces (Fig. 8-51). Most likely, it represents a hypersensitivity reaction to streptococcal infection, medication, sarcoidosis, tuberculosis, or other bacterial or fungal infections. Noninfectious disorders such as ulcerative colitis and regional ileitis have also been implicated.

Erythema nodosum is most often seen in children older than 10 years. The lesions begin as red, tender, slightly elevated nodules that develop into brownish-red or purplish-red lesions within a few days. The disorder usually lasts between 2 and 6 weeks, although recurrences are common.

Differential diagnosis includes cellulitis, insect bites, thrombophlebitis, ecchymoses, and vasculitis. The fact that lesions are symmetric, recurrent, and persistent helps exclude cellulitis and ecchymoses. Their pretibial and extensor location helps differentiate the lesions from

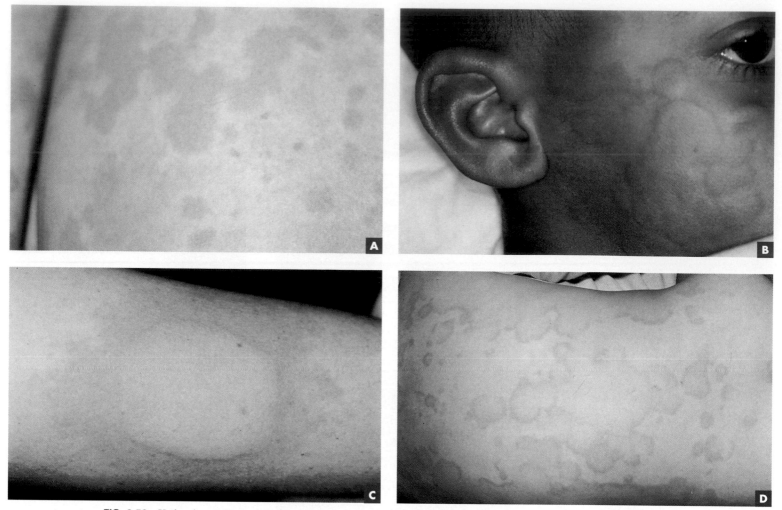

FIG. 8-52 Urticaria. *A*, Typical erythematous raised wheals are seen. *B*, The wheals on this child's face have red rims and lighter centers. *C*, This patient with cold-induced urticaria has a giant whitish wheal with an erythematous halo. *D*, Gyrate urticarial plaques have evolved from individual plaques that became confluent. (*A* and *C* Courtesy Dr. Douglas W. Kress, Children's Hospital of Pittsburgh.)

thrombophlebitis. Insect bite reactions are typically pruritic, and other exposed sites such as the arms, head, and neck may be involved. The deep-seated nature of the nodules in erythema nodosum should allow differentiation from the smaller, more superficial palpable lesions of cutaneous vasculitis.

Treatment should be directed toward the underlying cause. Nonsteroidal antiinflammatory agents may be effective in reducing pain, and bed rest is beneficial.

Urticaria

Urticaria, commonly known as *hives,* is characterized by the sudden appearance of transient, well-demarcated wheals that are usually intensely pruritic, especially when arising as part of an acute IgE-mediated hypersensitivity reaction (Fig. 8-52, *A*). Individual lesions usually last 1 to 2 hours, but they may persist up to 24 hours. They may have an edematous white center and macular red halo (Fig. 8-52, *B*) or the reverse—a red center with an edematous white halo. Size can vary from a few millimeters to giant lesions of over 20 cm in diameter (Fig. 8-52, *C*). Central clearing with peripheral extension may lead to the formation of annular, polycyclic, and arcuate plaques, simulating erythema multiforme and erythema marginatum (Fig. 8-52, *D*). The reaction may involve the mucous membranes and can spread to the subcutaneous tissue, producing woody edema known as *angioedema.*

Urticaria can be caused by a variety of immunologic mechanisms, including IgE antibody response, complement activation, and abnormal levels of or sensitivity to vasoactive amines. Most commonly, acute urticaria (lasting less than 6 weeks) is caused by a hypersensitivity reaction to food, drugs, insect bites, contact allergens, inhaled substances, or acute infections (especially beta-streptococcal infections and viral infections, including mononucleosis). Chronic urticaria (lasting more than 6 weeks) can be a sign of an underlying disorder such as occult infection (of the urinary tract, sinuses, or dentition), hepatitis B, or connective tissue disease (see Chapter 4).

Urticarial/Erythema Multiforme-Like Reaction

One relatively common acute clinical picture involves a constellation of urticarial lesions, periarticular swelling, and extremity angioedema in conjunction with acute upper respiratory infection or following use of sulfa-containing antibiotics or cefaclor. The urticaria is typically either nonpruritic or only mildly pruritic, and lesions evolve into target shapes or gyrate plaques simulating erythema multiforme, although they do not vesiculate (Fig. 8-53, *A* and *B*). With this eruption, painful migratory periarticular swelling is seen, especially involving wrists and ankles, and often associated with bluish discoloration of overlying skin. Migratory stocking-glove angioedema, which is also painful, is common; occasionally, facial edema is seen as well (Fig. 8-53, *C*). Symptoms wax and wane over 1 to 3 weeks until the condi-

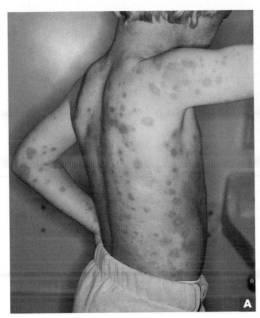
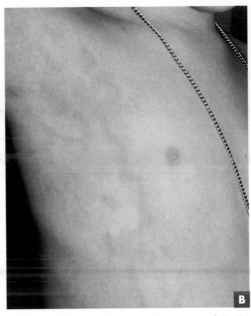
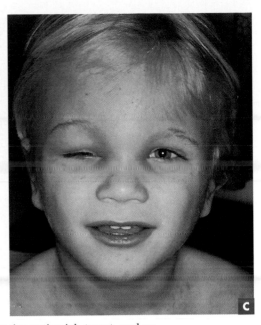

FIG. 8-53 Urticarial/erythema multiforme-like reaction to cefaclor. *A* and *B,* Extensive urticarial, target, and gyrate lesions are seen over the back, arms, and trunk. *C,* Facial edema involving the forehead was prominent in this child.

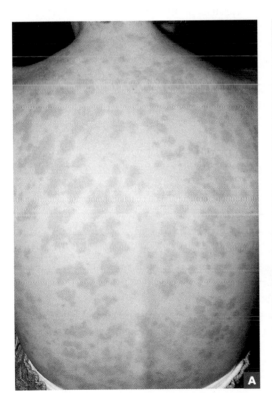
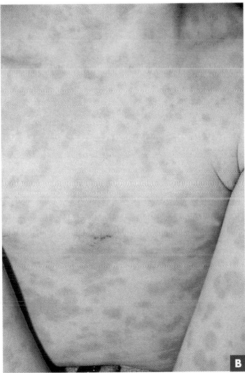
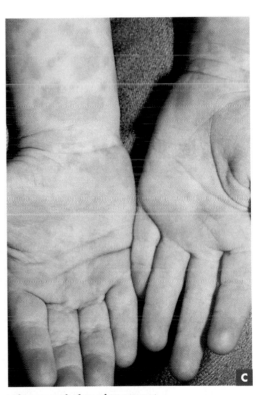

FIG. 8-54 Morbilliform drug eruption. *A* and *B,* This diffuse exanthum developed on the seventh day of treatment with amoxicillin for streptococcal pharyngitis. *C,* The palms and soles were also affected.

tion resolves. This appears to be a delayed hypersensitivity or "serum sickness-like" reaction, although some of the clinical features resemble those of vasculitic eruptions.

Drug Eruptions

Morbilliform Drug Eruption

Many different types of drug eruptions are seen in children. Morbilliform or maculopapular exanthems account for more than half of all cutaneous drug reactions. The rash is reminiscent of measles or other viral exanthems (see Chapter 12). Erythematous macules and papules, which may range from fine to blotchy, begin to erupt on the face and trunk within 5 to 14 days after starting a medication. They then spread to the extremities over 1 to several days (Fig. 8-54, *A* to *C*). The rash, which may be pruritic, is occasionally restricted to the extremities or appears acrally (distally) and spreads centrally. Lesions may become confluent and generally resolve over 1 to 2 weeks with the development of mild purpura and fine desquamation.

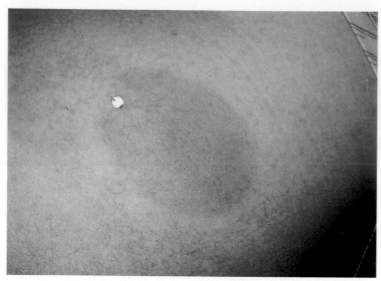

FIG. 8-55 Fixed drug eruption. This hyperpigmented patch with an erythematous border developed on the flank of an adolescent taking tetracycline.

Fixed Drug Eruption

Fixed drug eruptions occur repeatedly in the same cutaneous site after reexposure to the offending drug. Postinflammatory hyperpigmentation is usually marked and may be the only manifestation of the rash during remissions. Morphologically and histologically the target and bullous lesions of fixed drug reactions may be indistinguishable from erythema multiforme and may represent a localized form of EM (Fig. 8-55).

Henoch-Schönlein Purpura

Henoch-Schönlein purpura (HSP) is an inflammatory disorder with multiple predisposing conditions, characterized by a diffuse vasculitis involving the small, nonmuscular blood vessels of the skin, gastrointestinal tract, kidneys, joints, and rarely the lungs and central nervous system. Although the exact etiology is unclear, the common history of antecedent upper respiratory or gastrointestinal infection suggests a hypersensitivity phenomenon resulting in a localized or widespread vascular insult. Other factors including drugs, food, immunizations, and chemical toxins have been implicated, as well. Histologically, immune complex deposition in capillaries and postcapillary venules is associated with a leukocytoclastic vasculitis in the skin and other involved organs.

After a prodrome of headache, anorexia, and fever lasting 1 to a few days, patients may develop one or more of the following in any order: rash, abdominal pain, arthritis, and occasionally hematochezia. Cutaneous lesions consist of erythematous macules, urticarial papules, and purpuric papules and plaques that tend to appear in crops (Fig. 8-56, *A*

to *C*), each resolving over 5 to 7 days, although the total duration of this waxing and waning eruption may last anywhere from 1 to 8 weeks (average 2 to 3). Of affected children, 15% to 40% have one or more recurrences, usually within 6 weeks of resolution of the first episode.

Although in most children the initial crop consists of purpuric lesions distributed symmetrically below the waist (over the buttocks, lower abdomen, and lower extremities), in some this may be preceded by a generalized urticarial eruption that is minimally pruritic and waxes and wanes over 1 to several days before the appearance of purpura. Subsequent crops of purpura usually involve the extensor surfaces of the arms, cheeks (Fig. 8-56, *D*), and tips of the ears. The rash also may involve the trunk and genitalia. In unusually severe cases, skin necrosis may occur, heralded by the appearance of bullae.

Joint involvement consists of painful, tender periarticular swelling, especially involving the wrists, ankles, and knees. The overlying skin tends to be ecchymotic. Stocking-glove edema of the hands and feet is also common (Fig. 8-56, *E*). In young children, nonpruritic angioedema of the face, scalp, sacral, and/or genital areas (Fig. 8-56, *F*) may be prominent. These phenomena wax and wane as does the exanthem (see Chapter 7).

Gastrointestinal symptoms can precede, coincide with, or follow the appearance of cutaneous lesions. Segmental edema of the intestinal tract can cause crampy to colicky abdominal pain and may even serve as the lead point for an intussusception. Mucosal hemorrhage can be the source of gastrointestinal bleeding that can range from occult loss to massive hematochezia or hematemesis (see Chapter 10).

Up to 25% of patients develop nephritis between 1 and 8 weeks after onset of symptoms (peak 1 to 3 weeks). This is more common in older children, and it is usually mild and self-limited. It is first detected by finding evidence of hematuria and proteinuria on urinalysis. Occasionally, nephritis is severe and progressive (see Chapter 13). Central nervous system involvement is extremely rare, and its presence is usually heralded by severe headache, altered level of consciousness, and/or seizures following meningeal hemorrhage.

Treatment of HSP is generally supportive, although gastrointestinal, renal, and central nervous system vasculitis may respond to systemic corticosteroids.

The cutaneous lesions of HSP must be differentiated from acute bacterial, viral, and rickettsial infections (see Chapters 5 and 12). Negative blood cultures and classic findings on cutaneous examination and skin biopsy define HSP. Purpuric rashes associated with thrombocytopenia are more likely to be associated with petechiae and can be ruled out by a normal platelet count. Finally, vasculitic rashes may also be seen in collagen vascular disorders such as lupus erythematosus, mixed connective tissue disease, and dermatomyositis (see Chapter 7). These disorders can usually be excluded by the absence of other findings.

Bites, Stings, and Infestations

Insect and spider bites may be associated with a number of cutaneous and systemic reactions. Lesions are found on exposed areas of skin, particularly the lower legs, arms, head, and neck. During the warm summer months they also may appear on the trunk. Protected areas (including the buttocks, groin, and axillae) are invariably spared. When bites involve the face, they can cause significant pruritic swelling that, though erythematous, is nontender and nonindurated (Fig. 8-57).

Insect Bites

Insect bites, most commonly caused by mosquitoes, fleas, mites, and flies, tend to produce mild acute local reactions, including erythema,

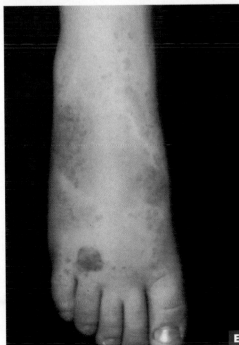
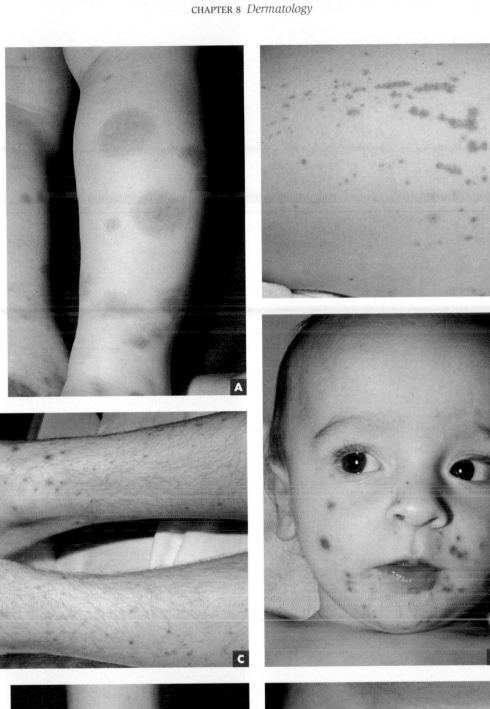
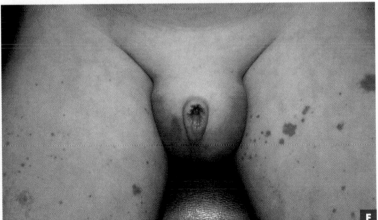

FIG. 8-56 Henoch-Schönlein purpura. *A,* Palpable purpuric macules, papules, and plaques are seen over the legs and heels of this toddler. *B* and *C,* These smaller purpuric papules are more typical and are seen initially over the buttocks, thighs, and ankles. *D,* Later crops may involve the upper extremities, trunk, and face. *E* and *F,* Edema of the extremities, genitals, and face may be impressive.

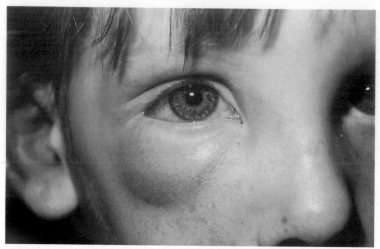

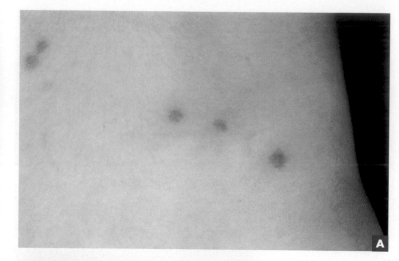

FIG. 8-57 Facial swelling caused by a mosquito bite. The area was pruritic, nontender, and nonindurated. (Courtesy Dr. Michael Sherlock.)

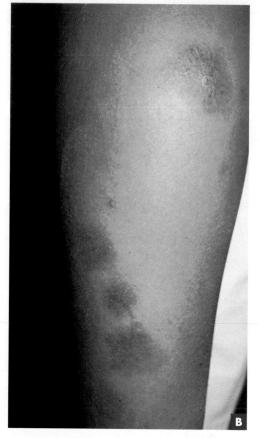

FIG. 8-58 Insect bites. *A,* Multiple erythematous papules with central puncta were the result of flea bites. *B,* Another child had an intense hemorrhagic reaction to flea bites. (*A* Courtesy Dr. Sylvia Suarez, Children's Hospital of Pittsburgh.)

edema, and urticarial papules, that are typically pruritic (Fig. 8-58, *A*). A tiny central crust or hemorrhagic punctum may be apparent on close inspection. Occasionally, patients develop more intense hemorrhagic reactions (Fig. 8-58, *B*).

Mosquito and mite bites occur only during the warm months of spring, summer, and fall. Flea bites occur year round, typically in households with pets. They are usually found on the lower legs above the sock line but can be more diffusely distributed on crawling infants and toddlers. Excoriation caused by scratching makes them prone to secondary impetiginization. On occasion the bites of grass or sand mites can produce frank blistering because the venom they inject contains a blistering agent (Fig. 8-48).

Biting flies include sand flies, blackflies, horseflies, and gnats. The bite itself causes immediate pain and is usually followed by the development of a painful papule that sometimes vesiculates centrally.

Spider Bites

Spider bites tend to provoke more intense inflammatory reactions than those of most insects. Commonly this consists of an area of erythema and induration that frequently becomes ecchymotic and is simultaneously painful and pruritic (Fig. 8-59). Less often, the lesions may vesiculate or even progress to develop central necrosis with eschar formation. The latter is particularly typical of the bite of the brown recluse spider.

Hymenoptera Stings

Bee, wasp, hornet, and yellow jacket stings typically produce a mild local reaction consisting of pain, erythema, and edema appearing within 2 hours after the sting. The honey bee leaves its stinger behind, embedded in the skin. Because this may continue to release venom for up to an hour, it should be removed as soon as possible using a horizontal scraping motion with a knife or fingernail. Grasping the stinger between forceps or two fingernails can inject more venom. There is some evidence that topical application of a paste of papain (meat tenderizer) mixed with water within minutes of the sting may reduce the severity of local reactions.

Hymenoptera stings commonly produce a late-onset increase in swelling that is more diffuse than the initial reaction and tends to peak in 48 to 72 hours. This is the result of a delayed hypersensitivity reaction, and it is described by patients as being both pruritic and painful (Fig. 8-60). Treatment is symptomatic.

In approximately 0.5% to 0.8% of the population, hymenoptera stings cause severe, acute, anaphylactic reactions within 15 minutes of the sting (see Chapter 4).

Papular Urticaria

Papular urticaria is a delayed hypersensitivity reaction to the bites of mosquitoes, fleas, bedbugs, or other insects. It usually occurs in infants

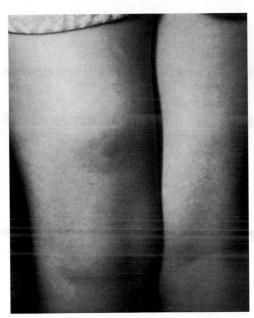

FIG. 8-59 Spider bites. A marked inflammatory response consisting of a central wheal with a wide erythematous halo is seen in this child.

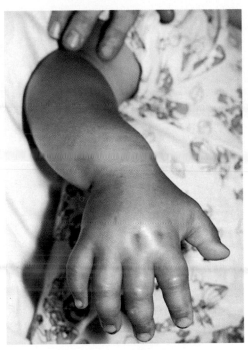

FIG. 8-60 Delayed hypersensitivity response to a bee sting. Marked swelling of the hand and fingers developed over 24 hours after a sting between the fingers.

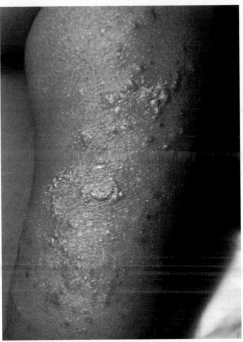

FIG. 8-61 Papular urticaria. This severe excoriated papular reaction developed in response to recurrent flea bites. (Courtesy Dr. Michael Sherlock.)

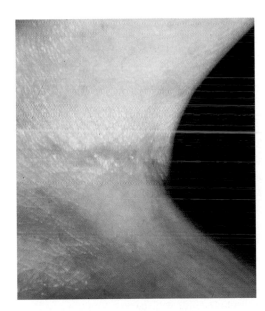

FIG. 8-62 Scabies burrow. This linear lesion in the finger web is characteristic of an itch mite burrow.

and children in the spring and summer months. Lesions consist of 3- to 10-mm urticarial wheals with a central punctum and are intensely pruritic. They tend to be grouped in clusters (Fig. 8-61) and are often excoriated or secondarily infected. They recur in crops, and each may persist for 2 to 10 days or longer.

General principles of therapy for insect bites consist of insect control, use of insect repellents, and application of topical corticosteroids supplemented by oral antihistamines for symptomatic relief. Parenteral administration of epinephrine, antihistamines, and corticosteroids combined with intensive supportive care may be lifesaving in anaphylactic reactions.

Infestations

Scabies

Scabies is a highly contagious infestation caused by the itch mite *Acarus scabiei*, which burrows under the skin. It is contracted by direct contact with other infested humans. The characteristic eruption appears 4 to 6 weeks after initial contact, and it is thought to represent a hypersensitivity reaction to the mites. Intensely pruritic papules, vesicles, pustules, and linear burrows appear in the finger and toe webs, the axillae, over the flexor surfaces of the wrists and elbows, around the nipples and waist, and over the groin and buttocks. The burrow, which is produced by the female mite, is the pathognomonic sign of scabies. It consists of a small, scaly linear papule with pinpoint vesicles at the ends (Fig. 8-62). In infants and toddlers the distribution differs, with the head; neck; trunk; palms; soles, dorsa, and instep portions of the feet; and lateral aspect of the wrists being more prominently involved (Fig. 8-63, *A* and *B*). This age group is also more prone to developing an intense nodular reaction to the mite (Fig. 8-63, *C*).

In many patients, excoriation, secondary infection, or even development of a widespread secondary eczematous eruption (as a result of scratching) alters the appearance of or masks the primary lesions, making diagnosis more difficult. Therefore scabies must be considered in any individual who has no history of atopic dermatitis but has severe pruritus and recent onset of an eczematous rash. The distribution of scabies in intertriginous areas and over the palms, dorsa, and soles of the feet helps to differentiate it from other insect bite reactions.

Although scabies can often be diagnosed clinically, an unequivocal diagnosis can be made with a skin scraping that shows a mite, mite eggs, or feces. The most important factor in obtaining a successful scraping is choice of site. Burrows and papules are most likely to be identified on the wrists, finger webs, feet, or elbows. A fresh burrow can be identified as a 5- to 10-mm raised mound with a small dark spot resembling a fleck of pepper at one end. This spot is the mite, and it can be lifted out of the burrow with a needle or the point of a scalpel

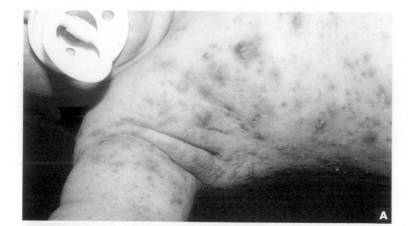

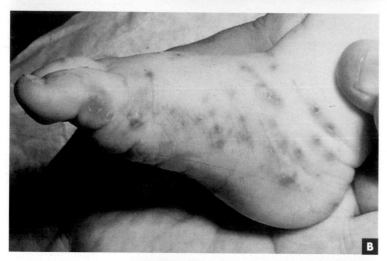

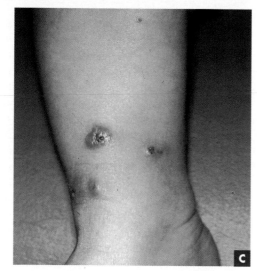

FIG. 8-64 Microscopic appearance of adult scabies mite. Note the small oval egg within the body.

FIG. 8-63 Infantile scabies. Widespread, pruritic, red papules, pustules, and vesicles are seen *(A)* over the trunk and axilla and *(B)* the dorsa and in-step portions of the feet, where burrows are also evident. Infants are also more likely to develop an intense nodular reaction to the mite *(C).*

Eradication of scabies necessitates topical application of lindane lotion to all household members (for varying periods of time, depending on age) and thorough cleansing of all dirty clothing, towels, and bedding. Permethrin 5% cream (Elimite) is a new product with similar efficacy and a superior safety profile, particularly in young children. Symptomatic therapy with oral antipruritic agents and topical steroids may be required long after the mites have been killed, that is, until the secondary reaction has subsided.

Lice

Three varieties of lice produce clinical disease in humans, and all can involve the scalp hair in children. Crab lice *(Phthirus pubis)* are transmitted primarily by sexual contact. They are short and broad, with claws spaced far apart to grasp the sparse hairs on the trunk, pubic area, and eyelashes (Fig. 8-65, *A*). They are typically found inhabiting the pubic hair and occasionally axillary hair and other body hair in adolescents and adults. Their bites produce bluish, pruritic papules that are distributed over the lower abdomen and upper thighs. Pruritus is intense, and a secondary eczematous rash may develop, particularly in the pubic area, as a result of scratching. Young children lacking pubic and axillary hair may develop scalp or eyelash infestations after close contact with infested adults. Body lice *(Pediculus humanus corporis)* generally live in bedding or clothing, and their eggs may be found in the seams of trousers or underwear. Bites produce urticarial papules, seen primarily over the waist, neck, shoulders, and axillae, which are usually obliterated by excoriations and secondary bacterial infection.

blade. If a scalpel is used to scrape the burrow, it is worthwhile to place a drop of mineral oil onto the skin to ensure adherence of the scrapings to the blade. The scrapings are placed on a slide, another drop of mineral oil is added, and a cover-slip is applied.

Mites are eight-legged arachnids easily visible under the scanning power of the microscope (Fig. 8-64). Care must be taken to focus through thick areas of skin scrapings so as not to miss camouflaged mites. The presence of eggs (smooth ovals, approximately one half the size of an adult mite) or feces (redish-brown pellets, often seen in clusters) is also diagnostic.

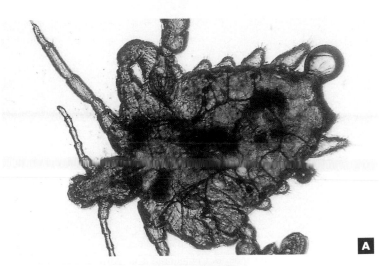

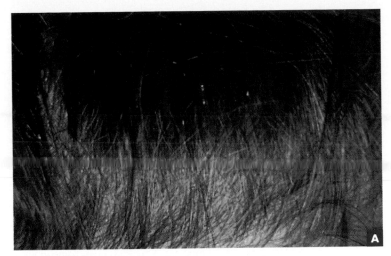

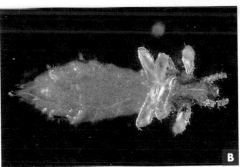

FIG. 8-65 Microscopic appearance of lice. *A*, The crab louse has a short, broad body, with claws spaced far apart. *B*, The head louse has a long, thin body, with claws spaced close together.

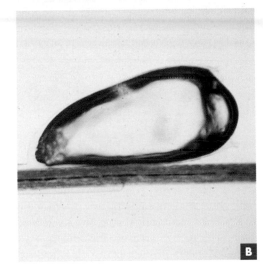

FIG. 8-66 Head lice. *A*, Nits appear as tiny white dots that adhere to the hair shafts. They are typically found 1 to 3 cm from the scalp above and behind the ears. *B*, Microscopic appearance of the nit of a head louse attached to a scalp hair. Microscopic examination distinguishes nits from hair casts and other artifacts. (*A* Courtesy Dr. Michael Sherlock.)

Head lice *(P. humanus capitis)* represent the most common cause of infestation in children. The lice are acquired by close physical contact; by sharing hats, combs, brushes, or scarves with an infested person; or by rubbing against upholstered furniture recently used by such a person. Head lice are long and thin, with claws spaced close together to grasp the more densely distributed scalp hairs (Fig. 8-65, *B*). Pruritus is the principal symptom, and the resultant scratching produces scalp excoriations that are vulnerable to secondary infection. Occipital adenopathy is common.

Nits are seen as oval, white 0.5-mm dots glued onto the hair shafts about 1 to 3 cm from the scalp (Fig. 8-66, *A*), particularly above and behind the ears. These are firmly attached to the hair and do not move along the hair shafts as do the hair casts for which they are frequently mistaken. Although nits may be seen along the entire length of the hair, they are deposited by the lice only near the scalp. Those far from the root indicate a span of perhaps months between infestation and examination. Nits are difficult to remove and may be nonviable shells. Patients adequately treated for lice still have non-viable shells attached to the hair. Removal is facilitated by use of a weak vinegar rinse (which is left on under a shower cap or towel for 15 to 20 minutes), followed by combing with a fine-toothed comb or cutting the hair close to the scalp. This is important because the persistence of dead nits is a common cause of misunderstanding by school health care workers who insist on retreating the children or sending them home from school. New or viable nits rarely recur in a previously treated child, and reports of lice resistant to treatment are rare and poorly documented. Active dis-

ease is present only if a viable organism or new nits attached close to the scalp are identified.

Diagnosis of pediculosis must be considered in patients with unexplained scalp pruritus. A careful search for the organism may permit a specific diagnosis. Lice are six-legged insects visible to the unaided eye; they are commonly found on the scalp, eyelashes, and pubic areas. They are best identified close to the skin or scalp, where they can be seen moving around and where their eggs are more numerous and more obvious. Diagnosis can be made either by identifying a louse or by plucking hairs and confirming the presence of nits by microscopic examination (Fig. 8-66, *B*).

Eradication of lice requires application of lindane shampoo to infested hair-bearing areas of all household members and cleaning measures similar to those specified for ridding the house of scabies. Special attention should also be given to hats, scarves, and coat collars.

Acne

Acne vulgaris, a disorder of the pilosebaceous apparatus, is the most common skin problem of adolescence. Lesions may appear on the face as early as age 8, although they usually begin to develop in the second decade of life during the onset of puberty. Other areas with prominent sebaceous follicles, including the upper chest and back, may be involved as well.

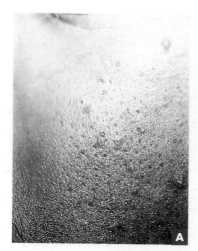
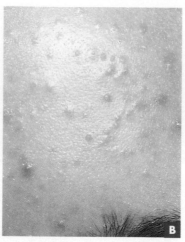
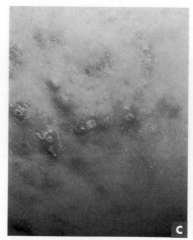
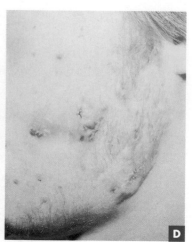

FIG. 8-67 *A,* Comedonal acne with open comedones, or blackheads, seen over the cheek. *B,* Comedonal acne with closed comedones, or whiteheads, on the forehead, accentuated by side lighting. *C,* Papulopustular acne with inflamed papules and pustules over the cheeks, which responded well to antibiotics. *D,* Cystic acne shows deep cysts with marked erythema that can cause severe scarring after the acne has resolved.

The exact pathogenesis of acne is unknown. However, abnormalities in follicular keratinization are thought to produce the earliest acne lesion, the microcomedone. In time, microcomedones may grow into clinically apparent open comedones (blackheads) (Fig. 8-67, *A*) and closed comedones (whiteheads) (Fig. 8-67, *B*). The entire process is driven by androgens, which stimulate sebaceous gland differentiation and growth, and the production of sebum. The proliferation of *Propionibacterium acnes* in noninflammatory comedones and the rupture of comedone contents into the surrounding dermis may trigger the development of inflammatory papules, pustules, and cysts (Fig. 8-67, *C*). Cystic acne is typified by nodules and cysts scattered over the face, chest, and back (Fig. 8-67, *D*). This form frequently leads to scarring.

Although therapy must be individualized, patients with mild to moderate comedonal and/or inflammatory acne respond well to a combination of topical retinoic acid, benzoyl peroxide, and antibiotics. Moderate to severe papulopustular acne warrants the use of oral antibiotics in combination with topical agents. Oral 13-cis retinoic acid, or isotretinoin should be reserved for patients with severe, scarring cystic acne recalcitrant to conservative measures.

Tumors and Infiltrations

Persistent lumps and bumps in the skin often raise fears of skin cancer. Fortunately, primary skin cancer is extremely rare in childhood, and most tumors and infiltrated lesions are benign. Hemangiomas and nevi, which can be regarded as tumors, are discussed in subsequent sections of this chapter.

Warts

Warts are benign tumors produced by human papilloma virus (HPV) infection of the skin and mucous membranes. In children they occur most commonly on the fingers, hands, and feet. The incubation period for warts varies from 1 to 6 months, and the majority of lesions disappear spontaneously over a period of 5 years. Local trauma promotes inoculation of the papilloma virus. Thus periungual lesions are common in children who bite their nails or pick at hangnails.

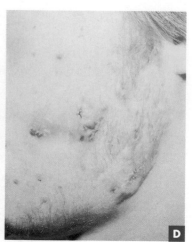

FIG. 8-68 Verruca vulgaris. Dry, rough, and crusty, these common warts usually involve the hands. The periungual distribution in this girl was due in part to her habit of picking at her cuticles.

Investigators have identified over 50 HPVs capable of producing warts, and many of these organisms produce characteristic lesions in specific locations. For instance, the discrete, round, skin-colored papillomatous (roughened) papules typical of *verruca vulgaris* (common warts) are produced by HPV types 2 and 4 (Fig. 8-68). The subtle, minimally hyperpigmented, flat warts *(verruca plana)* caused by HPV 3 are frequently spread by picking and scratching and thus may become widespread on the face, arms, and legs (Fig. 8-69).

Plantar warts (Fig. 8-70) are associated with HPV type 1. Although not proven, the spread of these warts probably occurs through contact with contaminated, desquamated skin in showers, pool decks, and bathrooms. Being much larger below the skin surface than is apparent from their external appearance, they often cause pain when the patient walks. Although lesions can be confused with corns, calluses, or scars,

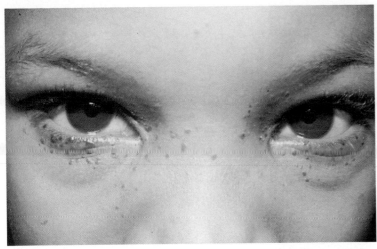

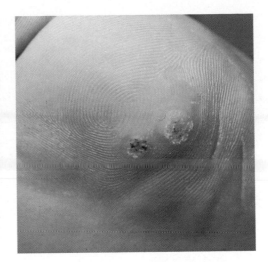

FIG. 8-70 Plantar warts. Two painful lesions are seen over the ball of the foot. Note how they interrupt the normal skin lines.

FIG. 8-69 Flat warts or verruca plana. These tiny, light brown warts are spread by scratching.

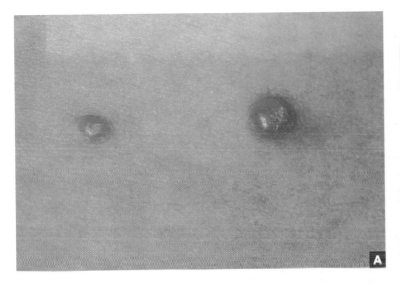

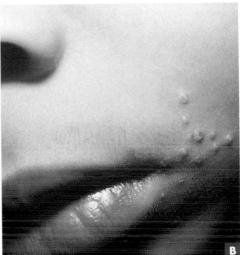

FIG. 8-71 Molluscum contagiosum. *A,* Close examination of these lesions reveals centrally umbilicated dome-shaped lesions. *B,* Lesions have spread on the face of this boy as a result of scratching. Note that some of these lesions have protruding white centers.

they can be distinguished by their interruption of the normal skin lines (dermatoglyphics). Characteristic black dots in the warts are thrombosed superficial capillaries.

Warts can also be found on the trunk, oral mucosa, and conjunctivae. Anogenital lesions *(condylomata acuminata)* are usually associated with HPV types 6 and 11, and the possibility of sexual abuse must be considered in children with lesions in this site (see Chapter 6).

Although warts are self-limited in most children, persistent, widespread lesions suggest congenital or acquired immunodeficiency. Warts may become a serious management problem in oncology and transplant patients who are chronically immunosuppressed.

Molluscum Contagiosum

Molluscum contagiosum is characterized by sharply circumscribed single or multiple skin-colored, dome-shaped papules with waxy surfaces.

They usually have umbilicated centers, although some lesions have protruding white centers (Fig. 8-71, *A* and *B*). This contagious disease is caused by a poxvirus. Lesions are found on the trunk, axillae, face, and genitals. They usually begin as pinpoint elevations of the skin and rapidly increase in size to 5 mm. The lesions are spread by scratching and thus are often arranged in a linear configuration (Fig. 8-71, *B*). Frequently a curdlike core can be expressed from the center; microscopic examination of this material reveals typical molluscum bodies. Destruction of lesions by curetting their cores or by application of a blistering agent and plastic tape that is peeled off in 3 days is curative, although many patients undergo spontaneous remission.

Milia

Milia (Fig. 8-72) are small (1 to 2 mm), whitish-yellow papules commonly seen on the face in neonates. They are firm and unlike pustules

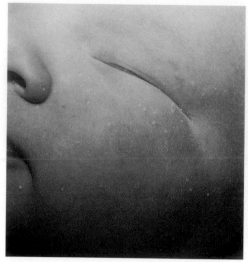

FIG. 8-72 Milia. Small, whitish-yellow papules found close to the skin surface, are particularly common around the eyes and midface.

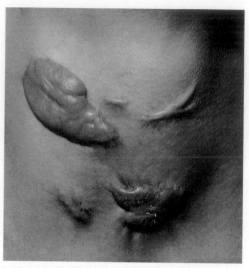

FIG. 8-73 Keloids. An abnormal reparative reaction to skin injury, keloids are characterized by proliferation of fibroblasts and collagen that extends beyond the margins of the original wound.

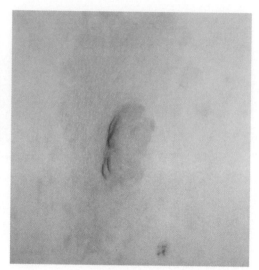

FIG. 8-74 Neurofibromatosis. Soft pink neurofibroma arising within a café-au-lait spot. Usually neurofibromas arise from normal skin.

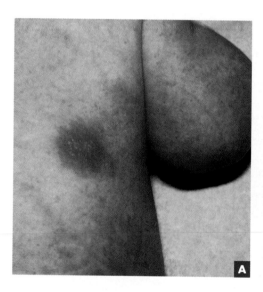

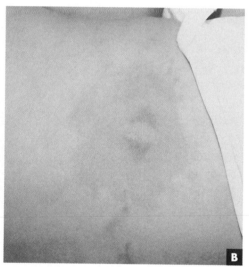

FIG. 8-75 Mastocytoma. *A,* The solitary brown plaque on this infant's back contained numerous mast cells on histopathologic examination. *B,* Darier sign. After firm stroking, a wheal-and-flare appears. This is diagnostic for mastocytoma.

are not easily removed by pressure. Milia consist of epithelial-lined cysts arising from hair follicles. They are persistent, although they may resolve spontaneously after months to years. They usually arise without any apparent cause, although they are often seen after skin injury, such as that caused by blistering eruptions or dermabrasion. They are a characteristic feature of the dystrophic form of epidermolysis bullosa (Fig. 8-89, *A*).

Keloids

Keloids are rubbery nodules or plaques that result from the proliferation of fibroblasts and deposition of collagen following injury to the skin (Fig. 8-73). They can be pruritic or tender, especially during the active growing phase, and they may extend well beyond the margins of the original wound. This latter trait distinguishes keloids from hypertrophic scars, which remain confined to the wound margins and flatten spontaneously within 6 months of the injury. Keloids may arise spontaneously or occur in a familial form. They are most common in African Americans, and occur most often on the ear lobes, upper trunk, and

deltoid areas. Fortunately, they are not seen on the mid-face. Keloids regress with intralesional steroid injections, alone or in combination with surgical excision. However, recurrences are common.

Neurofibromas

Neurofibromas are solitary or multiple growths of neural tissue, presenting as soft, skin-colored or pink dermal nodules (Fig. 8-74). The central portion of an early lesion is particularly soft, and fingertip pressure creates the illusion of pressing in a buttonhole. Von Recklinghausen disease (neurofibromatosis-1) is a syndrome characterized by the presence of multiple neurofibromas, café-au-lait spots, axillary freckling, and various systemic disorders. When considering this diagnosis, the clinician must remember that the neurofibromas usually appear after puberty, whereas in prepubertal children, café-au-lait spots are the most important cutaneous marker of von Recklinghausen disease (see Chapter 15). Solitary neurofibromas without other stigmata of neurofibromatosis occasionally develop in normal individuals.

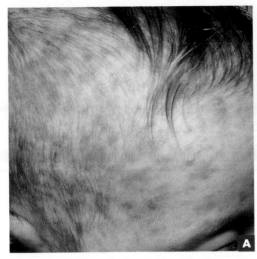

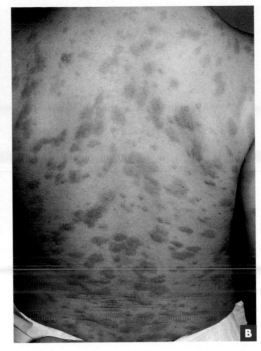

FIG. 8-76 Urticarial pigmentosa. *A,* Numerous reddish-brown lesions are seen on the scalp and forehead of this toddler. *B,* Marked hyperpigmentation developed in the truncal lesions of this child. *C,* This infant has a wheal-and-flare reaction after accidental rubbing.

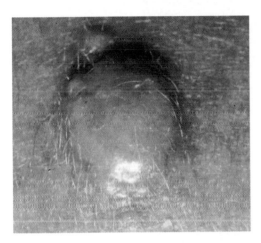

FIG. 8-77 Juvenile xanthogranuloma. This 1-cm, yellowish nodule located on the back of a 3-month-old infant is the result of infiltration and proliferation of histiocytes.

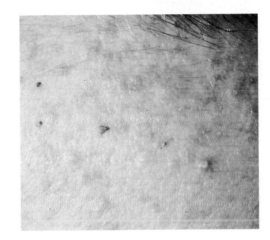

FIG. 8-78 Letterer-Siwe disease. The skin manifestations of the histiocytosis syndromes are similar and show infiltrated scaling papules with petechiae, resembling seborrheic dermatitis.

Mastocytosis

Cutaneous mastocytosis refers to a group of disorders characterized by dermal infiltrations of mast cells.

Mastocytoma

Isolated mastocytomas may be seen in infants. They usually appear as skin-colored or light brown, slightly indurated plaques, 1 to 2 cm in size (Fig. 8-75, *A*). Development of a wheal-and-flare after firm stroking of the lesion (Darier sign) confirms the diagnosis (Fig. 8-75, *B*). This is a response to the vascular effects of histamine released from infiltrating mast cells. Occasionally, enough histamine is released from a large mastocytoma to cause localized blistering or systemic symptoms of flushing, wheezing, or diarrhea. Mastocytomas can be located anywhere on the body and usually resolve by puberty.

Urticaria Pigmentosa

Urticaria pigmentosa is another form of cutaneous mastocytosis that presents with numerous small, brownish papules or plaques, most commonly on the trunk (Fig. 8-76, *A* to *C*). These may be present at birth, or they may appear later in childhood. The hyperpigmented macules over-

lying mast cell infiltrates also typically react to stroking with a wheal-and-flare (Fig. 8-76, *B* and *C*). Urticaria pigmentosa in children is usually limited to the skin and often resolves by adolescence. However, the bone marrow, gastrointestinal tract, and other organs may be involved. Rare systemic findings in children with urticaria pigmentosa include chronic diarrhea, gastric ulcers, flushing reactions, headaches, and failure to thrive. In infancy there is a tendency for lesions to blister, and rarely widespread erosions may result in dehydration and sepsis.

Juvenile Xanthogranuloma

Infiltration of the skin by other types of cells can also occur. An example is juvenile xanthogranuloma (JXG), in which local infiltration and proliferation of histiocytes form an isolated plaque or nodule or groups of small nodules (Fig. 8-77). These asymptomatic red or yellowish-brown lesions grow very rapidly in infants and young children but resolve spontaneously later in childhood. They are not associated with abnormalities of circulating lipids. In cases with multiple lesions there may be an associated ocular involvement; this is the most common cause of nontraumatic hyphema in children. Hence, ophthalmologic

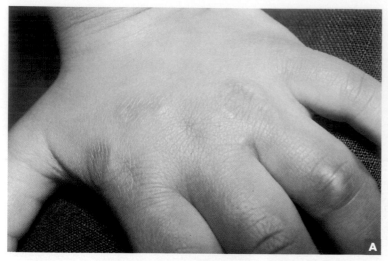

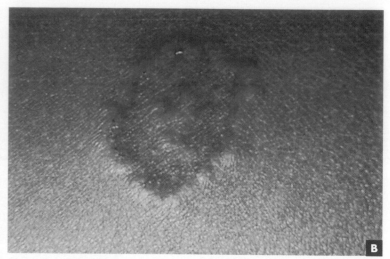

FIG. 8-79 Granuloma annulare. *A,* Three raised, indurated rings with intact overlying skin along with an early papular lesion on the ring finger are seen on this child's hand. *B,* This segmented ring is slightly excoriated because of scratching. (*B* Courtesy Dr. Michael Sherlock.)

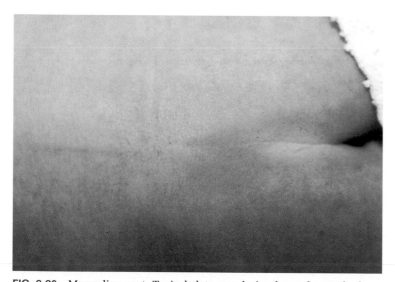

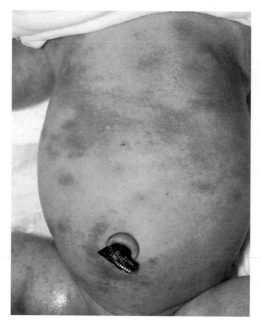

FIG. 8-81 Erythema toxicum neonatorum. Numerous yellow papules and pustules are surrounded by large intensely erythematous rings on the trunk of this infant.

FIG. 8-80 Mongolian spot. Typical slate-gray lesion located over the lumbosacral area of this black infant.

evaluation is important in patients with multiple or diffuse xanthogranulomas.

The Histiocytoses

The histiocytosis syndromes are more serious proliferative disorders of Langerhans cells. The group includes Letterer-Siwe disease, Hand-Schüller-Christian disease, and eosinophilic granuloma. Skin infiltration is most common in Letterer-Siwe disease. This entity begins in infancy with a diffuse papular, scaly eruption that differs from the usual seborrheic dermatitis by virtue of its associated infiltrated, crusted papules and petechiae (Fig. 8-78). Diagnosis is suggested by associated systemic manifestations such as hepatosplenomegaly and chronically draining ears. It is confirmed by skin biopsy, which shows characteristic Langerhans granules within the cytoplasm of infiltrating mononuclear cells (see Chapter 11).

Granuloma Annulare

When fully evolved, granuloma annulare is an annular eruption histologically characterized by dermal infiltration of lymphocytes around altered collagen. The lesion begins as a nodule or papule that gradually extends peripherally to form a ring. The initial papule and subsequent ring are raised and indurated, and in some cases the ring is broken into segments. The overlying epidermis is usually intact and the same color as the adjacent skin (Fig. 8-79, *A*). However, it may be slightly erythematous or even hyperpigmented. Most lesions are asymptomatic, although a few are mildly pruritic. In the latter instance, superficial excoriation caused by scratching may be noted (Fig. 8-79, *B*). Lesions are most commonly found on the extensor surfaces of the lower legs, feet, fingers, and hands, but other areas may be involved. They resolve spontaneously within a few months to several years, and no treatment is required. Their origin is unclear.

Granuloma annulare is most commonly confused with tinea cor-

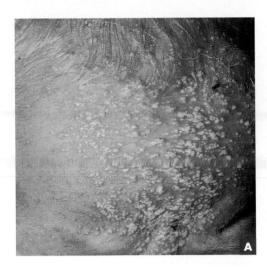

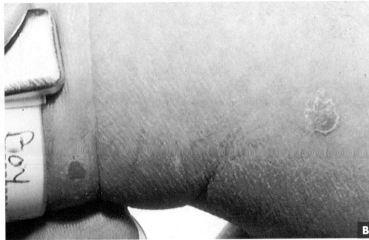

FIG. 8-82 Transient neonatal pustular melanosis. *A,* A myriad of tiny pustules dot the forehead and scalp of this neonate. *B,* When the pustules rupture, a pigmented macule surrounded by a collarette of scale remains.

poris or ringworm (Fig. 8-33). However, the thickened indurated character of the ring and the lack of an active microvesicular and scaling border enable clinical distinction.

Neonatal Dermatology

The skin of a newborn differs from that of an adult in several ways: it is thinner, less hairy, has fewer sweat and sebaceous gland secretions, and has weaker intercellular attachments. During the neonatal period, common rashes or skin abnormalities may develop that need to be differentiated from more serious cutaneous disorders. Transient phenomena include erythema toxicum neonatorum and transient neonatal pustular melanosis. More serious diseases include Letterer-Siwe disease (because it involves other organ systems) and staphylococcal scalded skin syndrome (because of potential fluid and electrolyte disturbances and life-threatening infection).

Mongolian Spots

Mongolian spots are flat, slate gray to bluish-black, poorly circumscribed macules. They are located most commonly over the lumbosacral area and buttocks (Fig. 8-80), although they can appear anywhere on the body. The spots range in size from 1 to 10 cm and may be single or multiple (see Fig. 6-31). Ninety percent of black infants, 81% of Asian infants, and 9.6% of white newborns have these macules, which contain accumulations of melanocytes deep within the dermis. There is no known risk of malignancy, and Mongolian spots usually fade without therapy by age 7.

Erythema Toxicum Neonatorum

Erythema toxicum neonatorum is a benign, self-limited, asymptomatic disorder of unknown etiology. It occurs in up to 50% of full-term in-

fants and has no racial or sexual predisposition. Lesions usually begin 24 to 48 hours after birth but may appear up to the tenth day of life. The disorder has been described as "flea-bite" dermatosis of the newborn, owing to the intense erythema with a central papule or pustule that resembles a flea bite (Fig. 8-81). Lesions are typically 2 to 3 cm in diameter, and there may be a few to several hundred on the back, face, chest, and extremities. The palms and soles are usually spared. A smear of material from a central pustule reveals numerous eosinophils; concomitant circulating eosinophilia is present in up to 20% of patients. The eruption fades spontaneously within 5 to 7 days. No treatment is necessary.

Differential diagnosis includes transient neonatal pustular melanosis, staphylococcal folliculitis, milia neonatorum, miliaria rubra, and herpes simplex (see Chapter 12). Infections can be excluded with a Gram stain, Tzanck smear, and cultures, when necessary.

Transient Neonatal Pustular Melanosis

Transient neonatal pustular melanosis (TNPM) is a self-limited dermatosis of unknown etiology. The rash usually presents at birth with 1- to 2-mm vesiculopustules or ruptured pustules that disappear in 24 to 48 hours, leaving pigmented macules with a collarette of scale (Fig. 8-82, *A* and *B*). Lesions may appear anywhere on the body but are most often seen on the neck, forehead, lower back, and legs. Wright stain of a pustular smear shows numerous neutrophils; Gram stain and culture are negative for bacteria. The hyperpigmentation fades in 3 weeks to 3 months. TNPM is a benign disorder and requires no therapy. Differential diagnosis is similar to that of erythema toxicum neonatorum.

Sebaceous Gland Hyperplasia and Neonatal Acne

Sebaceous gland hyperplasia is a common entity consisting of multiple 1- to 2-cm papules usually located over the nose and cheeks of full-term

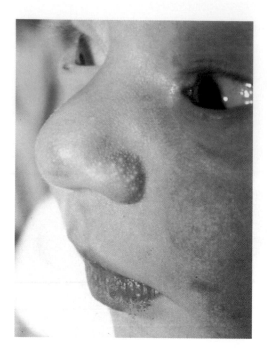

FIG. 8-83 Sebaceous gland hyperplasia. Note the yellowish papules on the nose of this infant.

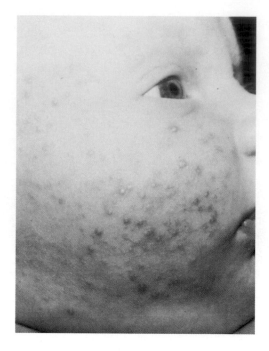

FIG. 8-84 Neonatal acne. Red papules and pustules are present over the nose and cheeks of this infant.

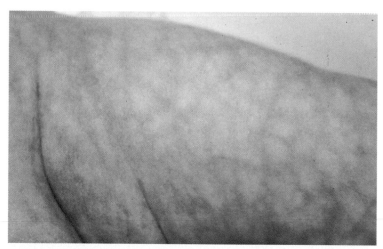

FIG. 8-85 Cutis marmorata. Note the reticulated bluish-purple mottling of this infant's thigh.

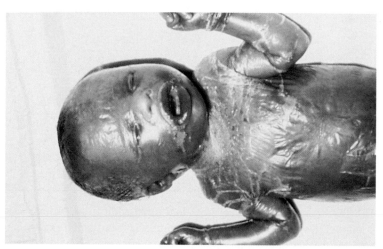

FIG. 8-86 Collodion baby. A shiny, transparent membrane covered this baby at birth; she later developed lamellar ichthyosis. Note the ectropion and eclabium (eversion and fissuring of the eyelid margins and lips).

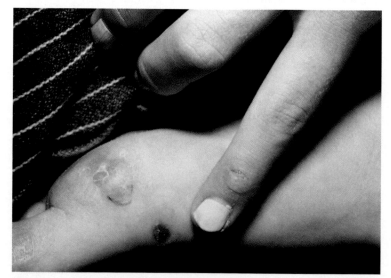

FIG. 8-87 EB simplex. Blisters form easily in pressure-bearing areas, particularly the hands and feet. Scarring does not occur.

infants (Fig. 8-83). It is a normal physiologic response to maternal androgenic stimulation of sebaceous gland growth. Lesions resolve spontaneously by 4 to 6 months.

Neonates can, however, develop acne vulgaris in the first few weeks of life. This condition is also thought to be secondary to stimulation of the sebaceous glands and induction of abnormal keratinization of the hair follicles by maternal androgens. Lesions consist of comedones, papules, and pustules usually located over the cheeks, forehead, and upper chest (Fig. 8-84). Neonatal acne usually resolves spontaneously over 4 to 8 weeks as the effects of maternal hormones dissipate. Though therapy is rarely required, use of 2.5% benzoyl peroxide and avoidance of topical oils may hasten resolution. The likelihood that these children will develop adolescent acne is unknown.

Cutis Marmorata

Cutis marmorata (Fig. 8-85) is a transient, netlike, reddish-blue mottling of the skin caused by variable vascular constriction and dilation. It is a normal response to chilling, and upon rewarming, normal skin

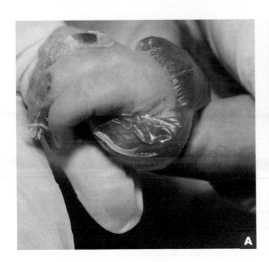

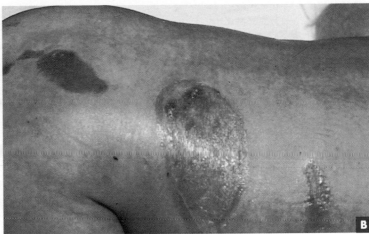

FIG. 8-88 Junctional EB. Widespread involvement was seen in this infant at birth. *A,* Note the erosions and the large, intact blister over the thumb and dorsum of the hand. *B,* Large denuded areas are evident over the back and buttocks.

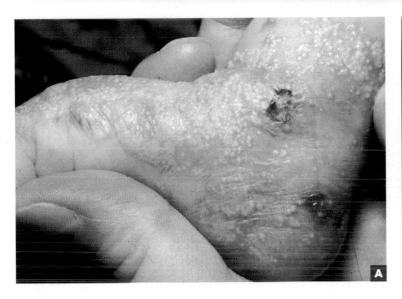

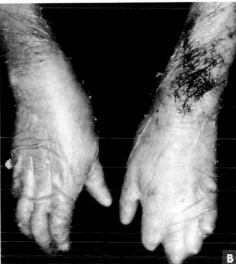

FIG. 8-89 Dystrophic EB. *A,* Blisters, erosions, and hundreds of milia are seen on the foot and ankle of this newborn. *B,* In this child with the recessive form of dystrophic EB, severe scarring encased the fingers, resulting in syndactyly.

color returns. The discoloration occurs primarily over the trunk and extremities in infants. In neonates the condition is benign. However, if mottling persists beyond 6 months of life, it may be a sign of congenital hypothyroidism.

Collodion Baby

In several variants of ichthyosis, particularly lamellar ichthyosis, the infant is born encased in a thick, parchmentlike scale known as a *collodion membrane* (Fig. 8-86). This dries and is shed in large sheets within 7 to 14 days. Significant secondary fluid, electrolyte, and heat losses can occur. Although scaling may resolve completely in some infants, most go on to develop cutaneous findings typical for the underlying ichthyosis (Figs. 8-8 and 8-9).

Epidermolysis Bullosa

Epidermolysis bullosa (EB) is a group of inherited mechanobullous disorders characterized by the development of blisters after mild friction or trauma. There are three general types: simplex, junctional, and dystrophic (scarring). These types are classified according to the level at which blister formation takes place. Each type has several subgroups, and all typically present with blistering in the newborn period.

Epidermolysis Bullosa Simplex

In EB simplex, blister formation takes place in the basal cell layer of the epidermis. On presentation, blistering can be mild or marked, generalized over the entire body, or localized to the hands and feet (Fig. 8-87). The disorder is inherited as an autosomal dominant trait. Although there is no scarring, secondary infection is a common complication.

Junctional Epidermolysis Bullosa

Junctional EB, inherited as an autosomal recessive trait, usually presents at birth with bullae and erosions in a generalized distribution. Blisters form at the junction of the epidermis and dermis (Fig. 8-88). The most common form is usually fatal within the first year because of sepsis and fluid loss. A milder subtype resembles generalized EB simplex.

Dystrophic Epidermolysis Bullosa

The scarring forms of EB are divided into dominant and recessive types. The plane of cleavage is in the upper portion of the dermis. In both, scarring occurs as the blisters heal, and milia are common (Fig. 8-89, *A*). The dominant form results in much less scarring than the recessive form; patients with the latter show retardation in growth and development, severe oral blisters, loss of nails; and sometimes syndactyly (Fig. 8-89, *B*).

Skin biopsies are helpful in distinguishing among the three general types of EB in neonates, and they are also helpful in determining prog-

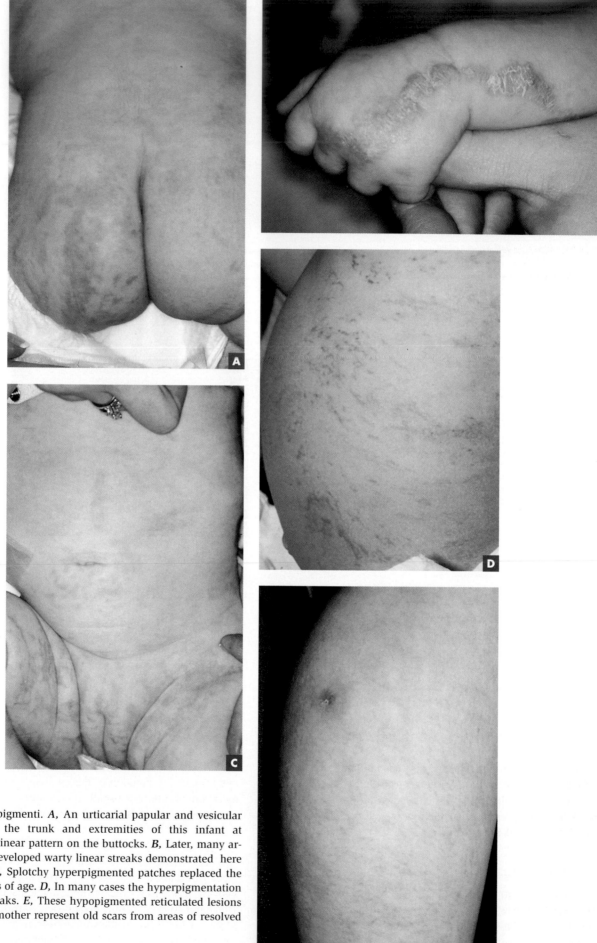

FIG. 8-90 Incontinentia pigmenti. *A,* An urticarial papular and vesicular eruption was noted on the trunk and extremities of this infant at 2 weeks of age. Note the linear pattern on the buttocks. *B,* Later, many areas of old inflammation developed warty linear streaks demonstrated here on the hand and wrist. *C,* Splotchy hyperpigmented patches replaced the warty lesions by 8 months of age. *D,* In many cases the hyperpigmentation appears in swirls and streaks. *E,* These hypopigmented reticulated lesions on the leg of this child's mother represent old scars from areas of resolved hyperpigmentation.

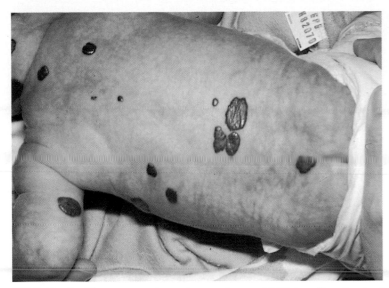

FIG. 8-91   Capillary or strawberry hemangiomas. Multiple soft, red, raised lesions dot the back and arms of this otherwise healthy 1-month-old.

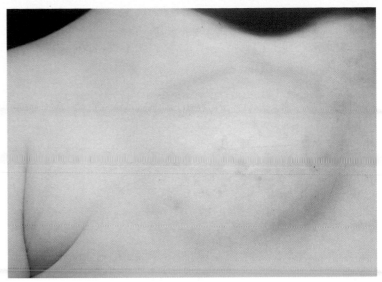

FIG. 8-92   Cavernous hemangioma. The vessels that make up this large, partially compressible lesion are deep beneath the skin surface but still impart a bluish hue to the overlying skin. Note the indistinctness of the margins.

nosis. Treatment is symptomatic and supportive. Genetic counseling is advisable.

Incontinentia Pigmenti

Incontinentia pigmenti (IP) is an X-linked, dominant disorder that affects the skin and may also involve the central nervous system, eyes, and skeletal system. It is seen predominantly in females and thus is thought to be fatal to males in utero. Clinically the disorder may present in any of three general phases, with some overlap. In the first phase, inflammatory vesicles or bullae appear initially on the trunk and extremities usually within the first 2 weeks of life (Fig. 8-90, *A*). New blisters then develop over the ensuing 3 months. At this stage a skin biopsy shows characteristic inflammation with intraepidermal eosinophils. Before the blistering phase ends, the second phase, marked by development of irregular, warty papules, supervenes (Fig. 8-90, *B*). These lesions resolve spontaneously within several months. A characteristic swirling or streaking pattern of brown to bluish-gray pigmentation on the trunk or extremities marks the third phase (Fig. 8-90, *C* and *D*). These pigmented whorls are usually located in different areas than those involved in the first two phases. The pigmentation lasts for many years and then gradually fades, leaving subtle, streaky, hypopigmented scars that may be the only residual cutaneous findings seen in affected mothers (Fig. 8-90, *E*), who should be carefully examined for these markers of IP.

A number of other systemic manifestations affecting various body systems are seen in patients with IP. Of IP patients, 30% have central nervous system abnormalities such as seizures, mental retardation, and spasticity. Ophthalmic complications, including strabismus, cataracts, blindness, and microphthalmia, are seen in 35% of IP patients. Pegged teeth and delayed dentition are seen in 65%. Cardiac and skeletal malformations also have been reported.

Differential diagnosis of IP in the blistering stage includes herpes simplex, bullous impetigo, and EB. Warts or epidermal nevi may mimic the warty phase. The swirled pigmentation of the third phase is very characteristic and not likely to be confused with other hyperpigmentation disorders. No specific therapy is required for IP, but genetic counseling is advisable.

Hemangiomas

Congenital vascular malformations termed *hemangiomas* are the most common neoplasms of childhood, occurring in 10% to 40% of all newborns. These lesions arise when islands of angioblastic tissue fail to reestablish normal communication with the vascular system. Hemangiomas can be divided into two groups—raised and flat—depending on their architecture. Although family members may be affected, hemangiomas are not thought to be inherited.

Hemangiomas: Capillary and Cavernous

The skin overlying a capillary hemangioma (sometimes called a *"Strawberry hemangioma"*) is usually normal or slightly red at birth. However, within the first few months of life there is marked vascular overgrowth resulting in bright red discoloration and definite elevation above the surrounding skin surface (Fig. 8-91). Lesions are soft, compressible, and usually range in size from 0.5 to 4 cm, although they can be much larger.

The vessels that comprise cavernous hemangiomas, another of the palpable forms, are located deep beneath the surface of the skin and appear bluish in color (Fig. 8-92). The borders of the lesion are usually indistinct, and it feels like a doughy mass that is only partially compressible. When placed in a dependent position, cavernous heman-

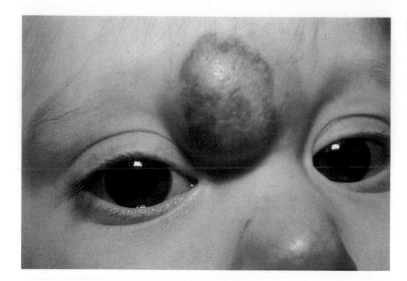

FIG. 8-93 Mixed hemangioma. The hemangioma on this child's nasal bridge has both capillary and cavernous components.

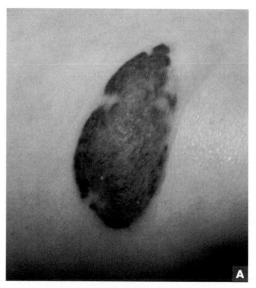
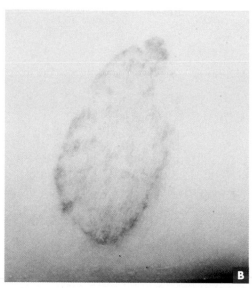
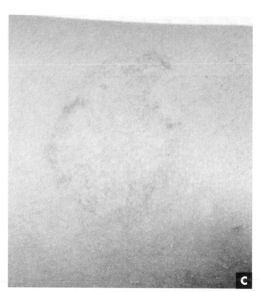

FIG. 8-94 Natural history of a capillary hemangioma. After growing for approximately 1 year, raised hemangiomas gradually involute. *A,* Appearance at 5 months. *B,* At 2 years. *C,* Almost total resolution at 5 years.

giomas enlarge as they fill with blood—a finding that helps differentiate them clinically from lymphangiomas. Combined capillary and cavernous hemangiomas are common as well (Fig. 8-93).

The natural history of raised hemangiomas is one of rapid growth for approximately 1 year, followed by a plateau period during which the lesion remains the same size. This is then followed by a period of slow involution (Fig. 8-94). Of raised hemangiomas, 50% disappear by age 7, and 90% are gone by age 9. In 40% of patients, the skin overlying the resolved lesion shows mild redundancy with telangiectasis.

Given the natural history of involution, watchful waiting is the best clinical approach unless the hemangioma involves a vital structure. Steroids or surgical intervention may be indicated if the lesion is life threatening (e.g., involves the airway) or interferes with vital functions (e.g., vision). Yellow pulsed dye laser therapy shows promising results. Complications such as ulceration, bleeding, or infection occur infrequently. Ulceration, which frequently hastens resolution of the lesion as it heals, can be treated with wet compresses and topical antibacterial ointments.

Vascular Malformations

Port Wine Stains

Port wine stains, named for their purplish-red color, are vascular malformations present at birth. Unlike capillary and cavernous hemangiomas, these lesions do not enlarge but tend to remain stable and flat. However, in adults, small angiomatous papules may develop within the lesion over time. The discoloration is due to permanent dilation of mature capillaries. Most commonly these lesions are located unilaterally on the face (Fig. 8-95). Port wine stains involving an extremity may be associated with local overgrowth of soft tissue and bone because of the abnormally rich blood supply. This results in hemihypertrophy, a phenomenon called the *Klippel-Trenaunay-Weber* syndrome. When a port wine stain involves the ophthalmic branch of the fifth cranial (trigeminal) nerve, it can be associated with vascular malformations of the ipsilateral meninges and cerebral cortex, a constellation termed the *Sturge-Weber syndrome.* Seizures, mental retardation, hemiplegia, and glaucoma are associated features (see Chapter 15).

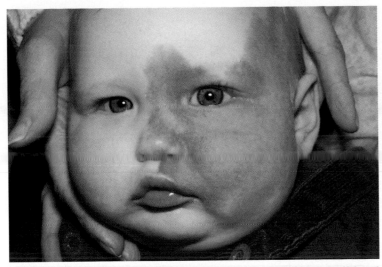

FIG. 8-95 Port wine stain. This infant has a characteristic purplish-red lesion covering nearly half of his face.

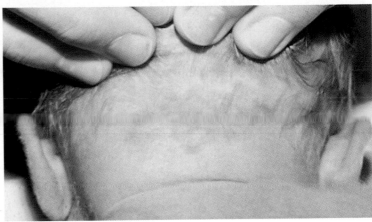

FIG. 8-96 Stork bite, or salmon patch. A typical, light red splotchy area is seen at the nape of the neck.

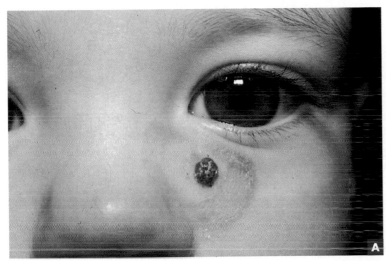

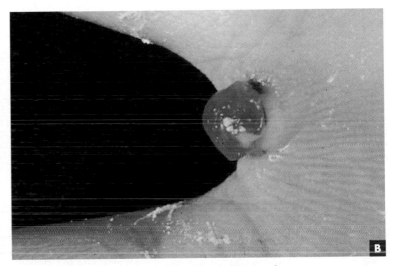

FIG. 8-97 Pyogenic granuloma. *A,* A raised hemorrhagic papule developed on this infant's cheek. *B,* Another rapidly growing, friable lesion is present between this child's fingers.

Salmon Patch (Stork Bite)

Another type of vascular malformation is the salmon patch (Fig. 8-96). This lesion is a normal variant seen in 40% of newborns and is usually located at the nape of the neck, the glabella, forehead, or upper eyelids. The patches represent distended capillaries and tend to fade within the first year of life. They may become more apparent during episodes of crying, breath-holding, or physical exertion.

Pyogenic Granuloma

Pyogenic granuloma is a common, benign, vascular tumor that resembles a small hemangioma. It is thought to be due to vascular overgrowth of granulation tissue after trauma or reaction to a foreign body such as a thorn, splinter, or piece of glass. It is seen in children and young adults, usually located on the face or an extremity, although on occasion the trunk and mucous membranes may be involved. Lesions are solitary, bright red, soft nodules that are often pedunculated. They average 5 to 6 mm in diameter; the surface is friable and bleeds easily

(Fig. 8-97, *A* and *B*). The rapid growth characteristic of these tumors can cause them to be confused with malignancies such as melanomas. Treatment consists of electrodesiccation of the blood vessels at the base. The lesion occasionally recurs, in which case repeat surgery is recommended.

Nevi and Melanomas

Nevomelanocytic nevus is a term used to describe a group of congenital and acquired pigmented lesions located in the dermis, which contain nevus cells derived from the neural crest. These nevus cells, like melanocytes in the epidermis, have the ability to synthesize melanin. The term *nevus* also refers to a group of congenital skin lesions composed of mature or nearly mature cutaneous elements organized in an abnormal fashion. Also known as hamartomas, these lesions may be comprised of almost any epidermal or dermal structures.

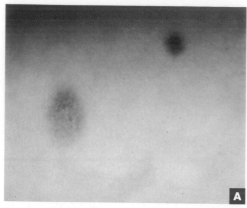

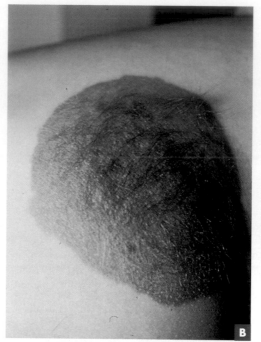

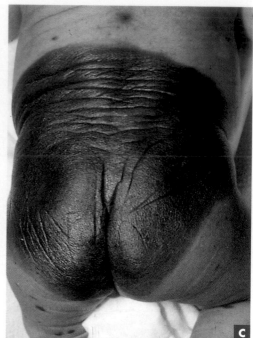

FIG. 8-98 Congenital nevomelanocytic nevi. *A,* Two small nevi with differing degrees of hyper-pigmentation seen on the thigh of this infant. *B,* During adolescence this nevus developed prominent hair and dark pigmented macules and papules within the borders of this congenital nevus. *C,* The giant nevus seen in this infant, covering the lower back and buttocks, is uniformly pigmented and has smaller satellite nevi.

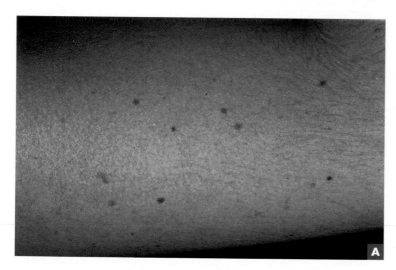

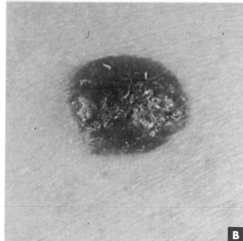

FIG. 8-99 Acquired nevomelanocytic nevi. *A,* Junctional nevi. These brown macules are flat on palpation. *B,* This typical compound nevus is raised, with a regular border and uniform pigmentation.

Nevomelanocytic Nevi

Congenital Nevomelanocytic Nevi

Congenital forms of nevomelanocytic nevi (CNN) consist of pigmented plaques often associated with dense hair growth. At birth, lesions may be tan or light pink, with only soft vellus hairs (Fig. 8-98, *A*). During infancy and childhood, the nevus darkens; the hair becomes more prominent; and small, dark macules or nodules may appear within the larger plaque (Fig. 8-98, *B*).

Giant CNNs covering large areas of skin (usually greater than 20 cm) are associated with a 2% to 15% lifetime risk of progression to melanoma (Fig. 8-98, *C*). Early treatment is recommended and consists of full-thickness excision followed by grafting. Some very large nevi may not be amenable to surgical management, however, and thus require impeccably close observation (facilitated by regular comparative photographs at 6- to 12-month intervals). Regular examinations should include careful palpation of the entire lesion because melanomas may arise deep within the nevus without visible surface change.

Small CNNs also may be associated with a higher than normal risk of developing melanoma, but the actual incidence is unknown. To date, there are no uniformly accepted guidelines for treatment. However, all CNNs must be differentiated from other congenital pigmented spots such as urticaria pigmentosa, lentigines, café-au-lait spots, and Mongolian spots.

Acquired Nevomelanocytic Nevi

Nevomelanocytic nevi acquired after birth are often referred to as *moles.* These begin to develop in early childhood as small, pigmented macules 1 to 2 mm in diameter, which are flat on palpation. At this stage, the nevus cells are limited to the epidermal-dermal junction and are called *junctional nevi* (Fig. 8-99, *A*). They then enlarge slowly and become papular or even pedunculated. In such elevated nevi, the nevus cells have proliferated into the dermis to become either intradermal or compound nevi (Fig. 8-99, *B*). During puberty, these lesions may darken noticeably and increase in size. However, normal nevomelanocytic nevi rarely exceed 1 cm in diameter. They tend to be located on sun-exposed areas and are seen less frequently on the soles, palms, legs, genitalia, and mucous membranes. Generally, nevi change slowly over months to years and warrant only observation.

Sudden enlargement of a nevus with redness and tenderness may occur because of infection of a hair follicle within the nevus or the rupture of a follicular cyst with acute foreign body inflammation. This may alarm the patient and necessitate dermatologic evaluation. Another,

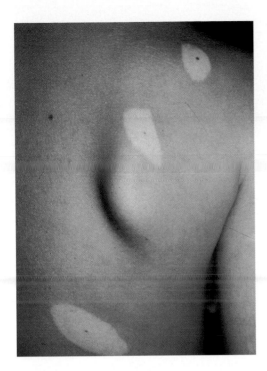

FIG. 8-100 Halo nevi. Large hypopigmented halos surround three relatively small nevi on the back of this boy.

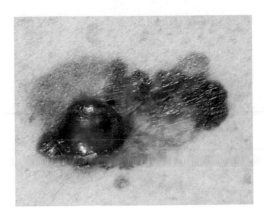

FIG. 8-101 Melanoma. This lesion shows the irregularity of outline, color, and thickness typical of a melanoma.

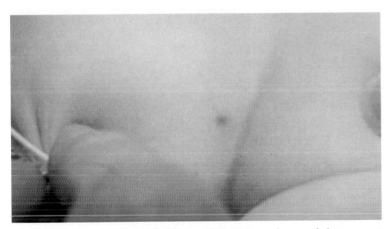

FIG. 8-102 Blue nevus. This blue nodule was made up of deep nevus cells; it was firm on palpation.

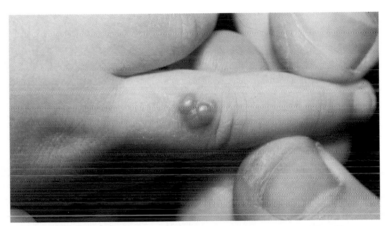

FIG. 8-103 Spitz nevus. This raised, red nevus grows rapidly.

slower change causing concern in patients is the appearance of a hypopigmented ring and mild local pruritus around a benign nevus. This is called a halo nevus (Fig. 8-100), and it is caused by a cytotoxic T-lymphocyte reaction against both the nevus cells and the innocent melanocytic bystanders. As a result, the nevus tends to disappear partially or completely, and the halo eventually repigments.

Nevi and Melanomas

As long as the clinical appearance of a nevus is typical, excision is unnecessary. However, a number of changes in pigmented lesions may portend the development of melanoma (Fig. 8-101). These include the following:

1. A change in size, shape, or outline, with scalloped, irregular borders
2. A change in the surface characteristics, such as development of a small, dark, elevated papule or nodule within an otherwise flat plaque; flaking, scaling, ulceration, or bleeding
3. A change in color, with the appearance of black; brown; or mixing of red, white, or blue
4. Burning, itching, or tenderness, which may be an indication of the body's immune reaction to malignancy

Fortunately, melanomas are still very rare in children. However, their incidence is increasing, and curative treatment is contingent on early diagnosis and prompt excision. A keen awareness of diagnostic features is important.

Melanomas in children may occur *de novo*, or they may develop within a giant congenital nevus, the latter being the most common source of this condition in children. Another cause of melanoma in the pediatric age group is transplacental transfer of maternal melanoma. Thus neonates born to mothers with a history of melanoma should be examined and followed carefully. Conversely, mothers of infants born with melanoma should be examined thoroughly for signs of the malignancy.

Differential diagnosis of childhood melanoma includes congenital and acquired nevocytic nevi; the blue nevus, a small, firm, blue papule consisting of deep nevus cells (Fig. 8-102); traumatic hemorrhage, especially under the nails or in mucous membranes; vascular lesions, such as pyogenic granuloma or angiokeratoma; and the Spitz nevus (benign juvenile melanoma), a red and rapidly growing nevocytic nevus (Fig. 8-103) that can be confused clinically and histologically with melanoma.

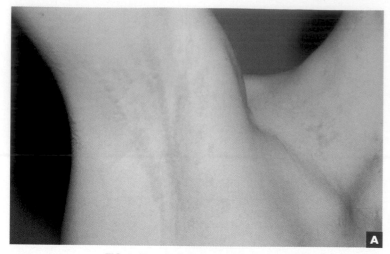
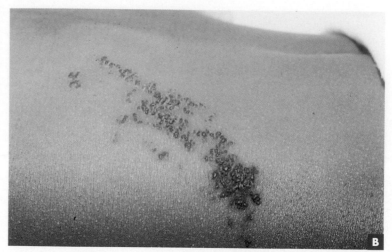

FIG. 8-104   Epidermal nevi. *A,* Light color in whites. *B,* Darker color in blacks. More extensive nevi may be associated with systemic abnormalities (epidermal nevus syndrome).

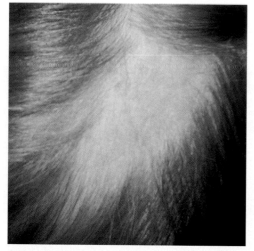

FIG. 8-105   Nevus sebaceous of Jadassohn. This yellowish, hairless plaque was present at birth.

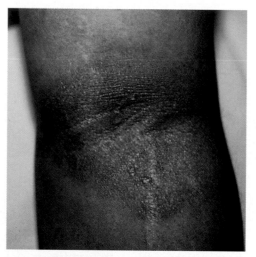

FIG. 8-106   Postinflammatory hyperpigmentation. This arose after chronic atopic dermatitis and trauma from persistent scratching.

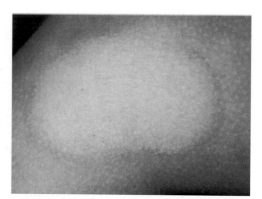

FIG. 8-107   Postinflammatory hypopigmentation. This reaction followed chronic dermatitis. Note the narrow rim of hyperpigmentation at the margin.

Hamartomatous Nevi

Hamartomatous nevi can be comprised of epidermal structures, hair follicles (nevus pilosis), apocrine and eccrine glands (apocrine and eccrine nevi), fibroblasts (connective tissue nevi), blood vessels (salmon patch, Fig. 8-96), and multiple components (nevus sebaceous).

Epidermal nevi are common in pediatric patients. They are composed of epidermal structures only and must be distinguished from nevus sebaceous (see following paragraph). The lesion may be present at birth or may develop during childhood and appears as a slightly hyperpigmented papillomatous or verrucous growth (Fig. 8-104, *A* and *B*). Verrucous changes are particularly common at puberty. It may be small and localized, linear, dermatomal, or generalized. The numerous clinical presentations are reflected in the number of descriptive synonyms: nevus verrucosus for localized disease, nevus unius lateralis for linear or unilateral involvement, and ichthyosis hystrix for bilateral involvement with irregular geometric patterns. Important associations with extensive epidermal nevi are seizures, mental retardation, and ocular and skeletal defects (see Chapter 15).

Nevus sebaceous of Jadassohn is characterized by a hairless, well-circumscribed, skin-colored or yellowish plaque located on the scalp, face, or neck (Fig. 8-105). The lesion is usually solitary and may be linear or round. It is present at birth, although at puberty, the plaque may become more verrucous, raised, and nodular (see Chapter 15). Histologically, epidermal proliferation is seen along with abortive hair follicles, sebaceous glands and apocrine structures. Approximately 10% to 15% of these nevi develop into secondary neoplasms, the most common being basal cell carcinoma, although other appendageal tumors have been reported. Long-term regular observation or prophylactic full-thickness excision is necessary.

Disorders of Pigmentation

Childhood disorders of pigmentation are usually of cosmetic importance only, although some pigmented lesions are markers of multisystem disease.

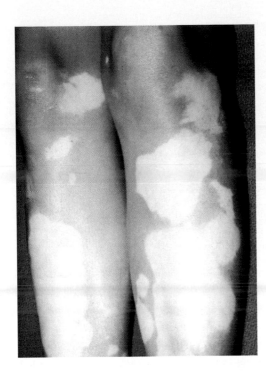

FIG. 8-108 Vitiligo. Completely depigmented patches are seen on the legs. Occasionally, macules of repigmentation arise from epidermal apendages within the white patches. A characteristic distribution helps to distinguish vitiligo from other causes of hypopigmentation.

Postinflammatory Pigmentary Changes

The most common pigmentation disorder is postinflammatory hyperpigmentation (Fig. 8-106) or hypopigmentation (Fig. 8-107). This follows inflammatory disorders of the skin, such as dermatitis, infection, or injury, and usually resolves spontaneously over a few months. Histologically, melanocytes are normal in these areas, although the dispersion of melanin and pigment to other cells is disturbed. Tinea versicolor may also present as hypopigmented patches covered with a fine scale, but KOH examination confirms the correct diagnosis by demonstrating typical "spaghetti and meatballs" organisms (Figs. 8-37 and 8-38). Postinflammatory hypopigmentation must be distinguished from vitiligo, in which there is a complete absence of pigment and usually no associated scaling or history of inflammation.

Vitiligo

In vitiligo (Fig. 8-108) there is a complete loss of pigmentation. Lesions are macular and usually are seen in a characteristic distribution around the eyes, mouth, genitals, elbows, hands, and feet. Spontaneous but slow repigmentation may occur in areas beginning around the openings of hair follicles, resulting in a speckled appearance. Histologically, melanocytes are absent in areas of vitiligo, and evidence suggests that they are destroyed by an autoimmune mechanism.

Ash Leaf Spots

White oval macules, termed *ash leaf spots* because of their shape, are a valuable early marker of tuberous sclerosis. These appear at birth or shortly thereafter as 1- to 3-cm macular lesions on the trunk. They are not as sharply demarcated or ivory white as the lesions of vitiligo, and their truncal distribution is different (see Chapter 15).

The identification of ash leaf macules may be enhanced, particularly in lightly pigmented individuals, by the use of a Wood light; this method of examination should be part of the assessment of any child who develops idiopathic seizures in infancy. The visible purple light emitted is absorbed by normal melanin in the skin. In a darkened room, areas of hypopigmentation or depigmentation appear bright violet, whereas normally melanized skin reflects little visible light and appears dull purple or black. In addition to tuberous sclerosis, Wood light examination also may be helpful in delineating the full extent of pigmentary changes in vitiligo and postinflammatory hypopigmentation.

Albinism

The term *albinism* refers to a heterogenous group of inherited disorders characterized by congenital hypopigmentation of the skin, eyes, and hair. It occurs in an X-linked ocular form (in which the skin appears clinically normal) and an autosomal recessive oculocutaneous form. In oculocutaneous albinism (OCA), both sexes and all races are affected equally. This form of the disorder is subdivided into a number of variants based on clinical findings and biochemical markers. Tyrosinase-negative and tyrosinase-positive subtypes have been identified based on the ability of plucked hairs to produce pigment when incubated in tyrosine. In classic tyrosinase-negative OCA, children are born without any trace of pigment. Affected individuals have snow-white hair, pinkish-white skin, and translucent or blue irises. Nystagmus is common, as is moderate to severe strabismus and poor visual acuity (see Chapter 19). Although children with tyrosinase-positive OCA may be clinically indistinguishable from their tyrosinase-negative counterparts at birth, they usually develop variable amounts of pigment with increasing age. Eye color may vary from gray to light brown, and hair may change to blond or light brown. Most black patients acquire as much pigment as light-skinned whites.

Because they lack the protection of melanin, patients with OCA are at high risk for early development of basal cell and squamous cell skin cancers. Hence they should be instructed in use of sunscreens and avoidance of excessive sun exposure.

Piebaldism

Piebaldism (partial albinism) is a rare autosomal dominant disorder characterized by a white forelock and a circumscribed congenital leukoderma. The typical lesions include a triangular patch of depigmentation and white hair on the frontal scalp. The apex of this patch points toward the nasal bridge (Fig. 8-109, *A*), and the patient may show hypopigmented or depigmented macules on the face, neck, ventral trunk, flanks, or extremities (Fig. 8-109, *B*). Within areas of decreased pigmentation, scattered patches of normal pigmentation or hyperpigmentation may appear. The lesions are stable throughout life, although some variability in pigmentation may occur with sun exposure. Special variants of piebaldism include Waardenburg syndrome, in which leukoderma is associated with lateral displacement of the inner canthi and inferior lacrimal ducts, a flattened nasal bridge, and sensorineural deafness, and Wolf syndrome, an autosomal recessive disorder associated with neurologic deficits.

Other Pigmentary Disorders

Café-au-lait spots are tan macules that can be an indication of neurofibromatosis (von Recklinghausen disease, see Chapter 15) or Albright syndrome, in which they are associated with polyostotic dysplasia. Most café-au-lait spots, however, occur in otherwise healthy individuals and vary from a few millimeters to over 10 cm in size. Borders are discrete but may be smooth or irregular. Swirled hyperpigmentation may be a marker of incontinentia pigmenti (Fig. 8-90, *C* and *D*), and diffuse hyperpigmentation may be seen in Addison disease and hemochromatosis. Peutz-Jeghers syndrome is manifest by lentigo-like pig-

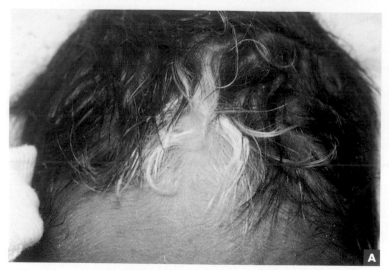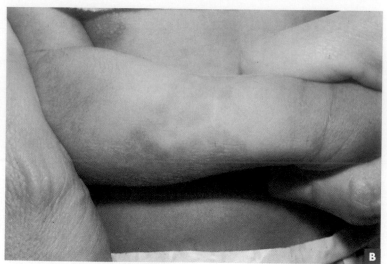

FIG. 8-109   Piebaldism. *A,* A white forelock overlies a depigmented patch of scalp and forehead. *B,* This infant also has a hypopigmented patch on his arm in which smaller areas of hyperpigmentation are seen.

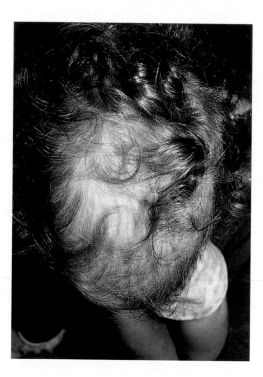

FIG. 8-110   Telogen effluvium. This toddler experienced sudden partial hair loss approximately 3 months after being hospitalized for pneumococcal sepsis. (Courtesy Dr. Alejandro Hoberman, Children's Hospital of Pittsburgh.)

mentation of the lips (see Chapter 17), oral mucosa, hands, and fingers and benign, small-intestinal polyps in children (see Chapter 10).

Disorders of the Hair and Nails

Diseases of the hair and nails make up an integral part of pediatric dermatology. Both hair and nails are composed of keratin produced by the epidermal hair follicles and the nail matrix. Some diseases are specific to these structures, whereas others affect the skin as well. In many cases important diagnostic clues to skin disease can be found in related abnormalities of the hair and nails.

The Alopecias

The most common diseases of the hair result in some degree of hair loss, or alopecia. Evaluation begins by determining whether scarring is

present. Nonscarring alopecia can be caused by growth defects causing the hair to be lost by the roots (effluvium) or by defects of the hair shaft causing breakage.

Alopecia Caused by Systemic Insult: Telogen and Anagen Effluvium

Normal hair cycles through a growth phase lasting 3 years or more (anagen phase) and a resting phase of 3 months (telogen phase), after which the hair is shed. The cycle then begins again. Telogen effluvium is one form of partial, temporary alopecia seen 3 months after a severe illness, surgery, or high fever. It rarely causes more than 50% hair loss. The initial systemic insult induces more than the usual 20% of hairs to enter the telogen phase, and 3 months later these hairs are shed simultaneously, producing marked thinning of scalp hair until new anagen hairs regrow (Fig. 8-110). Anagen effluvium is the sudden loss of the growing hairs (80% of normal scalp hairs) caused by the abnormal cessation of the anagen phase. The hair shafts taper and lose adhesion to the follicle. This type of hair loss is most common after systemic chemotherapy.

Alopecia Areata

Alopecia areata is a form of localized anagen effluvium presenting with round patches of alopecia that may be located anywhere on the scalp, eyebrows, lashes, or body. Occasionally, hair loss is diffuse or generalized. The injury causing cessation of growth is thought to be of immunologic origin. Clues to diagnosis include absence of inflammation and scaling in the involved areas of scalp, and the presence of short (3 to 6 mm), easily epilated hairs at the margins of the patch (Fig. 8-111, *A* and *B*). Under magnification these hair stubs resemble exclamation points because the hair shaft narrows just before its point of entry into the follicle. Another finding in many patients with alopecia areata is Scotch-plaid pitting of the nails, consisting of rows of pits crossing in a transverse and longitudinal fashion (Fig. 8-123). The clinical course of alopecia areata is difficult to predict. The disorder may resolve spontaneously; it may persist, with the appearance of new patches while the old patches regrow; or it may progress to total scalp or even generalized alopecia (alopecia totalis) that can be permanent (Fig. 8-111, *C*).

Trauma-Induced Alopecia
Trichorrhexis Nodosa
Alopecia caused by hair shaft breakage is due to a structural defect of the hair, and it is easily diagnosed by microscopic examination. The

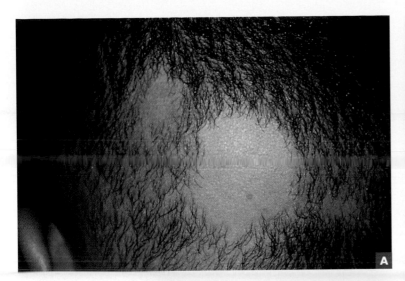

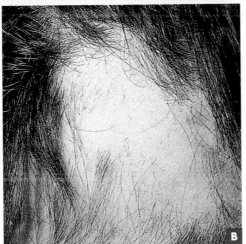

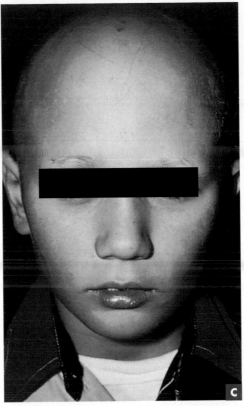

FIG. 8-111 Alopecia areata. *A,* Patches of complete hair loss with otherwise normal scalp are typical of this disorder. *B,* In this close-up, small broken hairs that pull out easily are seen at the margins. *C,* In this boy the disorder has progressed to alopecia totalis. Note that his eyebrows are involved as well. (*C* Courtesy Dr. Michael Sherlock.)

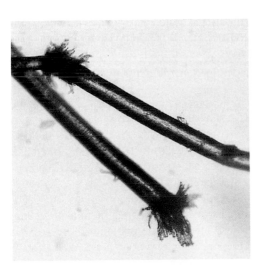

FIG. 8-112 Trichorrhexis nodosa. A brittle hair shaft defect usually caused by overmanipulation of the hair or chemical use. The frayed brown appearance is typical.

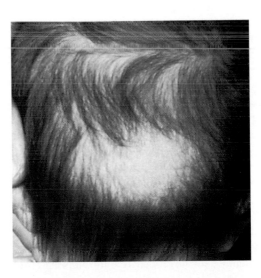

FIG. 8-113 Friction alopecia. Hair loss of the occiput resulted from rubbing of the head on sheets and pillows.

most common structural defect is acquired trichorrhexis nodosa. This defect presents at any age as brittle, short hairs that are perceived by the patient as nongrowing. On gentle pulling, many hairs are easily broken. Microscopically the distal ends of the hairs are frayed, resembling a broom (Fig. 8-112). Other hairs may have nodules, resembling two brooms stuck together. The fragility is caused by damage to the outer cortex of the hair shaft, resulting in a loss of structural support. Without this support, the weaker fibrous medulla frays like an electrical cord with broken insulation. This disorder is most common in blacks, arising from the trauma of combing tightly curled hairs. It is also seen after repeated or severe chemical damage to the cortex from hair straight-

eners, bleaches, and permanents. Because hair growth is normal, the disorder is self-limited and normal hairs regrow when the source of the damage is eliminated.

Other common causes of hair loss associated with shaft abnormalities include friction alopecia, traction alopecia, and trichotillomania. All are caused by external trauma and breakage of an otherwise normal hair shaft.

Friction Alopecia

Friction alopecia (Fig. 8-113) is common on the posterior scalp of infants, where the head rubs on the pillow or bed clothes. Although worrisome to parents, this disorder is self-limited. When severe or long-

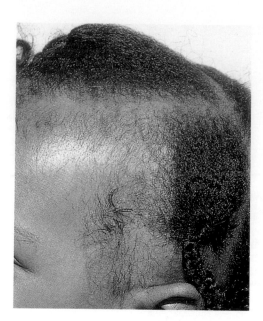

FIG. 8-114 Traction alopecia. The hair thinning and loss is due to excessive traction on the hairs as a result of tight braiding.

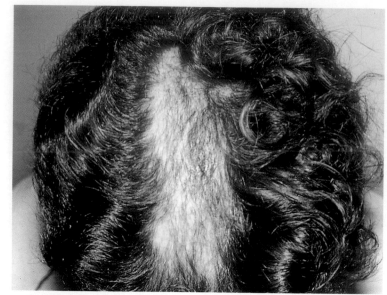

FIG. 8-115 Trichotillomania. This linear patch of sort broken hairs is typical of hair pulling.

standing, it should raise the question of neglect, suggesting that the infant is being left to lie in his or her crib for extended periods of time.

Traction Alopecia

Traction alopecia (Fig. 8-114) is common in young girls whose hairstyles, such as ponytails, pigtails, braids, or cornrows, maintain a tight pull on the hair shafts. This traction causes shaft fractures and follicular damage; if prolonged, permanent scarring alopecia can result.

Trichotillomania

Trichotillomania is a fairly common disorder seen in school-age children and adolescents that mimics many other types of alopecia. It presents with bizarre patterns of hair loss, often in broad, linear bands on the vertex or sides of the scalp where the hair is easily twisted and pulled out (Fig. 8-115). Rarely the entire scalp, eyebrows, and eyelashes are involved. The most important clue is the finding of short, broken-off hairs along the scalp, with stubs of different lengths in adjacent areas. This is caused by repetitive pulling and/or twisting of the hair, which fractures the longer shafts. Once broken, the hairs are too short to be rebroken until they grow longer.

Trichotillomania is often confused with alopecia areata because there are patches of hair loss with short hairs and involvement of the eyebrows and eyelashes. However, in trichotillomania, patches of hair loss are never completely bald, and the hair shafts are normal anagen hairs that are usually difficult to remove from the scalp. In addition, there are no associated nail abnormalities.

Parents and children usually deny vigorously that the alopecia could be caused by the child, and thus diagnosis rests on a high index of suspicion and recognition of the clinical findings. Although trichotillomania may occur in children with severe psychiatric disease, most cases are associated with situational stress (e.g., school phobia, marital or social problems) or habitual behavior.

Scarring Alopecia

Scarring alopecia in children is less common than nonscarring alopecia and may be caused by a number of disorders. Aplasia cutis congenita is an ulceration of the vertex of the scalp of a newborn that heals with a hairless scar. Morphea (localized scleroderma) may involve the scalp with indurated, hairless plaques. Scarring alopecia may also result from severe infection (e.g., inflammatory tinea capitis) or trauma, such as oil burns from hot-comb straightening of the hair. A scalp biopsy is often helpful in determining the cause of scarring alopecia.

Tinea Capitis Infections of the Hair and Scalp

Fungal infection of the hair weakens the shaft, causing breakage. This typically results in the development of multiple patches of partial alopecia. *Trichophyton tonsurans* is the organism responsible for over 95% of the scalp ringworm in the United States. For unknown reasons, infection is endemic among black school children, although it is occasionally found in whites. *Microsporum canis* (the dog and cat ringworm) accounts for a few cases of tinea capitis and shows no racial predilection.

There are a variety of clinical presentations of tinea capitis. In some patients, mild erythema and scaling of the scalp occur in association with partial alopecia (Fig. 8-116, A). In other cases, infection by endothrix, which invades the hair shafts, causes widespread breakage at the scalp creating a "salt-and-pepper" appearance, with the short residual hairs appearing as black dots on the surface of the scalp (Fig. 8-116, B). Occasionally, scalp lesions are annular, simulating tinea corporis. In yet other children, sensitization to the infecting organism results in more erythema, edema, and pustule formation. As the latter rupture, the area weeps and golden crusts form, simulating impetigo (Fig. 8-116, C). Some cases are characterized by patches of heaped-up scale in association with small pustules (Fig. 8-116, D). Less commonly, intense inflammation causes formation of raised, tender, boggy plaques or masses studded with pustules that simulate abscesses, termed *kerions* (Fig. 8-116, E). Unless treated promptly and aggressively with oral antifungal agents and in severe cases steroids, the latter may produce scarring and permanent hair loss. Incision and drainage are not indicated because loculations are small and septae thick. The more inflammatory forms are often associated with occipital, postauricular, and posterior cervical adenopathy. When pustules or weeping and crusting lesions involve the scalp or hairline, the infection is far more likely to be of fungal than bacterial origin.

Fungal infection of the scalp is readily confirmed by a KOH examination of infected hairs (Fig. 8-117). Hairs should be pulled from the

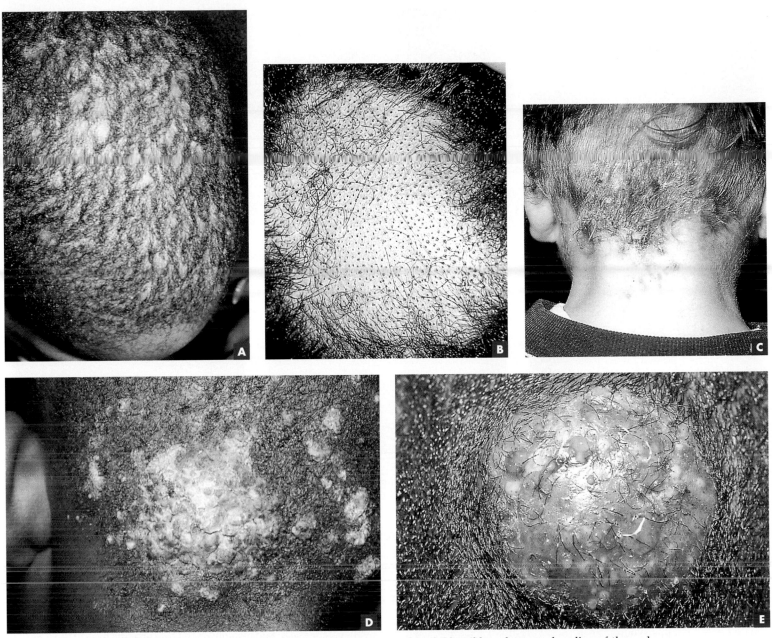

FIG. 8-116 Tinea capitis can present in many guises. *A,* In this child, mild erythema and scaling of the scalp are associated with spotty alopecia. *B,* Infiltration of hair shafts by endothrix has resulted in widespread breakage at the scalp, producing a "salt-and-pepper" appearance. *C,* Superficial papules and pustules have ruptured, producing a weeping, crusting lesion simulating impetigo. *D,* This variant of tinea is characterized by thick heaped-up scale. *E,* Kerion. A boggy mass has formed as a result of an intense inflammatory response. This child, seen relatively late in the course, had total alopecia over the involved area. Note that the lesion is studded with pustules.

scalp rather than cut so that the root is available for examination as well. A Wood light may also be useful in certain patients. Formerly, its most common use was in screening patients for fungal alopecia because the then-most-common causative organism, *Microsporum audouinii,* was easily identified by its fluorescence under Wood light. Today, *Trichophyton tonsurans,* which does not fluoresce, is the most common causative organism in the United States. Currently, only *M. canis,* which causes 5% of cases, fluoresces bright bluish-green.

Topical antifungal agents do not penetrate deeply enough to be effective in treatment of tinea capitis. Hence, oral antifungal agents (griseofulvin or ketoconazole) are administered over 2 to 4 months. This usually eradicates the infection. However, the risk of recurrence is high. Concurrent use of selenium sulfide shampoo (2.5%) reduces spore formation and shedding and thus may help minimize the risk of spread to siblings and classmates until oral treatment is complete.

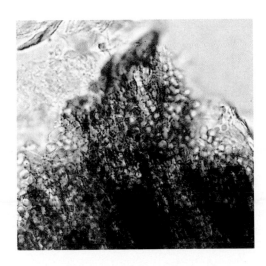

FIG. 8-117 Microscopic appearance of hair shafts infected with fungi. Note the tight packing of fungal arthrospores that cause hair shaft fragility and breakage (KOH mount for endothrix).

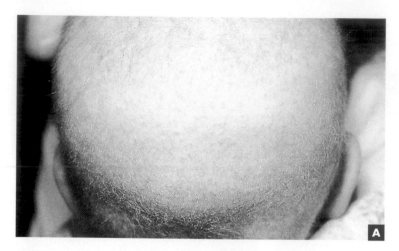

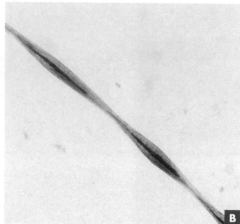

FIG. 8-118   Monilethrix. *A*, Short, broken hairs give the appearance of diffuse alopecia. *B*, Microscopically, periodic narrowing of this hair shaft is visible. Hairs are brittle and break off at constricted points near the scalp.

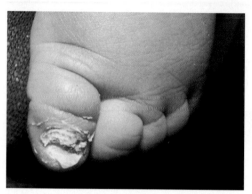

FIG. 8-119   Chronic paronychia with nail dystrophy caused by Candida infection.

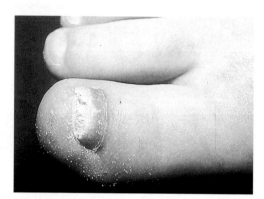

FIG. 8-120   Onychomycosis caused by a chronic dermatophyte infection of the nail plate in a 4-year-old boy. This is rare in prepubertal children.

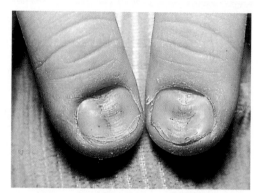

FIG. 8-121   Traumatic nail dystrophy. This teenager developed median nail dystrophy as a result of chronically picking at his nails.

Congenital and Genetic Disorders

Some structural defects of the hair shaft are congenital in origin or associated with heritable syndromes.

Monilethrix and Pili Torti

Monilethrix is a developmental hair defect that produces brittle, beaded hair. The condition is autosomal dominant, and clinical manifestations usually appear after 2 to 3 months of age, when the fetal or neonatal vellus hairs are replaced by abnormal beaded hairs (Fig. 8-118, *A*). The scalp is most severely affected, although hair on any part of the body can be involved. The disease is generally permanent. Microscopically there is regular, periodic narrowing of the hair shafts (Fig. 8-118, *B*). Breakage occurs in the constricted areas close to the scalp. Care must be taken not to confuse monilethrix with pili torti, another structural defect in which the hair shaft is twisted on its own axis. Pili torti may be localized or generalized and also appears with the first terminal hair growth of infancy. It may be associated with Menkes' kinky hair syndrome, an inherited defect of copper absorption, which also affects the central nervous, cardiovascular, and skeletal systems.

Disorders Affecting the Nails

Patients may seek the advice of a physician for nail disorders because of pain or cosmetic concerns. For the physician, knowledge of nail disorders is helpful in detecting clues to systemic disease.

Paronychia

Paronychia is a common childhood disorder. It presents as a red, swollen, tender nail fold, usually on the side or at the base of the nail. The acute form, with sudden swelling and marked tenderness, is often caused by bacterial invasion after trauma to the cuticle or after a dermatitis that has damaged the stratum corneum barrier (see Chapter 12). Chronic paronychia may involve one or several nails. There is usually an associated history of chronic dermatitis or frequent exposure to water. Tenderness is mild, and a small amount of pus can sometimes be extruded. There is often some degree of associated nail dystrophy (Fig. 8-119). The causative organisms are *Candida* species, usually *C. albicans*. This form resolves with the use of topical antimycotics and avoidance of water.

Onychomycosis and Nail Dystrophy

Onychomycosis, or fungal infection of the nail plate (Fig. 8-120), is rare in children before puberty. Thus nail dystrophy should not be treated as a fungal infection unless proven by microscopic examination or fungal culture. Dystrophic nails (Fig. 8-121) occur frequently as a complication of trauma or underlying dermatosis, such as psoriasis or atopic dermatitis.

Trauma

Trauma to the nail may cause subungual hemorrhage, resulting in a brownish-black discoloration. This is particularly likely following crush injuries. Usually the diagnosis is simple, unless trauma is subtle. When

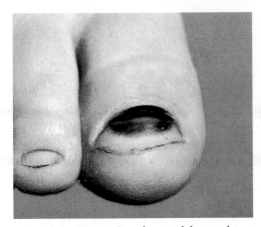

FIG. 8-122 Traumatic subungual hemorrhage. Discoloration because of traumatic hemorrhage under the toenail is common in children and athletic adults. It is a result of jamming the toe into the end of the shoe while running or stopping (turf toe).

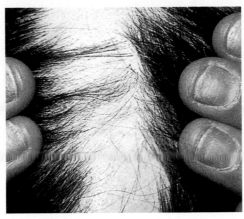

FIG. 8-123 Broad, shallow Scotch-plaid pitting of the nails associated with alopecia areata.

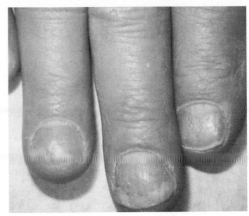

FIG. 8-124 Psoriatic nails. Psoriasis affecting the nails results in onycholysis and pitting.

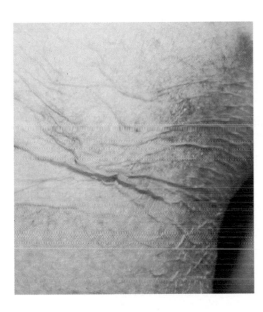

FIG. 8-125 Steroid-induced skin atrophy. Topical steroids may cause marked atrophy and fragility of the skin, especially if used under occlusion regularly for more than 1 month.

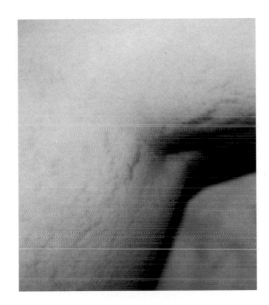

FIG. 8-126 Steroid-induced striae distensae. Prolonged use of potent fluorinated steroids may cause permanent striae distensae.

a large, painful hematoma is produced, this should be evacuated using electrocautery to relieve pain and reduce risk of infection. Pigmentation at the base of the great toenail, caused by jamming the toe into the end of the shoe at a sudden stop, is called *turf toe* and results in mild subungual hemorrhage (Fig. 8-122). This must be distinguished from melanoma. Hemorrhage can be identified by the presence of purplish-brown pigment in the distal nail and normal proximal outgrowth of the nail.

Nail Findings in Other Dermatologic Disorders

Nail disorders may provide clues to other dermatologic or pediatric syndromes. For example, alopecia areata is associated with a characteristic Scotch-plaid pitting of the nails (Fig. 8-123). Similarly, psoriasis affects the nails in a number of ways that may help to distinguish it from other scaling disorders. Psoriasis in the nail matrix results in scattered pits that are larger, deeper, and less numerous than those found in alopecia areata (Fig. 8-124). Psoriasis of the nail bed, especially under the distal nail, causes separation of the nail from the underlying skin (onycholysis) and oil-drop discoloration with heaped-up scaling. Onycholysis alone, without pits or discoloration, may be caused by

trauma, infection, nail-polish hardeners, or phototoxic reactions to drugs such as tetracycline.

Complications of Topical Skin Therapy

An important rule in medicine is "do no harm." To follow that rule, the physician must recognize the adverse effects of the therapies prescribed.

Topical Steroids

The most commonly used topical medications are steroids. These may be classified as high or low potency, according to their biological activity. Generally, fluorinated steroids are more potent than nonfluorinated steroids, and those in ointment bases are more active than those in cream or lotion bases. High-potency steroids should be used only for short periods of time or major side effects may develop. These side effects include skin atrophy (Fig. 8-125), telangiectases, and increased skin fragility; acneiform eruptions; permanent skin striae (Fig. 8-126);

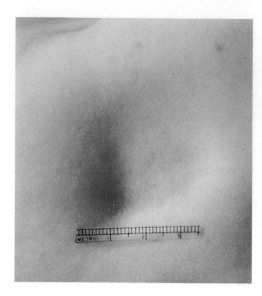

FIG. 8-127 Steroid-induced subcutaneous atrophy. Injection of steroids into fat instead of muscle often produces subcutaneous atrophy. Whereas in some cases this may resolve in 6 to 12 months, in others it can be permanent.

they develop. Further, all patients placed on high-dose steroids who have no past history of varicella should be alerted to return immediately for zoster immune globulin if they discover that they have been exposed to chickenpox.

Other Agents

Other complications from topical medications, such as contact dermatitis, can be easily prevented. Allergic contact dermatitis is frequently seen as a reaction to both prescribed and over-the-counter drugs. The most common allergens are neomycin, "-caine" topical anesthetics or antipruritics, and ethylenediamine (a preservative in many topical preparations). Anaphylaxis can occur even in response to topical medications, especially if applied to broken skin. Hence, obtaining a history of drug allergies is important before prescribing topical agents.

Fortunately, most complications of therapy can be avoided if the physician has clear knowledge of the disease, its treatment, and the pharmacologic agents being prescribed.

and masking or delayed recognition of infections and infestations such as tinea corporis and scabies.

Use of fluorinated steroids should be avoided on the face, genitals, or intertriginous areas because absorption is greater and side effects are more common. Accidental injection of steroids into fat on attempted intramuscular injection may cause permanent subcutaneous atrophy (Fig. 8-127). If the medication is applied to large areas, if the treated area is occluded, or if therapy is continued for a long period, adrenal suppression may result.

Secondary bacterial infections and viral infections such as chickenpox may also progress with unusual rapidity in children on widespread topical or systemic corticosteroids. Hence, patients should be instructed to look for early signs of secondary infection and return promptly if

BIBLIOGRAPHY

Hurwitz S: *Clinical pediatric dermatology*, Philadelphia, ed 2, 1981, WB Saunders.

Meneghini CL, Bonifazi E: *An atlas of pediatric dermatology*, Chicago, 1993, Year Book Medical Publishers.

Ruiz-Maldonado R, Parish LC, Beare JM: *Textbook of pediatric dermatology*, Philadelphia, 1989, Grune and Stratton.

Schachner LA, Hansen RC: *Pediatric dermatology*, ed 2, New York, 1995, Churchill Livingstone.

Weinberg S, Leider M, Shapiro L: *Color atlas of pediatric dermatology*, ed 2, London, 1990, McGraw-Hill.

Weston WL: *Practical pediatric dermatology*, Boston, ed 2, 1985, Little Brown.

9

Endocrinology

DAVID FINEGOLD

Clinical presentations of endocrine disease vary widely such that alterations in hormonal balance can result in children who are too fat, too thin, too short, too tall, or have distinctive dysmorphology. A steady discovery of new genes, mutations, and altered gene products has helped explain at the molecular level the clinical presentation of insufficient or excessive hormone secretion as well as altered hormone receptor activity. Despite the explosion of new information, the clinical presentations of abnormal endocrine states remain constant. The recognition of physical signs associated with these states continues to remain a cornerstone of correct diagnosis and treatment of these imbalances in the neuroendocrine axis. The following text emphasizes physical signs associated with normal endocrine maturation, as well as with states of hyposecretion and hypersecretion related to the neuroendocrine axis.

The Anterior Pituitary Gland

The human pituitary gland contains anterior and posterior regions that have substantially different functions. This chapter concentrates on the anterior section and its relationship to the release of hormones in endocrine glands. The anterior pituitary contains cells that secrete three types of hormones: corticotropin-related peptide hormones, glycoprotein hormones, and somatomammotropins. These compounds have great biologic potency and, with the exception of prolactin, are regulated through closed feedback loops and specific agonists and antagonists.

The **corticotropin-related peptide hormones** consist of adrenocorticotropic hormone (ACTH), alpha-melanocyte-stimulating hormone (α-MSH), and gamma- and beta-lipotropins (γ-LPH, β-LPH). These hormones are derived from a common precursor molecule, proopiomelanocortin, within whose amino-acid structure are contained their sequences. Within the subunit structure of β-LPH are the important neuroendocrine molecules alpha-, beta-, gamma-endorphin and enkephalin. After posttranslational processing from this large precursor molecule, the secretion of ACTH is regulated by the level of corticotropin-releasing factor (CRF) in the pituitary-portal plasma and by the level of plasma cortisol secreted from the adrenal gland, which has a negative feedback effect on further secretion of ACTH (Fig. 9-1). The relationship between ACTH and cortisol secretion has been well studied.

The **glycoprotein hormones** of the pituitary include follicle-stimulating hormone (FSH), luteinizing hormone (LH), and thyroid-stimulating hormone (TSH). Each of these hormones is composed of two dissimilar peptide subunits. The alpha chain is highly similar in structure among the three hormones. However, the beta chain is unique and confers specificity from one hormone to another. These three hormones also contain significant amounts of carbohydrate and sialic acid residues along with their basic amino acid structures. LH and FSH secretions are positively stimulated by gonadotropin-releasing hormone (GnRH).

The control of LH and FSH secretion is sensitive to the periodic nature of GnRH release. If GnRH periodicity is disturbed—either by increasing or decreasing the frequency of GnRH pulses or by continuously exposing the gonadotrophs to GnRH stimulation—LH and FSH secretion may be shut off. This knowledge has permitted the development of potent GnRH agonist analogues that are effective in the treatment of disorders such as central precocious puberty.

The primary action of FSH and LH is on the gonads. FSH directly stimulates gametogenesis in the testes and supports follicular development in the ovaries. LH stimulates Leydig cell function of the testes, producing testosterone, and acts to promote luteinization of the ovaries (Fig. 9-2). The negative feedback effect of sex steroids on LH and FSH production is dramatically emphasized in postmenopausal women, in young girls with Turner syndrome, or in patients with galactosemia, in whom marked elevations of these hormones occur. Inhibin is produced by the gonads and appears to inhibit FSH release.

TSH stimulates many aspects of thyroid function. These aspects include increasing the size of thyroid cells and the vascularity of the gland. Specific increases in the size of follicular epithelial cells and in the amount of colloid are easily determined. Moreover, TSH increases radioactive iodide uptake, thyroglobulin synthesis, and thyroxine and triiodothyronine release from the thyroid gland. Basic alterations in thyroid cell biochemistry also occur following TSH administration. The rate of TSH secretion appears to be determined by the level of circulating thyroid hormone and by the hypothalamic hormone, thyrotropin-releasing hormone (TRH). However, negative feedback of TSH secretion by circulating thyroid hormone occurs mainly at the pituitary level (Fig. 9-3).

The somatomammotropin hormones—**prolactin** (PRL) and **growth hormone** (GH)—have similar chemical structures and some overlap of their biologic activity. The amino acid sequences of both contain two or three disulfide bridges.

PRL acts directly on its target organs and does not require an intermediary secondary endocrine gland. PRL's only major function in humans is the initiation and maintenance of lactation. In contrast to the

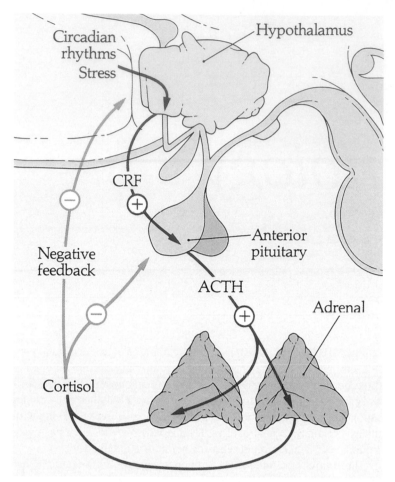

FIG. 9-1 Feedback regulation of ACTH at the level of the hypothalamus, pituitary, and adrenal glands.

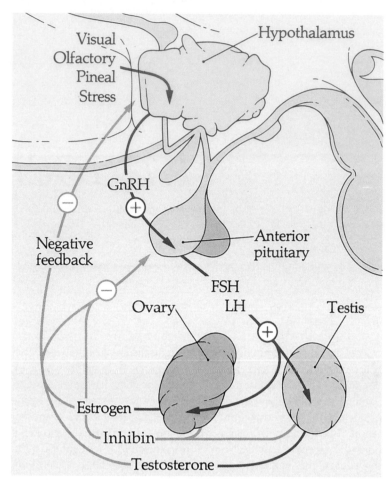

FIG. 9-2 Feedback regulation of LH and FSH at the level of the hypothalamus, pituitary, and gonads.

other anterior pituitary hormones, PRL appears to be under tonic stimulation. Chronic inhibition through hypothalamic secretory mechanisms appears to be the major regulator of unrestrained PRL secretion. Dopaminergic pathways and dopamine have potent PRL inhibitory properties, and dopamine appears to fit many criteria for the physiologic PRL inhibiting factor. Bromocriptine, a potent dopaminergic agonist compound, has been used to treat states characterized by PRL hypersecretion.

GH modulates complex metabolic processes. The basis of GH action involves multiple steps. Its obvious effects can be seen in hypopituitary children in whom it has been used for treatment.

The secretion of GH is modulated by the relative balance between the levels of GH-releasing hormone and somatostatin released by the hypothalamus. These hypothalamic polypeptides exert their effects by interacting with the transmembrane spanning receptor superfamily and result in GH secretion. The binding of GH to the GH receptor pro-

ceeds in an ordered fashion with GH binding initially to one GH receptor and then attracting a second GH receptor with resultant GH action. GH appears to generate direct effects via the GH receptor signal transduction pathway and secondary effects via insulin-like growth factor I (IGF-I). Further actions mediated by IGF-I involve the multiple IGF binding proteins, of which six have been described. There are four principal IGF binding proteins present in human plasma. IGFBP-3 appears to be GH dependent and approximates the concentrations of IGF-I plus IGF-II in plasma. IGFBP-3 concentration has been proposed as a screening study for GH deficiency. IGFBP-2 concentration appears to be increased in hypopituitarism and may also be elevated in patients with non–islet cell tumor hypoglycemia. IGFBP-1 circulates in a much lower molar concentration than IGFBP-3 and IGFBP-2, but does appear to be present in high concentrations in amniotic fluid and in the endometrium. IGFBP-1 concentration appears to have significant variation with feeding and fasting. Failure to elevate IGFBP-1 concen-

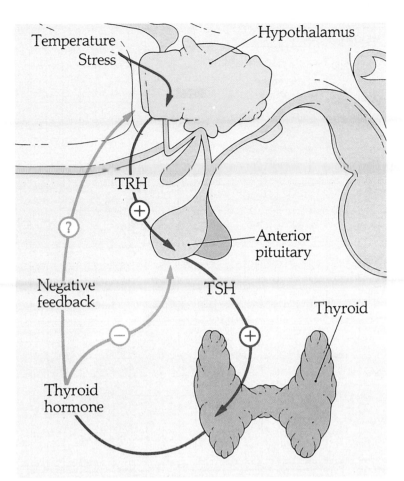

FIG. 9-3   Feedback regulation of TSH at the level of the hypothalamus, pituitary, and thyroid gland.

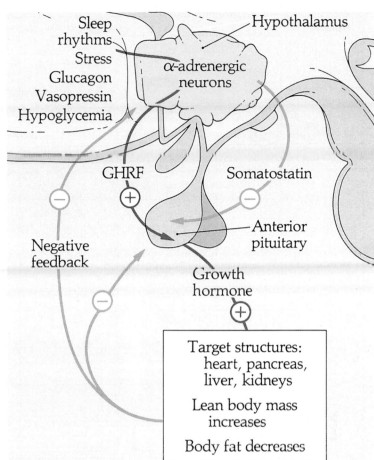

FIG. 9-4   Feedback regulation of GH at the level of the hypothalamus, pituitary, and target organs.

tration during fasting may be a sensitive diagnostic adjunct in children with hyperinsulinism.

GH stimulates an increase in lean body mass, as well as a marked increase in the size of the heart, pancreas, liver, and kidneys. It also has positive effects on carbohydrate, fat, and protein metabolism and causes a decrease in body fat. GH inhibits carbohydrate uptake by muscle. This diabetogenic effect of GH action has been well demonstrated and is a known complication of GH hypersecretion. On the other hand, hypoglycemia may be seen in patients who are GH deficient.

GH appears to mediate some of its effects on bone and linear growth via the somatomedins. These peptides have some structural similarity to proinsulin. Somatomedin C appears to mediate sulfate and phosphate incorporation into cartilage. Somatomedin C is identical to the peptide originally called IGF-I. GH is regulated on chronic and acute levels through a variety of mechanisms. A rapid fall in plasma glucose

concentration may elicit a brisk rise in GH secretion. However, hypoglycemia of slow onset may not activate GH secretion. Neural factors, such as sleep, stress, and alpha-adrenergic agonists may result in augmentation of GH secretion. Glucagon and vasopressin appear to cause hormonal augmentation of GH secretion. A fall in plasma somatomedin also may result in GH elevations (Fig. 9-4).

The anterior pituitary, with its diverse cell types and hormonal secretory patterns, controls many important biologic processes. Anterior pituitary hormone deficiencies cause subsequent deficiencies in the output of secondary endocrine glands. Consequently, specific aspects of growth and development are consistently disturbed by oversecretion or undersecretion of the pituitary. Particular alterations in physical appearance should alert physicians to an abnormality in the anterior pituitary and to subsequent secondary deficiencies (e.g., in the thyroid or adrenals).

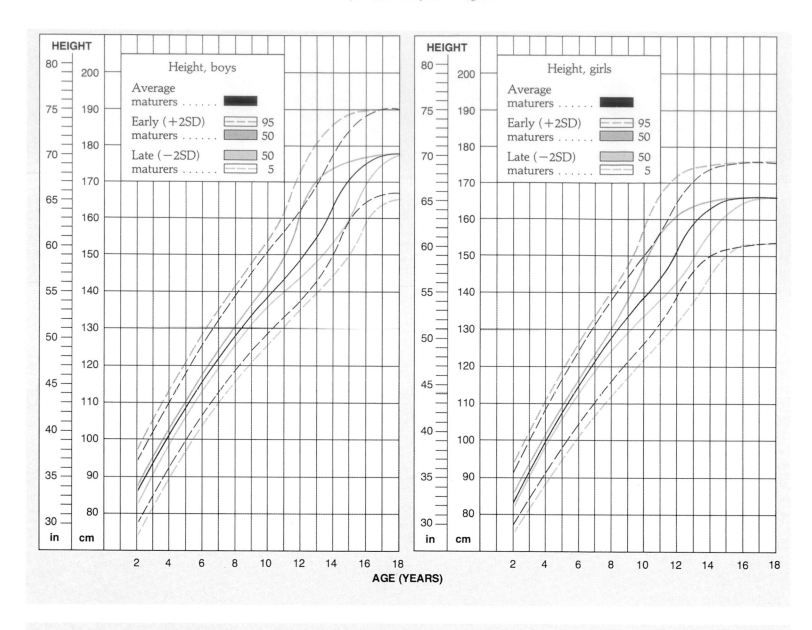

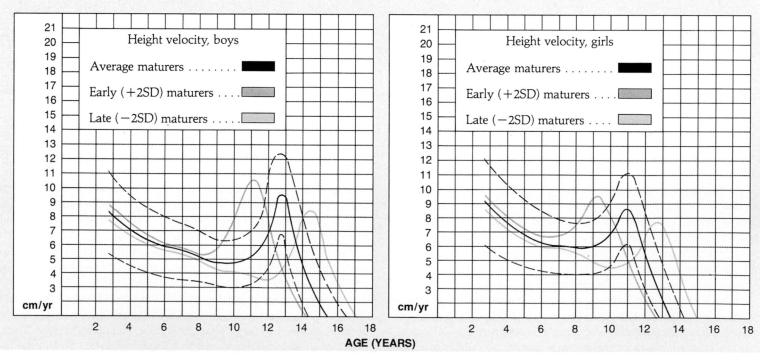

FIG. 9-5 Linear growth and growth velocity curves for boys and girls. (Modified from Tanner JM, Davies PSW: Clinical longitudinal standards for height and height velocity for North American children, *J Pediatr* 107:317-329, 1985.)

TABLE 9-1

Nonendocrine Causes of Short Stature

Familial short stature (genetic)
Constitutional delay of sexual development
Malnutrition and psychosocial factors
Systemic disease
  Pulmonary
    Cystic fibrosis
    Asthma
  Cardiac and circulatory
    Congenital heart disease (cyanotic and acyanotic)
    Acquired heart disease
  Renal
    Renal insufficiency
    Pyelonephritis (chronic)
    Renal tubular acidosis
  Gastrointestinal and hepatic
    Malabsorption
    Inflammatory bowel disease
    Hepatic insufficiency
  Neurologic
    Mental retardation with growth delay
  Musculoskeletal and connective tissue
    Chondrodystrophies
    Storage diseases
    Rickets
    Skeletal dysplasias
  Immunologic
    Immune deficiencies
Syndromes associated with short stature
  Chromosomal abnormalities
    Trisomies 13, 18, 21
    Turner syndrome
  Other syndromes
    Noonan
    Progeria
    Silver
    Cockayne
    Seckel

TABLE 9-2

Endocrine Causes of Short Stature

Thyroid hormone deficiency or resistance
Cortisol hypersecretion (Cushing syndrome)
Inborn errors of steroidogenesis—adrenal hyperplasias
  (untreated)
Precocious puberty (untreated)
  Central precocious puberty
  Male limited familial precocious puberty
  McCune-Albright syndrome
Disorders of the neuroendocrine GH axis
  Physical destruction of the pituitary and/or hypothalamus
  PIT-1 (transcription factors) mutations
  Somatostatin or GH-releasing hormone abnormalities
  GH gene mutations
  Laron syndrome types I and II (GH receptor or postreceptor
    defects)

Normal Growth

Normal growth occurs at a varying rate throughout the process of normal development. Moreover, wide variability exists in growth rates between individual children at different ages. Incremental growth rate is one of the most important elements in assessing whether a child has a pathologic abnormality of growth. As seen in Fig. 9-5, the growth velocity curve may be calculated as the first derivative of the linear growth curve. This manipulation illustrates the wide variability in growth rates at different ages. The curve also illustrates that in the first 2 to 3 years of life, growth is constantly decelerating. The growth velocity during infancy rapidly decelerates. Most children find their percentile track by 15 to 18 months of age. During the first 36 months of life, children who fall across percentiles in a downward fashion must be followed closely, and a decision must be made as to whether a detailed investigation regarding the cause is appropriate. The hand x-ray examination for bone age is uninformative before 18 months of life. Thus if a delayed bone age is suspected in the first 36 months of life, epiphyseal development should be estimated by hemiskeleton radiographic examination. During the latency years, a long period of constant growth occurs, followed by a sharp acceleration in growth velocity during adolescence. A growth rate below 4 to 5 cm per year for girls and boys between 4 years of age and adolescence is abnormal and should be investigated. This sharp increase in growth velocity is the harbinger of puberty. Adolescence is the only time during which the rapid growth of the infant is recapitulated.

Of those children with short stature and normal body proportions who are brought to their pediatrician for evaluation, only a few have growth failure of an endocrine origin. The differential diagnosis of children with short stature may be related to nonendocrine causes or endocrine alterations (Tables 9-1 and 9-2). The majority of short children who have organic illness suffer from major systemic diseases of cardiac, pulmonary, gastrointestinal, or renal origin. The most common cause of short stature in children is short parents. The genetic growth potential of a child is heavily determined by the growth achieved by both parents and by their relatives, and this information should be part of a careful history taken in evaluating short children. The heritability of height has been estimated to be as high as 0.64, rising to as much as 0.9 between identical twins. Determination of epiphyseal maturation, or bone age, is often helpful in evaluating children with short stature. Children who have genetically determined short stature generally have a bone age equivalent to their chronologic age. Those who have constitutional delay as a cause of short stature usually are of normal length at birth but develop mild growth deceleration in early childhood. Growth velocity is usually in the 3rd to 25th percentile for age. Puberty is delayed, as is the pubertal growth acceleration. A family history of "late bloomers" or delayed puberty is common. Bone age in constitutional delay is delayed, being more consistent with the child's height age rather than chronologic age.

Genetic syndromes (such as Turner syndrome or Down syndrome) are cases in which chromosomal abnormalities limit physical growth. Congenital disorders of bone mineralization and bone growth, such as the chondrodystrophies, also represent an important cause of short stature. Achondroplasia and at least some cases of hypochondroplasia have been explained by mutation in the gene encoding the fibroblast growth factor receptor–3 (FGFR-3). An aggressive endocrine investigation should be undertaken to ascertain the presence or absence of hypopituitarism and GH deficiency only after these other diseases have been eliminated from consideration.

Although deficiencies of anterior pituitary hormones, such as TSH or ACTH, may result in secondary hypothyroid and hypoadrenal states, these states tend to be milder than those of primary hypothyroidism or

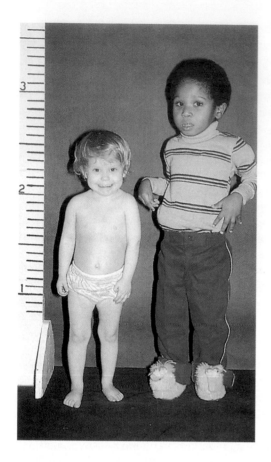

FIG. 9-6 The normal 3½-year-old boy is in the 50th percentile for height. The short 3-year-old girl exhibits the characteristic "Kewpie" doll appearance, suggesting a diagnosis of GH deficiency.

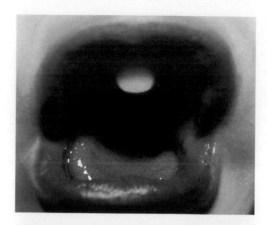

FIG. 9-7 The presence of a single central maxillary incisor should alert the clinician to investigate the possibility of GH deficiency. (Courtesy Dr. P. Lee, Pittsburgh.)

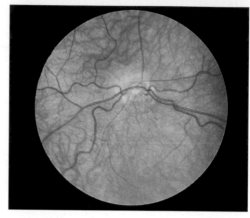

FIG. 9-8 Pale optic discs, suggesting optic atrophy, often are seen with septo-optic dysplasia. This finding also suggests pituitary endocrine deficiencies ranging from isolated GH deficiency to panhypopituitarism (Courtesy Dr. D. Hiles, Pittsburgh.)

Addison disease and thus their clinical signs are not as striking. The most striking feature of the panhypopituitary patient is growth retardation.

Endocrine Imbalances

Growth Hormone Deficiency

The phenotypic features of a child with GH deficiency are most striking. GH deficiency tends to be recognized by the characteristic features of normal body proportion and increased adiposity around the trunk and extremities. As seen in Fig. 9-6, GH-deficient children have delicate features; in boys with this disorder, the genitalia frequently are small. Children with hypopituitarism tend to have high-pitched voices compared with other children of the same age. After 10 years of GH treatment, the "Kewpie doll" appearance is no longer noticeable. In GH deficiency, the height age is delayed along with a significant delay in the bone age.

Children with a variety of midline defects have a higher incidence of hypopituitarism when compared with normal children. The child seen in Fig. 9-7 has a single central maxillary incisor—an example of a midline abnormality consistently associated with GH deficiency. Other physical findings suggestive of pituitary endocrine abnormalities include the syndrome of septo-optic dysplasia, with pale optic discs (Fig. 9-8), and children with cleft lip and cleft palate. These embryologic defects, presenting in infancy, also may be associated with significant risks of hypoglycemia. Recurrent protracted hypoglycemia may be an early presentation of hypopituitarism. The hypoglycemia is effectively treated with GH replacement therapy. Neonatal hypopituitarism should also be suspected in boys with microphallus and/or persistent hypoglycemia.

Although the diagnosis of GH deficiency is still challenging, knowledge of acquired and inherited forms of GH deficiency have expanded rapidly. Obviously, any trauma resulting in destruction of the pituitary gland regions of the hypothalamus that regulate secretion of GH may result in loss of GH secretion.

Short stature may be one of numerous phenotypic presentations of inherited alterations in the neuroendocrine axis. PIT-1 is a pituitary-specific transcription factor that is critical for pituitary development. This transcription factor is key in regulating the synthesis of prolactin and the beta subunit of thyrotropin. Mutations in PIT-1 have been identified in family members of individuals deficient in GH, prolactin, and TSH, who may also have severe mental retardation and short stature. This disorder may present as either a dominant or recessive inheritance pattern. Specific mutations resulting in loss of function of the GH gene product have also been identified. At least four forms of isolated GH deficiency caused by specific mutations have been identified. Types Ia and Ib appear to have an autosomal recessive inheritance. Type Ia is the result of deletions, frame shifts, and nonsense mutations that result in the absence of the GH gene product. Because of this absence, affected individuals often develop anti-GH antibodies when treated with GH. Type Ib is the result of splice-site mutations and low, but detectable, levels of GH are measurable. As would be expected, dwarfism is generally less severe in the Ib type, and treatment with exogenous GH is often successful. Idiopathic GH deficiency type II is inherited with an autosomal dominant pattern and seems to be the result of a splice-site dominant negative mutation. Type III GH deficiency is X-linked and is often associated with hypogammaglobulinemia.

Thyroid Gland Disorders

The thyroid gland is situated in the neck or, in rare cases, at the base of the tongue or in the mediastinum. Both overactivity and underactivity of the thyroid gland may be associated with a goiter; however, the signs of hyperthyroidism and hypothyroidism are dramatically different. Examination of the thyroid gland is an important step in the evaluation of a suspected abnormality in thyroid hormone release.

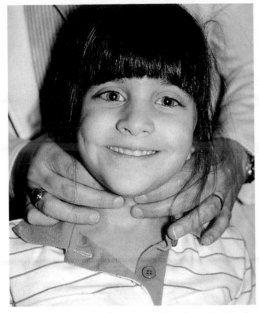

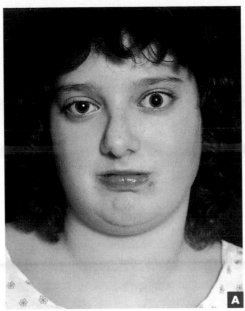

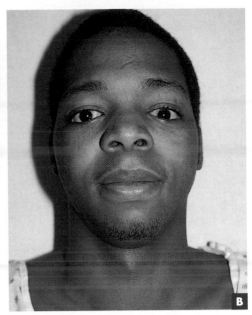

FIG. 9-9   Correct palpation of the thyroid gland is performed from behind the child.

FIG. 9-10   These patients with Graves disease illustrate mild thyromegaly and proptosis or ophthalmopathy. Ophthalmopathy is less dramatic in children than the eye disease seen in adult patients with Graves disease.

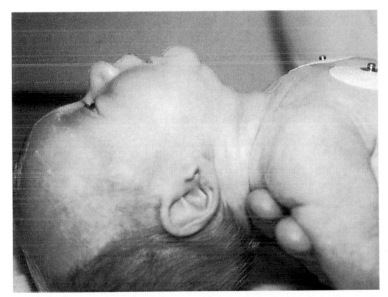

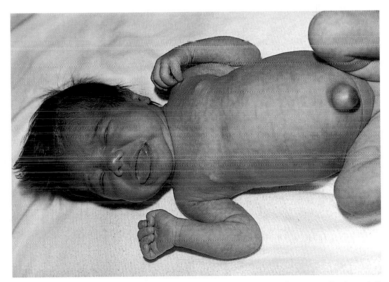

FIG. 9-11   Examination of the neonatal thyroid gland may be effectively performed by elevating the infant's trunk and allowing the head to drop back gently, as shown.

FIG. 9-12   A child with cretinism. (Courtesy Dr. T.P. Foley, Jr., Pittsburgh.)

As seen in Fig. 9-9, the thyroid gland usually can best be palpated with the examiner behind the patient. After identification of the cricothyroid cartilage, the second and third fingers are moved laterally along the trachea just medial to the sternocleidomastoid muscles. Two distinct lobes are palpable; the right lobe is usually greater in size than the left lobe. With a goiter present, these lobes may be quite easily identified. The texture of the gland will vary in hyperthyroidism and hypothyroidism, the former usually being soft and fleshy, and the latter usually firm or bosselated. Because the thyroid is directly supported by the trachea, having the patient swallow several mouthfuls of water will elevate and depress a palpable gland along with the trachea during the swallowing motion.

Most physicians are familiar with the symptoms associated with hyperthyroidism, or Graves disease. An acceleration in basal metabolism with concomitant tachycardia, weight loss, heat intolerance, and nervousness are characteristic. Exophthalmos, a characteristic eye finding of Graves disease, usually is less dramatic in children than in adults, but the appearance of proptosis can easily be appreciated (Fig. 9-10). The hyperthyroid gland can become quite large, as much as 3 to 4 times its normal size, and it is quite warm during palpation. A bruit often may be heard over a hyperthyroid gland.

Either congenital or acquired hypothyroidism may also produce a goiter. A goiter in an infant with congenital hypothyroidism suggests an enzymatic defect in thyroid hormone biosynthesis. To demonstrate a goiter in a newborn, the examiner's hand is placed gently under the back and shoulder blades of the infant, and the infant's trunk is raised from the bed (Fig. 9-11). As the head falls backward, the neck is elevated and a goiter, if present, will be displayed prominently. Because of neonatal thyroid screening, the coarse features of the congenital hypothyroid baby, referred to as a *cretin* (Fig. 9-12), are now a thing of

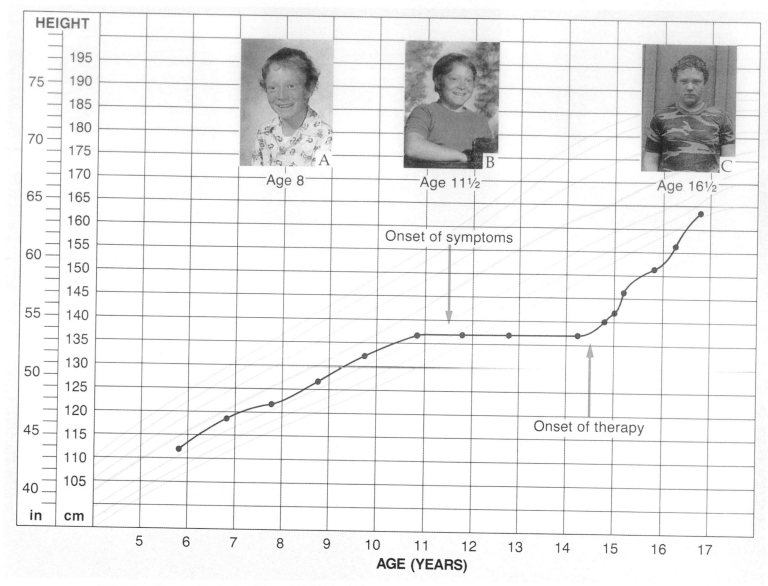

FIG. 9-13 The growth curve of this child with acquired hypothyroidism shows marked growth deceleration. Following thyroid replacement, significant catch-up growth occurs. The inserted photographs illustrate: *A,* The child before onset of acquired hypothyroidism. *B,* The change in body habitus associated with acquired hypothyroidism. *C,* Resolution following thyroid replacement at the indicated times.

the past. However, the broad nasal bridge, thick lips, and dull appearance characteristic of a cretin were seen regularly in endocrine clinics and pediatric offices not long ago because of the difficulty of making this diagnosis early. Careful retrospective evaluation of hypothyroid babies identified through neonatal thyroid screening has indicated that all such physical findings may be absent or too subtle to diagnose with certainty in the neonatal period. This uncertainty, in combination with the success of early treatment of congenital hypothyroidism, mandates continued neonatal thyroid screening.

Acquired hypothyroidism, most frequently caused by Hashimoto thyroiditis, may also present in a subtle fashion. Despite the subtlety of these clinical findings, the astute clinician will take note of dry skin, constipation, hair loss, depressed or delayed relaxation phase of deep tendon reflexes, and weakness of the child with acquired hypothy-

roidism. The most dramatic expression of acquired hypothyroidism may be a sharp deceleration in growth, as seen in the growth curve shown in Fig. 9-13. Following institution of thyroid hormone therapy, rapid growth occurs, returning the child to normal growth percentiles.

Turner Syndrome

Although genetic in origin (see Chapter 1), Turner syndrome must be included in any discussion of short stature. Although its nature need not be solely endocrine, Turner syndrome is a common diagnosis in short women seen in endocrine clinics. Some of the clinical presentations of Turner syndrome are shown in the pictures of young women reported in the original article by Turner (Fig. 9-14). The wide carrying angle (cubitus valgus), shieldlike chest, and webbed neck may be eas-

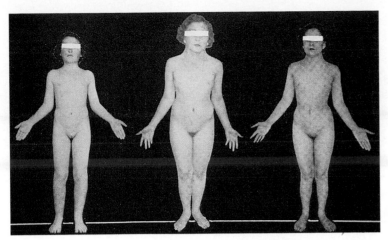

FIG. 9-14 Turner used this photograph in 1938 to describe the syndrome that bears his name. Note the clinical heterogeneity within the syndrome.

TABLE 9-3

Common Clinical Findings in Turner Syndrome

Skeletal Growth
  Disturbances
  Short stature
  Short neck
  Abnormal upper- to
    lower-segment ratio
  Cubitus valgus
  Short metacarpals
  Madelung deformity
  Scoliosis
  Genu valgum
  Characteristic facies—
    micrognathia,
    high-arched palate

Lymphatic Obstruction
  Webbed neck
  Low posterior hairline
  Rotated ears
  Edema of hands, feet
  Nail dysplasia
  Characteristic
    dermatographics

Germ Cell Defects
  Gonadal failure
  Infertility

Miscellaneous Defects
  Strabismus
  Ptosis
  Multiple pigmented nevi
  Cardiovascular anomalies
  Hypertension
  Renal and renovascular
    anomalies
  Hearing abnormalities

Associated Disorders
  Hashimoto thyroiditis
  Hypothyroidism
  Alopecia
  Vitiligo
  Gastrointestinal disorders
  Carbohydrate intolerance

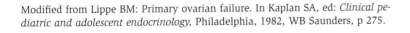

Modified from Lippe BM: Primary ovarian failure. In Kaplan SA, ed: *Clinical pediatric and adolescent endocrinology,* Philadelphia, 1982, WB Saunders, p 275.

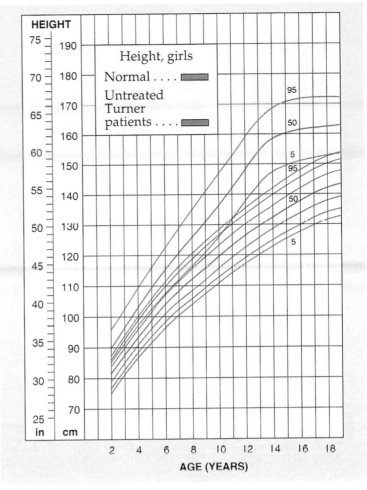

FIG. 9-15 Growth curve for Turner syndrome.

ily appreciated. A more comprehensive list of physical findings in patients with Turner syndrome is listed in Table 9-3. Turner syndrome should be suspected in any short girl presenting with pubic or axillary hair and absence of breast development and menses. Karyotyping is diagnostic in a clinical picture suggestive of Turner syndrome. Recent studies suggest that growth hormone treatment with or without weak androgenic steroids may significantly augment ultimate adult growth in girls with Turner syndrome. Growth charts for untreated girls with this syndrome are shown in Fig. 9-15.

Parathyroid Gland Dysfunction

Dysfunction of the parathyroid glands usually does not present a unique phenotype. A Chvostek sign (distortion of the face when the

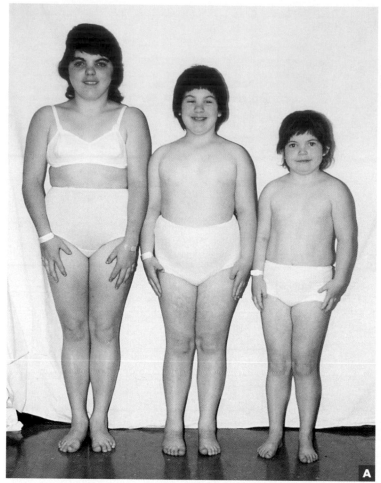

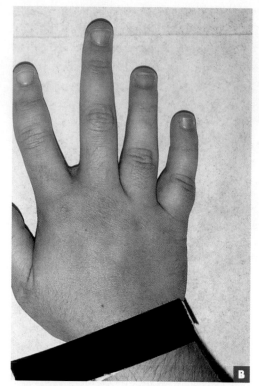

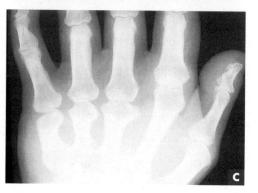

FIG. 9-16 *A,* Sisters with Albright hereditary osteodystrophy (pseudohypoparathyroidism). *B,* The short fourth metacarpal may easily be appreciated in this photograph. *C,* Radiograph of the hand illustrates the short fourth metacarpal seen in pseudohypoparathyroidism, as well as in other syndromes such as Turner syndrome. This child also has a short third metacarpal. (*A* and *B* courtesy Dr. J. Parks; *C* courtesy Dr. J. Medina, Pittsburgh.)

seventh nerve is stimulated with a reflex hammer) or Trousseau sign (cramping of the hand when a blood pressure cuff is elevated significantly above the systolic blood pressure) may be the only significant sign seen in an individual with hypocalcemia. However, Albright hereditary osteodystrophy syndrome (pseudohypoparathyroidism) is associated with a very characteristic phenotype. These patients may have a round facies, short stature, obesity, skin hyperpigmentation with irregular margins, and a short thick neck (Fig. 9-16, *A*). Shortening of the metacarpals and metatarsals is most common in the fourth digit (Fig. 9-16, *B* and *C*). These patients may have decreased intelligence and subcutaneous calcification, present with hypocalcemia and hyperphosphatemia, and characteristically have reduced phosphaturia when given exogenous parathyroid hormone. This phenotype has been explained by a variety of mutations in the guanine nucleotide–binding protein alpha-stimulating polypeptide (GNAS1) of the G protein signal transduction system. Mutations in the GNAS1 gene have also been implicated in McCune-Albright syndrome. The G proteins are coupled to the super-family of seven membrane-spanning receptors. When these receptors interact with their ligands, they generate a signal through an alteration in the state of their coupled G protein complex. G proteins consist of at least one stimulatory (G_s) and one inhibitory (G_i) complex, both of which are heterotrimers. Loss of function mutations in G_s-alpha

subunit results in the phenotype of Albright hereditary osteodystrophy syndrome, whereas gain of function mutations in G_s-alpha subunit results in McCune-Albright syndrome or has been identified in subsets of thyroid adenomas or somatotropinomas. The cause of the syndrome is probably heterogeneous, and further mechanisms will be found to contribute to this group of patients. The inheritance pattern is confusing, suggesting an autosomal dominant pattern, but evidence for autosomal recessive and X-linked families is also present in the literature. Albright hereditary osteodystrophy syndrome should be suspected in a short child with hypocalcemia and a history of similarly affected family members.

Adrenal Gland Dysfunction

Hyperfunction or hypofunction of the adrenal glands results in some of the most dramatic physical alterations of any endocrinologic disorder. Cushing syndrome, the phenotype resulting from excess glucocorticoid action, is seen in both endogenous and exogenous steroid exposure. Rounded facies, plethora, and a central obesity are characteristic of Cushing syndrome (Fig. 9-17). The so-called buffalo hump behind the neck has been described frequently. These children often may show centripetal obesity. Because of their excessive metabolism, muscle

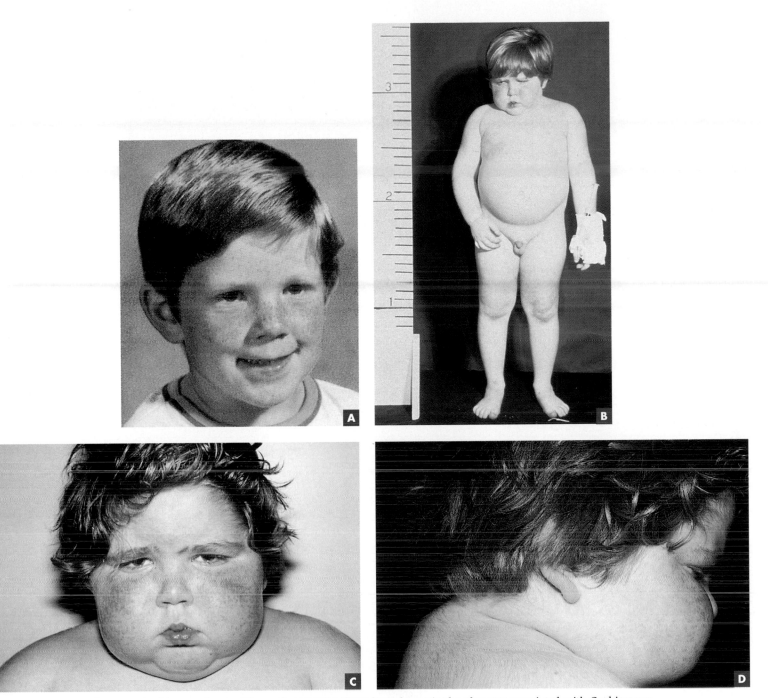

FIG. 9-17 Cushing syndrome. These photographs show how dramatic the changes associated with Cushing syndrome are and how rapidly they can occur. *A,* Patient before the onset of Cushing syndrome. *B,* Patient 4 months after *A* was taken. Note the centripetal obesity of the trunk compared with the extremities after the onset of Cushing syndrome. *C,* Moon facies is clearly demonstrated and should raise the diagnostic index of Cushing syndrome. In diagnosing Cushing syndrome, equally important to the physical manifestations shown here is the presence of growth failure. *D,* Buffalo hump. Excessive adipose tissue over the lower cervical and upper thoracic spine is characteristic of Cushing syndrome.

weakness and muscle wasting occur, resulting in comparatively thin extremities (Fig. 9-17, *B*). These children frequently are irritable and quite miserable. The skin is usually thinned and easily bruised. Hypertension and, ultimately, loss of bone mineral and osteoporosis occur with longstanding glucocorticoid exposure.

Endogenous Cushing syndrome may be caused by adrenal tumors, pituitary adenoma, or ectopic ACTH production. Elevated 24-hour urine free cortisol is the best test in the diagnosis of Cushing syndrome. The high- and low-dose dexamethasone suppression test remains the most important diagnostic study for differentiating between the causes of

Cushing syndrome. Following 2 days of baseline studies, dexamethasone is administered in a "low dose" of 0.005 to 0.006 mg/kg, or 0.25 mg, every 6 hours for 3 days in the older child or adult. Following the low-dose administration, a "high dose" of 0.02 to 0.025 mg/kg, or 2 mg, every 6 hours is administered for the last 3 days of the tests. The differential findings in the specific etiology of Cushing syndrome are listed in Fig. 9-18. Improvement in surgical technique has improved the outcome in the treatment of pituitary Cushing syndrome. Medical therapy for adrenal tumors or to suppress pituitary ACTH production is still inadequate.

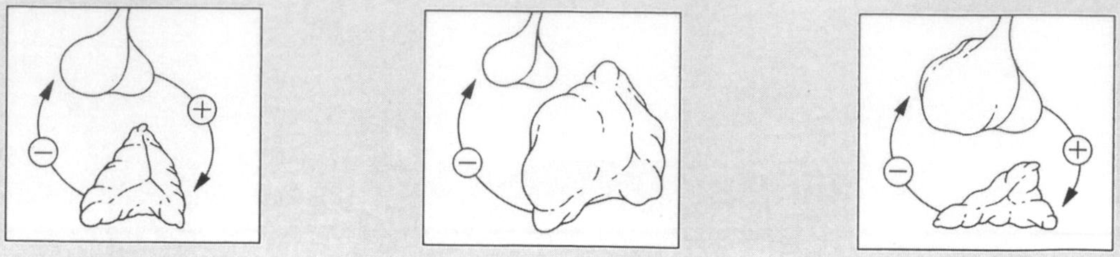

	Normal	Adrenal Tumor	Pituitary Hypersecretion
Plasma cortisol diurnal rhythm	10–25 µg% rhythmic	High no rhythm	High no rhythm
Plasma ACTH	Normal	Low	High
Plasma ACTH after adrenalectomy, on normal cortisol replacement	Normal	Low	High
Plasma glucocorticoid response to ACTH	3–5 fold rise	+, 0	+
Urinary glucocorticoid response to metyrapone	2–4 fold rise	0	+
Plasma glucocorticoid response to dexamethasone	Suppressed	No fall	Partial fall

FIG. 9-18   The differential diagnosis of Cushing syndrome as interpreted from the dexamethasone suppression test. (Modified from Williams RH: *Textbook of endocrinology,* ed 6, Philadelphia, 1981, WB Saunders, p 272.)

In striking contrast to the obesity seen with glucocorticoid excess, patients with Addison disease (glucocorticoid and mineralocorticoid deficiency) present with a thin body habitus and wasting of subcutaneous tissue (Fig. 9-19, *A*). There is little change seen in overall growth rate. Frequently a striking hyperpigmentation or bronzing of the skin occurs, with emphasis of this pigmentary change in flexor creases, in scars, and over the areolae of the nipples (Fig. 9-19, *B* through *D*). Vitiligo may occur as well. Frequently patients may be confused and weak. In far-advanced Addison disease vascular collapse is common. The decreased circulating plasma volume is reflected by the thinned narrow heart shadow seen on a chest radiograph (Fig. 9-19, *E*). If untreated, patients with Addison disease gradually weaken and die. However, replacement of glucocorticoid with cortisol and of mineralocorticoid with a compound such as 9-alpha-fludrocortisone (Florinef) allows the patient with Addison disease to lead a normal life. Tuberculosis was formerly the most common cause of Addison disease. Autoimmune de-

struction of the adrenal gland has now replaced tuberculosis as the most common cause of the disease. The clinical manifestations of Addison disease are less fully expressed in individuals who have either isolated ACTH deficiencies or hypothalamic alterations in corticotropin-releasing factor kinetics. This is well demonstrated in the girl with isolated ACTH deficiency seen before and after treatment (Fig. 9-19 *F* and *G*). Although she has the clinical wasting associated with Addison disease, her skin is pale as opposed to bronzed.

Sexual Maturation

Anomalies of Early Sexual Development

Sexual maturation begins in fetal life. With normal progression, a normal internal and external male or female genital anatomy is formed (Fig. 9-20). If normal progression of sexual development fails, however,

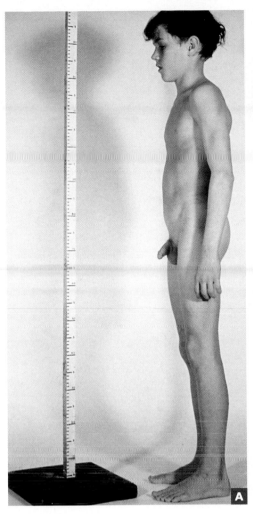

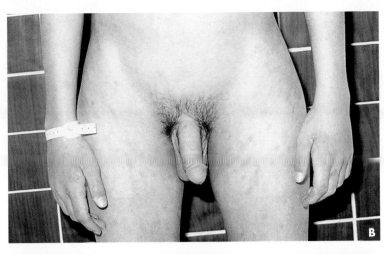

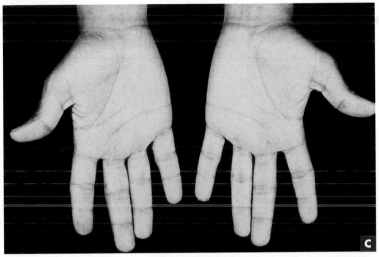

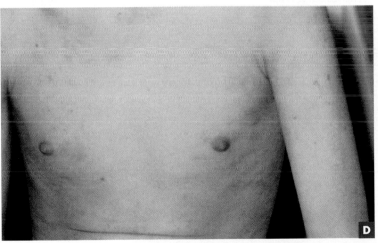

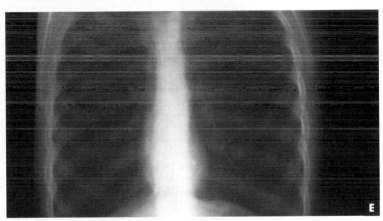

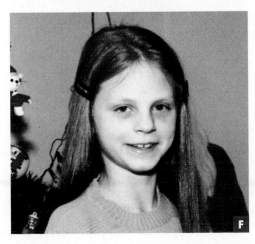

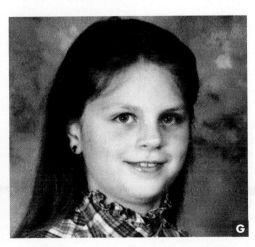

FIG. 9-19 *A,* This patient shows the thin habitus and ill appearance characteristic of Addison disease. *B* through *D,* Hyperpigmentation may be marked. *E,* Microcardia is characteristically seen on chest radiograph. *F,* Young girl with isolated ACTH deficiency shows wasting and pallor rather than excessive bronzing. *G,* The same girl after therapy. (*A* through *D* courtesy Dr. M. New; *E* courtesy Dr. J. Medina, Pittsburgh.)

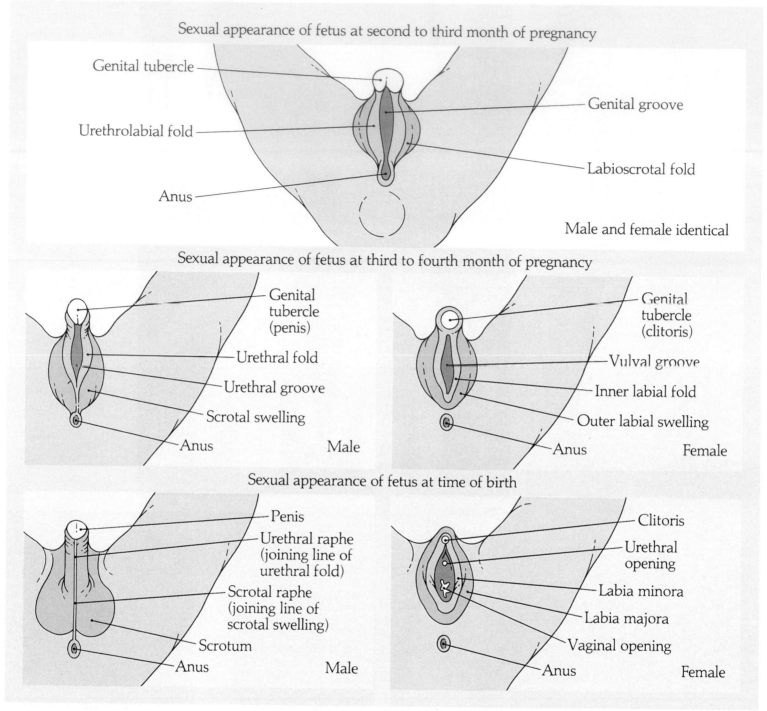

Sexual appearance of fetus at second to third month of pregnancy

Genital tubercle

Urethrolabial fold

Anus

Genital groove

Labioscrotal fold

Male and female identical

Sexual appearance of fetus at third to fourth month of pregnancy

Genital tubercle (penis)

Urethral fold

Urethral groove

Scrotal swelling

Anus   Male

Genital tubercle (clitoris)

Vulval groove

Inner labial fold

Outer labial swelling

Anus   Female

Sexual appearance of fetus at time of birth

Penis

Urethral raphe (joining line of urethral fold)

Scrotal raphe (joining line of scrotal swelling)

Scrotum

Anus   Male

Clitoris

Urethral opening

Labia minora

Labia majora

Vaginal opening

Anus   Female

FIG. 9-20   Schematic drawing demonstrating differentiation of normal male and female genitalia during embryogenesis.

children may be born with ambiguous genitalia (Fig. 9-21), which presents a difficult and urgent diagnostic problem for the obstetric/pediatric team. Children with ambiguous genitalia must be evaluated with urgency, and a diagnosis must be determined as quickly as possible. This provides the basis for an appropriate recommendation to parents regarding the sex of rearing and also for the rapid and appropriate institution of therapy in cases where medical intervention is necessary.

The classification of anomalous sexual development can be based on gonadal development. Some disorders of gonadal differentiation (such as Klinefelter syndrome, Turner syndrome, and their variants) may not necessarily present with anomalous external genitalia. True hermaphroditism, although rare, frequently may present with ambiguous genitalia at birth. Female pseudohermaphrodites (genotype XX) have ovaries, although they present with ambiguous external genitalia. The most com-

mon cause of female pseudohermaphroditism is virilizing adrenal hyperplasia. However, any androgen or synthetic progestin transferred from the maternal circulation, either exogenously administered to the mother or endogenously produced by the mother, may result in virilization of the fetal genitalia. Teratogenic factors also may have an effect on the development of the external genitalia. These factors are constantly being elucidated as new drugs are introduced. Male pseudohermaphrodites (genotype XY) have testes and ambiguous external genitalia. The causes of male pseudohermaphroditism are multiple and complex and reflect the complex biosynthetic and hormonal processes required to induce normal development of the male external genitalia. Testicular unresponsiveness to either human chorionic gonadotropin (HCG) or LH is an early developmental error that will affect external genital development. Inborn errors of testosterone biosynthesis at both adrenal and tes-

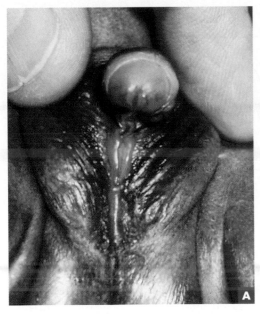
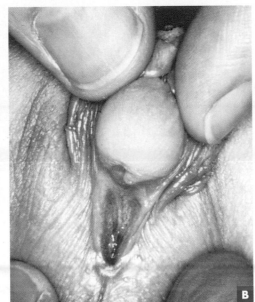
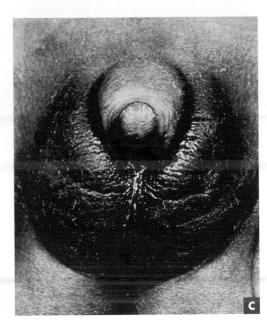
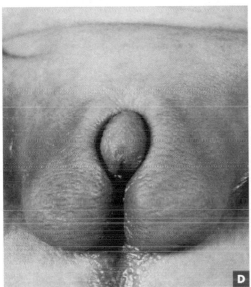
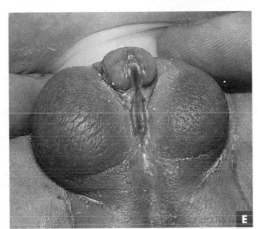

FIG. 9-21 Examples of ambiguous genitalia. These cases include (*A*) a true hermaphrodite and (*B* through *E*) congenital virilizing adrenal hyperplasia. (*B* through *D* courtesy Dr. D. Becker, Pittsburgh.)

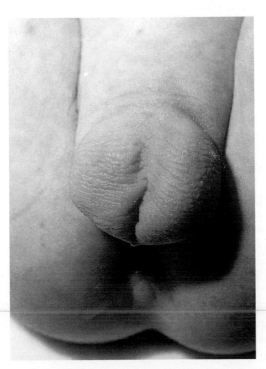

FIG. 9-22 Agenesis of the phallus. (Courtesy Dr. D. Becker.)

ticular levels also will interfere with external genital development, since the development of external genitalia in the male is induced by the effects of both testosterone and dihydrotestosterone. A deficiency in the hormone may induce these abnormalities, or a defect in the hormone receptor may affect development, with inadequate recognition of androgenic hormones resulting in feminization of normal males. This is seen in its most dramatic form in the syndrome of testicular feminization, where the genitalia show no ambiguity, although the gonads are testes, and the individual's karyotype is XY. Karyotypic abnormalities also may be associated with ambiguous genitalia.

The testis determining factor has been discovered to be the gene product of the SRY gene located at chromosomal region Yp11.3. SRY acts during a critical period in a pathway of gene expression resulting in formation of the normal testis. SRY appears to determine male sex through activation of the gene for Müllerian inhibiting substance, with resultant regression of the Müllerian structures. Significant loss of function mutations result in XY gonadal dysgenesis, whereas milder mutations may be associated with ambiguity of the external genitalia. Rare cases of ambiguous genitalia are unclassifiable, and the mechanisms associated with these disorders remain to be elucidated.

Some children born with anatomic variants, such as agenesis of the phallus (Fig. 9-22), may have neither a karyotypic nor a biochemical

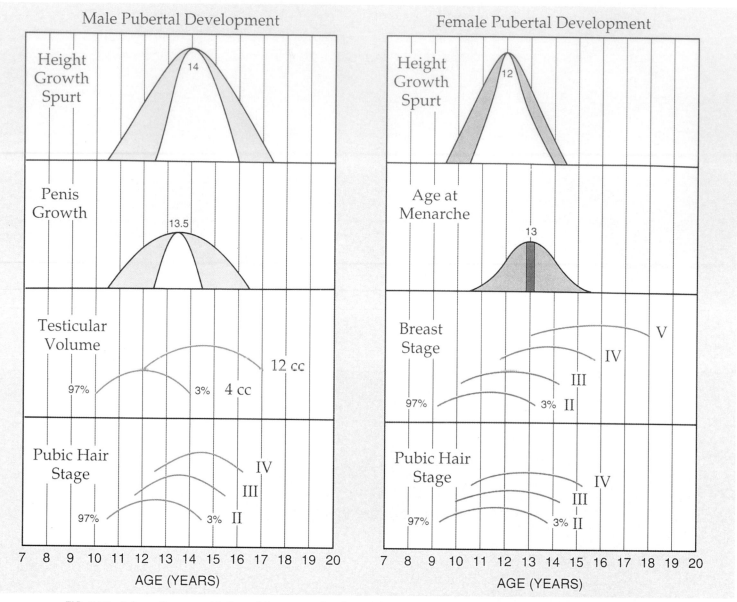

FIG. 9-23 Schematic representation of the onset of male and female puberty. (Modified from Johnson TR, Moore WM, Jeffries JE: *Children are different: development physiology,* ed 2, Columbus, Ohio, 1978, Ross Laboratories, Division of Abbott Laboratories, pp 26-29.)

defect but rather a developmental anomaly. These anomalies also may outlie the classification of ambiguous genitalia described above. Regardless, any child seen at birth with ambiguous genitalia should not receive a sex assignment until the appropriate sex of rearing may be properly assessed and assigned. An appropriate sex assignment must be based on the following considerations: potential for mature sexual function, potential fertility, and the long-term psychologic and intellectual impact on the child and family.

Development in Puberty

The pattern of timing of pubertal events for boys and girls is generally predictable (Fig. 9-23). However, for both boys and girls, the age of puberty varies in different regions of the world. In the United States, the onset of breast development and pubic hair growth occurs at approximately 10½ years of age, with menarche occurring at approximately 12½ years of age. However, considerable variations exist for any individual patient.

The Tanner Stages

Because the onset and progression of puberty are so variable, Tanner has proposed a scale, now uniformly accepted, to describe the onset and progression of pubertal changes (Fig. 9-24). Boys and girls are rated on 5-point scales. Boys are rated for both genital development and pubic hair growth, and girls are rated for breast development and pubic hair growth.

The stages for male genital development are as follows (Fig. 9-24, *A*):

Stage I (Preadolescent)—The testes, scrotal sac, and penis have a size and proportion similar to those seen in early childhood.

Stage II—There is enlargement of the scrotum and testes and a change in the texture of the scrotal skin. The scrotal skin also may be reddened, a finding not obvious when viewed on a black-and-white photograph.

Stage III—Further growth of the penis has occurred, initially in length, although with some increase in circumference. There also is increased growth of the testes and scrotum.

Stage IV—The penis is significantly enlarged in length and circum-

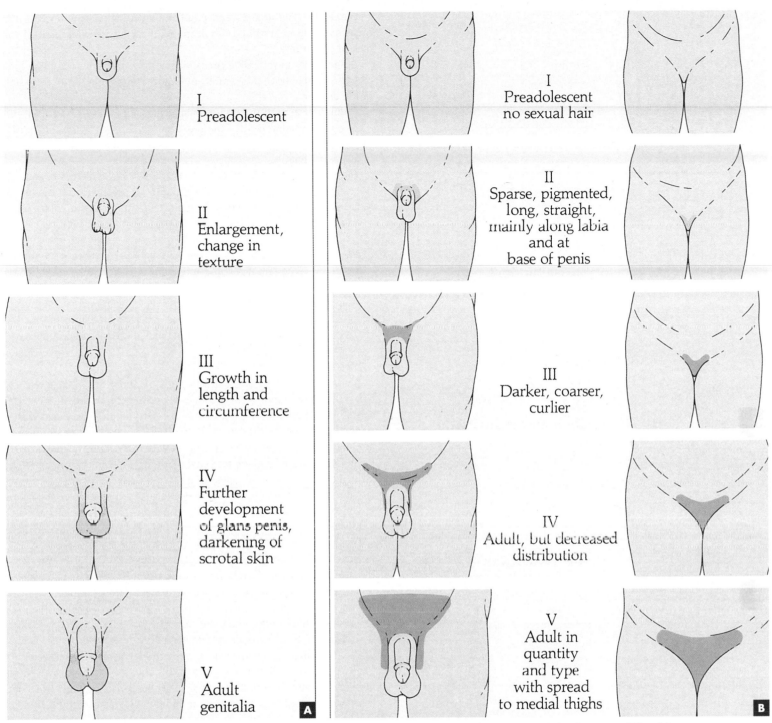

FIG. 9-24 Schematic drawings of male and female Tanner stages show: *(A)* male genital development, *(B)* pubic hair development, and *(C)* breast development. (Modified from Johnson TR, Moore WM, Jefferies JE: *Children are different: development physiology,* ed 2, Columbus, Ohio, 1978, Ross Laboratories, Division of Abbott Laboratories, pp 26-29.)   *Continued*

ference, with further development of the glans penis. The testes and scrotum continue to enlarge, and there is distinct darkening of the scrotal skin. This is difficult to evaluate on a black-and-white photograph.

Stage V—The genitalia are adult with regard to size and shape.

The stages in male pubic hair development are as follows (Fig. 9-24, *B*):

Stage I (Preadolescent)—Vellous hair appears over the pubes with a degree of development similar to that over the abdominal wall. There is no androgen-sensitive pubic hair.

Stage II—There is sparse development of long pigmented downy hair, which is only slightly curled or straight. The hair is seen chiefly at the base of the penis. This stage may be difficult to evaluate on a photograph, especially if the subject has fair hair.

Stage III—The pubic hair is considerably darker, coarser, and curlier. The distribution of hair has now spread over the junction of the pubes, and at this point the hair may be recognized easily on black-and-white photographs.

Stage IV—The hair distribution is now adult in type but still is considerably less than that seen in adults. There is no spread to the medial surface of the thighs.

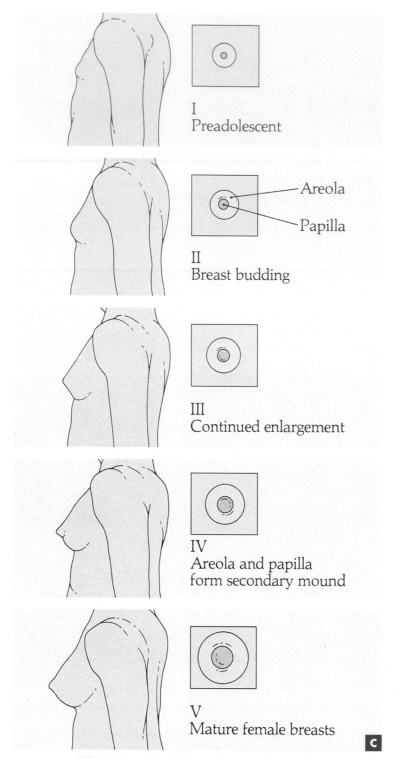

I
Preadolescent

II
Breast budding

Areola

Papilla

III
Continued enlargement

IV
Areola and papilla
form secondary mound

V
Mature female breasts

C

FIG. 9-24, cont'd   For legend see previous page.

Stage V—Hair distribution is adult in quantity and type and is described as an inverse triangle. There can be spread to the medial surface of the thighs.

In young women, the Tanner stages for breast development are as follows (Fig. 9-24, *C*):

Stage I (Preadolescent)—Only the papilla is elevated above the level of the chest wall.

Stage II (Breast Budding)—Elevation of the breasts and papillae may occur as small mounds along with some increased diameter of the areolae.

Stage III—The breasts and areolae continue to enlarge, although they show no separation of contour.

Stage IV—The areolae and papillae elevate above the level of the breasts and form secondary mounds with further development of the overall breast tissue.

Stage V—Mature female breasts have developed. The papillae may extend slightly above the contour of the breast as the result of recession of the areolae.

Pubic hair growth in females is staged as follows (Fig. 9-24, *B*):

Stage I (Preadolescent)—Vellous hair develops over the pubes in a manner not greater than that over the anterior abdominal wall. There is no sexual hair.

Stage II—Sparse, long, pigmented, downy hair, which is straight or only slightly curled, appears. These hairs are seen mainly along the labia. This stage is difficult to quantitate on black-and-white photographs, particularly when pictures are of fair-haired subjects.

Stage III—Considerably darker, coarser, and curlier sexual hair appears. The hair has now spread sparsely over the junction of the pubes.

Stage IV—The hair distribution is adult in type but decreased in total quantity. There is no spread to the medial surface of the thighs.

Stage V—Hair is adult in quantity and type and appears in an inverse triangle of the classically feminine type. There is spread to the medial surface of the thighs but not above the base of the inverse triangle.

Precocious Puberty

The Tanner classification has become an important instrument for communication among physicians, allowing a semiquantitative description of the pubertal progression of boys and girls. However, variations in the timing and normal progression of puberty often are associated with specific pathologic entities. A diagnosis of precocious or early development may be made if sexual maturation begins before age 8 for girls and before age 9 for boys. In girls the causes of isosexual precocity (development along lines of the same sex) are related to alterations in gonadal or central nervous system function. True precocious puberty follows an early onset of pulsatile LH and FSH secretion and the subsequent response of the ovary. Estrogen-secreting tumors of the ovary, however, will suppress development of normal LH and FSH secretion. McCune-Albright syndrome, polyostotic fibrous dysplasia with sexual precocity, has been associated with either central or peripheral causes of precocious puberty.

Long-standing hypothyroidism in girls may be associated with isosexual precocity and inappropriate secretion of gonadotropins. Galactorrhea also may occur in association with elevated prolactin levels.

Isosexual precocity in young boys also may be caused by central nervous system abnormalities or by peripheral dysfunction. However, intracranial neoplasms are more commonly associated with precocious puberty in boys as compared with girls. Adrenal or testicular neoplasms in young boys are unusual. Late-onset congenital virilizing adrenal hyperplasia also may result in isosexual precocity in boys. Treatment for precocious puberty is diagnosis specific. The discovery of the long-acting GnRH analogues has revolutionized the treatment of central precocious puberty in childhood. These analogues may be injected on a daily or monthly basis or given via nasal spray. The continuous stimulation to the pituitary gonadotropic cells effectively suppresses gonadotropin secretion and inhibits further pubertal development.

Premature Thelarche and Pubarche

Premature Thelarche. This condition may occur before expected pubertal development (Fig. 9-23). The breast tissue may appear unilaterally or bilaterally and may regress or persist (Fig. 9-25). Premature thelarche is a diagnosis of exclusion and cannot be made in the presence or progression of other pubertal signs. The ingestion of exogenous estrogens, such as oral contraceptives, should always be suspect in cases of breast enlargement. Neonatal breast enlargement secondary to maternal

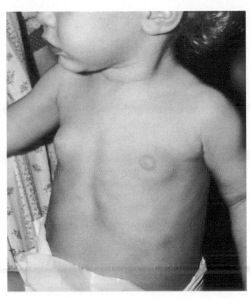

FIG. 9-25 Isolated breast enlargement in a toddler with premature thelarche.

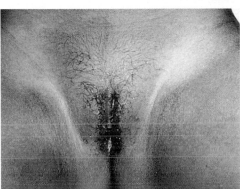

FIG. 9-26 Pubic hair development in a prepubertal girl with premature adrenarche.

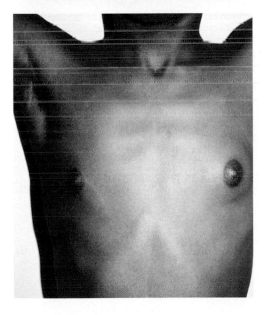

FIG. 9-27 Adolescent boy with asymmetrical breast enlargement.

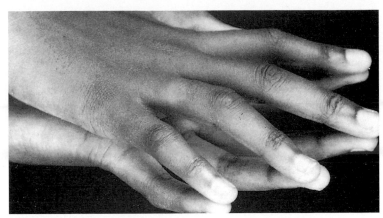

FIG. 9-28 Diabetic sclerodactyly is seen in this patient's inability to flatten the palms and fingers as he presses both hands together. (Courtesy Dr. A. Rosenbloom, Gainesville, Fla.)

ACTH stimulation testing. The presence of adrenal or gonadal tumors is best defined by imaging procedures, as well as blood and urine steroid level determination.

Adolescent Male Gynecomastia

Adolescent gynecomastia in the male is common, occurring in up to 40% of boys (Fig. 9-27). Breast development usually is mild and regresses with advancing puberty. However, in some cases breast development progresses to a female breast contour that corresponds to Tanner stage III or greater. This may become a profound psychologic burden and require surgical intervention. The differential diagnosis includes Klinefelter syndrome estrogen-secreting tumors. Small testes are associated with both conditions. Additionally, patients with Klinefelter syndrome exhibit a eunuchoid body habitus. Karyotyping and measuring of estrogen and gonadotropin levels can differentiate among these conditions.

Islets of Langerhans Diseases

Diabetes Mellitus

Diabetes mellitus represents one of the most common of the chronic diseases seen by the endocrinologist. Before the institution of aggressive insulin therapy, children with diabetes mellitus and short stature were seen frequently in endocrine clinics and represented instances of the Mauriac syndrome. This syndrome is characterized by poorly controlled diabetes, short stature, hepatomegaly, and sexual infantilism. This is now a very rare occurrence. In a carefully treated child with type I, or insulin-dependent, diabetes mellitus, growth rate should be indistinguishable from that of a normal child. However, one physical finding still frequently seen in diabetic patients is that of limited joint mobility. Fig. 9-28 shows the inability of a diabetic child to flatten the palms because of waxy thickened skin in the areas of the proximal and distal interphalangeal joints. Although this phenomenon is not as yet completely understood, it has been associated with poor diabetic control. The development of specific skin lesions, such as necrobiosis lipoidica diabeticorum, also may be associated with diabetes. Fig. 9-29 shows such a lipid-filled skin lesion, which may occasionally be seen in a child with type I diabetes.

hormones may occur in either sex. This condition regresses with time and may be confused with premature thelarche or precocious puberty.

Premature Pubarche. In contrast to premature thelarche, the appearance of pubic or axillary hair before expected pubertal development often is associated with a pathologic diagnosis (Fig. 9-26). Late-onset forms of adrenal hyperplasia and, more uncommonly, adrenal and/or gonadal tumors are seen in patients with premature pubarche and are reflected in the elevation of steroid hormones. Patients with late-onset forms of adrenal hyperplasia may be differentiated with

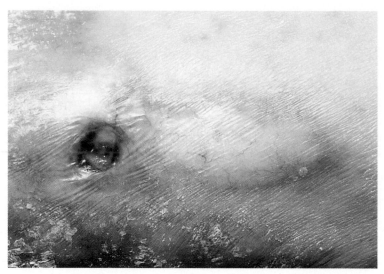

FIG. 9-29 Necrobiosis lipoidica diabeticorum is characterized by the presence of yellow waxy skin lesions that exhibit reddened components. Small areas of ulceration also may be seen. (Courtesy Dr. B. Cohen, Pittsburgh.)

TABLE 9-4

Postprandial Hypoglycemia

Postgastric surgery
Diabetes mellitus
Galactosemia
Hereditary fructose intolerance
Reactive or functional hypoglycemia

TABLE 9-5

Fasting Hypoglycemia

Increased substrate utilization
  Hyperinsulinism—endogenous
    Insulinoma
    Nesidioblastosis
    Autoimmune hypoglycemia
    Infants of diabetic mothers
    Beckwith-Wiedemann syndrome
    Leprechaunism
Decreased substrate production
  Inborn errors of carbohydrate metabolism
    Defects of gluconeogenesis
    Glycogen storage diseases
  Inborn errors of protein metabolism
    Maple syrup urine disease
    Methylmalonic aciduria
  Inborn errors of fat metabolism
    Systemic carnitine deficiency
    Carnitine acetyltransferase deficiency
    Hydroxymethylglutaryl CoA lyase deficiency
    Acyl CoA dehydrogenase deficiency
  Counterregulatory hormone deficiency
    Cortisol
    Thyroid
    Glucagon
    Growth hormone
    Catecholamines
  Ketotic hypoglycemia
  Hepatic and renal disease
  Extrapancreatic neoplasms
  Reye syndrome

TABLE 9-6

Drug-Induced Hypoglycemia

Insulin
Oral hypoglycemic agents
Ethanol
Salicylates
Propranolol
Miscellaneous other drugs
Akee fruit

Hypoglycemia

The differential diagnosis of hypoglycemia is broad and involves many systems. A useful classification divides hypoglycemic states into those associated with the postprandial period (Table 9-4), those that occur during a fasting or catabolic stress (Table 9-5), and iatrogenic or drug-induced hypoglycemias (Table 9-6). Specific syndromes associated with hypoglycemia may be diagnosed at first glance during the examination. The most striking of these is Beckwith-Wiedemann syndrome (Fig. 9-30),

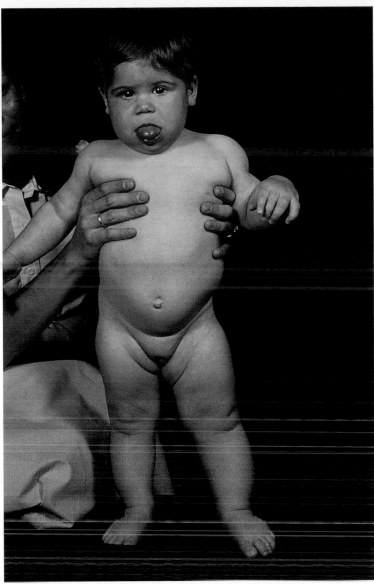

FIG. 9-30 Beckwith-Wiedemann syndrome. Note hemihypertrophy on the left side, along with the prominence of the tongue. (Courtesy Dr. D. Becker, Pittsburgh.)

which is associated with macrosomia, macroglossia, omphaloceles, hemihypertrophy, and embryonal tumors. Beckwith-Wiedemann syndrome has been mapped to chromosome 11p1.5. This region also contains the recently characterized sulfonylurea receptor gene (SUR). This gene is mutated in some families with recessively inherited hyperinsulinism. The hypoglycemia has been attributed to hyperinsulinism. These individuals may require aggressive treatment with diazoxide or may come to partial or complete pancreatectomy because of the severity of the hypoglycemia.

Another rare cause of hypoglycemia, which may be quickly diagnosed, is leprechaunism. A small, wizened infant presenting with severe recurrent hypoglycemia can readily be diagnosed as having leprechaunism. The cause of the hypoglycemia seems to be hyperinsulinism and an abnormal cellular response to insulin's action. In this case, however, the hyperinsulinism seems to be a state associated with an unusual response to insulin with hypoglycemia, as opposed to simple hyperinsulinism.

Summary

As seen in the illustrations, endocrine imbalances may result in dramatic alterations in a child's phenotype. These alterations should be readily recognized and thus direct the diagnostic approach. Careful attention to the appearance of children requiring evaluation by a physician should allow early diagnosis of endocrine disorders, resulting in prompt therapeutic intervention and in restoration of the child's appearance and overall state of well-being.

BIBLIOGRAPHY

DeGroot LJ, et al, eds: *Endocrinology*, ed 3, Philadelphia, 1995, WB Saunders.

Kappy MS, Blizzard RM, Migeon CJ, eds. *Wilkins the diagnosis and treatment of endocrine disorders in childhood and adolescence*, ed 4, Springfield, Ill, 1994, Charles C Thomas.

Lifshitz F, ed: *Pediatric endocrinology: a clinical guide*, ed 2, New York, 1990, Marcel Dekker.

Scriver CR, Beaudet AL, Sly WS, Valle D, eds: *The metabolic and molecular bases of inherited disease*, ed 7, New York, 1995, McGraw-Hill.

Wilson JD, Foster DW, eds: *Williams textbook of endocrinology*, ed 8, Philadelphia, 1992, WB Saunders.

10

Nutrition and Gastroenterology

J. CARLTON GARTNER JR.

Nutrition and gastroenterology are areas closely related to the daily activities of most pediatricians. As a world health problem, the cycle of diarrhea, poor nutrition, and consequent absorptive disorders causes untold harm. This chapter initially deals with nutritional assessment and malnutrition in children and then with some rarer nutritional deficiencies that may be diagnosed by careful examination and limited laboratory testing. This supplements material already available in standard textbooks. The gastroenterology section features conditions that may be diagnosed on clinical grounds, including cystic fibrosis, and includes several hepatic disorders based on our extensive experience at a transplant center.

Nutrition

Normal Nutrition

Any discussion of nutrition in infancy must begin with the normal requirements (Table 10-1). Fortunately, breast milk, the perfect infant food, exists worldwide. Breast milk has advantages beyond the issue of maternal-infant bonding (Table 10-2). The only supplements required are fluoride and vitamin D (in dark-skinned infants in a sunlight-deprived environment). In the latter part of the first year, babies fed exclusively breast milk may require additional iron. As a general rule, content and absorption of nutrients from breast milk are ideal for all infants, with the possible exception of the very low–birth-weight infant, who may have higher electrolyte, calcium, phosphorus, and vitamin requirements. Table 10-3 compares the major components of formula, cow's milk, and breast milk.

Nutritional awareness is mandatory for children's health-care workers, given the importance of growth and development. Each pediatric visit, whether for routine care or serious illness, should include a basic nutritional assessment. This process may include dietary, clinical, anthropometric, and detailed laboratory data. In a healthy child a brief dietary history (adequate formula in sufficient quantity) and a plot of height, weight, and head circumference on standard curves are sufficient. The ill child may require more careful assessment to clarify acute or chronic malnutrition and plan effective therapy.

Clinical Observations of Malnutrition

The clinical signs of chronic malnutrition are relatively easy to recognize. A cycle of recurrent gastrointestinal disturbances is the most common prodrome to undernutrition. Dehydration must be recognized early (dry mucous membranes, oliguria) before more serious complications ensue (e.g., depressed fontanelle, sunken eyes, diminished skin turgor) (Figs. 10-1 and 10-2). Rapid treatment and follow-up may interrupt the vicious cycle of malnutrition. Perhaps the most significant advance in world health in recent years is the use of oral rehydration solution (ORS) to treat gastroenteritis. Numerous studies have shown the advantages of this inexpensive, readily available mixture, which requires only potable water and appropriate dilution.

Clinical descriptions of malnutrition differentiate between marasmus (caloric deficiency with wasting of tissue) and kwashiorkor (protein deficiency with edema). More recently it has become evident that these conditions often overlap and have a similar pathogenesis. For both conditions, physical signs and descriptions help in patient evaluation and treatment. Malnourished children are often apathetic and have decreased physical activity. Marasmus is characterized by a marked weight-for-height reduction with emaciation, loss of subcutaneous fat, lusterless and sparse hair, and poor nail growth—producing a rather simian appearance (Fig. 10-3).

Classic kwashiorkor patients look well-nourished ("sugar babies") without wasting. The initial "moon face" of kwashiorkor is often mistaken for proper nutrition. The child is often edematous, which becomes strikingly apparent after nutritional repletion (Fig. 10-4). These children usually suffer acute protein deficiency in addition to preexisting caloric deprivation. Skin changes in kwashiorkor patients include hyperpigmentation and hypopigmentation with a scaly, weeping dermatitis that may ulcerate and desquamate (Fig. 10-5). The rash is often more prominent in areas that are chronically irritated (e.g., the infant groin and areas of peripheral edema). It resembles pellagra but is seen in areas that are not exposed to sunlight.

Failure to Thrive

In many areas of the world the gap between the well-nourished and the severely malnourished infant or child is filled by the problem com-

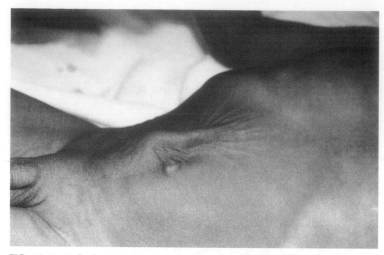

FIG. 10-1 Dehydration. Poor skin turgor is indicative of decreased extracellular volume. In this patient with severe dehydration, skin remains tented after release and retracts quite slowly.

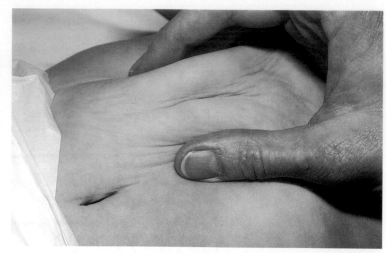

FIG. 10-2 Hypernatremic dehydration. The skin often has a "doughy" texture when the dehydration is associated with elevation of serum sodium.

T A B L E   1 0 - 1

Nutritional Requirements

Age	Calories (kcal/kg/day)	Protein (gm/kg/day)
0-12 months	100	2.5-3
1-7 years	75-90	1.5-2.5
7-12 years	60-75	1.5-2.5
12+ years	30-60	1.0-1.5

T A B L E   1 0 - 2

Advantages of Breast-Feeding

Convenience
No sterilization required
Maternal-infant bonding
Less frequent hospitalizations
Possible increase in IQ
Optimal absorption of nutrients, vitamins, and trace elements
Possible protection from allergen exposure
Less obesity

T A B L E   1 0 - 3

Comparison of Milks—Selected Components

Component	Breast milk	Formula	Whole cow's milk
Protein (g/dl)	1.2	1.5	3.3
Source	Human	Skim milk	Whey/casein
% calories	7	9	20
Fat (g/dl)	4	3.8	3.7
Source	Human	Soy/coconut	Butterfat
% calories	54	50	50
Carbohydrate (g/dl)	6.8	6.9	4.9
Source	Lactose	Lactose	Lactose
% calories	40	41	30
Osmolality (mEq/liter)	300	290	288
Renal solute load (mEq/liter)	87	90	226
Na^+ (mEq/liter)	7	9	24
K^+ (mEq/liter)	13	18	35
Ca^{++} (mg/liter)	340	440	1150
P (mg/liter)	140	300	920
Ca/P ratio	2.2	1.5	1.3
Iron (mg/liter)	0.5	0 or 12	1
Vitamin D (IU)	22	420	444
Fluoride (mg/liter)	0.01	0*	0.02

*Unless water is added to concentrate.

monly known as *failure to thrive*. Definitions of this condition are often vague, but failure to grow at an appropriate *rate* is a reasonable description. Generally, weight is affected first, with height and head circumference decrements occurring later. Although organic disorders are possible, in industrialized countries most of these children are categorized as having nonorganic problems related to the environment or parenting. A careful history and physical examination with selected laboratory tests usually can exclude disease states. The most important factor is a careful dietary history that includes volumes consumed,

formula dilution, amount of emesis, etc. Growth curves are helpful and often can prevent overinvestigation of children with normal variations in growth (Fig. 10-6).

Anthropometric Measurements and Laboratory Tests

After the initial clinical examination of the malnourished patient, anthropometric measurements should be made. These enable large groups of children to be followed sequentially, and they aid in distinguishing be-

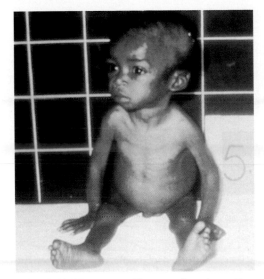

FIG. 10-3 Marasmus. Note profound wasting and sparse hair, producing a characteristic simian appearance.

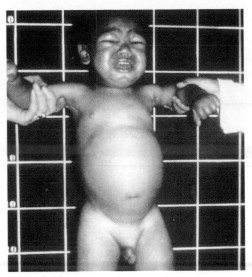

FIG. 10-4 Kwashiorkor. This patient has a typical "sugar baby" appearance with generalized edema. Note the periorbital and limb edema.

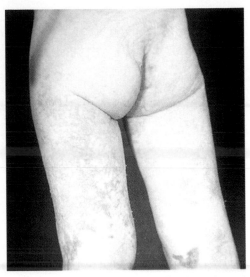

FIG. 10-5 The rash of kwashiorkor is scaly and erythematous, and may weep, especially in edematous areas.

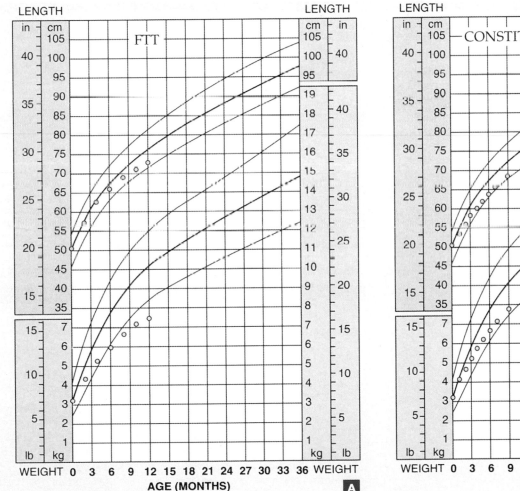

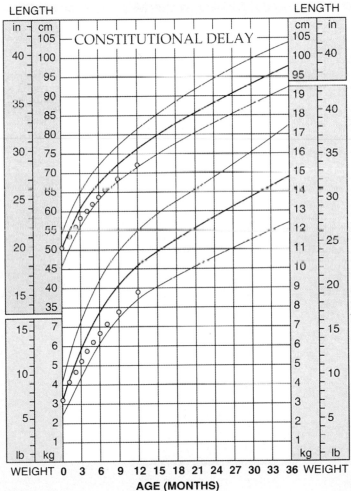

FIG. 10-6 Examples of growth curves. *A,* Typical failure to thrive with deceleration of weight gain. *B,* Slow growth but at a normal rate consistent with constitutional delay.

tween acute and chronic malnutrition and assessing the effects of protein or total calories. Using standard curves, such as 1976 National Center for Health Statistics charts, height-for-age deficit (actual height divided by expected height-for-age [50th percentile] × 100) and weight-for-height deficit (actual weight divided by expected weight-for-height [50th percentile] × 100) may be calculated. Diminished height for age most commonly reflects chronic undernutrition, whereas low weight for height may indicate more acute malnutrition. Nutritional status is graded using these two parameters (Table 10-4). In addition, measurements of triceps skinfold thickness and midarm muscle circumference

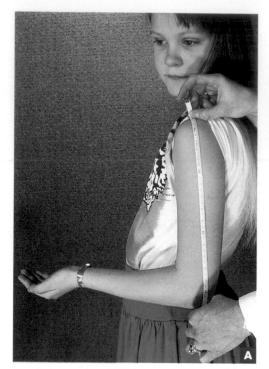
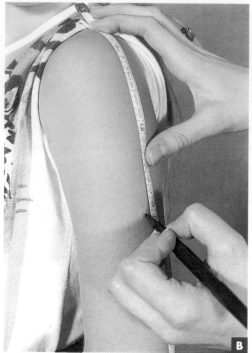
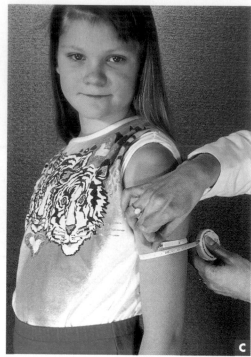

FIG. 10-7 Midarm circumference. *A,* Locate the midpoint of the arm with arm bent at 90-degree angle, tape at acromion and olecranon processes. *B,* Mark at midpoint. *C,* Make measurement at midpoint with arm hanging loosely.

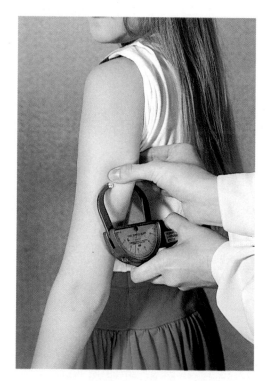

FIG. 10-8 Triceps skinfold. Grasp a vertical pinch of skin and subcutaneous fat. The caliper jaw is placed over the skinfold at the midpoint mark while maintaining grasp of skinfold. Make reading to nearest 1 mm without excessive pressure. Average three readings for the final result.

TABLE 10-4

Grading of Nutritional Status

Grade	Height for age	Weight for height
I	<95%	<90%
II	<90%	<80%
III	<85%	<70%

TABLE 10-5

Anthropometric Assessment of Nutritional Status

Measurement	Deficiency	Indicated deficiency
Weight for age	<90% of standard	Protein-calorie
Height for age	<95%	Protein-calorie
Weight for height	<90%	Protein-calorie
Triceps skinfold	<5%	Calorie
Midarm muscle	<5%	Protein

further delineate protein and calorie deficits (Table 10-5). The measurements must be done carefully (Figs. 10-7 and 10-8). When completed, the measurements are compared with standards (Walker and Hendricks, pp 17-23) and the predominant deficiencies can be defined.

Laboratory testing can be helpful in identifying some malnourished children. Not only is the degree of malnutrition confirmed, but certain specific deficiencies may be uncovered. Unfortunately, an inexpensive laboratory test for early malnutrition is not yet available. Amino acid nomograms may aid early diagnosis but are expensive and require a sophisticated laboratory. Decreases in body proteins are helpful but reflect normal body catabolism. Consequently, retinol binding protein ($t_{1/2}$ 12 hours) and transferrin ($t_{1/2}$ 9 days) indicate more current nutritional

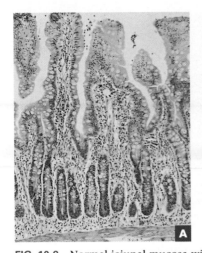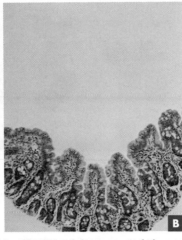

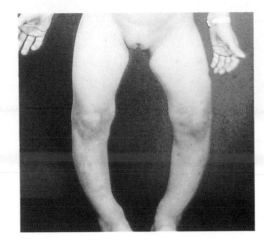

FIG. 10-10 Hypophosphatemic rickets marked by the obvious bowing.

FIG. 10-9 Normal jejunal mucosa with tall villi and deep crypts (A) complicating chronic diarrhea and malnutrition (B).

TABLE 10-6

Nutritional Deficiencies With Characteristic Physical Signs

Vitamin/mineral	Sign/symptom
Calcium, phosphorus, vitamin D	Rickets/osteomalacia
Vitamin A	Night blindness, xerophthalmia, Bitot spots, follicular hyperkeratosis
Vitamin C	Scurvy. bone lesions, bleeding
Vitamin E	Hemolytic anemia, peripheral neuropathy
Vitamin K	Petechiae, ecchymoses
Thiamine (vitamin B₁)	Beriberi: heart failure, increased intracranial pressure
Niacin	Pellagra: dermatitis (sun-exposed areas)
Riboflavin (vitamin B₂)	Angular stomatitis, cheilosis
Vitamin B₆	Anemia, dermatitis, neuropathy
Vitamin B₁₂	Anemia, neuropathy
Folate	Anemia
Iron	Anemia, koilonychia
Biotin	Rash, hair loss
Essential fatty acids	Rash, coagulopathy
Zinc	Rash (acrodermatitis), growth failure, delayed sexual development, ageusia
Copper	Bone changes, hypopigmentation, anemia, neutropenia
Selenium	Heart failure

status than the standard albumin (t½ 20 to 24 days). An additional aid in assessing lean body mass is a comparison of 24-hour creatinine excretion with standard norms for height (creatinine height index).

Because infection is a major cause of morbidity and mortality in the malnourished patient, a basic immunologic assessment is indicated. Total lymphocyte counts and skin tests are a minimal baseline, since the major effects are in the T-lymphocyte system.

Therapy

After clinical, anthropometric, and laboratory assessments are completed, decisions about aggressive nutritional repletion or mere maintenance therapy can be made. Obviously, patients with hypoproteinemia and major changes in weight for height will need more vigorous therapy. Parenteral nutrition should be considered for patients with profound injury to the gastrointestinal tract (Fig. 10-9). This advance in nutritional therapy continues to be perfected by better mixtures, less cumbersome and better tolerated catheters, and home total parenteral nutrition (TPN) using advanced programmable pumps. Recovery from intestinal injury is enhanced by intraluminal nutrition (which should be initiated as soon as possible). Industrialized countries fortunately have many modified and elemental formulas for children with acute or chronic digestive disturbances. Since malnutrition has profound effects on intestinal absorption, several of these formulas may be invaluable. It is important to know the specific content of each product used. High-osmolar formulas are often not tolerated, especially by the compromised small-bowel mucosa.

Before initiating nutritional therapy (or after a period of hyperalimentation), it helps to look for specific vitamin, mineral, and trace element deficiencies. The more common and previously well-described deficiencies are listed in Table 10-6. It is often difficult to assign individual findings, such as angular stomatitis, to specific deficiencies in a child with chronic, severe malnutrition. Several deficiencies, often seen in a hospital population, are discussed below.

Rickets (or osteomalacia in nongrowing bone) from vitamin D deficiency remains a world health problem. However, the increased survival of premature infants has led to biochemical rickets from calcium or phosphorus deficiency. Increased supplements of these minerals lead to reversal of the changes. The resurgence of breast-feeding, especially in dark-skinned or vegetarian populations, has produced clinical rickets. It should be noted that disorders of two other organ systems—liver and kidney—may produce clinical or biochemical osteomalacia. Poor bile flow and consequent malabsorption are the primary cause in hepatobiliary disorders. Additionally, end-stage renal disease with failure of renal hydroxylation of vitamin D₃ or renal tubular wasting of phosphorus may cause poor bone matrix formation.

In all of the above conditions that cause osteomalacia, the physical changes are similar: poor growth, curvature of weight-bearing bones (Fig. 10-10), widening of epiphyses, and costochondral beading (Fig. 10-11). Softening of the skull (craniotabes) is seen in infants. With ap-

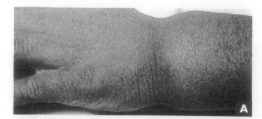

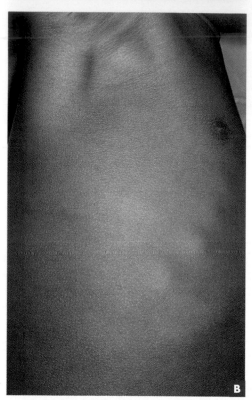

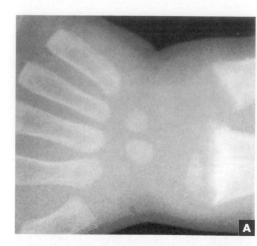

FIG. 10-11 Infantile rickets marked by widened wrists *(A)* and enlargement of the costochondral junction ("beading") *(B)*. The latter occurred as the result of a rapid growth spurt after liver transplantation.

FIG. 10-12 Radiograph of the wrist in a patient with rickets *(A)* shows irregularity and widening of the epiphyses in the distal radius and ulna. With appropriate therapy *(B)*, remineralization and healing occur.

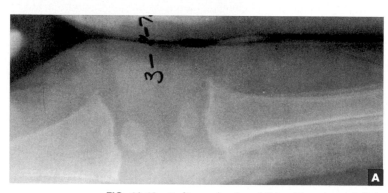

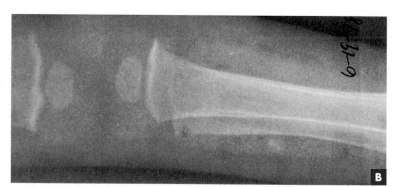

FIG. 10-13 Radiograph of a child with copper deficiency *(A)* reveals irregular epiphyses with spur formation, cloaking of metaphyses, periosteal new bone formation, and osteoporosis. After 3 months of intravenous copper *(B)*, the child demonstrates healing of the metaphyses.

propriate vitamin and mineral supplementation, radiographic healing occurs, followed by bony remodeling (Fig. 10-12).

Deficiencies of other fat-soluble vitamins (E, K, A) may occur as well. Clinical vitamin E deficiency can progress from absence of peripheral deep tendon reflexes to marked ataxia. Vitamin K deficiency, seen in patients with long-standing steatorrhea or liver disease, causes prolongation of the prothrombin time and can be associated clinically with easy bleeding and bruising. Vitamin A deficiency causes follicular hyperkeratosis, xerophthalmia, night blindness, and unusual shiny gray, triangular lesions on the conjunctivae (Bitot spots).

Parenteral nutrition has been lifesaving, especially for neonates with major intestinal disorders complicated by malnutrition. Unfortunately, as trial-and-error methods were used in early hyperalimentation, numerous deficiencies were uncovered during prolonged periods of alimentation. Examples of this include fatty acid deficiency with the typical scaly dermatitis, and zinc deficiency with alopecia, diarrhea, and acrodermatitis; these conditions are now rare. Before reformulation of our own hyperalimentation mixture several years ago, other unusual problems were uncovered. A child on hyperalimentation for 6 months developed irritability, bone pain, and decreased hair pigmentation.

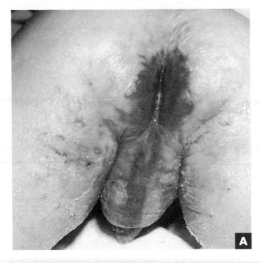

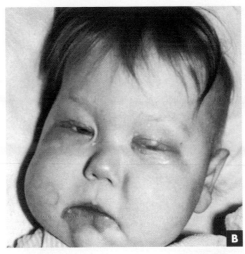

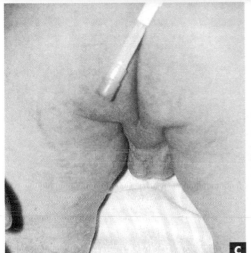

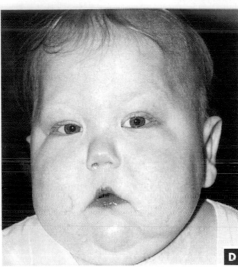

FIG. 10-14   Biotin deficiency. *A* and *B,* This child on chronic hyperalimentation developed dermatitis in perianal, perioral, and lid areas along with some thinning of hair. *C* and *D,* The rash has cleared dramatically after 4 days of biotin.

Anemia and progressive neutropenia ensued, and a skeletal survey and copper and ceruloplasmin determinations confirmed copper deficiency. Bone changes included osteoporosis, metaphyseal spurs, and periosteal new bone formation. Hematologic and then bone changes reversed with copper administration (Fig. 10-13). Another patient with short-gut syndrome on home hyperalimentation developed a peculiar weeping dermatitis in the perioral, perianal, and lid areas along with lethargy and malaise. Changes reversed in only 4 days when intravenous biotin was added (Fig. 10-14).

Conclusion

Careful nutritional assessment followed by detailed clinical examination can uncover specific nutritional deficiencies and delineate the severity and chronicity of malnutrition. These facts will then allow a more specific plan of nutritional repletion to be formulated using a combination of parenteral and enteral routes.

Gastroenterology

Disturbances of gastrointestinal (GI) function are common in pediatric practice, perhaps second only to respiratory symptoms as a reason for office visits. However, clues to specific disorders are uncommon. This section emphasizes the major symptoms that bring patients with GI disease to medical attention and defines entities that may be diagnosed by examination. Later in this section cystic fibrosis and liver disorders are also discussed.

Malabsorption

Malabsorption syndromes in pediatrics range from single sugars (lactase deficiency) to more complex multinutrient problems such as those associated with the short-gut syndrome. The physical signs usually are those of malnutrition. Most clinicians, however, suspect celiac disease when they see a child with "potbelly" and wasted extremities and buttocks. A gluten-free diet is prescribed, and the results are quite rapid and dramatic (Fig. 10-15). Because this is a lifelong condition, careful confirmation by repeated small intestinal biopsies is indicated.

Vomiting

Recurrent vomiting is a frequent symptom in childhood, most commonly associated with diarrhea (gastroenteritis).

Pyloric Stenosis
Early onset, a forceful projectile quality, continued hunger, and associated constipation are characteristic of hypertrophic pyloric stenosis.

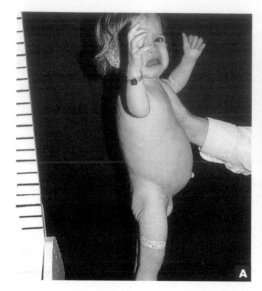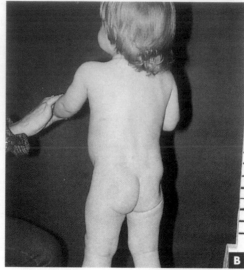

FIG. 10-15 Celiac disease. *A,* This child had a pot-belly, vomiting, and weight loss as her major symptoms and was originally thought to have psychosocial failure to thrive. When celiac disease was suspected, the child was placed on a gluten-free diet. Note the protruding abdomen and wasted buttocks. *B,* After 10 weeks on the diet the improvement is obvious.

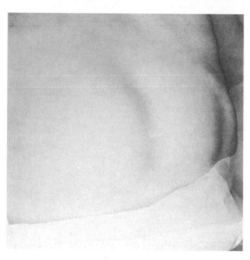

FIG. 10-16 Pyloric stenosis. The giant gastric waves are best seen just after a feeding.

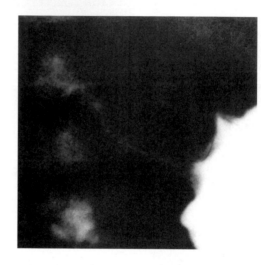

FIG. 10-17 This typical barium study in a patient with pyloric stenosis demonstrates a "stringlike" pyloric channel.

Giant gastric peristaltic waves and the typical firm pyloric olive are noted on examination (Fig. 10-16). In questionable cases, radiographs may confirm the diagnosis by demonstrating a stringlike pyloric channel (Fig. 10-17) Abdominal ultrasonography can also demonstrate the pyloric tumor.

Reflux

Gastroesophageal reflux is a common and usually self-limited condition beginning in early infancy. Many of these children have emesis even in the newborn nursery. Very characteristic are frequent episodes of emesis beginning immediately after feeding and continuing for several hours. Presentations of this disorder are multiple and include neurologic and/or behavioral abnormalities (Sandifer syndrome) characterized mainly by peculiar extension movements of the head and neck (Table 10-7). The problem usually lessens and gradually disappears by 1 year of age. Complicated reflux—failure to grow, aspiration, esophagitis, hemorrhage, apnea—is less frequent. Clinical diagnosis is sufficient in mild cases, but more persistent or difficult problems may require further diagnostic testing. Barium swallow is helpful but diagnostic of abnormality in only 50% of the cases. Twenty-four hour (or shorter) esophageal pH-probe measurements, esophagoscopy and/or biopsy, aspiration nuclear scans, and esophageal manometric studies may all be necessary before arriving at a final assessment. Additionally, psychophysiologic factors may predominate in the rumination syndrome.

TABLE 10-7

Presentations of Gastroesophageal Reflux

Regurgitation
  "Spitting," rumination
  Emesis
  Failure to thrive

Esophagitis
  Irritability
  Colic
  Hiccups
  Anemia
  Hematemesis
  Stricture
  Protein-losing
    enteropathy
  Melena, occult blood loss

Behavioral
  Dystonic posturing
  Sandifer syndrome

Respiratory
  Wheezing, asthma
  Recurrent pneumonia
  Aspiration
  Laryngospasm
  Apnea

Neurologic
  Seizure-like episodes

Other
  Clubbing of digits
  Sudden infant death
    syndrom or apparent
  life-threatening event

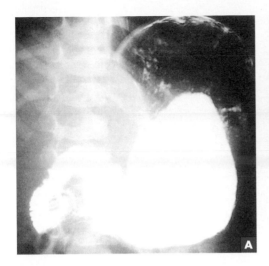

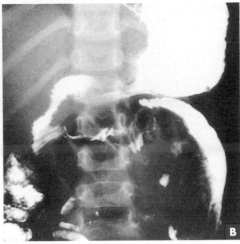

FIG. 10-18 Upper GI series demonstrates poor flow through the duodenum *(A)* and mass ef-fect of the hematoma displacing other loops of bowel *(B).*

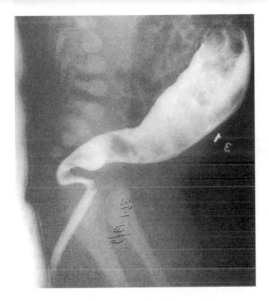

FIG. 10-19 The ta-pered transition zone to a normal-caliber colon is characteristic of Hirschsprung disease.

Constipation

Chronic constipation is usually functional and is often related histori-cally to problems at the time of toilet training. Overflow incontinence (encopresis) may result and is usually manageable by a period of catharsis and bowel "retraining" in preschool or young school-age chil-dren. Occasionally, major psychopathology is uncovered, especially in the older child, and appropriate intervention is necessary. Bladder dys-function with recurrent urinary tract infections may be associated with major long-standing constipation.

Examination of the child with constipation usually reveals palpable stool in the descending colon and rectum. If the history dates to early in-fancy and obstipation is present as well, one should consider Hirschsprung disease. Barium enema radiographic studies are usually diagnostic (Fig. 10-19), although rectal biopsy for ganglion cells and spe-cial stains is necessary for confirmation. In older children, rectal mano-metric studies may help separate organic from functional disorders.

Abdominal Pain

Recurrent abdominal pain (RAP), often vague and nonspecific, is found in as many as 25% of school-age children. Typically the pain is episodic, unrelated to meals, and centrally located in the abdomen; in addition, the child may appear pale. The definition includes the "rule of 3," that is, patient older than 3 years, with more than three episodes over at least 3 months. Despite careful evaluation, a precise cause is sel-dom determined. In one long-term follow-up study at the Mayo Clinic, the only condition that appeared to be missed, though rarely, was re-gional enteritis. Unfortunately, 20% of children with RAP are subjected to laparotomy. Less than 5% of these children will have an organic dis-order. The history and examination clues that warrant further investi-gation are listed in Table 10-8.

In addition to inflammatory bowel disease, peptic ulcer disease should be considered in patients with RAP. In children, clues may be nocturnal pain and occasionally emesis. The incidence is unknown but seems to be increasing, possibly based on better diagnostic techniques, such as endoscopy (Fig. 10-20). A major development in the diagnosis and treatment of ulcer disease is the relationship to infection with *Helicobacter pylori.* The majority of patients with duodenal ulcer dis-ease will be infected and have antral gastritis (Fig. 10-21). Treatment for this organism, usually with a combination of a bismuth preparation, metronidazole, and either tetracycline or amoxicillin, will lead to heal-ing of the ulcer. There is less evidence for an association with gastric ulcer disease and little evidence for an association with RAP. Although not yet fully established as a purely infectious disease, the thinking

In late stages these children regurgitate constantly and swallow in a self-stimulating fashion.

Therapy in mild cases includes frequent small feedings and mainte-nance of an upright position. This is usually accomplished by elevating the head of the crib and keeping the infant in a prone position. By in-creasing intraabdominal pressure, the "infant seat" actually worsens re-flux. The value of thickened feedings (rice cereal added to formula) is still debated, although infants seem to cry less on this regimen. Vari-able results have been obtained with drug therapy using bethanechol or metoclopramide. Persistent, complicated reflux requires surgery—usually a Nissen type of fundoplication.

Trauma

No discussion of pediatric differential diagnosis is complete without a mention of trauma or child abuse. The GI tract may figure in subtle forms of abuse: chronic diarrhea from laxative abuse and feigned bleed-ing episodes are reported (Munchausen syndrome by proxy). Likewise, vomiting may be induced by occult trauma or abuse. Blunt injury to the abdomen, such as that from a bicycle handlebar, may produce an intra-mural duodenal hematoma with partial or complete obstruction and a fullness or mass on radiographic abdominal examination (Fig. 10-18). Resolution usually takes place slowly, and parenteral nutrition may be required for a period of time. As with other suspicious injuries, skele-tal survey and detailed family evaluation are mandatory if the trauma is not explained by an obvious accident.

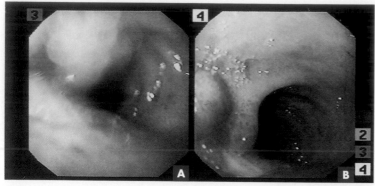

FIG. 10-20 *A,* Peptic ulcer. Two endoscopic views of the duodenum demonstrate the grayish-white base of an ulcer crater. *B* also demonstrates slightly erythematous, boggy tissue at the margin of the ulcer.

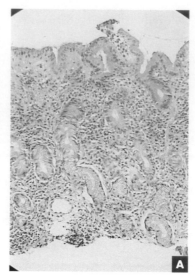
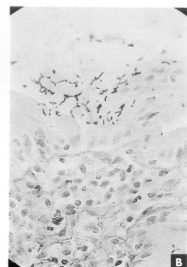

FIG. 10-21 Antral gastritis in a 9-year-old boy with abdominal pain and nausea for 1 week. *A,* Gastric biopsy with inflammatory infiltrate of plasma cells, neutrophils, and occasional eosinophils (H & E, ×25). *B,* Steiner silver stain (×400) demonstrates rod-shaped, spiral bacteria attached to the mucosa. Urease testing was positive, confirming infection with *Helicobacter pylori.*

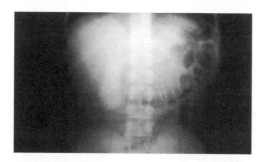

FIG. 10-22 Plain abdominal film demonstrates gallstones in this patient with sickle cell disease and abdominal pain.

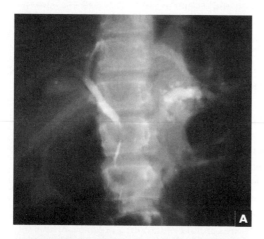

FIG. 10-23 Congenital pancreatic anomaly. This 12-year-old boy had recurrent abdominal pain for 10 years. *A,* Hematemesis prompted endoscopy and a retrograde cholangiogram, demonstrating an ectatic pancreatic duct. *B,* Operative cholangiogram defines a narrow duct just before entry into the duodenum. Division of the duct and anastomosis to the jejunum led to complete resolution of symptoms.

TABLE 10-8

Clues to Organic Disease in Recurrent Abdominal Pain

Weight loss
Nocturnal pain
Recurrent emesis
Regular school attendance
Easygoing personality
Stable home environment
Heme-positive stools
Abnormal physical examination findings—clubbing, perianal skin tags, abdominal mass
Abnormal screening laboratory test results—decreased albumin, increased ESR, anemia, increased lipase/amylase

ESR, erythrocyte sedimentation rate.

are the most common cause of pancreatitis in adults, congenital abnormalities may be more common in children (Fig. 10-23). Several studies demonstrate that trauma is the leading cause of acute pancreatitis in pediatric patients—at times related to abuse. Other causes in order of frequency are: idiopathic; biliary tract disease; drugs; infectious disease; congenital anomalies; and several "miscellaneous" disorders, such as penetrating peptic ulcer. The common presenting symptoms are abdominal pain, usually in the midepigastric area; nausea; and emesis associated with elevation of pancreatic enzymes (amylase/lipase). Chronic pancreatitis may be more subtle and at times may mimic RAP. Anatomic, hereditary, and idiopathic causes are much more common in chronic pancreatitis. Ultrasound and computed tomography (CT) have aided the diagnosis of pancreatitis and the treatment of complications, such as pseudocyst formation (Fig. 10-24).

The causes of acute abdominal pain in children are numerous. Appendicitis may not have the classic sequence in pediatric patients, and suspicion must be high in any acute illness. All too often, perforation

about peptic ulcer disease has undergone a radical shift in the last decade. Secondary ulcer disease may also be seen related to conditions such as systemic illness, collagen vascular disease, and drug therapy, especially nonsteroidal antiinflammatory agents.

Pancreatitis may also be seen in children, both as an acute condition and as a chronic, relapsing disorder. Although gallstones (Fig. 10-22)

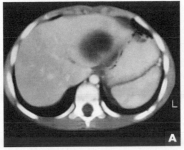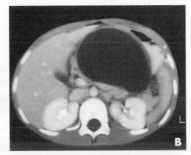

FIG. 10-24 Pancreatic pseudocyst. Abdominal pain and emesis led to CT scan in this patient who had a bicycle handlebar injury 2 weeks earlier. *A* demonstrates septation of the cavity, and *B* shows compression of stomach and pancreas by the cyst.

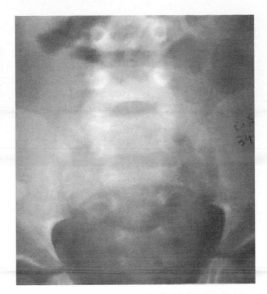

FIG. 10-25 An appendiceal fecalith can be seen in the right lower quadrant in this child with surgically proven acute appendicitis.

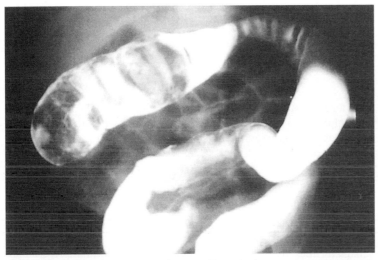

FIG. 10-26 Intussusception. Barium outlines the intussuscepted segment. Unfortunately, this lesion required laparotomy, because reduction did not occur during the barium enema.

TABLE 10-9	
GI Hemorrhage—Children Older Than 1 Year	
Upper	**Lower**
Esophageal varices	Colonic polyps
Gastric ulcers	Anal fissure
Gastritis	Intussusception
Duodenal ulcer	Meckel diverticulum
	Ulcerative colitis
	Regional enteritis
	Hemorrhoids

has occurred before the diagnosis, and an appendiceal fecalith may be a good though infrequent clue (Fig. 10-25).

Less than one third of patients with intussusception will have the classic triad: colicky pain, currant jelly stools, and an abdominal mass (Fig. 10-26). Neurologic symptoms, such as lethargy or seizure, are occasional clues to the diagnosis. Reduction by barium enema simplifies management of this disorder in most instances.

Hemorrhage

The etiology of GI hemorrhage usually requires detailed endoscopic and x-ray examination. In younger infants, particularly neonates, the diagnosis may remain unclear in more than 50% with a benign outlook. Generally, melanotic stools or frank hematemesis indicate upper gastrointestinal bleeding, whereas bright blood per rectum indicates loss from the lower gastrointestinal tract. Portal hypertension, often of extrahepatic origin, is suggested by splenomegaly, which may become evident only when volume status has been normalized after a recent hemorrhage. Other clues of chronic liver disease or colitis may be helpful. Perioral melanotic spots (Peutz-Jeghers syndrome) and other manifestations of intestinal polyposis syndromes (such as Gardner syndrome) can be detected by examination. The common disorders causing gastrointestinal hemorrhage are listed in Table 10-9 (see Chapter 17).

Diarrhea

Diarrhea in the pediatric patient is usually acute and infectious in etiology. Chronic persistent diarrhea (more than 2 weeks) is a more difficult problem. Early onset, poor growth, and malnutrition suggest a congenital or more serious disorder (chronic protracted diarrhea). Fortunately, most older infants and children have a postinfectious or even dietary cause. A carefully performed history and examination—especially related to growth, diet, and caloric intake—may prevent excessive investigation.

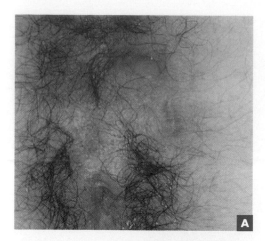

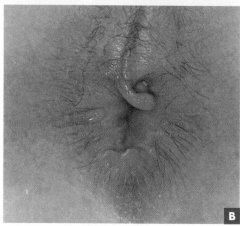

FIG. 10-27 *A,* In this patient with Crohn disease, the slightly raised, erythematous lesion eventually drained and represented a fistulous opening. *B,* Note a scar from previous incision and drainage. Perianal skin tags are common in Crohn disease and a good clue to diagnosis.

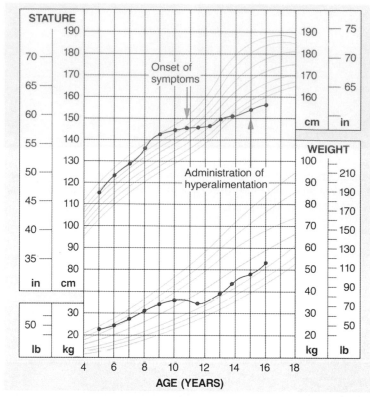

FIG. 10-28 Crohn disease. This growth curve demonstrates a falloff before onset of disease symptoms and continued poor growth through many exacerbations requiring steroid therapy. Home hyperalimentation has maintained weight gain.

Major clues to the etiology of diarrhea can be found when the stool is carefully examined. Small bowel diarrhea is usually watery and free of mucus. Unabsorbed sugar is easily detected by the Clinitest tablet, although heating and acidification are necessary if sucrose is present.

Stool pH also may be low (<5) in the presence of undigested carbohydrate. Excessive neutral fat (triglyceride) or split fat (fatty acid) supports the presence of malabsorption and can be easily detected. Neutral fat can be seen if several drops of water are added to the specimen. If 2 drops of 95% alcohol and 2 drops of stain (oil red-Sudan III) are added, smaller and more definite globules may be seen. Heating with acetic acid may be necessary to see split fat clearly under the microscope.

Infectious diarrhea often produces stools with blood or mucus. Stool leukocytes, another possible clue, can be seen more easily when 2 drops of water and 1 drop of methylene blue are added to a fresh stool smear before microscopic examination (Sondheimer). Whereas chronic diarrhea may be caused by malabsorption, chronic nonspecific or toddler's diarrhea is common and self-limited unless severe dietary restrictions are initiated. Stools are loose and often contain undigested fibers but no carbohydrate or fat. Occasionally, these children do better when placed on a diet containing unrestricted fat. The health beliefs of some parents, such as the benefits of low-fat, low-cholesterol foods, may contribute to the problem. Again, stool examination is helpful, especially a search for *Giardia lamblia* in children who are not thriving.

Inflammatory Bowel Disease

Crampy abdominal pain with mucus and blood suggests large-bowel involvement, and numerous clues may suggest chronic inflammatory bowel diseases such as Crohn disease or ulcerative colitis. Whereas clinical distinctions are at times blurred in these latter disorders, severe perianal disease with fistulae and fissures along with perianal skintags is more common in Crohn disease (Fig. 10-27). Additionally, poor growth before major GI symptoms often indicates Crohn disease (Fig. 10-28). Rectal disease is characteristic of ulcerative colitis, whereas perianal disease is less common. Histologically, Crohn disease is characterized by transmural inflammation with granuloma formation and skip areas. This deep inflammatory process accounts for the tendency to form fistulae and abscesses. Crypt abscesses are often seen in ulcerative colitis and help to distinguish this disorder from many other causes of acute colitis. Radiographically, Crohn disease may involve the entire bowel, with segmental narrowing, skip areas, and fistula formation (Fig. 10-29). Ulcerative colitis is a mucosal inflammation confined only to the large bowel (Fig. 10-30). Endoscopic findings are delineated in Figs. 10-31 and 10-32.

Osteoarthropathy, or clubbing in its mildest form, is seen in many conditions in which there is overt cardiopulmonary disease, such as cyanotic heart disease or lung disease, and in gastrointestinal diseases (especially Crohn) and liver disorders. Pathogenetic mechanisms are not clear, but shunting from right to left via pulmonary or abdominal vessels is a possibility. Earliest signs of osteoarthropathy are softening and loss of a normal angle at the base of the nail (Fig. 10-33).

Many rashes accompany inflammatory bowel disease, including erythema nodosum, erythema multiforme, papulonecrotic lesions, and ulcerative erythematous plaques. Perhaps the most characteristic rash is pyoderma gangrenosum. Initial lesions are papular, then become bullous, and finally are deeply ulcerated and necrotic. The most frequent locations are the cheeks, thighs, feet, hands, legs, and inguinal regions (Fig. 10-34).

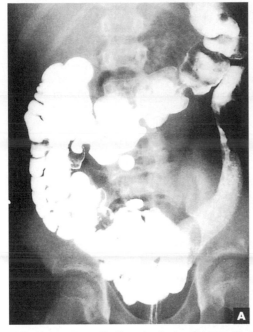
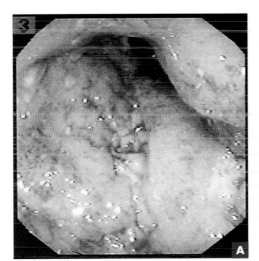
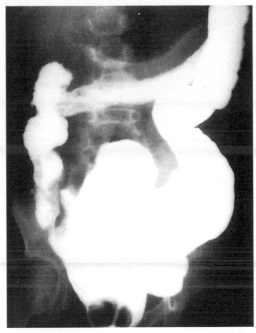

FIG. 10-29 X-ray findings in Crohn disease. *A,* Segmental narrowing of the left colon. *B,* A narrow and irregular terminal ileum.

FIG. 10-30 X-ray findings in ulcerative colitis. There is narrowing and loss of haustral markings, especially in the transverse colon. Mucosal irregularities are prominent in the right colon.

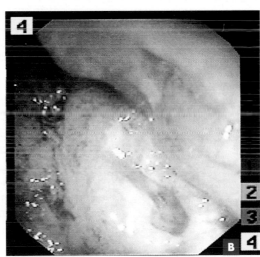
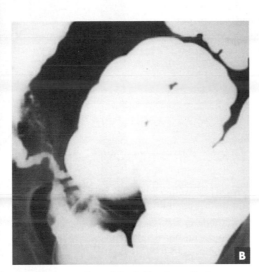
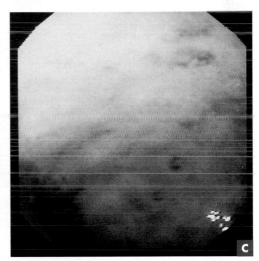

FIG. 10-31 Endoscopic findings in Crohn disease. *A* and *B,* Note deep linear, ulcerated fissure. *C,* Patchy colonic ulcers surrounded by normal mucosa.

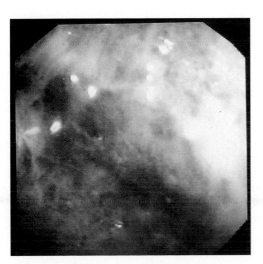
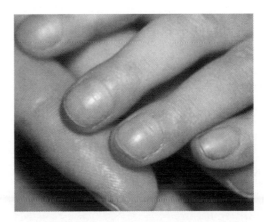

FIG. 10-32 Colonoscopic view of ulcerative colitis. The entire mucosa is inflamed and friable.

FIG. 10-33 Osteoarthropathy (clubbing). Note thickening and loss of the angle at the nail bed

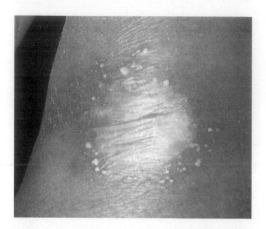

FIG. 10-34 Pyoderma gangrenosum associated with inflammatory bowel disease. Initial papulopustules coalesce to form a deep necrotic lesion.

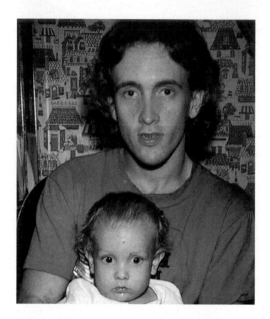

FIG. 10-36 Alagille syndrome. The child has intrahepatic biliary hypoplasia, butterfly vertebrae, and mild pulmonic stenosis. The father does not have liver disease, but he does have moderate pulmonic stenosis and poor growth. Note the narrow, thin face and pointed chin of both father and child.

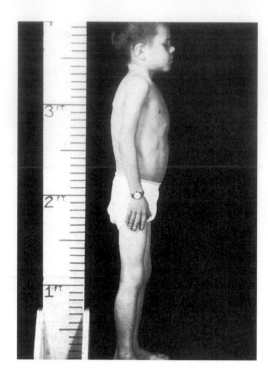

FIG. 10-35 Cystic fibrosis. This child presented with chronic cough. Note an increased AP chest diameter and overall poor nutrition, as well as clubbing.

TABLE 10-10

Obstructive Jaundice in the Neonate—Major Causes

Anatomic
  Biliary atresia, extrahepatic
  Biliary atresia, intrahepatic
    Syndromic (Alagille syndrome)
    Nonsyndromic
  Choledochal cyst
  Spontaneous perforation of bile duct
Hepatitis
  Idiopathic neonatal
  Other—cytomegalovirus, hepatitis B, etc.
  Toxic—sepsis, urinary tract infection, parenteral nutrition
Metabolic disorders
  Alpha$_1$-antitrypsin deficiency
  Cystic fibrosis
  Tyrosinemia
  Galactosemia
  Storage diseases—Niemann-Pick disease, etc.
  Other
Genetic and familial
  Familiar cholestasis (Byler disease)
  Chromosomal disorders (trisomy E)

Cystic Fibrosis

Cystic fibrosis is the most common inherited lethal disorder in whites, with predominantly pulmonary and GI manifestations. Clues to the diagnosis of cystic fibrosis are myriad and involve multiple systems. Few clinicians would fail to think of the diagnosis with meconium ileus, chronic cough, failure to thrive, and malabsorptive stools, so a few less common presentations are discussed here.

Edema in an infant who is breast-fed or on soy formula and consuming adequate calories should strongly suggest cystic fibrosis. As noted in the section on kwashiorkor, these infants often appear well fed but quite thin after fluid is diuresed. The older child with asthma or recurrent bronchitis should be examined closely for signs of chronic lung disease. Subtle increases in anteroposterior chest diameter, clubbing, and rather poor general nutrition make a sweat test mandatory (Fig. 10-35) (see Chapter 16).

Chronic Liver Disease

Infancy

Obstructive jaundice is the major clue to most hepatobiliary disorders in early infancy. Exceptions are metabolic or storage diseases (glycogen storage, Gaucher disease, etc.) in which organomegaly is the prominent finding. Neonatal obstructive jaundice has a large group of diagnostic possibilities—extrahepatic biliary atresia and neonatal "giant cell" hepatitis being the most common (Table 10-10). Although not specific, acholic stools are a sensitive marker of complete obstruction. Clues to individual disorders occasionally are present. Intrahepatic biliary atresia (biliary hypoplasia, paucity of bile ducts) is seen either in syndromic (Alagille syndrome) or nonsyndromic form. Peculiar facies (deeply set eyes, narrow chin), persistent posterior embryotoxon, pulmonary artery abnormalities, and butterfly vertebrae are characteristic of Alagille syndrome or arteriohepatic dysplasia (Figs. 10-36 and 10-37). This condition has been localized to chromosome 20. Many individuals have only a few features of the disorder; prognosis is variable. These patients often suffer from xanthoma formation and severe pruritus, which occasionally

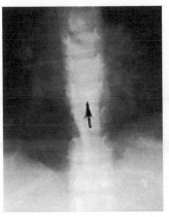
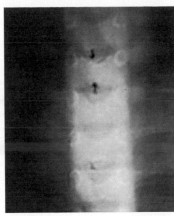

FIG. 10-37   These x-rays illustrate defects in the vertebral arches that lead to the "butterfly" appearance.

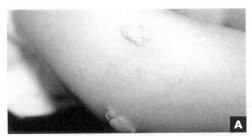
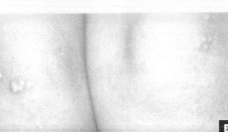
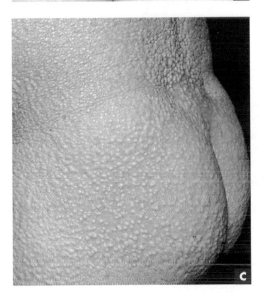

FIG. 10-38   Xanthomas in chronic liver disease. Characteristic areas in the early stages of disease are "pressure points" such as elbows *(A)* and knees *(B)*; later, xanthomas may become generalized *(C)*.

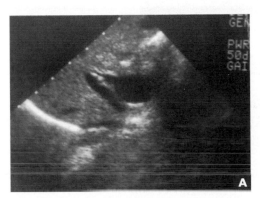
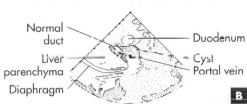
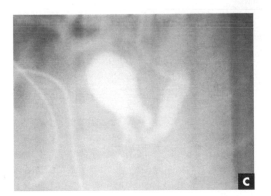

FIG. 10-39   Ultrasound of infant with obstructive jaundice demonstrates cystic structure below the liver *(A and B)*. Intraoperative cholangiogram in same patient defines cyst and gallbladder along with hepatic and cystic ducts *(C)*.

Normal duct
Duodenum
Liver parenchyma
Cyst
Portal vein
Diaphragm

are features of other chronic liver diseases (Fig. 10-38). The choledochal cyst is a surgically correctable cause of jaundice and may be palpable (Fig. 10-39).

Extrahepatic biliary atresia (EBA), with an incidence of 0.65 per 10,000 live births, is the most common cause of end-stage pediatric liver disease. Approximately 350 children are born with this condition in the United States every year. EBA may be associated with abnormalities of other organ systems, situs inversus viscerum, and polysplenia with or without congenital heart disease. Additionally, GI tract anomalies, such

as malrotation (Fig. 10-40) and vascular anomalies (Fig. 10-41), may rarely complicate initial surgery and later liver transplantation.

Childhood

Children with chronic liver disease and cirrhosis have many clinical features in common. The liver is usually firm and is often irregular and enlarged, although in late stages it may decrease in size. Splenomegaly follows portal hypertension. Portosystemic venous anastomoses lead to

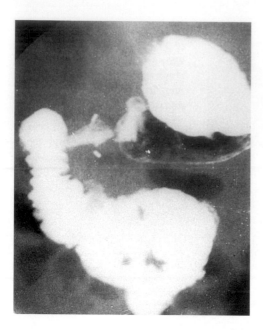

FIG. 10-40 Malrotation in biliary atresia. The duodenal "C" loop is not closed and is displaced to the right.

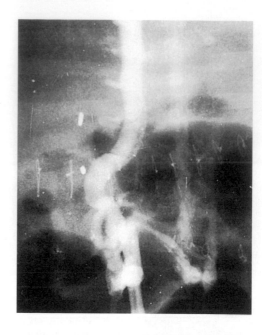

FIG. 10-41 Vascular anomaly in biliary atresia. The inferior vena cava is interrupted and continues as an azygous vein.

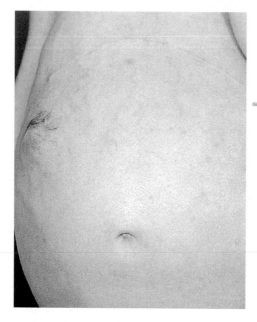

FIG. 10-42 Chronic liver disease/portal hypertension. This child had biliary atresia with good bile flow after a portoenterostomy procedure. Cirrhosis developed late, with physical signs of prominent abdominal veins and ascites.

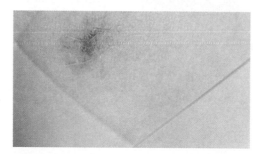

FIG. 10-43 Spider nevus. The vascular lesion blanches with compression by a glass slide, but it reappears when pressure is released.

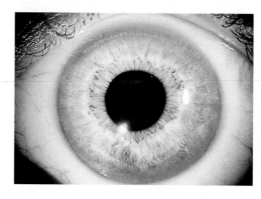

FIG. 10-44 Kayser-Fleischer ring appears as brownish discoloration in the posterior part of the cornea, as defined by slit-lamp examination. Early KF rings may be seen only by slit lamp and begin at the superior and inferior poles.

the development of dilated vessels in the abdominal wall (caput medusae) and gastrointestinal tract (varices, hemorrhoids) (Fig. 10-42). Ascitic fluid may form, and if present in sufficient quantity, produce flank dullness and a fluid wave. Ultrasonography may detect even smaller amounts of free fluid. Spider nevi, dilated vascular channels that disappear with pressure, are seen in normal adolescents but should suggest chronic liver disease if other historic or examination clues are present (Fig. 10-43).

Wilson disease is one of the chronic liver disorders that can be reversed with therapy. Presentations include hepatitis, neuropsychiatric disturbances, hemolytic anemia, and cirrhosis. The clinician must establish a diagnosis in any child older than 4 years with persistent

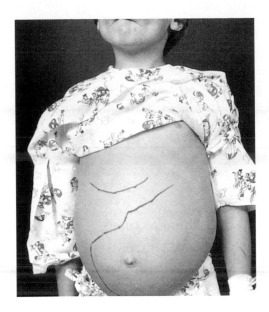

FIG. 10-45 Congenital hepatic fibrosis. This clinically well child had hematemesis and hypersplenism with normal liver function studies. Note massive splenic size and large left lobe of liver. Portosystemic shunting was effective therapy.

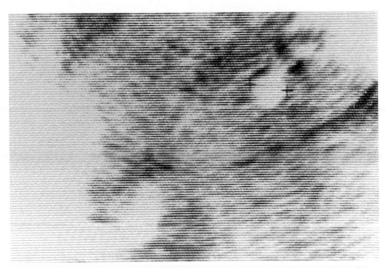

FIG. 10-46 Ultrasonogram of the kidney in a patient with congenital hepatic fibrosis reveals a cystic structure.

transaminase elevation. Serum ceruloplasmin is usually reduced and 24-hour copper excretion elevated. However, measurement of hepatic copper may be necessary in some patients. Kayser-Fleischer rings occasionally are visible without the use of a slit lamp (Fig. 10-44). Therapy with copper-chelating agents, such as penicillamine, must be initiated before irreversible cirrhosis develops. Both the chronic liver failure and the neurologic disorder may be effectively treated by transplantation.

Finally, one chronic hepatic disorder can usually be recognized by examination alone. The healthy-appearing child with massive splenomegaly and a large, firm left lobe of the liver with no stigmata of chronic liver disease except GI hemorrhage almost certainly has congenital hepatic fibrosis (Fig. 10-45). These children may suffer from part of the spectrum of polycystic kidney disease in childhood, and renal function studies are warranted (Fig. 10-46). Therapy for this condition may include shunting procedures for portal hypertension because liver function may remain normal indefinitely.

BIBLIOGRAPHY

Ament M: Diagnosis and management of upper gastrointestinal tract bleeding in the pediatric patient, *Pediatr Rev* 12:107-116, 1990.

Balistreri WF: Neonatal cholestasis, *J Pediatr* 106:171-184,1985.

Bithoney WG, Dubowitz H, Egan H: Failure to thrive/growth deficiency, *Pediatr Rev* 13:453-459, 1992.

Fitzgerald JF: Constipation in children, *Pediatr Rev* 8:299-302, 1987.

Gartner JC: Recurrent abdominal pain—who needs a workup? *Contemp Pediatr* 6:62-82, 1989.

Gryboski J: The child with chronic diarrhea, *Contemp Pediatr* 10.71-97, 1993.

Lake A: Recognition and management of inflammatory bowel disease in children and adolescents, *Curr Probl Pediatr* 18:379-437, 1988.

Macarthur C, Saunders N, Feldman W: *Helicobacter pylori*, gastroduodenal disease, and recurrent abdominal pain in children, *JAMA* 273:729-734, 1995.

Mews C, Sinatra F: Chronic liver disease in children, *Pediatr Rev* 14:436-443, 1993.

NIH Consensus Development Panel on *Helicobacter pylori* in peptic ulcer disease, *JAMA* 272:65-69, 1994.

Orenstein S: Gastroesophageal reflux, *Pediatr Rev* 13:174-182, 1992.

Orenstein S, Orenstein D: Gastroesophageal reflux and respiratory disease in children, *J Pediatr* 112:847-858, 1988.

Silber G: Lower gastrointestinal bleeding, *Pediatr Rev* 12:85-92, 1990.

Sondheimer JM: Office stool examination. a practical guide, *Contemp Pediatr* 7:63-82, 1990.

Steinberg W, Tenner S: Acute pancreatitis, *N Engl J Med* 330:1198-1210, 1994.

Suskind RM, ed: *Textbook of pediatric nutrition*, New York, 1981, Raven Press.

Suskind RM, Varma RN: Assessment of nutritional status of children, *Pediatr Rev* 5:195-202, 1984.

Walker WA, Hendricks KM: *Manual of pediatric nutrition*, Philadelphia, 1985, WB Saunders.

11

Hematology and Oncology

J. JEFFREY MALATACK ❦ JULIE BLATT
LILA PENCHANSKY

Hematology

The tools of the clinical pediatric hematologist have evolved over recent years, as techniques previously limited to research and laboratory settings have moved into the realm of normal investigation and therapeutics. Despite such advances, however, the core of hematologic diagnosis resides in a thorough medical history; physical examination; evaluation of the patient's peripheral blood, complete blood count (CBC), and reticulocyte count; and occasionally, bone marrow examination. In contrast to much of pediatric diagnosis, laboratory results carry a disproportionate weight in the evaluation of the patient with hematologic problems.

This chapter first highlights common hematologic conditions and selected rarer entities. In this context, peripheral blood smear and basic diagnostic tests are used to evaluate nonmalignant hematologic disease, including signs and symptoms of clotting abnormalities. Then attention is given to hematologic findings in leukemia and solid tumors.

Peripheral Blood Smear

The peripheral blood smear has two major functions. First, it provides confirmation of the values given on the standard Coulter counter printout, which may falsely report elevated white blood cell (WBC) counts resulting from the presence of nucleated red blood cells (RBCs). In addition, the presence of RBC fragments may result in falsely elevated platelet counts. Second, review of the peripheral smear allows the diagnostician to perform the differential WBC count at the same time as examination of RBC, WBC, and platelet morphology.

A systematic approach to the evaluation of the smear can maximize the amount of information extracted. First, the slide is scanned under low power, and an area is chosen in which the RBCs are just barely touching (Fig. 11-1). Areas in which the RBCs are too dense or too sparse are fraught with artifact. Under low power, mononuclear and polymorphonuclear cells are visible. By using the high-dry or oil lens, the examiner can observe normal RBC morphology. The normal RBC appears as a biconcave disc with an area of central pallor surrounded by an otherwise homogeneous red circle (Fig. 11-2). Beyond the new-born period, during which time it is larger, the RBC is about the size of the nucleus of a small lymphocyte.

After an evaluation of RBC morphology, a WBC differential count can be performed and the morphology of the cells assessed. A blood smear made from anticoagulated blood may have artifacts such as vacuolation of the WBCs. Finally, platelets should be scrutinized for number (each platelet found on a high-dry field represents approximately 10,000 to 15,000 platelets per mm^3).

Red Blood Cell

The RBC is the most ubiquitous of the blood's cellular components. Its primary function is to mediate the exchange of respiratory gases (oxygen and carbon dioxide) between the lungs and body tissues. This is accomplished by the critical biochemical features of its oxygen-carrying intracellular component, hemoglobin (Hgb). Hemoglobin's oxygen-binding sites are completely saturated by passage of the RBC through the lungs. As the cells circulate through the systemic capillaries, the hemoglobin releases 25% of its bound oxygen to the tissues. However, the amount of oxygen released in the tissue may be significantly increased under certain conditions (fever, acidosis, level of 2, 3-diphosphoglycerate), allowing some compensation for a decrease in hemoglobin. Nonetheless, a progressive decrease in the hemoglobin level eventually leads to tissue hypoxia, which triggers a release of erythropoietin. This induces an increase in RBC production, which brings the critical RBC mass back toward normal values.

Red Cell Production

RBC production usually occurs in the bone marrow, but under conditions of disease, it also can occur in extramedullary locations such as the spleen. For the first 48 hours after it has joined the peripheral circulation, a newly formed RBC, or reticulocyte, can be stained by a supravital dye for easy identification. Generally, the reticulocyte count is a reflection of the replacement of senescent RBCs. Since the RBC's life span is approximately 120 days, 0.83% of the RBC's mass must be replaced every day. Because reticulocytes maintain their staining characteristics

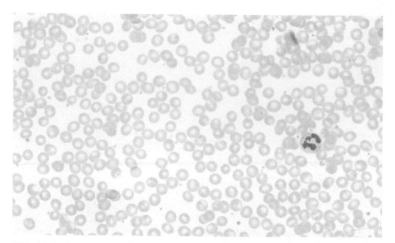

FIG. 11-1   Low-power (×100) magnification of a normal peripheral blood smear.

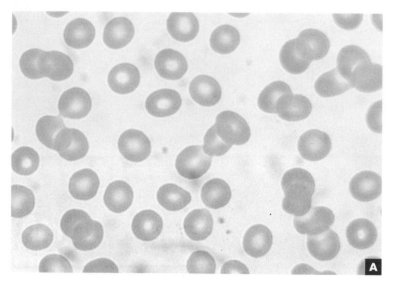

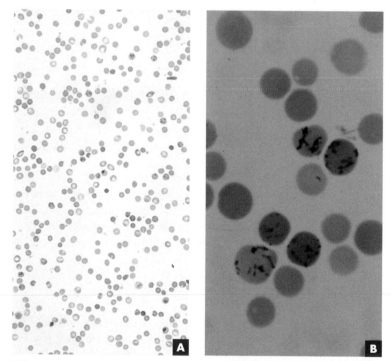

FIG. 11-3   *A,* Reticulocyte-stained peripheral blood smear in a patient with a high (18%) reticulocyte count. The darkly stained cells are reticulocytes. The patient had hemolytic anemia. *B,* Oil immersion view of reticulocyte-stained peripheral blood from the same patient. Higher power reveals reticulin staining of the RBCs.

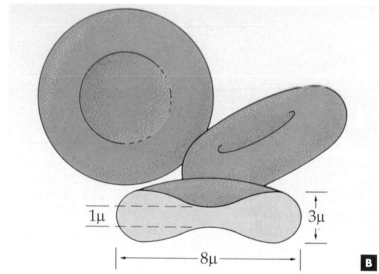

FIG. 11-2   High-power (×400) magnification of a normal peripheral blood smear *(A).* Schematic drawing of an RBC in two views demonstrates features of the normal biconcave disc *(B).*

for approximately 48 hours, the normal reticulocyte count (percentage of peripheral RBCs that are reticulocytes) is approximately 1.66%, ranging from 0.83% to 2.49%. This figure is 1% to 2% higher in menstruating women. Increased reticulocyte counts are also a reflection of increased RBC loss through hemolysis or hemorrhage. Decreased reticulocyte counts indicate decreased RBC production (Fig. 11-3).

Anemia

Increased RBC loss or decreased RBC production can result in an overall decrease in RBC mass below a critical level, leading to anemia. This is the most common abnormality of RBCs, and it is identified as a decreased hemoglobin level and decreased hematocrit. Recognition that a

child's hemoglobin level is too low requires knowledge of age, gender, and race-related normal values. At any given age, anemia is a value greater than two standard deviations below the mean (Table 11-1). For children 6 months of age until puberty, a hemoglobin level of less than 11 g/dl is a useful definition of anemia and an indication for evaluation. Alternatively, an inappropriate drop in the hemoglobin level may also be significant: the 5-year-old child who has a hemoglobin level of 11.5 g/dl but who, 1 month earlier, had a level of 13 g/dl, may require evaluation.

Severe anemia from any cause may elicit symptoms of fatigue, decreased appetite, and in extreme cases, shock, congestive heart failure, or even stroke. Physical examination of the anemic child may reveal pallor, although in the fair-skinned or very dark-skinned child this may be easily missed, even given an extremely low level of hemoglobin,

TABLE 11-1

Hemoglobin and Mean Corpuscular Volume Values at Various Ages

Age	Hemoglobin (g/dl)	MCV (fl)
Birth (cord blood)	16.5	108
1 to 3 days (capillary)	18.5	108
1 week	17.5	107
2 weeks	16.5	105
1 month	14.0	104
2 months	11.5	96
3 to 6 months	11.5	91
$\frac{1}{2}$ to 2 years	12.0	78
2 to 6 years	12.5	81
6 to 12 years	13.5	86
12 to 18 years—girls	14.0	90
boys	14.5	88
18 to 49 years—women	14.0	90
men	15.5	90

Modified from Dallman PR. In Rudolph A, ed: *Pediatrics*, ed 16, New York, 1977, Appleton-Century-Crofts.
MCV, Mean corpuscular volume.

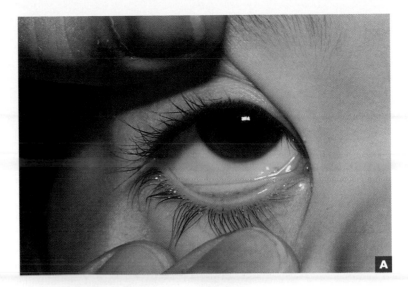

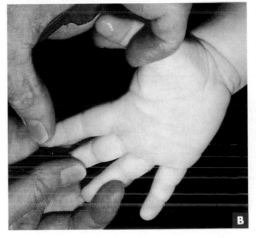

FIG. 11-4 *A,* Pale conjunctiva in a patient with severe anemia. *B,* Pale palmar creases in a child with a hemoglobin level of 4 g/dl.

unless palmar creases or conjunctivae also are examined for pallor (Fig. 11-4). Vital signs may be normal, but with severe anemia, the heart rate increases.

Before embarking on a workup in a child with a low hemoglobin level, it is worth considering whether the reported blood value is accurate. Reasons for inaccuracy include poor quality control in the use of the Coulter counter, dilution of blood drawn from venous lines, and falsely elevated values, particularly in neonates when the CBC is obtained by heel or finger stick. Anemia, when it does occur, may be an isolated finding, or it may be part of the spectrum of pancytopenia in which WBC and platelet levels also are decreased.

Conceptionally, anemia occurs as a result of one of the following:
1. Decreased bone marrow production of RBCs
2. Increased destruction of mature RBCs peripherally or of their precursors while they are still in the bone marrow (ineffective erythropoiesis)
3. Hemorrhage
4. Combinations of the above

Anemias resulting from decreased RBC production include microcytic anemia, pure red cell aplasia, and megaloblastic anemia. Hemolytic anemias, characterized by increased RBC destruction without evidence of blood loss or ineffective erythropoiesis, include RBC membrane defects, intracellular RBC defects, and extraRBC factors causing hemolysis.

Anemias Resulting from Decreased Red Cell Production

RBC morphology generally categorizes the type of anemia present and may suggest certain pathogenic mechanisms.

Hypochromic Microcytic Anemia

Hypochromic microcytic anemia represents the most common type of isolated failure of RBC production. Microcytosis exists when the mean corpuscular volume (hematocrit × 10 ÷ RBC number [in millions per mm³]) is low or when the RBCs themselves are smaller than the nuclei of the small lymphocytes. Hypochromia, a decrease in the concentration of intracellular content, is recognized when the mean corpuscular hemoglobin concentration (hemoglobin [in g/dl] × 10 ÷ hematocrit) is decreased or when the hemoglobinized rim of the RBC is less than two thirds the diameter of the entire cell. Normally, the ratio of RBC volume to the intracellular RBC content is homeostatically maintained. As the concentration of intracellular content decreases for any reason, the volume of the cell also decreases.

The differential diagnosis of hypochromic microcytic anemia includes iron deficiency, lead poisoning, thalassemia minor (alpha and beta types), thalassemia major (Cooley anemia), chronic infection, chronic inflammatory states, and sideroblastic anemia.

IRON DEFICIENCY ANEMIA

Iron deficiency anemia is the most common pediatric hypochromic microcytic anemia. Iron deficiency is only a laboratory finding, not a diagnosis. The causes of iron deficiency must be elucidated through a careful history and physical examination. Although poor nutrition is the most common cause, other causes such as hemorrhage or malabsorption also must be considered. Iron deficiency anemia occurs in infants whose rapidly increasing RBC mass outstrips the dietary iron intake. This lack of iron leads to failure of hemoglobin production and the formation of hypochromic microcytic cells. Since the normal full-term infant has adequate iron reserve to accommodate the increasing RBC

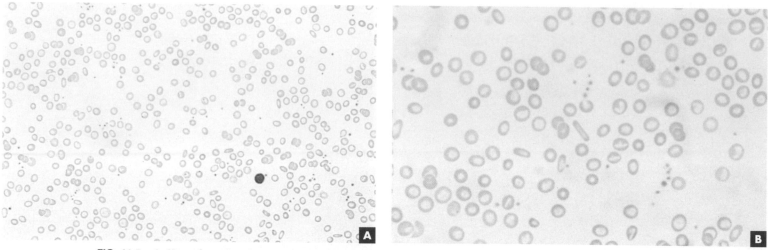

FIG. 11-5   *A,* Hypochromic microcytic anemia of iron deficiency anemia. This 16-month-old patient has a history of excessive milk intake. Note the marked central pallor of the RBC with a small rim of hemoglobin, as well as its small size in comparison with that of the adjacent small lymphocyte nucleus. *B,* Peripheral blood smear of a patient with iron deficiency. Frequent "cigar cells" can be seen in addition to the hypochromic microcytic RBCs.

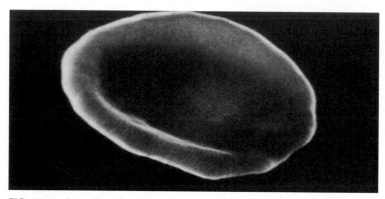

FIG. 11-6   Scanning electron microscope image of an iron deficient cell. Note the three-dimensional shape and curled edges.

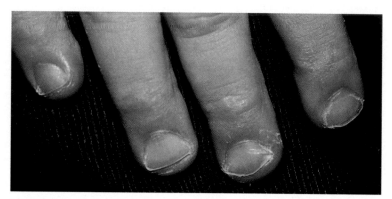

FIG. 11-7   Spooning of fingernails in child with iron deficiency anemia.

mass through the first 5 months of life, iron deficiency usually is not seen until the second half of the first year of life. It is detected most often in the 10- to 18-month-old child.

The typical clinical history is that of an infant fed non–iron-containing whole cow's milk who, from early infancy, takes large volumes of milk and little else. These children often are large, but their pallor belies their apparent robust size. Whole cow's milk not only is deficient in dietary iron but often leads to an enteropathic condition with gastrointestinal blood loss, exacerbating the child's iron-deficient status.

Fig. 11-5, *A,* shows the peripheral blood smear of a 16-month-old child who had been fed large amounts of whole milk from 3 months of age. The RBCs are microcytic and hypochromic. The number of platelets is characteristically increased (particularly when the enteropathic condition is present), although it may be normal or even decreased. In severe iron deficiency anemia, anisocytosis (varied size of RBCs) and poikilocytosis (varied RBC shape) may be prominent. Nonspecific abnormalities of RBC morphology, such as the presence of microovalocytes (cigar cells) (Fig. 11-5, *B*) or basophilic stippling (Fig. 11-11), may also occur. Bizarre RBC shapes are due to a three-dimensional change in structure when viewed in a two-dimensional plane of the light microscope. The microovalocyte of iron deficiency appears oval because op-

posite ends of the severely dehemoglobinized RBCs tend to curl up (Fig. 11-6). When viewed in two dimensions, the cell appears ovoid.

The condition of the child with iron deficiency may be asymptomatic despite a significant degree of anemia. However, when symptoms are present, irritability is the prominent finding. Children have also been shown to demonstrate decreases in Bayley IQ scores, as well as occasional peculiar physical findings such as "spooning" of the finger- and toenails (koilonychia) (Fig. 11-7) and glossitis.

Iron deficiency must be differentiated from thalassemia and lead poisoning. Although the patient history generally suggests the appropriate diagnosis, the distinction can be made, for the most part, on the basis of a few laboratory tests. Review of the peripheral smear (Fig. 11-5, *A*) should first confirm the presence of microcytosis or hypochromia, which, like the measurements of hemoglobin, are susceptible to technical errors. In thalassemia minor, the hemoglobin is generally not less than 9 g/dl; moreover, for a given degree of anemia, the mean corpuscular volume tends to be lower in the child with thalassemia than in the child with iron deficiency. These trends may be reflected in the Mentzer index, which mathematically relates the mean corpuscular volume to the RBC number (Mentzer index = mean corpuscular volume ÷ number of RBCs ÷ 10^6). Mentzer indices greater than 13.5 suggest iron deficiency, whereas values less than 11.5 indicate thalassemia minor. In

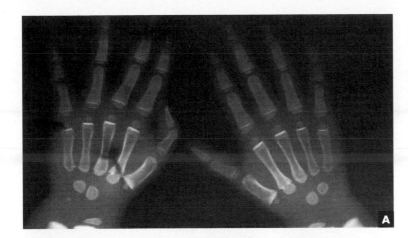

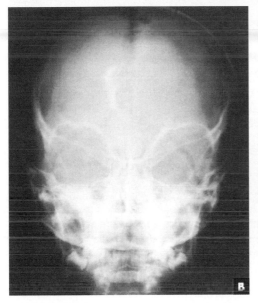

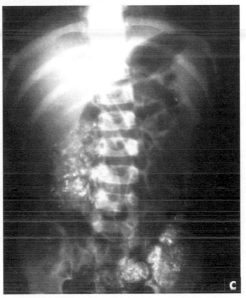

FIG. 11-8 *A,* Hand radiograph of a child with lead intoxication reveals marked linear increases in the density of the metaphyses. These should not be confused with the growth arrest lines seen after a variety of illnesses. *B,* Skull film of a patient with lead intoxication with encephalopathy. Note the split sutures indicative of increased intracranial pressure. *C,* Abdominal radiograph of a child with a history of pica and lead intoxication reveals radiodense, lead-containing paint chips scattered throughout the colon.

practice, the index has not been helpful, since most children with mild anemias may have intermediate index values. Other helpful clues to the diagnosis can come directly from the RBC number, since children with iron deficiency usually have a low RBC number, whereas thalassemia tends to produce RBC numbers greater than $5 \times 10^6/mm^3$. The RBC distribution width (standard deviation of red blood cell volume ÷ mean corpuscular volume × 100) is a reflection of the degree of anisocytosis and is significantly larger in iron deficiency than in thalassemia trait.

The clinical history—along with the results of the CBC; the differential, platelet and reticulocyte counts; and review of the peripheral smear—is sufficient for diagnosis in most instances of hypochromic microcytic anemia. Occasionally, other, more specific laboratory tests may be needed. If the evaluation before obtaining a specific test strongly suggests iron deficiency and the child does not live in an area where a high incidence of lead exposure occurs, a therapeutic trial of oral iron may be a reasonable approach. However, the physician is obliged to follow up on the patient until the blood count has returned to normal; improvement is not enough. The coexistence of lead poisoning and iron deficiency is well documented. Hence, partial response to iron therapy does not eliminate lead poisoning from diagnostic consideration.

Choosing between specific studies such as serum iron levels and total iron binding capacity (used together to calculate iron saturation) or ferritin and free erythrocyte protoporphyrin (FEP) is often a matter of personal preference. In addition, when the degree of anemia is mild, the results of any combination of tests may be equivocal. FEP has the advantage of screening for lead poisoning or porphyria. Ferritin is an acute phase reactant and may be elevated into the low normal range in a child with a concurrent inflammatory process. Iron saturation and ferritin levels have age-related normal values. Children up to age 15 have serum ferritin levels less than 10 μg/mg, indicating iron deficiency. Transferrin saturation confirms iron deficiency if it is under 12% for children 5 to 10 years old and under 16% for older children. FEP levels indicate iron deficiency if they are over 90 μg/dl RBC for infants and preschoolers up to age 4 years and over 70 μg/dl RBC for older children.

LEAD POISONING

Lead intoxication leads to microcytic anemia. However, nonhematologic manifestations of lead intoxication, particularly neurologic complications, often dominate the picture. The spectrum of clinical presentations of lead intoxication ranges from vague symptoms of abdominal pain, vomiting, malaise, and behavioral changes to acute encephalopathic conditions, with rapid progression to coma and death. Late physical findings may include papilledema. Significant radiographic changes also are seen in lead intoxication (Fig. 11-8).

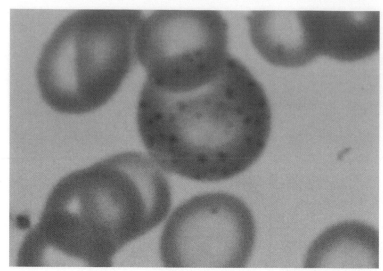

FIG. 11-9 Hypochromic microcytic anemia resulting from lead intoxication. Note the prominent basophilic stippling. This finding is not specific for lead intoxication but may be seen in thalassemia and treated iron deficiency.

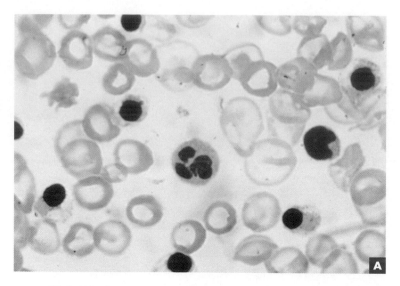

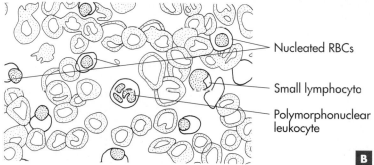

FIG. 11-10 Peripheral blood smear of a child with thalassemia major. Note the hypochromic microcytic anemia and prominent nucleated RBCs surrounding the polymorphonuclear cells and lymphocytes.

Lead intoxication occurs as a result of excessive environmental lead intake. Aerosolized and oral lead-containing environmental contaminants are major sources of lead intoxication. Although clearly a common mechanism in lead poisoning, pica, which is associated with the intake of flaking lead paint, represents neither the only nor the prevailing cause of lead intoxication. The finger-sucking behavior of children in homes where lead paint has become a part of house dust is perhaps a more important factor. A contaminated water supply resulting from old plumbing and deteriorating lead-containing soldered joints can cause lead intoxication in the infant (earlier than the usual "at risk" age).

Hematologic abnormalities of lead intoxication are a direct result of the effect of lead on several cellular enzymes involved in heme production. Lead inhibits these enzyme systems, impairing iron use and globin synthesis. Thus despite normal intracellular levels, iron is unable to be incorporated into heme, and hemoglobin production fails. Reduced hemoglobin production leads directly to microcytic hypochromic anemia. Basophilic stippling is a secondary and inconsistent hematologic manifestation of lead intoxication that occurs as a result of inhibition of yet another RBC enzyme, 5-pyrimidine nucleotidase. This enzyme normally removes nucleotide chains from the RBC after its nucleus has been extruded. In lead poisoning, these chains persist, and the nucleotide remnants stain blue on a normal Wright stain, causing a stippling of the RBC (Fig. 11-9). Although basophilic stippling is more prominent in lead intoxication, it is also present in thalassemia and treated iron deficiency. Its presence on the peripheral smear is nonspecific.

Differentiating lead intoxication from iron deficiency can, at times, be difficult. Also, lead intoxication and iron deficiency may coexist, further confusing the diagnosis. Lead poisoning and iron deficiency cause erythrocyte protoporphyrin to accumulate in blood. The FEP is elevated in both conditions, although extremely high levels are more common in lead intoxication. Further testing, such as determination of blood lead level, is necessary to determine the cause of elevated FEP levels. When suspicion of lead intoxication exists, a lead level should be determined. Recent information incriminating even low-level lead intoxication as a cause of disturbed cognitive function underscores the necessity for clinicians to consider this diagnosis. Silent lead intoxication with blood lev-

els of 15 µg/dl remains a significant pediatric health problem and may not be associated with the signs of chronic high-level lead poisoning previously described.

THALASSEMIA

Thalassemia is a term applied to a group of genetic disturbances decreasing hemoglobin production and leading to anemia and/or altered levels of the various hemoglobins in the blood.

Thalassemia trait is also responsible for hypochromic microcytic anemia. In patients with beta-thalassemia trait, hemoglobin electrophoresis usually reveals an increse in Hgb A_2 and Hgb F, whereas in patients with alpha-thalassemia trait the findings may be normal. This costly test probably is overused in the evaluation of hypochromic microcytic anemia. Hemograms on parents may be helpful if they show a microcytosis in at least one parent, further suggesting a diagnosis of thalassemia trait. If a diagnosis of thalassemia is suggested by any of the studies already discussed, both parents should have hemograms performed. Although the child may suffer from thalassemia trait, it is conceivable that both parents may also have thalassemia trait, and a subsequent child may be born with thalassemia major, a disease with serious implications regarding morbidity and mortality. Appropriate genetic counseling is indicated in this case.

Thalassemia major (Cooley anemia) causes hypochromic microcytic anemia that results from ineffective erythropoiesis caused by an imbalance between alpha- and beta-hemoglobin chain synthesis. The peripheral blood smear shows hypochromia, microcytosis, target cells, basophilic stippling, and often, large number of nucleated RBCs (Fig. 11-10). Beta-thalassemia major is associated with increased marrow activity, which is ineffectively attempting to correct the degree of

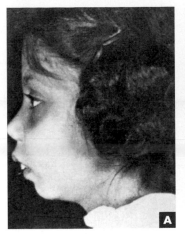 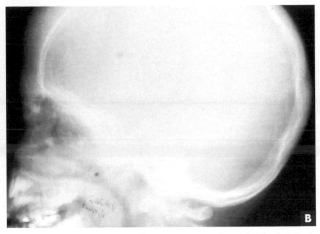

FIG. 11-11 *A,* Maxillary hyperplasia resulting from an increased marrow space in a child with thalassemia major. *B,* Skull radiograph of the same patient demonstrates an increased marrow cavity of the skull and facial bones.

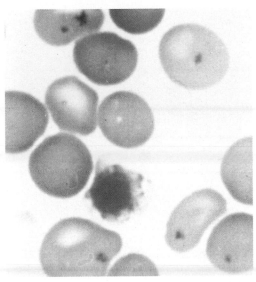

FIG. 11-12 Ringed sideroblast (iron-containing normoblast) on iron stain of the bone marrow. They are present in patients with sideroblastic anemia.

anemia. The increased marrow activity expands the marrow cavity, producing a characteristic bony hyperplasia evidenced by physical and radiographic findings (Fig. 11-11). Untreated patients with thalassemia major have chronic and severe anemia; marked hepatosplenomegaly; scleral icterus; and listlessness and may have high-output cardiac failure secondary to severe anemia. In addition, malocclusion may occur because of malar hypertrophy. This picture should not be confused with thalassemia trait, iron deficiency, or lead poisoning. Thalassemia major generally presents after the first 6 months of life at a time when beta-chain synthesis increases. Hydrops fetalis may result from alpha-thalassemia major. Ethnicity may be an important clue in the history: Beta-thalassemia trait tends to occur in patients of African or Mediterranean descent, whereas alpha-thalassemia trait tends to occur in blacks or Orientals. Thalassemia major is largely restricted to people of Mediterranean or Middle Eastern heritage.

CHRONIC INFLAMMATORY STATES

Chronic inflammatory states, such as chronic infection or collagen vascular diseases (particularly juvenile rheumatoid arthritis), may lead to hypochromic microcytic anemia. Although the symptoms of the child's primary illness usually clarify the diagnosis, there are occasionally cases in which a chronic subclinical infection (particularly of the urinary tract) may go undiagnosed. Differentiating a chronic inflammatory state from other causes of hypochromic microcytic anemia is usually more easily done on clinical than laboratory grounds. One laboratory study that may be of value is the serum ferritin determination. The ferritin is decreased in iron deficiency, whereas in chronic inflammatory states it is usually elevated.

SIDEROBLASTIC AND OTHER ANEMIAS

The sideroblastic anemias are characterized by the presence of a population of hypochromic microcytic cells in the peripheral blood as well as sideroblasts in the bone marrow (Fig. 11-12). The sideroblastic anemias, very rare in pediatrics, can be hereditary or acquired. The hereditary anemia is caused by a deficiency of an enzyme or enzyme activity required for hemoglobin production. The acquired form may arise secondary to drugs or toxins (lead being the most important of those in childhood), malignancy, or inflammatory endocrine disease, or it may be idiopathic.

Copper deficiency and chronic disease, although generally resulting in normocytic anemia, may occasionally cause a microcytic condition.

Macrocytic Anemia

Macrocytic anemia (mean corpuscular volume >100 fl on the Coulter indices) may be associated with decreased RBC production. Some patients with macrocytic anemia may have hemorrhage or hemolysis and a brisk reticulocytosis, which accounts for the large RBCs on the peripheral smear. Such causes of macrocytic anemia usually are easily recognized and differentiated from macrocytic anemia based on bone marrow failure. Macrocytosis is relatively uncommon in pediatric patients after the neonatal period (Table 11-1). The differential diagnosis of macrocytosis includes reticulocytosis, Down syndrome, pure red cell aplasia (which also may be normocytic), hypothyroidism, liver disease, and megaloblastic anemia.

MEGALOBLASTIC ANEMIA

These anemias constitute another group of conditions characterized by failure of adequate RBC production. Although the etiology of the megaloblastic anemias may vary, common morphologic abnormalities

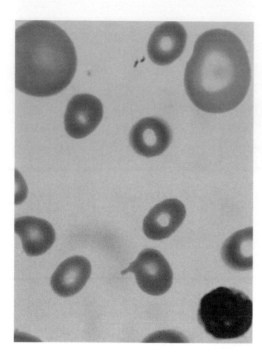

FIG. 11-13 Peripheral blood smear of a patient with megaloblastic anemia. Note the enlarged RBC (macrocyte) at the upper left. It is much larger than the normal small lymphocyte in the same field.

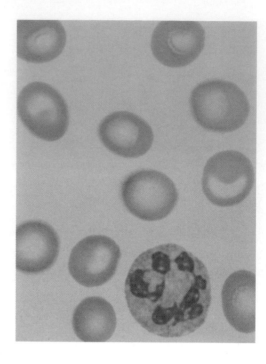

FIG. 11-14 Hypersegmented polymorphonuclear leukocyte in a patient with phenytoin-induced folate deficiency.

of the erythropoietic cells exist. The hallmark is the megaloblast, a nucleated marrow RBC with a lacy chromatin pattern and a dyssynchrony of maturation between cytoplasm and nucleus. The morphologic alterations are a direct result of decreased nucleoprotein deoxyribonucleic acid synthesis compared with cytoplasmic protein synthesis, which stems from a relative decrease in the factors needed in deoxyribonucleic acid replication, namely folate or cobalamin (vitamin B_{12}). From a morphologic standpoint, RBCs are the primary cells affected by megaloblastic changes.

On the peripheral blood smear, the RBCs are large in size (macrocytes), and they display a great deal of variation in their shapes (Fig. 11-13). These macrocytic cells are generally normochromic.

Although RBCs are primarily affected in megaloblastic anemia, all of the actively dividing marrow cells fail to have normal duplication of deoxyribonucleic acid and become involved in the pathologic process. Neutrophils are the second most likely cells to display morphologic abnormalities. These cells, like the RBCs, are large, and hypersegmentation of the nucleus is a pathognomonic finding (Fig. 11-14). Neutropenia is common. The more severe and prolonged megaloblastic anemias may lead ultimately to thrombocytopenia, with large bizarre platelets on the peripheral blood smear. Megaloblastic changes in each cell line are shown in Fig. 11-15.

Laboratory diagnosis requires the measurement of folate and vitamin B_{12} levels in the serum and RBCs. Because a typical Western diet is very unlikely to lead to folate or vitamin B_{12} deficiency, a low level of either should raise questions of altered bioavailability or peculiar diet. Goat's milk is folate deficient (though in recent years many canned goat's milk products are folate supplemented), and an infant on a goat's milk diet may become folate depleted over time. Fad diets are often not structured thoughtfully and may lead to folate deficiency.

When the diet is not peculiar, various drugs that decrease folate absorption (phenytoin) or interfere with folate metabolism (methotrexate) may lead to megaloblastic changes. A pathologic condition of the gastrointestinal tract may be the primary disease causing malabsorption of folate or vitamin B_{12} and secondary megaloblastic changes. Pernicious anemia is a specific cause of failure of vitamin B_{12} absorption because of the absence or deficiency of the intrinsic factor required for vitamin B_{12} absorption. Glossitis (Fig. 11-16) or angular stomatitis seen in vitamin B_{12} deficiency can be a helpful physical finding in the differential diagnoses.

Normocytic, Normochromic Anemia

The third morphologic subgroup of anemia includes those with normochromic and normocytic RBCs. These anemias are easily analyzed on the basis of an algorithm beginning with a reticulocyte count. These normocytic and normochromic anemias with low reticulocyte counts develop because of failed RBC production. The differential diagnosis of this group includes pure red cell aplasia, dyserythropoietic anemia, renal disease, infection, and drug-induced aplasia. When low-reticulocyte normocytic, normochromic anemia occurs in the presence of a decrease in WBCs and platelets, the diagnosis is more ominous and includes leukemia, aplastic anemia, and tumor infiltration of the marrow.

PURE RED CELL APLASIA

Pure red cell aplasia can be acquired or congenital. The congenital form (referred to variously as *congenital hypoplastic anemia, chronic idiopathic erythroblastopenia, chronic congenital aregenerative anemia, erythropoiesis imperfecta*, or Blackfan-Diamond syndrome) is characterized by onset of anemia by 6 months of age with a low absolute reticulocyte count. Approximately 25% of patients with pure red cell anemia have minor congenital anomalies, including thumb anomalies and/or a Turner phenotype (see Chapter 1). Some of the patients go

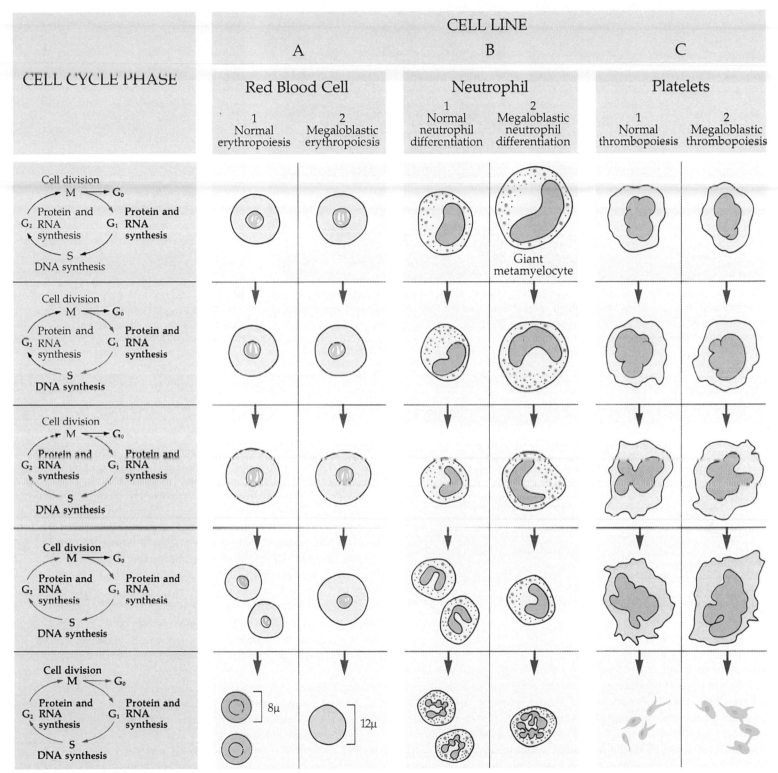

FIG. 11-15 Schematic comparison of normal cellular maturation and megaloblastic differentiation of three cell lines. The cell cycle phase is identified to the left of the figure. Note that megaloblastic cells fail to undergo replication of deoxyribonucleic acid and cellular division at the S and M phases, respectively, leading to large RBCs; hypersegmented polymorphonuclear leukocytes; and large, bizarrely shaped platelets.

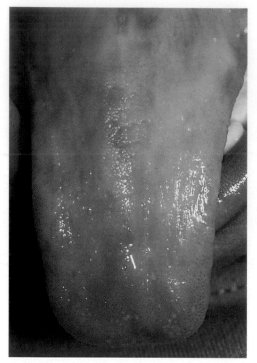

FIG. 11-16   Smooth, beefy tongue of a patient with vitamin B$_{12}$ deficiency. The patient depended on total parenteral nutrition for several years without vitamin B$_{12}$ supplementation.

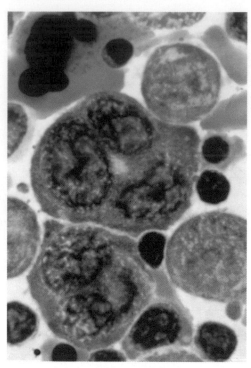

FIG. 11-17   Congenital dyserythropoietic anemia type III. Note the centrally located gigantoblast.

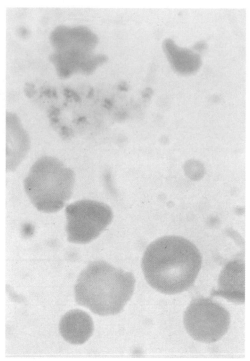

FIG. 11-18   Coombs-positive hemolytic anemia. Note the spherocytes and a large RBC with polychromasia, indicating the presence of regenerative anemia.

TABLE 11-2

Features Differentiating Pure Red Cell Anemia From TEC

RBC characteristic	Disease	
	Pure red cell anemia	TEC
Hemoglobin	Increased fetal	Normal fetal
Cellular antigen	I	I
Mean corpuscular volume	Increased	Normal
RBC enzyme activity	Normal or high	Low

into spontaneous remission; in others, remission may occur years after the onset of signs of the disease. The largest subgroup responds to corticosteroid therapy. The conditions of a final subgroup, steroid unresponsive, do not undergo remission. These patients remain transfusion dependent for the rest of their lives. Pure red cell aplasia often has an associated macrocytosis on the peripheral blood smear. However, it has been included in the discussion of normocytic, normochromic anemias because it may be normochromic, normocytic and must be distinguished from the most frequently acquired pure red cell aplasia, transient erythroblastopenia of childhood (TEC), which is normocytic and normochromic.

TEC occurs in 1- to 4-year-old children and appears 2 weeks to 2 months after a respiratory or gastrointestinal illness. Differentiating TEC from pure red cell anemia is important because TEC is transient and self-limited, whereas pure red cell anemia is chronic. Pure red cell anemia may be responsive to steroids when therapy is begun early in the course

of the disease. Fortunately, it has been noted that these RBCs have fetal characteristics, whereas the RBCs of TEC have age-appropriate characteristics (Table 11-2). The cause of TEC remains obscure. Human parvovirus B19, known to depress erythropoiesis especially in the fetus or patients with hemolytic anemia, has been implicated as the etiologic agent in TEC in only a minority of patients. TEC may occur after many different viral infections and most likely represents altered immunity from the infection that affects erythropoiesis.

Non–TEC-acquired pure red cell aplasia is rare in pediatrics. In adults, pure red cell aplasia is sometimes suspected on an autoimmune basis and is frequently associated with thymoma. Three types of non–TEC-acquired pure red cell aplasia have been recognized. Type I has a serum immunoglobulin G inhibitor of erythropoiesis and high erythropoietin levels. Type II has a low erythropoietin activity level and an erythropoietin immunoglobulin G antibody. Type III has no anti-erythropoiesis or antierythropoietin serum antibodies. Rather the defect appears intrinsic to the stem cell. Some of these children are preleukemic. Thymoma-associated pure red cell aplasia is extremely rare in children. Drugs, particularly chloramphenicol, have been responsible for a significant percentage of pure red cell aplasias.

The peripheral blood smear from a patient with pure red cell aplasia is often nonspecific (although it may show atypical lymphocytes as vestiges of a residual viral infection), and the bone marrow aspirate may rarely be more specific. It may demonstrate the vacuolated erythroblasts of the chloramphenicol effect or the multinucleated giant cells indicative of the rare congenital dyserythropoietic anemia (Fig. 11-17). Low reticulocyte normocytic, normochromic anemia with depressed WBCs and platelets is discussed in the section on pancytopenia.

Hemolytic Anemias

Normocytic, normochromic anemias with increased reticulocyte counts but without evidence of blood loss most likely result from he-

TABLE 11-3

Common RBC Hemolytic Disorders by Predominant Morphology

Spherocytes
  Hereditary spherocytosis
  ABO incompatibility in neonates†
  Immunohemolytic anemias with IgG- or C3-coated RBCs†
  Hemolytic transfusion reactions†
  Severe burns or other RBC thermal injuries

Bizarre Poikilocytes
  RBC fragmentation syndromes (microangiopathic and
    macroangiopathic hemolytic anemias)
  Hereditary elliptocytosis in neonates

Elliptocytes
  Hereditary elliptocytosis
  Thalassemia
  (Other hypochromic microcytic anemia)
  (Megaloblastic anemia)

Spiculated or Crenated RBCs
  Acute hepatic necrosis (spur-cell anemia)
  Uremia
  Abetalipoproteinemia

Prominent Basophilic Stippling
  Thalassemia
  Unstable hemoglobin levels
  Lead poisoning‡

Irreversibly Sickled Cells
  Sickle cell anemia
  Symptomatic sickle syndromes

Intraerythrocytic Parasites
  Malaria
  Babesiosis
  Bartonellosis

Target Cells
  Hgb S, C, D, and E
  Hereditary xerocytosis
  Thalassemia
  (Other hypochromic microcytic anemia)
  (Obstructive liver disease)
  (Postsplenectomy)

Nonspecific or Normal Morphology
  Embden-Meyerhof pathway defects
  HMP shunt defects
  Adenosine deaminase hyperactivity with low RBC ATP
  Unstable hemoglobin levels
  Paroxysmal nocturnal hemoglobinuria
  Dyserythropoietic anemia
  Copper toxicity (Wilson disease)
  Erythropoietic porphyria
  Vitamin E deficiency
  Hypersplenism

Modified from Nathan DG, Oski FA, eds: *Hematology of infancy and childhood*, ed 2, Philadelphia, 1981, WB Saunders.
ATP, Adenosine triphosphate; *HMP*, hexose-monophosphate shunt.
*Nonhemolytic disorders of similar morphology are enclosed in parentheses for reference.
†Usually associated with a positive Coombs test.
‡Disease sometimes associated with this morphology.

molytic processes. However, the reticulocyte count may not be elevated if it is measured within a few days of the onset of hemolysis. Patients with hemolytic anemia can suffer from any of the symptoms common to all anemias; in addition, they develop an indirect hyperbilirubinemia with or without clinical icterus. Other laboratory evidence of hemolysis is present, including increased levels of carboxyhemoglobin, lactate dehydrogenase, and serum glutamic-oxaloacetic transaminase and decreased levels of haptoglobin.

The differential diagnosis of hemolytic anemia rests largely in the recognition of specific morphologic abnormalities on the peripheral blood smear (Table 11-3) followed by appropriate specific laboratory tests.

Normocytic, Normochromic Anemia With
Elevated Reticulocyte Count and Spherocytes

COOMBS-POSITIVE HEMOLYTIC ANEMIA
Direct and indirect Coombs tests, which evaluate the patient's blood for the presence of anti-RBC antibody and complement on RBCs or in the serum, respectively, identify immunohemolytic anemia. The antibody- and complement-mediated RBC destruction produces spherocytes on the peripheral blood smear (Fig. 11-18). Coombs-positive hemolytic anemia in the newborn most often represents an isoimmune hemolytic anemia. This is caused by a maternal antibody that has crossed the placenta into the neonate, hemolyzing the newborn RBCs (i.e., maternal antibodies form to fetal RBC antigens when fetal blood gains entry into maternal circulation via a break in placental integrity). Maternal antibodies cross the placenta and cause fetal RBC hemolysis. In the majority of cases of isoimmune hemolytic anemia, the maternal antibody is directed at ABO or Rh RBC antigens. When Rh antigen is the antibody target, the blood smear does not show spherocytes.

HEREDITARY SPHEROCYTOSIS
Coombs-negative hemolytic anemia with spherocytes often represents hereditary spherocytosis, which is the most common cause of genetically determined hemolytic anemia in the white population. Hered-

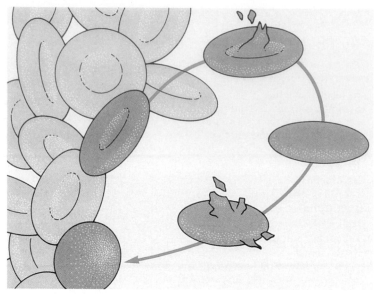

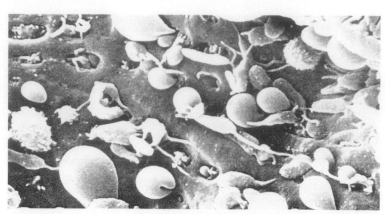

FIG. 11-20 RBCs being deformed as they traverse the microcirculation of the splenic sinusoids. (From Zucker-Franklin D, Greanes MF, Grossi CE, Marmont AM: *Atlas of blood cells,* Milan, Italy, 1981, Ermes.)

FIG. 11-19 Schematic drawing shows a developing spherocyte resulting from the process of repeated membrane fragmentation, loss, and repair.

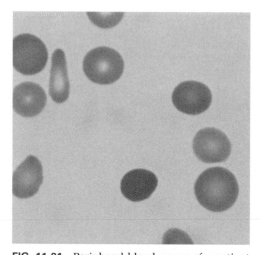

FIG. 11-21 Peripheral blood smear of a patient who underwent splenectomy for hereditary spherocytosis. Note the presence of small, perfectly round cells without an area of central pallor. The mean corpuscular hemoglobin concentration may be normal but often is increased in these patients. Reticulocytosis also may be prominent.

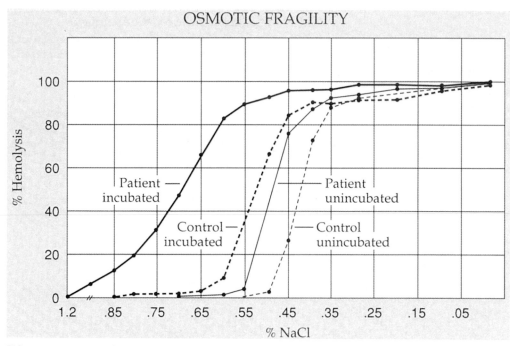

FIG. 11-22 Osmotic fragility of unincubated and incubated RBCs from a normal individual and from a patient with hereditary spherocytosis. The striking increase in fragility produced by the incubation of RBCs in hereditary spherocytosis is obvious.

itary spherocytosis is transmitted frequently as an autosomal dominant trait, and it is named for the peculiar appearance of the RBCs on the peripheral blood smear. The RBC membrane defect, which appears to result from inherent membrane instability, leads to loss of membrane. Membrane repair occurs, which decreases the normal RBC surface-to-volume ratio, causing the normal, bioconcave disc configuration to assume a more geometrically efficient spherical shape (Fig. 11-19). The direct consequence of this new morphology is a less pliable cell. The inability of this new cell to deform during transit through the splenic microcirculation leads to RBC destruction (Fig. 11-20). The characteristic smear may show increased numbers of spherocytes after splenec-

tomy, when spherocytes are less likely to be removed from the circulation (Fig. 11-21). Osmotic fragility testing (Fig. 11-22), used commonly in patients with suspected hereditary spherocytosis, is an excellent confirmatory test but is not pathognomonic for the diagnosis.

ELLIPTOCYTOSIS

Hereditary elliptocytosis (Fig. 11-23) is another membrane defect morphologically distinct from hereditary spherocytosis. However, the pathophysiology of RBC destruction is similar to that in hereditary spherocytosis. Also, like hereditary spherocytosis, hereditary elliptocytosis appears to be transmitted as an autosomal dominant trait. In most instances, hereditary elliptocytosis is a mild, well-compensated hemolytic

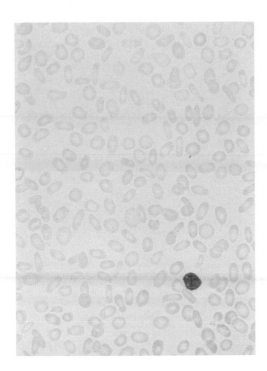

FIG. 11-23 Peripheral blood obtained incidentally from a 3-year-old child with elliptocytosis. Over 90% of the cells are elliptocytes. The child had a history of neonatal jaundice but had been well before and has been well since.

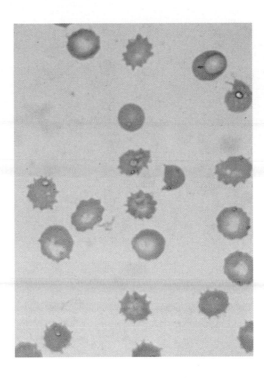

FIG. 11-24 Spiculated cells seen in a patient suffering from acute hepatic necrosis. The associated hemolytic anemia—spur-cell anemia—was severe.

anemia that is clinically insignificant unless splenic hypertrophy develops resulting from another disease process. The elliptocyte form bears only a superficial similarity to that of the "cigar cell" of iron deficiency anemia (Fig. 11-5). Unlike the cigar cells, the elliptocytes of hereditary elliptocytosis have normal size, have a normal mean corpuscular value, and are true elliptocytes. Elliptocytes also may be found in the peripheral blood smear of thalassemia or in megaloblastic anemia.

Hereditary stomatocytosis leads to still another morphologic defect. Its infrequency precludes a more lengthy discussion, but it is mentioned here for completeness.

ACANTHOCYTIC AND ECHINOCYTIC ANEMIA

A number of hemolytic anemias are characterized by spiculated RBCs referred to as *acanthocytes* or *echinocytes* (Fig. 11-24). Abetalipoproteinemia, which generally presents as a neurologic disorder with progressive ataxia, is also characterized by retinitis pigmentosa, fat malabsorption, and the absence of chylomicrons and very low-density and low-density lipoproteins. Roughly 50% to 90% of the RBCs on peripheral smear are acanthocytes, which develop as a direct result of the alterations of the serum lipids. Altered membrane lipid composition changes the fluidity of the RBC, which leads to the acanthocytic form. Malabsorption of fat-soluble vitamins in abetalipoproteinemia results in vitamin E deficiency, leaving the RBCs subject to oxidative injury. However, despite altered membrane fluidity and vitamin E deficiency, hemolysis in abeta-lipoproteinemia is mild.

Spur-cell anemia is another disorder characterized by acanthocytes. The hemolysis in this disorder, in contrast to abetalipoproteinemia, is brisk. Spur cell anemia develops in the setting of sudden and massive liver injury arising from any cause (e.g., hepatitis with acute yellow atrophy, shock liver, hepatic infarction). The hepatic decompensation leads to increased serum lipid and cholesterol levels, which lead, in turn, to increased RBC membrane cholesterol content, thus altering RBC membrane fluidity. Spiculated cells in lesser numbers can also be seen in uremia and anorexia nervosa as well as severe malnutrition. Probably the most frequent cause of spiculated RBCs on the peripheral blood smear is inadequate slide preparation. Thus when confronted with such a slide, review of repeated peripheral blood smears is prudent.

TARGET CELLS

Target cells draw their name from their targetlike appearance on the peripheral blood smear. They are often seen as a secondary response to a process that increases the RBC membrane or decreases the RBC content, leading to an increase in the surface-to-volume ratio of the RBCs (Fig. 11-25, *A*). In a dried smear, the excess surface accumulates and bulges outward in the area that is normally the RBC's central pallor, producing the characteristic target cell morphology. Liver diseases of any type (particularly obstructive hepatopathy), with their secondary alteration of serum lipids leading to membrane lipid loading, are well-known causes of target cell formation. Splenectomy decreases reticuloendothelial remodeling of reticulocytes, removes lipid-loaded RBC membranes, and leads to targeted RBCs. Mechanisms previously discussed, which decrease RBC intracellular content hypochromic microcytic anemia), also induce target formation. Finally, in a rare autosomal recessive condition, familial lecithin-cholesterol acyltransferase deficiency (characterized by anemia, corneal opacities, hyperlipidemia, proteinuria, chronic nephritis, and premature atherosclerosis), there are prominent target cells on the peripheral blood smear.

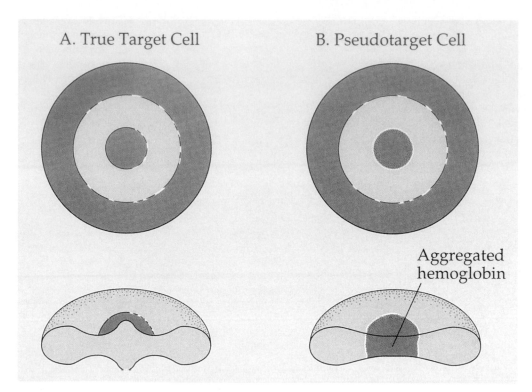

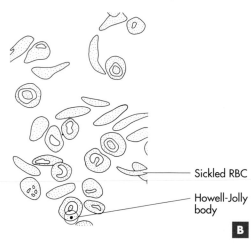

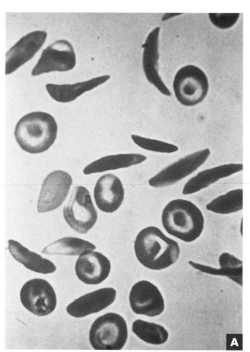

A. True Target Cell   B. Pseudotarget Cell

Aggregated hemoglobin

FIG. 11-25 Schematic depiction of the morphology of the true target cell *(A)* compared with that of a pseudotarget cell *(B)*.

Sickled RBC

Howell-Jolly body

FIG. 11-26 Peripheral blood smear of a black child with Hgb SS disease. Note the prominent targets and sickle cells, and the Howell-Jolly body.

In addition, target cells (or more accurately, pseudotarget cells) occur with various hemoglobinopathies. This happens more often in conditions associated with Hgb C, but also with Hgb S, D, and E (Figs. 11-26 and 11-27) because of aggregation of hemoglobin in the central region of the RBC (Fig. 11-25, *B*).

Intracellular Red Cell Defects
Hemoglobinopathies
Hemoglobinopathies often result in a characteristic and even diagnostic peripheral blood smear. They can be responsible for hemolysis resulting from unstable hemoglobin variants or altered (decreased) hemoglobin solubility.

UNSTABLE HEMOGLOBIN VARIANTS

Unstable hemoglobin variants, unlike most hemolytic hemoglobinopathies, rarely have a characteristic morphology—although basophilic stippling and Heinz bodies may be noted on special staining of the peripheral blood (Fig. 11-28). The Heinz bodies represent hemoglobin aggregates that have precipitated intracellularly. RBCs in Heinz body anemia usually are normocytic but may be hypochromic as a result of RBC splenic "pitting" of precipitated hemoglobin. Because the precipitated hemoglobin may be mistaken for reticulum, reticulocyte counts may be spuriously high. Methylene blue staining of RBCs after they have incubated for a few hours can demonstrate the Heinz bodies. Hemolysis may be mild (Hgb$_{Köln}$) or

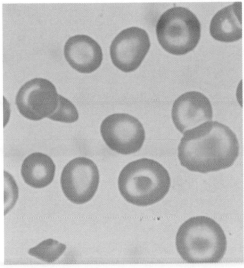

FIG. 11-27 Peripheral smear of sickle C (Hgb SC) disease with target cells. Sickled cells are less frequent in this disease than they are in Hgb SS disease.

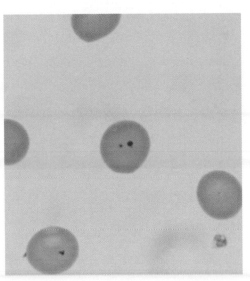

FIG. 11-28 "Heinz body prep" of a 2-week-old infant with brisk hemolytic anemia. Note the dark-staining material in two of the RBCs.

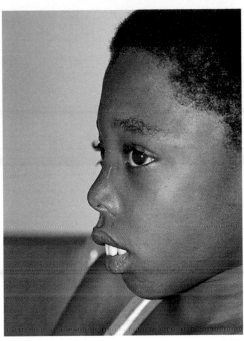

FIG. 11-29 Maxillary hyperplasia in a child with sickle cell anemia.

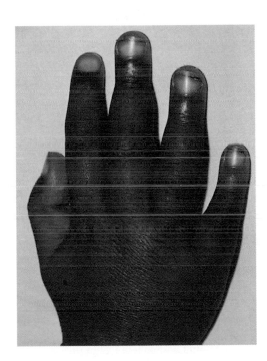

FIG. 11-30 Dactylitis (hand foot syndrome) in a 3-year-old girl with sickle cell disease. This syndrome, which primarily affects toddlers, is seen less frequently in older children after the bone marrow of the small bones of the hands and feet loses hematopoietic activity. This loss of marrow activity is due to cortical thickening from increased use of hands and weight bearing by the feet.

SICKLE CELL DISEASE

Of the hemoglobinopathies that have altered hemoglobin solubility, none is as well known or as ubiquitous as sickle cell anemia. Substitution of valine for glutamic acid at position six in the beta-chain of the hemoglobin molecule leads to the cross-linking of one beta-chain to a second hemoglobin molecule's beta-chain when the hemoglobin is in its deoxygenated state. This cross-linkage tips the solubility balance, leading to the sickling of the RBC (Fig. 11-26). Although sickle cell disease is seen predominantly in black patients, it is by no means exclusive to blacks, with Mediterranean and Middle Eastern peoples also being affected.

The clinical signs and symptoms of sickle cell anemia are due to decreased survival and altered rheology of the sickled RBC. As with any chronic hemolytic state, marrow cavity enlargement occurs, leading to maxillary hyperplasia and the so-called sickle cell facies (Fig. 11-29). Altered rheology, which occurs because sickle cells lose the ability to deform in the microcirculation (Fig. 11-20) leads to a logjam phenomenon, causing tissue infarction and painful crises. This same logjamming, also referred to as *vasoocclusive crisis*, when occurring in certain locations, gives rise to clinical manifestations such as dactylitis (Fig. 11-30) in the toddler, priapism (Fig. 11-31), splenic sequestration, and skin ulceration.

The vasoocclusive phenomenon also may lead to the two most life-threatening complications of sickle cell diseases: overwhelming infection with encapsulated organisms (most often pneumococcus) and stroke. The increased infectious risk in the sickle cell patient has multiple mechanisms, but by far the most important are splenic dysfunction related to congested blood flow and then, ultimately, splenic infarction. Stroke appears to occur only after larger cerebral arteries are damaged because of the effect of altered rheology and sickling in the vasa vasorum and on the nutrient layer of blood flow through these large cerebral vessels.

The peripheral smear of a patient with sickle cell disease is diagnostic of a sickling disorder (Fig. 11-26).

Sickle cell disease is an autosomal recessive disorder with the heterozygote having a significant but less than 50% proportion of hemoglobin of the sickle cell type. Heterozygous carriers of the sickle cell

brisk (Hgb$_{Bristol}$), or it may be induced by drugs such as sulfonamides (Hgb$_{Zurich}$).

Unstable hemoglobinopathies have an autosomal dominant pattern of inheritance, and affected individuals are heterozygotes. A homozygous state would, in most cases, be incompatible with life. Congenital Heinz body hemolytic anemia is an important cause of congenital hemolytic anemia. This condition, although frequently a persistent process in the older infant, has been observed to resolve. At least some of these self-limited cases may represent the presence of unstable gamma-hemoglobin, which normally disappears as the infant ages. The precipitate-unstable hemoglobin secondarily increases membrane fragility, leading to the hemolysis seen in this disorder.

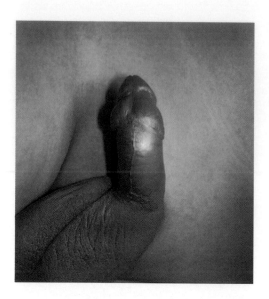

FIG. 11-31 Priapism in an adolescent. Erection had persisted for 12 hours, and had become extremely painful for the patient.

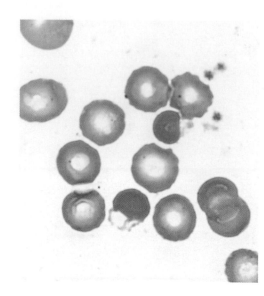

FIG. 11-32 Peripheral smear of patient with G6PD deficiency in the midst of a hemolytic episode. Note the blister cells with hemoglobin condensed in the remaining (nonblistered) portion of the cell.

gene, although suffering a number of difficulties (e.g., poor urine-concentrating ability, occasional episodes of renal papillary necrosis with hematuria), have normal life expectancies and are virtually free of any significant consequences of their heterozygous state.

An effective screening test—the sickle cell preparation—is widely available. It identifies the child with at least 20% Hgb S. It is not useful for distinguishing sickle cell disease from the heterozygous sickle cell trait. Additionally, it may fail to detect a hemoglobinopathy related to a hemoglobin other than hemoglobin S, and it may also fail to detect a neonate who has not yet started to synthesize significant amounts of hemoglobin SS.

HEMOGLOBIN C DISEASE

Though less common than sickle cell disease, disease associated with Hgb C is not rare in the black population. As in sickle cell disease, Hgb C disease occurs because of one amino acid change. The change, again like Hgb S, is at the sixth position of the beta-chain but is a lysine rather than a valine replacement. In its homozygous form, Hgb C disease is a mild disorder characterized by hemolytic anemia and splenomegaly. The tendency of Hgb C to aggregate into precipitates is responsible for the characteristic target (actually a pseudotarget, Fig. 11-25, *B*) morphology of the Hgb C homozygous and Hgb C trait (heterozygous) cells on the peripheral blood smear (Fig. 11-27). Vasoocclusive phenomena are not associated with this disease, although target cells are formed on the dried peripheral blood smear. However, Hgb C, when paired in a double heterozygous state with Hgb S, is associated with vasoocclusive phenomena, though less severely than Hgb SS.

Red Blood Cell Enzyme Abnormalities

Abnormalities of the RBC enzymes also may lead to hemolysis. Although almost any of the RBC enzymes involved in RBC glycolysis or free radical detoxification via the pentose shunt may be responsible for hemolysis, glucose-6-phosphate dehydrogenase (G6PD) deficiency is by far the most frequent. A second enzyme, pyruvate kinase (PK), when deficient, also leads to a hemolytic state. PK deficiency, although far less frequently seen than G6PD deficiency, is prevalent enough to deserve attention in this discussion. The blood smears of patients with RBC enzyme deficiency–induced hemolysis often are normal, although occasionally with G6PD deficiency, a suspicious morphology may be present (Fig. 11-32).

More than 370 variants of G6PD have been identified, for which enzyme activity may be normal, elevated, or severely deficient. Clinical syndromes may vary as well, with the degree of hemolysis paralleling

---

TABLE 11-4

Drugs Associated With Clinically Significant Hemolysis in G6PD Deficiency

Antimalarials
Pamaquine
Pentaquine
Primaquine
Quinocide

Antipyretics and Analgesics
Acetanilid
Aminopyrine
Antipyrine

Sulfa Drugs
N-Acetylsulfanilamide
Salicylazosulfapyridine

Sulfamethoxypyridazine
Sulfapyridine
Thiazolesulfone

Miscellaneous
Acetylphenylhydrazine
Fava beans
Nalidixic acid
Naphthalene
Phenylhydrazine
Toluidine blue

---

inversely the level of G6PD activity. In all instances, the hemolysis is due to the intracellular generation of free radicals and peroxides, which fail to be detoxified by the patient with G6PD deficiency.

Chronic hemolysis is extremely mild and subclinical in the common types. Triggered hemolysis associated with G6PD deficiency (Mediterranean type) is severe and abrupt and parallels inversely the severe enzyme deficiency. In contrast, triggered hemolysis with G6PD deficiency (A– type) may be severe but self-limited when the enzyme deficiency is mild. In addition, some agents that trigger hemolysis with G6PD deficiency (Mediterranean type) may be tolerated by patients with G6PD deficiency (A– type). A list of some of the drugs associated with clinically significant hemolysis in G6PD deficiency is provided (Table 11-4). Recent work has deemphasized the role of certain drug triggers. In many instances the infection being treated by certain drugs rather than the drugs themselves is responsible for the hemolysis.

PK deficiency is the second most prevalent enzyme abnormality of the RBC that leads to hemolysis; however, it is a far second, indeed, with one case of PK deficiency occurring worldwide for 500,000 cases of G6PD deficiency. Like G6PD deficiency, wide clinical variability exists with PK deficiency. Mild, fully compensated hemolytic anemia, as

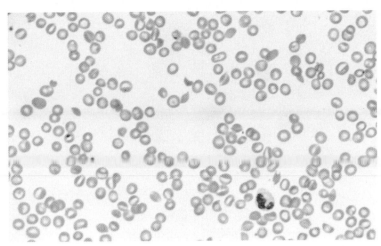

FIG. 11-33 Peripheral blood smear of a child with DIC secondary to meningococcemia. Note the RBC fragments and decreased platelet levels.

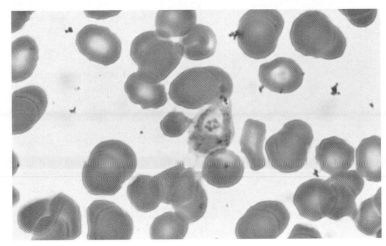

FIG. 11-34 Peripheral blood smear prepared by the so-called "thick prep" method. *Plasmodium vivax* malaria is seen intracellularly in the RBC in the center of the smear.

TABLE 11-5

Clinical Equivalent of Experimental DIC-Triggering Agents

Gram-negative septicemia
Necrotizing enterocolitis
Shock from any cause
Endothelial damage (virus, bacteria, rickettsia, heat stroke)
Trauma, burns
Ascitic fluid (La Veen shunt)
Hypoxia-acidosis, severe hyaline membrane disease

Malignancies (acute leukemia, neuroblastoma, rhabdomyo-sarcoma)
Dead fetal twin
Hemolysis transfusion reaction
Small-for-gestational-age-infant (placental infarct)
Purpura fulminans
Localized giant hemangioma

Modified from Corrigan JJ: Disseminated intravascular coagulopathy, *Pediatr Rev* 1(2):39-45, 1979.

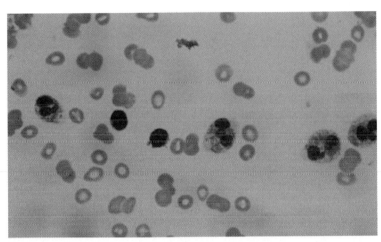

FIG. 11-35 Peripheral blood smear showing neutrophilia and increased band forms (shift to the left) in a child with pneumococcal sepsis.

well as severe neonatal hemolysis and hyperbilirubinemia, may occur. Hemoglobin levels range from 6 to 10 g/dl with normochromic anemia with normocytic or macrocytic indices, depending on the degree of reticulocytosis. The reticulocyte count can range from 5% to as high as 90% in the patient who has had a splenectomy. For the subgroup of patients with severe, transfusion-dependent disease, splenectomy may ameliorate or eliminate the need for transfusions. In addition to chronic hemolysis, PK deficiency may have triggered episodes (usually resulting from intercurrent infection).

Hemolysis Caused by ExtraRBC Factors

Microangiopathic Hemolysis

Hemolysis of RBCs can occur not only from intrinsic abnormalities of the RBCs but also from alterations in the RBC environment. Disseminated intravascular coagulation (DIC), which may be triggered by many differing pathologic conditions, has, as its common manifestation, the hemolysis of RBCs and utilization of platelets and clotting factors. Regardless of the trigger, production of fibrin in the microcirculation and fibrin deposition in capillaries cause shearing of the RBCs as they cross these capillary beds (Fig. 11-33). The clinical presentation of DIC is dom-inated by the clinical presentation of the original disease. In pediatrics, infection with shock is, by far, the most frequent cause of DIC. Patients may have petechiae, purpura, and persistent bleeding from venipunctures. Diseases known to trigger DIC are listed in Table 11-5.

Localized microangiopathic changes of the peripheral blood smear also may be seen without fully developed DIC. In these instances the fragmentation of the RBCs occurs during transit through the involved organ or tissue (e.g., kidney in hemolytic-uremic syndrome and hemangioma in Kasabach-Merritt syndrome).

Malaria

Malaria is the most frequent cause of hemolysis on a worldwide scale. The patient who contracts the disease after being fed on by the tropical *Anopheles* mosquito is parasitized within the RBCs with organisms at the merozoite stage (Fig. 11-34). The parasitization causes a clinical picture of intermittent fever, chills, and jaundice and may lead to encephalopathy, massive hemolysis with hemoglobinuria (black-water fever), and death. The cause of the hemolysis has been attributed to multiple mechanisms, including altered RBC osmotic fragility, membrane loss of negative surface charge, direct injury by the parasite, autoimmunity, splenic pitting, and hypersplenism.

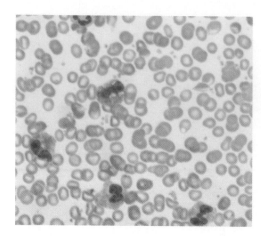

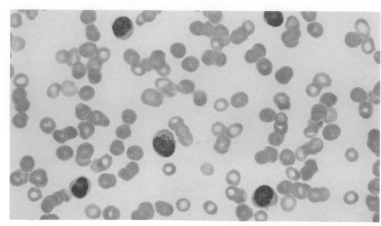

FIG. 11-36 Eosinophilia with an increase in WBC count. This patient suffered from a parasitic infection that triggered the increase in the number of eosinophils.

FIG. 11-37 Lymphocytosis seen in a peripheral blood smear from a child with pertussis.

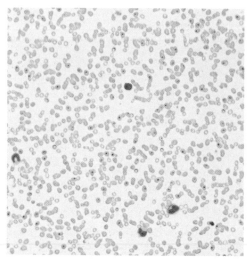

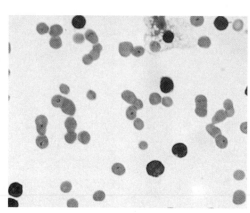

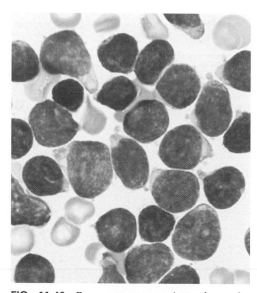

FIG. 11-38 Monocytosis in a child recovering from chemotherapy-related neutropenia.

FIG. 11-39 Peripheral blood smear of a child with acute lymphocytic leukemia. Note the decreased platelets on the smear and the absence of normal WBCs.

FIG. 11-40 Bone marrow aspirate from the child with acute lymphocytic leukemia whose peripheral blood is shown in Fig. 11-45. Note the monotonous pattern of the lymphoblastic cells (L-1).

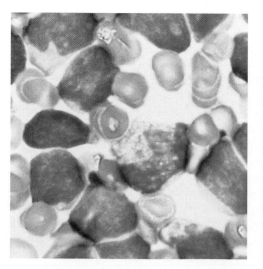

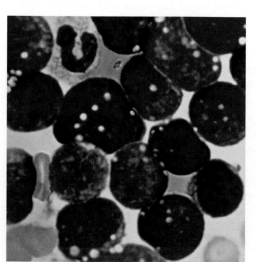

FIG. 11-41 Bone marrow aspirate shows L-2 lymphoblasts in another patient with acute lymphocytic leukemia. These lymphoblasts are larger and more heterogeneous in appearance than the L-1 lymphoblasts, and the nucleus to cytoplasm ratio is lower than that for L-1 lymphoblasts. The nucleoli are prominent.

FIG. 11-42 L-3 lymphoblasts represent the third morphologic presentation of acute lymphocytic anemia in this bone marrow aspirate. These lymphoblasts are large, deeply staining cells that often are vacuolated.

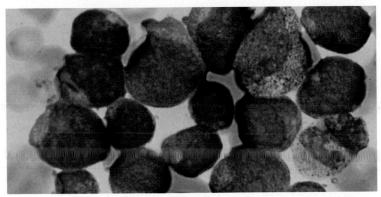

FIG. 11-43 Peripheral blood smear shows an Auer rod (red barlike figure in the cytoplasm) in a myeloblast of a patient with acute nonlymphocytic leukemia.

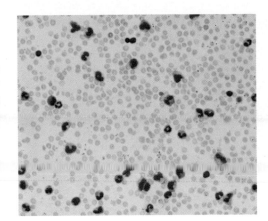

FIG. 11-44 Leukemoid reaction in a patient with pneumococcal sepsis. A higher magnification would reveal toxic granulations and Döhle bodies (see Fig. 11-50) in the polymorphonuclear leukocytes.

TABLE 11-6

Normal Leukocyte and Differential Counts*

	12 Months	4 Years	10 Years	21 Years
Leukocytes, total	11.4 (6.0-17.5)	9.1 (5.5-15.5)	8.1 (4.5-13.5)	7.4 (4.5-11.0)
Neutrophils, total	3.5 (1.5-8.5)	3.8 (1.5-8.5)	4.4 (1.8-8.0)	4.4 (1.8-7.7)
	(31%)	(42%)	(54%)	(59%)
Neutrophils, band forms	0.35	0.27 (0-1.0)	0.24 (0-1.0)	0.22 (0-0.7)
	(3.1%)	(3.0%)	(3.0%)	(3.0%)
Neutrophils, segmented	3.2	3.5 (1.5-7.5)	4.2 (1.8-7.0)	4.2 (1.8-7.0)
	(28%)	(39%)	(51%)	(56%)
Eosinophils	0.30 (0.05-0.70)	0.25 (0.02-0.65)	0.20 (0-0.60)	0.20 (0-0.45)
	(2.6%)	(2.8%)	(2.4%)	(2.7%)
Basophils	0.05 (0-10)	0.05 (0-0.20)	0.04 (0-0.20)	0.04 (0-0.20)
	(0.4%)	(0.6%)	(0.5%)	(0.5%)
Lymphocytes	7.0 (4.0-10.5)	4.5 (2.0-8.0)	3.1 (1.5-6.5)	2.5 (1.0-4.8)
	(61%)	(50%)	(38%)	(34%)
Monocytes	0.55 (0.05-1.1)	0.45 (0-0.8)	0.35 (0-0.8)	0.30 (0-0.8)
	(4.8%)	(5.0%)	(4.3%)	(4.0%)

From Altman PL, Dittmer DS, eds: *Blood and other body fluids,* Washington, DC, 1961, Federation of American Societies for Experimental Biology.
*Values are expressed as cells ×10³/µl. Mean values are given; ranges are in parentheses. Percent is for mean values.

White Blood Cells

Normal values for total WBC number and differential counts are age related (Table 11-6). Black patients may have lower granulocyte counts than whites of the same age. Leukocytosis and leukopenia are common pediatric problems. Generally, these are due to increases or decreases in specific types of WBCs. Few of the most common causes of neutrophilia (Fig. 11-35), neutropenia, eosinophilia (Fig. 11-36), lymphocytosis (Fig. 11-37), lymphopenia, or monocytosis (Fig. 11-38) are primary hematologic disorders. It is usually obvious from the clinical context which type of disease is operative in a given case. The pertinent history and physical findings related to increases or decreases in WBC numbers are outlined throughout this atlas.

Leukemia and Leukemoid Reactions

In some cases a leukocytosis may result from an increase in the number of immature rather than mature WBCs of any given cell line (a so-called shift to the left). Leukemia (Fig. 11-39) is the prototype, and Figs. 11-40 to 11-43 illustrate the varied appearances of blast cells. Fig. 11-44 shows a leukemoid reaction, which is characterized by a high WBC count (usually greater than 50,000/mm³) with an increase in the number of immature myeloid cells.

There are many causes of leukemoid reactions, including Down syndrome and sepsis. Leukemoid reactions must be distinguished from leukemia, and although this is definitively accomplished on the basis of a bone marrow aspirate, peripheral blood studies can facilitate a diagnosis. The leukocyte alkaline phosphatase level is increased in leukemoid reaction and decreased in chronic myelogenous leukemia. Another differential diagnostic consideration is that of leukoerythroblastosis (Fig. 11-45) in which increased numbers of immature granulocytes are accompanied on the smear by nucleated RBCs and RBC fragments, teardrops, target cells, and large platelets. This morphologic condition, in turn, has a long list of causes that includes the spectrum of myeloproliferative disorders ranging from myelofibrosis to chronic myelogenous leukemia, polycythemia vera, and essential thrombopenia.

Morphologic Abnormalities

With or without an absolute increase in the numbers of specific WBC subsets, there may be morphologic abnormalities in the WBC. In-

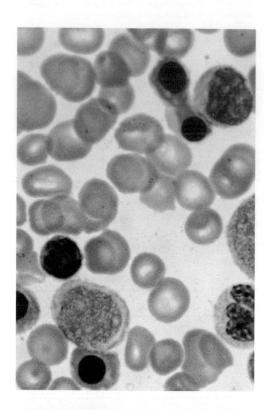

FIG. 11-45 Leukoery-throblastosis seen on a peripheral blood smear.

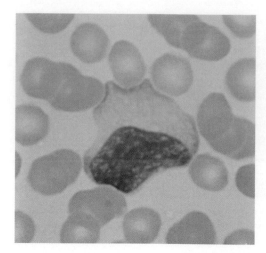

FIG. 11-46 Atypical lymphocyte from a patient with infectious mononucleosis. The nucleus is large, and the cytoplasm is abundant. Note that where the lymphocyte cytoplasm abuts a red cell, the lymphocyte deforms around it.

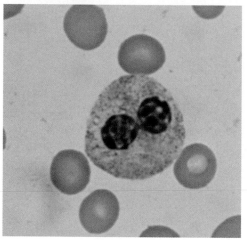

FIG. 11-47 Pelger-Huët anomaly. Note the uniform bilobed nucleus of the granulocyte.

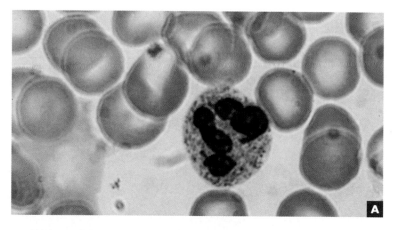

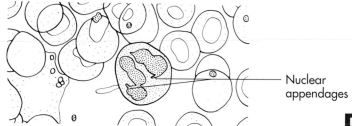

FIG. 11-48 Nuclear appendages, which can be seen normally in female polymorphonuclear leukocytes. An increase in appendages is seen in trisomy 13-15.

creased numbers of young lymphocytes that are not lymphoblasts often are accompanied by morphologic abnormalities, the most common of which is the atypical lymphocyte (Fig. 11-46). This is a large cell with an irregular plasma membrane that often "hugs" adjacent RBCs. Its nucleus also is large, and nucleoli may be visible. The abundant cytoplasm is typically basophilic and may contain vacuoles and azurophilic granules. Morphologic subtypes of atypical lymphocytes may occur, but clinically, their recognition is of little use. Although infectious mononucleosis comes to mind when atypical lymphocytes are seen, these lymphocytes are not specific and may be present in many other situations, especially viral illnesses.

Morphologic abnormalities of the granulocytic series, although less common, may provide clues to the diagnosis. The hypersegmented

neutrophil, which may be an early clue to vitamin B_{12} deficiency, has been noted previously (Fig. 11-14). This needs to be distinguished from familial hypersegmentation by looking at the peripheral smears of family members.

Neutrophil Abnormalities

Occasionally, mature neutrophils may be abnormally large in members of a given family—the so-called hereditary giant neutrophils. The Pelger-Huët anomaly (Fig. 11-47) is sometimes acquired as an adult and generally spurs a search for occult malignancy. However, it carries no such connotation in children. Increased numbers of nuclear appendages also may be seen in the neutrophils of patients with trisomy 13-15 (Fig. 11-48). These, however, may be difficult to distinguish from

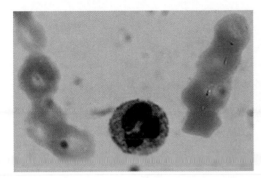

FIG. 11-49 Toxic granulations and a Döhle body are found in a child with sepsis. The Döhle body appears as a grayish-blue staining area, which is located at the inferior border of this cell.

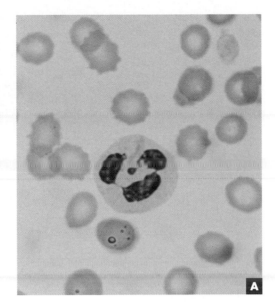

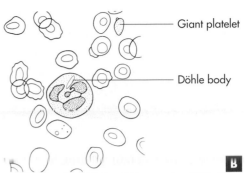

FIG. 11-50 May-Hegglin anomaly showing a Döhle body in the WBC and giant platelets that may be decreased in number.

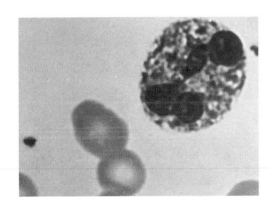

FIG. 11-51 Polymorphonuclear leukocytes with prominent granules characterize Reilly bodies as seen in Hurler syndrome.

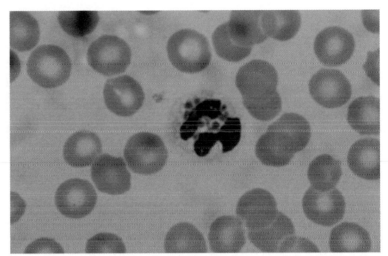

FIG. 11-52 Peripheral blood smear of a child with Chédiak-Higashi syndrome. (Courtesy Dr. William Zinkham, Baltimore.)

normal neutrophil "drumsticks," which are nuclear appendages that occur in 2% to 10% of neutrophils of normal girls.

Vacuoles can occur in any WBC for a variety of reasons, including artifact from anticoagulant agents, infections, or storage diseases. Certain types of inclusions, such as those seen in Gaucher disease, are limited to bone marrow histiocytes and are not detected on examination of the peripheral smear.

Toxic granulations, which are prominent azurophilic granules, are another common type of WBC inclusion. They are nonspecific but can be seen in viral and bacterial infections (Fig. 11-49). Toxic granulations must be distinguished from the hereditary dense granulation that may occasionally be present in the neutrophils of normal individuals. Döhle bodies, pale blue inclusions that usually are located peripherally in the

cytoplasm of neutrophils, may coexist with toxic granulations. Together with giant platelets, Döhle bodies are seen in patients with the dominantly inherited May-Hegglin anomaly (Fig. 11-50).

Reilly bodies, or Alder-Reilly bodies, are metachromatic prominent granules when stained with toluidine blue. When present in any WBCs, they are virtually pathognomonic of Hurler syndrome (Fig. 11-51). Coarse azurophilic neutrophilic granules that resemble Reilly bodies but are nonmetachromatic have been reported in Batten disease. Likewise, large greenish-brown neutrophil inclusions are characteristic of the patient with rare Chédiak-Higashi syndrome (Fig. 11-52). Such granules may appear in eosinophils and basophils as well.

WBCs also may acquire inclusions by engulfing particles from their surroundings. Erythrophagocytosis (Fig. 11-53) is a nonspecific finding

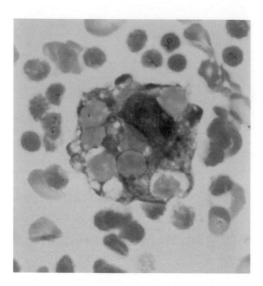

FIG. 11-53 Prominent erythrophagocytosis in which numerous RBCs are engulfed by WBC cytoplasm.

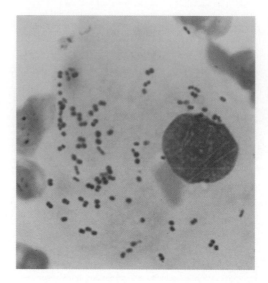

FIG. 11-54 Intracellular bacteria on Wright stain of a buffy-coat smear from a neutropenic patient. Note the numerous darkly stained bacteria in the cytoplasm.

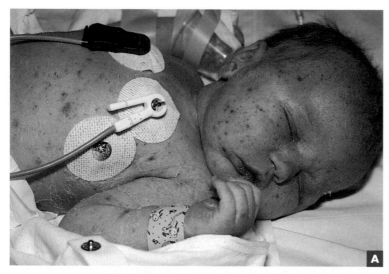

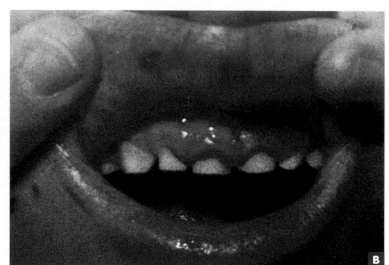

FIG. 11-55 *A,* Tiny petechiae and larger ecchymoses in an infant with severe immune thrombocytopenia. *B,* Purpura occurring on the oral mucosa or retina is called *wet purpura* and may suggest an increased tendency for major bleeding in the thrombocytopenic patient.

that is presumably immune mediated and seen in viral infections and primary diseases of the reticuloendothelial system. The LE cells of systemic lupus erythematosus are a diagnostically useful example of cellular phagocytosis, although in general, they are not seen on routine peripheral blood smears. Fig. 11-54 shows a buffy-coat preparation from a patient with suspected sepsis, demonstrating intracellular bacteria. In most of these WBC anomalies, the clinical diagnosis is often suspected on the basis of presenting signs and symptoms even before the hematologic abnormality is identified. One exception to this rule is the toddler with moderate to severe neutropenia that may be chronic yet benign. The conditions of many of these children are entirely asymptomatic, and the neutropenia is an incidental finding. However, chronic benign neutropenia is a diagnosis of exclusion. The differential diagnosis is reviewed elsewhere.

Bleeding Disorders

Excessive bleeding or bruising is a common complaint during childhood. The hematologic causes (to be distinguished from child abuse, trauma, vascular anomalies) fall into two categories: disorders of platelets and coagulopathies. The child with mucocutaneous bleeding

or purpura (petechiae or ecchymoses [Fig. 11-55]) is most likely to fall into the first; bleeding into deep tissue or joints is most likely to be a reflection of the second. There are exceptions to these guidelines. Patients with either problem may have bleeding precipitated by trauma or surgery and may develop hematuria, guaiac-positive stools, menorrhagia, or bleeding in the central nervous system. Frequent epistaxis, although possibly related to bleeding disorders, is more likely to have a nonhematologic cause such as nose picking, dry mucous membranes, or rarely, hypertension. Nonetheless, documentation of these problems or a positive family history usually calls for laboratory evaluation, which likely includes a CBC, differential count, platelet count, and a basic coagulation workup consisting of measurements of prothrombin time (PT) and partial thromboplastin time (PTT). Not all children with purpura are thrombocytopenic.

Platelet Disorders

A CBC and peripheral blood smear reveal a platelet count that, if normal, is 150,000/mm³ to 450,000/mm³. The smear does not give information regarding the diseases of platelet function that are less often seen, but it does confirm quantitative abnormalities. Clinically, thrombocytopenia may be inapparent until counts are significantly depressed

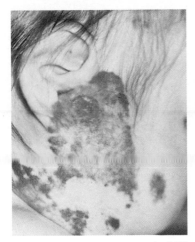

FIG. 11-56 Hemangioma of child with Kasabach-Merritt syndrome.

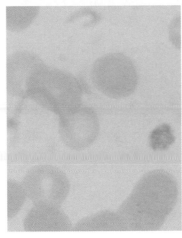

FIG. 11-57 Megathrombocyte in the peripheral blood of a patient with idiopathic thrombocytopenic purpura.

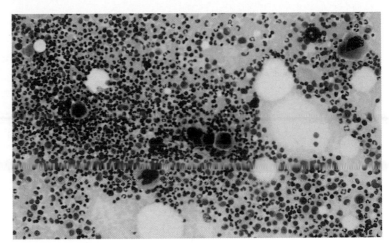

FIG. 11-58 Bone marrow aspirate with prominent megakaryocytes in idiopathic thrombocytopenia purpura. In children with thrombocytopenia—on the basis of decreased platelet production—megakaryocytes are decreased in number.

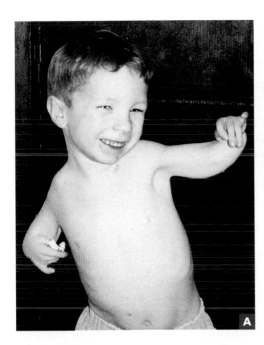

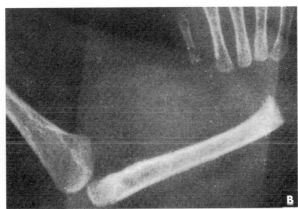

FIG. 11-59 *A,* Child with thrombocytopenia-absent radius syndrome. *B,* Radiograph of the same patient. Note the absence of radii.

below normal, and frank purpura is infrequently seen with counts greater than 20,000/mm³. It is important to ascertain that the decreased platelet number is not a spurious finding by repeating the test and reviewing the blood smear. The child whose peripheral blood smear is shown in Fig. 11-50 unfortunately underwent a splenectomy for presumed idiopathic thrombocytopenic purpura. However, the platelet count persistently was reported as less than 20,000/mm³, whereas the manually performed platelet count number was considerably higher. The Coulter counter had ignored these large platelets and incorrectly counted them as WBCs.

Isolated thrombocytopenia may result from decreased production or from increased destruction. The etiologies for the latter are numerous and include the idiopathic or immune thrombocytopenias, hypersplenism, DIC, consumption related to intracardiac defect or bypass surgery, washout from exchange transfusion, local microangiopathic disease (hemolytic uremic syndrome), or local thrombosis (renal vein thrombosis).

DIC has already been discussed as a cause of hemolysis and occurs most often in the pediatric age range as a secondary phenomenon related to shock in bacterial or, less frequently, viral sepsis (Fig. 11-36). DIC also is seen in Kasabach-Merritt syndrome when platelet con-

sumption occurs within the endothelial maze of massive strawberry and cavernous hemangiomas (Fig. 11-56).

The clinical setting often helps distinguish when thrombocytopenia is due to destruction as opposed to reduced production and identify the immediate reason for the pathophysiologic state. Some combination of peripheral blood smear, bone marrow aspirate, antiplatelet antibody testing, and therapeutic trial of intravenous high-dose gamma-globulin may define the diagnosis. The peripheral smear may reveal large platelets (megathrombocytes) (Fig. 11-57). The bone marrow may have abundant megakaryocytes (Fig. 11-58) and no infiltrative process. Antiplatelet antibodies may be present, and the patient may respond quickly to the gamma-globulin. All this may suggest idiopathic thrombocytopenic purpura. Isoimmune thrombocytopenia in the newborn occurs when fetal platelets cross the placenta into the maternal circulation and may, depending on the platelet antigens, trigger a maternal production of immunoglobulin G aimed at the foreign fetal platelet antigen. These antiplatelet antibodies can then cross the placenta and lead to infant thrombocytopenia.

Patients with isolated thrombocytopenia on the basis of failure of production have decreased or absent megakaryocyte precursors. Differentiation of the various causes of decreased production, such as

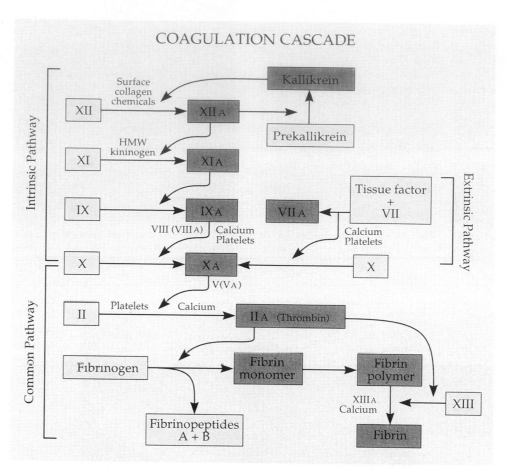

FIG. 11-60 PT measures the extrinsic and common pathways, whereas the PTT measures the intrinsic and common pathways.

thrombocytopenia-absent radius syndrome (Fig. 11-59) and amegakaryocytic thrombocytopenia, may rest on clinical findings. Patients with this syndrome may have a number of other congenital problems such as leukemoid reactions, congenital heart disease, and failure to thrive. Their thrombocytopenia frequently resolves as they grow older. Rarely, thrombocytopenia may be caused by a combination of decreased production and increased destruction. This can be seen in sepsis, collagen diseases, and Wiskott-Aldrich syndrome.

Qualitative or functional platelet defects may also lead to a bleeding diathesis. In the setting of normal platelet number and normal clotting studies, the possibility of poorly functioning platelets needs to be considered. The bleeding time, the value of which recently has been called into question, has traditionally been viewed in the child with a platelet count greater than 100,000/mm³ as the simplest and best test of platelet function, although it can also be abnormal in diseases of connective tissue (e.g., Ehlers-Danlos syndrome). The highly specialized tests necessary to confirm a diagnosis of platelet dysfunction are available in most large centers. Information in addition to that mentioned, which may point to a reason for platelet dysfunction, includes a history of drug exposure by direct ingestion by the patient or in some cases via breast-feeding (aspirin alone or as a component of another medication is the best known and affects platelet studies for the 7- to 10-day life of the platelet), history of uremia, hypothyroidism, hyperbilirubinemia, and inflammatory bowel disease. Von Willebrand disease is a relatively common disorder in which the bleeding time is generally increased with or without an increase in the PTT. Von Willebrand

disease usually is inherited in an autosomal dominant fashion, although it may also occur sporadically. It is not strictly a disorder of platelet function; rather, the disease is caused by an abnormality of the factor VIII molecule, which binds platelets to the endothelium. The tendency to bleed may vary from patient to patient and from time to time in any given patient. The condition is frequently asymptomatic, being detected when an abnormal bleeding time or PTT is noted as part of a preoperative screen or when mucosal bleeding such as menorrhagia is demonstrated. Hemarthroses generally are not seen in children with von Willebrand disease, even when the PTT is prolonged.

Coagulopathies

Coagulopathies occur when the circulating factors necessary for normal coagulation are deficient from lack of production or from excessive consumption. Coagulopathies can occur as genetic defects, as in the decreased production of normal procoagulants (hemophilia), or as acquired conditions resulting in depressed factor production (vitamin K deficiency, liver disease) or overutilization of factors (DIC).

Whatever the cause of coagulopathy, the measurement of the PTT and PT is the first step in clarifying the diagnosis. The clotting system is shown in Fig. 11-60. The PTT evaluates the intrinsic and common pathway, whereas the PT evaluates the extrinsic and common pathways. Values for these screening tests are age related so that normal newborns, especially premature infants, have prolonged PTs and PTTs compared with those of older children. These screening tests, although sensitive enough to detect the mild, moderate, or severe defi-

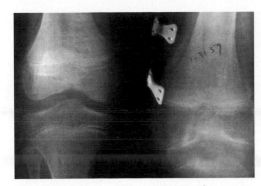

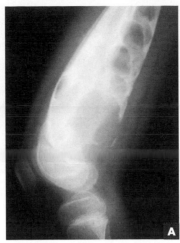

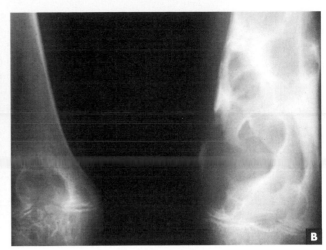

FIG. 11-61 Hemophiliac arthritis after recurrent hemarthroses. Note the widened joint space on the left knee compared with that of the normal right knee.

FIG. 11-62 *A,* Pseudotumor of the femur resulting from recurrent hemarthroses with subsequent bony destruction of the knee and adjacent bony structure. *B,* Note that the opposite knee also demonstrates early destructive changes in the distal femur and joint.

ciencies of hemophilia, are normal in carriers with approximately 50% factor levels.

Hemophilia A and B

Although deficiencies have been reported for every procoagulant, factor VIII deficiency (hemophilia A) and factor IX deficiency (hemophilia B) make up the majority of hemophilias. Because hemophilias A and B are transmitted in an X-linked recessive inheritance pattern, hemophilia is found nearly always in males. Hemophiliacs may have variable degrees of factor deficiency and commensurate levels of clinical disease. Patients with mild hemophilia have factor activity between 5% and 30% and, in general, suffer only from bleeding if they undergo surgery or suffer major trauma. Patients with moderate hemophilia have a factor activity of 1% to 5% and suffer localized hemorrhage in response to trauma. Finally, patients with less than 1% factor activity (the most frequent genotype) have spontaneous soft tissue hemorrhage or bleeding associated with only minor trauma.

Patients with hemophilia often present in the newborn period at the time of circumcision. Infants who escape clinical problems at that time generally do not present until 12 to 18 months of age—when they have become more mobile and minor trauma from falls precipitates bleeding. Although the clinical manifestations of hemophilia can affect any organ, the musculoskeletal, central nervous, and urinary systems predominate. The most common of the clinical manifestations include hemarthroses and soft tissue bleeding with intramuscular hematomas. Secondary hemophiliac arthropathy also may occur, with the knees, elbows, and ankles being the most commonly involved joints. Recurrent,

untreated hemorrhages may lead to contractures (Fig. 11-61) and painful arthritis (Fig. 11-62). Finally, intramuscular bleeding can cause compartment syndromes with secondary peripheral nerve palsies.

Decreases in clotting factor production may be acquired as well as inherited. Hepatic synthesis of clotting factors may be depressed in vitamin K–deficient patients. Vitamin K deficiency in the newborn may be suggested by cephalohematomas, bleeding from scalp or mouth sites, or intracranial hemorrhage, particularly if there has been inadvertent omission of prophylactic vitamin K administration, breast-feeding, antibiotics, or maternal ingestion of vitamin K inhibitors in the last trimester.

The PT and/or PTT may be prolonged for a variety of reasons other than hemophilia or depressed factor production. The presence of acquired inhibitors of in vitro coagulation (lupus anticoagulants), which most often are defined in a coagulation laboratory by "mixing" studies, is one such reason. Children who have received antibiotics, especially the penicillins, may develop inhibitors that may persist for even months after discontinuation of medication. Other drugs and viral infections have been implicated as well. Lupus anticoagulants rarely have been associated with thrombosis and even more rarely with bleeding events. About 10% of patients with systemic lupus erythematosus harbor such antibodies. DIC with consumption of clotting factors, as well as platelets, also prolongs the PTT and PT (Fig. 11-33).

Far less common than bleeding, thrombotic events may also occur. Once again, an inherited deficiency of anticoagulants (proteins C and S, antithrombin III) (Fig. 11-63) or an acquired alteration in normal co-

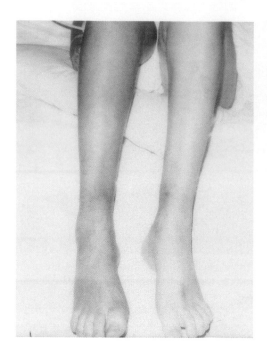

FIG. 11-63 Swollen, discolored leg in a child with deep venous thrombosis resulting from protein C deficiency. (Courtesy Dr. R. Kellogg.)

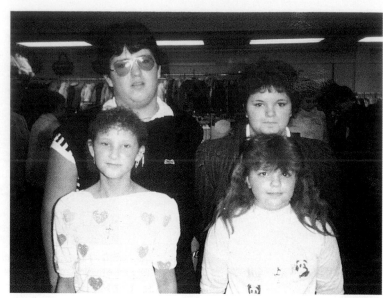

FIG. 11-64   Patient with Fanconi anemia (shortly after bone marrow transplantation) and her three siblings. The patient *(front left)* had a hemoglobin level of 3.5 g/dl, short stature, and increased skin pigmentation. Note the patient's diminutive size with respect to her more robust siblings.

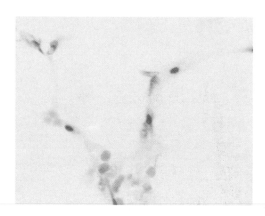

FIG. 11-65   Bone marrow biopsy of a patient with acquired aplastic anemia. Stromal marrow cells are present with virtually no hematopoietic cells.

agulation balance (paroxysmal nocturnal hemoglobinuria, tumors, nephrotic syndrome, deep catheter, dehydration, antiphospholipid antibodies, and medications) are possible.

Pancytopenia

Pancytopenia refers to a reduction in all three formed elements of the blood. In an analogous manner to anemia, pancytopenia is not a single disease entity but rather may result from a number of disease processes. Pancytopenia may occur from bone marrow failure or extramedullary cellular destruction (as seen in autoimmune disease, particularly systemic lupus erythematosus) or as a combination of depressed marrow function and increased cellular destruction. When pancytopenia is due to destruction of the formed elements of the blood, invariably there is another underlying disease. On the other hand, the pancytopenia resulting from bone marrow failure can be divided into genetically predisposed (constitutional) marrow failure syndromes, acquired marrow failure syndromes, and marrow replacement.

The most frequent of the constitutional marrow failure syndromes is Fanconi anemia. Fanconi anemia is a familial disorder marked by the association of pancytopenia and marrow hypoplasia with a variable constellation of congenital anomalies of the skin, skeleton, central ner-

vous system, and genitourinary tract (Fig. 11-64). Fragility of the chromosomes further characterizes this syndrome, and it occurs even in the absence of physical anomalies. Patients may have anemia very early in life but generally develop signs of marrow failure in midchildhood. The abnormal chromosomes are the most characteristic laboratory finding, and chromosome breaks, gaps, and rearrangements are common.

Acquired marrow failure syndromes (aplastic anemia) occur as a result of an insult to the bone marrow from a variety of sources, including drugs, toxins, solvents, and radiation, as well as autoimmune and postinfectious disorders. Nevertheless 50% of aplastic anemia cases have no apparent insulting agent and are idiopathic in origin.

The clinical course of aplastic anemia from any of these causes is that of inexorable bone marrow failure with anemia, thrombocytopenia, and leukopenia, leading ultimately to death from bleeding or infection if spontaneous recovery or successful intervention fails to occur.

Although the peripheral smear reveals a paucity of platelets and WBCs with a low reticulocyte count and normochromic and normocytic anemia, a marrow biopsy generally is needed to clarify the diagnosis (Fig. 11-65).

Marrow replacement, another cause of pancytopenia, occurs with a hematopoietic malignancy such as leukemia (Fig. 11-40) or from solid tumors invading the marrow (Fig. 11-66). A direct "crowding out" phenomenon and an alteration of the marrow "milieu" appear to contribute to marrow failure.

Oncology

Almost 7000 new cases of cancer in children younger than 15 years of age are reported in the United States each year, reflecting an annual incidence of approximately 10 in 100,000. Whereas mortality was once

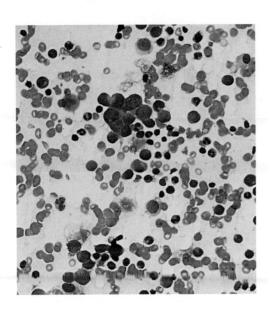

FIG. 11-66 Pseudorosettes (clumps of tumor cells) are particularly characteristic of a neuroblastoma metastasized to the bone marrow.

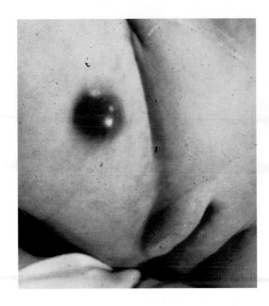

FIG. 11-67 Subcutaneous nodule in a child with neuroblastoma. Lesions, which occasionally may be seen with leukemia or other solid tumors, may be dark ("blueberry muffin") or skin colored. (From Pearson H: Tumors of the sympathetic nervous system. In Altman AJ, Schwartz AD, eds: *Malignant diseases of infancy, childhood, and adolescence,* ed 2, 1983, Philadelphia, WB Saunders.)

TABLE 11-7

Red Flags of Malignancy

Pallor, fatigue	Anorexia	Hepatomegaly
Petechiae	Poor growth	Splenomegaly
Fever, infection	Headache, vomit-	Abdominal mass
Bone pain, limp	ing, lethargy	Testiculomegaly
Weight loss	Lymphadenopathy	

TABLE 11-8

Groups at High Risk of Cancer

Hereditary cutaneous syndromes (xeroderma pigmentosum)
Neurocutaneous syndromes (neurofibromatosis)
Chromosomal abnormalities (Down syndrome, Bloom syndrome)
Hereditary or acquired immunodeficiency (ataxia-telangiectasia)
Autoimmune diseases
Congenital malformations or syndromes (hemihypertrophy, Beckwith-Wiedemann syndrome)
Sibling with cancer
History of prior cancer
Intrauterine (diethylstilbestrol) or postnatal (chemotherapy) agents
Drugs
Radiation
Metabolic diseases (alpha$_1$-antitrypsin deficiency)

the rule, it is now less than 40%. Thus the majority of children with cancer have a curable illness.

The job of recognizing the signs and symptoms of malignancy usually falls to the pediatrician or family practitioner. In this section, most of the common and some of the exotic presentations that should raise suspicion of childhood cancer are highlighted, with a view toward facilitating prompt referral to a pediatric oncologist. For details about specific cancers and their management, more comprehensive texts are recommended.

Signs and Symptoms

Red flags that signal malignancy—leukemias and solid tumors—may be detected in the course of history taking, physical examination, or review of a few basic laboratory tests (Table 11-7). These may be the direct effects of tumor (mass effects) or secondary to "humors" produced by cancerous or reactive cells (so-called paraneoplastic syndromes). The condition of a child with cancer may be entirely asymptomatic when routine physical examination suggests an abnormality. However, frequent nonspecific systemic complaints include fatigue, weight loss, fever (which may have a discernible pattern or an infectious source), and night sweats (most commonly but not exclusively associated with Hodgkin disease). Less common systemic complaints include diarrhea, failure to thrive, and pruritus (again, associated with Hodgkin disease). Among the more localizing complaints are headaches and vomiting, which are often but not always most prominent in the morning (brain tumors); constipation or voiding difficulty (pelvic tumors); hypertension (renal tumors, neuroblastoma, or pheochromocytoma); and bone pain and/or limp, which result from cortical lesions of primary bone or metastatic tumors or extensive intramedullary disease as in leukemia.

All of these complaints are more likely to have a cause that is not malignant. However, persistence (2 weeks is a reasonable though not absolute guideline) or undue severity may give these signs increased significance. Similarly, in the context of a number of predisposing, underlying diseases (Table 11-8), malignancy should be considered earlier. Certainly, children with a history of one cancer, by virtue of genetics or as a "late effect" of anticancer therapy, are at greater risk of a second cancer. Cancer in a parent or sibling, although heightening anxiety about the possibility of cancer in a child, is rarely by itself a major predisposing factor. The notable exception is the infant or toddler who has an identical twin with leukemia. In this child, the risk may be as high as 25%.

Specific physical findings may be sought when a particular diagnosis is suspected. For example, subcutaneous nodules should be looked for in infants with neuroblastoma (Fig. 11-67). However, even without knowledge about particular tumors, careful physical examination discloses signs of malignancy in addition to those mentioned. A list of such signs by organ system follows.

Skin

Examination of the skin should be complete. The clinician looks for cancerous lesions and cutaneous manifestations of extracutaneous can-

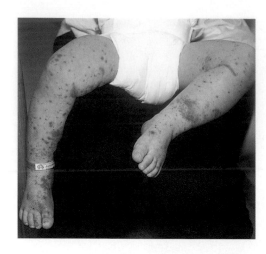

FIG. 11-68 Purpuric lesions in a child with neuroblastoma and tumor-related coagulopathy. Similar lesions may result from isolated thrombocytopenia.

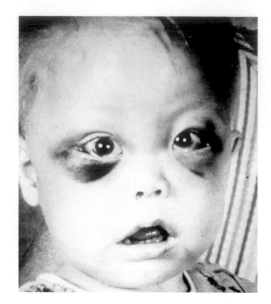

FIG. 11-69 Raccoon eyes, indicative of retroorbital tumor (usually neuroblastoma), may involve supraorbital or infraorbital areas. "Shiners" resulting from trauma or abuse may be part of differential diagnosis. (Courtesy H. Pearson, New Haven, Conn.)

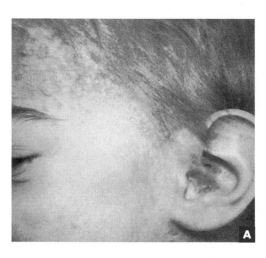

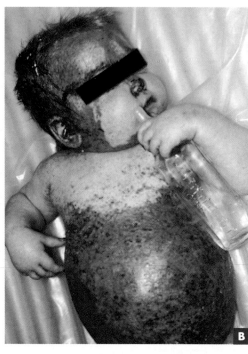

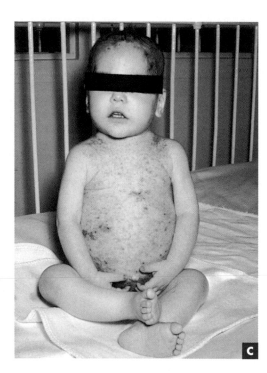

FIG. 11-70 *A,* Seborrhea in infant with histiocytosis X. Chronic ear damage is also seen. *B* and *C,* Hemorrhagic and papular rashes also are seen in some children with this group of diseases. (Courtesy Dr. P. Gaffney, Pittsburgh.)

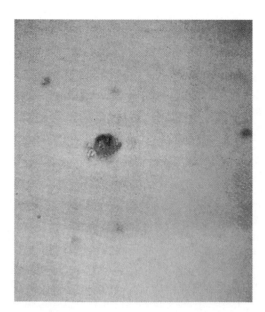

FIG. 11-71 Melanoma. In addition to location (see text), suspicious signs are a red-brown-black color that tends to be diffuse at the periphery, crusting, bleeding, pain, or itching.

cers and picks up signs of a variety of precancerous or cancer-associated diagnoses (Table 11-8). Even in white children, skin color may be deceptive. Thus pallor, a result of anemia, may be most readily appreciated by examination of subconjunctival or palmar creases (see section on hematology). Purpura, small petechiae, or large ecchymoses (see section on hematology) are commonly found on the lower extremities or at sites of trauma, but they should be sought elsewhere on the body, including on the retina or oral mucosa ("wet purpura"). Easy bruisability usually is due to thrombocytopenia, although patients with platelet counts greater than 20,000/mm³ may have no spontaneous bleeding tendency. Infrequently, purpura may result from coagulopathy without thrombocytopenia (Fig. 11-68). Bleeding at a particular location may suggest a more specific diagnosis. For example, racoon eyes (Fig. 11-69) are periorbital ecchymoses attributable to retroorbital tumor, notably neuroblastoma; isolated vaginal bleeding may be seen with rhabdomyosarcoma or yolk sac tumors arising in the vagina; and gross or microscopic hematuria is sometimes seen in children with Wilms tumor.

Seborrhea, which is usually a benign finding, may be one of the cutaneous manifestations of histiocytosis X (Fig. 11-70) (see Chapter 8),

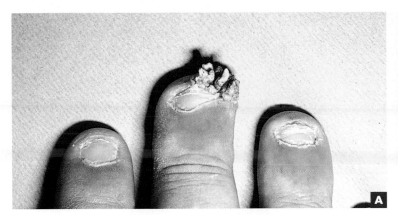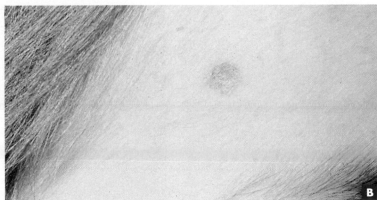

FIG. 11-72 *A,* Squamous cell carcinoma. *B,* Basal cell carcinoma on forehead of a 7-year-old boy who had received prophylactic cranial radiation as part of his treatment for acute lymphoblastic leukemia 5 years before he developed a second cancer. (*A* courtesy Dr. J. Zitelli, Pittsburgh; *B* from Pratt CB, Douglass EC: Management of the uncommon cancer of childhood. In Pizzo PA, Poplack DG, eds: *Principles and practice of pediatric oncology,* Philadelphia, 1988, JB Lippincott.)

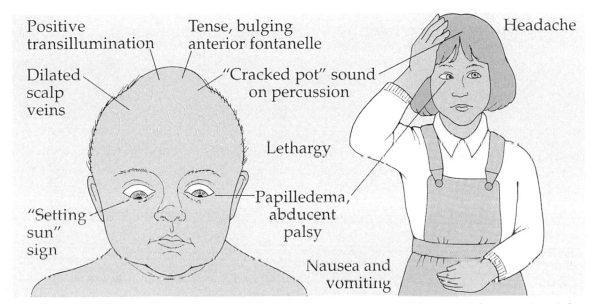

FIG. 11-73 Macrocephaly and superficial venous distension secondary to increased intracranial pressure in an infant with a glioma of the central nervous system. The older child may instead show changes in mental status, vomiting, or focal neurologic signs. (From Stein SC: *Brain tumors in children,* Resident and Staff Physician, 26:34-28, 1980.)

and this diagnosis should be suspected if seborrhea is unusually severe or persists despite standard treatment measures. Melanoma (Fig. 11-71), although extremely rare in childhood, is most likely to result from transformation of pigmented or junctional nevi. It should be considered when pigmented lesions change in size or color or develop irregular margins. These precancerous lesions should be removed prophylactically when they occur on the palms, soles, genitalia, anorectal mucosa, nail beds, or lower extremities. Squamous and basal cell carcinomas (Fig. 11-72) arise most often in the setting of heritable diseases such as xeroderma pigmentosum or basal cell nevus syndrome. Although Kaposi sarcoma has been described in only 1% of pediatric AIDS patients (predominantly in the adenopathic form), the increasing incidence of AIDS makes recognition of the cutaneous manifestations (see Chapter 4) important.

Head and Neck

Findings on the head, eyes, ears, nose, and throat examination may include macrocephaly, bulging fontanelle, and/or superficial venous distension resulting from increased intracranial pressure and hydrocephalus from primary or metastatic tumor involving the brain (Fig. 11-73). Chronic draining ears (Fig. 11-74) are seen with histiocytosis, and this diagnosis should be suspected when problems persist despite antibiotics. Inappropriate loosening of the teeth should also prompt concerns about histiocytosis. Otorrhea also may be seen with other head and neck tumors such as rhabdomyosarcoma.

Ocular Findings

Cat's eye reflex or leukokoria with an absent red reflex is characteristic of retinoblastoma (see Chapter 19) and should be sought as part

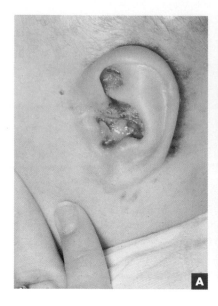

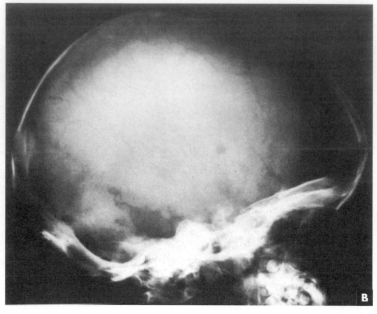

FIG. 11-74   *A,* Otorrhea in child with histiocytosis. *B,* X-ray film shows destruction of mastoid bone in same child. (*A* courtesy Dr. P. Gaffney, Pittsburgh.)

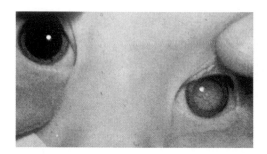

FIG. 11-75   Cat's eye reflex or leukocoria in child with retinoblastoma. (From Abramson D: Retinoblastoma, *CA* 32:130-140, 1982.)

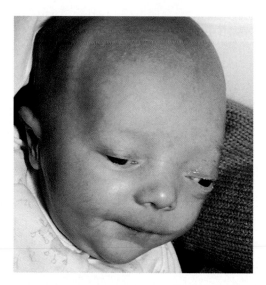

FIG. 11-76   Proptosis in child with retroorbital rhabdosarcoma. Note also, large head secondary to increased intracranial pressure. (Courtesy Dr. V. Albo, Pittsburgh.)

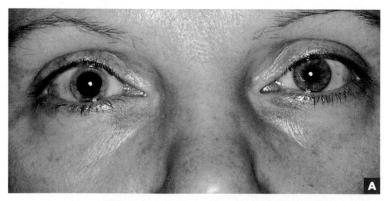

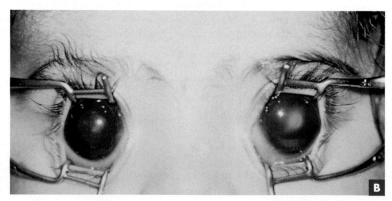

FIG. 11-77   *A,* Heterochromia iridis in adult who had Wilms tumor as a child. *B,* Aniridia. (*A* courtesy Dr. J. Roen, New York.)

of the routine physical examination in the neonate and young child. This is often best appreciated from a frontal photograph of the child (Fig. 11-75) and therefore may be brought to the attention of a physician by a parent. Strabismus (see Chapter 19), particularly when first seen after infancy, may be a sign of an orbital tumor or intracranial

pathologic condition and even if intermittent merits attention. Similarly, proptosis (Fig. 11-76), characteristic of orbital rhabdomyosarcoma or histiocytosis, also deserves attention.

Heterochromia (Fig. 11-77, *A*), usually a benign oddity, may be associated with Wilms tumor or with cervicothoracic neuroblastoma

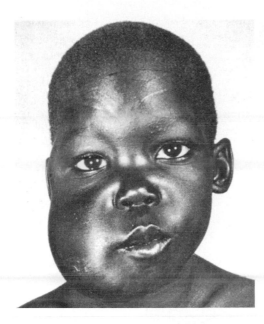

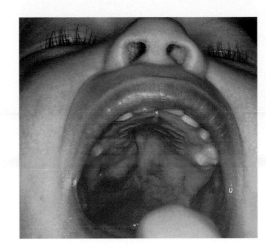

FIG. 11-78 Burkitt lymphoma of the jaw in African child. (Courtesy Dr. I. Magrath, Bethesda, Md.)

FIG. 11-79 Intraoral extension of intracranial rhabdomyosarcoma. The lesion was first detected by the child's dentist and was biopsied by an ear, nose, and throat specialist who did not suspect malignancy.

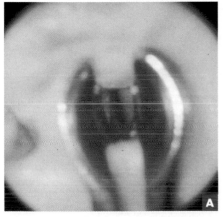

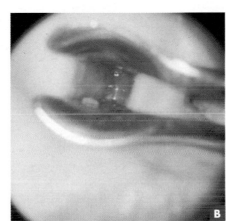

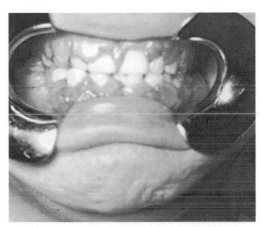

FIG. 11-80 Intranasal glioma occluding right nostril. The normal left nostril is also shown. (Courtesy Dr. S. Stool, Pittsburgh.)

FIG. 11-81 Gingival hyperplasia resulting from leukemic invasion of the gums. (From Bluefarb, SM: *Dermatology*, Kalamazoo, Mich, 1984, Upjohn.)

(preoperatively or postoperatively, when it occurs alone or as part of Horner syndrome). Aniridia (Fig. 11-77, *B*), when it occurs sporadically and not as an autosomal-dominant trait, also has been associated with Wilms tumor. Both eye findings in the infant or toddler should prompt appropriate diagnostic studies.

Orofacial Findings

Although masses such as the jaw lesion shown in Fig. 11-78 are likely to be referred early to an oncologist, intraoral (Fig. 11-79) or intranasal (Fig. 11-80) masses are more likely to masquerade as nonmalignant lesions, which may forestall correct diagnosis. These may be entirely asymptomatic, or they may cause local bleeding or difficulty swallowing or breathing. Gingival hyperplasia can be seen in children with leukemia, especially the acute myelomonocytic kind (Fig. 11-81).

Although most physicians look for cervical adenopathy, it is important to remember the other lymph node groups that may be involved by focal or generalized adenopathy in leukemias, lymphomas, or solid tumors. A schematic diagram depicting the major lymph node regions is presented in Fig. 11-82. Although large, rock-hard nodes that are fixed to the subcutaneous tissue are most convincing for malignancy, texture and size can be misleading. Because Hodgkin disease and non-Hodgkin lymphoma can occur concurrently with or after infectious

mononucleosis, a positive monospot test may be a false reassurance. Therefore persistent adenopathy, even in that setting, should be followed closely. The algorithms for workup of adenopathy and indications for biopsy are reviewed in Chapter 12.

In addition to examination of the lymph nodes, examination of the neck may disclose jugular venous distension, which may be subtle or fulminant and associated with varying degrees of facial fullness, plethora, and respiratory distress (Fig. 11-83) (see later description). Goiters or nodular thyroids with or without bruits may be seen in patients with thyroid carcinoma.

Chest

External examination of the chest may disclose obvious skeletal or other chest wall masses that may be asymptomatic or associated with localizing or pleuritic pain. Scoliosis has been associated with paravertebral tumors (Fig. 11-84). Respiratory distress may result from an intrathoracic process or abdominal distension from a mass or ascites. The superior vena cava syndrome, caused by obstruction of venous return to the heart through the superior vena cava by a mass lesion, also may result in wheezing, cough, and the plethora previously noted. In pediatrics, this syndrome is a medical emergency, most commonly caused

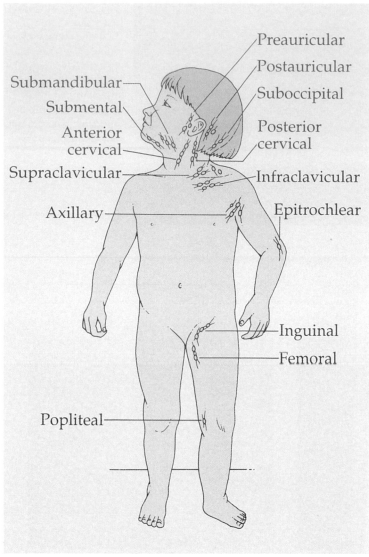

FIG. 11-82 Lymph node regions palpable on physical examination. Rarely, retroperitoneal nodes may become so enlarged that they are palpable.

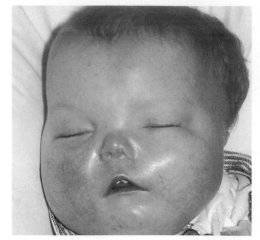

FIG. 11-83 Superior vena cava syndrome. Discoloration of the face and neck with venous distension. The mediastinal masses that produce these findings may pose considerable anesthetic risk.

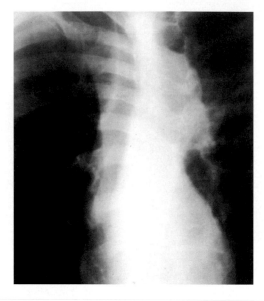

FIG. 11-84 Paravertebral mass and associated scoliosis.

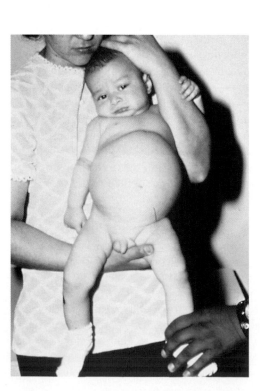

FIG. 11-85 Abdominal swelling with hepatosplenomegaly in child with neuroblastoma. (From Pearson H: *Malignant diseases of infancy, childhood, and adolescence,* ed 2, Philadelphia, 1983, WB Saunders.)

by non-Hodgkin lymphoma. However, such tumors often are asymptomatic. Neural tumors such as neuroblastoma or ganglioneuroma also may present as asymptomatic posterior or superior mediastinal masses on chest x-ray studies (Fig. 11-95). They often are detected on chest x-ray study performed for some other reason or as part of a staging workup in a child in whom cancer is suspected or diagnosed on the basis of some other findings.

Abdomen

An observant parent may be the first person to detect abdominal swelling or mass (see Chapter 17), which may result from hepatomegaly and/or splenomegaly (Fig. 11-85), the flank mass of Wilms tumor, the often more centrally located retroperitoneal neuroblastoma, other intraabdominal tumors, or ascites. Wilms tumor and neuroblastoma are the most likely diagnoses in children younger than 5 years. The former condition is commonly asymptomatic but occasionally may be diagnosed when hematuria is noted. Children with abdominal presentations of neuroblastoma often (although not always) look ill. Superficial venous distension (Fig. 11-86) may signal deep venous obstruction related to intraabdominal tumor. These findings, even when obvious, may be asymptomatic or associated with vomiting, diarrhea, constipation, respiratory embarrassment, or decreased urine output.

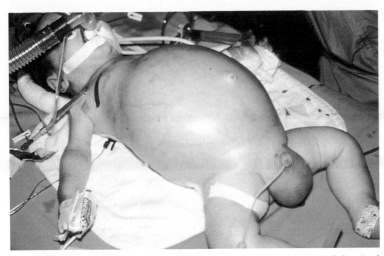

FIG. 11-86 Superficial venous distension in a child with intraabdominal tumor. (Courtesy Dr. D. Nakayama, Chapel Hill, NC.)

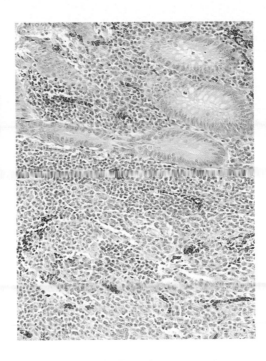

FIG. 11-87 Microscopic picture of the appendix, showing involvement with non-Hodgkin lymphoma. Malignant cells, predominating in the lower half of the slide, are large, with clear cytoplasm and irregularly shaped nuclei.

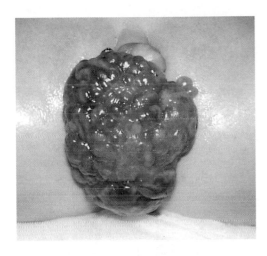

FIG. 11-88 Sarcoma botryoides in child with multiple congenital anomalies. Note the grapelike appearance of the lesion.

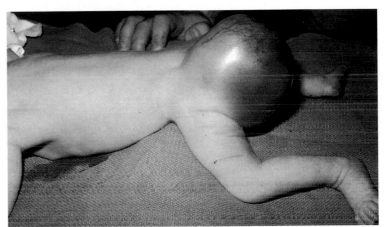

FIG. 11-89 Sacrococcygeal teratoma.

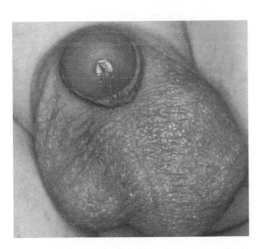

FIG. 11-90 Unilateral scrotal swelling in an infant with a left testicular mass.

Primary intestinal tumors, notably non-Hodgkin lymphoma, may masquerade as acute abdominal pain such as appendicitis (Fig. 11-87) or provide a lead point for intussusception. The pediatric surgeon, recognizing these possibilities, needs to send specimens for careful pathologic review.

Urogenital Tract

Involvement of the genitourinary system or perianal area by tumor may be reflected in the obstructive symptoms already described. Sarcoma botryoides (Fig. 11-88) is a subtype of rhabdomyosarcoma named for its grapelike appearance. Classically, it involves the vagina but may also involve the mucosal surfaces of other hollow organs such as the bladder or larynx. This tumor and sacrococcygeal teratoma (Fig. 11-89) usually are grossly apparent. However, both may present as intraabdominal or pelvic masses. The latter may need to be distinguished from a meningomyelocele and other spinal tumors, but as with these other diagnoses, it may cause peripheral neurologic abnormalities. As noted, Wilms tumor may present with asymptomatic hematuria.

Testicular enlargement (Fig. 11-90) (see Chapter 17) may be secondary to involvement by metastatic leukemia or lymphoma (in which case bilateral swelling may be seen) or to primary testicular tumors. Priapism (Fig. 11-31) is a rare, concomitant sequela of chronic myelogenous leukemia. Isosexual precocity, particularly in a boy, may be caused by a tumor of the central nervous system, gonads (ovaries or testes), or adrenal gland. Other endocrinopathic conditions such as Cushing syndrome, diabetes insipidus, and hypoglycemia also have been described as presenting manifestations of pediatric cancer. Particularly in the case of adrenal tumors (Fig. 11-91), early diagnosis contributes to curability.

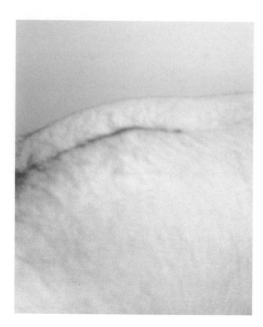

FIG. 11-91 Abdominal distension and hirsutism in a young girl with adrenocortical carcinoma. (Courtesy Dr. P. Lee, Pittsburgh.)

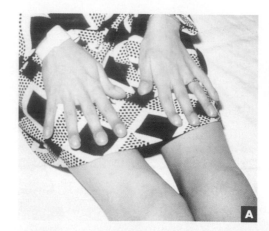

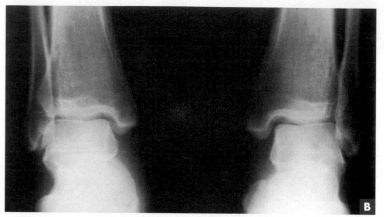

FIG. 11-92 Clubbing (*A*) and bone lesions (*B*) in a child with hypertrophic osteoarthropathy secondary to hepatocellular carcinoma not involving the lung. (Courtesy Dr. K.S. Oh, Pittsburgh.)

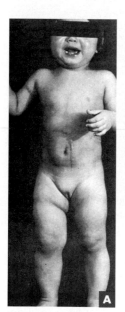

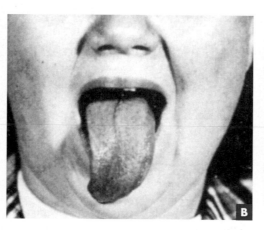

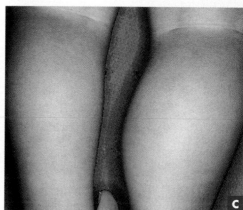

FIG. 11-93 *A* and *B*, Hemihypertrophy. *C*, Asymmetry resulting from soft tissue sarcoma of left calf. (*A* and *B* from Fraumeni JF, Geiser CF, Manning MD: Wilms' tumor and congenital hemihypertrophy: report of five new cases and review of literature, *Pediatrics* 40:886-899, 1967. *C* courtesy Dr. D. Nakayama, Chapel Hill, NC.)

Musculoskeletal System

Bone and joint manifestations of pediatric cancer are relatively common. Arthralgia, or full-blown arthritis, is a well-described (so-called juvenile rheumatoid arthritis–like) presentation of acute lymphocytic leukemia. Findings may be migratory and typically involve the knees, wrists, and fingers. Bone pain, as previously discussed, also is common. Hypertrophic osteoarthropathy, probably one of the paraneoplastic syndromes, has been described in children with hepatomas, not all of whom have advanced disease at the time of presentation (Fig. 11-92). Hemihypertrophy (Fig. 11-93) (see Chapter 9), or relative enlargement of one or more parts (usually the legs or feet) of one side of the body, has been associated with the subsequent development of a number of solid tumors and with leukemia and should be distinguished from hemiatrophy,

which is not a predisposing condition. A mass involving one extremity (Fig. 11-93, *C*) is not usually confused with hemihypertrophy. Deep vein thromboses may be caused by vessel compression by tumor or a paraneoplastic effect. Primary bone tumors are most commonly seen in adolescents and should be considered when patients experience persistent pain, even in the absence of objective findings.

Nervous System

Neurologic symptoms of pediatric cancer include headaches and vomiting. In addition, seizures or changes in mental status may be caused by primary or metastatic intracranial tumors or by metabolic abnormalities. Cranial nerve palsies (Fig. 11-73) may be localizing or false-localizing signs. Malignant and benign tumors of the central ner-

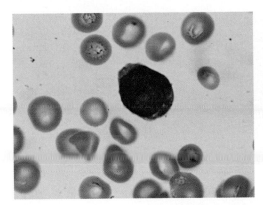

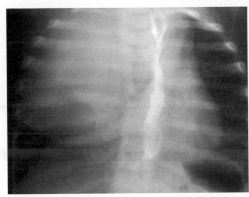

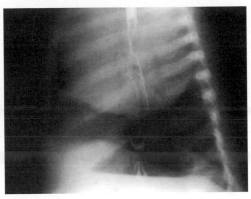

FIG. 11-94 Blasts in peripheral blood of a baby who also had hepatosplenomegaly and thrombocytopenia but who turned out to have a viral illness instead of leukemia.

FIG. 11-95 Posterior mediastinal mass in a child with neuroblastoma. Calcification, not present in this film, may be seen in 50% of cases. (Courtesy Dr. J. Medina, Pittsburgh.)

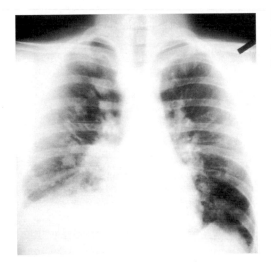

FIG. 11-96 Pulmonary nodules in an adolescent with metastatic sarcoma.

vous system may cause these symptoms. Medulloblastoma is one of the most common malignancies of the central nervous system in childhood and can present with any of these signs. In addition, because these tumors usually arise in the cerebellum, patients may have ataxia. Brain tumors, particularly those such as craniopharyngioma, that arise in the thalamus or hypothalamus can present with failure to thrive with or without abnormalities of sexual development (precocity or delay). Opsoclonus-myoclonus (dancing eyes, dancing feet) is a much talked about, infrequently seen, and poorly understood syndrome most closely associated with neuroblastoma. Spinal cord tumors or tumors that press on the cord may present with bowel-bladder dysfunction, paresthesias, and changes in gait. Pain on percussion over the vertebral column may be an early sign of cord compression and should be actively sought in the child with suspected cancer in whom it may be another of the oncologic emergencies.

Laboratory Aids to Diagnosis

Evaluation of Blood and Bone Marrow Specimens

In the case of leukemia, or occasionally solid tumors, a CBC ordered with differential and platelet counts may provide the first suggestion of malignancy, particularly in the child with persistent but minimal and nonlocalizing symptoms. Careful attention should be paid to abnormalities in the WBC count (which may be increased or decreased), he-

moglobin level, and platelet count. Although thrombocytopenia is commonly associated with leukemia, thrombocytosis can rarely be seen in that disease; it is characteristic of neuroblastoma or hepatic cancers, even when the bone marrow is not involved. Although blasts are not specific for leukemia (Fig. 11-94), their presence should hasten further workup. However, blasts in the peripheral blood never preclude the need to examine the bone marrow. Conversely, the absence of blasts does not rule out a diagnosis of leukemia, and a child who is subsequently found to have leukemia may have a CBC that is entirely normal at the time of presentation. Because multiple special studies, including flow cytometry and chromosomal analysis, are needed for evaluation of bone marrow specimens, a child who warrants a bone marrow workup should be referred to a pediatric oncologist.

Evaluation of Metabolic Abnormalities

Metabolic abnormalities may be a reason for morbidity and mortality. Therefore a battery of "tumor" chemistry tests also should be ordered in the child with a suspicion of cancer. These would include electrolyte, blood urea nitrogen, creatinine, uric acid, lactate dehydrogenase, calcium, and phosphorus levels, the results of which should be checked as soon as they are ready, as well as liver function tests. Even in children with primary or metastatic disease involving the liver, serum glutamic-oxaloacetic transaminase, serum glutamic-pyruvate transaminase, bilirubin, and alkaline phosphatase levels may all be normal. Although 24-hour urine collections can be used to measure the catecholamine metabolites homovanillic acid and vanillylmandelic acid in children with suspected neuroblastoma, in many hospitals, random urine samples can be tested with similar accuracy and much greater ease. Because it may take a prolonged period to get these results, further evaluation may need to be done without waiting.

Mediastinal Masses

The likely cause of mediastinal masses (see Chapter 17) depends to a certain extent on location. Tumors of the posterior mediastinum (especially when calcified on x-ray films) are commonly neurogenic (e.g., neuroblastoma or its benign counterpart ganglioneuroma [Fig. 11-95] or lymphoma). Tumors of the anterior mediastinum are thymomas, teratomas, or lymphomas. Middle mediastinal masses or hilar adenopathy is most likely to be leukemic or lymphomatous. Parenchymal pulmonary nodules, when tumor related, are likely to be asymptomatic and are most commonly related to metastatic sarcoma or Wilms tumor (Fig. 11-96). Neuroblastoma classically avoids the lung parenchyma until late in a disease's course. Pleural effusions, although relatively rare

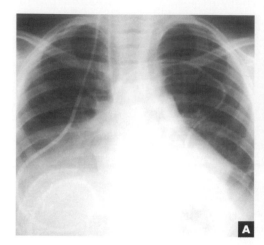

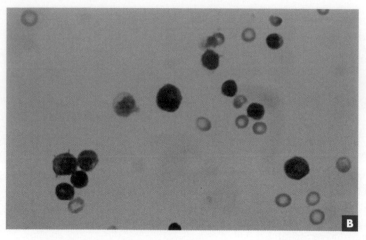

FIG. 11-97 *A,* Pleural effusions in a child with malignant lymphoma. *B,* Thoracentesis cytology of the same patient. Note the large cells with high nuclear to cytoplasmic ratios and fine nuclear chromatin.

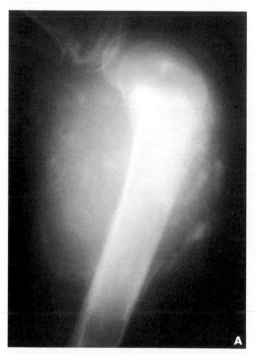

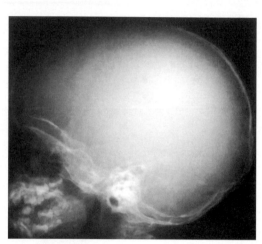

FIG. 11-99 Lytic lesions in child with leukemia. Similar lesions may result from metastatic solid tumors.

FIG. 11-98 *A,* X-ray film of a child with osteosarcoma shows soft tissue swelling, calcification, cortical bone destruction with increased osteodensity, and new bone formation (Codman triangle). *B,* Ewing sarcoma shows cortical destruction and soft tissue swelling of diaphysis of femur. (Courtesy J. Medina, Pittsburgh.)

in pediatric cancers, may be malignant, and cytologic testing should be considered if a diagnostic thoracentesis is done (Fig. 11-97).

Evaluation of Bone Pain

In evaluating bone pain (see previous section), plain radiographs often are ordered by the primary pediatrician. Frequent findings include the destructive lesions of primary bone tumors. Osteosarcoma most frequently occurs in the metaphysis of a long bone of the lower extremity, whereas Ewing sarcoma is more commonly a diaphyseal lesion (Fig. 11-98). Lytic or blastic lesions may be seen in patients with leukemia, lymphoma, and metastatic tumors (Fig. 11-99); metaphyseal lucencies and growth arrest lines are nonspecific findings of chronic dis-

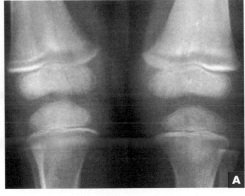

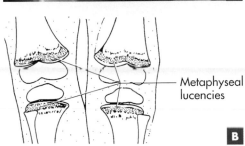

Metaphyseal lucencies

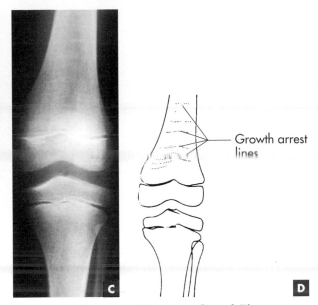

Growth arrest lines

FIG. 11-100 Metaphyseal lucencies *(A and B)* and growth arrest lines *(C and D)* in children with acute lymphocytic leukemia. (Courtesy Dr. J. Medina, Pittsburgh.)

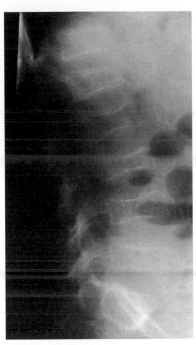

FIG. 11-101 Diffuse osteopenia in acute lymphocytic leukemia. This child was followed for many months by an orthopedist before an abnormal hemogram prompted referral to a hematologist.

ease but are most commonly associated with acute lymphocytic leukemia (Fig. 11-100). Diffuse osteopenia (Fig. 11-101) is presumably an effect of tumor-produced bone-resorbing factors. However, a normal plain film should never exclude the possibility of malignancy as a cause of bone symptoms. A bone scan or repeat plain film may be indicated after an arbitrary interval.

Specialized Techniques

The reasons for obtaining a chest x-ray film have been discussed. Whether more specialized radiographic studies such as intravenous pyelograms, sonograms, computed tomographic scans (always with and without contrast), and magnetic resonance imaging scans are ordered by the generalist or are not done until referral to a specialist is a decision that should depend on the following:

1. The degree of the child's illness and the timeliness of the studies obtained
2. Knowledge of how reliable the diagnostic radiology services are at a particular hospital
3. The ability to get good copies of the studies sent with the patient when he or she is ultimately transferred

Whether the child with suspected malignancy should have a tissue biopsy (other than a bone marrow) at the referring institution is also controversial. Under optimal circumstances, the surgeon should be familiar with the requirements of cancer operations, and adequate fresh tissue should be available with which to confirm a specific tumor diagnosis. It is often convenient for the biopsy to be done at the institution where the oncologist is located.

BIBLIOGRAPHY

Lanzkowsky P, ed: *Pediatric oncology: a treatise for the clinician,* New York, 1983, McGraw-Hill.

Miller DR, Pearson HA, Baehner RL, McMillan LW: *Smith's blood diseases of infancy and childhood,* ed 7, St Louis, 1995, Mosby.

Nathan DG, Oski FA: *Hematology of infancy and childhood,* ed 4, Philadelphia, 1993, WB Saunders.

Oski FA, Naiman JL: *Hematologic problems of the newborn,* ed 4, Philadelphia, 1993, WB Saunders.

Pizzo PA, Poplack DG, eds: *Principles and practice of pediatric oncology,* Philadelphia, 1989, JB Lippincott.

Wintrobe MM, et al: *Clinical hematology,* ed 8, Philadelphia, 1981, Lea & Febiger.

Zucker-Franklin D, Greanes MF, Grossi CE, Marmont AM: *Atlas of blood cells,* Milan, Italy, 1981, Ermes.

12

Pediatric Infectious Disease

HOLLY W. DAVIS ✦ RAYMOND B. KARASIC

*I*n selecting infectious diseases for presentation in an atlas format, we have chosen to emphasize common and serious disorders in which visual findings tend to be prominent. Modes of presentation, patterns of clinical evolution, and spectra of severity will be stressed. The following topics are covered: infectious exanthems, mumps, bacterial skin and soft tissue infections, infectious lymphadenitis, bacterial bone and joint infections, and congenital and perinatal infections. Because of its recent resurgence, we have added a new section on tuberculosis in childhood. This is designed to help practitioners who have seen few, if any, cases during decades of declining incidence to familiarize themselves with its modes of presentation and clinical and radiographic manifestations, thereby facilitating earlier recognition and diagnosis.

Human immunodeficiency virus infection is covered in Chapter 4.

Infectious Exanthems

Exanthematous disorders are numerous, commonly encountered, and because they have many similarities, often a source of clinical confusion. In establishing a diagnosis the clinician should attend not only to the basic character of the exanthem but also to its mode of spread, its distribution, the evolution of lesions, and the constellation of associated symptoms. In some of these illnesses the presence of a characteristic oral enanthem can be helpful in establishing the diagnosis.

Viral Exanthems

Along with mumps, three exanthems—measles or rubeola, rubella, and varicella—continue to be regarded as the usual childhood diseases. Although immunization has been responsible for causing a marked decrease in the incidence of measles, mumps, and rubella compared with their incidence in the prevaccine era, cases of measles (and less often mumps) still occur in children who are nonimmunized and in those whose immunity has waned. Although varicella remains a common illness, use of the recently licensed varicella vaccine is likely to lead to a decrease in the incidence of this disease, as well.

Rubeola (Nine-Day or Red Measles)

Measles is a highly contagious, moderate to severe acute illness with a typical prodrome and mode of evolution. Prodromal symptoms consist of fever, malaise, dry (occasionally croupy) cough, coryza, and conjunctivitis with clear discharge and marked photophobia (Fig. 12-1, *A*). One to two days after onset of prodromal symptoms, a pathognomonic enanthem (Koplik's spots) appears on the buccal mucosa (Fig. 12-1, *B*). The lesions consist of tiny bluish-white dots surrounded by red halos, which increase in number and then fade over a 2- to 3-day period. The exanthem is seen first on day 3 or 4, as the prodromal symptoms and fever peak in severity. It is a blotchy, erythematous, blanching, maculopapular eruption that appears at the hairline and spreads cephalocaudally over 3 days, ultimately involving the palms and soles (Fig. 12-1, *C* and *D*). Once generalized, the rash becomes confluent over proximal areas but remains discrete distally. Older lesions tend to develop a rusty hue as a result of capillary leak, and cease to blanch with pressure. Fading commences after 3 days, with clearing 2 to 3 days later. Fine, branny desquamation of the most severely involved areas may ensue. Generalized adenopathy may be present in moderate to severe cases.

During the acute phase of this illness, most patients are quite ill systemically. They are lethargic, have moderate to severe malaise and anorexia, and prefer to be left alone to sleep in a darkened room.

The incubation period for measles is 9 to 10 days, and patients are contagious from approximately 4 days before the appearance of rash until about 4 days after. The attack rate in exposed, susceptible people is greater than 90%. Morbidity is rather high and mortality not uncommon, especially in children of third-world countries. The peak season for measles is late winter through early spring. Potential complications (resulting either from extension of the primary infection or from secondary invasion by bacterial pathogens) include otitis media, pneumonia, obstructive laryngotracheitis, and acute encephalitis.

Rubella (German Measles)

Although rubella has little or no prodrome in children, adolescents, like adults, may experience 1 to 5 days of low-grade fever, mild malaise, adenopathy, headache, sore throat, and coryza. Fever, if present at all

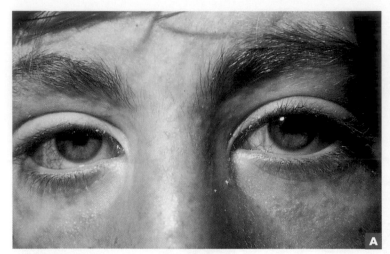

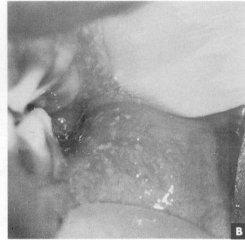

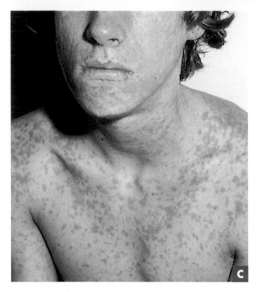

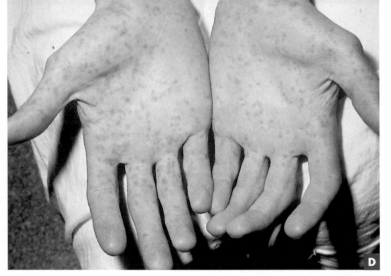

FIG. 12-1 Rubeola/measles. *A,* During and after the prodromal period, the conjunctivae are injected and produce a clear discharge. This is associated with marked photophobia. *B,* Koplik's spots, bluish-white dots surrounded by red halos, appear on the buccal and labial mucosa a day or two before the exanthem and begin to fade with onset of the rash. *C,* The measles exanthem is a blotchy, erythematous, blanching maculopapular eruption that appears at the hairline and spreads cephalocaudally over 3 days, ultimately involving the palms and soles *(D).* With evolution, lesions become confluent at proximal sites. (*A, C,* and *D* courtesy Dr. Michael Sherlock.)

in young children, is low grade and rarely lasts more than a day. The exanthem is a discrete, pinkish-red, fine maculopapular eruption, which, like measles, typically begins on the face and spreads cephalocaudally (Fig. 12-2, *A*). The rash becomes generalized within 24 hours, then begins to fade, clearing completely by 72 hours. Forchheimer's spots, an enanthem consisting of small reddish spots on the soft palate, are seen in some patients on day 1 of the rash and can be helpful in differential diagnosis (Fig. 12-2, *B*). Adenopathy, often generalized, is a common but not invariable feature. Occipital, posterior cervical, and postauricular nodes tend to be those most prominently enlarged. Arthritis and arthralgias are frequent in adolescent and adult female patients, beginning on day 2 to 3 and typically lasting 5 to 10 days. Large or small joints may be affected.

Many patients infected with rubella do not manifest this typical picture. Up to 25% of infected people are asymptomatic, yet are capable of transmitting the virus to others. In some, the rash may last only 1 day and it may involve only the trunk; in others, the exanthem is absent and the patient appears to have pharyngitis or an upper respiratory tract infection. Because many other viruses, including adenoviruses, coxsackieviruses, and echoviruses, can produce a rubella-like picture, serologic testing is necessary to establish the diagnosis. Such testing is important if the patient is pregnant or has been in contact with a pregnant woman or if arthritis is a prominent feature, simulating the picture of acute rheumatic fever or rheumatoid arthritis.

The incidence of rubella peaks in late winter and early spring, and the disease is contagious in patients from a few days before to a few

days after appearance of the exanthem. The incubation period ranges from 14 to 21 days. Complications are rare in childhood and include arthritis, purpura with or without thrombocytopenia, and mild encephalitis. The major complication results from spread of the virus to susceptible pregnant women and their fetuses, resulting in congenital rubella syndrome (see the section on Congenital and Perinatal Infections). When such an exposure is thought to have occurred, a specimen of blood should be obtained from the pregnant woman for the measurement of antibody. If antibody is present, immunity can be assumed; if antibody is absent, the woman should be retested in 3 to 4 weeks. If antibody is detected in the second specimen, infection has occurred and the fetus is at risk.

Varicella (Chickenpox)

Varicella in the normal host is a relatively benign, albeit highly contagious, illness caused by the varicella-zoster virus. A brief prodrome of low-grade fever, upper respiratory tract symptoms, and mild malaise may occur, followed rapidly by the appearance of a pruritic exanthem. Lesions appear in crops and evolve rapidly over several hours. Most patients have three crops, although some may have only one and others may have as many as five. Initial crops involve the trunk and scalp, and subsequent crops are distributed more peripherally; thus, the mode of spread is centrifugal. The presence of scalp lesions with the initial crop often is helpful in diagnosing the infection in a patient who presents early in the course of the disease. Lesions begin as tiny erythematous papules that rapidly enlarge to form thin-walled, superficial central

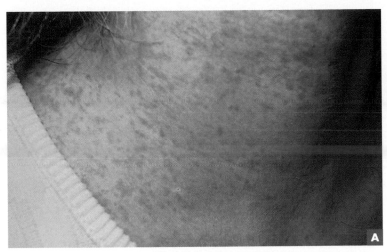
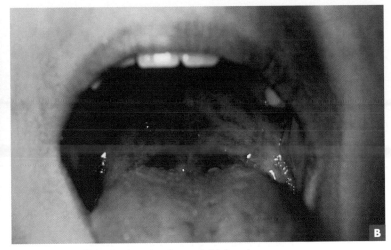

FIG. 12-2 Rubella/German measles. *A,* The exanthem of rubella usually consists of a fine, pinkish-red, maculopapular eruption that appears first at the hairline and rapidly spreads cephalocaudally. Lesions tend to remain discrete. *B,* The presence of red palatal lesions (Forchheimer spots), seen in some patients on day 1 of the rash, and occipital and posterior cervical adenopathy are findings suggestive of rubella. (Courtesy Dr. Michael Sherlock.)

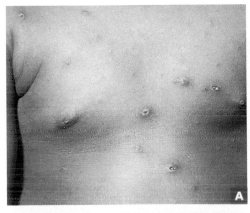
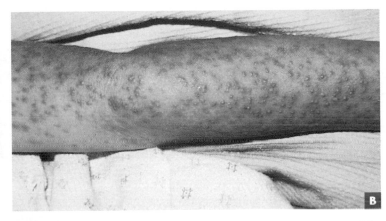
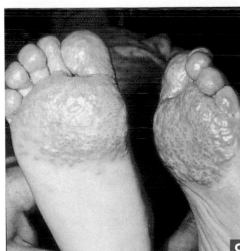
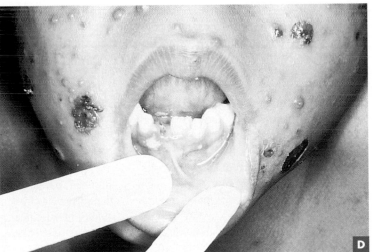

FIG. 12-3 Varicella/chickenpox. *A,* The characteristic finding of lesions in all stages of evolution is seen on the trunk of this child. Note the presence of papules, vesicles, and umbilicated and scabbed lesions, all within a small geographic area. *B* and *C,* In this child with underlying eczema, the first crop of vesicles appeared in clusters at sites previously affected by dermatitis. The flexor surface of his arm is covered with numerous discrete lesions, and vesicles are confluent over the plantar surface of his toes and on the balls of his feet. *D,* On mucosal surfaces, thin-walled vesicles may form, which rapidly rupture, forming painful shallow ulcers. (*B* and *C* courtesy Dr. Michael Sherlock; *D* courtesy Dr. Ellen Wald, Children's Hospital of Pittsburgh.)

vesicles surrounded by red halos. Vesicular fluid changes promptly from clear to cloudy; then drying begins, resulting in an umbilicated appearance. As the surrounding erythema fades, a central crust or scab is formed, which sloughs after several days. A hallmark of this exanthem is the finding of lesions in all stages of evolution within a relatively small geographic area of skin (Fig. 12-3, *A*). Generally, all scabs have sloughed by 10 to 14 days. Scarring usually does not occur unless lesions become secondarily infected. It is important to recognize that in patients with preexisting dermatologic problems, the lesions of varicella, like other viral exanthems, tend to appear first and cluster most heavily at sites of prior skin irritation, such as the diaper area or sites of eczematoid dermatitis (Fig. 12-3, *B* and *C*).

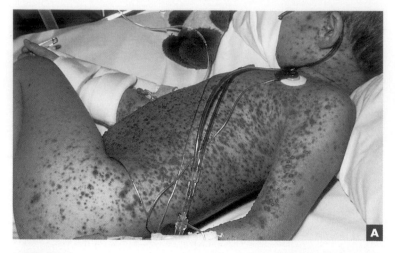

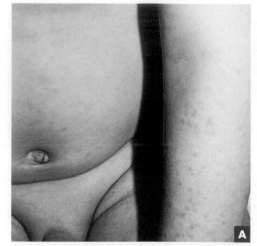

FIG. 12-5 Adenovirus. *A*, This discrete, erythematous, blanching maculopapular rash was generalized when first noted and occurred in association with pharyngitis and, *B*, a nonpurulent conjunctivitis. (Courtesy Dr. Michael Sherlock.)

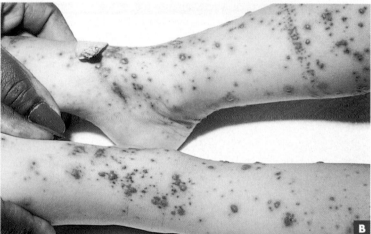

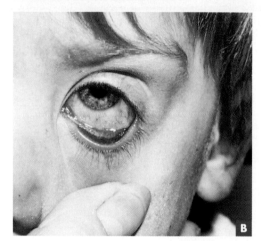

FIG. 12-4 Disseminated hemorrhagic varicella. *A*, In the immunocompromised child, skin lesions tend to be hemorrhagic and nearly confluent. *B*, Lesions also evolve more slowly than usual, remaining vesicular for a prolonged period.

An enanthem is commonly seen and consists of thin-walled vesicles that rapidly rupture to form shallow ulcers (Fig. 12-3, *D*). Other mucosal surfaces may be affected as well. Although skin lesions are pruritic, those on the oral, rectal, or vaginal mucosa and those involving the external auditory canal or tympanic membrane can be very painful, necessitating analgesia. Systemic symptoms generally are mild, although low-grade to moderate fever may be present during the first few days. In most cases, pruritus is the child's major complaint. In adolescents and adults the illness is more likely to be severe with prominent systemic symptoms and more extensive exanthematous involvement.

Varicella occurs year round, with peak incidences in late autumn and late winter through early spring. The period of communicability begins 1 to 2 days before the appearance of lesions and lasts until all lesions have crusted over. The incubation period ranges from 10 to 20 days, with high secondary attack rates in susceptible people. The most common complication in normal hosts is secondary bacterial infection of excoriated skin lesions. Such infection can range from impetigo to cellulitis. Other complications, though rare, include pneumonia, hepatitis, and encephalitis. The onset of these complications typically is heralded by a secondary fever spike concurrent with an increase in general systemic symptoms. In patients with encephalitis, an altered level of consciousness along with other signs of neurologic dysfunction occur. Reye's syndrome, an encephalopathy of unclear etiology, is a well-recognized but fortunately rare complication that can occur as a child is recovering from acute varicella. Repetitive pernicious vomiting is followed by an altered level of consciousness in which periods of lethargy alternate with periods of delirium or combativeness.

In the immunocompromised host with deficient cellular immunity, varicella is a severe and often fatal disease with central nervous system (CNS), pulmonary, and generalized visceral involvement. Skin lesions often are hemorrhagic and tend to remain vesicular for a prolonged period of time (Fig. 12-4). In the potentially compromised host who has not had varicella previously (including those on short-course high-dose steroids), parents must be forewarned of these dangers and instructed to notify their physician immediately of any possible exposure. This enables the administration of varicella-zoster immune globulin within 96 hours of exposure, thus reducing the severity of illness.

Adenovirus Infections

There are approximately thirty distinct types of adenoviruses capable of producing a variety of clinical illnesses, including conjunctivitis, upper respiratory tract infections and pharyngitis, croup, bronchitis, bronchiolitis and pneumonia (occasionally fulminant), gastroenteritis, myocarditis, nephritis, cystitis, and encephalitis. An exanthem occasionally accompanies other symptoms, and a variety of rashes have been described. The eruption may consist of discrete, nonspecific, blanching, maculopapular lesions or it may be morbilliform, rubelliform, or on occasion, petechial. Typically the rash is generalized when first noted. The most readily identifiable clinical constellation consists of conjunctivitis, rhinitis, pharyngitis, and a discrete, blanching, macu-

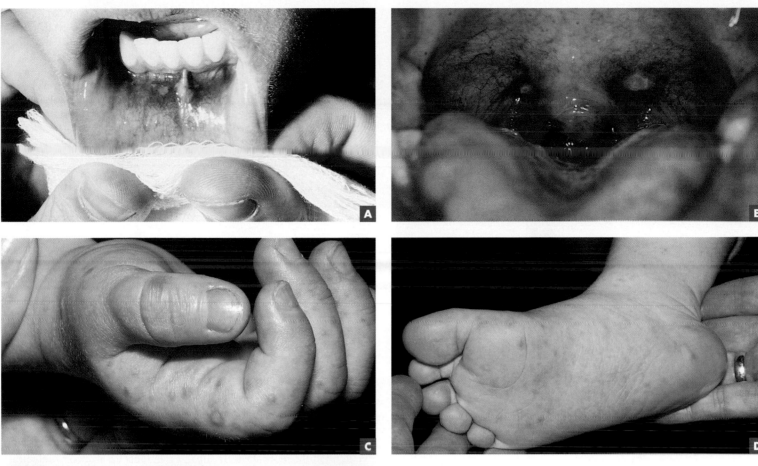

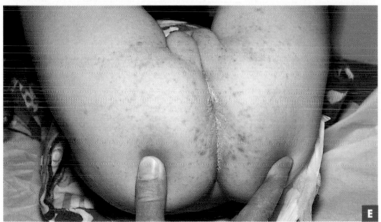

FIG. 12-6 Coxsackie hand-foot-and-mouth disease. The exanthem of this disorder is characterized by mildly painful, shallow, yellow ulcers surrounded by red halos. These may be found on the labial or buccal mucosa *(A)*, tongue, soft palate *(B)*, uvula, and anterior tonsillar pillars. When oral lesions occur in the absence of the exanthem, the resulting disorder is called *herpangina. C* and *D,* The exanthem of coxsackie hand-foot-and-mouth disease involves the palmar, plantar, and interdigital surfaces of the hands and feet, and *(E)* sometimes the buttocks. It consists of thick-walled, gray vesicles on an erythematous base.

lopapular rash (Fig. 12-5). Anterior cervical and preauricular lymphadenopathy, low-grade fever, and malaise are common associated findings. The peak season for adenovirus infections in temperate climates is late winter through early summer, and the infection is maximally contagious during the first few days of illness. The incubation period ranges from 6 to 9 days.

Coxsackie Hand-Foot-and-Mouth Disease

Of the enteroviruses, coxsackie group A16 produces the most distinctive exanthem, known as *hand-foot-and-mouth disease.* Patients may have a brief prodrome consisting of low-grade fever, malaise, sore mouth, and anorexia, during which lesions are absent. Within 1 to 2 days, oral lesions and soon skin lesions appear. The former consist of shallow, yellow ulcers surrounded by red halos. They are found on the labial and buccal mucosal surfaces, the gingivae, tongue, soft palate, uvula, and anterior tonsillar pillars (Fig. 12-6, *A*

and *B*). These enanthematous lesions usually are only mildly painful. Early in the illness, small vesicles may be seen on the palate or mucosal surfaces. The cutaneous lesions begin as erythematous macules on the palmar aspect of the hands and fingers, the plantar surface of the feet and toes, and the interdigital surfaces. Occasionally the buttocks may be involved as well. They evolve rapidly to form small, thick-walled, gray vesicles on an erythematous base (Fig. 12-6, *C* to *E*), which may feel like slivers, be pruritic, or be asymptomatic. More than 90% of patients with disease caused by coxsackie A16 have oral lesions and about two thirds have the exanthem. In those cases in which the cutaneous manifestations are absent, the process is called *herpangina* (caused by coxsackieviruses and other enteroviruses) and may resemble early herpes gingivostomatitis. However, coxsackie ulcers are less painful and are less often associated with the high fever and intense gingival erythema, edema, and bleeding typical of herpes (see Fig. 12-10).

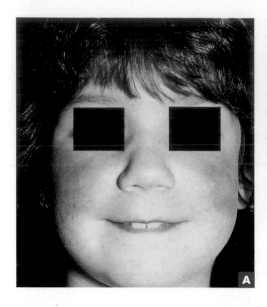

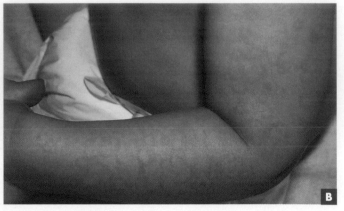

FIG. 12-7 Erythema infectiosum (fifth disease). *A*, On day 1, warm, erythematous, nontender, circumscribed patches appear over the cheeks. These fade on the following day, as *(B)* an erythematous, lacy rash develops on the extensor surfaces of the extremities. (Courtesy Dr. Michael Sherlock.)

Coxsackie hand-foot-and-mouth disease is highly contagious, with an incubation period of approximately 2 to 6 days. Symptoms last 2 days to 1 week. The peak season is summer through early fall.

Other enteroviral syndromes produced by the coxsackie group and by echoviruses include a mild, nonspecific febrile illness with myalgias, headache, and abdominal pain; generalized exanthems that may be maculopapular, vesicular, or urticarial; encephalitis, acute cerebellar ataxia, and myelitis; pleurodynia; myocarditis; hemorrhagic conjunctivitis; and gastroenteritis.

Erythema Infectiosum (Fifth Disease)

Erythema infectiosum is a mildly contagious illness, caused by parvovirus B19, that principally affects preschool and young school-age children. It occurs year-round, with a peak incidence in late winter and early spring. The disorder is characterized primarily by its exanthem; fever and constitutional symptoms are unusual. Occasionally, headache, nausea, myalgias, and peripheral polyarthralgias are reported. The rash begins on the face, with large, bright red, erythematous patches appearing over both cheeks (Fig. 12-7, *A*). These patches are warm but nontender and have circumscribed borders that usually are macular but may be slightly raised. They are easily distinguished from those of cellulitis and erysipelas (see Figs. 12-37, 12-38, and 12-40) by their symmetry and lack of tenderness and by the absence of high fever and toxicity. The facial lesions begin to fade on the following day, and a symmetrical, macular or slightly raised, lacy, erythematous rash appears on the extensor surfaces of the extremities (Fig. 12-7, *B*). Over the next day or so, the rash may spread to the flexor surfaces, buttocks, and trunk. Resolution occurs within 3 to 7 days of onset.

Studies have shown that the virus is transmitted primarily by respiratory secretions and—after transmission—replicates in red blood cell precursors in the bone marrow. It then may cause a biphasic illness, with fever and nonspecific symptoms accompanied by red blood cell suppression occurring approximately a week later, followed by the appearance of the exanthem characteristic of fifth disease 1 to 2 weeks hence. Viral shedding ceases before this latter phase. Although red blood cell suppression caused by parvovirus does not result in anemia in normal people, it can cause an aplastic crisis in patients with sickle cell disease, other hemoglobinopathies, and other forms of hemolytic anemia.

Roseola Infantum (Exanthem Subitum)

Roseola infantum is a febrile illness that primarily affects children between the ages of 6 and 36 months. The causative agent is human herpesvirus 6. The clinical course begins abruptly with rapid temperature elevation, which occasionally precipitates a febrile seizure. Anorexia and irritability are the major associated symptoms. Examination reveals no source for the fever, which usually is higher than 39°C. Administration of an antipyretic produces only a transient decrease in temperature, which then rises rapidly to its former height. Although most patients do not look toxic, many undergo a sepsis workup and lumbar puncture because of the combination of unexplained high fever and marked irritability. Fever persists for approximately 72 hours, whereupon the fever abruptly subsides. In most cases an erythematous, maculopapular exanthem appears simultaneously with defervescence, but in a small percentage of patients it develops 1 day before or after fever lysis. Lesions are discrete, rose-pink macules or maculopapules that begin first on the trunk and then spread rapidly to the extremities, neck, face, and scalp (Fig. 12-8). They may last several hours to a day or two before resolution.

Although cases occur year-round, roseola appears to be more common in late fall and early spring. Secondary cases are uncommon, except in institutional settings. The duration of communicability is unclear, but the incubation period is thought to be 10 to 15 days.

Infectious Mononucleosis

Infectious mononucleosis is an acute, usually self-limited illness of children and young adults caused by the Epstein-Barr (EB) virus. Transmission of EB virus can occur by intimate oral contact (i.e., kissing), sharing eating utensils, or transfusion. The incubation period usually ranges from 30 to 50 days, although it is shorter (14 to 20 days) in patients with transfusion-acquired infection.

In its most typical form, infectious mononucleosis is characterized by fever, fatigue, pharyngitis, lymphadenopathy, splenomegaly, atypical lymphocytosis, and a positive heterophil antibody response. Nevertheless, most young children with EB virus infection do not have classic mononucleosis; instead, they tend to have either a nonspecific illness, which is clinically indistinguishable from other common viral diseases, or—less frequently—subclinical infection.

Clinical Features of Mononucleosis. The illness often begins with a prodrome, which lasts from 3 to 5 days, consisting of fatigue, malaise, and anorexia, often in association with headache, sweats, and chills. Photophobia and edema of the eyelids and periorbital tissues may be noted in some patients. The acute phase usually is heralded by a fever, which may show wide daily fluctuations. Pharyngitis and cervical node enlargement then become apparent. The sore throat tends to increase in severity over several days before abating and may be associated with

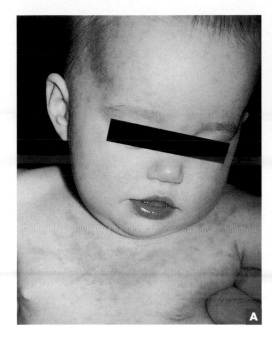

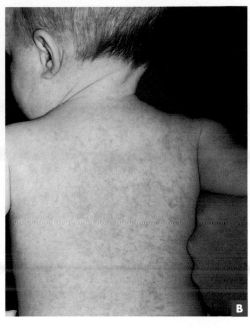

FIG. 12-8 Roseola infantum/exanthem subitum. *A* and *B,* The exanthem of this disorder usually appears abruptly after 3 days of high fever and irritability. It is characterized by discrete, rose-pink macules. It may be generalized at first or may start centrally and spread centrifugally. Scalp involvement is prominent.

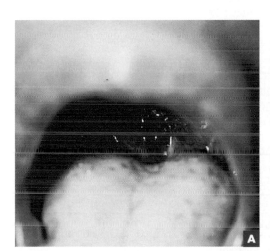

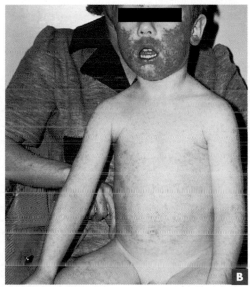

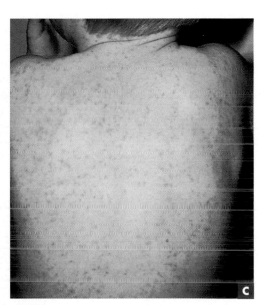

FIG. 12-9 EB virus mononucleosis. *A,* Severe pharyngotonsillitis is seen in this child, whose tonsils are markedly enlarged and covered with a gray exudate. The uvula is erythematous and edematous. *B* and *C,* In this child with EB virus mononucleosis, a diffuse, erythematous, maculopapular rash was part of the clinical picture. Lesions on his face are hemorrhagic and confluent as a result of prior irritation. (He had practiced shaving 2 days before.) Note also the swelling in the region of the tonsillar node and the fact that the child is mouth breathing as a result of adenoidal hypertrophy. (*B* and *C* courtesy Dr. Michael Sherlock.)

significant dysphagia. Tonsillar and adenoidal enlargement can range from mild to marked, and the tonsillar surface may vary in appearance from one of mild erythema to one of severe exudative inflammation with palatal and uvular edema (Fig. 12-9, *A*). Halitosis and palatal petechiae are common. Approximately one third of patients show severe pharyngeal manifestations. The anterior cervical lymph nodes are routinely enlarged, and posterior cervical adenopathy is characteristic. In classic cases the adenopathy becomes generalized toward the end of the first week. Involved nodes are firm, discrete, and mildly to moderately tender. Splenomegaly develops in approximately 50% of patients in the second to third week of illness; 10% have associated hepatic enlargement.

An exanthem is seen in 5% to 10% of patients with mononucleosis, although this percentage is greatly increased in patients treated with ampicillin for pharyngeal or respiratory symptoms. Usually an erythematous, maculopapular, rubelliform rash, the exanthem can be morbilliform, scarlatiniform, urticarial, hemorrhagic, or even nodular (Fig. 12-9, *B* and *C*).

Less common manifestations or complications of mononucleosis include pneumonitis with a pattern of a diffuse, atypical pneumonia; hematologic abnormalities such as direct Coomb's-test–positive hemolytic anemia and thrombocytopenia; icteric hepatitis; neurologic disorders such as acute cerebellar ataxia, encephalitis, aseptic meningitis, myelitis, and Guillain-Barré syndrome; and rarely, myo-

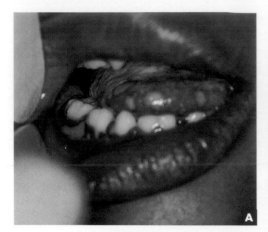
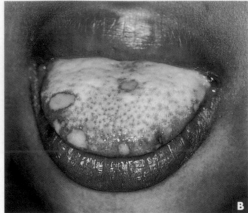
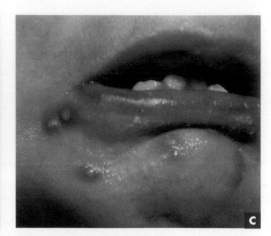

FIG. 12-10 Herpes simplex infections. *A,* Herpetic gingivostomatitis is characterized by discrete mucosal ulcerations and diffuse gingival erythema, edema and friability in association with fever, dysphagia, and cervical adenopathy. *B,* Numerous yellow ulcerations with thin red halos are seen on the patient's tongue as well. *C,* These thick-walled vesicles on erythematous bases were noted in this child who showed early findings of intraoral involvement, as well. (*C* courtesy Dr. Michael Sherlock.)

carditis and pericarditis. Neurologic and hepatic involvement occasionally can be fulminant, resulting in death. Other major complications include acute upper airway obstruction resulting from tonsillar and adenoidal hypertrophy and splenic rupture, which may occur spontaneously or as a result of minor trauma, repeated palpation, or the increase in intraabdominal pressure associated with defecation. Although younger patients are somewhat less subject to the less usual manifestations and complications of mononucleosis, they are more vulnerable to acute upper airway obstruction as a result of tonsillar and adenoidal hypertrophy. This is manifested by mouth breathing, retractions when recumbent, and sterterous snoring and apnea during sleep. Moreover, children under 5 years of age who show significant tonsillar and adenoidal enlargement during the EB virus infection are more likely to have secondary otitis media and, subsequent to resolution of the acute process, may suffer recurrent bouts of otitis media, tonsillitis, and sinusitis as a result of persistent tonsillar and adenoidal hypertrophy.

Diagnostic Methods. Several laboratory studies may be helpful in suggesting or confirming the diagnosis of infectious mononucleosis. A classic finding is a lymphocytosis of 50% or more, with at least 10% atypical lymphocytes. These atypical lymphocytes vary in appearance, in contrast to the monotonous forms seen with leukemia. There is considerable variability, however, in the degree of lymphocytosis and in its timing. Eighty percent or more of patients have mild elevations in liver enzymes early in their disease. Most commonly the diagnosis is confirmed by the finding of heterophil antibodies in the serum toward the end of the first week or at the beginning of the second week of illness. Currently, rapid slide tests, of which the Monospot is best known, are the most prevalent method of detecting heterophil antibodies. Although the presence of heterophil antibodies is highly specific for infectious mononucleosis, the sensitivity of the test is limited, in that only about 85% of adolescents (and a smaller percentage of younger children) with mononucleosis ever show measurable heterophil antibodies. Although EB virus infection can be confirmed by measuring specific EB virus antibody titers, such studies are usually reserved for patients with severe, prolonged, or atypical heterophil-negative cases of suspected EB virus infection.

Differential Diagnosis of Mononucleosis. In view of the multiple modes of presentation and the wide variability in severity of illness, clinical manifestations, and clinical course, there exists a broad range of differential diagnostic possibilities. In patients presenting with fever

and exudative tonsillitis, the principal diagnostic considerations include group A streptococcal pharyngitis, diphtheria, and other viral causes of pharyngitis. If lymphadenopathy and splenomegaly are the predominant features, the differential diagnosis includes cytomegalovirus infection, toxoplasmosis, malignancy, and drug-induced mononucleosis (caused by phenytoin, para-aminosalicylic acid, and diaminodiphenylsulfone). In patients with severe hepatic involvement, EB virus infection can simulate other forms of viral hepatitis as well as leptospirosis. Although the history and some aspects of the clinical picture may help in distinguishing one disease from another, specific serologic tests often are required to accomplish this.

Herpes Simplex Infections

The herpes simplex viruses produce infections that primarily involve the skin and mucous membranes, although in neonates, immunocompromised hosts, and, rarely, normal hosts, infection can result in disseminated disease and CNS involvement. Like other herpesviruses, herpes simplex virus—after producing initial (primary) infection—often enters a latent or dormant stage residing in local sensory ganglia; once latent, the virus can be reactivated at any time, causing recurrent infection. There are two distinct serotypes of herpes simplex virus, types 1 and 2. Herpes simplex type 1 is the more common pathogen and can produce a variety of clinical syndromes. In contrast, herpes simplex type 2 virus usually is a genital pathogen (see Chapter 18), although occasionally it is the source of oral lesions and is the usual agent associated with neonatal herpes (see the section on Congenital and Perinatal Infections).

Diagnosis of symptomatic herpes simplex infections often can be made on clinical grounds alone, particularly in cases of primary infection. When the diagnosis is in question, a Giemsa-stained (Tzanck) smear of scrapings obtained from the base of a vesicle (see Chapter 18) usually demonstrates ballooned epithelial cells with intranuclear inclusions and multinucleated giant cells when the lesion is herpetic. Viral cultures yield results in 24 to 72 hours. Acute and convalescent titers are less useful and are of no help during recurrences.

Primary Herpes Simplex Infections. Over 90% of primary infections caused by herpes simplex type 1 are subclinical; nevertheless, because the virus is ubiquitous, symptomatic primary infections are common. One of the most prevalent forms of primary infection is *herpetic gingivostomatitis.* Patients with this condition typically have high fever, irritability, anorexia, and mouth pain; infants and toddlers often drool

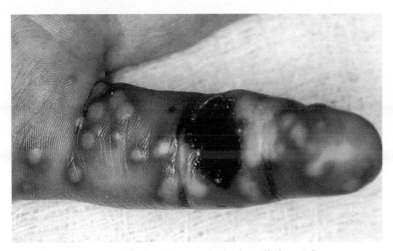

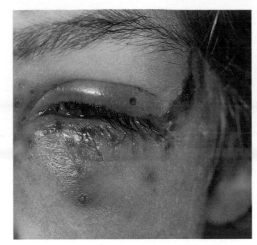

FIG. 12-12 Ocular herpes may only involve the lids and periorbital skin but can spread to involve the conjunctiva, cornea, and deeper structures, with devastating results.

FIG. 12-11 Herpetic whitlow. Grouped, thick-walled vesicles on an erythematous base that are painful and tend to coalesce, ulcerate, and then crust are the typical characteristics of an herpetic whitlow.

copiously. The gingivae become intensely erythematous, edematous, and friable and tend to bleed easily. Small yellow ulcerations with red halos are seen routinely on the buccal and labial mucosae, on the gingivae and tongue, and often on the palate and tonsillar pillars (Fig. 12-10, *A* and *B*). Within a short time, yellowish-white debris builds up on mucosal surfaces and halitosis becomes prominent. Thick-walled vesiculopustular lesions also may develop on the perioral skin (Fig. 12-10, *C*). The anterior cervical and tonsillar nodes are enlarged and tender. Symptoms last from 5 to 14 days, but the virus may be shed for weeks following resolution. The illness can vary from mild to marked in severity. Young children with prolonged high fever and intense pain may become dehydrated and ketotic and should be followed closely and hydrated as needed. The diffuseness of the ulcerations and mucosal inflammation and the intense gingivitis help to distinguish this disorder from herpangina (see Fig. 12-6) and exudative tonsillitis, as well as from other forms of gingivitis.

Primary herpetic infections involving the skin typically present with fever, malaise, localized lesions, and regional adenopathy. The skin lesions generally result from direct inoculation of previously traumatized skin, for example, at the site of an abrasion, burn, or small cut. The lesions consist of deep, thick-walled, painful vesicles on an erythematous base; they usually are grouped but may occur singly. As they evolve over several days, the vesicles become pustular, coalesce, ulcerate, and then crust over. As a result, the lesions may simulate those of bacterial infection, but the presence of grouped vesicles and the relative sparseness of bacteria on Gram stains of vesicular fluid support the clinical diagnosis of herpes, which can be confirmed by positive findings on Giemsa stain of scrapings from the base of the lesion or by viral culture.

Although the virus can infect any area of the skin, the lips and fingers or thumbs (as in *herpetic whitlow*) are the most common sites of involvement (see Figs. 12-10 and 12-11). Occasionally the eyelids and periorbital tissues are affected (Fig. 12-12); this can lead to keratoconjunctivitis, which is diagnosed on the basis of finding of characteristic dendritic ulcerations visible on slit-lamp examination (see Chapter 19). Because this complication carries a risk of causing permanent visual impairment, urgent ophthalmologic consultation is indicated whenever there is any suspicion of ocular herpetic infection.

Eczema Herpeticum (Kaposi's Varicelliform Eruption). Patients with atopic eczema and other forms of chronic dermatitis are at risk for a

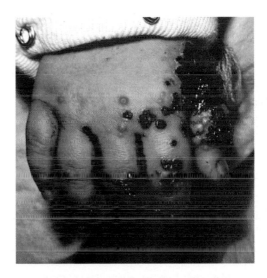

FIG. 12-13 Eczema herpeticum (Kaposi's varicelliform eruption). Primary herpes simplex infection in a child with underlying eczema produced crops of hemorrhagic vesiculopustular lesions limited to areas of preexisting dermatitis, which then ruptured and crusted. (Courtesy Dr. Michael Sherlock.)

particularly severe form of primary herpes simplex infection and thus should avoid contact with people with active herpetic infections. The illness is heralded by the onset of high fever, irritability, and discomfort. Lesions appear in crops and primarily involve areas of previously affected skin. Typically they evolve to form pustules, which rupture and form crusts over the course of a few days. Occasionally these lesions become hemorrhagic (Fig. 12-13). Multiple crops can appear over 7 to 10 days, simulating varicella. However, the slower evolution of lesions, the tendency of such lesions to become hemorrhagic, their concentration in eczematoid areas, and the persistence of fever and systemic symptoms for as long as 1 week help to distinguish this disorder from varicella. Severity ranges from mild to fulminant and is dependent in part on the extensiveness of the preceding dermatitis. When the area of involvement is large, fluid losses can be severe. There also is a significant risk of secondary bacterial infection. Up to 40% of cases are fatal.

Recurrent Herpes Simplex Infection. As mentioned earlier, following primary infection the herpes simplex virus becomes latent within the ganglia that lie in the region of initial involvement; reactivation of the latent virus results in localized recurrences at or near the site of previous infection. Fever, sunlight, local trauma, menses, and emotional stress are recognized triggers, and because the mouth is the major site of primary infection, labial and perioral lesions (cold sores) are

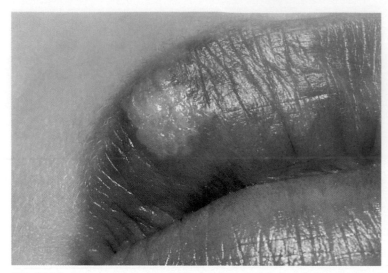

FIG. 12-14 Recurrent herpes labialis (cold sore). After a brief prodrome of burning, these grouped vesicles filled with yellow fluid erupted on this child's upper lip.

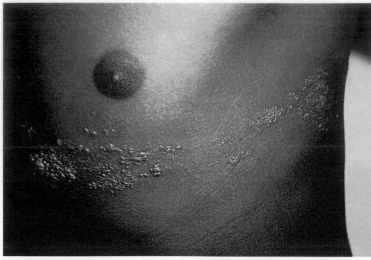

FIG. 12-15 Herpes zoster. The dermatomal distribution of these grouped vesicles is a hallmark of herpes zoster. The vesicles are rather thin walled and coalescent, and they lie on an erythematous base. (Courtesy Dr. Michael Sherlock.)

seen most commonly. Many patients report a prodrome of localized burning along with stinging or itching before the eruption of grouped vesicles. These vesicles contain yellow, serous fluid and often appear smaller and less thick walled than primary lesions (Fig. 12-14). After 2 to 3 days, the vesicular fluid becomes cloudy, and then crusts form. Although fever and systemic symptoms are absent, regional nodes may be enlarged and tender. The localization of the lesions to a small area helps to distinguish them from those of herpes zoster. Prodromal symptoms and discomfort help to distinguish recurrent herpes simplex from impetigo and contact dermatitis.

Herpes Zoster (Shingles)

The varicella-zoster virus, like other herpesviruses, takes up permanent, albeit generally quiescent, residence in its host after initial infection (i.e., varicella). Generally the virus lies dormant in the genome of sensory nerve root cells, but it can reactivate as herpes simplex does. Mechanical and thermal trauma, infection, and debilitation all have been postulated as triggers. In the reactivated form, herpes zoster, lesions consist of grouped, thin-walled vesicles on an erythematous base, which are distributed along the course of a spinal or cranial sensory nerve root (Fig. 12-15). They evolve from macule to papule to vesicle and then to a crusted stage over a few days. Hyperesthesia or nerve root pain may precede, accompany, or follow the eruption and does not correlate with the severity of the rash. Pain, if present at all in pediatric patients, rarely is severe and generally is short-lived, unless a cranial nerve dermatome is involved. Fever and constitutional symptoms may or may not be part of the picture, but regional adenopathy is common.

Thoracic dermatomes are involved in most patients, followed in frequency by cervical, trigeminal, lumbar, and facial nerve regions. Cranial nerve involvement may produce a puzzling prodrome consisting of severe headache, facial pain, or auricular pain with no evident cause, lasting up to several days before appearance of the eruption. Lesions appear unilaterally on the tonsillar pillars and uvula with involvement of the maxillary branch of the trigeminal nerve, on the buccal mucosa and palate with involvement of the

mandibular division, and on the face, cornea, and tip of the nose with involvement of the ophthalmic branch (see Fig. 20-45). When the geniculate ganglion is affected, vesicles are seen in the external auditory canal in concert with facial paralysis. Although varicella can be transmitted by patients with herpes zoster, contagion generally is less of a problem because most patients have lesions on areas that are covered by clothing and the oropharynx is not involved in most.

Gianotti-Crosti Syndrome

The eruption of Gianotti-Crosti syndrome, or papular acrodermatitis, though distinctive, often goes unrecognized (or is misdiagnosed). First described in association with anicteric hepatitis B, this exanthem has also been seen in association with other viral agents, including EB virus, coxsackieviruses, parainfluenza viruses, echoviruses, cytomegalovirus, and respiratory syncytial virus. Cases usually occur sporadically but occasionally occur in clusters. Most patients are between 1 and 6 years of age (range, 3 mo to 15 years).

A mild prodrome consisting of low-grade fever and malaise is typical and may be associated with generalized adenopathy, hepatosplenomegaly (especially with hepatitis B), upper respiratory tract symptoms, and diarrhea. Within a few days the first of several crops of lesions appears abruptly. They consist of discrete, firm, lichenoid papules with flat tops (Fig. 12-16, *A*) and range from 1 to 10 mm in diameter, tending to be larger in infants and smaller in older children. Papules can be flesh colored, pink, red, dusky, coppery, or purpuric. They are distributed fairly symmetrically over the extremities (including the palms and soles), buttocks, and face, with relative sparing of the trunk and scalp (Fig. 12-16, *B*), although the upper back may be involved. They tend to remain discrete but can become confluent, especially over pressure points (Fig. 12-16, *C*), and Koebner's phenomenon may be seen. Pruritus is unusual, and there is no associated mucosal enanthem.

The exanthem often clears within 2 to 3 weeks but can persist for 8 weeks or more. Results of laboratory studies are generally nonspe-

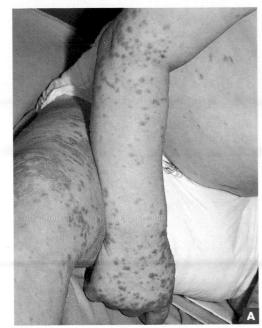
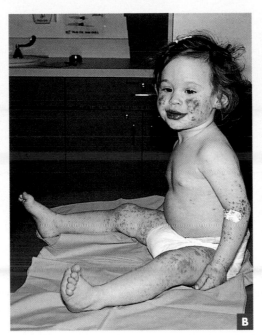
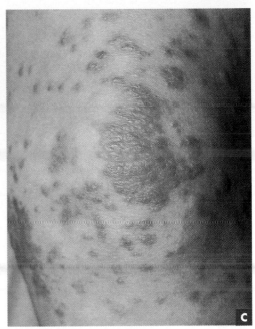

FIG. 12-16   Gianotti-Crosti syndrome. *A,* Lesions consist of raised lichenoid papules with flat tops which appear in crops and tend to remain discrete. *B,* This child shows the characteristic acral distribution, with lesions involving the extremities and face but with relative sparing of the trunk. *C,* Lesions can become confluent over pressure points such as the knee.

cific; however, liver function tests should be done, and if the results are abnormal, serologic studies for hepatitis B should be performed.

Treatment is symptomatic, and steroid creams are contraindicated because they may make the rash worse.

Bacterial Exanthems

Streptococcal Scarlet Fever

Although most commonly associated with pharyngitis and impetigo, the group A β-hemolytic streptococci are frequently the cause of an illness associated with a generalized exanthem known as *scarlet fever,* or *scarlatina.* The exanthem is produced by an erythrogenic toxin excreted by the streptococcus. Streptococcal infections occur year-round, although pharyngitis and scarlet fever have a peak incidence in winter and spring. Transmission requires close contact to permit the direct spread of large droplets, and those with nasal infection are particularly effective sources. Anal carriers as well as contaminated food sources also have been responsible for outbreaks. The incubation period for scarlet fever ranges from 12 hours to approximately 7 days. The disease is contagious during the acute period, and patients may transmit the organisms during active subclinical infection as well. An average of 50% of family members living with an index case will become secondarily infected, and up to half of these will have subclinical disease.

Once a severe illness associated with high morbidity and mortality, scarlet fever has become a much milder illness over the past several decades. In the classic case, which is seen less than 10% of the time, the patient experiences the abrupt onset of fever, chills, malaise, headache, sore throat, and vomiting; abdominal pain also may be a prominent complaint. Within 12 to 48 hours the exanthem appears and rapidly generalizes, usually beginning on the trunk and spreading peripherally, but sometimes spreading cephalocaudally. The face is flushed with perioral pallor (Fig. 12-17, *A*). The remaining skin becomes diffusely erythematous and is covered by tiny pinhead-sized papules, giving the appearance of a sunburn with goose bumps. The texture is sandpapery on palpation, and the erythema blanches with

pressure (Fig. 12-17, *B*). The skin may be pruritic, but it is not tender. Many patients also will have urticaria and dermographism. In severe cases, vesiculation may occur. Following generalization the rash becomes accentuated in skin folds or creases, and 1 to 3 days after its appearance, petechiae may appear in a linear distribution along the creases, forming Pastia's lines (Fig. 12-17, *C*). Examination of the oropharynx in the "textbook" case discloses large, very erythematous and edematous tonsils that often are covered by exudate, along with palatal erythema and petechiae (see Chapter 22). The uvula may be erythematous and edematous as well. The tongue also shows characteristic findings. During the first 2 days it has a white coating through which erythematous papillae project, resulting in a "white strawberry tongue" (Fig. 12-17, *D*). Subsequently the white coat peels, leaving a glistening red surface with prominent papillae, a "red strawberry tongue" (Fig. 12-17, *E*). Tender cervical adenopathy is seen in 30% to 60% of patients. Without treatment, the rash, fever, and pharyngitis resolve within 1 week; with treatment, improvement is relatively rapid. Desquamation occurs regardless of treatment and begins several days after onset, occurring in a cephalocaudal distribution (Fig. 12-17, *F* and *G*). The skin is shed in fine, thin flakes (in contrast to the thick flakes that characterize desquamation following staphylococcal exanthems [see Figs. 12-18 and 12-20]), and the extent of this process is directly proportional to the intensity of the exanthem.

Diagnosis is easy in the classic case, but the wide spectrum in the severity of the disease and in its manifestations can occasionally cause confusion. Fever may be absent or low grade, and malaise may be minimal. Pharyngitis may be mild (without exudate, petechiae, or marked erythema) or absent, even when the throat is the site of infection. In such cases, tongue findings may be absent as well. If streptococcal skin or wound infections are the primary site of infection, the oropharynx is normal. The appearance of the exanthem may vary also. In some children it is patchy but continues to be most prominent near skin folds (Fig. 12-17, *H*). An occasional child may have diffuse petechiae. Still others may present with fever or nasopharyngitis and urticaria as their initial manifestations. In dark-skinned children, erythema and perioral

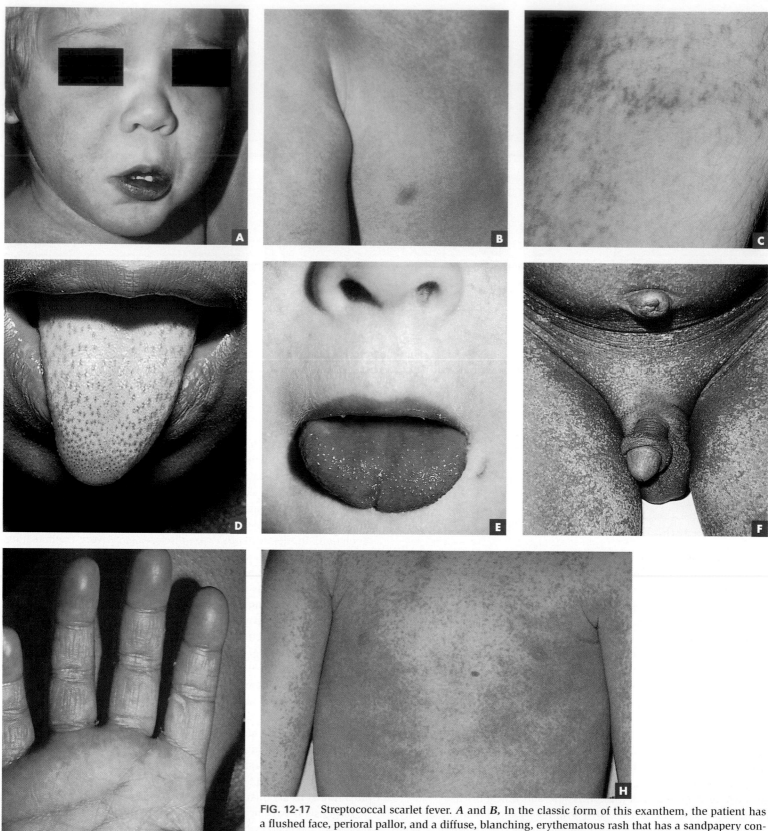

FIG. 12-17 Streptococcal scarlet fever. *A* and *B,* In the classic form of this exanthem, the patient has a flushed face, perioral pallor, and a diffuse, blanching, erythematous rash that has a sandpapery consistency on palpation. *C,* Within 1 to 3 days of onset, Pastia's lines may be noted. *D,* During the first 1 to 2 days the tongue has a white coating through which prominent erythematous papillae project. Then a few days after onset the white coat peels, leaving (*E*) the characteristic red strawberry tongue with glistening surface and prominent papillae. *F* and *G,* Desquamation occurs in fine, thin flakes as the acute phase of the illness resolves and is proportional to the intensity of the exanthem. *H,* There is a wide spectrum in severity and manifestations. In this child with streptococcal scarlet fever, the rash has a patchy distribution but is accentuated in the axillae and other creases. (*A, B,* and *F* courtesy Dr. Michael Sherlock.)

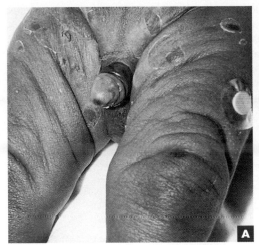
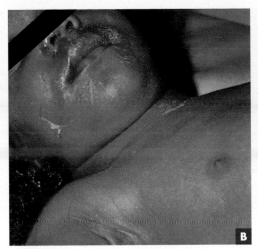
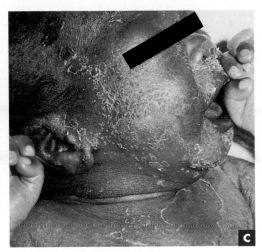

FIG. 12-18   Staphylococcal scalded skin syndrome. *A,* This infant shows evidence of epidermal separation and has numerous ruptured bullae over the inguinal region and thighs. *B,* In this older child, symptoms were mild and only the skin of the face, axillae, and perineum showed signs of epidermal separation. Note the evidence of a positive Nikolsky's sign on her upper lip and cheek, which resulted when she wiped her nose. *C,* A denuded area is evident on the upper chest, and thick flakes have begun to form on the face. Culture of the purulent nasal discharge was positive for *Staphylococcus aureus.* (Courtesy Dr. Michael Sherlock.)

pallor may be difficult to appreciate and the papules may be larger, thus producing a texture less like that of sandpaper.

The recognition of scarlet fever, followed by treatment with a 10-day course of penicillin or erythromycin, is important, not only to shorten the course of the illness but also to prevent rheumatic fever and pyogenic complications, the most common of which include adenitis, otitis, sinusitis, and peritonsillar and retropharyngeal abscesses. Therefore, in patients with fever or nasopharyngitis and urticaria and in children with scarlatiniform eruptions, a screening throat culture for group A streptococci should be obtained, regardless of the presence or absence of other symptoms. Poststreptococcal nephritis, however, is not prevented by antimicrobial therapy.

Staphylococcal Exanthems

Coagulase-positive staphylococci are ubiquitous organisms that are carried at any given time by approximately one third of the population. Although the hallmark of staphylococcal infection is the abscess, numerous forms of infection are seen, and at least three distinct generalized exanthematous disorders have now been identified: staphylococcal scalded skin syndrome; staphylococcal scarlet fever; and toxic shock syndrome. In each form the organisms at the primary site of infection release exotoxins, which then produce the characteristic rash. Transmission may occur by means of direct contact with persons who are infected or who are carriers. Sites of carriage include the nose, skin, axilla, perineum, hair, and nails. Spread of infection also may occur by means of airborne particles or through contact with contaminated objects or food. Draining skin lesions, nasal discharge, and contaminated hands constitute particularly important sources of transmission. Traumatic or surgical wounds, burns, insect bites, areas of preexisting dermatitis, viral skin lesions, and prior viral respiratory tract infection all serve as major predisposing conditions.

Staphylococcal Scalded Skin Syndrome. A disorder seen most commonly in infants and young children, staphylococcal scalded skin syndrome is caused by phage group II coagulase-positive staphylococci. The primary infection usually is mild, with purulent nasopharyngitis, conjunctivitis, impetigo, and infections of the umbilicus and circumcision sites seen most commonly. Rarely, sepsis, pneumonia, or other se-

vere invasive staphylococcal infections may precede the onset of the exanthem.

The infecting organisms produce an epidermolytic exotoxin, which is spread hematogenously and causes cleavage of the skin between the epidermis and the dermis. This process may begin within hours or days of the appearance of signs of the primary infection, and typically its onset is heralded by fever and irritability, often accompanied by vomiting. These symptoms are followed by the development of a diffuse erythroderma that spreads rapidly from head to toe and simulates the appearance of a sunburn. In contrast to streptococcal scarlet fever, the involved skin is tender, even to light touch. Within 1 to 3 days, thinwalled, flaccid, bullous lesions appear, which rupture soon after formation (Fig. 12-18, *A*). Simultaneously, larger portions of the epidermis begin to separate in sheets, and during this phase the placement of light lateral traction on the skin causes the epidermis to pull away from the dermis, leaving a raw, weeping surface; this separation of the skin in response to stroking is called *Nikolsky's sign* (Fig. 12-18, *B*). After exfoliation the surface gradually dries, forming large, thick flakes (Fig. 12-18, *C*).

There is a broad spectrum of severity for this syndrome. In severe cases the patient appears toxic and in considerable pain. The patient may shed large portions of skin, resulting in significant fluid losses that may be accompanied by difficulties with temperature regulation. In mild cases (Fig. 12-18, *B*) toxicity is absent and only localized areas of skin are denuded, with the face and perineum constituting the primary sites of shedding. The causative organism can be isolated from the site of primary infection, but it is absent—at least initially—from the bullae and from sites of skin separation.

Staphylococcal Scarlet Fever. Staphylococcal infection can result in an exanthem that initially is indistinguishable in appearance from that produced by group A β-hemolytic streptococci. The illness is characterized by fever, irritability, and moderate malaise, followed by the abrupt onset of a generalized erythematous rash, often of sandpapery consistency, with accentuation in the skin creases (Fig. 12-19, *A*). In contrast to the exanthem seen in streptococcal scarlet fever, the involved skin usually is tender, the tongue is normal, and there is no palatal enanthem. Evolution of lesions also differs, in that within 2 to

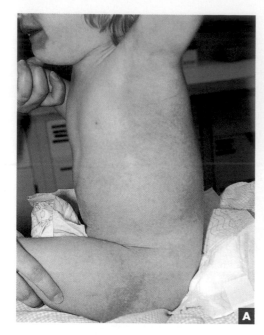

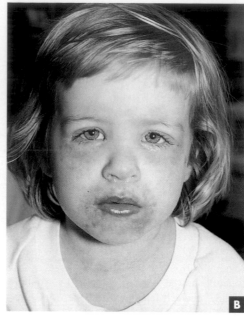

FIG. 12-19 Staphylococcal scarlet fever. *A,* In this patient, nasopharyngitis and purulent conjunctivitis antedated the development of a generalized sandpaper-like rash, which was tender to the touch. *B,* The skin in the periorbital and perioral areas has begun to crack, fissure, and weep serous fluid.

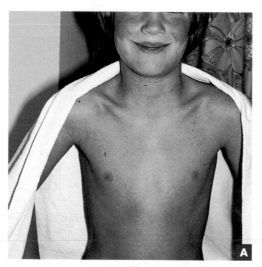

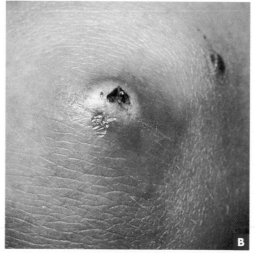

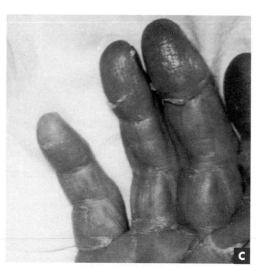

FIG. 12-20 Toxic shock syndrome. *A,* This young boy presented with diffuse erythroderma, fever, chills, myalgias, headache, vomiting, and orthostatic dizziness with mild widening of his pulse pressure. *B,* Examination disclosed an infected puncture wound of the knee, which grew *Staphylococcus aureus.* Though his illness was relatively mild, the association of gastrointestinal symptoms and orthostatic changes suggested TSS, which was confirmed by laboratory studies and by *(C)* subsequent desquamation. This begins periungually, and the skin is shed in thick casts. (*C* courtesy Dr. George Pazin, University of Pittsburgh Medical Center.)

5 days the skin begins to crack, fissure, and weep, especially in the perioral and periorbital areas and in the skin creases (Fig. 12-19, *B*). It is then shed in large, thick flakes over 3 to 5 days. Local skin and wound infections are common antecedents, and their presence often enables presumptive identification of staphylococci as causative agents early in the disease. However, when nasopharyngitis is the source of primary infection, the picture can be very difficult to distinguish from that of variants of streptococcal infection, in which the strawberry tongue and palatal petechiae often are absent. The same may be true if a local infection with lymphangitis is the source. In such cases the tendency for the staphylococcal rash to be tender may be the major clinical distinction, pending Gram's staining or culture results. Unless the primary infection is severe enough to warrant parenteral treatment, oral antimicrobial therapy is sufficient.

Toxic Shock Syndrome. Toxic shock syndrome (TSS) is the third syndrome of staphylococcal origin characterized by a generalized exanthem. It is seen in children and adults who have localized infections caused by coagulase-positive staphylococci of phage groups I or III and in menstruating women and girls whose vaginas are colonized with these organisms. In the latter subgroup of patients (who may not have a history of prior vaginal discharge), there is a strong correlation with tampon use, indicating that the impedence of normal menstrual flow or the presence of secondary abrasions may contribute to the development of this syndrome. Patients with non–menstrually associated TSS often have an obvious primary focus of infection in the form of a skin lesion, an abscess, or purulent conjunctivitis (Fig. 12-20, *B*).

In its full-blown form, TSS begins with a prodrome consisting of low-grade fever, malaise, myalgias, and vomiting. This is followed by

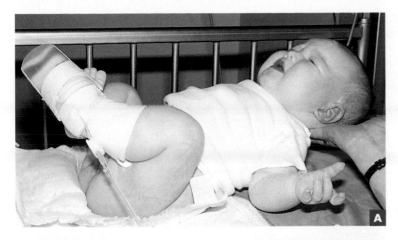

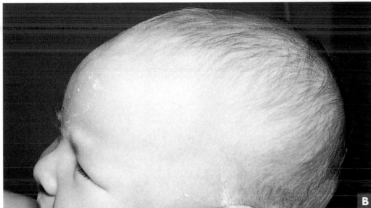

FIG. 12-21 Meningitis. *A,* Nuchal rigidity and a positive Brudzinski's sign are demonstrated. On attempted passive flexion of the neck, the infant grimaces with pain, neck stiffness limits flexion, and the knees and hips are flexed to reduce traction on the meninges. *B,* This infant also was found to have a bulging anterior fontanelle when sitting quietly, reflecting increased intracranial pressure.

an abrupt increase in fever, accompanied by chills, worsening myalgias, repetitive vomiting, abdominal pain, orthostatic dizziness, and weakness. Soon thereafter, patients show a diffuse erythroderma, mimicking a sunburn (Fig. 12-20, *A*). Conjunctivitis with photophobia, oropharyngeal erythema, and a strawberry tongue are common features. Subsequently severe watery diarrhea, hypotension, and oliguria may become prominent, accompanied by alterations in level of consciousness. This often necessitates massive volume replacement and vasopressor therapy. In severe cases, adult respiratory distress syndrome may develop. Many patients have muscle tenderness and weakness as well as diffuse abdominal tenderness without peritoneal signs. A small proportion show nonpitting edema of the face, hands, and feet. Over the ensuing days, petechiae and a secondary maculopapular rash may be noted, along with oral ulcerations. Desquamation is routine, usually beginning a week after onset of the rash. It is most prominent over the palms and soles and in the periungual areas, and the skin is shed in thick casts (Fig. 12-20, *C*). Parenteral antimicrobial therapy directed against *Staphylococcus aureus* is designed to eradicate any focus of infection and reduce the risk of recurrence.

Clinical and laboratory findings in severe cases point toward the existence of a process in which there is diffuse vascular leakage with third-spacing of fluids, electrolytes, and serum proteins. Secondary hypotension and hypoperfusion result in azotemia. Toxin-related hepatic changes may also be noted.

As recognition of TSS has increased, the existence of a wide spectrum of severity has become apparent. Mild cases mimic the picture of staphylococcal scarlet fever. Such patients tend to have smaller gastrointestinal losses and less difficulty with fluid shifts and attendant complications.

Meningococcal Exanthems

Neisseria meningitidis is capable of producing several clinical illnesses, two of which—acute meningococcemia and meningococcosis, or chronic meningococcemia—are characterized in part by a generalized exanthem. The organism is carried in the upper respiratory tract of humans who, though usually asymptomatic, nevertheless may transmit the organism via droplet spread of respiratory secretions. Most people so exposed become carriers and do not acquire clinical disease. Clinical illness is most common in children under 5 years of age, with a peak incidence between 6 and 12 months of age. A secondary peak of lesser magnitude is seen in adolescence. Susceptibility to disease appears to be related to a lack of bactericidal antibody or to a failure to produce antibody in response to infection. It is still unclear whether antecedent viral respiratory tract infection is a predisposing factor.

Although meningococcal infection occurs year-round, the peak season for these illnesses is late winter and early spring. Invasive disease occurs both endemically and epidemically. Persons who have intimate contact with infected patients, such as other members of the same household or persons in "closed communities" such as military barracks, dormitories, or daycare centers, are at highest risk of becoming secondarily infected. The incubation period after exposure ranges from 1 to 10 days, with most clinical cases developing in less than 4 days. Secondary attack rates range from 0.3% to 10% and are highest during epidemic outbreaks. Any mucosal surface is subject to infection, which may remain localized or may serve as the source of invasive disease.

Acute Meningococcemia. The two major invasive forms of meningococcal disease are meningitis and septicemia, which may occur singly or in combination. Patients usually experience a prodromal period ranging from a few hours to 5 days. During this phase, symptoms of upper respiratory tract infection or nasopharyngitis in association with fever are typical. Patients also may experience lethargy, headache, myalgias, arthralgias, and vomiting. After this, an abrupt change occurs, characterized by increased fever with chills (or occasionally hypothermia), worsening malaise, and progressive lethargy. In the 90% in whom meningitis is the primary manifestation, vomiting, irritability (often with a high-pitched cry in infants), and nuchal rigidity are prominent (Fig. 12-21, *A*). Infants may also have a bulging fontanelle (Fig. 12-21, *B*). Delirium, combativeness, stupor, and seizures also may develop. Although some of these patients also have meningococcemia, cutaneous manifestations are less likely to develop in them than in those without meningitis. Endotoxic shock and disseminated intravascular coagulation (DIC) also are unusual, and mortality is relatively low.

In contrast, approximately 10% of patients show a picture of overwhelming sepsis with little or no evidence of meningitis. In these patients the abrupt change in the clinical picture just described typically heralds the development of a rash in association with manifestations of shock, including mottling, distal coolness with decreased capillary refill or cyanosis, and either widened pulse pressure or frank hypotension. Up to 85% of these patients have cutaneous lesions involving the trunk and extremities. Such lesions may consist of tender pink macules; petechiae, which often are palpably raised; and purpura, which when present is most prominent on the extremities and may progress to form areas of frank necrosis (Fig. 12-22). The combination of purpura and shock is termed the *Waterhouse-Friderichsen syndrome* and has been associated in some but not all instances with adrenal hemorrhage and secondary adrenal insufficiency. Evolution may be fulminant, resulting in prostration within a few hours, or it may be slower, occurring over a

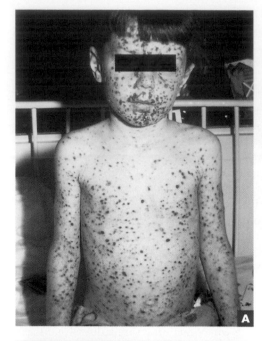

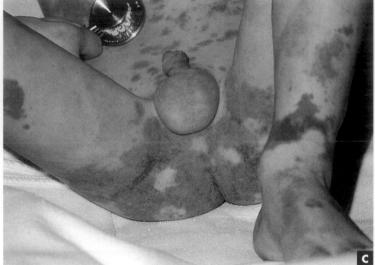

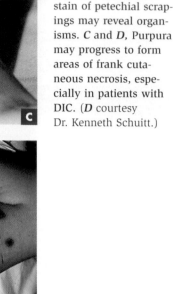

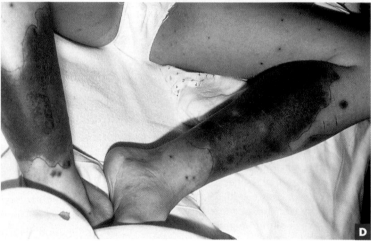

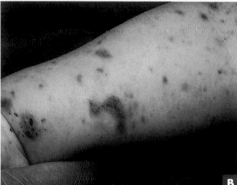

FIG. 12-22 Meningo-coccemia. *A,* This youngster manifests the generalized purpuric and petechial rash characteristic of acute meningococcemia. *B,* Petechiae are more apparent in this close-up of an infant. Gram's stain of petechial scrapings may reveal organisms. *C* and *D,* Purpura may progress to form areas of frank cutaneous necrosis, especially in patients with DIC. (*D* courtesy Dr. Kenneth Schuitt.)

period lasting up to 24 hours. The prognosis in patients with a short prodrome, fulminant progression, and early appearance of purpuric lesions is particularly poor. More than 60% of such patients have clinical evidence of hypotension and DIC on presentation, and approximately 50% have no leukocytosis, indicating that their immune system has been overwhelmed. Only about 20% of these patients have meningitis. Mortality in such patients approaches 40%, whereas only 3% of those showing slower progression die. Most deaths occur within 24 hours of presentation and result from a combination of circulatory collapse and congestive heart failure caused by endotoxic shock and myocarditis.

In many cases the diagnosis can be suspected clinically and is confirmed by laboratory findings. Gram-stained smears of petechial lesions and buffy coat preparations often will reveal gram-negative diplococci. Cultures of blood, cerebrospinal fluid (CSF), and petechial lesions should be performed unless the severity of illness precludes lumbar puncture. Counterimmunoelectrophoresis of urine, CSF, or blood may provide rapid confirmation. Because of the potential for deterioration, aggressive empiric antimicrobial therapy and vigorous supportive measures should be instituted promptly whenever meningococcemia is suspected.

There are numerous differential diagnostic possibilities, which include other forms of bacterial sepsis, bacterial endocarditis, Rocky Mountain spotted fever, and various other disorders characterized by thrombocytopenia. Some forms of septicemia caused by gram-negative bacilli initially may be clinically indistinguishable from meningococcal

septicemia. Similarly, *Haemophilus influenzae* type b septicemia as well as pneumococcal septicemia may be associated with the development of petechiae, though in these cases they are not palpable. The purpuric lesions of staphylococcal sepsis tend to become pustular early on, and the site of primary infection also helps distinguish infection with this organism. Adenoviral and streptococcal infections may produce petechial rashes but usually do not cause a septic picture. Other clinical characteristics help to identify patients with thrombocytopenia resulting from immune thrombocytopenic purpura, acute leukemia, and mononucleosis; the centripetal mode of spread of the petechial rash of Rocky Mountain spotted fever and the initial distribution and subsequent mode of spread of the lesions of Henoch-Schönlein purpura help to distinguish these illnesses. Differentiation can be particularly difficult in the case of a child presenting with high fever with no source other than that of an upper respiratory tract infection and a petechial rash. These findings may represent early nonfulminant meningococcemia, but they also can be part of the picture of viral illness or another bacterial process; in such cases observation or presumptive therapy may be necessary.

Meningococcosis (Chronic Meningococcemia). Meningococcosis, a disorder more indolent than acute meningococcemia, is defined as a meningococcal sepsis with a fever of greater than 1 week's duration, without meningitis. On average, symptoms last 6 to 8 weeks prior to diagnosis. In most cases, symptoms are intermittent; in all cases, they consist of fever and chills (without rigor) and are associated with an ex-

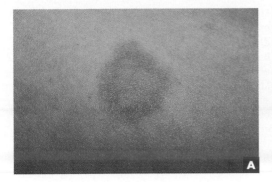
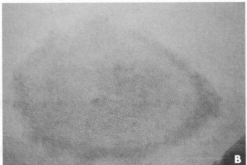

FIG. 12-23 Erythema Migrans. *A,* This 2- to 3-cm lesion is just starting to clear centrally. *B,* This larger plaque-like lesion had a bluish center the day before, which has faded to a pinkish hue. *C,* Central clearing is nearly complete, and within the erythematous border the puncta of two tick bites are evident. (*A* and *B,* Courtesy Dr. Sylvia Suarez, Children's Hospital of Pittsburgh; *C,* courtesy Dr. Ellen Wald, Children's Hospital of Pittsburgh.)

anthem in nearly 95% of cases. The rash waxes and wanes, often in association with the fever. Lesions may consist of tender erythematous, subcutaneous nodules, erythematous macules and papules, or petechiae, occurring singly or in combination. Urticarial lesions are seen occasionally. The feet, legs, upper arms, and trunk are the sites most commonly involved. Mild malaise and myalgias tend to accompany the fever, and headache and arthralgias also are common. In childhood cases, swelling of hands, feet, knees, and ankles may occur intermittently, without evidence of warmth or erythema, however, when the legs are involved, the child may refuse to walk.

The diagnosis of meningococcosis can be difficult because early blood cultures often are negative (although children are more likely than adults to have positive cultures) and skin lesions generally are negative for organisms, both on smear and culture. Throat culture usually is negative, as well. Leukocytosis is seen with the fever. The sedimentation rate may be normal or elevated. Thrombocytopenia is seen occasionally. Close follow-up and monitoring of the clinical course, combined with repeated blood cultures, is the best way to confirm the diagnosis. Of the patients whose infection goes undiagnosed and untreated, approximately one third ultimately suffer severe localized infection (after an average of 10 weeks of illness), with meningitis, carditis, nephritis, and ocular infection occurring most commonly.

Lyme Disease

Lyme disease is a multisystem, tick-borne infection caused by the spirochete *Borrelia burgdorferi.* Named for the eastern Connecticut community where it was first discovered two decades ago, Lyme disease was originally identified as a cause of chronic arthritis. Subsequent investigation has established the multisystem nature of the illness, which primarily involves the skin, heart, nervous system, and joints.

Transmission of Lyme disease occurs when a person is bitten by an infected *Ixodes dammini* tick (which, when not engorged, is about the size of the head of a pin). The *Borrelia* organisms for which the tick is a vector can be harbored by any feral or domestic animal, but the tick's preferred hosts and major reservoir for infection are the white-footed mouse during its nymph and larval stages and the white-tailed deer during its adult stage. Wooded, grassy areas heavily populated by deer are major sites of acquisition. The spread of deer from rural to suburban areas, along with heightened awareness of the problem, are responsible for the rising incidence of this disease, which is seen primarily in the summer and early fall.

After an incubation period of 3 to 31 days, the distinctive exanthem of Lyme disease, known as *erythema migrans,* appears. The rash begins as a red papule or macule at the site of the tick bite and often goes unrecognized. The lesion gradually enlarges (to a median size of 15 cm), forming a large plaque, which tends to clear centrally, giving it an annular configuration (Fig. 12-23).

Occasionally, instead of clearing, the central portion develops a bluish discoloration or becomes indurated or vesicular; rarely it necroses. The exanthem may be warm but is generally otherwise asymptomatic, although some patients report mild pruritus and burning or prickling sensations. Multiple secondary annular lesions or evanescent red blotches, which are smaller than the primary lesion, develop in about half of all patients with erythema migrans.

Although erythema migrans may be the sole manifestation of early Lyme disease, it is often accompanied by a flulike constellation of systemic symptoms that are probably the result of early hematogenous dissemination of the causative organism. These symptoms include fever (usually low grade but in some cases high spikes with chills), malaise and fatigue, headache sometimes accompanied by mild meningismus, and myalgias and arthralgias. Occasionally, nausea, vomiting, conjunctivitis, pharyngitis, a malar rash, and either regional adenopathy in association with the erythema migrans lesion or generalized adenopathy are seen.

Untreated, the erythema migrans lesion gradually resolves over 3 weeks and systemic symptoms often wax and wane over the course of several weeks. With treatment, the rash clears within several days and the systemic symptoms tend to resolve in 1½ to 4 weeks.

Other less common manifestations of early disseminated disease involve the nervous system and heart. Aseptic meningitis sometimes accompanied by focal neurologic signs and symptoms and unilateral or bilateral facial nerve palsy with or without CSF pleocytosis are the neurologic manifestations seen most often in pediatric patients. Optic neuritis, iritis, and keratitis are unusual. Carditis, characterized by varying degrees of atrioventricular block or myopericarditis, is rare in children.

The arthritis of Lyme disease is a late manifestation, seen in up to 50% of untreated patients. It is pauciarticular, involving large joints, especially the knee. Pain, warmth, and swelling are typical, but overlying erythema is unusual. The initial episode usually lasts about a week but can be prolonged. Thereafter, numerous recurrences may be experienced. Rarely, after a year, a chronic erosive arthritis may develop. Late neurologic manifestations include encephalitis, encephalopathy, ataxia, radiculoneuritis, and myelitis. The features of this later phase of Lyme

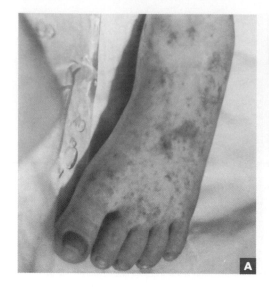
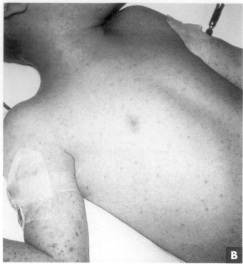

FIG. 12-24 Rocky Mountain spotted fever. *A,* The exanthem characteristic of this disease first appears distally on wrists, ankles, palms, and soles. It may be petechial from the outset, or it may start as an erythematous, blanching, macular or maculopapular eruption, which then becomes petechial as it spreads centripetally. *B,* In this child the rash has become generalized. Both petechial and blanching, erythematous lesions are present. (*A* courtesy Dr. Ellen Wald, Children's Hospital of Pittsburgh; *B* courtesy Dr. T. F. Sellers, Jr.)

disease are probably the result of a combination of ongoing infection and compromise of the patient's immune response.

In patients with erythema migrans, the diagnosis can be made solely on clinical and epidemiologic grounds, even in the absence of a clear history of a tick bite. Results of serologic studies generally are not helpful in making a diagnosis during the early stages of the illness (although an IgM enzyme immunoassay is now available that can increase the yield). Such studies can be valuable, however, for diagnosing the disease in patients with neurologic, cardiac, or joint manifestations, especially in those with no prior history of a tick bite or erythema migrans. In patients with neurologic complications, both CSF and serum specimens should be submitted for analysis. Because commercially available test kits have been found unreliable, antibody studies should be done at a reference laboratory and confirmed with a Western immunoblot test to ensure maximum accuracy.

Although antimicrobial treatment can be helpful in both early and late stages of the disease, therapy should be initiated as early as possible, because it not only hastens resolution of early symptoms, but also prevents later complications of the disease.

Rocky Mountain Spotted Fever

Rocky Mountain spotted fever is an acute, potentially severe exanthematous disease caused by *Rickettsia rickettsii*. These obligate intracellular parasites usually are transmitted to man by the bite of an infected tick, which injects organisms while it feeds on the host. Once injected, the organisms multiply in the endothelium of small blood vessels and are spread hematogenously, resulting in a widespread vasculitis characterized by focal inflammation and thrombosis with secondary vascular leakage. Because ticks are active during warm months, the peak seasons for this disorder are spring and summer. The incubation period ranges from 2 to 14 days, with an average of 4 to 8 days. Two thirds of cases occur in children under 15 years of age. Yearly outbreaks tend to occur in circumscribed geographic areas. Mortality is as high as 5% to

7% and often stems from failure to diagnose and treat the condition in its early phase.

Onset may be acute or gradual and is characterized by fever and headache. The headache, which may be frontal or generalized, typically is severe, unremitting, and unresponsive to analgesia. Headache may not be a major complaint in very young children, however. Other less constant symptoms include chills, anorexia, nausea and vomiting, sore throat, abdominal pain, diarrhea, arthralgias, and myalgias. Respiratory symptoms are uncommon. The spleen is enlarged in 30% to 50% of patients, but adenopathy is not prominent. The exanthem usually is noted on or about the third day of illness, but it may appear as late as the beginning of the second week.

In most patients, the characteristic appearance and mode of spread of the exanthem are the most helpful clue to clinical diagnosis. The rash begins on the wrists, ankles, palms, and soles, usually appearing as an erythematous, blanching, fine, macular or maculopapular eruption. It then spreads centripetally and becomes petechial (Fig. 12-24), although occasionally lesions are petechial from the outset. In some cases, the eruption is not prominent and may even be transient, making diagnosis difficult. Conjunctival injection, with photophobia and petechial hemorrhages, often develops simultaneously with the rash. Firm, nonpitting, nondependent edema, beginning in the periorbital region and then generalizing, tends to occur a few days after the onset of symptoms. In severe cases, CNS symptoms develop with disease progression and range in severity from restlessness, irritability, and anxiety to confusion, delirium, and coma, with or without seizures and focal neurologic signs. Myocarditis, DIC, renal failure, and cardiovascular collapse are features of advanced disease.

White blood cell counts are normal or low in the first few days and then tend to rise. Thrombocyotpenia is common. Other laboratory abnormalities include hyponatremia resulting from fluid shifts and renal losses; hypoproteinemia resulting from vascular and renal losses and hepatic dysfunction; abnormal liver function tests; and hyperkalemia with increasing cell death.

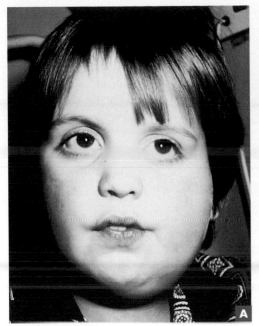

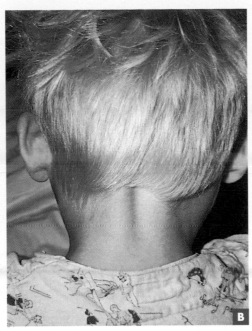

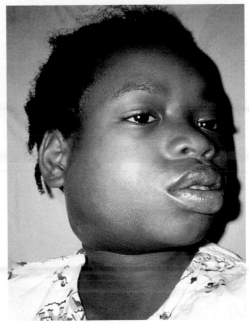

FIG. 12-25 Mumps. *A,* This young boy showed unilateral parotid swelling, which was indurated and moderately tender. Visually it was appreciated best in this view, which reveals swelling anterior and inferior to his left ear. *B,* Bilateral postauricular swelling (right greater than left) can be appreciated when the patient is viewed from behind. Secondary displacement of the auricle is evident. (*A* courtesy of Dr. G. D. W. McKendrik; *B* courtesy Dr. Michael Sherlock.)

FIG. 12-26 Suppurative parotitis. This patient had high fever, chills, and marked enlargement of the right parotid gland, which was severely painful and exquisitely tender. The overlying skin is erythematous, and purulent material was seen draining from Stensen's duct. (Courtesy Dr. Sylvan Stool, The Children's Hospital, Denver.)

Because there is no diagnostic test capable of providing prompt definitive results, and because the early institution of antimicrobial treatment is crucial to a favorable outcome, the diagnosis of Rocky Mountain spotted fever must be made on clinical grounds and as early as possible. The diagnosis should be suspected in any child with fever, headache, toxicity, and a centripetally spreading petechial rash, especially when the patient's history suggests or confirms an exposure to ticks. The *R. rickettsii* organisms are sensitive to both chloramphenicol and tetracyclines, and recovery is the rule if therapy is begun during the first week of illness. If treatment is delayed beyond the first week, however, the outcome may be unfavorable despite the institution of antimicrobial therapy and vigorous supportive measures. Subsequent serologic confirmation may be made using complement fixation tests or a variety of other assays. Immunofluorescent examination of skin biopsy specimens obtained 4 to 8 days from onset can provide earlier confirmation, but often this test is not readily available.

Mumps (Epidemic Parotitis)

Mumps is an acute viral illness that preferentially involves glandular and neural tissues. Although salivary glands, especially the parotid glands, are the most common sites of clinical involvement, the CNS and other glandular tissues may be affected as well. In as many as one third of patients the infection is subclinical. Peak incidence is in late winter and spring. The incubation period is 16 to 18 days, with the disease being contagious in patients from 1 to 7 days before the onset of clinical symptoms and for 5 to 9 days thereafter. Asymptomatic people also can transmit the virus.

Prodromal symptoms consist of fever, headache, malaise, and anorexia. In the typical case these symptoms are followed within 24 hours by the onset of an earache or face pain, which older children often can localize to the region of the pinna. Pain is aggravated by chewing and by stimulation of salivation (in particular, by sour foods).

Parotid swelling generally becomes noticeable within the next 24 hours, increases gradually over the next few days, and then abates over a similar period of time. Fever may persist for the duration of swelling but can disappear early in the course. On examination, an area of tender, indurated swelling, extending from the preauricular area through the subauricular space to the postauricular region, can be palpated (Fig. 12-25, *A*). With pronounced enlargement the pinna is pushed up and out (Fig. 12-25, *B*). The gland is mildly to moderately tender to palpation. The color of the overlying skin is normal. Intraoral examination may reveal erythema and edema of Stensen's duct. Bilateral involvement is usual, although one gland will tend to enlarge before the other, and up to 25% of symptomatic patients will have unilateral inflammation.

This "typical picture" is but one of many possible variants of clinical mumps. In some cases the parotid gland is spared and the submental or sublingual salivary glands may be the primary site of involvement. In the former instance, indurated swelling is found below the midportion of the mandible; in the latter case, bilateral submental swelling is seen externally and sublingual swelling noted intraorally.

Preauricular swelling and induration, the Stensen's duct abnormality, and the absence of prominent overlying erythema help to distinguish parotid swelling from cervical adenitis involving the tonsillar node. In confusing cases and in cases in which the submental or sublingual salivary glands are involved, closely simulating adenopathy, the patient can be given lemon juice to sip or a lemon wedge to suck. In patients with mumps, this results in a prompt enlargement of the affected gland and in pain as salivation is stimulated, whereas no such change is seen in patients with adenopathy. In cases of bacterial parotitis, the patient is likely to have high fever and to show signs of toxicity. The overlying skin is erythematous, with exquisite tenderness found on palpation (Fig. 12-26). Purulent drainage from Stensen's duct is usually seen when the gland is massaged.

Although it has been estimated that up to 75% of patients with mumps may have CSF pleocytosis, symptomatic meningoencephalitis is

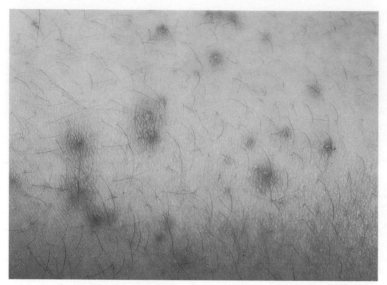

FIG. 12-27 Folliculitis. The extensor surfaces of the extremities and other hair-bearing areas are the most common sites of this superficial infection of hair follicles. Lesions begin at the base of a hair shaft as erythematous nodules and then evolve to form a central pustule with a thin, red rim.

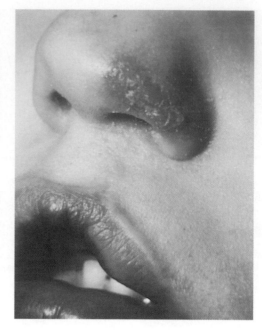

FIG. 12-28 Streptococcal impetigo. This impetiginous lesion has evolved from a papule to a vesicle that ruptured, producing this characteristic honey-colored crust. (Courtesy Dr. Michael Sherlock.)

seen only in about 10% of patients. CNS symptoms usually follow parotitis but can develop before or even in the absence of salivary gland involvement. There is a wide spectrum in the severity of these symptoms, ranging from isolated headache and malaise with fever to frank nuchal rigidity with nausea, vomiting, and severe alterations in sensorium. Fortunately, permanent sequelae are rare, although children recovering from severe mumps meningoencephalitis may not return to normal levels of school performance for up to 6 months or a year.

Mumps orchitis is much less common in boys than in men, who have 20% to 30% incidence. Orchitis usually follows salivary gland enlargement but may occur in its absence. Fever, chills, headache, nausea, vomiting, and lower abdominal pain are prominent and develop with the onset of painful, generally unilateral testicular swelling. Epididymitis is an invariable accompaniment. This process lasts 3 to 7 days. Oophoritis, seen in an occasional female patient, presents with a secondary temperature spike, nausea, vomiting, and severe lower abdominal pain and tenderness. Involvement may be unilateral or bilateral, and when unilateral and on the right side, it may be indistinguishable from appendicitis. Pancreatitis is an uncommon though potentially severe manifestation. Such patients tend to have sudden onset of excruciating epigastric pain in association with fever, chills, repetitive vomiting, weakness, and prostration. This, too, tends to last for 3 to 7 days. Thyroiditis, mastitis, bartholinitis, and dacryocystitis have been reported in isolated cases as well.

Bacterial Skin and Soft Tissue Infections

Superficial bacterial skin infections occur with a relatively high frequency in childhood. In most cases, the causative organisms are inoculated through a small wound such as a superficial cut, an abrasion, an insect bite, or a burn. Infection may occur at the time of the injury if the pathogen has colonized the site previously, or it may occur subsequently as the result of scratching, touching, or contamination with dirt. In some cases a preexisting dermatitis sets the stage for secondary infection by breaking down the skin barrier. The ever-present risk of infection in patients with preexisting dermatitis must be kept in mind, especially when steroids are prescribed.

Although most superficial infections are relatively minor in severity, diagnosis and proper treatment are important to reduce further spread of infection and to prevent its transmission to others. Deeper skin and soft tissue infections, although less common, have the potential for causing greater morbidity and even mortality. As with superficial lesions, inoculation from without is the most common mode of acquisition. In many instances, however, these infections represent metastatic foci of bacteremic spread.

Group A β-hemolytic streptococci and coagulase-positive staphylococci are the organisms most commonly responsible for skin and soft tissue infections. Both organisms commonly reside in the nasopharynx, and staphylococci routinely colonize the skin, a phenomenon that is less likely, though still possible, with streptococci. Both organisms are transmitted readily by carriers or persons with active naospharyngeal or skin infections. The fact that each pathogen produces relatively characteristic clinical features can help, to some extent, in making clinical diagnoses. Staphylococci, for example, are somewhat more likely to remain localized, stimulating suppuration and tissue necrosis, whereas streptococcal infection tends to spread along tissue planes and through lymphatics and thus is more commonly associated with secondary cellulitis, lymphangitis, and regional adenopathy.

Folliculitis

Folliculitis is a superficial infection or irritation of hair follicles. The scalp, face, extensor surfaces of the extremities, and buttocks are the most common sites of involvement. Patients with dry, atopic skin and keratosis pilaris (a condition in which follicles become blocked by keratin plugs) are particularly prone to this problem (see Chapter 8). Additional predisposing factors include seborrhea, excessive sweating, poor hygiene, and topical application of or contact with oils, tars, and adhesives. In each of these situations, obstruction of follicles occurs, setting the stage for inflammation and secondary infection. After occlusion, a superficial erythematous nodule develops around the hair. The lesion then evolves into a thin-walled central pustule with a narrow red rim (Fig. 12-27). The lesions may itch or burn and subsequently may drain and crust. Although it takes a given lesion 7 to 10 days to heal without treatment, multiple crops may occur. With scratching the infection may be spread to other areas, and secondary

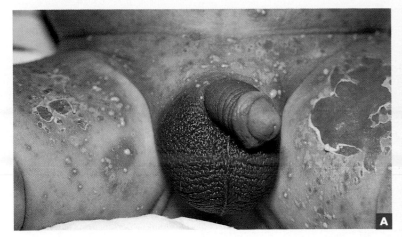

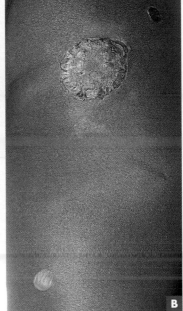

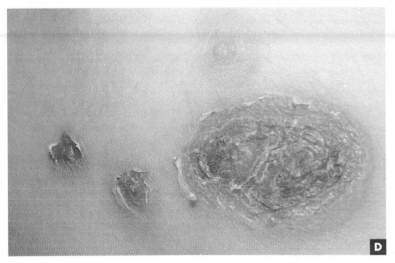

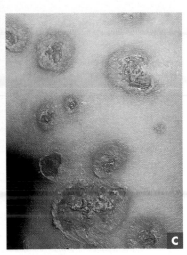

FIG. 12-29 Staphylococcal impetigo. *A,* This infant with staphylococcal diaper dermatitis has multiple small, thin-walled pustules that rupture rapidly and coalesce, leaving a shallow base and a superficial peeling rim. *B,* The various stages of bullous impetigo are evident in this child. An unruptured flaccid bulla is seen near an older lesion that has spread outward and crusted peripherally; just above that another bulla has just ruptured. *C,* In this child with staphylococcal impetigo, older lesions have central crusts with bullous rims that are spreading outward. *D,* The findings of long standing impetigo are seen in this youngster whose lesions are crusted in rings, resembling an onion. Note also the smaller satellites surrounding the larger primary lesion.

impetiginous lesions may develop. Coagulase-positive staphylococci are the pathogens usually identified, although other skin colonizers may participate. Oral antimicrobial therapy directed at the staphylococcus and treatment or avoidance of the predisposing condition are the measures indicated to eradicate the process.

On occasion the early lesions found in some forms of tinea capitis and tinea corporis may mimic folliculitis, although itching usually is more prominent in fungal infections and the surrounding rim of erythema tends to be wider. Tinea should be suspected, especially if folliculitis is localized to the hairline of the scalp (see Chapter 8). Older lesions, if present, may help in distinguishing between fungal and bacterial infections. Gram's staining, potassium hydroxide preparations, and cultures can be useful in evaluating questionable cases.

Impetigo

Impetigo is a superficial infection of the epidermis caused by streptococci, staphylococci, or both. Exposed portions of the body, including the face, extremities, hands, and neck, are the most common sites of involvement. Lesions teem with organisms and serve as a potential source of transmission to others. In temperate climates the disorder has a peak incidence in summer and early fall because of increased exposure of the body surface to insect bites, injury, and colonization by pathogenic organisms. In warm climates, impetigo is prevalent year-round. Although impetigo has traditionally been considered a streptococcal disease, recent evidence indicates that *Staphylococcus aureus* has eclipsed group A streptococcus as the predominant cause of impetigo.

In patients without preexisting dermatitis, lesions tend to be localized, but if the child has an antecedent condition such as eczema, the infection can spread rapidly to involve extensive areas.

In cases caused by group A streptococci alone, the lesion begins as a papule and evolves rapidly to become a small, thin-walled vesicle with an erythematous halo. The initially serous vesicular fluid becomes cloudy and the vesicle ruptures, forming a superficial honey-colored crust (Fig. 12-28). If the crust is lifted, a shallow, smooth, weeping, erythematous base is revealed. Secondary enlargement and tenderness of the regional lymph nodes are common.

The initial macules of primary staphylococcal impetigo may evolve rapidly to form small, thin-walled pustules (Fig. 12-29, *A*) or the larger flaccid bullae of bullous impetigo (Fig. 12-29, *B*). The latter contain slightly cloudy fluid and often are a centimeter or more in diameter. In either instance the pustules or bullae rupture rapidly, leaving a shallow erythematous base surrounded by a superficial peeling rim (Fig. 12-29, *B*). In patients with more long-standing or combined infection, lesions may crust centrally and enlarge centrifugally. This may result in the formation of a superficial central scab surrounded by a bullous rim or a dried lesion with multiple concentric rings resembling an onion slice (Fig. 12-29, *C* and *D*). Lesions may coalesce over time, and satellite lesions may form around larger primary lesions. Regardless of type, impetigo frequently is pruritic and the patient is stimulated to scratch, thereby spreading the infection to other sites or even inoculating the offending bacteria deeper into the skin.

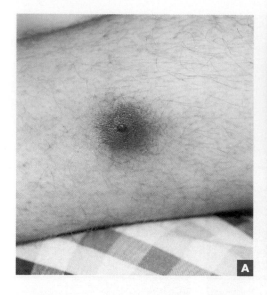

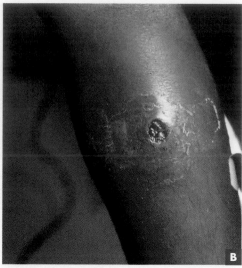

FIG. 12-30 Ecthyma. *A,* In focal ecthyma resulting from the inoculation of group A streptococci, the lesion initially consists of a central vesicle or pustule (that rapidly crusts over) on a painful, indurated, erythematous base. *B,* With progression a deep, widening ulcer forms, as seen in this child after removal of the overlying crust. (Courtesy Dr. Ellen Wald, Children's Hospital of Pittsburgh.)

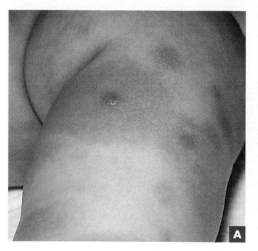

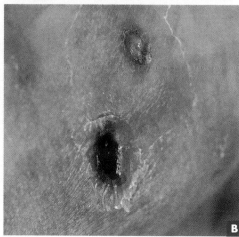

FIG. 12-31 Metastatic ecthyma. *Pseudomonas* septicemia may result in metastatic ecthymatous lesions that begin as pink macules, become hemorrhagic *(A),* and ultimately necrose centrally to form a black eschar *(B).* (Courtesy Dr. Ellen Wald, Children's Hospital of Pittsburgh.)

The possible source of the causative organisms may be the patient's own skin or nasopharynx or those of another infected person. In patients with facial and perinasal lesions, the nose is the most likely site of origin. Oral antimicrobial therapy is preferred for eradication and is a particularly important measure if the source of infection is the nasopharynx or if the lesions are extensive, although topical antibacterial therapy with mupirocin is effective for eradicating small numbers of lesions on the extremities and may reduce the spread of infection to others. If the patient has a predisposing dermatosis, this too must be treated.

On occasion, infection with other organisms can simulate the picture of impetiginous lesions. One form of tinea capitis produces lesions identical to those of streptococcal impetigo (see Fig. 8-116, *C*). Hence, if small pustules and golden-crusted lesions are seen on the scalp or at the hairline, Gram's staining and potassium chloride preparations are indicated to ensure correct diagnosis. *Candida* organisms can produce tiny pustules, which rupture and have a superficial peeling rim, at times simulating staphylococcal infection in the diaper area. However, in candidal diaper dermatitis, lesions are smaller (pinpoint in size), pustules are more evanescent, the inflammation is more diffuse, and the erythema more intense than is the case in staphylococcal impetigo (see Fig. 8-40). In confusing cases a potassium hydroxide preparation or Gram's staining can be used to clarify the etiology.

Ecthyma

Ecthyma is an ulcerative skin infection that penetrates more deeply than impetigo to involve the dermis. The disorder is most prevalent in tropical climates. Poor hygiene, insect bites, and trauma are the major predisposing factors, accounting for the fact that the lower extremities and the buttocks are the usual sites of involvement. Initially, lesions may resemble impetigo, consisting of a vesicle or a pustule on an erythematous base, which then ruptures and crusts over. In ecthyma, however, the lesions are painful and the crusts harder, thicker, and more adherent than they are in impetigo; the surrounding area of erythema is indurated. The ulcerative base beneath the crust gradually deepens and enlarges. Unroofing the crust uncovers a round, deep, punched-out ulcer with raised borders (Fig. 12-30). The size of the lesions ranges from 0.5 to 3 cm. Without treatment these lesions take weeks to heal, leaving a circumscribed scar.

In most cases, ecthyma is the result of direct inoculation of organisms through the skin, with group A β-hemolytic streptococci being the usual pathogen. On occasion, staphylococci or *Pseudomonas* organisms may be the cause; when infecting a small wound, the latter organism is more likely to produce a central abscess that exudes a greenish or bluish purulent exudate when its crust is lifted. *Pseudomonas* septicemia also may result in metastatic ecthymatous lesions, which begin as pink macules, evolve into hemorrhagic papules, and then necrose

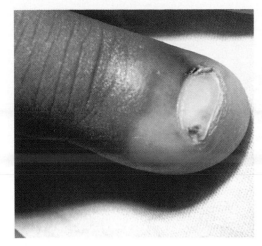

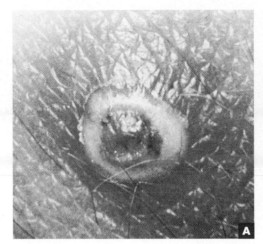

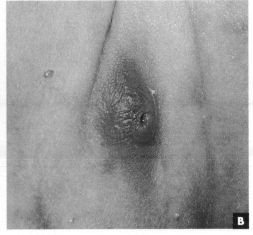

FIG. 12-32 Paronychia. Chewing on a hangnail predisposed this child to the development of a paronychia. Initially, erythema developed near the hangnail and was followed rapidly by suppuration.

FIG. 12-33 Furuncle. *A,* In this well-developed furuncle, the abscess has burrowed to the surface and the skin has thinned centrally and begun to necrose. There is a wide surrounding rim of erythema and induration. *B,* This furuncle located on the neck of a young infant had spontaneously ruptured and drained earlier in the day but was beginning to enlarge again. (*A* courtesy Dr. Bernard Cohen, Johns Hopkins Hospital.)

centrally to leave a dark eschar on an erythematous base (Fig. 12-31). Subsequently, ulceration occurs, associated with deep necrosis. This metastatic form of ecthyma is distinguished easily from primary cases by virtue of the formation of multiple lesions and the presence of systemic signs of sepsis.

Abscesses of the Skin and Soft Tissues

Abscesses are localized collections of purulent material, which are buried in a tissue, an organ, or a confined space. They result from the deep seeding of pyogenic organisms, which, in the case of abscesses involving the skin and its appendages, usually are coagulase-positive staphylococci. As the area of inflammation expands outward, central necrosis occurs and the process tends to produce an increase in pressure, with resultant pointing toward the surface or spread along tissue planes and further local tissue destruction. Drainage is essential for healing, because the abscess contents provoke a continuing inflammatory response and antimicrobials are generally unable to penetrate to the necrotic center of the lesion. Abscesses of the skin and soft tissues are categorized in part according to the site of involvement and in part according to the structure involved. The types most commonly encountered in childhood are discussed in the following sections.

Paronychia (Periungual Abscess)

A paronychia is a relatively superficial abscess that develops under the cuticle or along the nail fold of a finger or a toe. It occurs as the result of staphylococci and occasionally streptococci gaining access through a traumatized hangnail or through lesions created by clipping a cuticle or by chewing on the fingers. Occasionally an ingrown toenail is the predisposing condition; in such cases the nail, which usually was cut improperly, grows laterally into the nail fold, lacerating the soft tissue and setting the stage for infection. In typical cases, erythema, pain, and tenderness develop at the site of injury and are followed rapidly by suppuration (Fig. 12-32). The infection then advances from the portal of entry around the nail fold, and if treatment is delayed, it can burrow beneath the base of the nail, creating a subungual abscess (onychia). Occasionally, secondary lymphangitis may develop. Drainage is accomplished readily by undermining the involved portion of the cuticle and nail fold with a scalpel blade. Unless secondary complications have developed, subsequent soaking usually is sufficient to promote healing, although oral antistaphylococcal agents hasten the process.

Abscesses of Skin Appendages

Furuncle. A furuncle, or boil, is a perifollicular dermal abscess that is usually caused by coagulase-positive staphylococci, perhaps in concert with other skin flora. It may be the result of extension of superficial folliculitis or of direct inoculation via minor trauma. Hairy areas subject to friction or maceration are particularly vulnerable. Skin contact with occlusive agents such as oils, tars, and adhesives is another common predisposing factor. The incidence of furuncles is much higher in older children and adolescents than it is in younger children.

The lesion begins as a small dermal nodule around a hair follicle, which initially may produce mild discomfort and itching. As it gradually enlarges, pain worsens and is aggravated by touching and motion of the involved area. With expansion, the overlying skin becomes reddened, central necrosis begins to occur, and with increased inflammation and pressure, the infection begins to seek egress. In the case of most furuncles, the abscess burrows toward the surface of the skin, which becomes thinned and shiny as the abscess becomes fluctuant (Fig. 12-33, *A*). Application of warm compresses can hasten this process. At this point, incision and drainage are indicated. Without intervention, spontaneous drainage of bloody purulent material ultimately occurs in most cases and the patient experiences prompt relief of pain (Fig. 12-33, *B*). In areas such as the nape of the neck or the upper back, where the overlying skin is thick enough to resist external pointing, the process may take a path of lesser resistance, burrowing outward from the center through the subcutaneous tissues and along fascial planes. If this process is not interrupted by early surgical intervention, the result is a gradual formation of a *carbuncle,* which consists of an extremely painful, exquisitely tender multilocular mass of interconnected dermal and subcutaneous abscesses, with multiple points of partial drainage at the skin surface. Carbuncle formation often is accompanied by fever, chills, and increasing malaise, and there is a significant risk of secondary bacteremia. Even with treatment, sloughing and extensive scarring tend to result.

Hidradenitis Suppurativa. In hidradenitis suppurativa, an apocrine gland is the site of infection and abscess formation. Hence, localization in these cases is limited to the axillae, perineum, and areolae and the

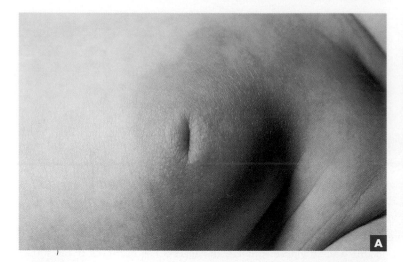

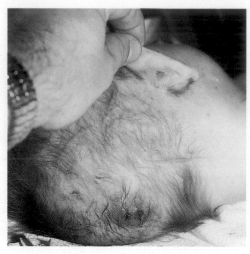

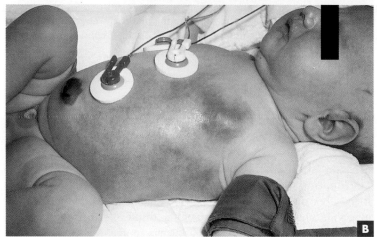

FIG. 12-34 Breast abscess. *A,* The typical manifestations of a breast abscess are seen in this neonate—swelling, induration, tenderness, warmth, and erythema. With compression, pus could be expressed from the nipple. *B,* This infant was not brought to the hospital until subcutaneous rupture and extensive cellulitic spread had occurred. She was febrile, toxic, irritable, and listless on presentation.

disorder only affects young people after the onset of puberty. Occlusion, maceration, and poor hygiene are major predisposing factors, fostering inflammation of the gland with resultant obstruction and providing a favorable environment for the multiplication of staphylococci and anaerobic bacteria. As the inflammatory process expands, the gland ultimately ruptures and an abscess forms. In contrast to the perifollicular furuncle, this infection is deeper and slower to localize and suppurate. It begins as a firm, mildly tender nodule that enlarges very gradually, becoming increasingly uncomfortable and tender to the touch. Recurrences of this disorder are considerably more common than are recurrences of furuncles.

Abscesses of Special Sites

The breasts, scalp, and perianal areas are three specific sites of abscess formation of particular importance in pediatrics. Breast and scalp abscesses are discussed in the following section. Perirectal abscesses are described in Chapter 17.

Breast Abscess. Breast abscesses occur with a small but significant frequency in pediatric patients, with incidence peaks in the neonatal and· pubertal age-groups. The incidence is highest in newborns at greater than 31 weeks' gestation at the time of birth, due in part to physiologic hypertrophy of breast tissue as a result of stimulation by

maternal hormones. Colonization of the skin or the nasopharynx with potentially virulent organisms (*S. aureus* or coliforms) during birth or in the nursery is another important predisposing factor. Up to 25% of affected infants have overt staphylococcal diaper dermatitis at the time of presentation. Minor local trauma also is thought to be a predisposing factor. Most cases occur during the second or third week after birth, but infection may occur as late as 8 weeks of age. The problem first manifests as swelling and tenderness of the affected breast. Unilateral involvement is the rule. With time, local warmth and overlying erythema become evident and it may be possible to express a purulent discharge from the nipple (Fig. 12-34, *A*). Axillary adenopathy may be present as well. Only 25% of infants have low-grade fever, and other systemic symptoms are uncommon unless treatment is delayed. Depending on the time of presentation, a firm, tender, nonfluctuant nodule may be found on palpation or the mass clearly may be fluctuant, indicating suppuration and necrosis. In the former instance, parenteral antibiotic therapy and close monitoring for progression are indicated. In the latter instance, prompt surgical incision and drainage are required. Broad-spectrum antimicrobial coverage should be provided pending culture results. Commonly recovered organisms include *S. aureus, Escherichia coli, Salmonella* species, *Streptococcus agalactiae, Proteus mirabilis,* and mixed flora. Delay in diagnosis and institution of treatment can result in subcutaneous rupture and cellulitic spread with secondary bacteremia (Fig. 12-34, *B*). Delay in surgical drainage of fluctuant lesions also can result in permanent loss of breast tissue, which in girls can produce a cosmetically deforming breast asymmetry that is first noted at puberty.

Breast abscesses may be seen again after puberty. Minor trauma, cutaneous infections, epidermal cysts, and duct blockages appear to be the common antecedent conditions. The clinical picture is similar to that seen in infants. Coagulase-positive staphylococci are the usual offending organisms.

Scalp Abscess. As is the case with breast abscesses, pyogenic infections of the scalp are particularly common in the neonatal period. Trauma is the predominant predisposing factor, and in neonates these abscesses commonly develop at sites where scalp leads were inserted for fetal monitoring during labor. Affected infants occasionally are found to have staphylococcal diaper dermatitis, as well. In most cases, the infection is localized and consists of a tender nodule with overlying

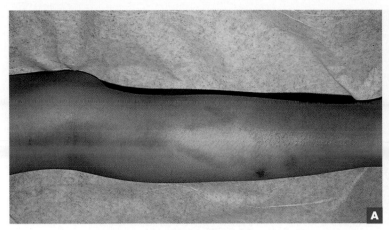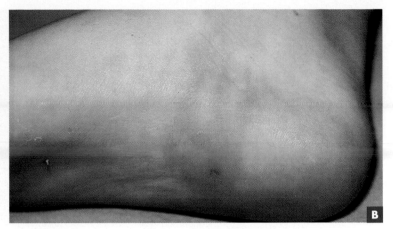

FIG. 12-36 Lymphangitis. *A,* An insect bite was the source of inoculation of group A streptococci in this child, who subsequently suffered secondary cellulitis and lymphangitis. The erythematous streaks coursing up the leg were tender and slightly indurated. *B,* Three distinct lymphangitic streaks are seen coursing up the instep from an area of cellulitis surrounding a puncture wound of the foot. *Pseudomonas* was the causative organism.

erythema (Fig. 12-35). The nodule commonly is fluctuant at the time of presentation, enabling prompt incision and drainage. Staphylococci and coliforms are the major pathogens recovered. Because of the neonate's immunologic immaturity, antimicrobial therapy also is recommended and in most cases can be administered orally. On rare occasions, infection is extensive and takes the form of a necrotizing fasciitis (see later discussion). In these patients and in the rare infant with a localized abscess and systemic symptoms, parenteral broad-spectrum antibiotic treatment (pending culture results) is indicated, in addition to incision, drainage, and debridement.

When scalp abscesses are encountered in older children, care should be taken to determine the responsible pathogen. Although staphylococci may be the source, invasive fungi are more likely to be the responsible organisms. These fungi produce a thick-walled, boggy, multilocular abscess termed a *kerion* (see Fig. 8-116, *D*). Gram's staining and potassium chloride preparations of purulent contents and of pulled hairs are important, because even though incision and drainage is the treatment of choice for abscesses of bacterial origin, oral antifungal and steroid therapy is indicated for the treatment of a kerion.

Lymphangitis

Inflammation of lymphatic channels is actually a secondary manifestation of infection at a distal site. The phenomenon is the result of invasion of lymphatic vessels by pathogenic organisms, which then spread along these channels toward regional lymph nodes. Group A β-hemolytic streptococci, by virtue of elaborating fibrinolysins and hyaluronidases, are the most common source of lymphangitis, although overt lymphangitis may also develop in wounds infected by staphylococci and *Pseudomonas* organisms. Clinically, erythematous, irregular linear streaks (which may be tender) are seen extending from the primary site toward the draining regional nodes (Fig. 12-36). The primary site may be an infected wound or an area of cellulitis. Systemic symptoms consisting of fever, chills, and malaise are often, but not invariably, present. Without appropriate antimicrobial therapy, cellulitis may develop or extend and necrosis and ulceration may occur, with the attendant risk of bacteremia. Culture and Gram's stain of material from the primary site will aid in the selection of antimicrobials; however, presumptive initial therapy is necessary pending culture results.

Erysipelas

Group A β-hemolytic streptococci are the source of erysipelas, an unusual and distinctive infection involving a localized area of the dermis and superficial lymphatics. The causative organisms usually are found in the upper respiratory tracts of afflicted patients and are inoculated through a break in the skin that may elude detection on presentation. Hematogenous seeding has been postulated in some cases. Systemic symptoms are prominent and precede the appearance of the characteristic skin lesion. The onset is abrupt and is heralded by fever and chills, often in association with nausea, vomiting, and headache. This prodrome is followed by the appearance of an intensely painful skin lesion that consists of a circumscribed, raised plaque that is usually deep purplish-red but which may be red or even pink (Fig. 12-37). The raised border, although irregular, is well demarcated and spreads centrifugally. Red lymphatic streaks may advance ahead of it toward the regional nodes. On close inspection the skin is seen to be edematous and may have a thickened peau d'orange character (see Fig. 12-37, *C*). On palpation it is found to be indurated, hot, and exquisitely tender. With evolution, small surface blebs containing yellow fluid may form. The face is the site most commonly involved, with the trunk, neck, and extremities being less frequent areas of localization. Patients may become bacteremic, with the development of metastatic foci of infection. Infants are at particular risk for systemic spread. The clinical picture of erysipelas is so characteristic that streptococcal infection can be presumed and parenteral antimicrobial treatment initiated. Cultures of tissue aspirate from the advancing border of the lesion and cultures of the nose and throat typically are positive for group A streptococci, as are blood cultures in septic patients.

Cellulitis

Cellulitis is an infection of bacterial origin, and subcutaneous loose connective tissue is the primary site of inflammation. With progression, the process extends centrifugally through the subcutaneous tissue and also may ascend to involve the lower dermis. Although cellulitis may develop anywhere on the body, it occurs most commonly on the extremities and face. There are three major modes of origin:

1. Extension from a wound.
2. Hematogenous seeding.
3. Extension from a deeper infection.

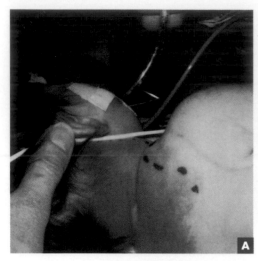
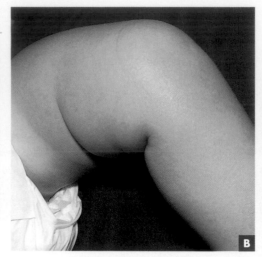
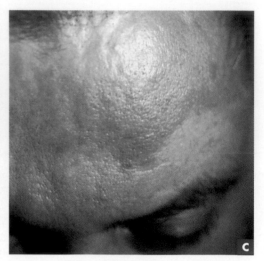

FIG. 12-37 Erysipelas. *A,* This 6-week-old infant had fever, lethargy, irritability, and hypotension in association with erysipelas. The purplish-red lesion was raised, indurated, and tender. The border, though irregular, was sharply demarcated from the adjacent skin. Cultures of blood and tissue aspirate grew group A streptococci. *B,* The sharply circumscribed area of erysipelas on this toddler's leg was pink. On close inspection, one can see that the skin has a peau d'orange quality. *C,* This is seen more clearly in a close-up of an adolescent's forehead. (*C* courtesy of Dr. James Ferante.)

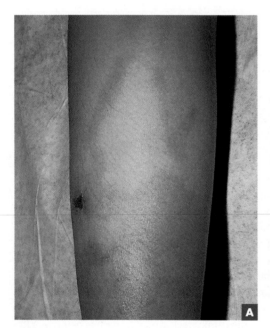
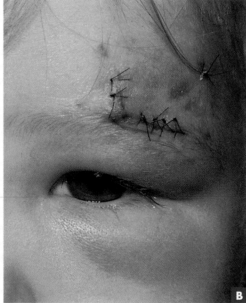

FIG. 12-38 Wound-related cellulitis. *A,* The infected mosquito bite that served as the source of cellulitis in this child can be seen on the left. The area of erythema was indurated and tender. Note that the skin is smooth and the borders fade gradually into the adjacent normal skin. *B,* Mild erythema and edema are evident in the periorbital area of an infant whose laceration from a dog bite had been sutured 48 hours earlier. The edematous areas were indurated and tender.

Clinically, cellulitis is characterized by painful, tender, indurated subcutaneous swelling. The overlying skin is smooth, warm, often shiny, and usually erythematous (see Fig. 12-38). Occasionally it is pink or has a violaceous hue. In contrast to erysipelas, the margins or borders of both the edema and erythema are indistinct, fading imperceptibly into the surrounding tissues. Before therapy, rapid extension is the rule. Systemic symptoms are common, particularly if infection is due to hematogenous spread or to extension from deeper sites. In such cases, fever, chills, malaise, and headache are typical. Toxicity may be marked when hematogenous seeding is the source.

Wound-Related Cellulitis

Extension of infection from an external wound such as a puncture, laceration, abrasion, or insect bite is perhaps the most common source of cellulitis, particularly in school-age children and adolescents. Mild local erythema immediately surrounding a wound, an impetiginous le-

sion, or a pustule may have been noted before the abrupt onset of increased pain and the rapid evolution of subcutaneous inflammation that herald the development of cellulitis. In most cases the primary lesion is readily identifiable at the time of presentation (Fig. 12-38), but in some instances it may no longer be detectable. Occasionally, secondary infection of a preexisting dermatitis may result in a cellulitis that spreads with frightening speed (Fig. 12-39). Group A streptococci and coagulase-positive staphylococci are the organisms recovered most commonly in these circumstances. *Pseudomonas* organisms and mixed flora may be responsible for cellulitis occurring secondary to puncture wounds of the foot (see Fig. 12-36, *B*). Although rapid peripheral spread, overt lymphangitis, and regional adenitis are regarded as highly characteristic of streptococcal infection, this same picture may be seen in patients with cellulitis caused by any of these wound-related pathogens. Fever and other systemic symptoms may be present with this form of cellulitis, but they are more likely to occur with cellulitis

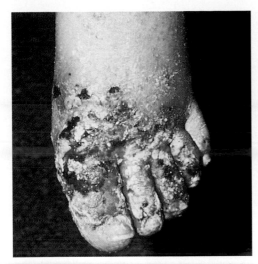

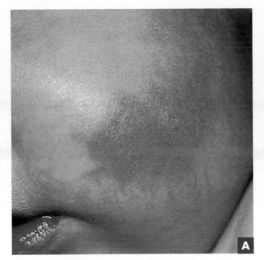

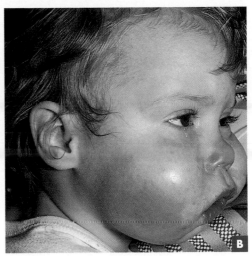

FIG. 12-39 This patient with cellulitis of the foot had been on topical steroid therapy for contact dermatitis for about 48 hours when he experienced the explosive onset of swelling, redness, and pain. Impetiginous changes are apparent, as well. (Courtesy Dr. Michael Sherlock.)

FIG. 12-40 Hematogenous cellulitis. *A,* This small erythematous patch with indistinct borders appeared on this infant's cheek shortly after the onset of fever, irritability, and anorexia. On palpation it was found to be indurated and tender. Blood culture was positive for *H. influenzae* type b. *B,* In this toddler, the evolution of buccal cellulitis due to *H. influenzae* was fulminant, resulting in unusually dramatic swelling.

due to hematogenous seeding or to extension of inflammation from deeper structures.

Hands, feet, and extremities are the most common sites of wound-related cellulitis. This necessitates close assessment and monitoring for further spread and for secondary neurovascular compromise. Inward spread to tendon sheaths of a hand or a foot can have disastrous consequences; hence, cellulitis involving these structures must be treated aggressively and clinical status must be monitored very closely. When an extremity is encircled by cellulitis, swelling and increased pressure can result in neurovascular compromise and extensive secondary damage distally if the area is not surgically decompressed.

Gram's staining and culture of material obtained from the primary wound or of tissue aspirate obtained from the center and margin of the inflamed area may be helpful in identifying the specific pathogen. For aspiration to be successful, a large syringe must be used to provide high-pressure suction and prior injection of nonbacteriostatic saline may be necessary. Blood cultures should be obtained in all patients with systemic symptoms. Prompt treatment is essential to prevent further spread and complications. Antimicrobial therapy often has to be selected empirically, pending culture results. Coverage for penicillinase-producing staphylococci is essential.

Major differential diagnostic considerations include angioedema resulting from insect bites and delayed hypersensitivity reactions to Hymenoptera stings. The former is pruritic and nontender and often has an identifiable central punctum (see Fig. 8-57); the latter tends to be simultaneously pruritic, mildly painful, and mildly tender (see Fig. 8-60). Both are unassociated with systemic symptoms or with adenopathy or lymphangitis. The history, lack of erythema, presence of ecchymotic discoloration, and absence of systemic symptoms all help to distinguish swelling due to trauma.

Hematogenous Cellulitis

Hematogenous seeding is another common source of cellulitis, particularly in infants and young children. Although young infants may show

the sudden onset of sepsis, followed soon by the appearance of cellulitis, older infants, toddlers, and preschool-age children commonly have antecedent upper respiratory tract symptoms. This prodrome is followed by the sudden development of a high fever that begins nearly simultaneously with the appearance of a nondescript area of swelling. Often this swelling is localized in the periorbital region (see Chapter 22), but at times it may be located over a cheek, the neck, or an extremity. The overlying skin rapidly becomes pink, red, or violaceous as the area of edema spreads and becomes indurated. Irritability, anorexia, and signs of toxicity become increasingly marked, in most cases prompting presentation for medical care within 24 hours. *H. influenzae* type b was once a likely source of this picture, but with widespread use of the Hib vaccine, the incidence of *H. influenzae* cellulitis has plummeted. *Streptococcus pneumoniae* as well as group B streptococci (in infants under 3 months of age) are other responsible pathogens.

H. influenzae type b appears to be the sole pathogen responsible for cellulitis of the cheek, also termed *buccal cellulitis*. In this form of cellulitis, a type limited exclusively to infants, the swelling, induration, and erythema are located over the midcheek near the mandibular ramus (Fig. 12-40). Localized erythema of the underlying buccal mucosa is a common associated finding. The systemic symptomatology and exquisite tenderness help to distinguish it from "popsicle panniculitis," which results from cold injury. The latter is characterized by the formation of a mildly tender, discrete, indurated, disc-shaped, subcutaneous mass located at the angle of the mouth, with reddish-purple discoloration of the overlying skin (Fig. 12-41). Systemic symptoms, induration, and tenderness also help to distinguish hematogenous cellulitis at other sites from sympathetic swelling caused by sinusitis (see Fig. 22-60) and from angioedema resulting from insect bites (see Fig. 8-57).

Because of the severity of the illness associated with buccal cellulitis and the inevitability of bacteremia with its attendant risks, expeditious evaluation and treatment are warranted. Blood cultures are positive in a very high percentage of patients and may be supplemented by culture of tissue aspirates from the area of cellulitis. Counterimmuno-

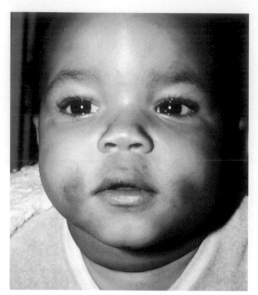

FIG. 12-41 Popsicle panniculitis. This older infant who had become fond of popsicles had bilateral areas of purplish-red swelling just lateral to the corners of his mouth. He was otherwise well. On palpation, masses could be appreciated that were mildly tender, discrete, indurated, and disc shaped. These were localized areas of fat necrosis caused by cold injury. (Courtesy Dr. Michael Sherlock.)

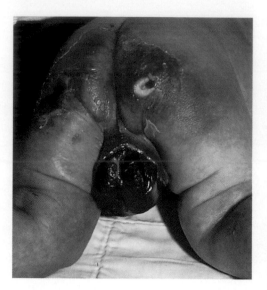

FIG. 12-42 Necrotizing fasciitis. The extent of cellulitis and tissue necrosis is evident in this child who is recovering from necrotizing fasciitis caused by group A streptococci. On presentation he was thought to have cellulitis but was more ill systemically and appeared much more uncomfortable than would be expected. Furthermore, on presentation the area of induration extended well beyond the overlying erythema. (Courtesy Dr. Michael Sherlock.)

electrophoresis also may be helpful. High-dose antimicrobial therapy should be administered parenterally, and agents selected that ensure coverage for β-lactamase–producing *Haemophilus* organisms.

Cellulitis Due to Extension of Infection from Deeper Structures

Though less common than the other forms, cellulitis resulting from extension of infection and inflammation from deeper structures may also occur. This possibility necessitates paying close attention to examination of underlying structures in evaluating any patient with evidence of cellulitis. Dental abscesses (see Fig. 20-49) and acute sinusitis (see Fig. 22-60) may underlie facial cellulitis. Osteomyelitis may produce secondary cellulitic changes in overlying soft tissues, especially after subperiosteal extension (see later discussion). Suppurative lymphadenitis and subcutaneous rupture of skin, scalp, and breast abscesses are other common sources (see Fig. 12-34, *B*). Fever, toxicity, and other systemic symptoms are not unusual with this form of cellulitis. Antecedent history along with the findings on careful examination usually will result in identification of this type of cellulitis and in recognition of the primary source.

Necrotizing Fasciitis

Variously termed *necrotizing fasciitis* or *cellulitis, synergistic cellulitis* or *gangrene, necrotizing erysipelas, streptococcal gangrene,* and more recently *flesh-eating* or *killer strep infection,* this dreaded disorder is a severe, deep, necrotizing soft tissue infection, which at a minimum involves subcutaneous tissues and fascial sheaths and often extends to underlying muscle. This process spreads relentlessly along fascial planes, producing edema, vascular thrombosis, and ever-widening necrosis, resulting in extensive soft tissue destruction. Deep surgical and traumatic wounds are major predisposing factors, although injection sites, cutaneous ulcers, abscesses, and omphalitis may serve as the initiating condition. Diabetics with vascular disease are at especially increased risk. The extremities, perineum, buttocks, trunk, and abdominal wall are the most common sites of involvement. Causative organisms include virulent strains of group A β-hemolytic streptococci, *S. aureus, Pseudomonas aeruginosa, E. coli,* and mixtures of aerobes, anaerobes, and facultative gram-negative rods.

Moderate to severe systemic symptoms are prominent clinically and, along with fever, usually precede the appearance of cellulitic changes. The local area of inflammation initially may resemble ordinary cellulitis, with nonraised, indistinct margins and localized subcutaneous edema with overlying erythema. However, on careful palpation, it often is possible to appreciate that the edema and induration are deeper and far more extensive than the overlying erythema, and the induration is unusually firm in consistency. Pain is remarkably severe early on, and the lesion is exquisitely tender. With progression, the overlying skin itself may become edematous, simulating erysipelas. Later it changes from red or purple to a patchy grayish-blue, and surface bullae, often filled with hemorrhagic fluid, may appear. At this point, numbness and decreased sensitivity to pain may be noted centrally. With further evolution, central necrosis or cutaneous gangrene supervenes (Fig. 12-42). If anaerobes are involved, crepitance may become evident clinically or subcutaneous emphysema may be visible on radiographs.

As the localized process evolves, systemic symptoms increase. Signs of poor perfusion, pallor, and mottling often are accompanied by grunting respirations and by alterations in level of consciousness, including disorientation, obtundation, and seizures. This picture may culminate in frank prostration, often in association with generalized edema. Common laboratory findings in advanced cases include anemia resulting from hemolysis and marrow suppression, proteinuria, hypoproteinemia, hypocalcemia resulting from saponification of necrotic fat, and hyponatremia. Blood and wound cultures are routinely positive.

Mortality ranges from 8% to 70%, depending on the series, and morbidity and disfigurement are common in survivors. Delays in diagnosis and inadequate surgical debridement are major factors in cases with poor outcome.

Early recognition is crucial to ensure appropriate intervention and improve prognosis. This can be particularly difficult in patients with cases resembling ordinary cellulitis that initially abate in response to antimicrobial therapy before worsening. Necrotizing fasciitis should be suspected in any patient with cellulitis (particularly around a deep wound) or omphalitis who has unusually severe pain and systemic symptoms that are out of proportion to local findings. This can enable surgical exploration before advanced skin changes and loss of sensation appear, signaling that necrosis already is extensive. If such changes are present, this process must be presumed. In early cases, findings yielded by examination of frozen sections of biopsy material may confirm the diagnosis. Incision and passage of a probe also can be helpful. If the probe passes easily along fascial planes, the diagnosis is confirmed. Control necessitates wide excision with extensive exposure and debridement of all necrotic tissues, in combination with broad-spectrum

	TABLE 12-1			

Infectious Causes of Generalized or Prominent Cervical Adenopathy

Disorder	Site of adenopathy	Character of nodes	Other features	Laboratory findings
EB virus mononucleosis	Anterior and posterior cervical, or generalized	Soft to firm, discrete, mildly to moderately tender	Pharyngitis; splenomegaly (50%); rash (15%); fever, malaise, fatigue	Atypical lymphocytosis; + Monospot (80% >4 yr); + EB virus titers; may have abnormal LFTs
Cytomegalovirus infection	Generalized or cervical	Soft to firm, discrete, mildly tender	Fever, malaise, fatigue; occasionally hepatosplenomegaly	Atypical lymphocytosis; abnormal LFTs; urine + for CMV on culture; + CMV titers
Toxoplasmosis	Generalized or cervical	Smooth, firm, mildly tender	Myalgias, fatigue, coryza; occasionally splenomegaly and maculopapular rash	Atypical lymphocytosis (frequent); + *Toxoplasma* titers
Brucellosis	Generalized or cervical and axillary	Discrete, may be mildly tender or nontender	History of contact with sick farm animal or ingestion of raw milk; afternoon fever and chills; sweats, malaise, headache and backache, arthralgia; splenomegaly; lasts weeks and may become chronic with metastatic abscesses	Normal or decreased WBC with lymphocytosis; + cultures and serologic tests
Rubella	Anterior and posterior cervical	Soft to mildly firm, discrete, mildly tender or nontender	Fine, discrete maculopapular rash; Forchheimer spots on palate	+ Rubella titer
Streptococcal pharyngitis	Anterior cervical	Soft to mildly firm, discrete, tender	Pharyngitis or nasopharyngitis; headache, malaise; abdominal pain; may have palatal petechiae and/or scarlatiniform rash	+ Throat culture for group A β-hemolytic streptococcus
Herpes simplex	Anterior cervical and submandibular	Soft to mildly firm, discrete, mobile, tender	Gingival erythema and edema with discrete mucosal ulcers; high fever	+ Viral culture (diagnosis usually made on clinical grounds)
Coxsackievirus herpangina	Anterior cervical	Soft to mildly firm, discrete, mobile, slightly tender	Discrete ulcers on labial mucosa, gingiva, tongue, and tonsillar pillars; may have vesicles on palms and soles	+ Viral culture (diagnosis usually made on clinical grounds)
Adenovirus	Anterior cervical and preauricular	Soft to mildly firm, discrete, mobile, mildly tender	Nonspecific pharyngeal inflammation, occasionally with exudate; may have conjunctivitis	+ Viral culture

antimicrobial therapy (guided in part by Gram staining results). Aggressive supportive measures are important as well.

Infectious Lymphadenitis

Lymph nodes respond to both systemic and local infections with increased cellular multiplication and activity, clinically manifested as enlargement and tenderness. If enlargement and degree of inflammation are mild, this often is called *reactive adenopathy*. Nodes usually are 2 cm or less in diameter, and they are discrete, slightly firm or rubbery, and mobile. Discomfort and tenderness are mild. However, if enlargement is marked and inflammation is pronounced, the phenomenon is termed *adenitis*. In this condition, the lymph node itself is infected. Nodes usually exceed 2 to 3 cm in diameter, and overlying soft tissues may become edematous, making it difficult to distinguish exact margins. With progression, the overlying skin often becomes erythematous

and may become adherent, reducing mobility. Discomfort and tenderness are usually, but not always, marked. Depending on the causative organism, suppuration may occur.

Adenopathy may be generalized or regional, but adenitis tends to be localized to a single node. Whereas adenitis is invariably infectious in origin, adenopathy also may be a feature of collagen vascular disease or it may be of neoplastic origin. Malignant nodes usually are very firm or hard, but occasionally they are rubbery. They also may be discrete, but not infrequently, they are matted and often appear fixed or poorly mobile. Tenderness is unusual. Depending on the type of malignancy, the adenopathy may be isolated to one region or it may be generalized and associated with hepatosplenomegaly and with systemic symptoms of anorexia, fatigue, weight loss, night sweats, and bone pain. Many of the infectious diseases associated with generalized or cervical adenopathy have been discussed earlier in this chapter. Some of the distinguishing features of the adenopathy characteristic of these disorders are given in Table 12-1. Neoplastic diseases are discussed in Chapter 11.

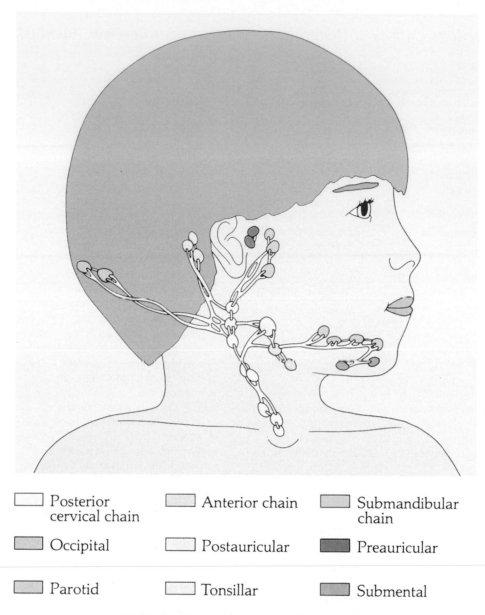

	Posterior cervical chain		Anterior chain		Submandibular chain
	Occipital		Postauricular		Preauricular
	Parotid		Tonsillar		Submental

FIG. 12-43   The superficial cervical lymph nodes.

In this section we concentrate on the manifestations and causes of focal lymphadenitis. Almost any organism capable of infecting tissue can produce adenitis; hence the number of potential pathogens is large. Assessment is facilitated by knowledge of the patterns of lymphatic drainage, the differential diagnostic possibilities of an inflammatory mass in a given region, and the varying clinical characteristics of adenitis produced by individual organisms.

By definition, infection of a lymph node is a secondary phenomenon occurring as a result of drainage through lymphatic vessels to a regional node. Identification of the primary source, when possible, is important in narrowing the list of potential causative organisms. In many instances, close examination of those areas whose lymphatics drain to the affected region reveals the site of inoculation. However, it is not uncommon for the primary site to have healed by the time adenitis becomes clinically manifest. In these cases, careful history-taking concerning prior distal wounds or inflammation, as well as about any possible environmental exposures, may disclose the identity of the

probable pathogen. This can be particularly important in cases caused by organisms not readily grown on culture and in those cases in which previous administration of antibiotics has suppressed the causative organism, resulting in negative cultures.

The Superficial Regional Lymph Nodes

The Cervical Lymph Nodes

The cervical nodes, being numerous and draining multiple structures, are particularly common sites of acute adenitis (Fig. 12-43). In addition to infections of the upper respiratory tract, those of the skin of the face, the scalp, conjunctivae, teeth, gingivae, ears, and neck all may serve as primary sites of infection. Nasal and oropharyngeal infections drain to the tonsillar and anterior cervical nodes (Fig. 12-44). Superficial facial infections and facial cellulitis may drain to the anterior cervical chain or to the preauricular or submental nodes. The occipital, posterior cervical, preauricular, and postauricular nodes receive lym-

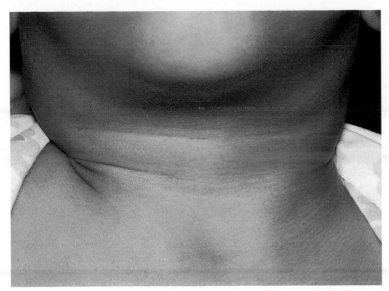

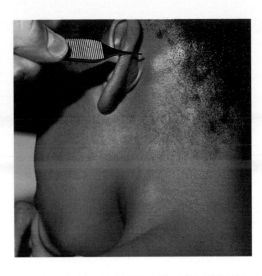

FIG. 12-45 Acute postauricular lymphadenitis. This child had folliculitic and crusted scalp lesions and a tender 1.5-cm postauricular node with overlying erythema. The initial suspicion of bacterial infection was not confirmed. A potassium chloride preparation and fungal culture identified tinea capitis as the primary process.

FIG. 12-44 Cervical adenopathy. Bilateral enlargement of the tonsillar nodes in this child was associated with viral pharyngitis.

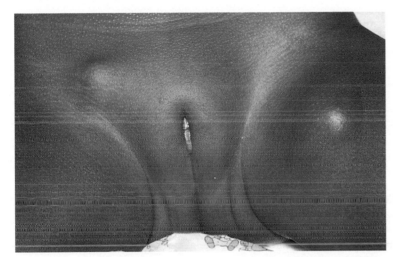

FIG. 12-46 Subacute lymphadenitis of a right inguinal and left femoral node resulted in dramatic swelling in this toddler. Atypical mycobacteria were found to be causative.

phatic drainage from nearby portions of the scalp, and thus may become inflamed and enlarged in connection with secondary infection of seborrhea, impetigo, wound infections, tinea capitis, or head lice infestation (Fig. 12-45). Conjunctival infections may result in adenitis of the preauricular node. The teeth, gingivae, and tongue are drained by lymphatics coursing to the submental and submandibular nodes, which can be secondarily involved in cases of dental abscess, gingivitis, and stomatitis. Infections of the external auditory canal and the auricle may drain to the preauricular or postauricular nodes, while those involving the neck may affect the anterior or posterior cervical chain.

Although the number of potential causative organisms is high, an individual pathogen often can be implicated by the findings from a careful history-taking and physical examination. Differentiation also must be made from other masses that may be present in the cervical region, many of which are congenital and subject to secondary infection, simulating adenitis. Many of these and their clinical characteristics are summarized in Table 12-2.

The Axillary and Epitrochlear Lymph Nodes

More than a dozen nodes occupy the axilla. Those in the anterior pectoral portion drain the breast and chest wall, those in the lateral or midportion receive drainage from the hand and arm (see Fig. 12-50, *C*), and those in the posterior subscapular region drain portions of the back. The epitrochlear node receives lymphatic vessels from the fingers, hand, and skin of the forearm, but it is a much less common site of adenitis than are the axillary nodes. Wound and skin infections, cellulitis, and herpes zoster are major sources of axillary adenitis in childhood.

The Inguinal Lymph Nodes

The inguinal nodes are divided into two groups by Poupart's ligament, with those above the ligament called *inguinal nodes* and those below it termed *femoral* nodes (Fig. 12-46; see Fig. 12-48). The inguinal group receives lymphatics from the external genitalia, anus, umbilicus, lower abdomen and back, buttocks, and upper thigh, and also may drain the lower leg. Thus, in addition to wound and skin infections, perianal, intraabdominal, and genital infections may serve as sources of inguinal adenitis. The femoral nodes primarily drain the foot and lower leg. The popliteal nodes receive drainage from the foot and lower leg, but like the epitrochlear nodes, they are unusual sites of adenitis.

Having contrasted the general features of acute lymphadenitis with those of adenopathy, as well as having discussed the regions of involvement and their likely sources, we now can look at the characteristics of adenitis produced by the various causative organisms.

Acute Suppurative Lymphadenitis

Group A β-hemolytic streptococci and coagulase-positive staphylococci are responsible for causing most cases of acute lymphadenitis, regardless of anatomic region. Together they account for up to 80% of cases of cervical adenitis alone. In recent years, staphylococcal infections have surpassed streptococcal infections in frequency. Other than culture of a specimen obtained by needle aspirate, there is no way to distinguish between the two clinically, as the clinical picture for both consists of sudden, painful, and rapid enlargement, usually of a single node. The involved node is firm and exquisitely tender and may range

TABLE 12-2

Differential Diagnosis of Cervical Adenopathy/Adenitis

Type of mass	Usual site	Character	Time of appearance
Lymphangioma	Preauricular, submental, sub-mandibular, supraclavicular	Soft, compressible; transilluminates; margins often indistinct; may enlarge with crying or straining; nontender unless infected	Birth to 2 years
Hemangioma	Preauricular, postauricular; may occur along or under sterno-cleidomastoid	Soft, compressible; margins often indistinct; enlarges with crying, straining, and dependency; nontender unless infected	Birth to 1 year; gradually enlarges during first year, then regresses
Branchial cleft cyst	Preauricular, at mandibular angle, along anterior border of sterno-cleidomastoid, suprasternal	Discrete; usually has overlying or nearby pore or fistula, which may retract with swallowing; nontender unless infected	Present at birth; often not noticed until infection produces enlargement, pain, and overlying erythema with or without drainage
Thyroglossal duct cyst	Midline, often at level of hyoid or just below	Discrete; usually has overlying pore or fistula; moves with tongue movement	Present at birth; often not noticed until infection produces enlargement, pain, and overlying erythema with or without drainage
Dermoid cyst	Midline, often submental or suprasternal	Discrete, smooth; doughy or rubbery; nontender; does not retract with swallowing	Infancy/childhood
Laryngocele	Just lateral to midline along anterior border of sternocleido-mastoid	Soft, compressible, may gurgle on compression; enlarges with straining or crying; nontender unless infected; may have associated stridor or hoarseness; air-fluid level may be seen on x-ray	Infancy/childhood
Esophageal diverticulum	Paratracheal, usually on the left	Soft, compressible; enlarges with crying or straining; nontender; may have history of dysphagia or aspiration	Infancy/childhood
Sialadenitis	Preauricular, extending under and behind ear; submandibular, submental	Firm; mildly tender when viral; exquisitely tender when suppurative, with pus exuding from orifice; pain increased with eating, especially sour foods; elevated serum or urine amylase level	Any age
Teratoma	Midline or paramedian	Solitary; firm with irregular border; rapid increase in size; calcifications may be seen on x-ray	Infancy/childhood
Thyroid goiter	Isthmus (midline) and lobes (paratracheal)	Diffuse enlargement; usually smooth contour and soft consistency, occasionally nodular; moves with swallowing	Occasionally neonatal (with maternal ingestion of iodides); childhood in endemic areas (iodine-deficient water); childhood/adolescence in familial cases
Graves' disease	Isthmus (midline) and lobes (paratracheal)	Diffuse enlargement; smooth contour and soft consistency; moves with swallowing; associated signs of thyrotoxicosis and exophthalmos	Childhood/adolescence
Hashimoto's thyroiditis	Isthmus (midline) and lobes (paratracheal)	Diffuse enlargement; distinct contours; firm or rubbery; surface may be irregular; may have neck soreness and dysphagia; may have symptoms of mild hyperthyroidism	Childhood/adolescence
Thyroid carcinoma	Usually in lateral lobe or at junction of isthmus and lobe	Solitary mass; firm or hard and differs in consistency from rest of gland; may have associated adenopathy; may have past history of irradiation	Childhood/adolescence

TABLE 12-2

Differential Diagnosis of Cervical Adenopathy/Adenitis—cont'd

Type of mass	Usual site	Character	Time of appearance
Leukemia	Any cervical node or nodes	Firm to hard; often enlarges rapidly; may be fixed or matted; nontender; often other regions involved; often hepatosplenomegaly; may have fever, anorexia, weight loss, bone pain, pallor, petechiae	Any age
Non-Hodgkin's lymphoma	Spinal accessory, supraclavicular	Firm to hard; enlarges rapidly; may be fixed or matted; nontender; often other regions are involved; may have fever, anorexia, weight loss, bone and joint pain	5-15 years
Hodgkin's disease	Anterior or posterior cervical, preauricular, supraclavicular	Firm, occasionally rubbery; slow growing; may be mobile, fixed, or matted; nontender; often otherwise asymptomatic; may have fever, malaise, weight loss, night sweats, and hepatosplenomegaly	Usually >5 years
Rhabdomyosarcoma	Nasopharyngeal, parotid, anterior or posterior cervical	Primary nasopharyngeal: symptoms of enlarged adenoids; later serosanguineous nasal discharge, weight loss, cranial nerve deficits, and secondary node enlargement Primary parotid or cervical: hard, painless, nontender mass	Any age, but more common in early childhood

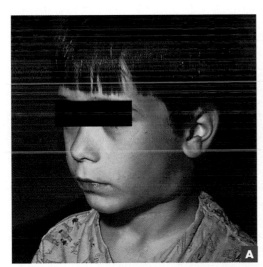
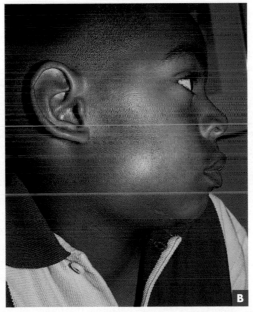
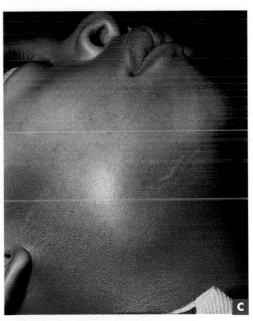

FIG. 12-47 Acute suppurative lymphadenitis. *A,* This youngster was seen within 24 hours of the onset of painful enlargement of the left tonsillar node. There was mild overlying edema, and the node was markedly tender. *B* and *C,* This boy had massive enlargement of the tonsillar node with overlying edema and mild erythema. The node was exquisitely tender, but there was no evidence of fluctuance. Group A β-hemolytic streptococci grew from his throat culture. The absence of preauricular swelling helps differentiate adenitis from parotitis. (*A* courtesy Dr. Michael Sherlock.)

in diameter from 2 to 6 cm (Fig. 12-47). Within 24 to 72 hours the overlying soft tissue becomes edematous and the skin erythematous. As many as 50% of patients may be febrile, and some appear toxic; bacteremia develops in a small percentage. Left untreated, suppuration occurs during the next several days and is detectable as central fluctuance. Simultaneously, thinning of the overlying skin may be noted as the process points toward the surface (Fig. 12-48). Occasionally the abscess may point inward, rupturing into the soft tissues and dissecting along tissue planes with potentially catastrophic effects. Prompt institution of antimicrobial therapy that empirically covers *S. aureus* can significantly alter this course. When high-dose oral therapy is started before the development of overlying cellulitic changes, such changes may be prevented and enlargement halted, followed by regression. Even patients with swelling and erythema at the start of therapy may not progress to suppuration. Patients with high fever and toxicity require parenteral treatment, as do children who fail to improve on oral medication. Suppuration necessitates incision and drainage.

Cervical nodes, especially the tonsillar and anterior cervical ones, are the most common sites of adenitis caused by streptococci or staphylococci. Patients usually are young children, with a peak incidence between 1 and 4 years of age. Many have a history of antecedent rhinitis, often associated with impetiginization of the anterior nares and anterior cervical adenopathy. Cough, anorexia, vomiting, and fever also may be present. These findings may persist or they may clear before the onset of adenitis. In older children, a recent episode of pharyngitis may be reported and in a small percentage adenitis develops in association with a peritonsillar abscess (see Fig. 22-71).

Secondarily infected dermatitis, insect bites, impetigo, and wound infections may precede the onset of adenitis in other patients, in which case the node affected depends on the primary site. These infections, as well as cellulitis, are common antecedents of axillary and inguinal adenitis caused by streptococci and staphylococci. Primary sources may be evident at the time adenitis develops, but often they have healed. It is also important to remember that invasive forms of tinea capitis may closely mimic streptococcal and staphylococcal infection, both in the appearance of the primary lesion and in the character of the secondary adenitis, although progression to suppuration is unusual.

Although streptococci and staphylococci are the predominant pathogens causing acute lymphadenitis, occasionally anaerobic bacteria—including *Actinomyces*—are responsible. The vast majority of cases caused by anaerobes are secondary to dental disease, including dental abscesses, gingivitis, and stomatitis; as a result, the submental or submandibular nodes are more likely to be affected. On occasion the adenitis appears simultaneously with facial cellulitis stemming from a dental abscess (see Chapter 20).

Actinomycotic adenitis, though unusual, has a distinctive clinical course. Enlargement of the affected node is gradual, and on palpation it is firm and lumpy, has an irregular border, and is mildly to moderately tender. Over time the center blackens and necroses, and a chronic draining sinus may form. Microscopic examination of the discharge discloses characteristic sulfur granules.

Mycobacterial Lymphadenitis

After decades of declining incidence in developed countries, the incidence of tuberculosis has begun to rise over the past several years (see the section on tuberculosis); hence, *Mycobacterium tuberculosis* as well as nontuberculous or atypical mycobacteria (especially *Mycobacterium avium-intracellulare*) continue to be important causes of lymphadenitis. Recognition of mycobacterial lymphadenitis is important, because its management is considerably different from that for lymphadenitis caused by other bacteria. Both groups of mycobacteria cause similar clinical findings. Nodal enlargement is gradual and persistent. The node is slightly to mildly tender, and initially there is little or no sign of warmth or overlying inflammation (Fig. 12-49, *A*; see Fig. 12-46). After a few weeks the node becomes adherent to the overlying skin, which in turn becomes thickened and tense, with overlying reddish or reddish-purple discoloration (Figs. 12-49, *B* and *C*). Suppuration may occur several weeks to months after onset and may result in rupture through the overlying skin with the formation of a chronically draining sinus. The risk of chronic drainage may be increased if aspiration or incision and drainage are attempted. Although the local clinical findings are similar, there are historical and other differences that can help to distinguish tuberculous lymphadenitis from atypical mycobacterial lymphadenitis.

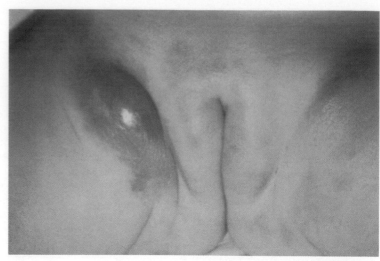

FIG. 12-48 Acute suppurative lymphadenitis. Increased pain and erythema, thinning of the overlying skin, and fluctuance on palpation signal that central necrosis has occurred. (Courtesy Dr. Michael Sherlock.)

Tuberculous Lymphadenitis

Children with tuberculosis may be of any age and frequently have a positive history of exposure to an infected adult.

Tonsillar and submandibular nodes are common sites of tuberculous lymphadenitis because of the lymphatic extension that occurs from paratracheal nodes. Supraclavicular nodes are affected as the result of drainage from apical lesions. The posterior cervical chain is another common area. Axillary, inguinal, and femoral nodes are more likely sites of enlargement if drainage is coming from a primary skin lesion. The ipsilateral preauricular node enlarges if the conjunctiva is the site of inoculation. Usually a group of nodes in one region is involved if lymphatic spread is the cause. If hematogenous dissemination is the source, involvement is frequently bilateral and may be generalized; in patients with protracted hematogenous dissemination, generalized adenopathy may be characterized by massive enlargement. The latter usually have systemic symptoms (see the section on Tuberculosis).

Initially, lymphoid hyperplasia develops as tubercles form, then necrosis and caseation supervene. Early on, nodes are firm discrete, and nontender; but with progression they tend to become matted and adherent to the overlying skin, which often becomes discolored, thickened, and scaly. Without treatment, spontaneous drainage ultimately occurs, leaving a draining sinus.

Chest radiographs reveal findings suggestive of tuberculosis in 75% of patients; the sedimentation rate exceeds 30 mm/hr in up to 80%; and the PPD test is positive, usually with more than 10 mm of induration. Treatment of tuberculous adenitis is pharmacologic, with excision reserved for cases with chronic drainage (see the section on Tuberculosis).

Adenitis Due to Atypical Mycobacteria

Patients with atypical mycobacterial adenitis usually are under 4 years of age and are unlikely to have a history of exposure to tuberculosis. A submandibular, submental, preauricular, anterior cervical, inguinal, or epitrochlear node may be the site of involvement. Bilateral adenitis and generalized adenopathy do not occur, and systemic symptoms are rare. Chest radiographic findings rarely are abnormal; only one third of patients have elevated sedimentation rates; and the PPD test is intermediate or positive, with induration ranging from 5 to 10 mm. Atypical mycobacteria invariably are resistant to multiple drugs, hence excisional biopsy generally is the treatment of choice.

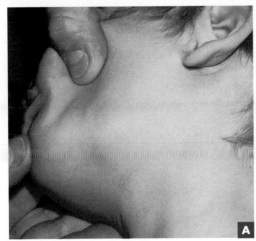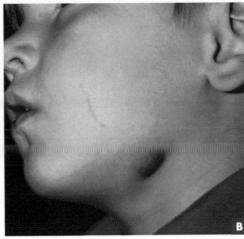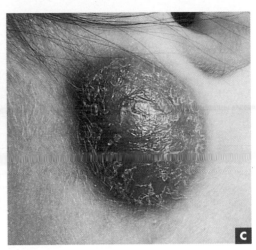

FIG. 12-49 Mycobacterial adenitis. *A,* Early in the course of adenitis caused by *Mycobacterium tuberculosis* or atypical mycobacteria, enlargement of the node is gradual, tenderness is mild, and there is little or no sign of warmth or overlying inflammation. *B,* After a few to several weeks the overlying skin becomes thickened, tense, discolored, and adherent to the node. *C,* This preauricular node was fluctuant, indicating suppuration. (Courtesy Dr. Michael Sherlock.)

Spontaneous regression can occur, however, making observation a reasonable course if suppuration or drainage has not occurred.

Adenitis Associated With Animal or Vector Contact

In many children, acute local lymphadenitis results from inoculation of a pathogen by means of an animal scratch or bite, from the bite of an insect vector transmitting a pathogen from an animal host, or from contact with a contaminated animal carcass. In some of these disorders, systemic symptoms are prominent; in others the local adenitis is the primary manifestation.

Pasteurella Multocida Adenitis

Suppurative adenitis caused by *P. multocida* may occur in patients who develop local infection at the site of a scratch or bite inflicted by a dog or cat. Soon after the manifestations of local infection appear at the primary site (usually within 24 hours), a regional node enlarges and becomes tender. Overlying swelling and redness are common, and suppuration may occur early. This picture is clinically indistinguishable from that of adenitis due to streptococci or staphylococci, but often *P. multocida* infection can be suspected on the basis of the history. Axillary and inguinal nodes are the most common sites of involvement. Systemic symptoms are unusual.

Cat Scratch Disease

Although low-grade fever may occur in about 25% of affected patients, adenitis is a primary feature of cat scratch disease, which is due to a pleomorphic bacillus that is seen in Warthin-Starry silver–stained sections of biopsied nodes. Recent studies indicate that *Rochalimaea henselae,* a gram-negative rickettsial bacterium, is the causative agent in most cases of cat scratch disease. Ninety percent have a history of either an antecedent cat scratch or of contact with cats, especially kittens. Although inoculation via a cat scratch is the most common means of infection, splinters, puncture wounds, and dog scratches also have been implicated. Incidence is highest in fall and winter in temperate climates, with cases occurring with equal frequency year-round in tropical areas. Most patients are in the 5- to 14-year age range, but family clusters that include younger children and adults have been reported.

Symptoms begin 3 to 30 days after inoculation, with 7 to 12 days being the most common interval. A red papule or series of papules is commonly noted at the site of inoculation (Fig. 12-50, *A* and *B*). Shortly thereafter, one or more regional nodes enlarge, becoming mildly painful and tender (Fig. 12-50, *C*). Involved nodes are firm, and overlying warmth and mild redness may develop within a few days of enlargement. In order of frequency, axillary, cervical, submandibular, preauricular, epitrochlear, and inguinal nodes have been reported as sites of involvement. In cases involving a preauricular node, associated conjunctivitis is common and points toward conjunctival inoculation as the source. Discomfort generally subsides in 4 to 6 weeks, but the node may remain enlarged or may fluctuate in size for months. Suppuration occurs in about one third of patients.

Diagnosis is made primarily on the basis of history, clinical picture and course, and/or findings yielded by an excisional biopsy specimen. An indirect fluorescent antibody test for detecting antibody to *Rochalimaea* species is currently available through the Centers for Disease Control and may be a useful adjunct for making the diagnosis of cat scratch disease. If infection is suspected, expectant follow-up is recommended. Most authorities believe aspiration is preferable to incision and drainage if suppuration occurs, because of concerns that the latter procedure may lead to prolonged drainage and scarring. In protracted or atypical cases, excisional biopsy is suggested.

Tularemia

Francisella tularensis may produce an illness in which adenitis is prominent and occurs in concert with systemic symptoms. Rabbits, hares, muskrats, and voles serve as endemic sources of this pathogen. Children may acquire the glandular or ulceroglandular form of the disease by handling or skinning dead animals, after an animal bite (especially that of a cat that hunts rabbits), or occasionally from the bite of an insect that serves as a vector for the pathogen. The incubation period ranges from 1 to 21 days. Onset is abrupt and characterized by fever, chills, headache, myalgias, vomiting, and possibly photophobia. Within 2 days, axillary, epitrochlear, or inguinal adenitis is noted, and soon thereafter a painful papule appears distal to the involved node at the site of inoculation. This ruptures within 1 to 2 days, forming a central ulcer with a raised edge. The involved node is firm and tender and

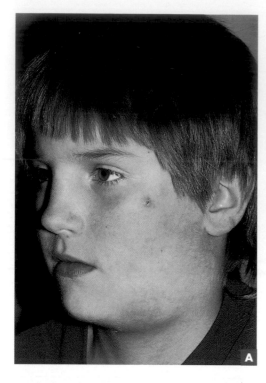

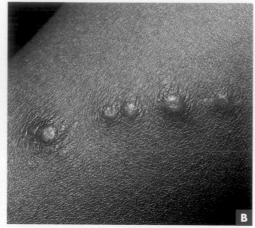

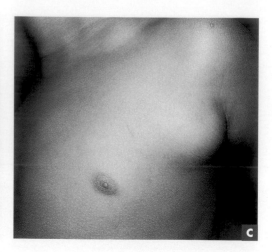

FIG. 12-50 Cat scratch disease. *A,* This boy presented with mildly painful "swollen glands." The left preauricular and tonsillar nodes were enlarged, firm, and mildly tender. An ulcerated papule, evident on his left cheek, was the site of a scratch inflicted by one of his kittens 2 weeks before. *B,* A line of papules is seen on the forearm of a 3-year-old at the site of a scratch inflicted by his new kitten 3 weeks before presentation. *C,* Marked enlargement of an ipsilateral axillary node had prompted his visit. The node was firm and only mildly tender. (*A* courtesy of Dr. Kenneth Schuit.)

may be associated with overlying erythema. Generalized adenopathy and hepatosplenomegaly may be noted in some patients, and in the second week of illness a blotchy, erythematous maculopapular rash (or occasionally a vesicular, pustular, or nodose exanthem) may appear. Without treatment, fever may persist for 2 to 3 weeks and the ulcer may take as long as a month to heal. The diagnosis is suggested by history, clinical picture, and course and is confirmed by serologic tests. Streptomycin is the treatment of choice.

Bubonic Plague

Now rare in developed countries, bubonic plague continues to sporadically afflict people who live or hunt in areas where infection is endemic in the wild rodent population. It is usually transmitted by means of a flea bite, but on occasion inoculation occurs through a break in the skin as a result of handling an infected carcass. Thus, inguinal and axillary nodes are the most common sites of bubo formation. The incubation period ranges from several hours to 10 days and ends with the abrupt onset of high fever, chills, malaise, weakness, and headache. Pain in the area of a regional node precedes rapid nodal enlargement. The node is fixed, firm, and exquisitely tender with overlying edema. Purplish discoloration is common. The inoculation site may appear normal, or it may be manifested as a skin abscess. Rapid progression of systemic symptoms occurs, with the patient appearing toxic and apprehensive and often manifesting delirium and signs of neurologic dysfunction. DIC and septic shock may supervene if treatment is not instituted promptly. If infection is suspected, the node should be aspirated to obtain material for culture, blood cultures should be performed, and broad-spectrum parenteral antibiotic therapy instituted.

General Approach to Diagnosis of Lymphadenitis

Because of the wide range of pathogens that can produce lymphadenitis, meticulous care must be taken during the clinical assessment. The history-taking should include questions concerning antecedent and current signs and symptoms, which may include prior wounds such as cuts, bites, punctures, splinters, or scratches distal to the inflamed node. Exposure to other ill persons or to animals, as well as recent

travel, should be determined. Questions also must be asked about the presence or absence of systemic symptoms and about the rapidity of the evolution of the adenitis itself. A history of past problems and medication intake is important as well. Physical examination must include precise measurement of the size of the inflamed node, in addition to inspection of overlying soft tissue and palpation to determine contour, consistency, and degree of tenderness. The region drained by the involved node must be inspected for clues as to the probable primary source of infection. Finally, close attention should be paid to the child's general status and to other portions of the reticuloendothelial system, such as to other nodal regions as well as to the liver and spleen.

With the preceding information, the specific pathogen may be evident on clinical grounds alone or the differential diagnostic possibilities may be considerably narrowed, permitting confirmation using a minimum of laboratory tests. Close follow-up is important for all children treated as outpatients, to monitor their clinical course and response to therapy.

Bacterial Bone and Joint Infections

Osteomyelitis

The anatomy and physiology of growing bone place children at particular risk for bacterial infection; in fact, 85% of cases of osteomyelitis occur in children under 16 years of age. In most series the highest incidence has been found to occur in infancy, with a secondary peak between 8 to 12 years. Among infants, males and females are affected with equal frequency, but among older children, males predominate in a ratio of 2–3 to 1. The advent of antimicrobial therapy and advances in diagnostic techniques have significantly altered the course of the disease and the outcome. Mortality has decreased from 25% in the preantibiotic era, to 1% to 2%; morbidity has declined from 50% to less than 15%.

S. aureus and β-hemolytic streptococci are the most commonly identified pathogens in all age groups. Gram-negative organisms account for a small percentage of cases. *Salmonella* species are of particular importance in children with sickle hemoglobinopathies, and

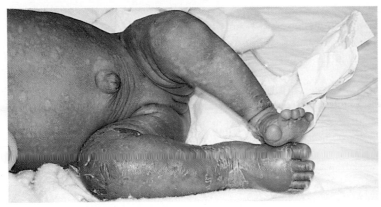

FIG. 12-51 Acute hematogenous osteomyelitis in infancy. Swelling of the entire leg and foot with overlying erythremia is evident in this 2½-month-old infant who had rapid extension of osteomyelitis of the tibia.

Pseudomonas organisms often are isolated in cases resulting from puncture wounds of the foot. In 15% to 20% of cases no causative organism is identified, often as a result of suppression by prior antibiotic therapy.

Once bacteria become established within bone, they stimulate an inflammatory response with the formation of exudate. As this collects, local pressure increases, promoting extension outward and causing further vascular stasis and thrombophlebitis. The resultant ischemia causes local bone necrosis. With further progression, dead bone can form a sequestrum surrounded by purulent material, which becomes inaccessible to antimicrobial penetration.

An appreciation of the anatomic and physiologic features of bone in general and of growing bone in particular is essential to an understanding of the pathophysiology of osteomyelitis in children. Nutrient vessels enter the diaphysis from the periosteum and extend to the metaphysis (or, in flat and irregular bones, to the area adjacent to the epiphysis), where terminal arterioles form loops and empty into larger sinusoidal veins. This area is one of sluggish, somewhat turbulent blood flow, which is prone to thrombosis and which serves as an ideal site for bacterial deposition in the face of bacteremia. Because they are devoid of phagocytic macrophages, the sinusoidal veins lack a major line of defense against bacteria.

In infants under 8 to 12 months of age, numerous additional factors facilitate the extension of infection, once it is present. Because the epiphyseal plate has not fully formed, the nutrient arterioles penetrate into the epiphysis; hence, rupture of infection into the adjacent joint is common. The cortex of the infant's metaphysis is thin and the trabeculae are fewer in number, facilitating penetration outward to a more loosely attached periosteum, as well as extension toward the diaphysis. Thus infants are far more likely to have extensive involvement, even with early diagnosis (Fig. 12-51). Once the epiphyseal growth plate has formed, it serves as a relatively effective barrier to joint extension, and the frequency of secondary septic arthritis is thereby substantially reduced, although sympathetic joint effusions are not uncommon. An exception to this is hematogenous osteomyelitis involving the proximal metaphysis of the humerus or femur and of the distal fibula, where the synovium of the adjacent joint inserts so as to include the metaphysis within the joint.

There are two major mechanisms through which bones become infected. Hematogenous spread accounts for more than 50% of cases affecting children. Areas of rich blood supply and sluggish flow are most vulnerable to bacterial seeding; hence the metaphyseal portions of long bones and the subepiphyseal portions of flat and irregular bones are the usual sites of such involvement. Trauma may be a predisposing factor, perhaps by virtue of producing local small-vessel occlusion with sec-

ondary stasis, anoxia, and necrosis, which makes the site more vulnerable to the deposition of hematogenously spread pathogens. Children with sickle hemoglobinopathies are particularly susceptible to hematogenous osteomyelitis as a result of their vulnerability to bacteremia and sepsis, and because their bones are predisposed to vascular sludging and infarction.

Spread from a contiguous focus of infection accounts for most of the remaining cases of osteomyelitis affecting children. Infections of fracture sites, surgical wounds, and puncture wounds as well as extension of infection from an adjacent site of cellulitis or an abscess serve as the predisposing conditions, with localization dependent on the original site of injury or infection.

While important in adults, peripheral vascular disease is rarely a predisposing condition in children. If this does occur in a young person, the patient usually is an adolescent with long-standing diabetes mellitus; the small bones of the hands or feet are the most common sites of involvement.

In addition to categorization by mode of spread or acquisition, osteomyelitis is further subdivided into acute, subacute, and chronic forms according to duration of symptoms. Of these, the acute form is by far the most common. The major clinical finding in each form is localized bone pain, which typically is constant, progressively more severe, exacerbated by movement; it commonly wakes the patient from sleep. The overlying soft tissues appear normal or may be warm, mildly swollen, and occasionally erythematous, but in contrast to the findings in cellulitis, these findings are often subtle and induration is unusual. Spasm of overlying muscles is often intense, adding to discomfort, and the adjacent joint may be held in flexion. Beyond these common features there is a wide range of clinical expression. Appreciation of this spectrum is important to ensure early diagnosis, thus resulting in a more favorable outcome.

Acute Osteomyelitis

Acute Hematogenous Osteomyelitis. In the acute hematogenous form of osteomyelitis, the mode of presentation and the clinical findings are age dependent, although most patients present within 1 week of onset of symptoms.

Infants under 6 months of age often have no systemic signs of infection. However, a small percentage have low-grade fever and a few may show a frankly septic picture. Early on, irritability and anorexia are the major manifestations. Within a few days, evidence of pain on movement or of decreased use of a limb may be noted (pseudoparalysis). At this time or soon after, localized soft tissue swelling develops. This often extends rapidly to involve the entire extremity, reflecting rapid spread of infection in the underlying bone (Fig. 12-51). For the same reason, tenderness also is diffuse. Furthermore, multiple bones may be involved. Careful attention must be given to joint examination because of the high risk of early joint extension and secondary septic arthritis.

In children 8 months to 2 years of age, fever and signs of toxicity are common although not universal. A history of or persistent signs of antecedent upper respiratory tract or skin infection are present in over 50% of cases. In many patients, systemic symptoms consist primarily of fever and irritability in association with refusal to walk, a limp, or decreased use of an extremity. A small percentage present with more severe systemic symptoms, including chills, lethargy, irritability, anorexia, vomiting, and dehydration. At this age children often are unable or unwilling to point to the site of discomfort, but on observation may be found to avoid moving the involved extremity or to hold a particular joint in flexion *consistently*. Soft tissue swelling and warmth may be noted overlying a metaphysis, but this often is subtle or absent in early cases and it is undetectable in cases in which the proximal femur

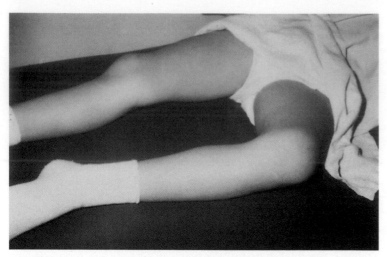

FIG. 12-52 Acute osteomyelitis. Fever, hip and thigh pain, and refusal to walk were the chief complaints in this 5-year-old child with osteomyelitis of the proximal femur. On inspection she lay still, holding the left leg externally rotated and flexed at the hip and knee. This same position also is adopted by children with acute arthritis of the hip.

is involved. Comparative circumferential measurements of suspected areas and painstaking care in first eliciting the child's cooperation, and then in palpating for evidence of muscle spasm or point tenderness, are well worth the effort if osteomyelitis is suspected. Even then, focal tenderness may be difficult to detect early in the course.

Children over 2 years of age with acute osteomyelitis are usually febrile but rarely toxic. They are more likely to complain of and point to a specific site of pain, and point tenderness generally is easy to elicit unless presentation is very early. Older patients describe the pain as deep, intense, and constant. Signs of adjacent joint flexion and of nearby muscle spasm are common (Fig. 12-52), but again, overlying soft tissue swelling may be subtle. Unless a sympathetic effusion has developed, the adjacent joint may be passively moved through its full range of motion, although this will exacerbate the pain.

If bones other than the long bones of the extremities are the site of infection, the clinical picture can be especially confusing. Osteomyelitis of the pelvic bones can mimic numerous other conditions. Although fever and an abnormal gait are the most common presenting complaints, lower abdominal and groin pain, hip or buttock pain, sciatica, and thigh pain (with swelling) can each be prominent early complaints in individual patients. Often the initial clinical picture is more suggestive of appendicitis, pelvic abscess, or infection of the hip or femur than of pelvic osteomyelitis. To establish the diagnosis, a high level of suspicion and great care in examination are necessary. In patients presenting with abdominal complaints, the absence of rebound tenderness, lesser prominence of gastrointestinal symptoms, onset of pain in the lower abdomen rather than in the periumbilical region, and normal findings on rectal examination can help to distinguish the process from that of acute appendicitis. Furthermore, while most patients have pain on hip motion in one or more planes, range of motion is either normal or only slightly limited, and with careful examination, point tenderness usually can be detected.

Acute Osteomyelitis Due to Contiguous Spread. Acute osteomyelitis resulting from the contiguous spread of infection must be suspected in patients with prior puncture wounds, deep lacerations, surgical incisions, open fractures, abscesses, or cellulitis who experience a sudden onset of increased pain at the wound site. This pain is perceived as deep, severe, and constant and is aggravated by movement. In these cases, soft tissue cellulitis is a common associated finding and fever is

usual. If extension of primary soft tissue infection is the source, the patient's condition often may have worsened clinically after a period of improvement in response to antimicrobial therapy or the patient may have failed to show the expected response to therapy.

Diagnostic Methods in Acute Osteomyelitis. Standard radiographic and laboratory studies are of somewhat limited use in the diagnosis of acute osteomyelitis. The sedimentation rate is elevated in the vast majority of patients and exceeds 40 mm/hr in about 80%. This finding is helpful primarily in confirming that an inflammatory process is the source of symptoms. White blood cell counts, though sometimes elevated with a left shift in differential, may be normal in as much as 50% of patients and thus are less useful.

Radiographic changes lag behind the clinical manifestations and can be subtle. The first noticeable radiographic change, seen about 3 days after the onset of symptoms, is the presence of deep soft tissue swelling displacing fat lines adjacent to a metaphysis (Fig. 12-53, *A*). In the ensuing days the swelling increases to obliterate fascial planes and then extends to involve subcutaneous tissues. These soft tissue changes can be very difficult to appreciate whenever osteomyelitis involves bones of the trunk or pelvis; however, in cases of pelvic osteomyelitis, clouding of the obturator foramen, distortion of the fascial planes around the adjacent hip, or even displacement of the bladder may be detectable. If a sympathetic joint effusion is present or if rupture into the adjacent joint has resulted in secondary septic arthritis, joint space widening or bony displacement may be evident (Fig. 12-53, *B*). Bony changes are not visible radiographically in untreated patients until 7 to 10 days after onset. These changes consist of periosteal elevation followed by focal evidence of bony lysis and, subsequently, by sclerosis or new bone formation at the margins of the lytic lesion (Fig. 12-53, *C* to *E*). The radiographic appearance of bony changes can be significantly delayed in patients who are being treated with an antibiotic for infection at another site, and early diagnosis of osteomyelitis and the institution of appropriate antimicrobial therapy may completely prevent development of these findings.

Technetium scanning has provided a better means of early identification and localization of sites of acute osteomyelitis. It can show abnormalities as early as 24 to 48 hours after the onset of symptoms, revealing discrete areas of increased uptake (Fig. 12-54, *A*). The procedure has been particularly useful as a diagnostic adjunct in cases of pelvic and vertebral osteomyelitis in which the mode of presentation has simulated the clinical picture of another condition (Fig. 12-54, *B*; see Fig. 12-57, *C*). It also can be helpful in distinguishing osteomyelitis from cellulitis, septic arthritis, and acute bony infarcts. In cellulitis, intense deep soft tissue uptake with faint diffuse uptake in underlying bone is seen; in septic arthritis, the scan may be normal, or if the condition is accompanied by overlying cellulitis, the scan may show increased periarticular soft tissue uptake; in early infarcts, uptake is decreased. Scans also are helpful in delineating additional areas of involvement in the small percentage of patients with multiple sites. Standard radiographs remain important, however, in identifying fractures and malignancies, which may simulate the appearance of osteomyelitis on bone scans. Bone scans have the additional limitation of an occasional false-negative reading, possibly due to local ischemia. Whenever suspicion remains high on clinical grounds, a repeat technetium scan or a gallium scan (which identifies purulent exudate) should be considered or aspiration should be performed.

Vigorous attempts must be made to isolate the causative organism in order to optimize therapy on the basis of known sensitivities and a determination of bactericidal levels. Aspiration of the site of maximal tenderness or maximal uptake as revealed by bone scan can be very useful, in that it provides material for Gram's stain and culture. In cases

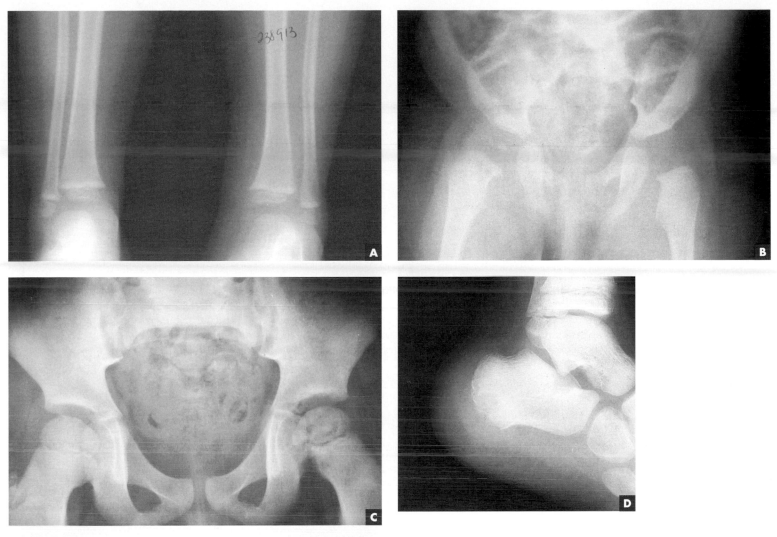

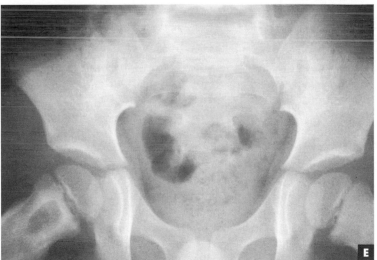

FIG. 12-53 Acute osteomyelitis. Radiographic changes lag behind the clinical manifestations in osteomyelitis. *A*, The first noticeable change, occurring about 3 days after onset, is deep soft tissue swelling, seen here adjacent to the metaphysis of the distal tibia on the left. *B*, In this neonate a radiolucency is evident in the proximal metaphysis of the right femur, which also is displaced upward and laterally. On aspiration of the hip, purulent fluid was obtained, confirming the suspicion of rupture of the infection into the hip and of secondary septic arthritis. *C*, The epiphysis and proximal metaphysis of the left femur have a moth-eaten appearance in this older child. *D*, Deep and superficial soft tissue swelling overlie the radiolucent lesion of the calcaneus in this boy who acquired *Pseudomonas* osteomyelitis after a puncture wound of the heel. *E*, The late changes of a lytic lesion with sclerotic margins are seen in the right femoral metaphysis of this child who was completing his course of therapy. (*A* courtesy Dr. Jocelyn Ledesma-Medina; *B*, *C*, and *E* courtesy Dr. Roderigo Dominguez; *D* courtesy Dr. Ellen Wald, Children's Hospital of Pittsburgh.)

in which purulent material is obtained, operative drainage should be considered strongly. Even in the absence of exudate, flushing the aspirating needle with culture media often will enable isolation of the causative organism. Blood cultures are positive in more than 50% of patients with acute hematogenous osteomyelitis and should be performed in all suspected cases.

Complications of osteomyelitis include secondary septic arthritis with resultant joint damage, epiphyseal injury with long-term morbid-ity resulting from impaired bone growth, progression to chronic osteomyelitis (now seen in less than 4% of cases), and rarely pathologic fractures. The rate of complications is highest in young infants who often have extensive bony involvement and secondary septic arthritis by the time the diagnosis is made. Care in clinical assessment and aggressive attempts to confirm the diagnosis of acute osteomyelitis as early as possible are as important in ensuring a good outcome and minimizing complications as are adequate antimicrobial therapy and recognition of

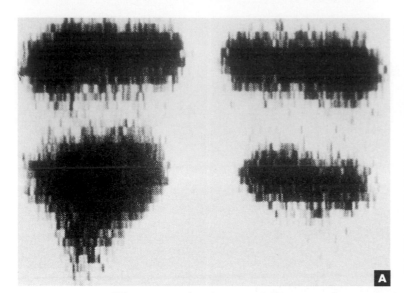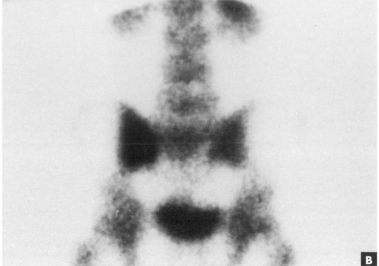

FIG. 12-54   Technetium scan findings in acute osteomyelitis. *A*, In this radionuclide scan, selectively increased uptake is seen in the proximal right tibial metaphysis. The uptake in the epiphyses is normal, reflecting active bone growth. *B*, This youngster showed a puzzling picture of abdominal pain suggestive of an acute abdomen. A bone scan was obtained after other studies were unrevealing. The increased uptake in the right sacroiliac area helped to identify osteomyelitis as the source of symptoms. (Courtesy Dr. Ellen Wald, Children's Hospital of Pittsburgh.)

the need for surgical intervention. Close collaboration between the primary care physician and orthopedic surgeon is essential to ensure that optimal decisions are made regarding the route and duration of pharmacotherapy and the need for and timing of surgical intervention, if indicated.

Subacute Osteomyelitis

Approximately 10% of cases of hematogenous osteomyelitis have an insidious onset and a subacute course, often characterized by mild to moderate local pain in an extremity, with or without swelling. Fever is unusual, and other systemic symptoms are absent. Typically the patient has had symptoms for a few to several weeks before presentation. In some instances this subacute course appears to be related to partial suppression of the infection by antibiotics that have been administered for infection at another site (such as for otitis media, tonsillitis, or impetigo). In these patients, pain may abate during the period of antimicrobial therapy, only to worsen once they stop taking the medication. In other cases in which antibiotics have not been prescribed, reduced bacterial virulence is postulated. Local tenderness is evident and overlying soft tissue swelling may be noted on examination. By the time diagnosis is made, multiple sites are involved in as many as 20% of patients. However, secondary sites may not be symptomatic.

Although white blood cell counts usually are normal, the sedimentation rate is elevated in most (but not all) patients. Blood cultures rarely are positive. Radiographs may show one of several possible findings. In children seen within a few weeks of onset who have taken antibiotics, radiographic findings may simulate the deep soft tissue swelling characteristic of early acute osteomyelitis. Other radiographic configurations include an isolated metaphyseal radiolucency surrounded by reactive bone (Brodie's abscess), a metaphyseal radiolucency with loss or disruption of cortical bone simulating a tumor, an excessive cortical reaction in the diaphysis simulating an osteoid osteoma, and multiple layers of subperiosteal new bone overlying the diaphysis, at times mimicking the appearance of Ewing's sarcoma (Fig. 12-55). Although a bone scan is not of great use in distinguishing subacute osteomyelitis from a primary bone tumor, it can be very help-

ful in revealing other sites of involvement. Because the long course, clinical picture, and radiographic findings of this infection often are indistinguishable from those of a neoplastic process, biopsy generally is required to establish the diagnosis and to isolate the causative organism. In the vast majority of cases, coagulase-positive staphylococci are found. Surgical curettage, immobilization, and antimicrobials are the mainstays of treatment.

Chronic Osteomyelitis

With the advent of antimicrobial therapy and improvements in diagnostic techniques, chronic osteomyelitis has become relatively rare in countries where there is ready access to medical care. Delay in diagnosis, inadequate antimicrobial or surgical therapy, and unusually resistant organisms are the major factors now associated with its development. Pathophysiologically, extensive necrosis, sequestrum formation as a result of bone death, and decompression caused by fistulization through the overlying soft tissues are characteristic findings (Fig. 12-56). Patients continue to be troubled by local pain of varying severity and by chronic draining sinuses. Aggressive surgical curettage and long-term antimicrobial therapy are required to achieve resolution, but despite this, permanent functional disability and deformity are not uncommon once osteomyelitis has become chronic.

Juvenile Discitis and Vertebral Osteomyelitis

Inflammation of an intervertebral disc space in childhood is a puzzling disorder, both in terms of its exact pathophysiology and its mode of presentation. Before the third decade of life, vascular channels penetrate through the vertebral end-plates and communicate with the intervertebral disc. Thus it is thought that hematogenously spread organisms are more likely to alight in the disc spaces of children and adolescents, whereas thereafter they may lodge in vascular arcades adjacent to the subchondral plate of the vertebra itself. This factor has been used to explain the higher frequency of discitis in children and the relative infrequency of acute vertebral osteomyelitis before adulthood. However, differences in the clinical picture, the less frequent isolation of pathogens, and evidence that immobilization alone is effective in

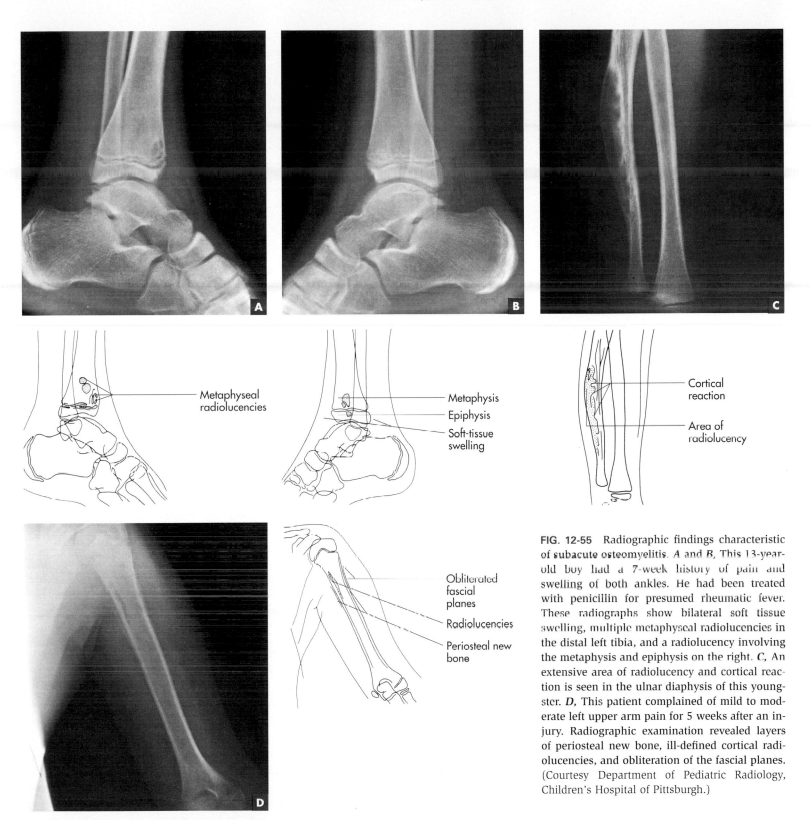

Metaphyseal
radiolucencies

Metaphysis
Epiphysis
Soft-tissue
swelling

Cortical
reaction

Area of
radiolucency

Obliterated
fascial
planes

Radiolucencies

Periosteal new
bone

FIG. 12-55 Radiographic findings characteristic of subacute osteomyelitis. *A* and *B*, This 13-year-old boy had a 7-week history of pain and swelling of both ankles. He had been treated with penicillin for presumed rheumatic fever. These radiographs show bilateral soft tissue swelling, multiple metaphyseal radiolucencies in the distal left tibia, and a radiolucency involving the metaphysis and epiphysis on the right. *C*, An extensive area of radiolucency and cortical reaction is seen in the ulnar diaphysis of this youngster. *D*, This patient complained of mild to moderate left upper arm pain for 5 weeks after an injury. Radiographic examination revealed layers of periosteal new bone, ill-defined cortical radiolucencies, and obliteration of the fascial planes. (Courtesy Department of Pediatric Radiology, Children's Hospital of Pittsburgh.)

treating discitis—while antimicrobial therapy is required in vertebral osteomyelitis—have led to speculation that disc space inflammation may be due to a low-grade viral or bacterial infection.

Known predisposing conditions in adults include urinary tract infections, pelvic inflammatory disease, and bowel and urinary tract surgery; in children they include upper respiratory tract infection, gastroenteritis, and genitourinary infection. The importance of antecedent trauma is unclear. Hematogenous spread may occur through the valveless veins of Batson's plexus or via the vertebral branches of the posterior spinal arteries. In both discitis and vertebral osteomyelitis, coagulase-positive staphylococci are the organisms most commonly isolated, followed by streptococci, gram-negative enteric pathogens, and corynebacteria. The lumbar spine and the lower thoracic spine are the most common sites of involvement for both entities.

The clinical picture of discitis, which is seen predominantly in children under 4 years of age, is dominated by pain and progressive limp.

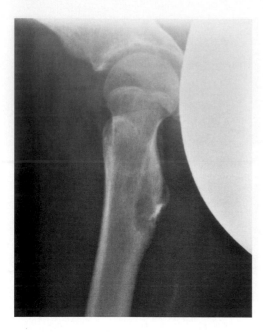

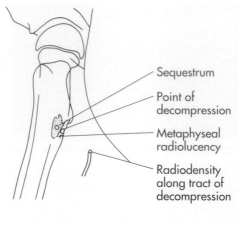

Sequestrum

Point of
decompression

Metaphyseal
radiolucency

Radiodensity
along tract of
decompression

FIG. 12-56 Chronic osteomyelitis. Inadequate initial treatment resulted in progression to chronic osteomyelitis in this child. In this radiograph, taken 6 months after the onset of symptoms, a radiodense sequestrum is seen within the metaphyseal radiolucency. The process also had begun to decompress into the soft tissues of the thigh. (Courtesy Department of Pediatric Radiology, Children's Hospital of Pittsburgh.)

Often the pain is perceived as a focal back pain that progressively worsens in severity. In a few instances it may be perceived as primarily worse in the flank, abdomen, or hip. It is constant; may be aggravated by sitting, standing, or movement; and typically is worse at night. Children who are too young to describe their pain may initially be irritable and refuse to walk or even sit. In some cases, increased irritability has been noted during diaper changes. Adoption of an abnormal posture is a frequent finding. Most commonly this posture is one of exaggerated lumbar lordosis, but in some cases the lumbar spine may be held stiff and straight. Toddlers may assume a knee-chest position. Fever often is present during the first week or two of symptoms, but it may be absent and often is low grade. Other systemic symptoms are unusual. Occasionally, abdominal distension is prominent, raising suspicion of intraabdominal pathology.

Failure to remember that vertebrospinal pathology may result in a limp or refusal to walk, and thus failure to examine carefully the backs of such patients, often results in long delays in diagnosis. Such examination may reveal paravertebral muscle spasm with guarding and exquisite focal tenderness, although in some cases tenderness may be vague or absent. Resistance to flexion and extension of the spine are common, and in the young may simulate meningeal signs. The loss of normal lumbar lordosis or the presence of local scoliosis may be noted early on. Pain on straight-leg raising and hip motion also may be encountered.

The sedimentation rate is elevated unless symptoms have been present for many months, but white blood cell counts are elevated only during the first few weeks. Specific radiographic changes do not appear until 2 to 6 weeks after onset, at which time disc space narrowing becomes evident. In ensuing weeks, irregularities of the adjacent vertebral end-plates become apparent. A technetium scan can reveal focal increased uptake as early as 1 week after the onset of symptoms. Culture of biopsy specimens of the disc space, when obtained early in the course, may yield an offending organism but commonly is negative after a few weeks of symptoms. Blood cultures rarely are positive. Most patients improve symptomatically with immobilization alone, and the process appears to resolve after several weeks of casting.

The clinical picture of vertebral osteomyelitis, seen in older children and adolescents, usually is one of the insidious onset of progressively worsening back pain that is constant, aggravated by movement, and increasingly resistant to analgesics. Usually fever is absent or low grade.

Occasionally the onset is acute, with fever and generalized systemic symptoms accompanying the abrupt appearance of pain. In the rare cases encountered in young children, onset usually is acute and the clinical picture dominated by abdominal or flank pain, with associated tenderness and often guarding. In some patients, paraspinous or spinous process tenderness, back stiffness, an exaggerated lumbar lordosis, and pain on leg motion or lower extremity weakness may be noted (Fig. 12-57). Laboratory findings in this setting are similar to those seen in children with discitis, with the exception that blood cultures obtained in the acute phase generally are positive. Early radiographic findings also are similar, but frank destructive lesions of the vertebral body are seen after the appearance of disc space narrowing. Cultures of operative biopsy specimens usually yield *S. aureus*. Antimicrobial therapy is necessary to achieve clinical resolution, and surgical debridement is more likely to be required.

Septic Arthritis

Bacterial invasion of the synovial membrane with resultant septic arthritis is a condition with a high potential for long-term morbidity. Release of lysosomal enzymes by attracted leukocytes, abscess formation, the development of granulation tissue, and ischemia resulting from increased intraarticular pressure act in concert to damage the articular surface and to promote synovial fibrosis and bony ankylosis. Early diagnosis and treatment are essential to prevent or at least minimize the extent of irreversible damage. This is hindered in many cases, however, by the fact that both the clinical picture and laboratory findings overlap with those seen in patients with viral and other forms of acute arthritis.

Septic arthritis is a disorder primarily affecting young children, with two thirds to three fourths of cases occurring in patients under 5 years of age. Males are affected twice as often as females. Ninety percent of cases are the result of hematogenous seeding in the course of bacteremia, and although in most cases the affected joint becomes the primary site of localization, it is not uncommon for septic arthritis to develop in a child with bacterial meningitis or pneumonia, often manifesting early in the course of treatment. As many as 40% of patients have a history or signs of an antecedent upper respiratory tract infection at the time of diagnosis. This is especially common in cases caused by *H. influenzae* type b. This organism was a major cause of septic

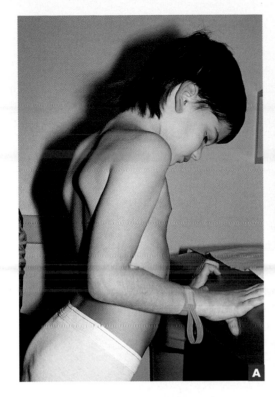

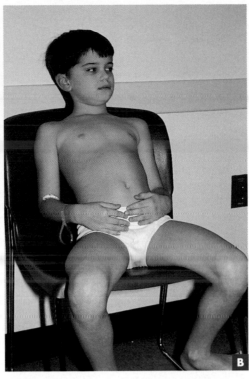

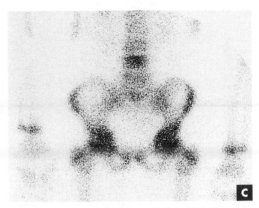

FIG. 12-57 Vertebral osteomyelitis. This 10-year-old boy had a 2-week history of intermittent fever, malaise, and steadily worsening lower back and left hip pain, exacerbated by movement. *A* and *B*, He had an exaggerated lumbar lordosis and extreme limitation of flexion, both standing and sitting. The straight leg–raising test also accentuated his pain. *C*, Bone scan revealed selectively increased uptake in the L4 vertebral body. (*C* courtesy the Department of Pediatric Radiology, Children's Hospital of Pittsburgh.)

TABLE 12-3

Relative Frequency of Pathogens in Septic Arthritis According to Age

Neonate	1 month–2 years	2-5 years	>5 years
S. aureus	Group A streptococci	*S. aureus*	*S. aureus*
Group B streptococci	*S. pneumoniae*	Group A streptococci	Group A streptococci
Gram-negative enteric pathogens	*N. meningitidis*	*N. meningitidis*	*N. gonorrhoeae*
	H. influenzae type b	*S. pneumoniae*	*P. aeruginosa*
	P. aeruginosa	*H. influenzae* type b	
	Salmonella species		

arthritis in toddlers before the widespread use of the Hib vaccine, but now its incidence is relatively low. Streptococcal skin and soft tissue infections may antedate septic arthritis caused by this pathogen. In older children and adolescents, gonococcal urethritis, vaginitis, and cervicitis assume importance as antecedents to hematogenous seeding (see Fig. 18-37, *D*). Prior trauma also may be a predisposing factor and is reported in a significant number of cases. In approximately 10% of patients, the septic arthritis is secondary to rupture of a primary osteomyelitis into the joint space. Direct penetrating injury accounts for a small percentage (see Chapter 21).

Bacterial pathogens are isolated in 65% to 75% of patients, either from synovial fluid, blood, or both. The relative frequency of pathogens varies considerably with patient age, as shown in Table 12-3. Children with sickle hemoglobinopathies occasionally suffer *Salmonella* septic arthritis. Failure to isolate an organism can be explained in some instances by suppression caused by prior antibiotic administration.

The knee, hip, elbow, and ankle are the joints most commonly affected. The wrist and shoulder are involved less often, with other joints being rare sites of septic arthritis. Only a single joint is affected in more than 90% of patients. *Neisseria gonorrhoeae* is the organism most com-

monly associated with multiple joint involvement, but other pathogens may be responsible, particularly coagulase-positive staphylococci and also *H. influenzae* type b. The hip and shoulder joints, if involved, are particularly prone to damage because clinical signs may be subtle and thus diagnosis often is delayed. Further, because the synovium inserts distal to the epiphysis of the proximal humerus and femur, compromise of the blood supply to the epiphysis is more likely to occur as a result of increased intraarticular pressure.

The typical clinical picture of hematogenous septic arthritis is one of a young child who presents with moderate to high fever and signs of toxicity, in association with severe localized joint pain, overlying swelling, and marked limitation in range of motion. The fever may be quite acute in onset or it may have been present for a few days, but the child tends to be seen soon after the onset of joint symptoms. Variations in this picture depend in part on the age of the patient, the joint involved, the causative organism, and the duration of symptoms. Infants and toddlers cannot describe focal pain and thus they tend to present with fever and irritability, the latter aggravated by movement. Refusal to bear weight or decreased use of an extremity may or may not have been noted by the family. When a knee, ankle, wrist, or elbow is

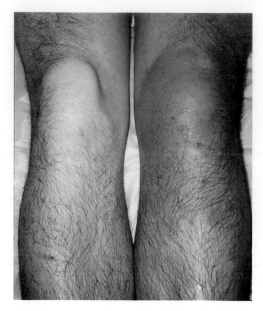

FIG. 12-58 Septic arthritis. This adolescent boy awoke suddenly at 3 A.M. with severe knee pain. By 8 A.M. he was febrile and had marked swelling with overlying erythema and extreme limitation of movement. Examination of joint fluid revealed gram-positive cocci in chains, with a white blood cell count of 24,000/mm³. Cultures were positive for group A streptococci. (Reprinted from the clinical slide collection on Rheumatic diseases ©1991, 1995. Used by permission of the American College of Rheumatology.)

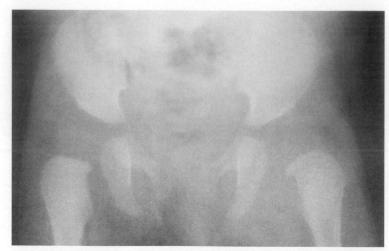

FIG. 12-59 Radiographic findings characteristic of septic arthritis. Although radiographs may be normal early on, joint space widening can be detected in most cases. In this infant who showed fever, toxicity, and refusal to move the left leg, capsular swelling and lateral displacement of the proximal left femur are readily apparent. (Courtesy Dr. Roderigo Dominguez, University of Texas.)

involved, local swelling and warmth usually are evident (Fig. 12-58). However, early on the swelling may be subtle and high fever may make any warmth hard to distinguish. Surface erythema often is absent. Whenever a hip is involved, swelling and warmth are not evident externally and pain may be referred to the knee or thigh. Often the position adopted by the patient is the best diagnostic clue. To minimize intraarticular pressure and pain, the child prefers to lie still with the knee and hip flexed and with the hip externally rotated (see Fig. 12-52). In cases of septic arthritis of the shoulder, subtle swelling may or may not be evident, but the shoulders may not be held at the same level and the arm on the involved side is held against the chest to splint the joint.

Septic arthritis of the sacroiliac joint (see Fig. 12-54, *B*), which accounts for about 1% of cases, can present a particularly confusing picture, often mimicking hip or intraabdominal disease. Only one third of patients have an acute presentation, and the remainder have a subacute course. Buttock pain, limp, and fever are the most common presenting complaints. As much as one third of patients complain of unilateral radicular pain. Findings of lower abdominal and rectal tenderness in association with normal hip motion may fool the examiner who fails to recognize that leg and buttock pain necessitate meticulous examination of the lower back. Such an examination will reveal tenderness over the involved sacroiliac joint, and pelvic compression will replicate the pain, as will hyperextension of the ipsilateral hip with the patient supine and dangling his or her leg over the edge of the table.

Limitation of joint motion and evidence of pain on motion are perhaps the most valuable clinical clues to the diagnosis of septic arthritis. Limitation usually is severe unless presentation occurs very early, and motion provokes marked discomfort. In young patients with fever and decreased use of an extremity but without clear-cut swelling, localization often is possible if, after careful inspection and palpation for bony tenderness, each joint is gently moved while the examiner carefully guards the other joints, without touching them. Diagnosis can be particularly difficult in neonates and very young infants, who may be afebrile and often have no systemic symptoms. In such cases, decreased use of an extremity often is the earliest clue. Pain on motion usually is evident, however, even before the appearance of localized swelling.

When septic arthritis is the result of rupture of a focus of osteomyelitis into a joint, distinction between the two processes can be very difficult to establish clinically. Focal pain generally is of longer duration, but because most cases occur in infants under 8 months of age, this clue often is unavailable. In older children the hip, shoulder, and ankle are the major sites of this secondary form of septic arthritis. These children usually have a history of prolonged focal pain, antedating a brief period of respite, followed by the sudden return of pain that is markedly aggravated by joint motion. In the days following a penetrating joint injury, a sudden increase in pain and swelling should prompt immediate suspicion of secondary septic arthritis.

Because of the high cost of delays in diagnosis in terms of morbidity, any child with fever, acute onset of pain, and limited motion of a joint should be presumed to have septic arthritis until proved otherwise. These findings should prompt expeditious diagnostic investigation. Plain radiographs with comparison views should be obtained without delay and inspected carefully for even subtle signs of joint space widening or capsular distension, although findings may be normal in early cases. If the hip is the suspected site of pathology, lateral and upward displacement of the femoral head may be noted along with displacement of the gluteal fat lines (Fig. 12-59). A bone scan is perhaps the best method of evaluating the child with suspected septic arthritis of the sacroiliac joint and is also useful in identifying patients with underlying osteomyelitis.

Arthrocentesis should be considered early, as examination of joint fluid is the study most likely to yield definitive results. A heparinized syringe should be used to prevent spontaneous clotting. Positive findings on Gram's stained specimens are particularly helpful; cultures are positive in 60% or more of cases. Pleocytosis is common, with two thirds of patients having a white blood cell count of more than 50,000/mm³. It is crucial to remember, however, that there is considerable overlap with nonbacterial arthritis in terms of the cell counts, differential counts, and protein and glucose levels found on examination of synovial fluid. Thus septic arthritis cannot be ruled out if these values are within the normal range.

Peripheral white blood cell counts and sedimentation rate may add suggestive evidence, but again there is overlap with viral arthritis. As

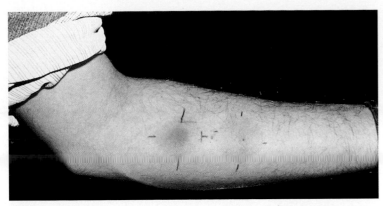

FIG. 12-60 Positive tuberculin skin test. This adolescent boy became infected as a result of living with and helping to care for a grandfather whose chronic "smoker's cough" was ultimately discovered to be a manifestation of chronic cavitary tuberculosis. He had a greater than 15-mm induration. (Courtesy Dr. Kenneth Schuitt.)

many as 20% of patients have white blood cell counts under 10,000/mm³, although most have a significant leftward shift. The sedimentation rate may be markedly elevated, but it is under 40 mm/hr in as many as 45% of patients. Blood cultures are positive in up to 40% of cases. Counterimmunoelectrophoresis studies may be helpful in identifying the responsible pathogen before culture results are available and in cases in which cultures prove negative.

Diagnosis thus is dependent on assessment of the assembled data, including clinical course, physical findings, and results of multiple laboratory studies. Even with negative findings on Gram's stain, empiric antimicrobial therapy selected to cover the most likely pathogens (see Table 12-3) should be started, pending culture results, in patients in whom septic arthritis is deemed likely on the basis of the available findings. As is true of osteomyelitis, collaboration between pediatric and orthopedic colleagues is essential, for drainage of infected material is essential to ensuring a good outcome.

Any disorder associated with acute arthritis must be considered as part of the differential diagnosis. In some instances the clinical picture of an obvious viral or vasculitic syndrome enables differentiation. The polymigratory picture of acute rheumatic fever and the much less acute onset of juvenile rheumatoid arthritis help to distinguish these conditions. Adenopathy, visceromegaly, anemia, and radiographic changes help distinguish malignant joint infiltration.

Tuberculosis

After decades of steady decline, tuberculosis has shown a disturbing increase in incidence in the United States over the past several years. This appears to be related to a combination of factors: the HIV epidemic (which predisposes to the reactivation of prior infection and to the development of active and rapidly progressive disease with new infection); a decline in the services of departments of public health; the rise in the homeless population and of barriers in access to health care; and an increase in the immigration of people from places where tuberculosis is prevalent. Worldwide, famine, war, and natural disasters that create large numbers of refugees; crowded living and working conditions;

and sweat-shop–type labor practices involving long working hours and the employment of child laborers spawn conditions that favor the acquisition of tuberculosis and its spread. In addition, poor compliance with long treatment regimens had led to increased transmission of ever-more-resistant organisms. High-risk groups in the United States include people from ethnic and racial minority groups, especially of low socioeconomic status living in overcrowded conditions in populous urban areas; immigrants and foreign-born adoptees from Southeast Asia, China, Latin America, Haiti, and eastern Europe; the homeless; migrant workers; elderly persons living in nursing homes; prisoners in correctional institutions; HIV-positive or immunosuppressed people; children in close contact with adults in these groups; and health care professionals. Most are located in seven states—California, Florida, Georgia, Illinois, New York, South Carolina, and Texas (border states or states with large immigrant populations or large pockets of people living in extreme poverty).

Transmission

Tubercle bacilli are transmitted from person to person, with the usual source an adult or adolescent with active pulmonary, especially cavitary, disease. When the infectious adult or teenager coughs, sneezes, or laughs, infected mucous droplets containing a myriad of organisms are propelled into the air and, once airborne, can be inhaled by those around them. Children with primary tuberculous disease rarely transmit infection because they have a relatively small number of organisms, if any, in endobronchial secretions and are rarely able to cough forcefully enough to expel them.

Infants and toddlers living with or in close contact with an infectious adult and adolescents and young adults helping to care for infectious people are at especially high risk for infection. Thus, parents, grandparents, older siblings, nannies and sitters, housekeepers, and boarders are the major sources of transmission to children. Less often, teachers, school bus drivers, coaches, and nurses have been source cases.

The portal of entry in more than 98% of instances is the lung; it is estimated that the inhalation of as few as one to three bacilli in a single aerosolized droplet can result in infection. Rarely a superficial skin or mucous membrane lesion may be the site of inoculation. Congenital infection can occur if a pregnant woman experiences lymphohematogenous spread during gestation or has tuberculous endometritis. Health care professionals are at particular risk when handling specimens of infected secretions or body fluids and contaminated syringes or instruments such as lavage tubes and bronchoscopes.

Pathogenesis

Once the organism has gained entry, there is a silent period of incubation lasting from 3 to 10 weeks. The larger the inoculum, the shorter the incubation period and the more severe the signs and symptoms of the primary infection. The end of the incubation period is marked by the development of hypersensitivity to the organism, as manifested by a positive PPD skin test (Fig. 12-60) and the onset of fever of 1 to 3 weeks' duration. During this time, the patient's inflammatory response intensifies in the *primary complex*, which has three components: (1) the primary focus or site at which the bacilli have lodged (usually a subpleural alveolus, which can be at any site in either lung), (2) the inflamed lymphatics which drain the area, and (3) inflamed regional lymph nodes. Macrophages migrate to the primary focus, transform into epithelioid cells, and gather into clusters, forming a tubercle. If the host's immune response is effective, the lesion is walled off, then gradually resolves and disappears. If the host response is less effective,

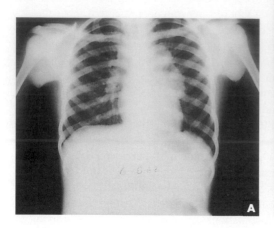
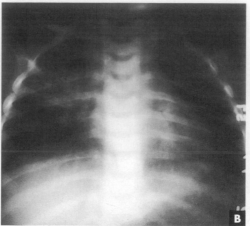
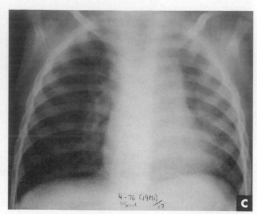
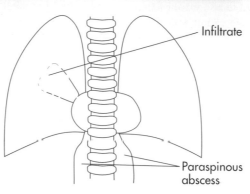

Infiltrate

Paraspinous
abscess

FIG. 12-61 Primary pulmonary tuberculosis. *A,* Marked enlargement of hilar nodes without a pulmonary infiltrate is seen in this asymptomatic child. She was tested as part of a contact investigation, and this chest x-ray was obtained because her skin test was positive. *B,* A hazy infiltrate involving a segment of the right upper lobe is seen extending from the hilum to the pleura. This child also has tuberculous spondylitis with a paraspinous abscess, the shadow of which is seen below the diaphragm. *C,* In this boy who presented with a pneumonic clinical picture, a hazy infiltrate occupies the entire left upper lobe. (*A* and *B* courtesy Dr. Jocelyn Medina; *C* courtesy Dr. Richard Towbin, Children's Hospital of Pittsburgh.)

bacilli multiply and the primary focus can caseate centrally. Thereafter, organisms in the lesion can travel along lymphatics to regional nodes, provoking more inflammation along the track and in the nodes. Infection can then spread by way of other lymphatics to more distant nodes—most commonly the paratracheal, anterior cervical, and abdominal nodes. New foci may heal, become dormant with the risk of later reactivation, or progress.

Affected nodes that enlarge and caseate can cause numerous complications. For example, hilar nodes pressing on an adjacent bronchus set up inflammation in its wall, leading to partial obstruction as the result of a combination of compression and edema collection. Occasionally the inflammatory process damages the cartilaginous rings, resulting in secondary collapse. In other cases it progresses to perforate the bronchial wall, releasing caseous material into the lumen, which may form an obstructive plug or provoke the formation of granulation tissue, or the organisms released from the caseous material may then travel through the airways to infect other parts of the lung. Rupture of a caseous subpleural primary focus or node results in pleural effusion. Enlarged caseous subcarinal nodes may compress the esophagus, causing dysphagia or rupture into it and producing a bronchoesophageal fistula. Infected nodes can compress the subclavian vein, resulting in edema of the ipsilateral upper extremity, compress the recurrent laryngeal or phrenic nerves, rupture into the mediastinum, or erode into adjacent blood vessels, setting the stage for miliary spread. The host's ability to mount an effective response to inhibit replication of tubercle bacilli and contain the primary infection depends on several factors. Very young children, malnourished children, adolescent girls, pregnant women, and immunodeficient or immunosuppressed people are at particular risk for progression of disease. Recent infection, especially with pertussis or viruses such as measles, influenza, and varicella, also increases the susceptibility to tuberculous infection and progression. Ge-

netic selection for resistance in populations living in endemic areas and acquired resistance appear to be somewhat protective.

Clinical Forms of Tuberculosis

Infection without Disease
Patients with this preclinical form of tuberculosis have a positive skin test reaction but no clinical signs and symptoms of disease and normal chest x-ray study findings. Although many of these children never manifest signs of primary infection, if the infection goes unrecognized and untreated, they have a 5% to 10% chance of reactivation of their tuberculosis later in life; thus they serve as a major reservoir. Other patients in this category simply have been identified very early and will go on to suffer clinical disease without treatment.

Tuberculous Disease
Patients who have evidence of tuberculosis on chest x-ray or clinical signs and symptoms of pulmonary or extrapulmonary infection are said to have disease. The risk of developing disease after infection exceeds 40% for infants, is 24% to 25% for children between 1 and 10 years of age, and is 15% for those between 11 and 15 years of age.

Primary Pulmonary Tuberculosis. The symptoms of primary pulmonary tuberculosis, which are typically insidious in onset, are often attributed to viral illness. Some children have low-grade fever with no apparent source, together with mild anorexia and decreased activity. Others may have associated rhinorrhea, nasal congestion, and pharyngeal erythema and are mistakenly thought to have a viral upper respiratory tract infection. On occasion, erythema nodosum may develop in concert with the fever. Chest examination is generally normal, even in patients with abnormal chest radiographs. Rarely children present with a more dramatic "pneumonic" mode of onset, with high fever, tachy-

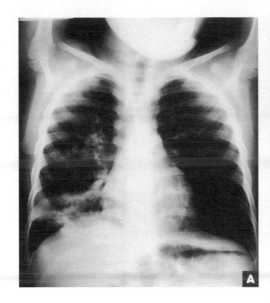

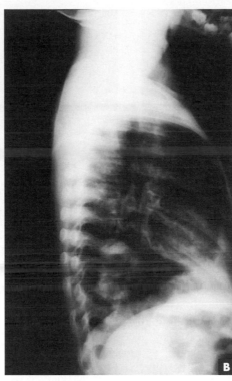

FIG. 12-62 Progressive primary pulmonary tuberculosis. This 8-year-old girl initially had fever, cough, and mild tachypnea. She was treated with antibiotics for presumed bacterial pneumonia but showed only partial clinical improvement. A repeat x-ray obtained a month later showed progression. A PPD test was then done and was positive. She has a collapse-consolidation lesion involving the right lower lobe, with a primary cavity. (Courtesy Dr. Ellen Wald, Children's Hospital of Pittsburgh.)

pnea, and signs of toxicity. In such cases the clinical findings are those characteristic of lobar pneumonia, with rales, rhonchi, and bronchial breath sounds heard on auscultation and dullness noted on percussion. Patients with either mode of onset tend to show improvement over a few days to a few weeks, though some may be noted to tire easily and be slightly less active than usual. Without specific treatment, some develop low-grade afternoon fevers weeks later that may persist for as long as a few months.

Radiographic findings characteristic of primary pulmonary tuberculosis may be limited to enlarged hilar (Fig. 12-61, *A*) or carinal nodes (seen best on lateral views); faint, cloudy infiltrates which extend to the pleura (Fig. 12-61, *B*); or a lobar infiltrate (Fig. 12-61, *C*) in patients exhibiting the "pneumonic" picture. Infiltrates contain the primary complex and, like it, can be located anywhere in either lung.

ENDOBRONCHIAL TUBERCULOSIS. When enlarged nodes cause bronchial obstruction (usually 3 to 6 months after infection, and most commonly in children under 2 years of age), focal hyperaeration or fan-shaped, segmental parenchymal *collapse-consolidation infiltrates* are seen (see Fig. 12-62). The latter consist of the primary focus and secondary inflammation and atelectasis. Sometimes narrowing of a bronchial lumen is noted. Infants affected by this endobronchial process often have a harsh, paroxysmal cough which mimics that of pertussis, along with wheezing and rhonchi noted on auscultation. The cough is often worse when the infant is lying supine than when prone. Respiratory distress may be noted during the course of an intercurrent infection. Older children generally have no cough but can manifest the auscultatory findings. With or without treatment, consolidation-collapse lesions can reexpand and resolve, clear with residual calcification of the primary complex and regional node (Ghon complex), or go on to scarring, with progressive contraction of the involved pulmonary segment in association with bronchiectatic changes. Calcification may persist, or start re-

sorbing within a few years. Occasionally, it progresses to ossification and formation of true bone.

PLEURAL EFFUSION. Rupture of a caseous subpleural, primary focus or lymph node can also occur 3 to 6 months after initial infection, but this usually occurs in school-age children. The caseous material provokes an intense pleural reaction with the formation of a proteinaceous effusion. This can be localized or generalized. Pleural effusion can also result from hematogenous spread or from direct extension of infection from a subpleural focus. Clinically development of pleural effusion is heralded by the abrupt onset of fever, chest pain, and shortness of breath and manifested by decreased chest wall movement and decreased breath sounds, dullness to percussion, and egophony on examination. When the effusion is massive, respiratory distress is evident. Pleural fluid is usually clear or slightly cloudy, greenish-yellow, often blood tinged, very high in protein, and usually low in glucose. Leukocytes predominate early, lymphocytes, later, with counts ranging from 300 to 10,000 cells/mm^3. Bacilli are present in very small numbers. Radiographs may show clouding of a lower lung field with obliteration of the diaphragm or, in the event of massive effusion, total "white-out" of the lung with mediastinal shift.

PROGRESSIVE PRIMARY PULMONARY TUBERCULOSIS. Progressive primary pulmonary tuberculosis occurs in infants and young children whose primary focus steadily enlarges, caseates, liquefies, and empties its bacilli-laden contents into a bronchus. The organisms then disseminate through the airways to the rest of the lung, setting up new foci of infection. Clinically these patients have remittant fever, cough, apathy, and malaise, along with anorexia and weight loss. Over time they begin to appear listless and chronically ill. Wet rales may be heard over the site of the primary cavity. Radiographically a small cavity is seen at the site of primary focus, along with a collapse-consolidation lesion (Fig. 12-62) and later diffuse infiltrates. On rare occasion, a large

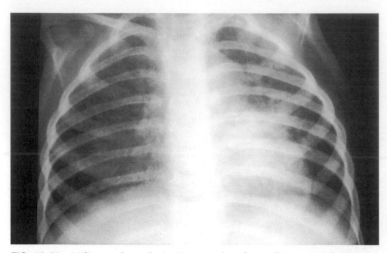

FIG. 12-63 Miliary tuberculosis. Two weeks after miliary spread, this infant's lung fields are symmetrically dotted with tiny tubercles. (Courtesy Dr. Richard Towbin, Children's Hospital of Pittsburgh.)

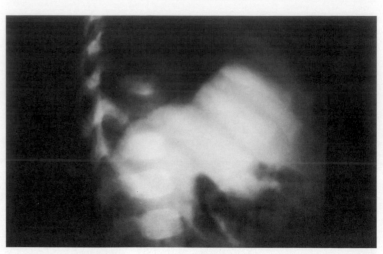

FIG. 12-64 Tuberculous spondylitis. Extensive bony destruction of the T12 vertebral body along with mild collapse of T11 is seen. (Courtesy Dr. Jocelyn Medina.)

caseous, primary focus can cause a pneumothorax, bronchopleural fistula, or caseous pyothorax if it ruptures into the pleura, or it may rupture into the mediastinum, after which caseous material may track upward to the supraclavicular fossa.

Lymphohematogenous Spread and Miliary Tuberculosis. Miliary tuberculous occurs when bacilli are disseminated from an involved node of the primary complex by means of the bloodstream to distant sites. In some patients this is clinically occult and occurs early during the incubation period or shortly thereafter. Major sites of seeding include the pulmonary apices, spleen, and superficial nodes. In some cases, evidence of resulting metastatic lesions is seen 2 to 4 months later, when the child has a nonspecific illness characterized by low-grade fever and fatigue, splenomegaly, and generalized adenopathy, sometimes associated with papulonecrotic skin lesions. Others remain asymptomatic and their metastatic lesions may either remain dormant or reactivate years later.

Acute miliary spread occurs in some patients (usually within 6 months of infection) when a caseous node ruptures directly into a vessel. Organisms in seeded foci may die, set up new foci that are then walled off and become dormant, or may progress, expand, and cause further complications. Miliary disease may be detected incidentally in an infant or child who undergoes chest radiography as part of evaluation for low-grade fever without an apparent source. Other children experience insidious progression of symptoms following intercurrent measles, influenza, or pertussis; still others may have a more abrupt onset of fever, tachypnea, lethargy, and weakness accompanied by hepatosplenomegaly. Within a few weeks, symmetric tubercles of uniform size are seen throughout the lung fields (Fig. 12-63) and rustling breath sounds can be heard on auscultation. Skin lesions, which may be nodular, purpuric, or papulonecrotic, may appear as well.

Still other children exhibit a process known as *protracted hematogenous spread,* which involves repeated episodes of release of organisms into the bloodstream. These patients have high sustained or spiking fever, leukocytosis (with counts up to 40,000/mm³), and marked, generalized, nontender adenopathy, and they look quite ill. Within a few weeks, mottled pulmonary lesions of varying size are seen. Polyserositis and multiple bony lesions tend to develop, along with crops of papulonecrotic skin lesions, which form after each episode of seeding.

Extrapulmonary Tuberculosis

TUBERCULOSIS MENINGITIS. Following lymphohematogenous or miliary spread, caseous foci may develop in the brain and meninges. Fifty per-

cent of infants and children with miliary tuberculosis go on to develop meningitis. Extension of infection or rupture of one of these foci into the subarachnoid space results in tuberculous meningitis, which usually develops within 3 to 6 months of initial infection in children under 6 years of age. The resulting exudate is thick and gelatinous. It infiltrates meningeal and cerebral vessels, causing vasculitis with secondary occlusion and infarction; it impedes CSF flow and resorption, often resulting in a communicating hydrocephalus; and it collects at the base of the brain, impinging on the optic chiasm and the third, sixth, and seventh cranial nerves.

Often preceded by a viral illness or head injury, the onset of symptoms is usually gradual, beginning with anorexia, fever, pronounced apathy, irritability, and emotional lability, often with headache. Within a week or two, drowsiness, vomiting, meningismus, a sluggish pupillary response, and cranial nerve palsies supervene, often accompanied by hyperreflexia and seizures. Confusion, disorientation, dysarthria, tremors, and athetosis are other findings that may be seen during this phase. Untreated, the child progresses to coma, the syndrome of inappropriate antidiuretic hormone, opisthotonic or decerebrate posturing, Cushing's triad, and death. CSF pressure is usually elevated, and the fluid is clear (though often xanthochromic); cell counts range from 50 to 500 cells/mm³, with leukocytes predominating early and lymphocytes later. The protein content is elevated (often markedly), and glucose levels are usually low. Early diagnosis and the institution of antituberculous therapy can significantly reduce morbidity and mortality, but even with treatment, complications are common in survivors.

SKELETAL TUBERCULOSIS. Skeletal tuberculosis is an extrapulmonary manifestation seen in 1% to 6% of children with untreated primary infection; it becomes clinically evident within 6 months to 3 years after the initial infection. Very young children are at greatest risk because of the high rate of blood flow through their growing bones. It can start as a metaphyseal endarteritis following hematogenous seeding; it can develop by means of extension from lymphatics, especially from a paravertebral node to a vertebra; or it can arise as the result of direct local or hematogenous spread from a neighboring bone.

Formation of granulation tissue and caseation characterize the inflammatory process, which ultimately results in pressure necrosis and the formation of a cold abscess, which can then rupture into an adjacent joint or surrounding soft tissues (see Fig. 12-61, *B*). The vertebrae, bones about the knee and hip, and, in infants, the phalanges, are the most common sites involved. Other than the phalanges, involvement of

TABLE 12-4

Risk Factors for Positive PPD Test

Degree of induration that represents a positive test	Risk factors
≥5 mm of induration	Known close recent contact with an infected patient
	HIV positive
	Chest x-ray showing old healed lesions
≥10 mm of induration	High-risk racial or ethnic group
	Less than 2 years of age
	Diabetes mellitus
	Currently taking steroids or immunosuppressive agents
	Malignancy
≥15 mm of induration	No risk factors

non–weight-bearing bones is unusual. As is often the case with osteomyelitis, a history of antecedent trauma before the onset of symptoms is frequently obtained. Fever is absent or low grade, unless the lesions develop as part of the process of protracted hematogenous spread. Pain is often relatively mild in comparison with that associated with bacterial osteomyelitis.

Tuberculous spondylitis usually involves the vertebral bodies of two or more thoracic vertebrae but can affect lumbar vertebrae as well. Clinically, nocturnal pain, manifested by crying in the night and restless sleep; low-grade fever; and later postural change (stiff back, kyphosis) and gait disturbance (with all weight-bearing joints kept slightly flexed) are prominent (patients with lumbar disease adopt a wide-based stance and gait). Pain may be localized to the back or referred to the chest or abdomen. When cervical vertebrae are affected, pain may be localized to the neck or referred to the occiput or arms; the child may have difficulty holding up his or her head, and torticollis is often present. Occasionally an opisthotonic posture is adopted. On examination, severe paraspinous muscle spasm, marked limitation of flexion, pain on percussion, and hyperreflexia with clonus may be evident. When there is an associated paraspinous abscess, swelling and fluctuance may be noted adjacent to the site of maximal tenderness. Initially radiographs show slight disc space narrowing; subsequently this is followed by mild wedging and partial collapse of the vertebral body. Later, bony destruction (Fig. 12-64) and ultimately pancake collapse of the vertebral body occur, resulting in kyphotic angulation—Pott's disease. Complications include paravertebral, psoas, and retropharyngeal abscesses as well as neurologic abnormalities secondary to associated spinal cord compression (which, because the spinal canal widens caudally, is more likely the higher the level of the vertebrae involved), inflammation, and vasculitis.

Involvement of bones about the knee results in pain, stiffness, and limp, which can be intermittent. Limitation of motion varies depending on the extent of associated synovial inflammation. Unilateral thigh or knee pain and limp are the most common modes of presentation of acetabular or proximal femoral disease.

The dactylitis seen in infancy is characterized by painless fusiform swelling of the fingers or toes. Radiographically, affected phalanges, and sometimes metacarpals, initially show fusiform enlargement and increased density. Later, cystic changes are seen.

TUBERCULOUS PERICARDITIS. Seen in less than 5% of children with progressive pulmonary tuberculosis, tuberculous pericarditis can result from direct invasion of organisms from an adjacent infected lymph node, from rupture of an adjacent primary focus into the pericardial sac, or from lymphatic spread from subcarinal nodes. A hemorrhagic exudate collects and may progress to tamponade. Patients tend to have low-grade fever, anorexia, and rarely chest pain. On examination a pericardial friction rub is usually apparent; with large effusions, heart sounds are diminished and a narrow pulse pressure is noted.

TUBERCULOUS ADENITIS. Tuberculous adenitis is discussed in the earlier section Infectious Lymphadenitis.

TUBERCULOSIS IN ADOLESCENCE. Adolescents may suffer a primary infection or experience reactivation of earlier disease. The latter is more likely if the primary infection occurred after 7 years of age. The period of the adolescent growth spurt, especially in girls of low socioeconomic status, is the time when the risk of the reactivation or the development of progressive primary disease is greatest. With reactivation, the new lesion develops in the same lobe as the old primary complex and tends to remain localized; there is a relatively low risk of hematogenous spread or extension to regional nodes because of prior development of hypersensitization. Affected patients have cough and fever, often accompanied by chest pain, and may exhibit hemoptysis. Anorexia with weight loss and easy fatigability are common. Chest findings may be normal early on, but moist rales may be heard over the apices after cough or on end-expiration. Small round or wedge-shaped infiltrates or linear streaks with mottling may be evident on chest x-ray. This and progressive primary disease can rapidly become chronic cavitary disease within a few years if appropriate treatment is not instituted.

With progression, weight loss and fatigue increase and an early morning cough productive of increasing amounts of sputum becomes bothersome. Daily fevers and night sweats are common, and an appearance of chronic illness supervenes. Wet rales, bronchial breath sounds, wheezing, and dullness to percussion are typical physical findings. Radiographs may reveal mottling, patchy infiltrates, segmental or lobar opacification, and cavitary changes, which may be unilateral or bilateral.

Tuberculin Testing

The gold standard of skin testing for tuberculosis is the Mantoux test with 5 tuberculin units (0.1 ml) of purified protein derivative (PPD). This is injected intradermally on the volar surface of the forearm, with the needle bevel up and oriented perpendicularly to the long axis of the arm. After injection, which when done properly, raises a weal, the 27-gauge needle should be left in for a few seconds to prevent leakage from the injection site. The test should be read by a health care professional 48 to 72 hours later; this is done by measuring the diameter of any induration that develops at the site, again at a right angle to the long axis of the arm (Fig. 12-60). The test is rarely negative in infected children; anergy is seen only in those who have overwhelming infection or are immunosuppressed and is occasionally seen in a child with an intercurrent viral infection. Use of multiple puncture tests as screening tools should be abandoned, because they cannot be standardized and can cause a high rate of false-positive results on subsequent PPD testing as the result of a booster phenomenon.

Recently, interpretation of a positive test has been changed on the basis of associated risk factors (Table 12-4).

Case Finding

The most efficient and cost-effective means of identifying infected children is through contact investigation of persons known to be in close contact with an adolescent or adult with pulmonary tuberculosis. Conversely, if a child is found to be positive, his or her household members and others in close contact should be tested to find the source case.

Because of the low prevalence of tuberculosis in most parts of the United States, routine yearly skin testing is not indicated. However, children from high-risk groups should be tested yearly and all new immigrants should undergo PPD testing.

Diagnosis

Most children with tuberculosis are diagnosed by means of skin testing as a result of contact investigations prompted by identification of an infectious adult. Cultures remain essential, however, for diagnosis and for the management of patients with infection and disease. However, in young children with primary pulmonary tuberculosis, sputum is unavailable for culture, the yield from early-morning gastric aspirates is only about 40%, and the yield from specimens obtained by bronchoscopy is often not much better. Hence, cultures of sputum and gastric aspirates from the source case adult, which have a much higher yield, are often the best means of obtaining the organisms and testing their susceptibility to antituberculous drugs, thereby guiding selection of the drug regimen.

Other specimens that can be used for cultures include pleural fluid and preferably a pleural punch biopsy specimen from patients with pleural effusion; CSF from patients with meningitis; lymph node biopsy specimens or aspirates from patients with adenitis; bone marrow biopsy or liver biopsy specimens from patients with miliary disease or protracted hematogenous spread; joint fluid or synovial biopsy specimens from patients with tuberculous arthritis; and skin biopsy specimens from patients with cutaneous lesions.

Treatment Principles

Appropriate therapy with antituberculous drugs prevents the development of disease in children who have infection without disease, and it halts the progression and prevents complications in those with primary pulmonary disease. Treatment has also proved very effective in managing progressive pulmonary and extrapulmonary forms of tuberculosis and in reducing their morbidity and mortality. Further, it dramatically reduces the risk of subsequent reactivation. In infectious adults and adolescents, therapy is aimed not only at managing the disease, but at rendering the person noninfectious as quickly as possible.

Tubercle bacilli thrive in large numbers in the well-oxygenated environment of an open pulmonary cavity but replicate much more slowly, sometimes intermittently, or become dormant in caseous lesions and within macrophages. Naturally resistant organisms are routinely found in patients with large populations of organisms. Therefore, agents are selected for their ability to kill (bactericidal) organisms in differing environments and to prevent the development of secondary drug resistance (bacteriostatic). The choice and number of drugs and duration of therapy are determined by the stage and severity of the disease at diagnosis, by epidemiologic data regarding the likelihood of drug resistance, and if available, results of cultures and susceptibility testing. The course of therapy must be lengthy (even with new shorter regimens) to ensure that slowly growing bacilli are eliminated and to give the patient's own host resistance time to kill organisms that persist, despite therapy. This necessitates close follow-up and the support of health care workers to facilitate compliance; in some cases, direct supervision of medication administration is necessary.

Children who have been exposed to an infectious adult, even those with negative PPD tests, are treated with a single drug for 3 to 4 months, then undergo another PPD test. If the test is again negative, medication is stopped. A single agent, taken for 9 months, usually suf-

fices in eradicating infection in patients who have infection without disease. Children with primary pulmonary tuberculosis are treated first with a combination of three drugs for 2 months, then with two drugs to complete a 6- to 9-month course. Those with milder forms of extrapulmonary disease are treated similarly, but for 9 to 12 months. Patients with tuberculous meningitis and those suspected of having resistant organisms are treated initially with four medications, pending the results of susceptibility tests, and treatment is continued for a minimum of 12 months.

Administration of corticosteroids in concert with antituberculous agents decreases the severity of the inflammatory response and attendant vasculitis, and thereby reduces morbidity and mortality in patients with severe complications, such as meningitis, miliary disease with alveolar-capillary block, massive pericardial and pleural effusions, and marked hilar adenopathy that produces respiratory embarrassment.

Congenital and Perinatal Infections

Numerous pathogens that produce relatively mild or even subclinical disease in children and adults can cause severe disease with devastating sequelae in children who acquire such infections prenatally or perinatally. Toxoplasmosis, rubella, cytomegalic inclusion disease, herpes simplex infection (the TORCH diseases), and congenital syphilis are well-known sources of pathology. In addition, sepsis, meningitis, pneumonia, and other infections caused by numerous perinatally acquired bacterial pathogens are the cause of significant neonatal morbidity and mortality, especially in infants born prematurely. Because of the breadth of this subject and because of limitations of space, we have elected to limit discussion to three disorders that tend to produce distinctive physical findings.

Congenital Toxoplasmosis

Toxoplasma gondii is an intracellular protozoan that is acquired primarily from the consumption of infected raw or undercooked meat, or from the ingestion or inhalation of oocysts excreted in cat feces. Occasionally, transmission occurs by means of transfusion or organ transplantation. Although most cases of postnatal infection are thought to be subclinical, a mononucleosis-like syndrome and cervical adenopathy have been identified as clinical features, and it may well be that in many cases the clinical picture simulates a viral illness and thus the true cause goes unrecognized.

Prenatally acquired infection has the potential to cause serious harm to the developing fetus. It is estimated that in the United States 1 to 2 per 1000 live-born infants have congenitally acquired toxoplasmosis. Maternal infection during pregnancy results in fetal infection less than 50% of the time, however. The risk of transmission to the fetus increases as gestation advances, but the severity of fetal injury is greater the earlier the infection occurs during pregnancy. Major sites of involvement are the CNS, retina, choroid, and muscles. Seventy percent of congenitally infected infants appear normal at birth, about 10% to 20% are overtly symptomatic, and approximately 10% have detectable chorioretinitis without other abnormalities (see Chapter 19). Infected infants without signs of disease and those with mild chorioretinitis alone are at risk for progressive ocular and, on occasion, CNS involvement if the infection is not diagnosed and treated. In many instances, however, the diagnosis is not suspected until signs of visual impairment, strabismus, or developmental delay prompt careful ophthalmologic and neurologic assessment.

In severely affected infants, the clinical picture may closely simulate that of other congenital infections, especially cytomegalovirus. These

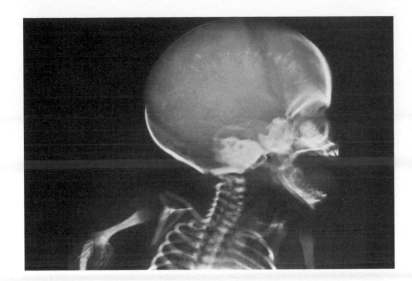

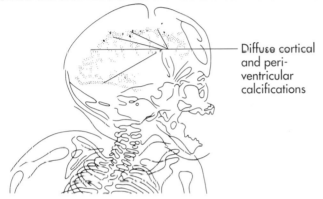

FIG. 12-65 Congenital toxoplasmosis. Microcephaly, ventricular dilatation, and cerebral calcifications were prominent findings in this infant with severe congenital toxoplasmosis. (Courtesy Department of Pediatric Radiology, Children's Hospital of Pittsburgh.)

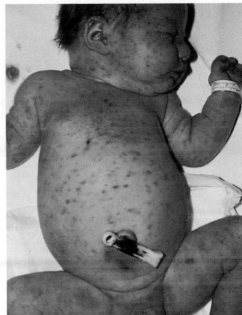

FIG. 12-66 Congenital rubella. This newborn had the full-blown picture of the "expanded rubella syndrome," including a generalized blueberry muffin rash, diffuse petechiae, hepatosplenomegaly, the early onset of jaundice, and neurologic depression. (Courtesy Dr. Michael Sherlock.)

infants tend to be small for gestational age, may be microcephalic or hydrocephalic, develop early-onset jaundice, have hepatosplenomegaly and diffuse adenopathy, and often are covered with petechial and purpuric lesions or with a generalized maculopapular rash. Seizures are common in these infants, as is a CSF pleocytosis with an increased protein content and xanthochromia. Skull radiographs may reveal diffuse cortical calcifications, in contrast to the periventricular pattern seen in cytomegalic inclusion disease (Fig. 12-65). Interstitial pneumonitis and myocarditis may be prominent features, as well. These infants are at high risk of suffering severe neurodevelopmental sequelae, if they survive. Other infants may appear normal initially but may rapidly develop signs of neonatal myocarditis with minimal CNS manifestations, although they, too, may have cerebral calcifications, as do many infants with apparently isolated chorioretinitis.

Diagnosis is best confirmed by IgM fluorescent antibody testing or, in patients presenting with ocular findings later in infancy, by the Sabin-Feldman dye test. Treatment with pyrimethamine and triple sulfa or sulfadiazine for 4 weeks appears to interrupt the infection and prevent the progression of ocular and CNS injury.

Congenital Rubella

Despite its usually mild manifestations when acquired postnatally, prenatal infection with rubella virus is a far from benign process. Intrauterine death, variable constellations of congenital anomalies, and

severe perinatal illness may result. The mother may or may not have symptomatic illness. In the viremic phase the virus is transmitted to the placenta, and then in most instances to the fetus. If the fetus becomes infected, mitotic activity is reduced and focal cytolysis and vascular injury occur, resulting in congenital malformations. The earlier in gestation the infection occurs, the greater the potential for injury. Of fetuses infected during the first 8 weeks, 39% will spontaneously abort or be stillborn, 25% will have gross anomalies noted at birth, and 36% will appear normal. Ultimately 85% of all liveborn infants infected during the first 8 weeks are found to have sequelae. Infections in the ensuing 12 weeks pose a gradually decreasing risk of causing anomalies, and those occurring thereafter do not cause defects. The most commonly encountered anomalies are central diffuse cataracts, congenital heart disease (patent ductus arteriosus, pulmonary artery stenosis, pulmonary valvular stenosis), and sensorineural deafness (usually bilateral, occasionally unilateral), seen singly or in combination.

There is thus a wide range of clinical manifestations. Some infants at risk are normal. Some appear normal at birth but later are found to have hearing loss. Some are small for gestational age and at birth have evidence of congenital heart disease and ocular anomalies, including microphthalmia, glaucoma, cataracts that may be central or diffuse, and pigmented retinopathy (see Chapter 19). Although usually present at birth, ocular findings may be missed unless a careful ophthalmologic examination is performed. Many of these infants manifest jaundice within 24 hours of birth and have hepatosplenomegaly and diffuse adenopathy as well.

Ten to twenty percent of liveborn infants with congenital rubella manifest signs of severe disseminated infection at or shortly after birth. In addition to early jaundice, hepatosplenomegaly, and adenopathy, they often show signs of myocarditis with ischemic changes on electrocardiograms, interstitial pneumonitis, thrombocytopenia with petechiae and purpura, and CNS dysfunction that may range from lethargy and hypotonia to frank meningoencephalitis. Radiographs may reveal bony abnormalities consisting of metaphyseal lucencies and irregular epiphyseal mineralization. In some cases a rubelliform rash or a characteristic raised, bluish, papular eruption, termed a *blueberry muffin rash*, may be evident as the result of dermal erythropoiesis (Fig. 12-66). Most of these severely affected infants are microcephalic, in addition to being small for gestational age. Survivors of this "ex-

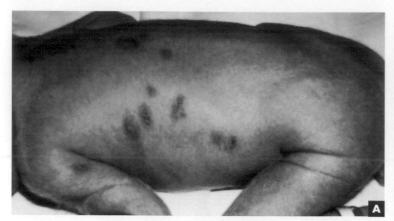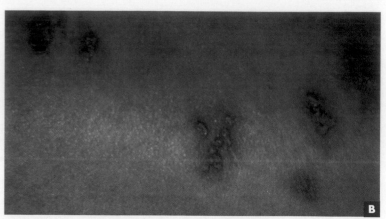

FIG. 12-67　Neonatal herpes simplex type 2 infection. *A* and *B*, Although normal at birth, fever, lethargy, and decreased feeding suddenly developed in this infant at 6 days of age. On examination, multiple grouped vesicular lesions were noted on the trunk and scalp. The liver and spleen were markedly enlarged and very firm. He had a fulminant course resembling that of septic shock and died within 24 hours. (Courtesy Dr. Michael Sherlock.)

panded rubella syndrome" are highly likely to be deaf and show significant psychomotor retardation.

In a small percentage of infants with congenital rubella, delayed manifestations may surface. These include anemia toward the end of the first month and the insidious onset of interstitial pneumonitis and the appearance of a chronic, generalized rubelliform exanthem at 3 to 4 months of age. Still later, immunodeficiency may be detected. Feeding difficulties, chronic diarrhea, and failure to thrive are common.

Infants with congenital rubella are chronically and persistently infected and tend to shed live virus in urine, stools, and respiratory secretions for up to a year. Hence, they should be isolated when in the hospital and kept away from susceptible pregnant women when sent home. Diagnosis can be confirmed by viral culture and specific IgM titers.

Neonatal Herpes Simplex Infection

Infants born vaginally to mothers with genital herpes simplex type 2 are at significant risk for acquisition of the infection. Typically the mother is asymptomatic and the infant appears totally normal at birth. Signs of infection may develop any time within the first 4 weeks but usually appear 4 to 8 days postpartum. Infection may be localized to the skin, eye, mouth, or CNS, or it may be systemic. In the latter instance, onset begins with fever or subnormal temperature in association with lethargy, poor feeding, vomiting, and jaundice. The liver and spleen are enlarged and often are remarkably firm. Respiratory distress supervenes, followed by a picture that is indistinguishable from that of septic shock with DIC. Approximately three fourths of affected infants have typical herpetic skin or mucosal lesions (Fig. 12-67). The scalp and face are the sites most commonly involved. Occasionally lesions are limited to the conjunctiva or to the oral mucosa. In the absence of these lesions, accurate diagnosis is extremely difficult. Mortality is high, exceeding 50%, but has been reduced by early recognition and systemic antiviral therapy. Nevertheless, morbidity remains high in survivors. The prognosis is relatively good for infants with localized skin, eye, or oral involvement. The survival rate is better in those with localized CNS disease than in those with systemic infection, but severe morbidity results in both.

Less frequently, infections may occur prenatally as a result of ascent from the lower genital tract through ruptured membranes or as a result of maternal viremia. In the event of prenatal acquisition, the infant may die in utero or may be born with jaundice, skin lesions, and signs of systemic infection.

BIBLIOGRAPHY

Barton LL, Feigin RD: Childhood cervical lymphadenitis: a reappraisal, *J Pediatr* 84:846-852, 1974.

Barton LL, Friedman AD: Impetigo: a reassessment of etiology and therapy, *Pediatr Derm* 4:185-188, 1987.

Bingham PM, Galetta SL, Athreya B, Sladky J: Neurologic manifestations in children with Lyme disease, *Pediatrics* 96:1053-1056, 1995.

Cherry JD: Newer viral exanthems, *Adv Pediatr* 16:233-286, 1969.

Chesney PJ, Davis JP, Purdy WK, Wand PJ, Chesney RW: Clinical manifestations of toxic shock syndrome, *JAMA* 246:741-748, 1981.

Clain A: *Demonstrations of physical signs in clinical surgery*, ed 17, Bristol: 1986, John Wright-PSG.

Committee on Infectious Diseases, American Academy of Pediatrics: *Report of the Committee on Infectious Diseases—the 1988 red book*, ed 21, Evanston, Ill., 1988, American Academy of Pediatrics.

Committee on Infectious Diseases, American Academy of Pediatrics: *1994 red book*, Elk Grove, Ill., 1994, American Academy of Pediatrics.

Dich VQ, Nelson JD, Haltalin KC: Osteomyelitis in infants and children, *Am J Dis Child* 129:1273-1278, 1975.

Feigin RD, Cherry JD: *Textbook of pediatric infectious disease*, ed 3, Philadelphia, 1992, WB Saunders.

Fleisher G, Ludwig S, Campos J: Cellulitis: bacterial etiology, clinical features and laboratory findings, *J Pediatr* 97:591-593, 1980.

Hanshaw JB, Dudgeon JA, Marshall WC: *Viral diseases of the fetus and newborn*, ed 2, Philadelphia, 1985, WB Saunders.

Hurwitz S: *Clinical pediatric dermatology*, ed 2, Philadelphia, 1993, WB Saunders.

Krugman S, Katz SL, Gershon AE, Wilfert CM: *Infectious diseases of children*, ed 9, St. Louis, 1992, Mosby.

Lascari AD, Bapat VR: Syndrome of infectious mononucleosis, *Clin Pediatr* 9:300-30-4, 1970.

Leibel RL, Fangman JJ, Ostrovsky MC: Chronic meningococcemia in childhood, *Am J Dis Child* 127:94-98, 1974.

Mandell GL, Douglas RG Jr, Bennet JE: *Principles and practice of infectious diseases*, ed 4, New York, 1995, Churchill Livingstone.

May M: Neck masses in children: diagnosis and treatment, *Pediatr Ann* 5:517-535, 1976.

Morrey BF, Bianco AJ, Rhodes KH: Septic arthritis in children, *Pediatr Clin North Am* 6:923-934, 1975.

Nixon GW: Acute hematogenous osteomyelitis, *Pediatr Ann* 5:65-81, 1976.

Rapkin RH, Bautista G: *Haemophilus influenzae* cellulitis, *Am J Dis Child* 124:540-542, 1972.

Salzar JC, Gerber MA, Goff CW: Long-term outcome of Lyme disease in children, *J Pediatr* 122:591-593, 1993.

Season EH, Miller PR: Primary subacute pyogenic osteomyelitis in long bones of children, *J Pediatr Surg* 11:347-353, 1976.

Shapiro ED: Lyme disease. In Burg FD, Ingelfinger JR, Wald ER, Polin RA: eds: *Current pediatric therapy*, ed 15, Philadelphia, 1996, WB Saunders.

Starke JR, Jacobs RF, Jereb J: Resurgence of tuberculosis in children, *J Pediatr* 120:839-855, 1992.

Steere AC: Lyme disease, *N Engl J Med* 321:586-596, 1989.

Toews WH, Bass JW: Skin manifestations of meningococcal infection, *Am J Dis Child* 127:173-176, 1974.

Tofte RW, Williams DN: Toxic shock syndrome: evidence of a broad clinical spectrum, *JAMA* 246:2163-2167, 1981.

Wannamaker LW, Ferrieri P: Streptococcal infections—updated, *DM* Oct pp 1-40, Oct 1975.

Wilson HD, Haltalin KC: Acute necrotizing fasciitis in childhood, *Am J Dis Child* 125:591-595, 1973.

13

Nephrology

DEMETRIUS ELLIS

The manifestations of renal and genitourinary disorders range from readily apparent gross structural abnormalities to subtle abnormalities of the urinary sediment. In this chapter, examples of physical findings, as well as characteristic urinary findings and radiographs, are used to demonstrate the broad spectrum of these disorders in the pediatric population.

Essentials of Medical History and Physical Examination

The medical history and physical examination often provide clues implicating a renal or genitourinary disorder. Congenital but often nonheritable genitourinary disorders are diagnosed with an increasing frequency by high-resolution ultrasonography during the second and third trimesters and may include obstructive disorders, such as posterior urethral valves, multicystic dysplasia, polycystic kidney disease, "prune belly syndrome," or renal agenesis. Oligohydramnios and fetal compression signs reflect reduced urine production associated with some of these disorders and may result in early postnatal death as a result of associated pulmonary underdevelopment. Unilateral and, less frequently, bilateral cystic dysplasia is the most common cause of abdominal mass in newborns. A large placenta may be a telltale sign of congenital nephrotic syndrome of the Finnish type in which severe proteinuria precedes birth. Failure to urinate during the first 24 hours of life should prompt evaluation for obstruction of the kidneys, ureters, or bladder. Urinary tract infection (UTI) should be a consideration in all febrile infants, particularly during the first 2 weeks of life, even in the presence of documented sepsis, meningitis, or other sources of infection. Urinary tract anomalies, including vesicoureteral reflux and megaureters distending the abdomen, are common in infants and young children with well-documented UTI. Children with true polyuria or polydipsia, rather than urinary frequency, may have a renal concentrating defect, such as nephrogenic diabetes insipidus, or salt-losing nephropathy, such as nephronophthisis.

Failure to thrive, lethargy, or irritability and recurrent emesis are common manifestations of renal disease in infants and may be associated with metabolic acidosis and other electrolyte disturbances. Occasionally, the renal disorder is discovered because of deliberate studies obtained upon discovering dysmorphic features, imperforate anus, vertebral abnormalities, fetal alcohol syndrome, or other disorders that have a renal component.

Family pedigrees may facilitate the diagnosis of congenital or heritable disorders such as cystinuria, cystinosis, oxaluria, and polycystic kidney disease and thereby lead to a variety of preventive measures before children become symptomatic. Hypertension in infants without aortic coarctation is most often a result of a renovascular disorder, such as renal venous thrombosis (infants of diabetic mothers, hyperviscosity syndrome, dehydration), arterial thrombosis (caused by embolism in patients with ventricular septal defect or patent ductus arteriosus or a result of umbilical artery catheterization), or renal artery stenosis. Asphyxia at birth or severe dehydration, sepsis, or shock may lead to acute tubular necrosis and oliguric renal failure.

Hypertension in the older child may cause headache, dizziness, recurrent emesis, epistaxis, or visual disturbances. In severe cases secondary congestive heart failure may occur, particularly if there is a history of oliguria, impaired renal function, or glomerulonephritis. Renal disorders account for most cases of hypertension, particularly in the preadolescent child in whom primary or essential hypertension is rare. The presence of café-au-lait spots, neurofibromas, fibrous-angiomatous lesions of the skin, thyroid enlargement, abnormal pulses, or bruits over the renal arteries or major vessels may point to a specific diagnosis.

Gross or microscopic hematuria is the most common reason children are referred to outpatient pediatric nephrology clinics. The medical history is critical to pinpointing the correct cause of hematuria because it facilitates the elimination of a large number of possibilities. These possibilities include complications in the neonatal period necessitating umbilical artery line placement that may result in renal or aortic occlusive disease, bronchopulmonary dysplasia managed with loop diuretics leading to hypercalciuria or nephrocalcinosis, use of medications that lead to tubulointerstitial nephritis or coagulopathies, congenital heart disease leading to subacute bacterial endocarditis (SBE) with secondary immune complex renal disease or thromboembolic disease, hemophilia, thalassemia, sickle cell disease, and other thrombotic or hemolytic disorders. The social history is particularly important in newborns because it may suggest child abuse, trauma, or Munchausen syndrome by proxy as the cause of the hematuria. Fever without an apparent source and symptoms of frequency, dysuria, back pain, or nocturia may suggest a UTI. The presence of hematuria or renal failure in other family members may suggest polycystic kidney disease, whereas a similar history together with neurosensory hearing loss may indicate Alport syndrome. Menarche is at times confused with hematuria.

In children with gross hematuria with or without flank or abdominal pain and absence of urinary casts or significant proteinuria to sug-

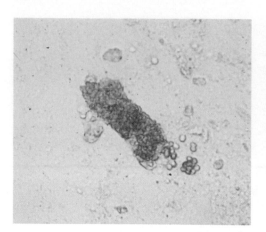

FIG 13-1 Red blood cell cast from a patient with poststreptococcal glomerulonephritis. These casts are almost always associated with glomerulonephritis or vasculitis and virtually exclude extrarenal disorders of bleeding.

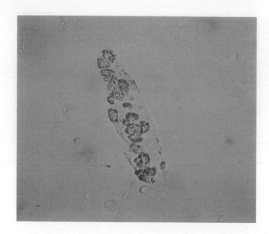

FIG. 13-2 White blood cell cast from a patient with chronic glomerulonephritis.

gest a glomerulonephritis, a family history of nephrolithiasis or a history of high dietary intake of salt, dairy products, or vitamins suggests hypercalciuria. Apart from hematuria with urinary casts, an acquired glomerulonephritis may be indicated by a history of an antecedent pharyngitis or concurrent infection, pallor, edema, rapid weight gain, arthritis, or arthralgia together with a purpuric or malar rash, which may suggest a diagnosis of Henoch-Schönlein purpura, systemic lupus erythematosus, or petechiae associated with hemolytic uremic syndrome. A history of direct or indirect trauma may explain the hematuria in the active and otherwise healthy adolescent.

Failure to grow in the absence of an obvious nutritional deficit may be a sign of a chronic renal disorder in any child. Evaluation of such a disorder should include a careful urinalysis, complete blood cell count, and measurement of BUN, serum creatinine, bicarbonate, alkaline phosphatase, calcium, and phosphorus levels.

Glomerular Disorders

Nephritis and Nephrosis

In children suspected of having a glomerular disease, the urinary sediment can provide important clues that may expedite the diagnosis and help formulate therapeutic plans. A classic example of nephritic syndrome is that of acute poststreptococcal glomerulonephritis, in which the urinalysis reveals variable levels of proteinuria and granular red (Fig. 13-1) and, less frequently, white (Fig. 13-2) blood cell casts. On the other hand, the urine of children with classic nephrotic syndrome, such as minimal change disease, shows heavy proteinuria (> 40 mg/m²/hr), free fat droplets and oval fat bodies, and little or no hematuria or other sediment abnormalities.

Unlike patients with nephrotic syndrome, those with acute nephritic syndromes are usually hypertensive, have darkly colored urine, and have a depressed glomerular filtration rate. Several disorders exhibit features of both nephritis and nephrosis. The nephrotic syndrome in childhood is generally the result of one of five primary disorders: minimal change disease, mesangial proliferative glomerulonephritis, focal glomerulosclerosis, membranous nephropathy, and membranoproliferative glomerulonephritis. Minimal change is the most common, account-

ing for more than 70% of all cases of nephrosis in children. It is so named because of its virtually normal light microscopic histology, negative immunofluorescence, and fusion of epithelial cell foot processes on electron microscopy. Laboratory features include selective proteinuria, normal complement levels, decreased IgG levels and increased IgM levels. Minimal change nephrotic syndrome is relatively benign, with more than 95% of patients maintaining adequate renal function.

Mesangial proliferative nephrosis exhibits diffuse proliferative changes with negative or variable deposition of mesangial IgG, IgM, and C3. It represents about 10% of nephrosis cases in childhood. Serum complement levels are normal, but hematuria is common.

Focal glomerulosclerosis accounts for 10% to 15% of nephrotic syndromes in childhood. It demonstrates focal and segmental sclerosis, with IgM and C3 deposition within affected glomeruli. Hematuria, pyuria, poorly selective proteinuria, and normal C3 levels are characteristic of laboratory features. The majority of children with mesangial proliferation or focal glomerulosclerosis progress to renal failure about 6 years after the onset of the disease.

Membranous glomerulopathy is an unusual cause of nephrotic syndrome in children, and it has unique histopathologic changes seen by microscopy. Capillary walls appear thickened, and the basement membrane has argyrophilic spikes on special staining. Immunoglobulin G deposits can be seen within the capillary walls, and electron microscopy shows subepithelial deposits. Protein excretion is variably selective, the serum C3 value is normal, and patients are prone to renal vein thrombosis. Ultimate renal function is maintained in 50% to 70% of children with this disorder.

Membranoproliferative glomerulonephritis is subdivided into two main types. Type I has lobular changes along with the mesangial proliferative changes and subendothelial deposits seen on electron microscopy. Hematuria is common, and the serum C3 level is intermittently low. More than half of patients avoid chronic dialysis. Type II disease has C3 capillary and mesangial immune deposits. Hematuria, persistently reduced serum C3 levels, and the presence of C3 nephritic factors are laboratory features of type II. The disorder is also known as *dense deposit disease* because of enhanced osmiophilic staining observed by electron microscopy. Unlike type I, almost all patients with Type II disease progress to end-stage renal disease.

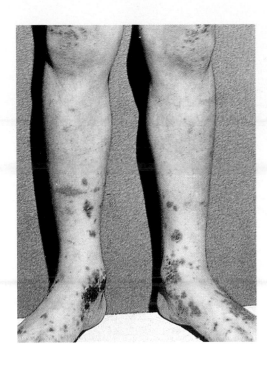

FIG. 13-3 Older child with severe Henoch-Schönlein purpura vasculitis resulting in cutaneous necrosis just below and anterior to the right malleolus.

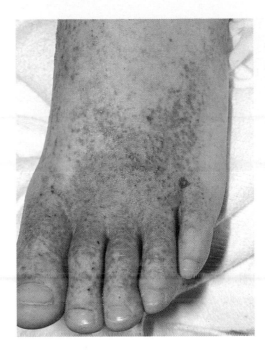

FIG. 13-4 The typical vasculitic rash of Henoch-Schönlein purpura is evident in the dorsum of the foot of this 15-year-old youngster. He went on to develop rapidly progressive glomerulonephritis and pulmonary hemorrhage that were managed by pulse methylprednisolone.

Acute Glomerulonephritis

The most common causes of acute glomerulonephritis in children include poststreptococcal or postpneumococcal glomerulonephritis, IgA nephritis, Henoch-Schönlein purpura, and hemolytic uremic syndrome. In some instances, these disorders may have an aggressive clinical course characterized by oliguria, hypertension, and rapid reduction in glomerular filtration rate, in which case the designation of rapidly progressive glomerulonephritis (RPGN) is given. The renal biopsy in such patients often demonstrates cellular or acellular crescents and inflammatory infiltrates. Several other chronic glomerulonephritides, such as membranoproliferative glomerulonephritis and membranous glomerulopathy, may also evolve into RPGN.

In addition to the clinical symptoms, the antinuclear antibody titer, streptococcal titers, quantitative serum immunoglobulin concentrations, and C3 and C4 levels often are helpful in differentiating several of the glomerulonephritides. Serum complement levels are particularly helpful because only a few of these conditions are associated with depressed complement levels. In poststreptococcal glomerulonephritis, the complement levels are only transiently reduced and return to normal concentrations within 8 weeks after onset of the renal symptoms.

A typical situation is that of a child 3 to 10 years of age, whose symptoms during the preceding few days include mild periorbital edema, headache, and decreasing urine output. The urine is described as being smoky or tea colored. Medical history reveals that 2 weeks earlier the patient experienced a febrile illness with painful pharyngitis for which he or she received no medical attention. Clinical examination reveals a blood pressure of 140/105 mm Hg, mild periorbital edema, and tenderness on palpation of the kidneys. A urinalysis shows the following values: 2+ protein, 3+ blood, and an SG of 1.020. Red blood cell casts (Fig. 13-1) are seen on urinalysis. Laboratory studies are consistent with mild renal insufficiency. Also found are a protein excretion of 1.1 g/24 hours, a low plasma C3 level, and elevated streptozyme and anti-DNAase B-titers, evidence that strongly implicates a streptococcal infection in the pathogenesis of the glomerulonephritis. Generally, complete and spontaneous recovery of all renal abnormalities occurs within 5 weeks with conservative management, although hematuria may persist for about 1 year or longer.

Chronic Glomerulonephritis

White blood cell casts may be seen in the urine sediment of patients with acute or chronic glomerulonephritis and vasculitis, as well as pyelonephritis and other disorders resulting in tubulointerstitial nephritis. The cast shown in Fig. 13-2 occurred in a child with systemic lupus erythematosus whose only symptom was mild back pain. Urinalysis demonstrated 2+ protein, microhematuria, pyuria without bacteria, and red and white blood cell casts. Diagnosis was confirmed by immunologic findings including low serum C3 and C4 levels, a positive fluorescent antinuclear antibody titer, and antibodies against double-stranded DNA. Renal biopsy revealed diffuse proliferative lupus nephritis. Note that formation of tubular casts is aided by diminished urine flow, high urinary solute concentration, and the hyaline matrix of plasma- and tubule-derived protein in which cells become embedded. Several acute glomerular syndromes may progress to chronic glomerulonephritis. In the final stages, many such patients develop hypertension and severe renal failure (uremia). On renal ultrasonography, the kidneys appear small and fibrosed.

Henoch-Schönlein Purpura

Three weeks after a respiratory infection, a 2-year-old boy experienced symptoms of generalized malaise, abdominal pain, periorbital edema, and difficulty walking "as if his legs were hurting." One day later he developed an ecchymotic, purpuric rash, the characteristic clinical manifestation of Henoch-Schönlein purpura. The rash covered the extensor surfaces of the extremities and the buttocks but spared the trunk. Individual lesions faded over 1 week, but new lesions appeared or recurred over several weeks. Other cutaneous manifestations of the vasculitic lesions in this disorder are shown in Figs. 13-3 and 13-4.

Some patients initially develop an urticarial-type eruption that subsequently becomes macular or maculopapular. Occasionally, younger patients develop an angioneurotic-like edema of the scalp, face, or dorsum of the hands or feet. Of children with Henoch-Schönlein purpura, 90% have a prodrome consisting of an upper respiratory infection 1 to 3 weeks before the onset of symptoms and 80% have melena, hematemesis, and/or arthritis mostly involving the ankles and knees. About half of the patients have renal involvement ranging from simple microhematuria and a variable degree of proteinuria to oliguria and re-

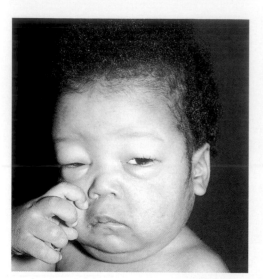

FIG. 13-5 Marked eyelid edema in a 2-year-old boy with minimal change disease and nephrotic syndrome. Eyelid edema in any child should prompt the performance of urinalysis rather than the presumption of allergy.

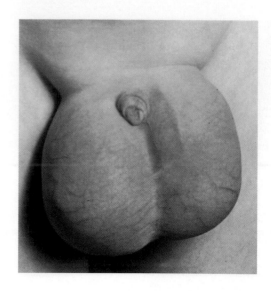

FIG. 13-6 Severe scrotal edema in a 6-year-old boy with nephrotic syndrome.

nal failure. In contrast to adults, use of multiple medications is rarely related to the onset of this condition in children.

There are no distinct biochemical features of this condition. Some patients have leukocytosis and an elevated serum IgA level. In the absence of severe proteinuria, hypoalbuminemia and edema are often a result of protein-losing enteropathy. Platelet counts and coagulation studies are normal. The skin rash is essential for the diagnosis of Henoch-Schönlein purpura because the renal abnormalities may otherwise closely resemble a similar disorder known as IgA nephropathy (Berger disease).

Nephrotic Syndrome

Children with nephrotic syndrome rarely have an underlying systemic illness or a history of drug intake and thus are designated as having primary or idiopathic nephrotic syndrome. Patients with poststreptococcal glomerulonephritis, Henoch-Schönlein purpura, IgA nephritis, or systemic lupus erythematosus, as well as rare patients treated with nonsteroidal inflammatory agents, lithium, colchicine, and other drugs, may also be associated with nephrotic-range proteinuria (i.e., ≥ 40 mg/m²/hr).

Minimal change disease is the single most common cause of idiopathic nephrotic syndrome in childhood. Generalized edema and rapid weight gain are characteristic features of this condition, with the former showing a predilection for the eyelids, pleural spaces, abdomen, scrotum, and lower extremities (Figs. 13-5 and 13-6). Although edema per se usually provokes few complaints from most patients, at times it may be disfiguring, and it may produce skin induration and breakdown, or interference with respiratory, genitourinary, or gastrointestinal function. Symptoms may occasionally be confused with allergic edema. However, the findings of severe proteinuria, hypoalbuminemia, and hypercholesterolemia usually lead to correct diagnostic and treatment measures.

Of special interest is nephrotic syndrome presenting in the newborn period or in the first 2 to 3 months of life. Acquired immunodeficiency syndrome (AIDS) has recently been added to the list of systemic diseases underlying infantile nephrotic syndrome and is increasingly recognized as a cause of this disorder in infants and young children. Focal glomerulosclerosis is the most common underlying histopathologic lesion.

Hematuria

Isolated gross or microscopic hematuria is probably the most common symptom prompting nephrologic assessment in children. Many such children have symptomless microscopic hematuria often detected during routine office visits or physical examinations required before participation in sport activities. Because of the large number of conditions associated with persistent hematuria in children, several algorithms have been devised to aid in the systematic evaluation of this condition (Fig. 13-7).

History and clinical symptoms may point toward trauma, viral or bacterial cystitis, drug-induced hematuria, or other causes. Detection of the most common causes of hematuria, including glomerulonephritis or UTI, can be readily achieved by the finding of cellular casts in a carefully performed examination of the urinary sediment or by appropriate bacterial cultures. Moreover, the absence of red blood cells in a child with positive o-tolidine reagent color change on the dipstick may lead to the correct diagnosis of conditions associated with rhabdomyolysis or hemolysis. Once these simple measures are undertaken, biochemical techniques are used to investigate renal function, hyperexcretion of metabolites resulting in nephrolithiasis (Fig. 13-8), hemoglobinopathies, bleeding diathesis, or immunologic assessment of an underlying glomerulonephritis. Measurement of calcium and creatinine concentrations in a single voided urine sample also should be included in the minimal initial assessment of asymptomatic hematuria, since hypercalciuria is found in a large proportion of such children. Identification of possible disorders by such methods may help determine the need for further assessment. Thus the finding of a nephritic sediment obviates the need for any radiologic procedures, whereas the presence of a single well-documented UTI in a child under 8 years of age may be an indication for imaging procedures. In the absence of any physical signs such as an abdominal mass to suggest Wilms tumor or neuroblastoma, malignancies of the kidney or urinary tract rarely present with isolated gross or microscopic hematuria. Renal ultrasonography coupled with Doppler evaluation of the renal vessels is useful in screening for the presence of tumor, polycystic kidney disease, or renal venous thrombosis in infants. Computed tomography or nuclear magnetic resonance techniques may provide detailed anatomic resolution of such masses.

ALGORITHM FOR DIAGNOSIS OF HEMATURIA

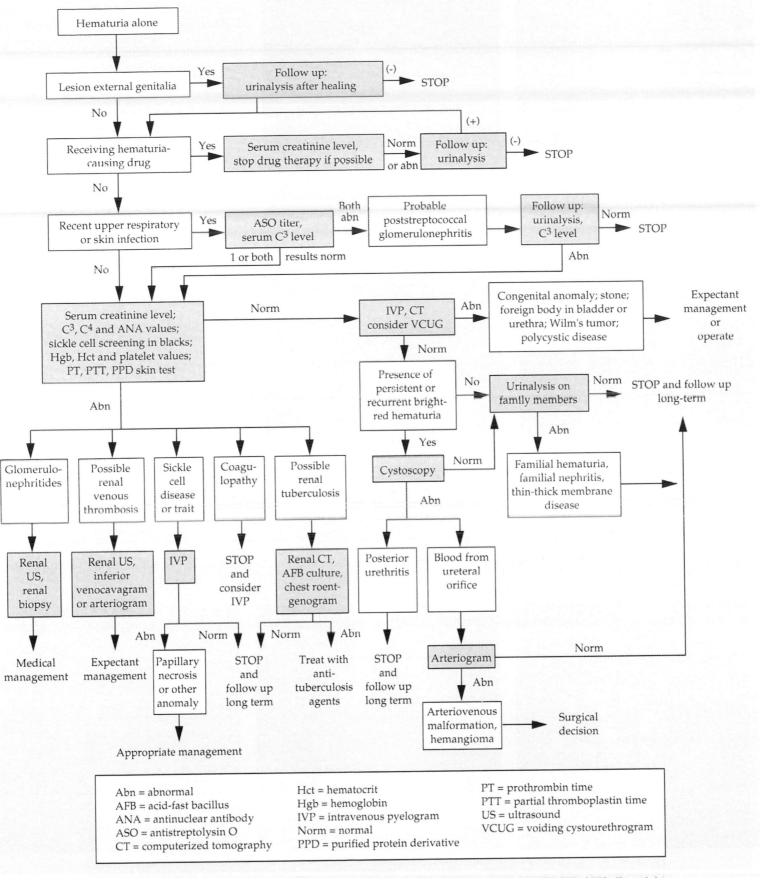

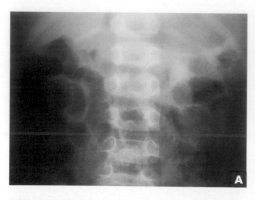

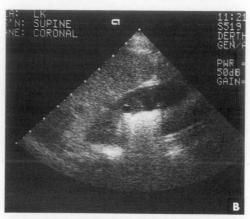

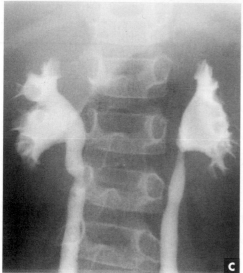

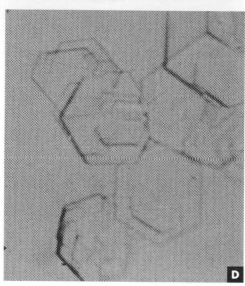

FIG. 13-8 A 6-year old boy, born of a consanguineous marriage, presented with diffuse abdominal pain, oliguria, and mild renal failure. *A,* Plain film of the abdomen showed a slight opacity in the area of the left kidney. *B,* Renal ultrasound demonstrated a distinct shadow produced by the calculus. *C,* An intravenous pyelogram showed the relatively radiolucent stone within the left renal pelvis. Multiple small calculi produced the dilation and partial obstruction of both ureters. *D,* The pathognomic flat hexagonal crystals found in the urine aided the diagnosis of cystinuria.

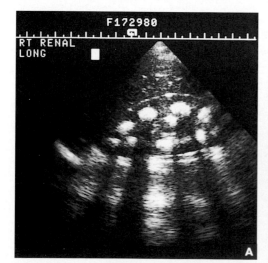

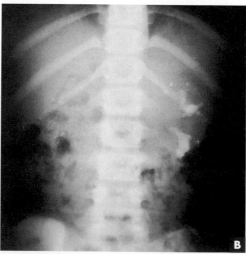

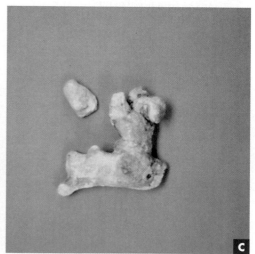

FIG. 13-9 *A,* Renal ultrasound demonstrates severe nephrocalcinosis in an 8-year-old girl who failed to thrive and showed familial type I renal tubular acidosis. Notice the multiple echogenic shadows produced by the calcium deposits within the renal parenchyma. *B,* A staghorn calculus in the left renal pelvis of another child with renal tubular acidosis. *C,* Appearance of calculus removed at operation. The shape of the calculus generally conforms to the pelvocaliceal system.

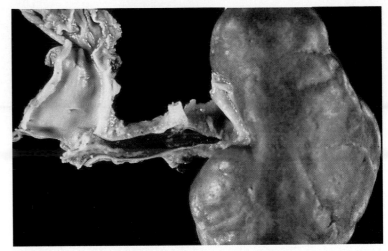

FIG. 13-10 A 12-year-old boy with ulcerative colitis, who died following a bout of severe diarrhea and dehydration. Apart from dural sinus thrombosis, the left renal vein contained this partially organized clot.

TABLE 13-1

Evaluation of Nephrolithiasis

Clinical History
Family history of nephrolithiasis
Immobilization or other protracted illness or stress
High dietary purine intake
Excessive salt or calcium ingestion
Large and infrequent meals
Excessive intake of vitamins or over-the-counter medications
Symptoms of UTI or history of pyelonephritis
Source and calcium content of drinking water
Polyuria or polydipsia

Physical Diagnosis
Band keratopathy and other signs of hyperparathyroidism
Elfin facies and other features of Williams syndrome

Radiologic Studies
Ultrasound—especially sensitive in identifying renal calculi and nephrocalcinosis
KUB—for the identification of ureteral stones; radiopaque stones include calcium oxalate and cystine
Intravenous urography—identifies urologic abnormalities and confirms obstruction; especially helpful in detecting radiolucent calculi such as uric acid, urates, matrix, and xanthine
^{125}I–hippurate scan—may provide differential renal function or suggest obstruction in children in whom an intravenous pyelogram poses high risk

Urinary Studies
Urinalysis—may reveal pyuria or bacteriuria, inability to lower urinary pH or to concentrate the urine, or flat hexagonal crystals pathognomonic of cystinosis
Urine culture
Screening with cyanide-nitroprusside (cystinosis)
Timed urine collections on two or more occasions for determination of the following values: creatinine, sodium, potassium, calcium, phosphorus, magnesium, oxalate, citrate, cystine, and uric acid

Biochemical Studies
Creatinine, BUN, electrolytes, total CO_2, albumin, calcium, phosphorus, magnesium, and uric acid; plasma parathyroid hormone levels if indicated
Chemical analysis of gravel or stones

Invasive cystography or arteriography is rarely necessary in the evaluation of structural lesions underlying isolated hematuria in children. A technetium 99^m dimercaptosuccinic acid (DMSA) renal scan may disclose renal scars suggestive of chronic pyelonephritis in children with or without vesicoureteral reflux. Finally, a renal biopsy may be helpful in making a definitive diagnosis in cases of suspected renal parenchymal disease manifested by hematuria.

Pediatric Nephrolithiasis

The diagnosis of nephrolithiasis should be entertained in any child with acute onset of flank or abdominal colicky pain. In children, renal colic is poorly localized and is often described as diffuse abdominal pain. Small stones may produce no pain at all and are detected only after an episode of gross hematuria, pyuria, or UTI. Thus a strong index of sus-

picion is required on the part of the clinician so that appropriate diagnostic studies are undertaken. Relatively few children pass gravel or stones, and the kind of crystals found in the urine are rarely of diagnostic value. Although dietary phytate is a more common cause of endemic stones in the Far East and UTI is more common in Europe, metabolic disorders predominate in children with nephrolithiasis in the United States. The clinical history and laboratory evaluation often reveal the cause of the stones. Biochemical analysis of the calculus is therefore of little diagnostic importance. One diagnostic approach to pediatric nephrolithiasis is shown in Table 13-1.

The most common calculus found in children consists of calcium oxalate. Such calculi frequently occur in children with idiopathic hypercalciuria, which may be silent or may be manifested by painless microscopic or recurrent gross hematuria for many years before frank nephrolithiasis occurs. Hypercalciuria is found in 35% of all children evaluated for hematuria. Screening for hypercalciuria may be done using a single voided urine specimen; a fasting calcium to creatinine ratio exceeding 0.21 is highly suggestive of this condition, which may then be confirmed by a 24-hour urine collection having a calcium content ≥ 4 mg/kg body weight. The nonabsorptive form of hypercalciuria appears to have an autosomal dominant inheritance underlying a renal tubular defect and net loss of calcium independent of the amount of dietary calcium ingested. The absorptive form may be associated with increased serum concentrations of calcitriol resulting in increased fractional absorption of calcium at the intestinal level. Premature infants who have been given high doses of furosemide to control fluid retention associated with bronchopulmonary dysplasia may develop hypercalciuria, nephrolithiasis, and nephrocalcinosis. Other disorders predisposing to nephrolithiasis include hyperparathyroidism, cystinuria (Fig. 13-8), hyperoxaluria, defects of purine metabolism and distal (type I) renal tubular acidosis (Fig. 13-9). UTIs and obstructive uropathy are also important. Laboratory studies and the radiologic location and appearance of the stone often provide clues as to the cause and treatment of the nephrolithiasis.

Apart from available medical therapies and traditional surgical techniques, specific conditions may be treated by newer modalities, such as extracorporeal shock-wave lithotripsy and stone fragmentation through pulse laser energy.

Renal Venous Thrombosis

Volume depletion secondary to diarrhea or vomiting (Fig. 13-10), hypotension, hypercoagulable or hyperviscosity states (hematocrit more

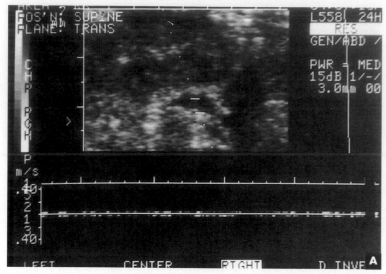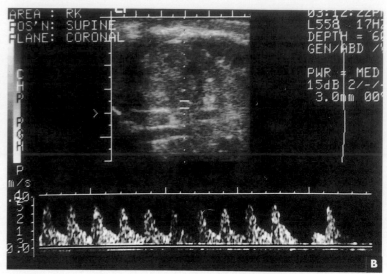

FIG. 13-11 Renal venous thrombosis. A plethoric 2-day-old infant of a diabetic mother (hematocrit 75%) was found to have an abdominal mass in the right abdomen on routine physical examination. Laboratory evaluation disclosed hematuria and thrombocytopenia without elevation in BUN or serum creatinine concentrations. *A,* Notice the absence of venous pulsations in the lower panel on the Doppler study of the right renal vein while arterial pulsations remained intact. *B,* Subsequent serial renal ultrasound studies showed a progressive reduction in the size of the right kidney despite recanalization of the venous thromboses.

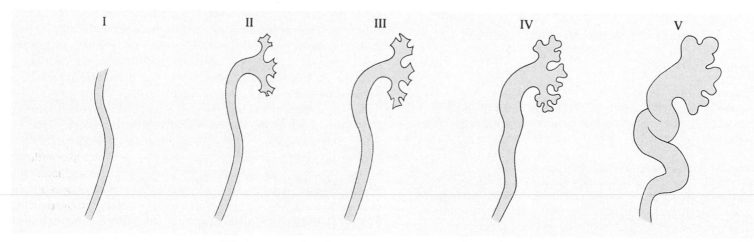

FIG. 13-12 Grades of vesicoureteral reflux, schematically presented.

than 65%), or indwelling catheters in the vicinity of the renal veins especially predispose infants to renal vein or intrarenal venous thrombosis. Older children with severe nephrotic syndrome are also prone to this disorder. Among children, 75% of all cases of renal venous thrombosis occur in the first month of life, and 50% of all cases are bilateral. The typical clinical features of renal vein thrombosis are a palpable renal mass in 60% of infants and hematuria and thrombocytopenia, which occur in more than 90% of the patients. Renal function may be normal, particularly in unilateral renal vein thrombosis or in bilateral disease that does not result in oliguria. The renal ultrasound is the diagnostic procedure of choice, particularly when coupled with Doppler examination of the renal and adjacent major vessels (Fig. 13-11).

Vesicoureteral Reflux

Vesicoureteral reflux is a congenital condition in which the normal valve mechanism of the ureterovesicular junction is impaired, leading to reflux of bladder urine into the ureter or kidneys. In a young child with UTI, such reflux of infected urine is a major risk factor for the development of pyelonephritis, renal scarring, and chronic renal damage.

The severity of vesicoureteral reflux is assessed by the findings on voiding cystourethrograms, and classified according to the following international grading system (Fig. 13-12):

Grade I—reflux into the ureter only (Fig. 13-13).

Grade II—complete reflux into the ureter, pelvis, and calyces without any dilation of the structures (Fig. 13-14).

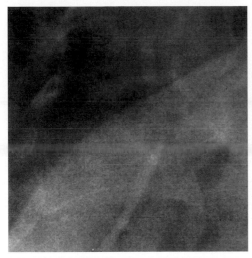

FIG. 13-13 Grade I reflux: cystourethrogram shows reflux only into the ureter.

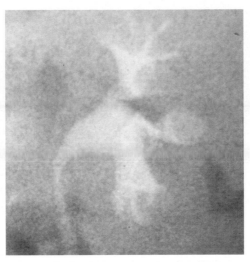

FIG. 13-14 Grade II reflux: cystourethrogram shows complete reflux into the ureter, pelvis, and calyces; no dilation.

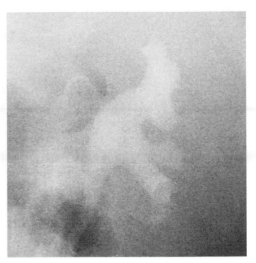

FIG. 13-15 Grade III reflux: cystourethrogram shows complete reflux with mild dilation of the ureter and renal pelvis but only slight blunting of the calyces.

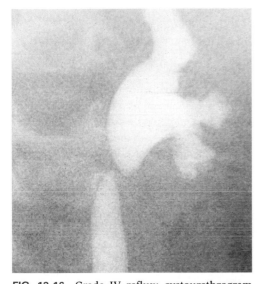

FIG. 13-16 Grade IV reflux: cystourethrogram shows complete reflux with moderate dilation of the ureter, pelvis, and calyces; complete obliteration of sharp angle of fornices.

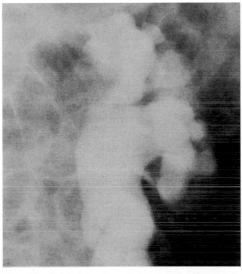

FIG. 13-17 Grade V reflux: cystourethrogram shows gross dilation of the ureter, pelvis, and calyces; obliteration of the papillary impressions of the calyces.

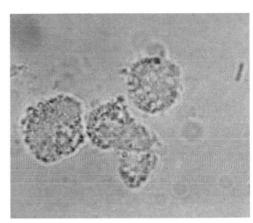

FIG. 13-18 High-power view of unspun urine shows several white blood cells and a rodshaped organism, suggestive of bacterial cystitis.

Grade III—complete reflux with mild dilation or tortuosity of the ureter, and mild dilation of the renal pelvis but only slight blunting of the calyceal fornices (Fig. 13-15).

Grade IV—complete reflux with moderate dilation of the ureter, renal pelvis, and calyces; complete obliteration of the sharp angle of the fornices with maintenance of the papillary impressions of the calyces (Fig. 13-16).

Grade V—gross dilation and tortuosity of the ureter with gross dilation of the renal pelvis and calyces, obliteration of the papillary impressions of the calyces (Fig. 13-17).

Grades I through III have a high rate of spontaneous resolution, and patients with such findings may be placed on suppressive an-

tibiotic regimens to ensure maintenance of sterile bladder urine. Grades IV and V are generally associated with significant anatomic abnormalities of the ureteral orifice, and they often require surgical correction.

Bacterial Cystitis

Young children whose symptoms include an acute onset of fever, emesis, dysuria, suprapubic pain, and a urinary sediment such as that shown in Fig. 13-18 should be suspected of having bacterial cystitis. By far the most common organism cultured from patients with acute or chronic urinary tract infections is *Escherichia coli; Pseudomonas* or *Pro-*

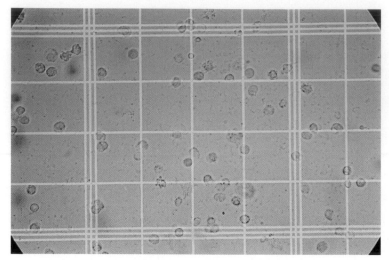

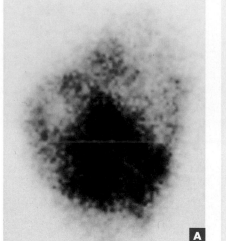

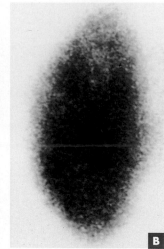

FIG. 13-19 Enhanced urinalysis using a Neubauer hemocytometer (×200) showing numerous white blood cells (>10 WBC/mm³) indicative of a UTI.

FIG. 13-20 Dimercaptosuccinic acid (DMSA) scan. The image in *A* is abnormal, with numerous filling defects indicative of pyelonephritis, whereas the image in *B* is normal.

TABLE 13-2

Sensitivity, Specificity, and Predictive Values of Standard Vs. Enhanced Urinalysis

	Standard			Enhanced		
	Cx +*	**Cx −†**	TOTAL	**Cx +**	**Cx −**	TOTAL
Test +	21	5	26	27	2	29
Test −	11	661	672	5	664	669
TOTAL	32	666	698	32	666	698
Sensitivity	65.6%			84.5%		
Specificity	99.2%			99.7%		
Positive predictive value	80.8%			93.1%		
Negative predictive value	98.4%			99.3%		
Prevalence	4.6%			4.6%		

From Hoberman A, Wald ER, Perchansky L, et al: Enhanced urinalysis as a screening test for urinary tract infection, *Pediatrics* 91(6):1196-1199, 1993.
*Cx+, Culture positive, >50,000 CFU/ml.
†Cx−, Culture negative.

teus organisms occasionally are found, particularly in patients with abnormal genitourinary anatomy.

The modern day dipstick test detects nitrite (produced by urinary pathogens by conversion of dietary nitrates) and leukocyte esterase (released by polymorphonuclear leukocytes present in urine). When both tests are positive, both the positive and negative predictive values are nearly 100% accurate in predicting UTI. Although these are good screening tests in older children with symptomatic or asymptomatic bacteriuria, they are impractical in infants because of stool contamination resulting in an increased rate of false-positive samples. Screening infants for UTI has markedly improved with the use of enhanced uri-

nalysis. Unlike standard urinalysis performed in uncentrifuged urine obtained by catheterization or suprapubic aspiration in which prediction of UTI is based on >5 white blood cells and any number of bacteria per high-power field, enhanced urinalysis consists of counting white blood cells in such a urine sample in a Neubauer hemocytometer (Fig. 13-19) and counting bacteria in a Gram stained smear. UTI is then predicted based on the finding of >10 white blood cells per mm³ plus any number of bacteria present in 10 oil fields examined. Based on results from the Children's Hospital of Pittsburgh (Table 13-2), enhanced urinalysis is more sensitive (84.5% vs. 65.6%) and has a higher predictive value (93.1% vs. 80.8%) than standard urinalysis in predicting UTI in febrile infants.

Although the diagnosis of UTI is established by appropriate urine cultures, the site of infection may not be apparent when considering the symptoms or urinalysis findings alone. DMSA scanning (Fig. 13-20) performed during a febrile, well-documented UTI is the earliest and most sensitive test available for detecting children with pyelonephritis at risk for developing renal scarring, as well as for detecting children with previous renal scars. Renal ultrasonography and intravenous pyelography, although less reliable, also may be useful in health care centers in which DMSA scanning is unavailable. We currently recommend that children under 8 years of age with abnormal DMSA scans undergo standard micturition cystourethrography under fluoroscopic monitoring to obtain the best baseline anatomic definition and to assess bladder capacity and emptying. If vesicoureteral reflux is found, future monitoring may be done by nuclear voiding cystourethrography, which limits radiation exposure. Such studies usually define structural abnormalities leading to obstructive nephropathy or vesicoureteral reflux and are essential in planning the medical and surgical management of these patients.

Developmental and Hereditary Disorders

Developmental Abnormalities

The number of congenital malformations associated with renal abnormalities is too large to discuss individually in this chapter. Renal abnormalities should be suspected in any child with one or more congenital abnormalities. In this chapter, only a selected number of syndromes are considered in which renal abnormalities are serious, relatively common, and easily diagnosed by the physical findings.

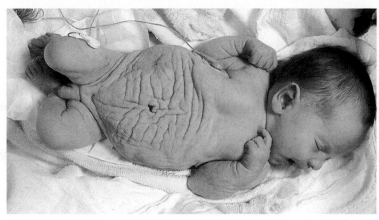

FIG. 13-21 Newborn with prune-belly syndrome shows the characteristic wrinkled and redundant skin covering the abdominal wall. On palpation, no abdominal muscular tissue or muscular tone could be detected.

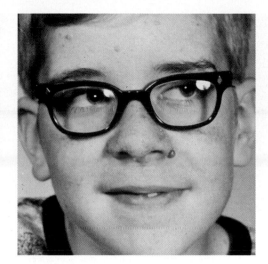

FIG. 13-22 This 6-year-old patient with tuberous sclerosis demonstrates characteristic papules distributed across the bridge of the nose and the nasolabial folds. He was originally diagnosed as having polycystic kidney disease because of abdominal distension and bilateral renal enlargement before the onset of any skin lesions.

Prune-Belly Syndrome (Eagle-Barrett Syndrome)

This syndrome usually consists of the absence of abdominal musculature, renal and urinary tract abnormalities, and cryptorchidism (Fig. 13-21). Boys are affected more severely and 20 times more frequently than girls. Although there is generally no ureteral obstruction, the ureters are dilated and tortuous, and 75% exhibit reflux. The bladder is enlarged despite low renal pelvic and intravesical pressures. Infection is common because of urinary stasis.

The major determinant of prognosis in these patients is the degree of associated cystic renal dysplasia. Intestinal malrotation is a common associated abnormality; anomalies of the limbs and heart may occur, but these are uncommon. Infertility in males is universal even when it is possible to surgically place the testes into their normal intrascrotal position. Libido and orgasm, however, remain normal. Early orchiopexy may improve the chances for fertility and prevent testicular neoplasia.

Tuberous Sclerosis

Tuberous sclerosis is a neurocutaneous syndrome inherited as an autosomal dominant trait with marked variability of expression. The full syndrome is characterized by myoclonic seizures, mental deficiency, foci of intracranial calcifications, depigmented "ash leaf" cutaneous patches, and pathognomonic skin lesions that are fibroangiomatous nevi (adenoma sebaceum). The latter may be present during the first year of life but may go unnoticed until the age of 4 to 7 years when they take the form of discrete yellowish papules distributed along the bridge of the nose and the nasolabial folds (Fig. 13-22). Patients with tuberous sclerosis may have hamartomas in many organs and tissues. Renal angiomyolipoma causing genitourinary symptomatology may suggest the diagnosis of polycystic kidney disease (PKD) in patients with minimal skin or central nervous system involvement (Fig. 13-23). Although small asymptomatic cysts are common in autopsy cases of tuberous sclerosis, large renal cysts may be discovered early in infancy and suggest the diagnosis of autosomal dominant PKD. Hypertension and renal insufficiency may further confuse the diagnosis. In such instances the diagnosis of tuberous sclerosis is confirmed by family history and the development of other features of the syndrome.

Imperforate Anus

Because of common embryologic origins and the anatomic proximity of the genitourinary and lower gastrointestinal tracts, children with

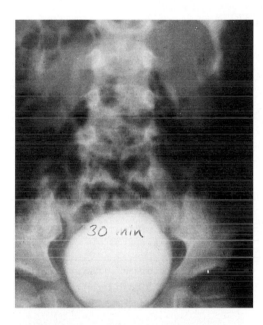

FIG. 13-23 Intravenous pyelogram of the patient in Fig. 13-22 shows enlarged kidneys with the collecting system stretched and distorted by multiple soft-tissue masses, later found to be renal angiomyolipoma.

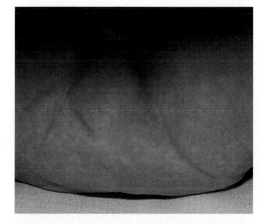

FIG. 13-24 Imperforate anus. This newborn boy has an absent median raphe and anal atresia. On further study he was found to have agenesis of the right kidney, severe dysplasia in the left kidney, and a communication of the blind-ended rectal pouch and the prostatic urethra.

imperforate anus have a high incidence of genitourinary and lower spinal abnormalities. A high imperforate anus (at or above the supralevator muscle) (Fig. 13-24) is associated with a 50% incidence of genitourinary anomalies, mainly unilateral renal agenesis, neurogenic bladder, or vesicoureteral reflux. In boys, one usually finds a fistulous

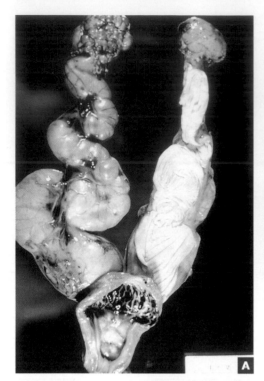

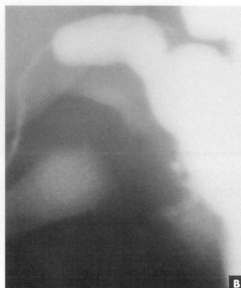

FIG. 13-25 *A,* Autopsy findings of a newborn with posterior urethral valves. Notice the marked enlargement and tortuosity of the ureters and the small, thick-walled, muscular bladder. *B,* An antemortem voiding cystourethrogram shows the markedly dilated proximal urethra typical of this condition.

communication between the blind end of the rectal pouch and the prostatic urethra. In girls, the rectum often communicates with the vagina or posterior fourchette. All children with imperforate anus should undergo evaluation of the genitourinary tract with renal ultrasound and voiding cystourethrography and must be monitored for UTI.

Posterior Urethral Valves

The most common obstructive lesions of the lower urinary tract in male infants are posterior urethral valves. Such folds traverse the urethra from a point just distal to the verumontanum to the proximal limit of the membranous urethra and obstruct urinary flow with consequent enlargement of the prostatic urethra, hypertrophy of the bladder neck, trabeculation of the bladder, and significant dilation of the upper urinary tract. Infants with posterior urethral valves may experience renal failure and profound electrolyte imbalance. Older children may have

abdominal masses, voiding disturbances, or infection. Diagnosis is made radiologically by voiding cystourethrography (Fig. 13-25) and confirmed endoscopically. Although urinary diversion is frequently required, some patients can be treated directly with transurethral valve ablation. Surgery is usually successful in achieving urinary drainage, but in many cases associated renal dysplasia may lead to chronic renal failure during infancy or childhood.

Crossed Renal Ectopy

Children with the developmental anomaly of crossed renal ectopy generally have an abdominal mass or hematuria following minor trauma. Obstruction at the ureteropelvic junction is common. The location of the ectopic kidney may be cryptic, as in the pelvic region, and can be best demonstrated by a renal radionuclide scan. Crossed renal ectopy, renal agenesis, and/or duplication of the collecting system are

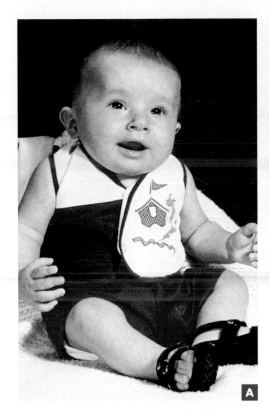

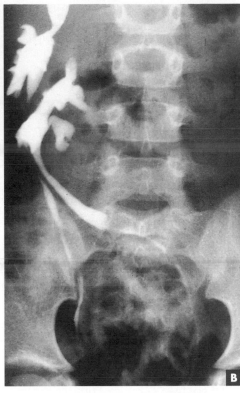

FIG. 13-26 An infant with Klippel-Feil syndrome (*A*) demonstrates a short neck (fused cervical vertebrae) and nonfunctioning right thumb caused by lack of tendons to this digit. Intravenous pyelogram (*B*) reveals crossed renal ectopia of the left kidney, whereas the ureter from the left kidney crosses the midline and inserts into the left side of the trigone.

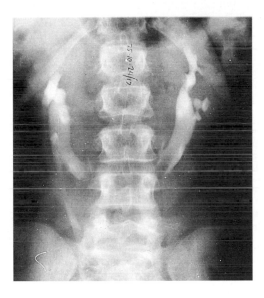

FIG. 13-27 Horseshoe kidney. This excretory urogram was performed as part of the evaluation for gross hematuria following abdominal injury in the child. Notice the unusual and oblong configuration of the collecting system resulting from fusion of the lower renal poles.

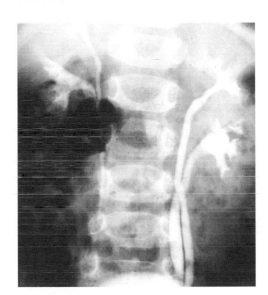

FIG. 13-28 Excretory urogram shows bilateral duplication of the urinary collecting system. This child has recurrent UTI as a result of vesicoureteral reflux in the ureter from the left lower pole. Ureteral duplication is incomplete on the right side (Y-type).

often found in association with Klippel-Feil syndrome (Fig. 13-26), but have also been associated with cervicothoracic vertebral anomalies and Müllerian duct aplasia in girls.

Horseshoe Kidney

Horseshoe kidney results from fusion of the lower renal poles during development (Fig. 13-27). Although generally asymptomatic, patients with horseshoe kidney may have (1) hematuria after trauma to the pelvic area; (2) a midline abdominal mass; or (3) a ureteropelvic junction obstruction, a common associated finding in this condition.

Duplication of the Urinary Collecting System

Duplication of the urinary collecting system is one of the most common of all genitourinary abnormalities. It is sometimes familial and more common in girls than in boys. About 30% of the duplications

are bilateral (Fig. 13-28) but with much variation in the extent of duplication. This condition occurs when the kidney is penetrated by two separate ureteral buds during nephrogenesis. When present, vesicoureteral reflux usually occurs in the ureter from the lower pole, whereas ureteral obstruction occurs almost exclusively in the ureter from the upper renal segment. Reflux into a duplicated system is unlikely to resolve spontaneously. These associated problems may predispose patients to recurrent infection or hydronephrosis necessitating surgical correction.

Hereditary and Metabolic Disorders

Polycystic Kidney Disorders

A useful classification and overview of the renal cystic disorders of childhood has been devised (Kissane, 1990). Only four of the most

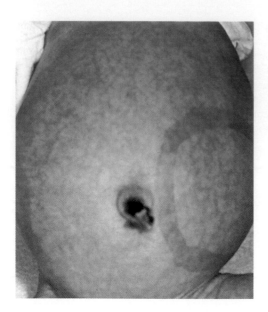

FIG. 13-29 This infant with infantile polycystic kidney disease shows marked abdominal distension and bilaterally enlarged kidneys, as indicated by the outlined area.

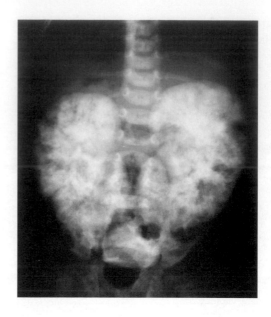

FIG. 13-30 Intravenous pyelogram of the patient in Fig. 13-29 shows the characteristic mottled nephrogram, with brushlike medullary opacification secondary to retention of contrast material in dilated cortical and medullary collecting ducts.

TABLE 13-3

Syndromes Associated With Cystic Kidneys

Syndrome	Inheritance*
Meckel-Gruber	ar
Jeune thoracic dystrophy	ar
Short rib polydactyly	ar
Zellweger cerebrohepatorenal	ar
Tuberous sclerosis	ad
von Hippel-Lindau	ad
VATER association	ni
Retina renal dysplasia	ar
Ivemark	ar
Fryns	ar
Trisomy 21, 13, or 18	—
Oral-facial-digital, type I	XL
Laurence-Moon-Bardet-Biedl	ar
Kaufman-McKusick	ar
Hypothalamic hamartoma	ni?
Lissencephaly	Variable
Prune-belly	ni?
Ehlers-Danlos	Variable
Branchio-oto-renal	ad
Roberts	ar
DiGeorge	Variable
Smith-Lemli-Opitz	ar
Turner	—
Noonan	—

From Zerres K: *Human Genetics* 68:104-135, 1984.
ar, Autosomal recessive; *ad*, autosomal dominant; *ni*, not inherited; *XL*, X-linked.

common and most important forms of PKD are presented here. Although autosomal dominant PKD (ADPKD) and cystic renal dysplasia are far more common (1/1000 population), autosomal recessive PKD (ARPKD, 1/40,000 population) is a much more serious disorder during childhood. Cystic renal dysplasia has no defined inheritance pattern and is often associated with other syndromes. Nephronophthisis, or medullary cystic disease complex, although less common than the other three disorders, is an important cause of end-stage renal disease

in childhood. Renal cystic disease also may be an important component of numerous syndromes (Table 13-3) that are not discussed in this chapter.

Autosomal Recessive

With the exception of the most severe manifestations of ARPKD, prenatal diagnosis by renal ultrasonography usually is unreliable until the second half of pregnancy. This disorder has variable expression, so that the severity of the cystic malformation often determines the age and mode of presentation. About 85% of cases begin during infancy. Oligohydramnios and associated pulmonary hypoplasia may result in life-threatening respiratory difficulties and talipes in the neonate, whereas abdominal masses and hypertension are common indications in later infancy; hepatic enlargement, portal hypertension, growth failure, and progressive renal insufficiency occur more commonly in the school-age child. Pancreatic cysts are rare and usually do not produce digestive difficulties. Hyponatremia often occurs in infancy and may relate to nonosmotic release of vasopressin, particularly in the setting of pulmonary disease, excessive renal salt wasting, extracellular volume contraction, and inadequate dietary salt replacement.

Congenital hepatic fibrosis is always present in this condition and may predominate over kidney involvement in some of the patients. Hypersplenism and hematemesis are frequent in such patients. Liver pathology may be similar in other autosomal recessive syndromes associated with PKD (Table 13-3).

It has become increasingly apparent that the ultrasonographic findings in ARPKD are not specific and may resemble those of ADPKD, particularly after infancy. Because of this and because the signs and symptoms can occur at various ages with either disorder, ARPKD has replaced the former designation of "infantile PKD." The abnormal gene is located on chromosome 6, but unlike ADPKD parental involvement is rare. Thus a normal renal ultrasound in both parents supports the diagnosis of ARPKD rather than ADPKD.

In children with ARPKD the cysts are initially small but can enlarge with age to produce palpable flank or abdominal masses (Fig. 13-29). The condition may be differentiated from bilateral hydronephrosis of any cause by thorough radiologic evaluation, which may include sonography, cystography, and intravenous pyelography. The intravenous pyelogram in Fig. 13-30 shows a characteristic mottled nephrogram, with the retention of the contrast material in dilated medullary and cortical collecting ducts producing brushlike medullary opacification with streaks radiating to the outer portion of the kidney. This correlates well with the pathologic findings in such kidneys of cystic dilation localized

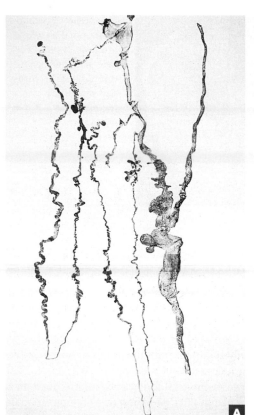

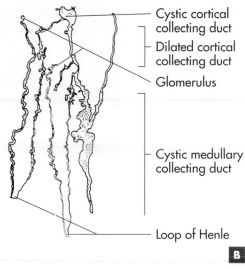

FIG. 13-31 *A* and *B,* The cystic areas are apparent in the microdissected nephron tree shown in this photograph. (Courtesy Dr. G. Fetterman, Pittsburgh.)

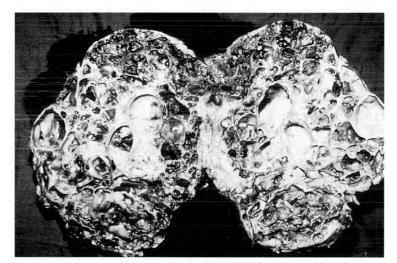

FIG. 13-32 Autosomal dominant (adult type) polycystic kidney disease. Notice replacement of normal renal parenchyma by fluid-filled cysts.

to the medullary and cortical collecting ducts. This localization is best demonstrated by isolated nephron microdissection (Fig. 13-31).

Autosomal Dominant

ADPKD is one of the most common inherited disorders and accounts for 10% of all patients with end-stage renal disease in the United States. Two gene mutations present on the short arm of chromosome 16 account for the majority of individuals with ADPKD, with the ADPKD1 gene comprising 90% of the cases and an even greater fraction of the more symptomatic individuals. Even within ADPKD1 families there is much variability in the phenotypic expression of the many extrarenal manifestations and in the severity of the renal disease or its clinical course. With current high-resolution renal ultrasonography, up to 90%

of one half of the presumed gene carriers under age 20 years will have detectable cysts. The false-negative ultrasonographic diagnosis for ADPKD in this age group is 8%. Compared with children with less than 10 cysts at the time of diagnosis of ADPKD, those with more than 10 cysts have a similar creatinine clearance but are more likely to complain of flank or back pain or urinary frequency and have a greater incidence of palpable kidneys, inguinal hernias, palpitations, hypertension, and urinary concentrating defect. Pathologically the cysts become very large and asymmetrical and involve all parts of the nephron (Fig. 13-32).

Because of the psychologic and practical (insurability, participation in sports) implications, it is recommended that an ultrasonographic diagnosis be pursued only in children at risk of developing ADPKD who manifest hypertension or those participating in contact sports who may be at risk for recurrent gross hematuria that may adversely affect the renal prognosis. Genetic linkage analysis may be done for prenatal diagnosis and family planning purposes or may be limited to individuals with a family history of PKD who are asymptomatic, have a nondiagnostic ultrasound, and wish to donate a kidney.

Except for children with enlarged kidneys and large cysts detected in infancy, renal failure or nephrolithiasis caused by ADPKD rarely occurs in childhood. Similarly, extrarenal manifestations, including rupture of intracranial aneurysm, colonic diverticula, or symptomatic mitral valve prolapse, are rare. Children with acute onset of "thunder clap" headache or neurologic symptoms that suggest impending rupture or compression of an intracranial aneurysm should undergo urgent magnetic resonance angiography.

Liver cysts may occur in ADPKD but are rarely associated with liver dysfunction or portal hypertension. A liver biopsy may help to differentiate ADPKD from ARPKD because congenital hepatic fibrosis is also found in ARPKD and is present only rarely in ADPKD.

Cystic Renal Dysplasia

Pathologically, abnormal renal morphogenesis includes processes leading to both deficient parenchyma (hypoplasia) (Fig. 13-33) and ab-

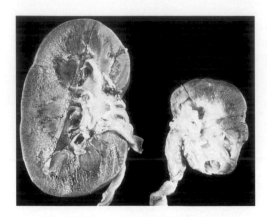

FIG. 13-33 Unilateral renal hypoplasia/dysplasia. In contrast to the normal right kidney, the left is markedly small. The parenchyma in the upper pole is normal but microscopic examination of the lower pole showed several morphologic features of dysplasia.

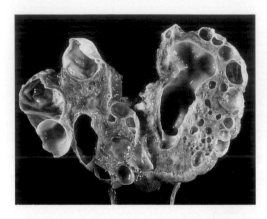

FIG. 13-34 Bilateral cystic renal dysplasia. Multiple cysts of variable size are seen throughout the cortex and medullary regions.

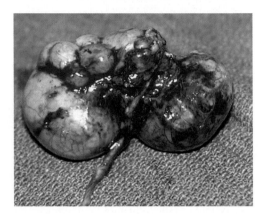

FIG. 13-35 A less severe form of multicystic renal dysplasia involving mainly the midportion of the kidney.

normally differentiated parenchyma (dysplasia) (Figs. 13-34 and 13-35). These conditions often coexist and, despite the presence of cysts, the kidneys may be too small to appreciate by bimanual examination (i.e., bracing the flank and back with the fingers of one hand while gradually producing deep abdominal compression with the other hand). When bilateral, these renal disorders are frequently detected during the first few weeks of life. The infant usually demonstrates poor weight gain, pallor, emesis, and tachypnea. Many of the early symptoms are secondary to metabolic acidosis resulting from renal insufficiency. The amount of urine output bears little relationship to the degree of renal failure as reflected by the serum creatinine level and BUN concentration. Collectively these conditions constitute the most common cause of chronic renal failure in children.

Patients with renal hypoplasia often have gastrointestinal, central nervous system, cardiac, and pulmonary abnormalities, but other abnormalities of the genitourinary tract are rarely present. Obstruction of the gastrointestinal or genitourinary tracts is commonly found in patients with dysplasia. Less common anomalies may include Down syndrome, tracheoesophageal fistula, ventricular septal defect, and lumbosacral dystrophies.

Cystic dysplasia may be a major component of several syndromes with distinct additional malformations (Table 13-3). Many of these syndromes have defined inheritance patterns. The overall risk for siblings of children with isolated forms of dysplasia or hypoplasia is usually less than 10%, but it may be higher if one of the parents has renal agenesis or a kidney that is affected by the same process. Pediatricians should be aware of several of the more common syndromes described in the paragraphs that follow.

MULTICYSTIC DYSPLASIA

Multicystic dysplasia is the most common cystic disorder in children and the most common cause of abdominal mass in newborns. It is usually unilateral. In typical cases there is complete loss of the renal architecture, and microscopically there are primitive ducts, fibrosis, and islands of cartilage representing the distinctive features of dysplasia. The condition may be discovered by prenatal sonography, or it is often diagnosed during the neonatal period after palpation of a "lumpy" intraabdominal mass of variable size that often transilluminates. Because atresia of the ureter is usually present, urine output and renal function depend on the presence of bilateral involvement and the degree of associated renal dysplasia. Very large multicystic kidneys can interfere with respiration or produce mechanical intestinal compression. Radionuclide scanning, renal ultrasonography, and retrograde urography are usually sufficient to establish the diagnosis.

The unaffected contralateral kidney is usually hypertrophied and has normal corticomedullary differentiation and no evidence of obstruction. Obstructive disorders, such as posterior urethral valves, urethral atresia, or ureteroceles obstructing a duplicated ureter draining the upper pole (especially in girls with wetness between episodes of normal voiding) may be associated with morphologic features of dysplasia. Biliary dysgenesis (congenital hepatic fibrosis) rarely has been associated with renal dysplasia.

Because a large percentage of multicystic kidneys spontaneously involute and are rarely the cause of hypertension, infection, or tumor development, the prevailing opinion is that unilateral and asymptomatic multicystic kidneys do not need to be removed. However, correction of any associated obstructive abnormalities that may be present in the contralateral kidney is of vital importance.

JUVENILE NEPHRONOPHTHISIS OR MEDULLARY CYSTIC DISEASE

Juvenile nephronophthisis and medullary cystic disease share similar morphologic features including prominent tubulointerstitial fibrosis and cysts that vary in number and size. The cysts are not prominent in most children, prompting the diagnosis of nephronophthisis, particularly if the disorder is autosomally inherited. The cysts usually enlarge with advancing renal failure. Juvenile nephronophthisis accounts for 2.4% of all children with end-stage renal disease in the United States. Polyuria and polydipsia as a result of a concentration defect and, at times, severe salt wasting are prominent clinical features. An ultrasound or abdominal CT scan may reveal normal-sized or small kidneys and loss of corticomedullary differentiation with or without medullary cysts. Hepatic fibrosis is probably the most important manifestation associated with juvenile nephronophthisis. Adults with this disorder have more prominent renal cysts and an autosomal dominant inheritance; thus it may be more aptly designated as medullary cystic disease.

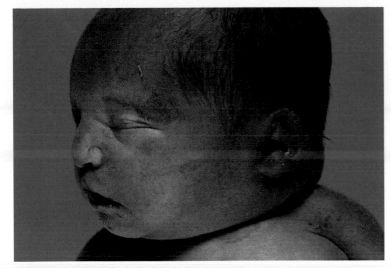

FIG. 13-36 Potter facies. This infant with bilateral multicystic dysplasia died at 12 hours of age with pulmonary insufficiency. The altered facies produced by the fetal compression syndrome of oligohydramnios includes small, posteriorly rotated ears, micrognathia, a beaked nose, and wide-set eyes. (Courtesy Dr. T. Macpherson, Magee-Women's Hospital, Pittsburgh.)

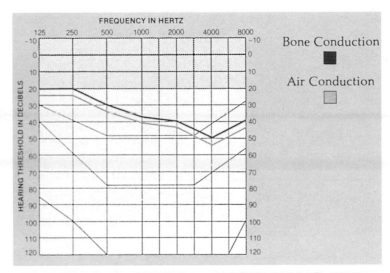

FIG. 13-37 In Alport syndrome, a loss of high-frequency auditory perception may be found in 40% of patients. Because the hearing deficit may be most marked at frequencies between 4000 and 8000 Hz, it may be initially detected only by audiometric testing.

Potter Sequence

Potter sequence can occur in any renal cystic or dysplastic disorder severe enough to produce oligohydramnios or anhydramnios. Oligohydramnios leads to a complex syndrome of fetal compression. Although chronic leakage of amniotic fluid may cause oligohydramnios, it most commonly occurs secondary to decreased fetal urine formation because of renal agenesis or severe underlying renal structural disorders. In the extreme example of renal agenesis the virtual absence of amniotic fluid during fetal life leads to pulmonary hypoplasia and fetal compression, which consequently results in abnormal positioning of the hands and talipes and altered facies characterized by abnormally small, posteriorly rotated ears; a small chin; a beaked nose; and unusual facial creases (Fig. 13-36). Such newborns have what is known as *Potter sequence*, and they usually die of respiratory insufficiency secondary to the severe associated abnormalities of pulmonary development.

Alport Syndrome

Alport syndrome, or hereditary progressive nephritis, is characterized by recurrent hematuria, progressive renal failure, and neurosensory deafness. It is transmitted by autosomal dominant inheritance with variable penetrance. The majority of affected individuals have an abnormal type IV collagen as a result of an abnormal X-linked gene present on chromosome 13, known as the COL4A5. However, a number of mutations have been defined that modify the clinical expression of the disease. The classic clinical presentation is persistent or recurrent hematuria that may be recognized early in childhood. Proteinuria is absent or mild in the early stages of the disease but increases as the disease progresses. The course is commonly one of slowly progressive renal failure, often accompanied by hypertension that is more severe in boys than in girls. The majority of patients with Alport syndrome have neither deafness nor ocular defects, but loss of high-frequency auditory perception occurs in as many as 40% of patients and thus may be used as a clinical marker in family studies (Fig. 13-37).

Alport syndrome must be differentiated from the many benign forms of childhood hematuria, including thin glomerular basement membrane disease, and other progressive glomerular disorders. Diagnosis relies on careful family history, audiologic or ocular abnormalities, re-

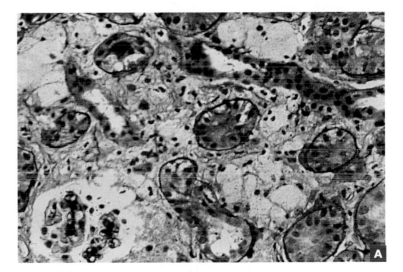

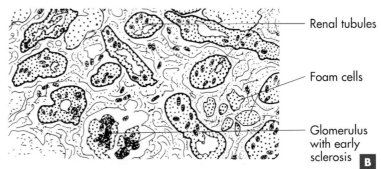

FIG. 13-38 *A* and *B*, Renal biopsy of a 6-year-old boy with high-frequency hearing loss and persistent hematuria and proteinuria reveals multiple aggregations of foam cells and areas of glomerular sclerosis.

nal histopathologic features such as the presence of foam cells and glomerular sclerosis on light microscopy (Fig. 13-38), and ultrastructural alterations of the glomerular capillary basement membrane (Fig. 13-39). There is no specific treatment for this disorder; progressive end-stage renal disease is managed with dialysis and renal transplantation.

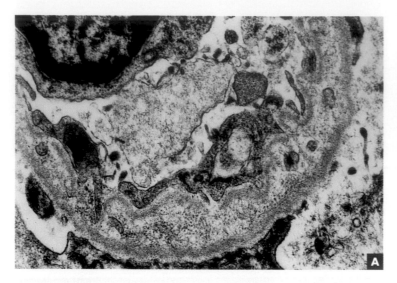

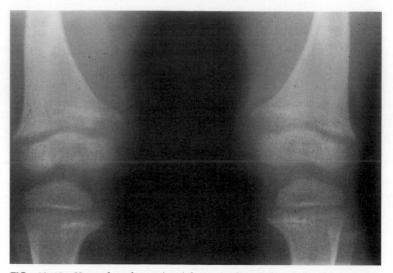

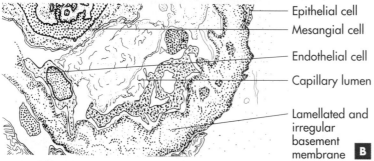

Epithelial cell

Mesangial cell

Endothelial cell

Capillary lumen

Lamellated and
irregular
basement
membrane B

FIG. 13-39 *A* and *B,* Ultrastructural studies on renal tissue from the patient in Fig. 13-38 reveal the characteristic lamellation and irregularities of the glomerular basement membrane, diagnostic of Alport syndrome.

FIG. 13-40 Hypophosphatemic rickets. Radiograph of the knees of a 2-year-old girl with bow legs. Note the widened space between the metaphyses and epiphyseal ossification center, cupping and splaying of the metaphyses of the femur and tibia, and an overall decreased density of bone. (Courtesy Dr. M. Goodman, Children's Hospital of Pittsburgh.)

Hypophosphatemic Rickets

Rickets is a disturbance of growing bone in which defective mineralization of the matrix leads to an abnormal accumulation of uncalcified cartilage and osteoid. Hypophosphatemic vitamin D–resistant rickets is an X-linked inherited disorder that, unlike other forms of childhood rickets, is clinically characterized by normal muscle tone and strength, absence of tetany or convulsions, growth failure, and the predominance of rachitic changes in the lower extremities. Biochemical differentiation consists of hypophosphatemia, normal plasma calcium and bicarbonate levels, normal parathyroid hormone and 1,25-hydroxyvitamin D levels, a plasma 1,25-dihydroxyvitamin D concentration that is low for the level of hypophosphatemia, and absence of aminoaciduria. The pathogenesis of the disorder is believed to involve a renal tubular phosphate leak that is accompanied by an inappropriately low 1,25-dihydroxyvitamin D synthesis by renal tubular cells. The characteristic radiologic features of hypophosphatemic rickets, as in all forms of childhood rickets, include early widening of the spaces between the end of the metaphyses of long bones and an overall decrease in bone density (Fig. 13-40).

The objective of treatment is to promote healing of the rickets and increase growth velocity through normalization of serum phosphorous and alkaline phosphatase concentrations while avoiding hypercalcemia, hypercalciuria, hyperoxaluria, and hyperparathyroidism. These goals are best accomplished by the judicious combined use of oral phosphate and calcitriol. Because nephrocalcinosis and eventually decreased glomerular filtration rate may occur in association mainly with phosphate supplements, regular biochemical and renal ultrasonographic monitoring is essential in determing the lowest amounts of oral phosphate and calcitriol doses that achieve the treatment objectives while minimizing the complications.

Cystinosis

Cystinosis is an autosomal recessive metabolic disorder characterized by the intralysosomal accumulation of cystine in most body tissues. After degrading intracellular protein, the cystinotic lysosomes are unable to transport cystine into the cytoplasm because of a recently discovered defect in the specific lysosomal transport system for this amino acid. In its nephropathic form, the disease causes global proximal tubular dysfunction (Fanconi syndrome) and progressive glomerular damage. The clinical manifestations of this renal tubular dysfunction include failure to thrive, renal tubular acidosis, and rickets, which results from persistent urinary losses of bicarbonate and phosphorus. Also associated with this disorder are low–molecular weight proteinuria and glycosuria.

Cystinotic children show a number of clinical features not obviously related to the renal abnormalities. The majority have blonde hair and a fair complexion; this, in association with growth failure and rickets, results in a strikingly similar appearance between unrelated patients. Clinical diagnosis is established by ophthalmologic examination, which detects a characteristic peripheral retinopathy, and by slit-lamp examination, which detects the deposition of crystalline material in the conjunctiva and cornea. Diagnosis is confirmed by the finding of cystine crystals in the bone marrow of affected patients (Fig. 13-41) and by the presence of elevated levels of cystine in fibroblasts or peripheral leukocytes.

Treatment of nephropathic cystinosis consists of correction of the metabolic abnormalities induced by the tubular dysfunction. Patients thus receive alkali, phosphorus, potassium supplements, and often vitamin D analogues. Despite such therapy, renal function progressively deteriorates, and most patients require end-stage renal disease therapy in the first decade of life. There is no specific treatment available for

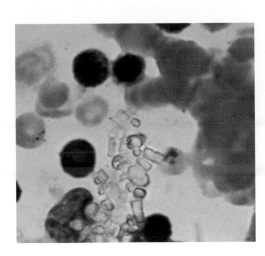

FIG. 13-41 Diagnosis of cystinosis is often confirmed by the finding of cystine crystals in bone marrow aspirate from affected individuals, as seen here.

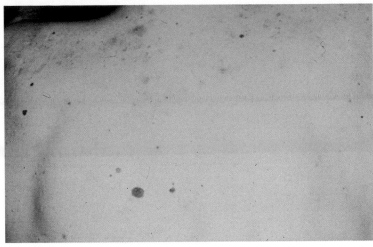

FIG. 13-42 Fabry disease. The small, reddish-purple papules are angiokeratomata. This young man had hematuria and minimal proteinuria but no renal insufficiency.

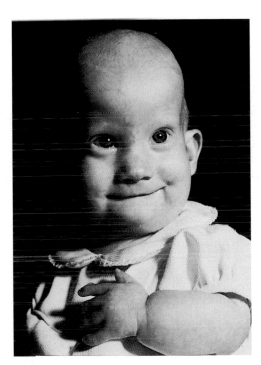

FIG. 13-43 Brachycephaly, short stubby fingers, alopecia, and short stature in a 2-year-old girl with Jeune syndrome and moderate renal failure.

this metabolic disorder. Treatment with cysteamine delays but does not prevent multiorgan injury. Patients with this condition may benefit from synthetic growth hormone because growth failure may persist despite successful kidney transplantation.

Angiokeratoma Corporis Diffusum (Fabry Disease)

The diagnosis of Fabry disease is usually made in childhood by recognition of its characteristic dermal telangiectasias, especially over the trunk (Fig. 13-42). This is one of the renal X-linked disorders for which prenatal diagnosis is possible through measurement of alpha-galactosidase (ceramide trihexodase A) in amniotic fluid cells or chorionic villi or by gene analysis. The absence of this enzyme leads to lysosomal accumulation of an abnormal neutral glycosphingolipid in the vascular smooth muscle of the glomeruli, heart, sympathetic ganglia, and skin. Peripheral nerve involvement results in limb paresthesias and pain. Thrombosis and hemorrhage in these vessels may result in myocardial or cerebrovascular ischemia, and progressive renal failure is usually preceded by hypertension, proteinuria, and hematuria.

Jeune Syndrome

Because many of the children born with Jeune syndrome have severe and usually lethal pulmonary agenesis, the condition is also known as *asphyxiating thoracic dystrophy*. However, many children overcome the early respiratory difficulties and may exhibit a small thoracic cage, brachycephaly, short limbs, abnormal radiologic features of the pelvic bones, and a variety of renal manifestations ranging from mild to moderate glomerular or tubular changes to microcystic renal dysplasia (Fig. 13-43). At the Children's Hospital of Pittsburgh, we have successfully transplanted four uremic children with Jeune syndrome

and have noticed marked improvement in their growth and bone disease, as well as excellent neurologic and intellectual development.

Drash Syndrome

Drash syndrome is characterized by Wilms tumor, male pseudohermaphroditism, and nephropathy. Although most children with this condition have an abdominal mass, there may be a history or clinical evidence of edema, reflecting the severe proteinuria. Because 70% of such children have nephrotic syndrome in the first month of life, they are often misdiagnosed as having congenital or Finnish-type nephrotic syndrome. However, instead of the typically microcystic proximal tubule, widened Bowman space, and mesangial proliferation found in the latter disorder, the characteristic lesion is that of diffuse mesangial sclerosis (Fig. 13-44). This progressive disorder leads to hypertension, hyperkalemia that is disproportionate to the reduction in glomerular filtration rate (hyporeninemic hypoaldosteronism), and progression to re-

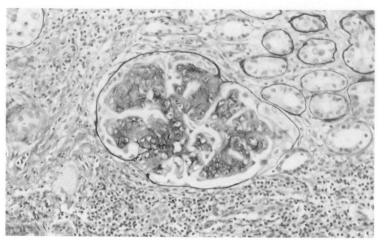

FIG. 13-44 Distinctive glomerular lesion of diffuse mesangial sclerosis in Drash syndrome. Notice the spongy and "solid" appearance of the mesangium without proliferative changes and the obliteration of the capillary lumina. Interstitial inflammation and dilated tubules also are apparent.

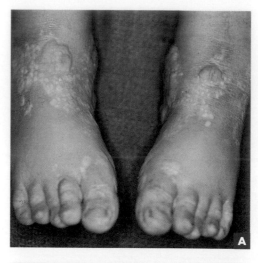

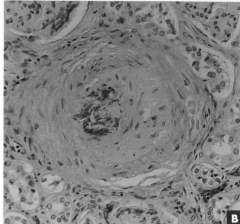

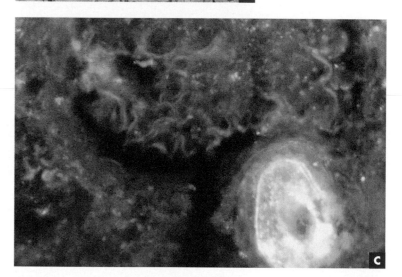

FIG. 13-45 *A,* Large xanthomatous subcutaneous deposits of cholesterol in the dorsal aspect of the feet of a 5-year-old boy with Alagille syndrome. *B,* Renal failure occurred secondary to diffuse renal arteriolar occlusion in lipid-laden endothelial cells and macrophages. *C,* Striking autofluorescence of the lipids is seen within such occluded vessels.

nal failure at 1 to 4 years of age. Despite the absence of ambiguous genitalia, the phenotypically female youngster whose biopsy is shown in Fig. 13-44 had an XY karyotype and absence of testes, ovaries, fallopian tubes, and uterus on abdominal laparotomy performed at the time of renal transplantation.

Alagille Syndrome

The main components of Alagille syndrome, which is also known as *arteriohepatic dysplasia,* are absence of intrahepatic bile ducts leading to cholestatic jaundice, unusual facies, posterior embryotoxon, vertebral defects, and pulmonary artery hypoplasia. Children with this condition have high circulating concentrations of total cholesterol, phospholipids, triglycerides, pre-beta and beta lipoproteins, and elevated apolipoproteins. Thus large lipid accumulations in the skin and other tissues are common (Fig. 13-45, *A*). Various renal abnormalities have been increasingly appreciated in association with Alagille syndrome. In one recent report, 18 of 26 such patients had glomerular lesions characterized by mesangial lipidosis. Although severe renal dysfunction is uncommon, children surviving advanced stages of liver failure may also develop severe renal failure. The latter may occur in association with liver failure ("hepatorenal syndrome") or may result from marked occlusion of renal arteries by lipid-laden or foam cells as shown in Fig. 13-45, *B* and *C.*

Renovascular Hypertension

Renal Artery Stenosis

Although only 5% of pediatric hypertension is caused by renal artery stenosis, detection of this abnormality is particularly important because a cure usually can be achieved. The basic pathophysiology of all renovascular hypertension involves activation of the renin-angiotensin-aldosterone system. If a lesion in the minor or major branches of the renal artery significantly decreases renal perfusion pressure, it causes an increased renin release from the affected kidney. The high plasma renin activity leads to increases in angiotensin II levels with subsequent increases in total peripheral vascular resistance. This also leads to increased adrenal aldosterone production with resultant renal sodium and water retention and expansion in extracellular fluid volume.

Renovascular hypertension should be suspected in any hypertensive child with the physical finding of high-pitched bruits heard in the flank or abdominal areas or when stigmata of syndromes associated with arterial abnormalities are present (e.g., homocystinuria, Marfan syndrome, and the phakomatoses). Patients with renovascular hypertension may show abnormalities on intravenous urography (delayed appearance of contrast in the affected kidney, difference in renal length, ureteric notching), abnormalities on radionuclide renal scans, or elevated plasma renin activity. Renal arteriography together with selective renal vein renin sampling is the definitive diagnostic procedure for all pediatric patients with suspected renovascular hypertension.

Intrinsic diseases of the renal artery include fibromuscular dysplasia, thrombotic and embolic lesions, aneurysms, arteritis, and arte-

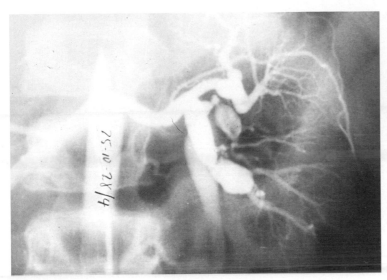

FIG. 13-46 Arteriogram of a 12-year-old patient with malignant hypertension shows multiple areas of stenosis alternating with aneurysmal dilation in the distal segment of the renal artery, characteristic of fibromuscular dysplasia.

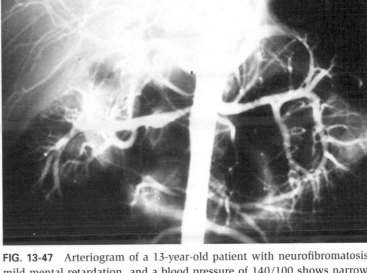

FIG. 13-47 Arteriogram of a 13-year-old patient with neurofibromatosis, mild mental retardation, and a blood pressure of 140/100 shows narrowing of the renal artery close to its origin from the aorta, in contrast to the distal involvement of fibromuscular dysplasia.

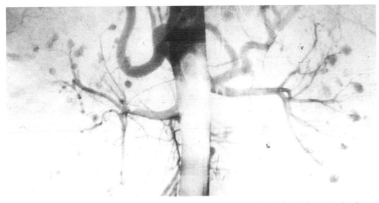

FIG. 13-48 This arteriogram is from a 12-year-old girl with weight loss, fever, abdominal pain, and malignant hypertension. Note the diagnostic features of renal involvement with polyarteritis nodosa, characterized by multiple thrombi and aneurysms.

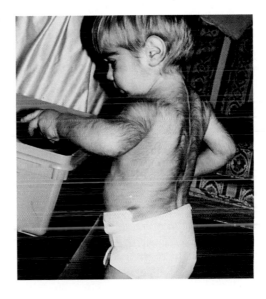

FIG. 13-49 A 2-year-old boy with generalized hirsutism secondary to treatment with cyclosporine.

riosclerosis. The lesions of fibromuscular dysplasia involve multiple areas of stenosis alternating with aneurysmal dilation in the distal two thirds of the main renal artery (Fig. 13-46). Pheochromocytoma and neurofibromatosis may also be associated with renal artery disease. Although difficult to differentiate from fibromuscular dysplasia histologically, the narrowing of the renal artery associated with neurofibromatosis generally begins within 1 cm of the origin from the aorta, distinguishing it from distal involvement of fibromuscular dysplasia (Fig. 13-47). The majority of pediatric patients with polyarteritis nodosa have renal involvement with hypertension, which leads to arterial lesions characterized by multiple thrombi and aneurysms (Fig. 13-48). Such arteriographic findings are diagnostic in the child with hypertension accompanied by weight loss, fever, and systemic manifestations of diffuse arteritis.

Correction of renovascular hypertension caused by intrinsic disease of the renal artery includes surgical revascularization of the kidneys or dilation of discrete stenoses by transluminal angioplasty. Diffuse arteritis, which may cause renovascular hypertension in children with underlying systemic diseases, is treated medically with corticosteroids, immunosuppressives, or anticoagulants depending on the nature of the primary disease process. Young children with bilateral renal artery stenosis together with coarctation of the abdominal aorta represent a most challenging management problem. The small caliber vessels and possible scarring in the vessel walls render bypass or reconstructive surgery a most difficult task. Transluminal angioplasty is also ineffective in most cases. This problem has been successfully managed by staged bypass of the coarctation and autotransplantation of one kidney, followed by autotransplantation of the remaining kidney at a later time.

Hirsutism

Although there are many endocrinologic causes of hirsutism, a number of drugs used in children with renal disorders are capable of producing this condition. Marked hirsutism generally accompanies the use of minoxidil or diazoxide, which are potent antihypertensive agents causing direct relaxation of arteriolar smooth muscle. Cyclosporine, used widely to combat tissue allograft rejection after organ transplantation, has a dose-dependent effect on hair growth (Fig. 13-49). Hirsutism and alteration in body image may be a major determinant of drug compliance, particularly in adolescent girls undergoing organ transplantation.

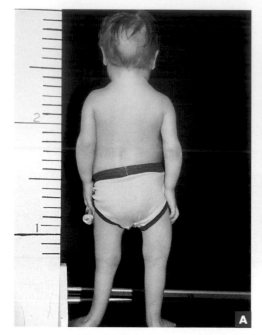

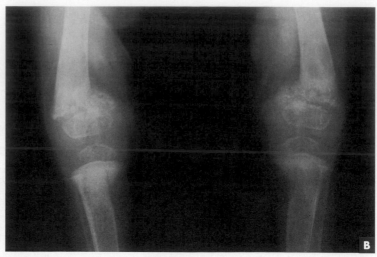

FIG. 13-50 Autonomous hyperparathyroidism and severe renal osteodystrophy in a 6-year-old boy with renal failure caused by posterior urethral valves. *A*, Bossing of the occiput. *B*, Radiograph shows distal femoral and proximal tibial areas, as well as subperiosteal erosion of the cortical bone and active rickets in the epiphyseal ossification centers.

Chronic Renal Failure

Renal Osteodystrophy

Renal osteodystrophy, or "renal rickets," is the osseous manifestation of chronic renal failure and results primarily from two major pathologic processes: (1) relative deficiency of 1,25-dihydroxyvitamin D, which leads to impaired mineralization of cartilage and bone, resulting in rickets and osteomalacia; and (2) an excess of parathyroid hormone, which leads to osteitis fibrosa cystica, the classic bone disease of primary hyperparathyroidism. In any given patient each of these pathologic processes may occur with varying severity, giving a wide range of clinical and radiologic presentations. In children, renal osteodystrophy is clinically characterized by growth retardation, bone pain, and deformity of long bones. The radiologic features in children include increased thickness and fraying of the radiolucent zone in the region of growth plates, subperiosteal erosion of the cortices of long bones and phalanges, and changes in bone density including osteoporosis, osteosclerosis, or coarsening of the trabecular pattern of long bones (Fig. 13-50) or, rarely, brown tumors (Fig. 13-51).

Prevention or treatment of this disorder consists of hormone replacement and aggressive medical control of the mineral imbalance, metabolic acidosis, and malnutrition. When the glomerular filtration rate decreases below 50 ml/min/1.73 m^2, these children are begun on commercially available 1,25-dihydroxyvitamin D$_3$, which is normally synthesized by healthy kidneys. Calcium carbonate preparations also are given to reduce intestinal absorption of dietary phosphate while simultaneously providing calcium supplementation and intestinal acid-neutralizing capacity, which helps to control the metabolic acidosis and hydrogen deposition in bone.

Anemia of Renal Failure

Severe anemia in chronic renal failure is caused by the inability of the damaged kidneys to secrete sufficient amounts of erythropoietin. In untreated children with end-stage renal failure, the hemoglobin levels are often lower than in adults (5 to 7 g/dl), and severely limit the tolerance to physical activity. Good overall nutrition and replacement of folic acid and other erythroactive water-soluble vitamins lost through dialysis treatments only partially obviate the need for blood transfusions. Thus many patients develop the facial features and radiographic appearance of Cooley anemia (Fig. 13-52). Utilization of recombinant erythropoietin has resulted in a marked improvement in the quality of life while preventing hemosiderosis, allergic reactions, infections, and other risks associated with frequent blood transfusions.

Growth Failure

Growth failure remains a major problem for children receiving dialysis and may persist following successful renal transplantation. Recombi-

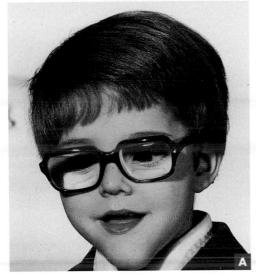 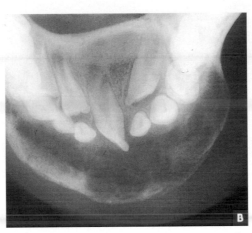

FIG. 13-51 *A,* This 5-year-old boy with moderate renal failure secondary to obstructive uropathy was admitted for evaluation of loose teeth, marked protrusion of the mandible, and exploration of a radiolucent mandibular tumor. *B,* Surgery was canceled after biochemical evaluation was consistent with renal osteodystrophy. Biopsy revealed a brown tumor resulting from intense osteoclastic activity and bone resorption. Medical treatment resulted in regression of the tumor and the prognathia, bone remineralization, strengthening of the dental ridge, and dental preservation.

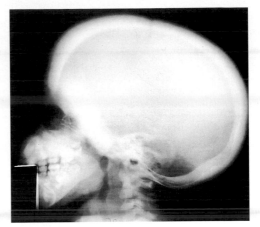

FIG. 13-52 Facial and radiologic features of the anemia of renal failure and extramedullary erythropoiesis in the same child shown in Fig. 13-51. Notice the thickened cranial table with the brushlike projections.

nant human growth hormone therapy has been extremely efficacious in promoting growth of such children before renal transplantation. Precautions may be needed if growth hormone therapy is continued after renal transplantation. This agent is effective even in children with normal concentrations of secretional endogenous growth hormone.

BIBLIOGRAPHY

Alagille D, Estrada A, Hadchouel M, et al: Syndromic paucity of interlobular bile ducts (Alagille syndrome or arteriohepatic dysplasia): review of 80 cases, *J Pediatr* 110:195-200, 1987.

Brewer ED, Benson GS: Hematuria: algorithms for diagnosis, *JAMA* 246:877-880, 1981.

Frick GM, Gabow PA: Hereditary and acquired cystic disease of the kidney, *Kidney Int* 46:951-964, 1994.

Gilli G, Berry AC, Chantler C: Syndromes with a renal component. In Holliday MA, Barratt TM, Vernier RL, eds: *Pediatric nephrology,* ed 2, Baltimore, 1987, Williams & Wilkins.

Goldraich NP, Goldraich IH: Update on dimercaptosuccinic acid renal scanning in children with urinary tract infection, *Pediatr Nephrol* 9:221-226, 1995.

Grupe WE: Relapsing nephrotic syndrome in childhood, *Kidney Int* 16:75-85, 1979.

Habib R, Dommergues JP, Gubler MC, et al: Glomerular mesangiolipidosis in Alagille syndrome (arteriohepatic dysplasia), *Pediatr Nephrol* 1:455-464, 1987.

Harms E: Prenatal diagnosis of inborn errors of metabolism with renal manifestations, *Pediatr Nephrol* 1:540-545, 1987.

Jensen JC, Ehrlich RM, Hanna MK, et al: A report of four patients with the Drash syndrome and a review of the literature, *J Urol* 141:1174-1176, 1989.

Kaplan BS, Kaplan P, Rosenberg HK, et al: Polycystic kidney disease in childhood, *J Pediatr* 22:867-880, 1989.

Kaplan MR: Hematuria in childhood, *Pediatr Rev* 5:99-105, 1983.

Kissane JM: Renal cysts in pediatric patients: a classification and overview, *Pediatr Nephrol* 4:69-77, 1990.

Laufer J, Boichis H: Urolithiasis in children: current medical management, *Pediatr Nephrol* 3:317-331, 1989.

McCrory WW: Glomerulonephritis, *Pediatr Rev* 5:19-25, 1983.

Sibley RK, Mohan J, Mauer SM, Vernier RL: A clinicopathologic study of forty-eight infants with nephrotic syndrome, *Kidney Int* 27:544-552, 1985.

Stapleton FB: Idiopathic hypercalciuria: association with isolated hematuria and risk for urolithiasis in children, *Kidney Int* 37:807-811, 1990.

Strauss J, Abitbol C, Zilleruelo G, et al: Renal disease in children with the acquired immunodeficiency syndrome, *N Engl J Med* 321:625-630, 1989.

West CD, McAdams AJ: The chronic glomerulonephritides of childhood. Parts I and II, *J Pediatr* 93:1-12, 167-176, 1978.

Zerres K: Genetics of cystic kidney diseases, *Pediatr Nephrol* 1:397-404, 1987.

14

Urologic Disorders

MARK F. BELLINGER

M any urologic abnormalities in children become manifest by findings evident on physical examination. Although some clinical presentations are unique, many disorders of different causes may present similar physical findings. Differential diagnosis is central to an appreciation of pediatric urologic disorders.

Physical Examination

Examination begins with a general overview of the patient. Hemihypertrophy, congenital scoliosis, facial or external ear deformities, and multiple congenital anomalies may be associated with urologic disorders. Abdominal examination begins with inspection for visible masses, followed by gentle palpation. Enlarged kidneys are usually palpable as upper abdominal or flank masses. An enlarged bladder or lesion of gynecologic origin may be palpable as a midline mass arising out of the pelvis. Abdominal masses should be characterized as cystic or solid; smooth, lobulated, or irregular; fixed or mobile; and tender or nontender. The groin should be examined for inguinal or mobile gonads. The lower back should be examined for hair tufts, clefts, sinus tracts, or other signs of spinal dysraphism. A general neurologic examination and testing of the anal wink, bulbocavernosus reflex, and lower extremity reflexes should be performed, especially if neurovesical dysfunction is suspected. The bulbocavernosus reflex is assessed by a brisk squeeze of the glans penis or clitoris or a tug on an indwelling Foley catheter. A positive response, which indicates an intact sacral reflex arc, is indicated by reflex contraction of the anal sphincter and bulbocavernosus muscle. Absence of the reflex strongly suggests the presence of a sacral neurologic lesion.

Genital examination involves inspection and palpation. The penis should be of appropriate size. Stretch length can be determined by using a tongue blade pressed against the pubic symphysis as the penis is gently stretched alongside it and the position of the tip of the glans marked for measurement. A concealed or "buried" penis may result from circumcision or may be a congenital finding. In some cases this is merely due to a thick suprapubic fat pad that will resolve with time, whereas in other cases the tethering may be due to dysgenetic fascial attachments that will require surgical correction. It may be difficult to determine the difference between the two. The foreskin should be examined for adhesions to the glans, and the meatus should be examined for size and location. The presence of chordee or a suggestion of its presence should be noted. The size and character of the scrotum and the location and size of the testes are determined. Retractile testes should come well into the dependent portion of the scrotum when the room is warm and the patient is relaxed. If it is difficult to determine whether the testes are retractile, cryptorchid, or normal, a repeat examination may be helpful. In the female patient, the introitus should be inspected to confirm a normal size and location of the clitoris, the urethral meatus, the vaginal introitus, and hymenal ring. Labial swelling or adhesions, vaginal or urethral discharge, or posterior displacement of the introitus with a short perineal body should be noted. The appearance and position of the anus should be noted. Rectal examination should be performed to assess sphincter tone or to help characterize abdominal or pelvic masses.

Antenatal Urinary Tract Dilation

Detection of urinary tract dilation (hydronephrosis) in the fetus is common, either during screening for a fetal anomaly or as a serendipitous finding (Fig. 14-1). Once detected, hydronephrosis in the fetus demands postnatal evaluation, particularly because many cases of hydronephrosis, even of a significant degree, are not detected by physical examination of the neonate. Because the most severe cases present as an abdominal or flank mass, a distended bladder, or generalized increase in abdominal girth and thus will lead to immediate uroradiologic evaluation, most questions surround those infants with modest fetal hydronephrosis and a normal postnatal physical examination. All infants with fetal urinary dilation should have postnatal sonography. Sonography should be done 3 to 10 days after delivery to allow increased urine production to "fill out" dilated systems that may be relatively decompressed in the immediate postnatal period. When early postnatal sonography is normal (spontaneous resolution of fetal hydronephrosis occurs in up to 20% of cases) (Fig. 14-2), follow-up sonography should be performed at several months and at 1 year, since delayed reappearance of dilation has been reported.

When postnatal hydronephrosis is documented, complete radiographic evaluation is indicated. If dilation is severe, renal function poor, or coexistent anomalies demand it, evaluation should be performed as soon as possible. If the infant is in stable condition (particularly when the lesion is unilateral or moderate in degree with good renal function), evaluation should be delayed for 4 to 6 weeks to allow improved glomerular filtration, making contrast or radionuclide studies more accurate. Voiding cystourethrography is an integral part of the evaluation

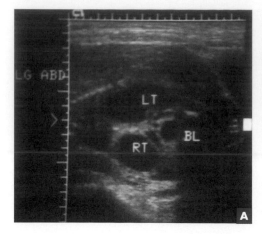

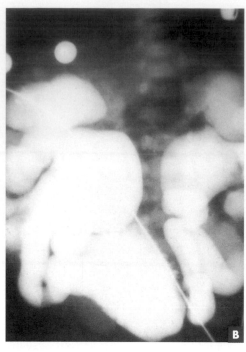

FIG. 14-1 *A*, Fetal ultrasonography performed to assess gestational age revealed bilateral fetal hydronephrosis and a distended bladder. *LT*, Left kidney; *RT*, right kidney; *BL*, bladder. *B*, Voiding cystourethrogram reveals posterior urethral valves and severe bilateral vesicoureteric reflux.

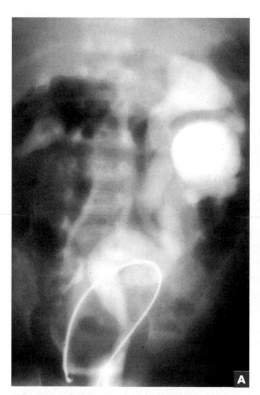

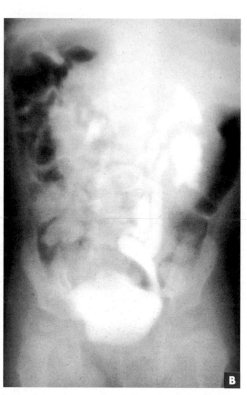

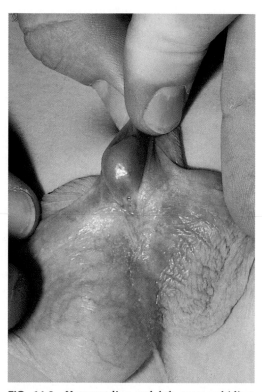

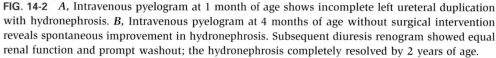

FIG. 14-2 *A*, Intravenous pyelogram at 1 month of age shows incomplete left ureteral duplication with hydronephrosis. *B*, Intravenous pyelogram at 4 months of age without surgical intervention reveals spontaneous improvement in hydronephrosis. Subsequent diuresis renogram showed equal renal function and prompt washout; the hydronephrosis completely resolved by 2 years of age.

FIG. 14-3 Hypospadias and left cryptorchidism in a neonate found to have mixed gonadal dysgenesis with a mosaic karyotype.

of every infant with hydronephrosis and should be the first study performed in all cases to rule out both infravesical obstruction and vesicoureteric reflux (Fig. 14-1, *B*). Subsequent evaluation with either intravenous urography, radionuclide scan, or both may be appropriate to assess function and document whether true obstruction or mere dilation is present. When nonobstructive dilation is found, long-term follow-up may document gradual resolution of the hydronephrosis (Fig. 14-2).

Cryptorchidism in the Neonate

Cryptorchidism occurs in approximately 3% of full-term boys and 33% of prematures. It is not unusual to observe gradual testicular descent in a premature infant. Cryptorchidism is associated with many syndromes but rarely with urinary tract anomalies. The exception is congenital monorchism, which may be associated with ipsilateral renal agenesis. Renal sonography is indicated. Hypospadias associated with even unilateral cryptorchidism should raise the question of intersex, and kary-

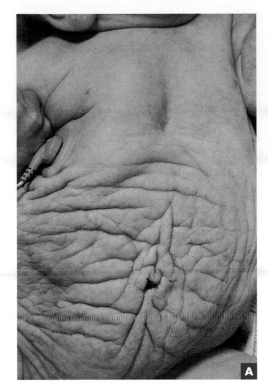

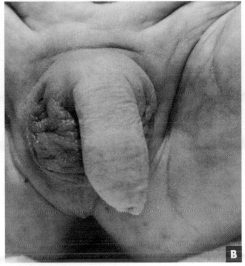

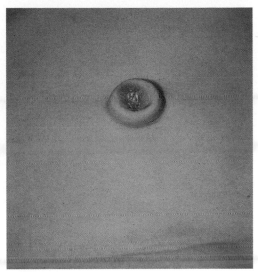

FIG. 14-5 Patent urachus in a girl with recurrent umbilical drainage and inflammation.

FIG. 14-4 *A,* Classic appearance of prune-belly syndrome in a neonate. *B,* Empty scrotum of the same infant.

otype should be determined in the neonate (Fig. 14-3). When bilateral nonpalpable testes are present in infancy, endocrinologic evaluation may determine whether functional testicular tissue exists. The infant with cryptorchidism should be monitored closely, with hormonal or surgical treatment undertaken between 6 and 12 months of age.

Prune-Belly (Eagle-Barrett Triad) Syndrome

This unique syndrome has a fascinating constellation of physical findings and occurs almost exclusively in boys at a rate of 1 in every 35,000 to 50,000 live births. The triad includes abnormal abdominal musculature (variable degrees of muscular laxity, which may be asymmetric), abdominal cryptorchidism, and very "floppy" urinary tracts with vesicoureteric reflux (Fig. 14-4). Plain abdominal film demonstrates the bell-shaped thorax and abdomen, and the typical prune-belly refluxing ureter, with distal ureteral tortuosity, is revealed by voiding cystourethrogram. Associated with the syndrome in most patients are prostatic hypoplasia and dimples on the lateral aspects of the knees thought to be secondary to an exaggerated cross-legged position in utero. Gastrointestinal and cardiac anomalies occur in a proportion of patients, but the factor that most determines longevity is the presence and degree of renal dysplasia.

Anomalies of the Urachus

The urachus extends from the bladder dome to the umbilicus and is usually a vestigial structure during extrauterine life. Several lesions may result from persistence of the urachus: patent urachus, vesicourachal diverticulum, urachal cyst, and alternating urachal sinus. Patent ura-

chus results when the urachal lumen fails to obliterate and the bladder communicates with the umbilicus (Fig. 14-5). Umbilical drainage, inflammation, or infection may result. The differential diagnosis includes persistent omphalomesenteric duct. Voiding cystourethrography is important in making this diagnosis and excluding infravesical obstruction. Urachal cysts may become infected and present in infancy through adulthood with suprapubic or infraumbilical pain, tenderness, a palpable mass, or inflammation. Urinary tract infection with irritative voiding symptoms may result. Sonography or computed tomography are diagnostic. Urachal diverticula usually are inconsequential.

Hydronephrosis

Ureteropelvic Junction Obstruction

Lesions of the ureteropelvic junction (UPJ) are a common cause of hydronephrosis. UPJ obstruction may present as antenatal hydronephrosis, neonatal flank mass, urinary tract infection, or recurrent abdominal pain in the older child and adolescent. In many cases of significant obstruction the kidney may not be palpably enlarged. UPJ obstruction may be documented by sonography or intravenous pyelography and confirmed by retrograde pyelography (Fig. 14-6, *A*). Voiding cystourethrography is important, particularly in infants because vesicoureteric reflux may coexist. In some cases reflux is the primary lesion, with the UPJ kink as a secondary lesion (Fig. 14-6, *B*). Not all hydronephrotic kidneys are truly obstructed, and in borderline cases diuresis renography (nuclear medicine) or percutaneous antegrade pressure perfusion studies (Whitaker test) may be necessary to determine whether surgical intervention is warranted. Some dilated but nonobstructed infant kidneys spontaneously return to a normal or near-normal appearance with time (see previous discussion).

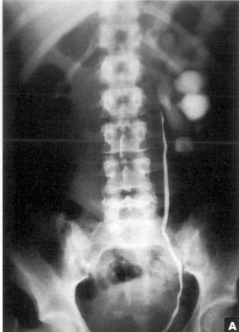
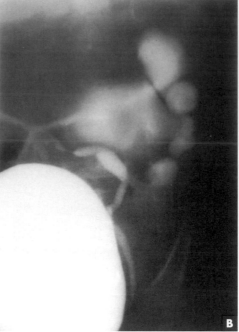

FIG. 14-6 *A,* Retrograde ureterogram defines obstruction at the ureteropelvic junction. *B,* The co-existence of vesicoureteric reflux and UPJ obstruction is seen in this voiding cystourethrogram.

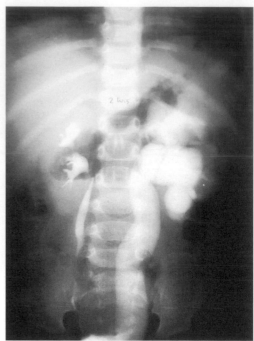

FIG. 14-7 Left megaureter with hydronephrosis.

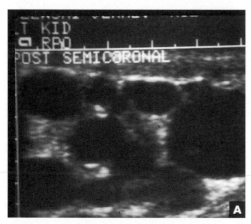
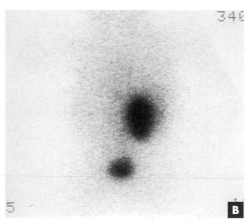

FIG. 14-8 *A,* Ultrasound examination of a multicystic kidney. *B,* Nuclear medicine scan of a nonfunctional left multicystic dysplastic kidney (posterior view). The top blot represents the right kidney and the lower one is the bladder.

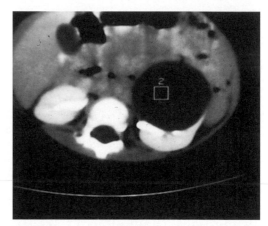

FIG. 14-9 Computed tomography of a huge left renal cyst, which presented as a left upper quadrant abdominal mass.

Megaureter

The term *megaureter* is descriptive of a large ureter, with or without hydronephrosis (Fig. 14-7). Megaureter may be the result of massive vesicoureteric reflux or obstruction at the ureterovesical junction, or it may be nonobstructive. Experience with neonatal megaureter has shown that many of these lesions, if studied by diuresis renography or Whitaker protocols, are nonobstructive and will resolve spontaneously. True obstructive megaureters require excision of the abnormal distal ureter and tapered reimplantation. A nonrefluxing megaureter is thought to be due to either local neurologic or, more likely, muscular abnormalities of the distal ureter that interfere with normal peristalsis. Megaureters are usually discovered on antenatal sonography or they present as a urinary tract infection. Calculi may form in them.

Multicystic Renal Dysplasia

Multicystic renal dysplasia (see Chapter 13) is the second most common cause of renal enlargement in the neonate and may be discovered by antenatal sonography, serendipitously, or during the evaluation of an abdominal mass. Multicystic renal dysplasia must be differentiated from hydronephrosis, and the combination of sonography and radionuclide scan is diagnostic (Fig. 14-8). Because contralateral vesicoureteric reflux is common, voiding cystourethrography should be performed in all patients to detect reflux into the solitary functioning kidney. A percentage of multicystic kidneys (at least 15% but perhaps much higher) spontaneously involute as determined by follow-up sonography, and there is still debate about the indications for nephrectomy. The Urology Section of the American Academy of Pediatrics has instituted a registry for longitudinal follow-up of these patients.

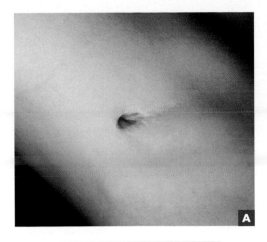

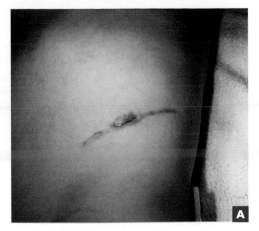

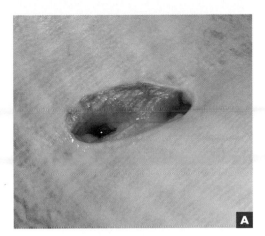

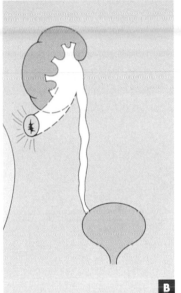

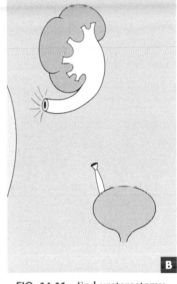

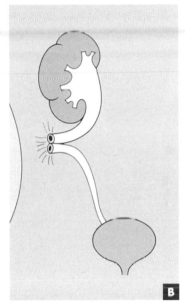

FIG. 14-10 Cutaneous pyelostomy.

FIG. 14-11 End ureterostomy.

FIG. 14-12 Loop ureterostomy. Note double-barreled stoma.

Simple Renal Cysts

Simple cysts were thought to be rare in children until the advent of high-resolution ultrasound technology. They are now frequently detected, albeit much less commonly than in adults, in whom the incidence increases with age. As a result, the traditional admonition to surgically explore all cysts in children has been replaced with the policy of radiographic evaluation similar to that in adults. Simple cysts should be treated as benign. Most cysts are discovered serendipitously while evaluating the urinary tract for infection-related symptoms, but large cysts occasionally present as abdominal masses. Radiologic evaluation usually includes sonography, but computed tomography (Fig. 14-9) and even cyst puncture for aspiration and contrast studies may be used to confirm the nature of the cyst. The differential diagnosis includes cystic Wilms tumor, multilocular cystic dysplasia, duplication anomaly with hydronephrosis, and adult polycystic disease.

Cutaneous Urinary Diversion

Although permanent urinary diversion in children is rarely performed in this age of intermittent catheterization and urinary tract reconstruction, temporary diversion still has an important role in difficult situations. Understanding the anatomic relationships of urinary stomas is an integral part of caring for children with diversions.

Cutaneous pyelostomy. The renal pelvis is marsupialized to the skin (Fig. 14-10). This is an uncommon diversion except in small infants with severe hydronephrosis and compromised renal function.

End ureterostomy. A single stoma is created, which usually requires using the distal ureter (Fig. 14-11).

Loop ureterostomy. A double-barreled stoma is created, allowing access to both the proximal and distal ureter (Fig. 14-12).

Intestinal diversion. An isolated segment of bowel is interposed between the skin and ureters. The normal continuity of the intestinal tract is restored (Fig. 14-13).

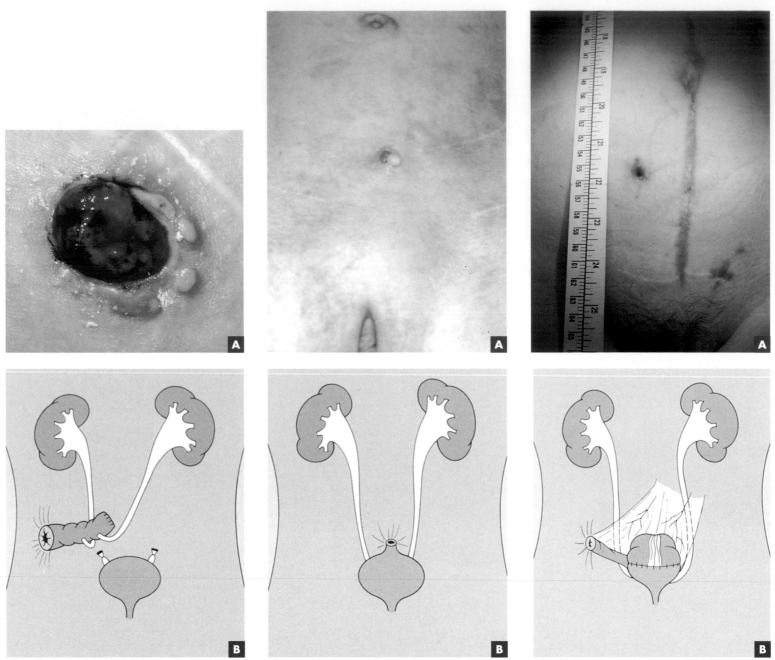

FIG. 14-13 Ileal conduit.   FIG. 14-14 Cutaneous vesicostomy.   FIG. 14-15 Appendicovesicostomy.

Cutaneous vesicostomy. This is probably the most commonly created temporary diversion in children, usually done in cases of urethral valves, neuropathic bladder, prune-belly syndrome, and occasionally severe vesicoureteric reflux. It is basically a vesicocutaneous fistula, and in the small infant it is simply covered with a diaper (Fig. 14-14).

Appendicovesicostomy. This is a continent diversion intended to allow intermittent catheterization of the bladder when urethral access is difficult (Fig. 14-15).

Nephrostomy. This percutaneous or operatively placed catheter is a temporary urinary diversion or upper tract access for contrast or manometric evaluations (Fig. 14-16).

Exstrophic Anomalies

Classic Exstrophy

Bladder exstrophy occurs in approximately 1 of every 40,000 live births. It predominates in boys and is thought to result from premature rupture of the cloacal membrane. The infant usually is otherwise healthy. Examination reveals a red mucosal surface of varying size on the suprapubic abdominal wall, which is the entire bladder opened as a book. On the inferior bladder surface the trigone and ureteral orifices are visible, freely effluxing urine. The penis is epispadiac and lies dorsally tethered against the bladder. When the penis is retracted downward, the entire mucosal surface of the urethra is seen to be

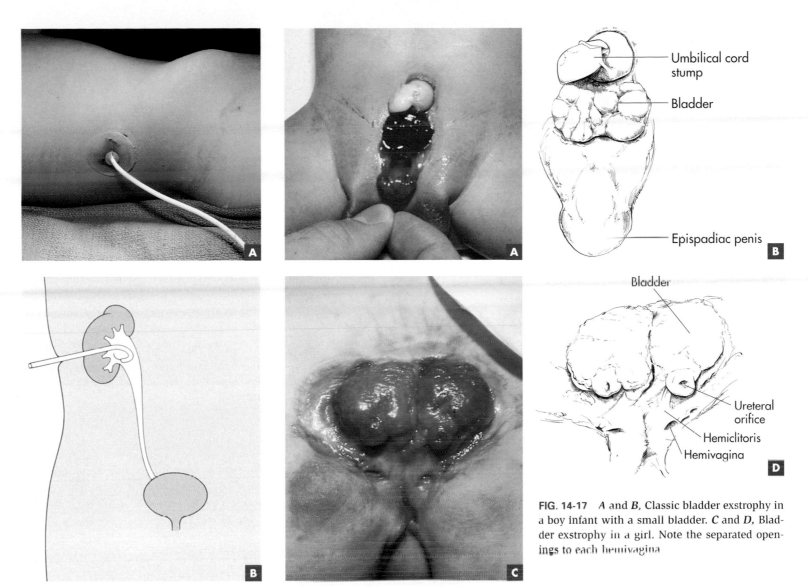

FIG. 14-16 Nephrostomy.

FIG. 14-17 *A* and *B*, Classic bladder exstrophy in a boy infant with a small bladder. *C* and *D*, Bladder exstrophy in a girl. Note the separated openings to each hemivagina

splayed open (Fig. 14-17, *A*). In severe cases the penis may be bifid or rudimentary, and gender assignment may be questionable. The scrotum may be normal or bifid, and testes may be undescended. Inguinal hernias are common. The pubic symphysis is widespread. In girls, a hemiclitoris and duplicate vagina are common (Fig. 14-17, *B*). The delicate bladder surface should be kept moist until urologic consultation is obtained. Prompt upper tract evaluation and neonatal closure are routine. Pelvic osteotomy may be necessary to achieve successful closure.

Cloacal Exstrophy

Cloacal exstrophy is a rare anomaly (1 in 200,000 births). It represents an embryologic mishap similar to that resulting in classic exstrophy, except that rupture of the cloacal membrane occurs before the urorectal septum has completed its descent to separate the hindgut from the bladder. The resulting constellation is severe, with long-term survival little better than 50% in most cases. Most children have a large omphalocele, and a majority have myelomeningocele and hydrocephalus. Examination of the exstrophic mucosa reveals that the bladder is di-

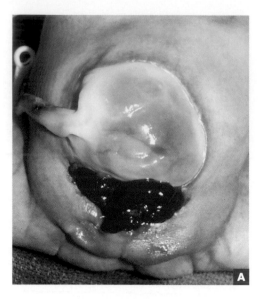

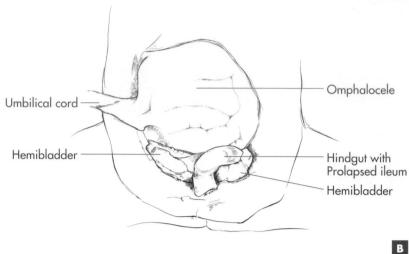

FIG. 14-18   Cloacal exstrophy.

Umbilical cord

Hemibladder

Omphalocele

Hindgut with
Prolapsed ileum

Hemibladder

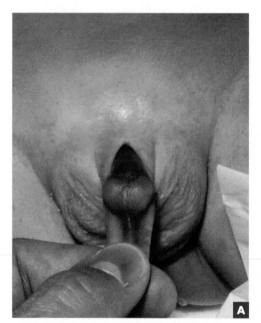

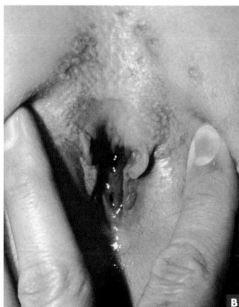

FIG. 14-19   *A,* Penopubic epispadias with incontinence in a boy infant. *B,* Epispadias in a girl reveals a patulous urethra and widespread hemiclitoris.

vided into two widely separated halves, with a strip of bowel mucosa in the middle. This strip is the ileocecal segment, usually accompanied by a long, prolapsed tubular structure, which is the terminal ileum (Fig. 14-18). Separate orifices enter the appendix and a short, blind colon. The anus is imperforate. The genitalia are usually hypoplastic and widely separate, and gender assignment is almost universally female. A multigender-specialty approach should be taken to the infant with cloacal exstrophy.

Epispadias

Epispadias represents the opposite end of the spectrum of exstrophic anomalies. Approximately 55% of patients are boys with penopubic epispadias and incontinence. These boys have a radiographically widened pubic symphysis and a broad spadelike penis with the urethra opened fully on its dorsal surface. The penis usually is tethered dorsally, and the patient is usually incontinent (Fig. 14-19, *A*). A small percent of boys demonstrate continence and penile or balanitic epispadias. In girls, incontinence usually is accompanied by a very wide urethra

and a bifid clitoris (Fig. 14-19, *B*). The cosmetic appearance of the genitalia in both genders can be improved by genitoplasty, but the larger problem is incontinence, which is accentuated by small bladder capacity. Staged surgical correction is the rule. Sonography and voiding cystourethrography should be performed in all cases.

Urinary Retention

Acute urinary retention in infants and children is usually voluntary and associated with severe acute cystitis, urethritis, meatitis (in boys), or vaginitis. In boys, urethral valves (anteroposterior), urethral stricture (congenital, traumatic), and meatal stenosis with meatitis (Fig. 14-20, *A*) should be considered. Retention in girls may be caused by severe labial adhesions or uncommon lesions such as a prolapsed ureterocele. Bladder or urethral calculus (Fig. 14-20, *B*) can be ruled out by a plain abdominal film and ultrasound examination. Severe constipation may coincide with retention, as may acute neurologic changes associated with spinal cord injury or transverse myelitis. Intermittent catheteriza-

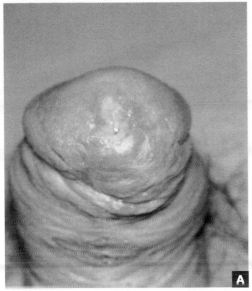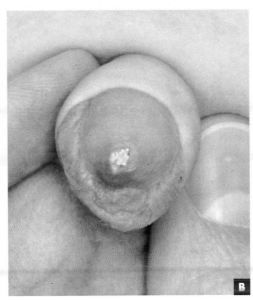

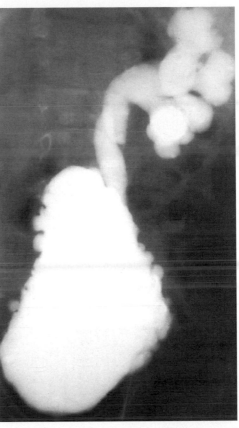

FIG. 14-20 *A,* Urinary retention secondary to severe chronic balanitis (balanitis xerotica obliterans). *B,* Urinary retention secondary to an impacted urethral calculus.

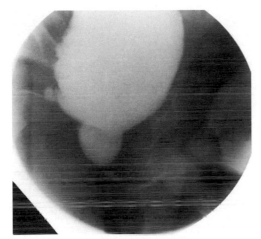

FIG. 14-22 Voiding cystourethrogram of a boy with Hinman-Allen syndrome shows severe dilation of the prostatic urethra thought to represent urethral valves. Severe bilateral hydronephrosis resulted from vesicoureteric reflux.

FIG. 14-21 Severe bladder trabeculation and vesicoureteric reflux in a child with myelomeningocele.

tion is extremely valuable in managing the bladder until diagnostic evaluations can be completed.

Neurovesical Dysfunction

Neurovesical dysfunction in childhood may be either congenital (meningocele, myelomeningocele, intradural lipoma, diastematomyelia, sacral agenesis) or acquired (trauma, transverse myelitis, spinal cord tumor). Independent of etiology, the evaluation and management of the child with neurovesical dysfunction are extremely important to preserve renal function, prevent renal damage from infection, and provide social continence. The pediatrician caring for an infant with neurovesical dysfunction should ensure that periodic evaluation of the child's urinary tract is carried out. This evaluation may include radiographic or urodynamic studies and should be repeated several times during the first year of life or after injury and at least yearly thereafter. Danger signs may include infection, fever, or a change in a normal pattern of bladder or bowel continence (Fig. 14-21).

Uninhibited bladder contractions and uncoordinated voiding are seen in various other neurologic conditions and may also result in bladder dysfunction severe enough to cause not only incontinence or retention of urine but also upper tract deterioration. Multiple sclerosis and other demyelinating diseases are examples. Severe cerebral palsy is frequently associated with incontinence, and when bladder dysfunction is severe, upper tract deterioration may result.

Nonneurogenic Vesical Dysfunction

The "nonneurogenic neurogenic bladder," or what is termed *Hinman-Allen syndrome,* is a little-known but very important entity that may result in incontinence and renal failure. This syndrome represents a learned disorder of micturition and usually presents as day and night incontinence, fecal soiling, and urinary tract infection. Many children display behavioral problems. The syndrome seems to be at the far end of the spectrum of the frequency or urgency syndrome common in childhood. Most children have urinary urgency to the point of inconti-

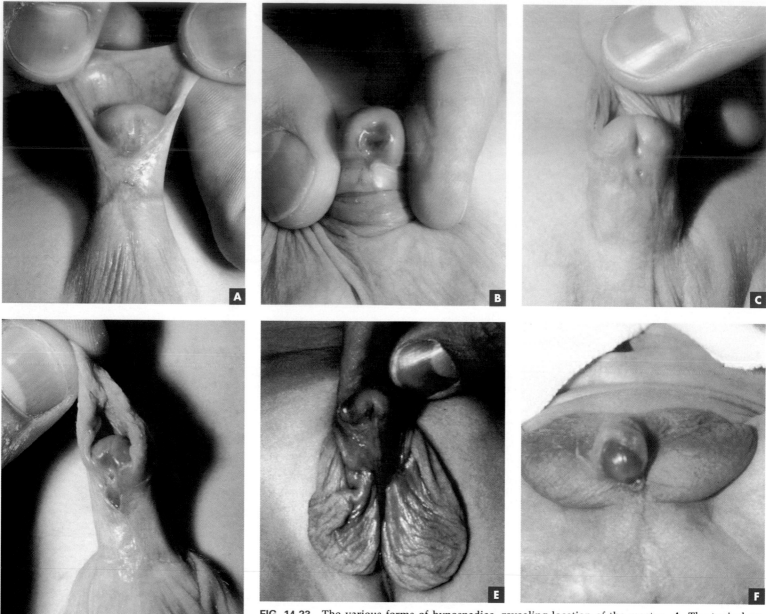

FIG. 14-23 The various forms of hypospadias, revealing location of the meatus. *A,* The typical appearance of the "dorsal hood" prepuce seen in association with hypospadias. *B,* Glanular hypospadias. *C,* Subcoronal hypospadias. *D,* Midshaft hypospadias. *E,* Scrotal hypospadias with bifid scrotum but without chordee. *F,* Perineal hypospadias with chordee.

nence, although overflow incontinence from a full bladder may also occur (the lazy bladder syndrome). On occasion, the child has disordered micturition without symptoms of incontinence and may have urinary tract infection or renal failure. The diagnosis of dysfunctional voiding is one of exclusion, made after ruling out occult neuropathy, since the uroradiographic findings often mimic neurovesical dysfunction (Fig. 14-22). If child and family are cooperative, bladder retraining using a timed, double-voiding regimen may be effective, frequently augmented with biofeedback. In severe cases, intermittent catheterization may be necessary to reverse hydronephrosis. When renal function is in jeopardy and patient cooperation is minimal, temporary urinary diversion may be appropriate. Many children with this disorder require behavioral or psychologic therapy in combination with thoughtful urologic management.

Anomalies of the Male Genitalia

Hypospadias

Hypospadias is a common anomaly that occurs in approximately 1 in 250 male births. The configuration of the urethra varies from mild glanular hypospadias to a severe perineal hypospadias with chordee. In describing the appearance of the hypospadiac penis, it is important to refrain from nonspecific terms such as *first-degree* and *minimal.* Proper definition of the anomaly should give an accurate description of the location of the meatus (glanular, coronal, subcoronal, distal shaft, midshaft, proximal shaft, penoscrotal, scrotal, perineal) and the presence or absence of chordee (Fig. 14-23). If hypospadias is associated with cryptorchidism, the karyotype should be determined. Voiding cystourethrography is not indicated in hypospadias except in severe le-

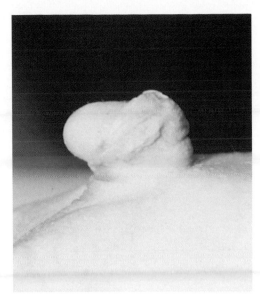

FIG. 14-24 Chordee not associated with hypospadias.

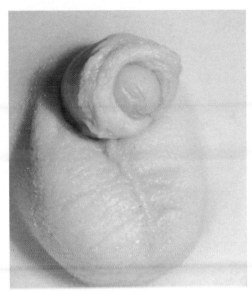

FIG. 14-25 Mild counterclockwise penile torsion.

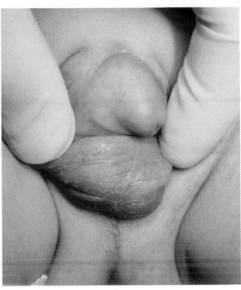

FIG. 14-26 Webbed penis.

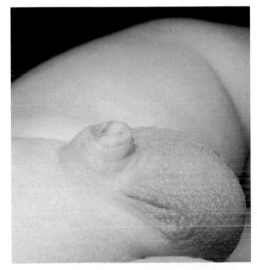

FIG. 14-27 Buried penis after circumcision.

sions or in boys with a history of urinary tract infection. Renal sonography is likely to be abnormal in boys with proximal hypospadias. Infants with hypospadias should not be circumcised because the dorsal preputial skin may be necessary for penile reconstruction. Repair is usually undertaken at 1 year of age.

Chordee

Chordee without hypospadias occurs much less frequently than chordee with hypospadias. Chordee may be a minor problem related to skin tethering, or it may be due to a congenitally short urethra, in which case surgical correction requires division of the urethra and interposition of a skin tube. If chordee is suspected in the neonate, circumcision should be delayed until examination under anesthesia and artificial erection can determine whether either circumcision or repair is appropriate (Fig. 14-24).

Penile Torsion

Torsion of the penis may be congenital or acquired. Congenital torsion may be severe and related to anomalous development of the corporal

bodies, but most commonly, it is mild and related to dysgenetic subcutaneous fascia (Fig. 14-25). Acquired torsion may occur after circumcision.

Webbed Penis

This minor anomaly is easily corrected with a V Y scrotoplasty (Fig. 14-26). Webbing is caused by the transposition of scrotal skin onto the ventral penile shaft at the penoscrotal junction. The ill effects are purely cosmetic in nature.

Buried Penis

Buried penis may occur as a primary finding in the neonate, but it is most common after circumcision (Fig. 14-27). Buried penis is usually the result of a thick suprapubic fat pad; it resolves with normal development. In severe cases, dysgenetic subcutaneous fascial bands bind the penis down. In general, penile stretch length should be measured and confirmed to be normal. The child should then be observed. Buried penis after circumcision may be similar to congenital buried penis, and observation may be the rule. In this situation, removal of more skin might leave the penile shaft skin deficient. If caused by a severe phimosis that covers the glans completely, surgical intervention may be necessary to open the phimotic ring and remodel the shaft skin.

Postcircumcision Lesions

Meatal Stenosis

Relative meatal stenosis is common after circumcision, secondary to mild recurrent meatitis. Mild to moderate stenosis usually is asymptomatic, but dysuria, strangury, or deflection of the urinary stream may bring the child to a physician's office. Mere examination of the meatus is insufficient to document stenosis, and the urinary stream should be observed for a thin or upward stream or for bulging of the meatus (Fig. 14-28). Meatotomy in the office under local anesthesia is curative.

Meatal Bridges

These unusual lesions appear to result from meatal stenosis in which the ventral aspect of the meatus recanalizes, leaving a bridge of skin that may cause dysuria or deflection and spraying of the urinary stream (Fig. 14-29).

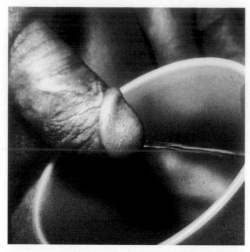

FIG. 14-28 Observation of the urinary stream in suspected meatal stenosis reveals a full stream.

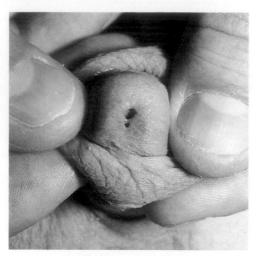

FIG. 14-29 Meatal bridge.

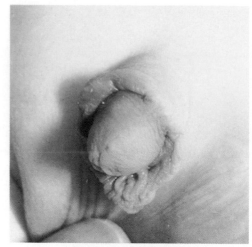

FIG. 14-30 Preputial adhesions after circumcision.

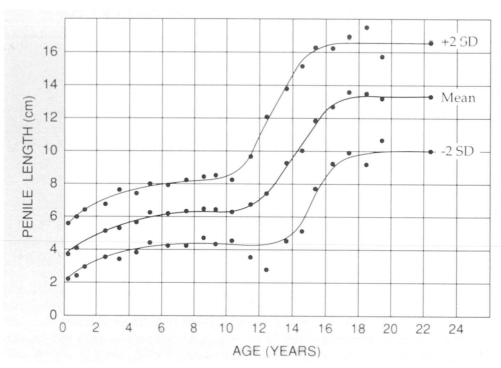

FIG. 14-31 Cumulative frequency curves of penile length for age. (From Lee PA, Mazur T, Danish R, et al: Micropenis. I, Criteria, etiologies, and classification. *Johns Hopkins Med J* 146:156-163, 1980.)

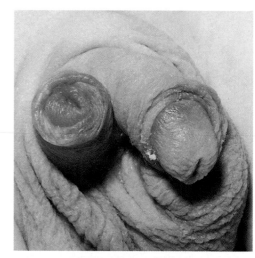

FIG. 14-32 Diphallus.

Preputial Adhesions

Fibrinous adhesions are a result of incomplete retraction of the prepuce during normal development or after circumcision. These adhesions resolve spontaneously with normal hygiene and development. Fibrous adhesions after circumcision result when the free edge of the circumcision adheres to the glans penis and, not properly cared for, grows onto the glans. The resulting bridge of skin may cause penile torsion or trap smegma, causing recurrent inflammation or infection (Fig. 14-30).

Microphallus

Microphallus (micropenis) is a small, normally formed penis more than two standard deviations below the mean (Fig. 14-31), which is thought to result from a disorder in the synthesis, metabolism, or use of testosterone. It is important to obtain an accurate penile stretch length and corporal shaft diameter. Karyotype, follicle-stimulating hormone (FSH), luteinizing hormone (LH), and testosterone levels should be measured in addition to a diagnostic human chorionic gonadotropin (HCG) stim-

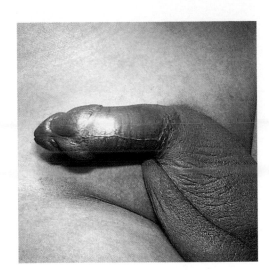

FIG. 14-33 Priapism.

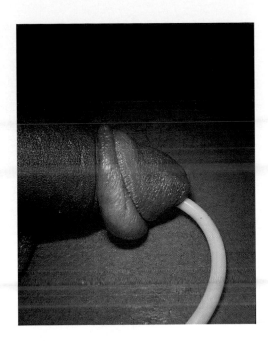

FIG. 14-34 Paraphimosis. Catheterized patient with edematous prepuce proximal to the glans.

ulation test. Although a great deal of controversy exists about the long-term outlook for penile growth at puberty and about the appropriateness of female gender reassignment in infancy, most authors suggest a diagnostic trial of testosterone for 3 months before making a final decision about gender of rearing.

Diphallus

Diphallus is a rare entity usually associated with severe deformities of the lower urinary tract and genitalia. Complete evaluation of the upper and lower urinary tract is mandatory. In most cases of diphallus, one penis is dominant in erectile and urethral function, but in some, the bladder is septate or duplicated, and each phallus plays a significant role (Fig. 14-32).

Priapism

Priapism is a persistent painful erection in which the corporal bodies are firmly erect but the glans is soft (Fig. 14-33). The shaft and preputial skin may become very edematous, and the pain of priapism usually is severe. Priapism in children usually is related to an underlying disease state as opposed to the more common idiopathic variety seen in adults. It is most frequently associated with sickle cell disease but may be seen in relation to pelvic malignancy, leukemia, blunt perineal trauma, or secondary to acute spinal cord injury. Sickle cell–related priapism should initially be treated as any other sickle cell crisis, with oxygenation, exchange transfusion, and alkalinization. Surgical therapy may be necessary to irrigate the corpora cavernosa or perform vascular bypass.

Acute Balanitis and Posthitis

These inflammatory lesions (balanitis = glans, posthitis = prepuce) are most common in uncircumcised boys with infection from the entrapped smegma beneath the foreskin. Usual treatment involves slight dilation of a snug preputial opening, warm baths, and a broad-spectrum antibiotic for a few days if the process is severe. Candidiasis or other causes should be treated appropriately.

Paraphimosis

Phimosis describes the inability to retract a tight, scarred prepuce. If a tight prepuce is retracted over the glans to the level of the corona, a tourniquet is essentially applied to the distal shaft and glans, and ischemia may result (paraphimosis) (Fig. 14-34). Treatment may involve manual compression of the glans and edematous prepuce to allow reduction of the tight band. In severe cases a "dorsal slit" must be performed, surgically dividing the phimotic band. Circumcision may be appropriate after an episode of paraphimosis.

Lesions of the Scrotal Contents

The testis is an ovoid structure lying in a vertical plane in the scrotum in which it is quite mobile, moving up and down with cremasteric contraction and relaxation. Posterior and slightly lateral to the testis lies the epididymis, which may be closely applied to the body of the testis or attached by a somewhat longer mesoepididymis. The appendix testis and appendix epididymis are small embryologic remnants attached to the upper anterior testis or head of the epididymis. These structures are not palpable in the normal state and are not constant findings in all boys.

Acute Scrotum

The acute scrotum is a urologic surgical emergency until proven otherwise. It is most imperative to rule out torsion of the spermatic cord. The most important aspects of evaluating the patient with an acute scrotum are history and physical examination. The nature of the onset of pain and swelling is important, as is a history of dysuria, fever, hematuria, previous urinary tract infection, urethral instrumentation, or perineal trauma. Examination of the scrotum starts with the normal testis, while observing the involved testis for its size, location, and anatomic orientation. The skin and wall of the scrotum are examined for edema, inflammation, and fluctuation. Mobility of the testis should be assessed, as should the presence or absence of a cremasteric reflex ipsilateral to the involved testis. Laboratory evaluation includes urinalysis, white blood cell count, and testicular flow scan if appropriate. The bottom line is expeditious evaluation with a liberal approach to exploration if the diagnosis is uncertain.

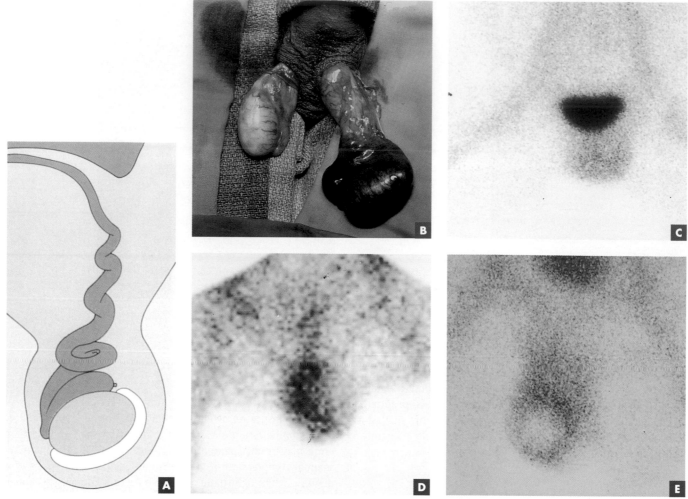

FIG. 14-35 *A,* Torsion of the spermatic cord. *B,* Surgical exploration and detorsion of left spermatic cord. Right testis also shows bell-and-clapper deformity. *C,* Nuclear blood flow scan showing normal flow to both testes. The dark area above the scrotum is the bladder full of radionuclide, which is excreted in the urine. *D,* Nuclear blood flow scan showing increased flow to the right testis resulting from epididymitis. *E,* Nuclear blood flow scan showing the classical "bulls-eye" configuration of a missed torsion of the right testis.

Torsion of the Spermatic Cord

Torsion of the spermatic cord is the most significant condition that must be excluded in cases of scrotal pain and swelling (Fig. 14-35). Because the testis deprived of its normal blood supply has at most a few hours before irreversible injury destroys spermatogenic potential, acute swelling of the scrotum is a diagnostic and surgical emergency until torsion has been adequately excluded as a cause. Torsion may occur at any age.

Antenatal torsion is thought in most cases to represent extravaginal torsion or torsion of the entire scrotal contents including the covering tunics. It occurs during descent of the testis and usually presents at birth as a firm, nontender mass high in the scrotum or at the scrotal inlet. Frequently there is fixation to the overlying skin as a part of the inflammatory response. Although a point of current controversy, the classic teaching has been that these testes are not salvageable, and that it is more important for the contralateral testis to have normal scrotal fixation and not be prone to asynchronous torsion. Although "salvage" of a testis after antenatal torsion is unlikely, acute torsion can occur during delivery and may be a reversible situation. A scrotal mass at birth should thus be considered a surgical emergency until

proven otherwise. If observation is chosen because the involved testis appears unsalvageable, most pediatric urologists now feel that delayed exploration of the contralateral testis should be undertaken to ensure that a "bell-and-clapper" deformity does not predispose the solitary testis to later torsion.

Intravaginal torsion (within the tunica vaginalis) may occur at any age. Most patients have acute, painful swelling of the scrotum, and many also have lower abdominal pain, nausea, and vomiting. It is not unusual for a boy to awaken with pain, but torsion also can occur after scrotal trauma or during almost any activity. On occasion, torsion has a much more insidious onset as a dull scrotal pain of subacute nature. Dysuria is usually absent, and urinalysis is normal, but leukocytosis may develop rapidly. Examination may vary depending on the time elapsed after the acute episode. Most patients are very uncomfortable. The scrotum is reddened and swollen, with the testis elevated because of foreshortening of the spermatic cord. The contralateral testis may have a more transverse orientation than normal. In the acute stage, a hydrocele may develop. The testis may have an abnormal orientation, with the epididymis located in an abnormal position. The cremasteric reflex usually is absent, and elevating the testis to the pubic

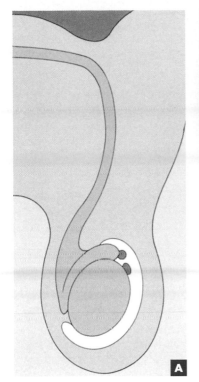

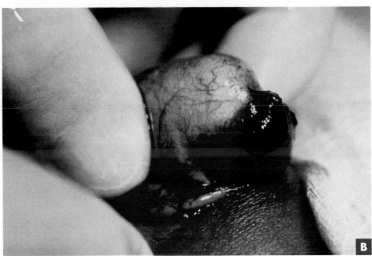

FIG. 14-36 *A,* Torsion of appendix testis or epididymis. *B,* Operative findings after torsion of an appendix epididymis.

symphysis increases pain (negative Prehn sign). When inflammation has progressed, the scrotum becomes a firm, homogeneous mass in which all anatomic landmarks are lost.

If torsion is suspected, attempting to detorque the cord by gentle twisting in either direction may allow the cord to untwist, at least partially. If detorsion occurs, relief of pain is instantaneous. Nuclear blood flow scanning, if immediately available, may be helpful in many instances. A normal nuclear medicine scrotal scan shows identical flow to both testes (Fig. 14-35, *C*). When the scrotum contains an inflammatory process, blood flow is increased on the involved side (Fig. 14-35, *D*), whereas in the presence of an acute torsion, blood flow is diminished. A "missed" torsion, in which the scan is performed several hours or days after torsion occurs, appears as a central area of diminished flow surrounded by a halo of increased activity (Fig. 14-35, *E*). Color flow Doppler imaging has proven to be a viable alternative to nuclear medicine imaging but requires more technical skill and a great deal of patient cooperation, since the transducer must be placed directly on the inflamed scrotum. In situations involving scrotal trauma, the Doppler studies add valuable information about the anatomy of the scrotal contents (i.e., intratesticular hematoma or ruptured testis).

Torsion of Testicular Appendages

The appendix testis and appendix epididymis are embryologic remnants that are normally undetectable on routine examination. Torsion of an appendix, which can occur in the early pubertal age group, may be difficult to differentiate from torsion of the spermatic cord. Early after the onset of acute scrotal pain, a small tender mass may be palpable on the upper anterior surface of the testis or epididymis (Fig. 14-36, *A*). In light-skinned children, the swollen, dark, infarcted appendage may be visible through the scrotal skin (the "blue dot" sign of Dresner) (Fig. 14-36, *B*). In later presentations the entire testis and scrotum may become inflamed and indistinguishable from torsion of the spermatic cord.

Epididymitis

Epididymitis may be secondary to bacterial infection, reflux of sterile urine into the ejaculatory ducts, or ectopic insertion of a ureter into the seminal vesicle or vas deferens. The clinical presentation of epididymitis may be indolent or acute, as with torsion. Fever often accompanies epididymitis, and the urinary sediment may reflect infection. Examina-

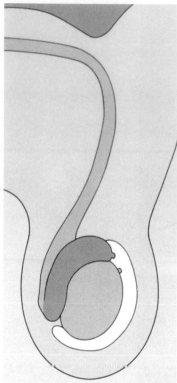

FIG. 14-37 Epididymitis.

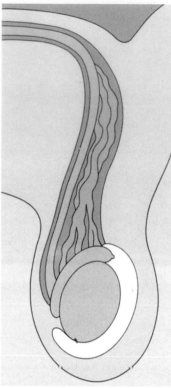

FIG. 14-38 Varicocele.

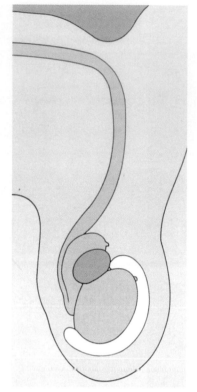

FIG. 14-39 Spermatocele.

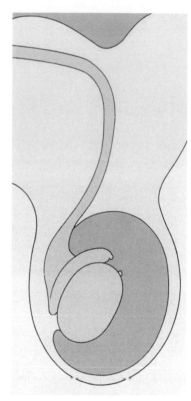

FIG. 14-40 Hydrocele.

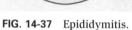

tion of the scrotum in early stages demonstrates a tender, slightly swollen epididymis (Fig. 14-37), but later the entire scrotal contents are replaced by an inflammatory mass. The cremasteric reflex is present, and elevation of the testis on the pubis may relieve pain (Prehn sign). A radionuclide scan demonstrates increased blood flow. If torsion of the spermatic cord cannot be excluded, surgical exploration must be carried out promptly. All children with epididymitis should undergo complete upper and lower urinary tract radiographic evaluation after resolution of the acute process.

Chronic Scrotal Swelling

Varicocele

A varicocele consists of dilated veins of the pampiniform plexus of the spermatic cord (Fig. 14-38). Varicoceles occur primarily on the left side and rarely before puberty. They may be bilateral. The postulated causes of varicocele vary from hormonal to hydrostatic. The postulated cause of testicular injury from varicocele varies from hormonal deficiencies to temperature effects. Most varicoceles decompress in the supine position. Those that do not decompress, or those that present with acute onset on either side, may lead to concern about lesions in the kidney or retroperitoneum causing obstruction to venous outflow. Most varicoceles are asymptomatic and are noted by the child incidentally or discovered on routine examination. Pain secondary to varicocele is uncommon.

Infertility is found in approximately 33% of adults with varicoceles, and because semen analyses are not generally available in children, controversy has arisen over the proper management of adolescents. It is common practice to ablate varicoceles in patients with testicular atrophy or bilateral varicocele. In patients with minimal or no testicular atrophy, a luteinizing hormone–releasing hormone (LHRH) stimulation test may demonstrate hormonal deficiencies, giving reason for correction.

Spermatocele

Spermatoceles are common in adults, and they are recognized frequently in adolescents as well. They are painless cystic masses located in the epididymis or testicular adnexa separate from the testis (Fig. 14-39). They vary in size but are usually less than 1 cm in diameter. They are mobile, transilluminate, and do not change in size. Spermatoceles contain sperm and are retention cysts of the epididymis or tubules of the rete testis. Excision is not recommended in routine cases because of the potential for scarring of epididymal tubules and subsequent infertility.

Hydrocele

Hydroceles are fluid accumulations within the tunica vaginalis or processus vaginalis (Fig. 14-40). They may be small or large, are usually painless even if they are large, and may be tense enough to obscure palpation of the testis. They transilluminate. Simple scrotal hydroceles are common in neonates and usually resolve spontaneously over several months. If the processus vaginalis remains patent, a communicating hydrocele results and may present with periodic increase and decrease in scrotal size. If a segment of processus vaginalis fails to obliterate, a hydrocele of the cord may result. This cystic, nontender mass in the groin may need to be differentiated from a sarcoma of the spermatic cord by exploration.

Lesions of the Female Genitalia

Labial adhesions are common in the prepubertal age group. They represent fusion of the labia minora, postulated to be caused by inflammation of the thin vaginal mucosa that simply adheres in the midline. Fusion begins posteriorly and may progress until almost complete fusion results (Fig. 14-41). On inspection, the vaginal introitus may be

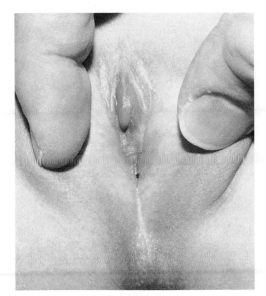

FIG. **14-41** Labial adhesions. Only a small opening remains anteriorly.

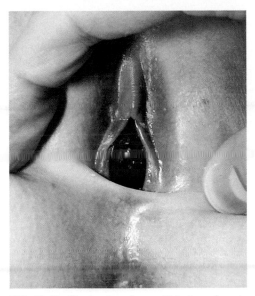

FIG. **14-42** Urethral prolapse. This is a chronic case in which the initial hemorrhagic nature of the acute prolapse has resolved with observation, leaving a protuberant, edematous urethra.

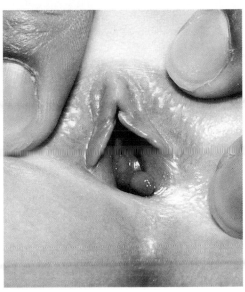

FIG. **14-43** A small polyp of the posterior vaginal fourchette.

closed with the exception of a small anterior opening. Severe fusion may be associated with dysuria, postvoid dribbling as the urine voided into the vagina drains out, or urinary tract infection. Although most adhesions lyse spontaneously as puberty approaches and the vaginal epithelium cornifies, problems of hygiene and discomfort bring many girls to the physician for evaluation and treatment.

Labial fusion must be separated mechanically. This is usually performed easily in the office, after application of a lidocaine ointment to the introitus. Lysis should be followed by the application of estrogen cream to the area for several days to thicken the vaginal mucosa. Unfortunately, many physicians think that mere application of estrogen will cure the problem. This is untrue. After lysis, simple hygiene should prevent recurrence.

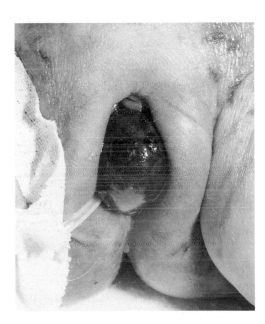

FIG. **14-44** Prolapsed ureterocele. The catheter enters the urethra.

Urethral Prolapse

Prolapse of the urethra occurs almost exclusively in black girls. Its cause is unknown. The presentation is usually bloody spotting, with occasional mild dysuria. Examination reveals a reddened or dark circumferential prolapse of the urethra with an otherwise normal introitus (Fig. 14-42).

Urethral Polyps

Small polyps may originate from the urethral meatus or hymenal ring (Fig. 14-43). These usually are thin mucosal tags that cause no symptoms and require no specific treatment. Fleshy polyps or multiple polyps should be examined closely and biopsied to exclude malignancy such as sarcoma botryoides (see Chapter 11).

Prolapsed Ureterocele

Prolapse of a large ureterocele through the urethral orifice should be considered in the differential diagnosis of all interlabial masses in infants and children (Fig. 14-44). Ureteroceles are cystic dilations of the distal ureter, which are located in the bladder or urethra and may prolapse through the urethral meatus as reddened or even necrotic mu-

cosal surfaces. A prolapsed ureterocele, unlike urethral prolapse, will not present a symmetric orifice but rather an asymmetric protrusion through the urethra. Catheterization alongside the prolapse may locate the lumen of the urethra. Prolapse of a ureterocele may be associated with a palpable distended bladder or flank mass (hydronephrosis). Ultrasound examination of the bladder and kidneys demonstrates unilateral or bilateral hydronephrosis or hydronephrosis of a segment of a complete ureteral duplication, usually the upper pole of an obstructed renal unit. Voiding cystourethrography with intravenous urography or radionuclide studies and occasionally direct puncture of the ureterocele with contrast injection may be appropriate to define the anatomy of the malformation.

Paraurethral Cysts

Cystic lesions of the paraurethral or vaginal mucosa may be found on routine examination and are usually asymptomatic. They rarely cause

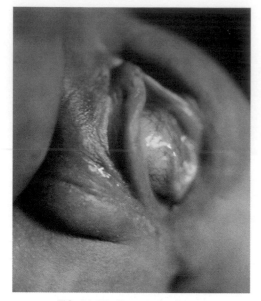

FIG. 14-45 Paraurethral cyst.

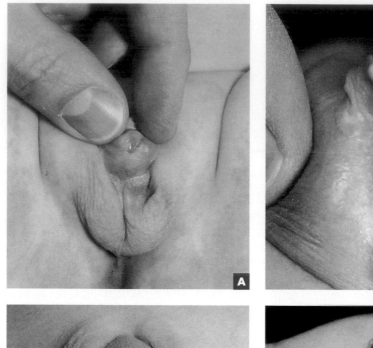

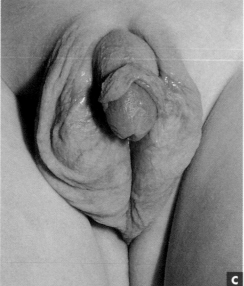

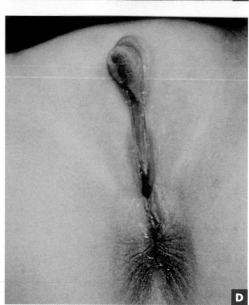

FIG. 14-46 Examples of conditions manifesting as ambiguous genitalia. *A,* Congenital adrenal hyperplasia. *B,* Mixed gonadal dysgenesis. *C,* True hermaphrodism. *D,* Posteriorly displaced urogenital sinus.

voiding symptoms and occasionally present in older girls as palpable interlabial masses. Normal mucosa overlies the cyst, which usually displaces the urethral meatus slightly from the midline. Most cysts rupture spontaneously, but aspiration or marsupialization may be necessary (Fig. 14-45).

Congenital Obstruction of the Vagina

Vaginal obstruction may occur as a result of an imperforate hymen, vaginal atresia or septa, or urogenital sinus malformation. Fusion anomalies of the müllerian structures may result in a septate vagina or bicornuate uterus with one obstructed segment. Neonates may have abdominal masses or urinary retention, girls with didelphia or bicornuate uterus may have pelvic pain or menstrual irregularities at puberty. Examination of the infant may reveal a distended vagina with a bulging hymenal membrane. If a vaginal septum or atresia is the cause of the obstruction, external genital examination may be normal and a complete pelvic examination with vaginoscopy may be necessary. Ultrasound examination of the pelvis may be helpful. All girls with uterine or vaginal anomalies should undergo sonographic or intravenous

pyelographic evaluation of the upper urinary tract given the high incidence of upper tract anomalies in this group. This is particularly important in girls with unilateral renal agenesis.

Ambiguous Genitalia

The human genitalia begin as undifferentiated structures that early in gestation are identical in both genetic genders. The combined effects of genetic, hormonal, and local influences modify the structure and function of the genitalia to produce genital structures appropriate to the genetic gender of the individual (see Chapter 9,). When abnormal development takes place, genitalia of indeterminate nature may result. The recognition of abnormal genitalia is the first step in the evaluation of intersex. The combination of hypospadias and unilateral cryptorchidism should be considered as representative of intersex until proven otherwise. Examination of the genitalia in suspected intersex cases should include assessment of phallic length and diameter, presence or absence of gonads and their size, assessment of labioscrotal and perineal anatomy, rectal examination, ultrasound examination of the

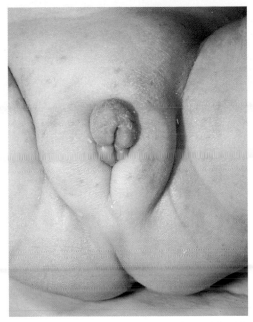

FIG. 14-47   Ambiguous genitalia in a girl with a high imperforate anus.

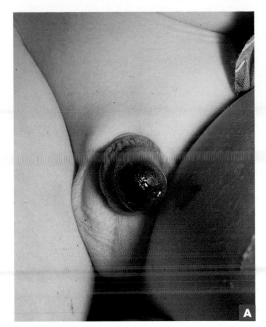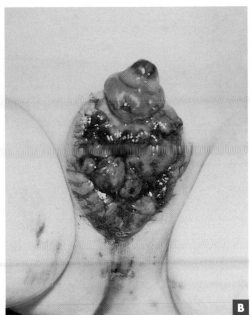

FIG. 14-48   *A,* Trauma to the glans penis from a falling toilet seat. A common injury that usually is best served by observation unless the urethra is disrupted. *B,* Perineal trauma. The testes were injured, but the urethra was intact.

pelvis, and flush genitogram (urethrogram) to delineate urethral or vaginal structures. A full genetic and endocrine evaluation should be carried out as well (Fig. 14-46).

Genital Ambiguity Associated With Imperforate Anus

The embryologic deformity that produces a high imperforate anus in girls occasionally also influences the formation of the external genitalia by presumed local factors. The end result may be genitalia that appear to be masculinized (Fig. 14-47).

Genital Trauma

Injury to the genitalia may be the result of minimal trauma or may be a part of multiple trauma. Although genital trauma may not be life-threatening, proper management may be very important to the later well-being and psychosocial development of the patient. This is particularly important in children. Trauma to the penis or scrotum should always raise the question of urethral injury (Fig. 14-48, *A*). This is easily ruled out in the emergency room or x-ray department by injecting contrast (intravenous contrast in case of extravasation into vascular struc-

tures) through the urethral meatus, using a blunt-tipped syringe or a small catheter. Once urethral injury has been excluded, urethral catheterization can be performed safely. Scrotal trauma mandates close evaluation of the testes, and if injury is discovered, examination and repair should be performed in the operating room (Fig. 14-48, *B*). Scrotal and testicular trauma is not uncommon in breech delivery, when the scrotum is the presenting part. Prompt urologic assessment should be sought. Ultrasound examination of the testes may be helpful if massive edema or hematoma preclude thorough examination. If injury is suspected, surgical exploration is the most conservative approach.

BIBLIOGRAPHY

Belman AB, Kaplan GW: *Genitourinary problems in pediatrics*, Philadelphia, 1981, WB Saunders.

Gillenwater JY, Grayhack JT, Howards SS, Duckett JW, eds: *Adult and pediatric urology*, St. Louis, 1987, Mosby.

Kelalis PP, King LR, Belman AB, eds: *Clinical pediatric urology*, Philadelphia, 1985, WB Saunders.

Lee PA, Mazur T, Danish R, et al: Micropenis. I, Criteria, etiologies, and classification, *Johns Hopkins Med J* 146:156-163, 1980.

Williams DI, Johnston JH, eds: *Paediatric urology*, London, 1982, Butterworth.

15

Neurology

HENRY B. WESSEL

Neurologic Examination

The primary objective of the neurologic examination is to determine the functional integrity of the central nervous system (CNS) and peripheral nervous system (PNS), detecting and localizing the sites of neurologic dysfunction. Techniques and interpretation of the pediatric neurologic examination are based largely on knowledge of normal growth and development. The examination is preceded by a thorough history of the presenting problem, including timing and mode of onset; course; and a past medical history that focuses on the antenatal, perinatal, and neonatal periods for possible prior insults (e.g., bleeding, infection, hypoxia, drugs, trauma). Abnormalities of birth weight; the need for resuscitation after delivery; early neonatal problems with hypoglycemia, hypocalcemia, or severe jaundice; and abnormalities in activity or difficulty feeding shortly after birth often serve as red flags. This is followed by a detailed history of behavior, growth, and development with attention to evidence of delay, slowing, cessation, or regression of developmental milestones and any possible association with prior illness or trauma. A family history of neurologic, neuromuscular, or developmental problems is also important.

The traditional systematic neurologic evaluation proceeds from assessment of mental status and language functions through evaluation of cranial nerves, gross motor function, muscle strength, gait and station, balance and coordination, sensory systems, and deep tendon reflexes. It is applicable to older children and adolescents without significant modification from the evaluation geared to the adult. Tools essential to the neurologist include the reflex hammer, bright penlight, ophthalmoscope, and stethoscope. For evaluation of the primary sensory modalities of light touch, pain, temperature, and vibration, wisps of cotton, sterile pins, glass test tubes (to hold hot and cold water), and a tuning fork (256 Hz for children and young adults, 126 Hz for older persons) are used. A collection of small, common objects (e.g., coins, buttons, keys) to be identified by feel alone are useful for assessment of stereognosis.

Neurologic examination of the younger child requires flexibility and a gentle, staged approach. The first stage consists of observation, much of which can be done while taking the history as the infant sits in the parent's lap or while the toddler or older child plays with toys provided by the examiner. The child's level of alertness and interest in people and the environment are assessed. Facies, head shape, body habitus, spontaneous movements, position, and posture, along with spontaneous vocalizations and quality and pitch of cry in infants, are noted. In the child old enough to walk, stance and gait, as well as the ability to run, stoop and recover, climb onto a stool, and rise from the floor (where developmentally appropriate), are observed. These observations provide a good general impression of the child's developmental level and abilities.

Much of the remainder of the neurologic examination also lends itself to play, and in phase two a more detailed assessment of mental status, language, handedness, and fine and gross motor skills is performed by engaging the child in play. A selection of rattles, keys, spinning and mechanical toys, dolls, cars, small blocks, noise makers, tennis balls, hand puppets, crayons, and picture books supplement the traditional instruments. If further observation of gait is needed, the examiner can have the child walk to or with the parent. Children older than 4 years love to show what they can do when asked to walk on their heels or toes, hop, or do tandem gait along a line. Pat-a-cake games are popular for testing rapidly alternating movements with young children. Then with the child comfortable and rapport established, the hands-on examination is initiated with the child still dressed and in the parent's lap. Trying to catch the otoscope light as it is shown over various parts of the body can precede following the light with the eyes and looking at it. For infants and toddlers, following a face or spinning toy is still better for testing extraocular movements (Fig. 15-1). Having a parent jingle keys at the child's eye level and asking the child to look at the sound while looking in the child's eyes facilitates the ophthalmoscopic examination in older preschool and young school-age children (Fig. 15-2). Asking young children to make faces, stick out their tongues, and blow up balloons are other helpful techniques in assessing cranial nerves.

Tone is assessed by observing resistance to passive motion. Then active motion and motion against resistance are checked. Older preschoolers and school-age children love showing their muscles, and push-pull games can be used to test muscle strength, especially when the children's efforts are admired. Deep tendon reflexes can often be tested at this time with only the shoes off. These are normally brisk, or 3+, in the young infant, becoming 2+ by 6 months of age. If directly tapping on the tendon seems upsetting to the child, it may help to place a finger over the tendon to be percussed and tap that. In infants and toddlers, it is often easier to elicit the ankle jerk by placing a finger over the ball of the child's foot and gently dorsiflexing it before percussing the Achilles tendon (Fig. 15-3). Preschoolers and young children love having the examiner express surprise and pleasure when reflexes are elicited.

Finally the parent is asked to help undress the child, and the remainder of the examination proceeds with the parent providing re-

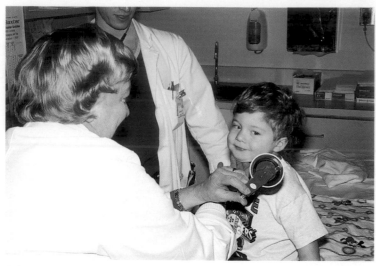

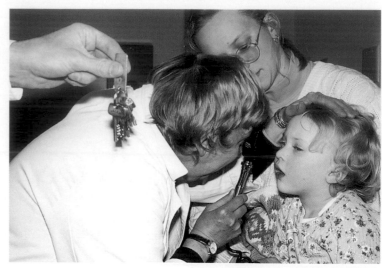

FIG. 15-1   Testing extraocular motion. Older infants and toddlers tend to be captivated by spinning or sparkling toys and readily follow the objects, making it easy to test such motion.

FIG. 15-2   Ophthalmoscopic examination. Having a parent hold and jingle keys at the child's eye level and asking the patient to look at the sound enhances the child's ability to focus, facilitating good visualization of the retina in young children.

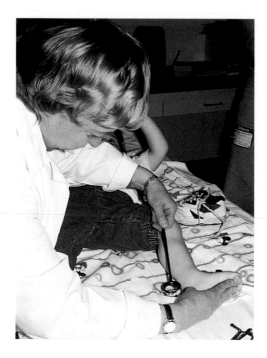

FIG. 15-3   Achilles reflex. Gently dorsiflexing the foot before percussing the Achilles tendon makes it easier to elicit this reflex.

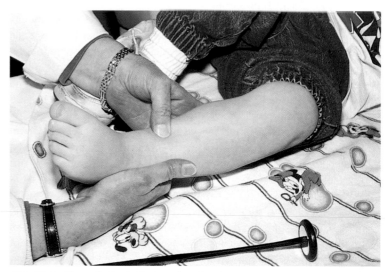

FIG. 15-4   Oppenheim technique for checking the Babinski response. Running the thumb down the medial surface of the tibia produces a more interpretable response in infants and toddlers because it avoids stimulation of a plantar flexion or withdrawal response.

assurance and assistance as needed. During this stage, head circumference is measured in the infant and toddler, and the head, midline of the neck and back, and skin are carefully examined for abnormalities. Muscles are inspected for symmetry, extremity circumference is measured a set distance from a bony landmark if asymmetry is suspected, and abnormal muscle movements are noted. The appropriate disappearance or persistence of primitive reflexes is determined in infants (see Chapter 3). The Babinski reflex is difficult to elicit and interpret during the first year because stroking the sole of the foot may simply stimulate withdrawal or plantar flexion. Using the Oppenheim technique—running the thumb down the medial surface of the tibia—gives a more interpretable response (Fig. 15-4). Evaluation of sensation is difficult in the younger child and is generally limited to appreciation of light touch and pin prick. These may be assessed with minimal discomfort using a partially unbent paper clip.

Neurologic examination of the newborn is highly specialized. The essential components of the neonatal examination include assessment of gestational age, growth patterns, dysmorphic features, motor tone, postures, spontaneous activity, cry, respiratory patterns, brainstem reflexes, response to bright light, response to noxious stimuli, developmental reflexes, and deep tendon reflexes (see Chapter 2). Normal findings vary with gestational age. The immaturity of the newborn's CNS, with functioning largely at a subcortical reflex level, may conceal all but the most severe neurologic deficits, hence the often deceptively normal examination of the newborn with hydranencephaly.

The most prevalent neurologic disorders in childhood are related to CNS infection, ingestions, congenital malformations, perinatal insults, trauma (including abuse), progressive neurodegenerative or neuromuscular processes, and metabolic disorders. This chapter concentrates on selected neurologic disorders accompanied by physical signs that can be detected on visual inspection.

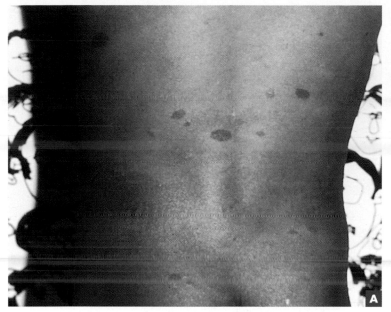

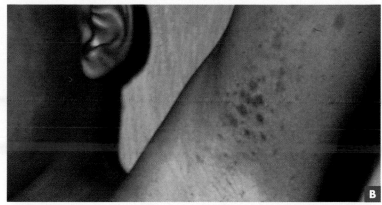

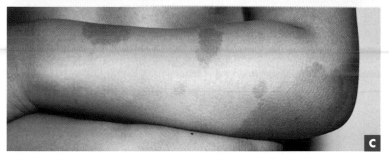

FIG. 15-5 Neurofibromatosis-1. Clinical manifestations of cutaneous pigmentary abnormalities. *A,* Most common are multiple café-au-lait spots over the trunk. *B* and *C,* Also seen are axillary freckling and extensive areas of hyperpigmentation. (Courtesy Dr. Michael Sherlock.)

Neurocutaneous Syndromes

The neurocutaneous syndromes or phakomatoses are congenital, often inherited disorders with prominent cutaneous and neurologic manifestations. The simultaneous involvement of the skin and nervous system, both derivatives of embryonic ectoderm, suggests that these disorders may be caused by an unknown abnormality of the embryonic epiblast. Although the clinical and pathologic features of the phakomatoses are diverse, these syndromes share a propensity for malformations and hamartomatous tumors of multiple organs. Among the more frequently encountered phakomatoses are neurofibromatosis, tuberous sclerosis, Sturge-Weber syndrome, ataxia telangiectasia, and linear sebaceous nevus.

Neurofibromatosis 1

Neurofibromatosis 1, or NF-1 (previously known as von Recklinghausen neurofibromatosis), is the most common of the neurocutaneous syndromes. NF-1 affects about 1 in 4000 individuals. Although usually inherited as an autosomal dominant disorder, as many as 50% of cases may be sporadic. The NF-1 gene has been localized to chromosome 17. Characteristic clinical manifestations include multiple hyperpigmented skin macules (café-au-lait spots), intertriginous freckling, multiple skin neurofibromas, and iris hamartomas (Lisch nodules). Associated abnormalities may include optic gliomas, other CNS tumors of glial or meningeal origin, neurofibromas of spinal or peripheral nerves, pheochromocytoma, macrocephaly, cognitive impairment, and bony abnormalities. Diagnostic criteria for NF-1 are summarized in Table 15-1.

Multiple café-au-lait spots, the most frequently encountered cutaneous abnormality, are brown hyperpigmented macules, usually most numerous over the trunk (Fig. 15-5, *A*). Other abnormalities of cutaneous pigmentation may include axillary or inguinal freckling or extensive areas of hyperpigmentation (Fig. 15-5, *B* and *C*). Hyperpigmented skin lesions almost always precede neurologic symptoms. However, they

TABLE 15-1

Diagnostic Criteria of Neurofibromatosis-1

Diagnostic criteria are met if two or more of the following are found:

- Six or more café-au-lait macules over 5 mm in greatest diameter in prepubertal children and over 15 mm in greatest diameter in postpubertal individuals
- Two or more neurofibromas of any type or one plexiform neurofibroma
- Axillary or inguinal freckling
- Optic glioma
- Two or more Lisch nodules (iris hamartomas)
- A distinctive osseous lesion such as a sphenoid dysplasia or thinning of long bone cortex with or without pseudoarthrosis
- A first-degree relative (i.e., parent, sibling, or child) with Neurofibromatosis-1 according to these criteria

are not necessarily present at birth and may be inconspicuous in early childhood, becoming more prominent at puberty.

Although multiple café-au-lait spots are a clinical hallmark of NF-1, they may also occur as an autosomal dominant trait unassociated with the other features of neurofibromatosis. Genetic investigations in such families have excluded linkage to the NF-1 locus on chromosome 17, indicating a distinct genetic disorder. Multiple café-au-lait spots are a prominent feature of McCune-Albright syndrome, the additional manifestations of which include skeletal dysplasia and endocrine abnormalities. The café-au-lait spots seen in McCune-Albright syndrome are often large and have irregular ("coast of Maine") margins in contrast with the smooth ("coast of California") borders characteristic of the hyperpigmented lesions of NF-1. Café-au-lait spots may be encountered in tuberous sclerosis and neurofibromatosis 2 (NF-2) but are seldom prominent. Café-au-lait spots, typically four or less in number, are pres-

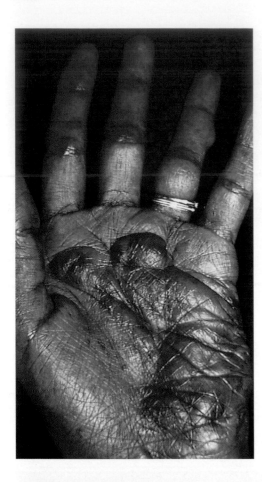

FIG. 15-6 Neurofibromatosis-1. Extensive plexiform neurofibroma of the palm. (Courtesy Dr. Michael Sherlock.)

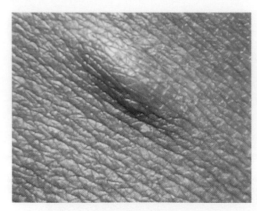

FIG. 15-7 Neurofibromatosis-1. Subcutaneous neurofibroma along the course of a nerve trunk. (Courtesy Dr. Michael Sherlock.)

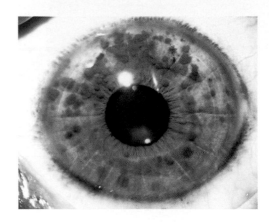

FIG. 15-8 Neurofibromatosis-1. Pigmented hamartomas of the iris (Lisch nodules).

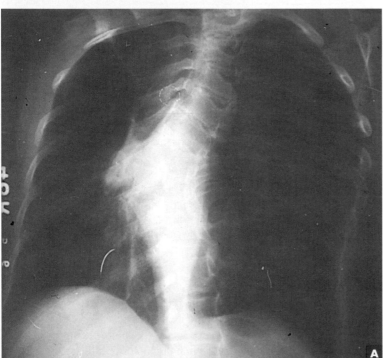

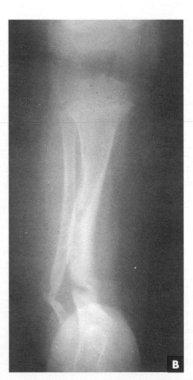

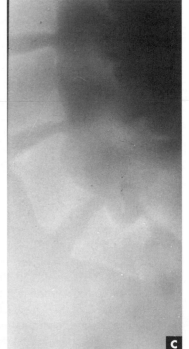

FIG. 15-9 Neurofibromatosis-1. Radiographic manifestations of skeletal abnormalities. *A,* Severe angular scoliosis and vertebral dysplasia. *B,* Congenital bowing and pseudarthrosis of the tibia and fibula. *C,* Scalloping of the posterior margins of the vertebral bodies resulting from dural ectasia. (Courtesy Department of Radiology, Children's Hospital of Pittsburgh.)

ent in about 10% of the general population and are not by themselves a sign of disease.

Additional cutaneous manifestations of NF-1 may include extensive plexiform neuromas at the terminal distribution of nerve fibers (Fig. 15-6) or small subcutaneous nodules—neurofibromas—scattered along the course of nerve trunks (Fig. 15-7).

Pigmented hamartomas of the iris, termed *Lisch nodules,* are found in over 90% of patients with NF-1 who are 6 years of age or older; they occur in nearly one third of younger patients (Fig. 15-8). They do not occur in normal individuals. These hamartomas are asymptomatic and

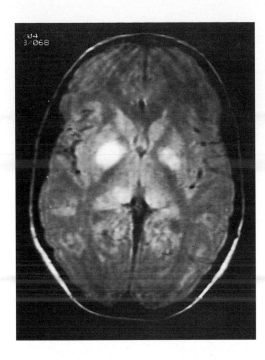

FIG. 15-10 Neurofibromatosis-1. MRI T2-weighted image demonstrates high signal areas in the region of the globus pallidus bilaterally. (Courtesy Division of Neuroradiology, University Health Center of Pittsburgh.)

TABLE 15-2

Diagnostic Criteria of Neurofibromatosis-2

- Bilateral eighth nerve masses seen with appropriate imaging techniques (e.g., CT, MRI) or
- A first-degree relative with Neurofibromatosis-2 and a unilateral eighth nerve mass or two of the following:
  - Neurofibroma
  - Meningioma
  - Glioma
  - Schwannoma
  - Juvenile posterior subcapsular lens opacity

do not correlate with the extent or severity of other manifestations. However, they are helpful in establishing the diagnosis.

Skeletal abnormalities are found in 51% of affected individuals. The characteristic findings (Fig. 15-9) include the following:

1. Severe angular scoliosis with dysplasia of the vertebral bodies
2. Defects of the posteriorsuperior wall of the orbit
3. Congenital bowing and pseudarthrosis of the tibia, fibula, femur, or clavicle
4. Disorders of bone growth associated with elephantoid hypertrophy of overlying soft tissue
5. Erosive bony defects produced by contiguous neurogenic tumors
6. Scalloping of the posterior margins of the vertebral bodies corresponding to saccular areas of dilation of the spinal meninges

Magnetic resonance imaging (MRI) scans frequently show areas of increased signal intensity on T2-weighted images of the globus pallidus, brainstem, or cerebellar white matter (Fig. 15-10). Believed to represent hamartomas, these regions of abnormal signal intensity do not appear to correlate with neurologic dysfunction. However, their presence helps confirm the diagnosis of NF-1. Computed tomography (CT) seldom demonstrates corresponding abnormalities.

Neurofibromatosis 2

Neurofibromatosis 2, or NF-2 (also known as *bilateral acoustic neurofibromatosis*), is a distinct genetic disorder characterized by autosomal dominant inheritance of bilateral acoustic neuromas with a penetrance of over 95%. The NF-2 gene is probably located on chromosome 22. Symptoms usually first appear in the teens or early twenties, when pressure on the vestibulocochlear or facial nerve complex results in impaired auditory discrimination, hearing loss, tinnitus, unsteadiness, or facial weakness. Presenile lens opacities, found in half the patients examined, may precede the onset of symptoms referable to acoustic neuroma. Other Schwann cell tumors of cranial nerves, spinal roots, or spinal cord, as well as multiple CNS tumors of meningeal or glial origin, may develop. Cutaneous manifestations such as café-au-lait spots, cutaneous neurofibromas, and intertriginous freckling are less common in NF-2 than in NF-1. Diagnostic criteria for NF-2 are summarized in Table 15-2.

TABLE 15-3

Diagnostic Features of Tuberous Sclerosis

Primary features (only one required for definitive purposes)	Secondary features (two required for presumptive diagnosis)
Shagreen patch	Hypopigmented macules (ash-leaf
Ungual fibroma	spots)
Retinal hamartoma	Gingival fibromas
Facial angiofibroma	Bilateral polycystic kidneys
(adenoma sebaceum)	Cardiac rhabdomyoma
Subependymal glial	Cortical tubers (by MRI)
nodules (by CT or MRI)	Radiographic "honeycomb" lungs
Renal angiomyolipomata	Infantile spasms
	Myoclonic, tonic, or atonic
	seizures
	First-degree relative with tuberous sclerosis
	Giant cell astrocytoma

Modified from Gomez MR, ed: *Tuberous sclerosis*, New York, 1979, Raven.

Tuberous Sclerosis

Tuberous sclerosis is an autosomal dominant neurocutaneous disorder in which the more prominent features include seizures (96%), mental retardation (60%), intracranial calcification (49%), tumors of various organs (including the brain, heart, liver and kidneys), and cutaneous lesions. The abnormal gene is located near the ABO locus on the long arm of chromosome 9. Seizures are the most frequent presenting complaint. The reported prevalence of the disorder is 1 in 150,000, although it may be an underestimate, since manifestations can be inconspicuous. Diagnostic features are summarized in Table 15-3.

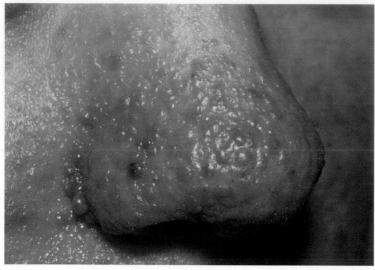

FIG. 15-11 Tuberous sclerosis. This adolescent boy had adenoma sebaceum in a characteristic malar distribution. Lesions were especially prominent over his nose.

FIG. 15-12 Tuberous sclerosis. Ash-leaf spot, an oval depigmented nevus with irregular borders. (Courtesy Dr. Michael Sherlock.)

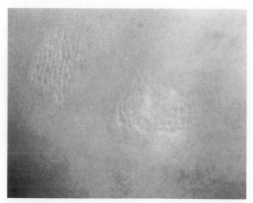

FIG. 15-13 Tuberous sclerosis. Shagreen patch. This plaque of thickened skin with a cobblestone texture is distinctive but is one of the less common cutaneous manifestations. (Courtesy Dr. Michael Sherlock.)

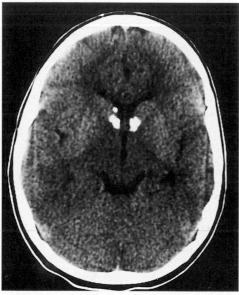

FIG. 15-14 Tuberous sclerosis. This CT scan through the foramina of Monro shows the multiple periventricular calcific deposits characteristic of this disorder. (Courtesy Division of Neuroradiology, University Health Center of Pittsburgh.)

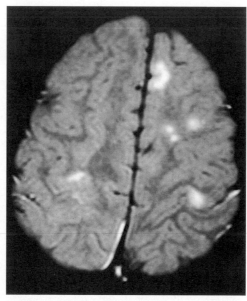

FIG. 15-15 Tuberous sclerosis. MRI demonstrates multiple cortical tubers that appear as areas of increased signal intensity in this T2-weighted image. The signal abnormalities arise predominantly within the white matter subjacent to the tuber. (Courtesy Division of Neuroradiology, University Health Center of Pittsburgh.)

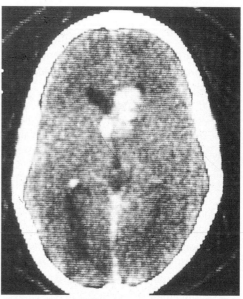

FIG. 15-16 Tuberous sclerosis. CT scan demonstrates a large subependymal astrocytoma, which intermittently obstructed the ventricular system, producing episodic symptoms of increased intracranial pressure. (Courtesy Division of Neuroradiology, University Health Center of Pittsburgh.)

The characteristic skin lesion of tuberous sclerosis is the angiofibroma (adenoma sebaceum). These are seen as erythematous papules distributed over the nose and malar region of the face (Fig. 15-11). Approximately 40% of children with tuberous sclerosis demonstrate these lesions by 3 years of age.

Ovoid depigmented nevi with irregular borders, termed *ash-leaf spots*, are another common cutaneous manifestation (Fig. 15-12). These generally appear earlier than adenoma sebaceum and may be present at birth. They are detectable by 2 years of age in over half of affected children. They resemble vitiligo but differ in that they are not completely devoid of melanin. In fair-skinned infants, these nevi may be demonstrable only under Wood light.

Another valuable cutaneous marker is the shagreen patch, a plaque of thickened skin with a cobblestone or orange-peel texture (Fig. 15-13). Histologically, the shagreen patch is a connective tissue nevus.

Additional dermatologic manifestations of tuberous sclerosis include periungual and dental fibromas and macular areas of hyperpigmentation. Recognition of the cutaneous features can suggest an etiologic diagnosis in some patients with mental retardation or seizures.

In patients with tuberous sclerosis, CT scans often demonstrate intracranial calcifications that appear as multiple scattered areas of increased density adjacent to the walls of the lateral and third ventricles (Fig. 15-14). CT is superior to MRI for demonstration of small calcifications. No relationship has been established between the extent of

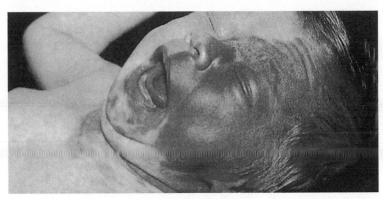

FIG. 15-17 Sturge-Weber syndrome. Nonelevated purple cutaneous hemangioma in a trigeminal distribution, including the ophthalmic division.

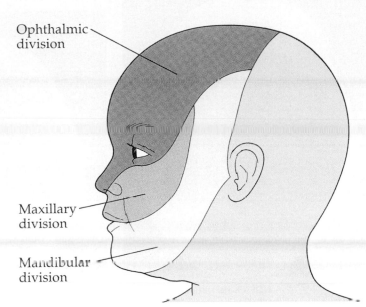

FIG. 15-18 Sturge-Weber syndrome. Cutaneous distribution of the division of the trigeminal nerve. Only patients with facial vascular nevi (port-wine stains) that involve the ophthalmic division are at risk for associated neuro-ocular symptoms.

periventicular calcification and clinical severity as judged by developmental function or seizure frequency. CT may also demonstrate asymptomatic but typical intracranial calcifications in individuals who lack external manifestations of the disorder. This can help identify subclinical cases and improve the accuracy of genetic counseling in affected families.

The characteristic gross abnormality of the brain is the presence of multiple gliotic nodules (hamartomas) of varying size, which constitute the tubers for which this disorder is named. These are located over the convolutions of the cerebral hemispheres and beneath the ependymal lining of the lateral and third ventricles. Heterotopic nodules of identical structure may be found in the cerebral white matter as well. Although cortical tubers are rarely apparent on CT scans, they are readily identified by MRI studies (Fig. 15-15). Severely affected patients have a greater number of cerebral cortical lesions detected by MRI scans, suggesting that MRI may be useful in predicting eventual clinical severity in young children with newly diagnosed tuberous sclerosis. Tumors may arise from cortical or subependymal tubers, complicating the course of the disease by producing increased intracranial pressure and other symptoms associated with intracranial mass lesions (Fig. 15-16).

Visceral lesions associated with tuberous sclerosis include cardiac rhabdomyoma, renal hamartoma and mixed embryonal tumor, and hepatic hamartoma. The cardiac rhabdomyoma is usually asymptomatic, but occasionally an affected newborn may have obstructive congestive heart failure. Renal lesions are often unimportant functionally but can produce albuminuria or hematuria. Chronic renal failure and malignant transformation of renal tumors are quite rare. Hepatic hamartoma is clinically insignificant.

Sturge-Weber Syndrome

The cardinal manifestations of Sturge-Weber syndrome are as follows:
1. A vascular nevus or port-wine stain over the face that involves the cutaneous distribution of the ophthalmic division of the trigeminal nerve
2. Ipsilateral leptomeningeal angiomatosis with associated intracranial calcifications
3. A high incidence of mental retardation and ipsilateral ocular complications

The vascular nevus (Fig. 15-17) is usually present at birth and consists of a pink-to-purple macular cutaneous hemangioma. Only patients with lesions involving the cutaneous distribution of the ophthalmic division of the trigeminal nerve (i.e., forehead and upper eyelid) are at risk for associated neuro-ocular complications (Fig. 15-18). Repeated ophthalmologic and CT examination are indicated only in this high-risk group.

The coincidence of seizures and facial vascular nevus should suggest the diagnosis of Sturge-Weber syndrome, which can be confirmed by CT scan (Fig. 15-19). These scans may be normal at birth but subsequently show areas of gyriform contrast enhancement corresponding to the leptomeningeal angiomatosis. Serial examinations often demonstrate progressive ipsilateral cerebral atrophy. Additional findings may include serpiginous calcifications of brain parenchyma underlying vascular malformations of the pia. These intracranial calcifications are first seen on CT scan but become evident on plain skull films by the end of the second decade.

Associated ocular abnormalities are often encountered. Buphthalmos or coloboma may be present at birth, and glaucoma frequently develops in infancy or later childhood (Fig. 15-20). Dilated vessels in the sclera, conjunctiva, and retina are common, whereas angiomatous malformations of the choroid occasionally occur.

The estimated incidence of facial cutaneous angioma is 1 in 5000, and the estimated frequency of the complete syndrome is 1 in 30,000. Among patients with the complete syndrome, seizures occur in 90%, and contralateral hemiparesis eventually develops in one third. Although most cases are sporadic, genetic determination has not been

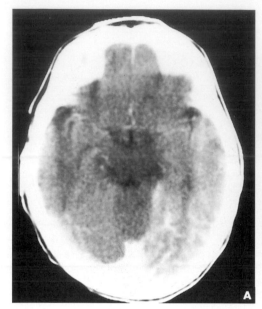
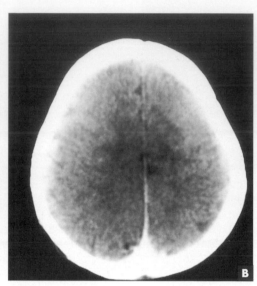
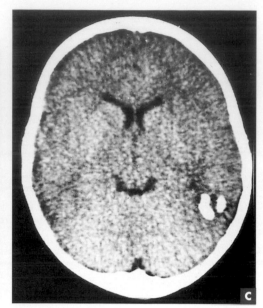

FIG. 15-19 Sturge-Weber syndrome. Although the CT scan is usually normal at birth, findings such as gyriform contrast enhancement, seen here in the left occipital, temporal, and parietal lobes *(A)* and associated hemispheric atrophy may be observed as early as 4 months of age *(B)*. Serpiginous parenchymal calcifications may be found in the older child. *(C)*. (Courtesy Division of Neuroradiology, University Health Center of Pittsburgh.)

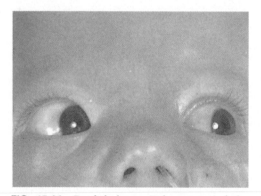
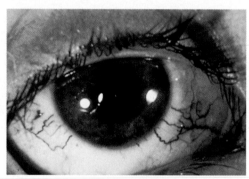
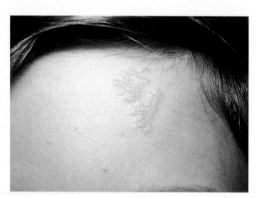

FIG. 15-20 Buphthalmos. Enlargement of the cornea of the right eye is evident. This is one of the associated ocular findings in Sturge-Weber syndrome. (From Booth IW, Wozniak ER: *Pediatrics*, Baltimore, 1984, Williams & Wilkins.)

FIG. 15-21 Ataxia telangiectasia. Such telangiectases in the bulbar conjunctiva usually develop between 3 months and 6 years of age.

FIG. 15-22 Linear nevus sebaceus of Jadassohn. This yellowish-tan, waxy-appearing lesion became elevated at puberty and was associated with seizures and mental retardation.

ruled out. There are, however, no reported cases of direct transmission from parent to child.

Ataxia Telangiectasia

Ataxia telangiectasia is a multisystem, autosomal recessive degenerative disorder characterized by ataxia, oculocutaneous telangiectasia, immunodeficiency, and a high incidence of neoplasia. The nature of the basic underlying defect is unknown. Ataxia is the usual presenting feature, and the course of the neurologic disturbance is rather stereotypic. Tremors of the head may be seen before 1 year of age, and unsteadiness of gait is evident when the child first walks. Progressive global ataxia and slurred, scanning, dysarthric speech are typical during the early school-age years. Loss of deep tendon reflexes and impairment of position and vibratory sensation are evident by the end of the first decade. Adolescence is marked by choreoathetosis, dystonic posturing, gaze apraxia, and progressive dementia.

The characteristic cutaneous manifestations of this disorder appear by 6 years of age. Telangiectases first appear on the bulbar conjunctivae (Fig. 15-21) and develop later over the malar regions, ears, antecubital fossae, neck, and upper chest.

Neuropathologic changes are widespread, with the cerebellum being the site of maximal degeneration. Loss of Purkinje and basket cells, thinning of the granular cell layer, and mild changes in the molecular layer are characteristic findings.

Systemic manifestations include major defects in cellular and humoral immunity. Deficiencies of immunoglobulins A and M are characteristic and together with impaired cellular immunity contribute to susceptibility to the recurrent sinus and pulmonary infections that mark this disorder (see Chapter 4).

Linear Sebaceous Nevus

The nevus sebaceus of Jadassohn is usually present at birth, manifesting as a yellowish-tan, waxy linear lesion (Fig. 15-22) that contains a papillo-

TABLE 15-4

Causes of Macrocephaly

Early Infantile (Birth to 6 Months)	Late Infantile (6 Months to 2 Years)	Early to Late Childhood (After 2 Years)
Hydrocephalus (progressive or arresting)	Hydrocephalus (progressive or arresting)	Hydrocephalus (arrested or progressive)
Induction disorders (congenital malformations)	Space-occupying lesions	Space-occupying lesions
Spina bifida cystica, cranium bifidum, Chiari malformations (types I, II, and III), aqueductal stenosis, holoprosencephaly	Tumors, cysts, abscesses	Preexisting induction disorder
Mass lesions	Postbacterial or granulomatous meningitis	Aqueductal stenosis, Chiari Type I malformation
Neoplasms, A-V malformations, congenital cysts	Dysraphism	Postinfectious
Intrauterine infections	Dandy-Walker syndrome, Chiari Type I malformation	Hemorrhagic
Toxoplasmosis, cytomegalic inclusion disease, syphilis, rubella	Posthemorrhagic	Megalencephaly
Peri- or postnatal infections	Trauma or vascular malformation	Proliferative neurocutaneous syndromes
Bacterial, granulomatous, parasitic	Subdural effusion	Familial
Peri- or postnatal hemorrhage	Increased intracranial pressure syndrome	Pseudotumor cerebri
Hypoxia, vascular malformation, trauma	Pseudotumor cerebri	Normal variant
Hydranencephaly	Lead, tetracycline, hypoparathyroidism, steroids, excess or deficiency of vitamin A, cyanotic congenital heart disease	
Subdural effusion	Primary skeletal cranial dysplasia (thickened or enlarged skull): osteogenesis imperfecta, hyperphosphatemia, osteopetrosis, rickets	
Hemorrhagic, infectious, cystic hygroma	Megalencephaly (increase in brain substance)	
Normal variant (often familial)	Metabolic CNS diseases: leukodystrophies (e.g., Canavan, Alexander), lipidoses (Tay-Sachs), histiocytosis, mucopolysaccharidoses	
	Proliferative neurocutaneous syndromes: von Recklinghausen, tuberous sclerosis, hemanigiomatosis, Sturge-Weber	
	Cerebral gigantism	
	Soto syndrome	
	Achondroplasia	
	Primary megalencephaly	
	May be familial, and unassociated or associated with abnormalities of cellular architecture	

From Gabriel RS: *Malformations of the central nervous system.* In Menkes JH, ed: *Textbook of child neurology,* ed 2, Philadelphia, 1980, Lea & Febiger.

matous excess of sebaceous glands. This nevus may be found on the scalp, face, neck, trunk, or extremities. With time, the lesion becomes unsightly. This phenomenon and a 15% to 20% risk of malignant degeneration have led practitioners to recommend early surgical excision. Although this lesion usually occurs as an isolated abnormality in otherwise normal individuals, an association with seizures and mental retardation has been reported. The risk of associated neurologic abnormalities is greatest when the cutaneous lesion is located in the midfacial area.

CNS Malformations

Malformations of the CNS are a leading cause of neurologic and developmental disability in infants and children. Although CNS malformations are not necessarily accompanied by external dysmorphic features, disturbances of cranial volume, abnormalities of head shape, and skin lesions overlying the dorsal midline should alert the physician to the possibility of associated CNS dysmorphogenesis.

Macrocephaly

Macrocephaly is a head circumference greater than two standard deviations above the mean for age, gender, and gestation. It is a phenomenon that can be caused by a myriad of conditions (Table 15-4), including excessive accumulation of cerebrospinal fluid (CSF) (hydrocephalus); intracranial mass lesions (tumors, subdural effusions); thickening or enlargement of the skull (primary skeletal dysplasias); and a true increase in brain substance (megalencephaly) such as that seen in Soto syndrome, achondroplasia, neurocutaneous syndromes, and certain lipidoses, leukodystrophies, and mucopolysaccharidoses. Primary megalencephaly may occur as a benign familial trait.

Evaluation of the child with a head that is abnormally large or appears to be growing at an excessive rate should include the following:
1. Serial measurements of head circumference
2. Measurement of the parents' head circumferences and exploration of family history for evidence of macrocephaly or neurologic and cutaneous abnormalities
3. Developmental history

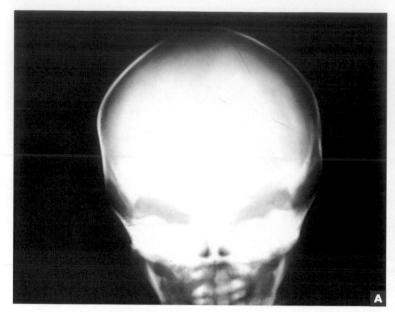
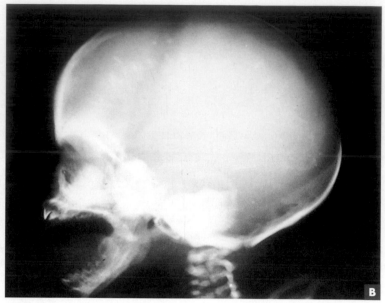

FIG. 15-23   Macrocephaly. Frontal *(A)* and lateral *(B)* radiographs reveal bilaterally symmetric, paraventricular cerebral calcifications in association with cranial enlargement in an infant with congenital cytomegaloviral infection. (Courtesy Department of Radiology, Children's Hospital of Pittsburgh.)

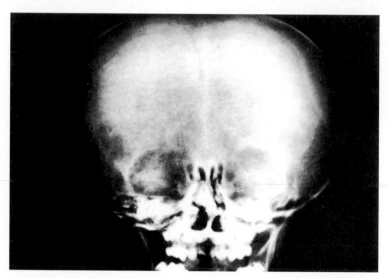

FIG. 15-24   Macrocephaly. Plain skull radiographs allow detection of primary skeletal dysplasias. In this case, note the mosaic rarification of the cranial vault and multiple wormian bones characteristic of osteogenesis imperfecta. (Courtesy Department of Radiology, Children's Hospital of Pittsburgh.)

4. Careful examination for evidence of increased intracranial pressure, developmental delay, skeletal dysplasia, abnormal transillumination, cranial bruits, ocular abnormalities, or organomegaly

Plain skull radiographs may provide evidence of increased intracranial pressure (see Fig. 15-37), identify intracranial calcification (Fig. 15-23), or detect primary skeletal dysplasias (Fig. 15-24). CT or MRI scans allow assessment of ventricular size and permit detection of intracranial mass lesions and chronic subdural effusions. CT is the method of choice for demonstrating intracranial calcification and detecting fresh blood.

Hydrocephalus

Hydrocephalus is an imbalance between CSF production and resorption of sufficient magnitude to result in a net accumulation of fluid within the ventricular system. Impaired CSF resorption may occur secondary to obstruction of CSF pathways within the ventricular system (noncommunicating hydrocephalus) or as a result of obstruction of the subarachnoid space (communicating hydrocephalus). Hydrocephalus secondary to CSF overproduction is rare but does occur in some cases of choroid plexus papilloma (see Fig. 15-44). Noncommunicating hydrocephalus is often due to aqueductal stenosis or congenital malformations of the fourth ventricle and accompanies tumors or vascular malformations of the posterior fossa, which compress the cerebral aqueduct or obstruct outflow from the fourth ventricle. Causes of communicating hydrocephalus include intracranial hemorrhage, meningitis, cerebral venous or dural sinus thrombosis, and diffuse infiltration of the meninges by malignant cells.

The clinical manifestations of hydrocephalus in infancy are stereotypic. The head is excessively large at birth or grows at an abnormally rapid rate, becoming macrocephalic over the first few months. The forehead is disproportionally large, and the face appears small in relation to the calvarium. The scalp is thin and glistening; its veins are distended, often becoming strikingly dilated when the infant cries. The anterior fontanelle is large, tense, and nonpulsatile, and the sutures are excessively wide (Fig. 15-25). Divergent strabismus, abducens nerve paresis, and impaired upward gaze are important ocular findings. With severe hydrocephalus, there may be involuntary, forced, conjugate, downward deviation of the eyes so that the inferior half of the iris is hidden by the lower eyelid, producing the "sunsetting" sign (Fig. 15-25, *B*). Neurologic abnormalities include developmental delay, persistence of early infantile automatisms, and spasticity and hyperreflexia of the lower extremities. CT or MRI scans demonstrate enlargement of the ventricular system and thinning of the cortical mantle and may provide additional anatomic information concerning the etiology (Fig. 15-26).

Infantile hydrocephalus must be distinguished from other causes of macrocephaly in infancy such as chronic subdural hematoma, expanding porencephalic cyst, and certain degenerative disorders that may produce abnormal enlargement of the head (see Table 15-4). In prema-

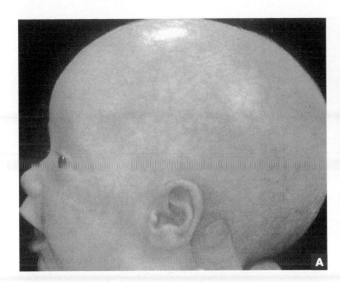

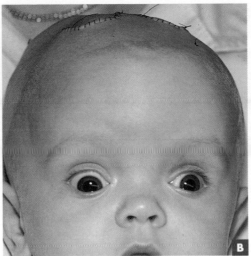

FIG. 15-25 Infantile hydrocephalus. *A,* Characteristic enlarged head, thinning of the scalp, distended scalp veins, and a full fontanelle. *B,* Paresis of the upward gaze is seen in an infant with hydrocephalus resulting from aqueductal stenosis. It appears more apparent on the right. This phenomenon is often termed the *sunsetting sign.* (*A* From Booth IW, Wozniak ER. *Pediatrics,* Baltimore, 1984, Williams & Wilkins; *B* Courtesy Dr. Albert Biglan, Children's Hospital of Pittsburgh.)

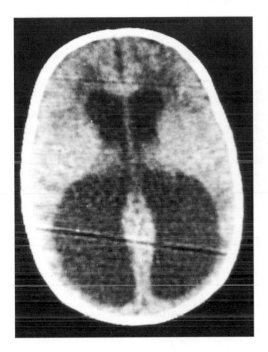

FIG. 15-26 Infantile hydrocephalus. CT scan demonstrates a dilated ventricular system and thinning of the cortical mantle. (Courtesy Division of Neuroradiology, University Health Center of Pittsburgh.)

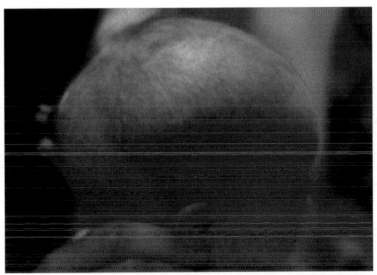

FIG. 15-27 Dandy-Walker malformation. Transillumination demonstrates a posterior fossa cyst. Note also the bulging occiput, prominent scalp veins, and enlargement of the head. (Courtesy Dr. Michael J. Painter, Children's Hospital of Pittsburgh.)

ture infants with suspected hydrocephalus, the normally rapid postnatal head growth must be taken into account.

Dandy-Walker Malformation

The Dandy-Walker malformation is a primary developmental abnormality characterized by progressive cystic enlargement of the fourth ventricle beginning early in fetal life. This is accompanied by enlargement of the posterior fossa and upward displacement of the tentorium, torcula, and transverse sinuses. Associated hydrocephalus is almost universal, and may be present at birth or may develop later, during infancy or childhood. Of affected individuals, 60% show signs of hydrocephalus and increased intracranial pressure by 2 years of age.

Clinical manifestations of Dandy-Walker malformation are variable and depend on the severity and rate of progression of the associated hydrocephalus. A child with a symptomatic condition often has an un-usually prominent bulging occiput in addition to the usual findings of hydrocephalus. In children under 1 year of age, transillumination of the skull effectively demonstrates the posterior fossa cyst (Fig. 15-27). Ataxia, nystagmus, and cranial nerve deficits may also be prominent.

Plain skull radiographs demonstrate posteroinferior enlargement of the cranial vault, thinning and ballooning of the occipital squama, and upward displacement of the torcula. CT or MRI scans confirm the presence of a large posterior fossa cyst, a small cerebellar remnant, and associated hydrocephalus (Fig. 15-28).

Hydranencephaly

Hydranencephaly is a severe anomaly of the brain characterized by the absence of the cerebral hemispheres despite intact meninges and a normal skull. Affected children often appear deceptively normal at

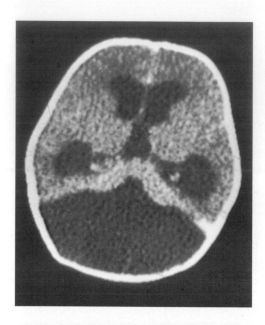

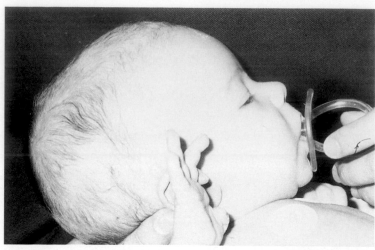

FIG. 15-28 Dandy-Walker malformation. CT scan shows a posterior fossa cyst, a small cerebellar remnant, and associated hydrocephalus.

FIG. 15-29 Hydranencephaly. Patient, age 3 weeks, has a deceptively normal appearance with little to suggest a severe brain abnormality.

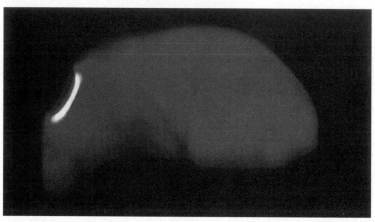

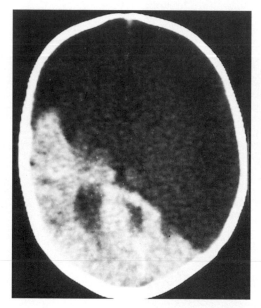

FIG. 15-30 Hydranencephaly. Transillumination of the skull lights up the entire calvarium, suggesting the diagnosis.

FIG. 15-31 Hydranencephaly. CT scan demonstrates replacement of the cerebral hemispheres by a large, water-dense cavity with residual islands of brain tissue in regions of the occipital poles and right inferior temporal lobe. (Courtesy Division of Neuroradiology, University Health Center of Pittsburgh.)

birth, with little to suggest the presence of a severe brain abnormality (Fig. 15-29). Since newborns function at a subcortical reflex level, even complete absence of the cerebral hemispheres may not interfere with normal reflexes. However, within the first few weeks of life, developmental arrest, decerebration, hypertonia, and hyperreflexia become apparent in the infant with hydranencephaly. Most of these infants do not live beyond 6 to 12 months, although survival for several years is occasionally reported. Seizures are common, and progressive enlargement of the head may complicate nursing care.

The diagnosis may be suggested if, on transillumination of the skull, the entire calvarium is lit up (Fig. 15-30). However, severe hydrocephalus and bilateral subdural hygromas may present a similar appearance.

CT scan demonstrates a large, water-dense cavity replacing the cerebral hemispheres with islands of residual brain tissue at the base (Fig. 15-31). To distinguish this disorder from massive bilateral subdural hygromas, cerebral angiography is required to confirm absence of the cerebrum.

Microcephaly

Microcephaly is a head circumference more than two standard deviations below the mean for age, gender, and gestation. Apart from cases resulting from premature closure of the sutures (generalized craniosynostosis), microcephaly reflects an abnormally small brain and can be a symptom of any disorder that impairs brain growth (Table 15-5). The neurologic manifestations range from minor (e.g., poor fine motor skills, mild intellectual impairment) to profound (e.g., decerebration, chronic vegetative state). Diagnostic evaluation should include the family history, prenatal history, search for associated congenital anomalies, karyotyping, amino acid screening, and serologic studies for intrauterine infection. Plain skull radiographs can detect craniosynostosis, whereas CT scan is useful in identifying intracranial calcifications. MRI is preferred for delineation of recognizable patterns of CNS dysmorphogenesis.

Occult Spinal Dysraphism

Development of the human nervous system begins early in the third week of gestation with the proliferation of ectodermal cells in the dor-

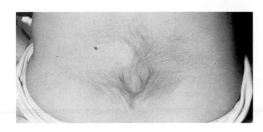

FIG. 15-32 Occult spinal dysraphism. Note the hairy patch over the lumbar region, here associated with diastematomyelia. (Courtesy Dr. Michael J. Painter, Children's Hospital of Pittsburgh.)

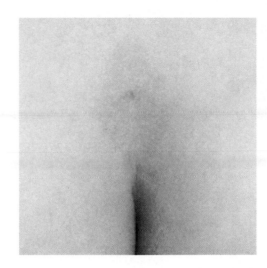

FIG. 15-33 Occult spinal dysraphism. Sacral sinus tract associated with intraspinal dermoid tumor. (Courtesy Dr. Michael J. Painter, Children's Hospital of Pittsburgh.)

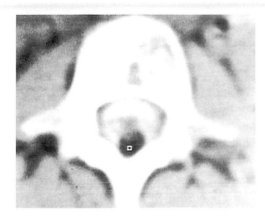

FIG. 15-34 Occult spinal dysraphism. CT scan demonstrates an intraspinal lipoma in a child with a subcutaneous lipoma over the lumbar spine.

Intraspinal lipoma

TABLE 15-5

Causes of Microcephaly

Genetic Defects	Antenatal Irradiation
Autosomal recessive defects	
Autosomal dominant defects	**Exposure to Drugs and Chemicals During Gestation**
	Ethyl alcohol exposure (fetal alcohol syndrome)
Disorders of Karyotype	Phenytoin exposure
Trisomies	Trimethadione exposure
Deletions	Methyl mercury exposure
Translocations	
	Maternal Phenylketonuria
Intrauterine Infections	
Rubella	**Perinatal Insults**
Cytomegalic inclusion disease	Traumatic insults
	Anoxic insults
Toxoplasmosis	Metabolic insults
Congenital syphilis	Infectious insults
Herpes virus infections	

sal midline to form the neural plate. By the end of the fourth week, the neural plate has invaginated and then fused in the midline to form the neural tube. The cerebrum, diencephalon, midbrain, and brainstem develop from the rostral portion of the neural tube. The caudal portion separates from the overlying ectoderm, forming the precursor of the spinal cord, and is surrounded by mesodermal elements destined to form the vertebral bodies and supporting soft tissue structures. Midline spinal cord and vertebral skeletal defects, termed *spinal dysraphism*, result from defective closure of the caudal neural tube. Abnormal neural tube closure beginning early in the embryologic sequence produces dysraphic states involving neural and skeletal elements (myelomeningocele), whereas closure defects occurring later produce congenital anomalies restricted to the posterior elements of the vertebrae (spina bifida occulta).

Occult spinal dysraphism is a defect of intermediate severity in which vertebral anomalies are associated with underlying intraspinal tumors or developmental abnormalities. Its presence is often betrayed by cutaneous abnormalities centered over the midline of the back, such

as a hairy patch (Fig. 15-32), skin tag, port-wine stain, hemangioma, subcutaneous lipoma, or sinus tract (Fig. 15-33). Patients with such skin lesions overlying the lumbosacral spine should have spinal radiographs taken. If these reveal underlying vertebral abnormalities, neuroradiologic investigations are indicated because early surgical intervention can prevent the development of progressive neurologic deficits. Common intraspinal lesions include dermoid tumors, intraspinal lipomas (Fig. 15-34), and diastematomyelia (Fig. 15-35).

Although some patients with occult spinal dysraphism may show signs of neurologic dysfunction and talipes equinovarus from birth, most develop symptoms insidiously after a symptom-free interval. Dysfunction usually begins at around 3 years of age, but many do not develop problems until school age or adolescence. Presenting complaints may include back or leg stiffness, clumsiness, mild weakness or numbness of the lower extremities, or problems with bladder dysfunction.

Objective findings may consist of decreased tone and deep tendon reflexes in the lower extremities; patchy decreases in sensation; and foot deformities consisting of broadening and shortening, deepening of

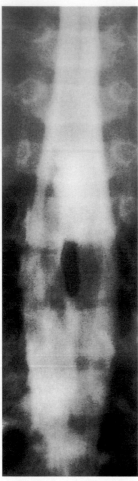

FIG. 15-35 Diastematomyelia. This 6-month-old infant had progressive inturning of and plantar flexion of the left foot and a slightly deviated gluteal cleft. On myelogram, her spinal cord splits at L1, coursing around a bony spur at L2, and then rejoins at L4-5. She also had complete spinal dysraphism of L2-4 and partial dysraphism at L1 and L5.

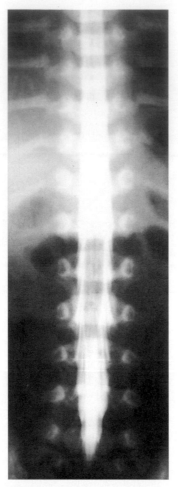

FIG. 15-36 Tethered cord resulting from a tight filum terminale. On myelography, the conus medularis is pulled down to L3-4 by a tethered filum terminale, the upper portion of which is thickened. Presenting symptoms included weakness of plantar flexion, eversion of the feet, and bladder dysfunction. (Courtesy Dr. Charles Fitz, Children's Hospital of Pittsburgh.)

the arch, and contractures of the toes. Associated tethering of the spinal cord may be present in infancy, but often these patients tend to develop symptoms during a period of rapid growth with back, leg, or buttock pain; signs of lower limb spasticity; and on occasion, bowel and bladder dysfunction. This presumably is due to progressive deformation of the tethered cord, which is not free to "ascend" normally within the spinal canal as the rate of linear growth of the vertebral column outpaces that of the spinal cord (Fig. 15-35). Tethering of the spinal cord by an anomalous filum terminale (Fig. 15-36), producing similar signs of progressive neurologic dysfunction, can occur in the absence of associated cutaneous abnormalities, vertebral defects, or intraspinal tumors.

Increased Intracranial Pressure

The cranial cavity is occupied by the brain, blood, and CSF. An increase in the volume of any of these compartments, unless accompanied by a concomitant decrease in one or both of the other compartments, results in increased intracranial pressure. Increased intracranial pressure can result from a wide variety of disorders and is itself hazardous. Recognition of associated signs and symptoms permits early diagnosis and prompt intervention to forestall progressive brain injury or catastrophic neurologic deterioration.

Primary Signs and Symptoms

The clinical manifestations of increased intracranial pressure vary with age. In infants, examination of the anterior fontanelle allows reliable assessment of intracranial pressure. In the normal, quiet infant held in an upright or sitting posture, the anterior fontanelle is flat or slightly concave. Under these conditions, an anterior fontanelle that bulges above the contour of the calvarium and that is excessively firm on palpation is always abnormal. Because the cranial sutures are not fused in infants and young children, increased intracranial pressure rapidly produces separation of the bony plates of the skull. In infants, this can be detected by palpation; in older children, skull radiographs may be needed to identify widened cranial sutures (Fig. 15-37, *A*). Prominent convolutional markings on the inner table of the skull (Fig. 15-37, *B*) are a less useful radiographic sign because they are frequently seen on skull radiographs of normal children. However, when secondary to increased intracranial pressure, they are preceded by suture diastasis and changes in the sella turcica (Fig. 15-37, *C*). An excessive rate of head growth is a prominent feature of chronically increased intracranial pressure in infants and children up to 3 years of age. Associated findings may include frontal prominence and distended scalp veins. If the ability to accommodate for increased intracranial pressure by expansion of the calvarium is exceeded, other symptoms appear. These may include listlessness, irritability, poor feeding, vomiting, failure to thrive, paresis of upward gaze (see Fig. 15-25, *B*), increased tone, hyperactive stretch reflexes, and a high-pitched cry. Papilledema is uncommon.

In older children and adults, the most consistent clinical features of increased intracranial pressure include headache, vomiting, visual disturbances, and papilledema. Headaches are of variable severity. They may be constant or intermittent and generalized or localized to frontal, temporal, or occipital head regions. In some, but by no means all cases, they recur on early arising or awakening and are accompanied by vomiting. The headaches may be exacerbated by sneezing, coughing, or straining. Vomiting resulting from increased intracranial pressure is no different than vomiting from other causes. It is seldom projectile and is not necessarily accompanied by headache.

Horizontal diplopia (double vision) secondary to paralysis of one or both abducens nerves is the most common visual disturbance. Initially, double vision may occur only on lateral gaze toward the side of the paretic lateral rectus muscle. This may be intermittent and may not be accompanied by limitation of ocular motility sufficient to be seen by the examiner. With progression, diplopia becomes constant and is present even with the eyes in the primary position, and an internal strabismus results (Fig. 15-38). Selective vulnerability of the sixth cranial nerve to increased intracranial pressure may be explained by its long intracranial course and proximity to rigid structures. Other visual disturbances may include transient obscurations, visual field deficits, and impaired upward gaze.

Sustained intracranial hypertension produces papilledema, a passive swelling of the optic disc (Fig. 15-39). The observation of papilledema in a child with headache, vomiting, or visual disturbances confirms the presence of increased intracranial pressure. The absence of venous pulsations or the presence of associated flame-shaped hemorrhages can help distinguish papilledema from other causes of blurred optic disc margins.

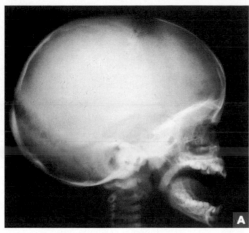
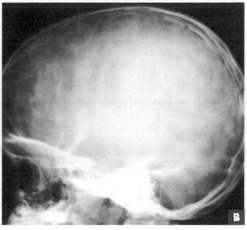
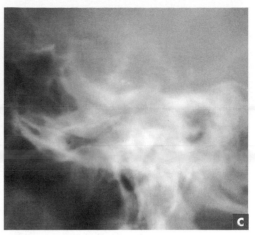

FIG. 15-37 Findings of increased intracranial pressure that may be seen on standard skull radiographs. *A,* Widening of the cranial sutures. *B,* Prominent convolutional markings on the inner table of the skull (beaten silver skull). *C,* Erosion of the sella turcica, in this case resulting from a craniopharyngioma. (*A* Courtesy Department of Neuroradiology, University Health Center of Pittsburgh. *B* and *C* Courtesy Dr. Jocelyn Medina.)

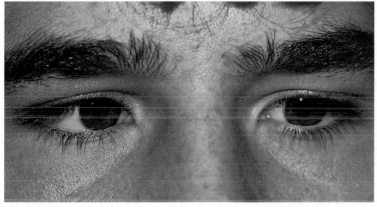

FIG. 15-38 Left abducens (sixth cranial nerve) palsy. This boy presented with headaches and diplopia and was found to have papilledema and a left abducens palsy. Note that his left eye cannot move past the midline on the left lateral gaze. (Courtesy Dr. Kenneth Cheng, Children's Hospital of Pittsburgh.)

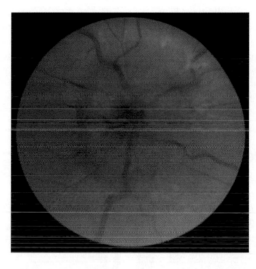

FIG. 15-39 Papilledema. Fundus photograph shows blurring of the optic disc margin, elevation and hyperemia of the optic nerve head, and distension of the retinal blood vessels. (Courtesy Dr. Kenneth Cheng, Children's Hospital of Pittsburgh.)

Increased intracranial pressure may be accompanied by changes in personality and behavior, deteriorating school performance, decreased appetite and activity, and alterations in level of consciousness.

Causes

Causes of increased intracranial pressure include cerebral edema, mass lesions, trauma, CNS infections, pseudotumor cerebri, and hydrocephalus.

Cerebral edema (Fig. 15-40), an expansion of brain volume resulting from an increase in brain content of water and salt, is a response of brain tissue to a variety of insults. Vasogenic cerebral edema results from the alterations in vascular permiability produced by brain tumor, trauma, abscess, and hemorrhage. Cytotoxic cerebral edema, caused by swelling of brain cells (neurons and glia), usually results from infection, hypoxia, ischemia, or toxins.

Intracranial mass lesions (e.g., tumor, hemorrhage, abscess, vascular malformations) produce increased intracranial pressure by occupying

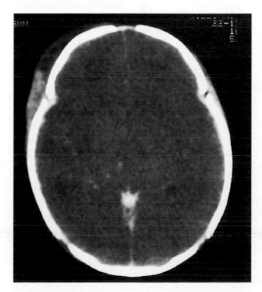

FIG. 15-40 Cerebral edema. CT performed 24 hours after severe hypoxic-ischemic injury. Note the obliteration of the cerebral ventricles, the loss of gray-white differentiation, and the homogeneous "ground-glass" appearance. (Courtesy Department of Neuroradiology, University Health Center of Pittsburgh.)

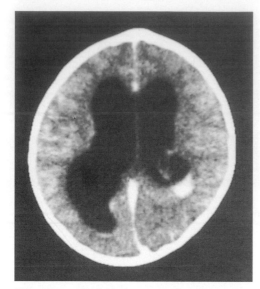

FIG. 15-41　Choroid plexus papilloma. CT of an infant with excessively rapid head growth. There is an enhancing mass within the body of the left lateral ventricle and associated ventricular enlargement (hydrocephalus) secondary to excessive secretion of CSF by the tumor. (Courtesy Dr. Michael Painter, Children's Hospital of Pittsburgh.)

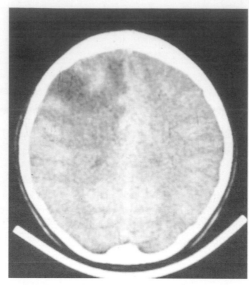

FIG. 15-42　Hemispheric oligodendroglioma. CT scan of a patient with seizures demonstrates a low-density mass lesion in the right frontal lobe. (Courtesy Dr. Michael Painter, Children's Hospital of Pittsburgh.)

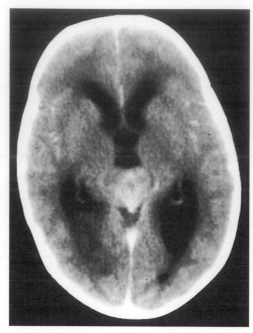

FIG. 15-43　Pineal region tumor. CT scan of a patient with headache, lethargy, vomiting, and paresis of upward gaze shows an enhancing mass lesion in the pineal region and severe obstructive hydrocephalus. (Courtesy Department of Neuroradiology, University Health Center of Pittsburgh.)

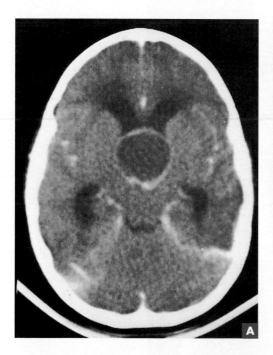

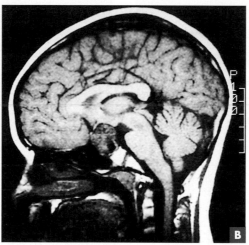

FIG. 15-44　Craniopharyngioma. *A,* CT scan shows a large, spherical suprasellar mass, obliteration of the third ventricle, and associated hydrocephalus. *B,* MRI scan provides superior visualization of the anatomic relations of this tumor to the optic chiasm and hypothalamus. (Courtesy Department of Neuroradiology, University Health Center of Pittsburgh.)

space, causing cerebral edema, obstructing CSF pathways, and altering blood flow. Choroid plexus papillomas, by secreting an excess of CSF, cause communicating hydrocephalus (Fig. 15-41). Although astrocytomas of the cerebral hemispheres (Fig. 15-42) often present with seizures or contralateral motor difficulties, symptoms of increased intracranial pressure are the initial manifestations in 37% of cases and are present at the time of diagnosis in 80%. Pineal region tumors (Fig. 15-43) frequently obstruct the third ventricle or cerebral aqueduct, producing signs and symptoms of increased intracranial pressure accompanied by *Parinaud syndrome* (impairment of the upward gaze with preservation of

the downward gaze and retraction-convergence nystagmus with attempted upward gaze) resulting from compression of the periaqueductal gray (see Fig. 15-25, *B*). Hypothalamic region tumors such as craniopharyngioma (Fig. 15-44) present with growth retardation or failure of sexual maturation accompanied by visual field defects resulting from compression of the optic chiasm. Hydrocephalus occurs in 25% of cases.

Headache and vomiting accompanied by disturbances of gait and coordination are frequent presenting manifestations of posterior fossa tumors such as cerebellar astrocytoma, medulloblastoma, and ependymoma. Midline tumors involving the cerebellar vermis can produce

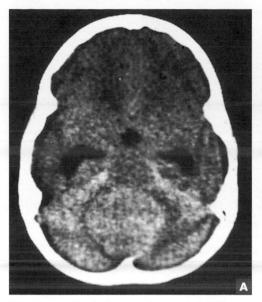

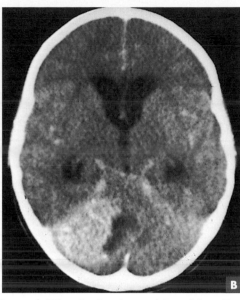

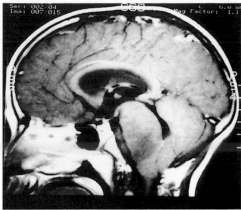

FIG. 15-45 Cerebellar neoplasms. *A,* Midline ependymoma filling the fourth ventricle and invading the cerebellar vermis. *B,* Glioblastoma of the right cerebellar hemisphere. (*A* courtesy Dr. Michael Painter, Children's Hospital of Pittsburgh. *B* Courtesy Department of Neuroradiology, University of Health Center of Pittsburgh.)

FIG. 15-46 Brainstem glioma. This 6-year-old girl had a 2 to 3 month history of personality change, decreased school performance, intermittent urinary retention and constipation; a 3-week history of ataxia and vague upper back pain; and a 6-day history of severe frontal headache with vomiting after breakfast. She had diplopia secondary to left sixth nerve palsy, nystagmus, right facial weakness, slurred speech, dysphagia with drooling, torticollis, an unbalanced gait with a tendency to list to the left, dysmetria greater on the left, and bilateral papilledema. Her MRI scan showed marked enlargement of the pons resulting from a mass lesion extending into the brainstem and compressing the fourth ventricle, causing hydrocephalus. (Courtesy Dr. Charles Fitz, Children's Hospital of Pittsburgh.)

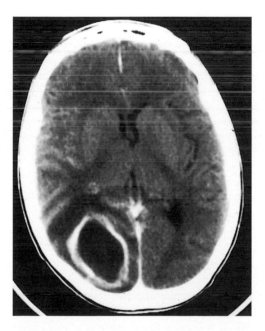

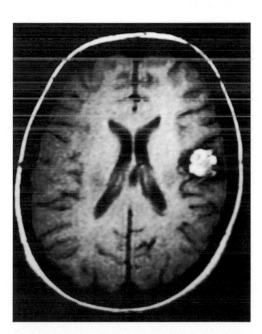

FIG. 15-47 Brain abscess. CT scan demonstrates a low-density mass lesion with an enhancing rim and surrounding edema in an immunosuppressed patient with an *Aspergillus* abscess. Bacterial abscesses and neoplasms can present a similar CT appearance. (Courtesy Department of Neuroradiology, University Health Center of Pittsburgh.)

FIG. 15-48 Intracranial hemorrhage. Enhanced MRI scan demonstrating a cerebral hemangioma with associated old hemorrhage. (Courtesy Dr. Michael Painter, Children's Hospital of Pittsburgh.)

truncal ataxia (Fig. 15-45, *A*), whereas mass lesions of the cerebellar hemispheres often cause unilateral limb ataxia and horizontal nystagmus (Fig. 15-45, *B*). The cardinal manifestations of brainstem glioma (Fig. 15-46) are cranial nerve palsies associated with contralateral hemiplegia and ataxia. Increased intracranial pressure is not an early feature.

Brain abscesses (Fig. 15-47) are uncommon in the absence of predisposing factors such as chronic otitis or sinusitis, chronic pulmonary infection, dental abscesses, cyanotic congenital heart disease, or immunosuppression. Unless accompanied by prodromal symptoms of fever, headache, lethargy, and malaise, brain abscesses may be impossible to distinguish from other intracranial mass lesions on clinical grounds.

Spontaneous intracranial hemorrhage (Fig. 15-48) secondary to rupture of a vascular malformation or arterial aneurysm is rare in the pediatric population. Leakage of small amounts of blood into the subarachnoid space produces symptoms (e.g., fever, headache, stiff neck) that mimic bacterial meningitis. In such cases, the correct diagnosis may be first suspected when lumber puncture yields grossly bloody fluid. The presentation of large subarachnoid hemorrhages is cata-

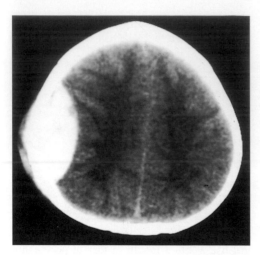

FIG. 15-49 Epidural hematoma. In this patient, blunt head trauma was followed by vomiting, progressive obtundation, and decreased movement of the left arm and leg. The CT scan showed a large, lens-shaped epidural hematoma over the right hemisphere. (Courtesy Department of Neuroradiology, University Health Center of Pittsburgh.)

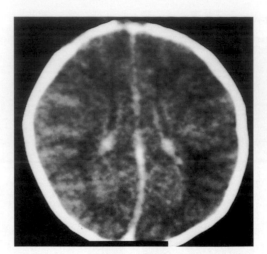

FIG. 15-50 Bacterial meningitis in an infant with fever, lethargy, nuchal rigidity, and a tense, distended fontanelle. The CT scan shows contrast enhancement of the cortical gyri and ependyma of the lateral ventricles. (Courtesy Department of Neuroradiology, University Health Center of Pittsburgh.)

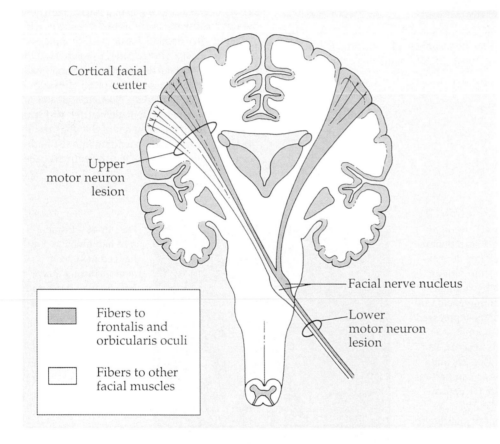

FIG. 15-51 Central motor control of the facial muscles. The portion of the facial nerve nucleus that supplies the lower half of the face receives predominantly crossed fibers originating from the opposite cerebral hemisphere; the portion that innervates the upper half receives fibers from both cerebral hemispheres. (Modified from Haymaker W: *Bing's local diagnosis in neurological diseases,* ed 15, St Louis, 1969, Mosby.)

Cortical facial center

Upper motor neuron lesion

Facial nerve nucleus

Lower motor neuron lesion

Fibers to frontalis and orbicularis oculi

Fibers to other facial muscles

strophic, with sudden onset of excruciating headache followed by collapse and evidence of increased intracranial pressure.

Head trauma results in increased intracranial pressure by provoking cerebral edema or causing intracranial hemorrhage. The modes of presentation of cerebral contusion, subdural hematoma, and posttraumatic cerebral edema are discussed in Chapter 6. The features of epidural hematoma (Fig. 15-49) in childhood, which differ from those encountered in adults, are emphasized here. Infants and young children with epidural hematoma frequently suffer no immediate loss of consciousness after the traumatic event. Associated linear skull fractures are less common than in adults, and the source of bleeding into the epidural space is generally ruptured epidural veins rather than lacerations of the middle meningeal artery. Hence the evolution of symptoms is slower, and the typical adult picture of immediate loss of consciousness, followed by a brief lucid interval and then collapse, is not

seen until adolescence. Often, persistent lethargy and intermittent vomiting are the only initial signs. Some affected children and adolescents, in addition to lethargy, demonstrate a slowed reaction time, especially when responding to questions (as if there is a processing delay) on early assessment. Severe headache, papilledema, and localizing signs may not emerge for several hours to several days. Once neurologic signs and symptoms appear they may progress rapidly to coma and death or evolve slowly over several days before producing brainstem compression.

Bacterial meningitis (Fig. 15-50) produces increased intracranial pressure by causing cerebral edema and impairing reabsorption of CSF. Signs and symptoms are discussed in Chapter 12. Although cerebral edema and intracranial hypertension may complicate the course of viral encephalitis, the usual presentation is with seizures, behavioral change, and altered level of consciousness.

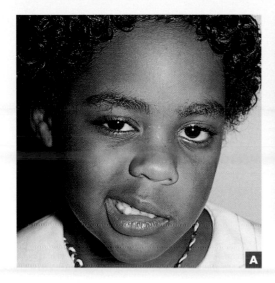

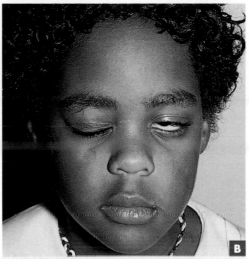

FIG. 15-52 Peripheral facial weakness. Flaccid weakness of the entire left face resulting from a lesion of the left facial nerve. *A,* Flattening of the nasolabial fold and inability to retract the corner of the mouth. *B,* Inability to fully close the eye.

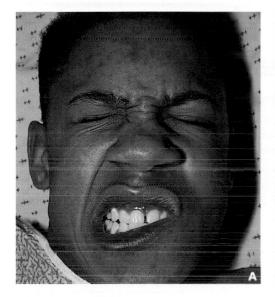

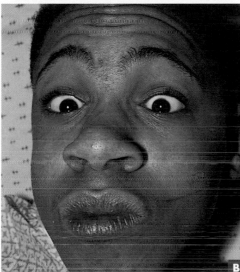

FIG. 15-53 Central facial weakness. *A* and *B,* Weakness of the left face with relative sparing of the upper portion secondary to a lesion of the right cerebral hemisphere. There is flattening of the nasolabial fold and inability to retract the corner of the mouth, but the ability to close the eye and wrinkle the forehead is preserved.

Continued

Pseudotumor cerebri is a syndrome of increased intracranial pressure that occurs in the absence of hydrocephalus or an intracranial mass. Pseudotumor cerebri is associated with the use of certain drugs (e.g., steroids, tetracycline, vitamin A, oral contraceptives), occurs as a complication of otitis media or sinusitis, and can be caused by a variety of endocrine and metabolic disturbances. However, in many instances it is idiopathic. The presenting symptom is headache. Papilledema is the rule and abducens nerve palsy is common (see Figs. 15-38 and 15-39). There may be associated nausea and vomiting, but most children do not appear acutely ill. Progressive papilledema may lead to optic atrophy, and treatment is essential to prevent loss of vision. Pseudotumor cerebri is a diagnosis of exclusion. A CT or an MRI scan must be done to rule out hydrocephalus or a mass lesion. Examination of the cerebrospinal fluid is unremarkable apart from increased opening pressure.

Facial Weakness

The cortical motor center controlling the muscles of facial expression is located in the lower third of the precentral gyrus (Fig. 15-51). Motor fibers arising in the cerebral cortex travel through the corona radiata, internal capsule, and cerebral peduncle into the pons, where the majority decussate to supply the facial (seventh) nerve nucleus on the op-

posite side. Some fibers, destined to terminate in the portion of the facial nerve nucleus that innervates muscles in the upper half of the face, do not decussate. Thus whereas the portion of the facial nerve nucleus that supplies the lower half of the face receives predominantly crossed fibers originating from the opposite cerebral hemisphere, the portion that innervates the frontalis muscle and the orbicularis oculi muscle has bilateral supranuclear control.

Peripheral Facial Weakness

A lesion of the seventh nerve nucleus or emergent facial nerve results in flaccid weakness of the entire face on the same side. On the affected side the face is smooth, with flattening of the nasolabial fold; drooping of the corner of the mouth; and inability to smile, frown, retract the corner of the mouth, wrinkle the forehead, or close the eye (Fig. 15-52). Causes of peripheral facial weakness include infection, trauma, hypertension, a cerebellopontine angle mass, tumors of the pons, and acute idiopathic paralysis (Bell palsy).

Central Facial Weakness

With a lesion above the level of the facial nerve nucleus (i.e., an upper motor neuron lesion), there is weakness of the lower part of the face on

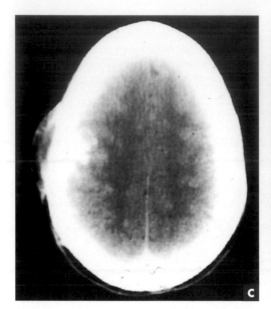

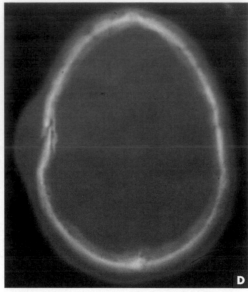

FIG. 15-53, cont'd *C* and *D,* CT scans show the depressed fracture of the temporal bone that was responsible for this central facial palsy.

TABLE 15-6

Clinical Features of the Muscular Dystrophies

	Duchenne	Becker	Fascioscapulohumeral	Limb-girdle	Myotonic
Inheritance	X-linked recessive	X-linked recessive	Autosomal dominant	Autosomal recessive	Autosomal dominant
Age of onset	Early childhood	Late childhood, adolescence	Variable: childhood through early adult life	Childhood to early adulthood	Highly variable
Pattern of weakness	Pelvic girdle, shoulder girdle	Pelvic girdle, shoulder girdle	Face, shoulder girdle	Pelvic girdle, shoulder girdle	Face, distal limbs
Rate of progression	Rapid	Slow	Very Slow	Variable	Variable
Associated features	Pseudohypertrophy of calves	Pseudohypertrophy of calves	None	Pseudohypertrophy rare	Myotonia
Systemic features	Mental retardation, abnormal electrocardiogram, cardiomyopathy	Occasional mental retardation	None	None	Frequent mental retardation, heart block, cataracts, premature balding, testicular tubular atrophy, diabetes

the opposite side but relative sparing of the upper portion of the face. The ability to wrinkle the forehead (frontalis muscle) and to voluntarily close the eyes (orbicularis oculi muscle) is preserved (Fig. 15-53).

Neuromuscular Disorders

Weakness is the most common presenting symptom of neuromuscular disease. If time is taken to determine the ways in which the weakness interferes with normal activities and uncover the types of tasks that the patient finds difficult, the distribution and severity of muscle weakness can be predicted from the clinical history. Determining the mode of on-

set and pattern of progression of the symptoms is essential in the differential diagnosis and selection of diagnostic studies. Since many neuromuscular disorders are genetically determined, a complete family history must be obtained.

Essential components of the physical examination of patients with neuromuscular disease include inspection, palpation, percussion, evaluation of the deep tendon reflexes, and assessment of muscle strength. Inspection can reveal muscle wasting and atrophy (or conversely hypertrophy), abnormal spontaneous activity, and abnormal resting postures. Palpation permits assessment of muscle consistency, determination of muscle tone (with observation of resistance to passive motion), and detection of muscle tenderness. Percussion is useful in detecting

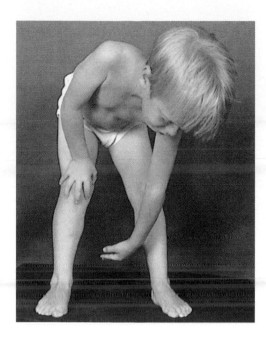

FIG. 15-54 Duchenne muscular dystrophy. This child, age 5, has difficulty rising from the floor. Unilateral hand support on the knee is required to get erect.

myotonia. Assessment of muscle strength includes individual muscle testing and functional evaluation. The strength of individual muscles is recorded using a standardized system such as the following:

0	No contraction
1	Flicker or trace contraction
2	Active movement with gravity eliminated
3	Active movement against gravity
4	Active movement against gravity and resistance
5	Normal power

Functional evaluation of muscle strength is accomplished by observing the patient rising from the floor, rising from a chair, stepping onto a stool, climbing stairs, walking on the heels, hopping on the toes, and raising the arms above the head. This evaluation permits rapid detection of proximal weakness of the hips and shoulders and distal weakness of the legs.

Duchenne Muscular Dystrophy

The muscular dystrophies are genetically determined disorders characterized by progressive degeneration of skeletal muscle, usually after a latency period of seemingly normal development and function. The various clinical types of muscular dystrophy are traditionally classified on the basis of patterns of inheritance, distribution of initial weakness, age of onset of clinical manifestations, and rate of progression (Table 15-6).

Duchenne muscular dystrophy, affecting 1 in 3500 male births, is characterized by X-linked recessive inheritance; early onset; symmetric and initially selective involvement of pelvic and pectoral girdles; pseudohypertrophy of the calves; very high levels of activity of certain serum enzymes, notably creatine kinase; and relentless progression leading to wheelchair confinement by adolescence and death from cardiorespiratory insufficiency by age 20 years.

Duchenne muscular dystrophy is caused by a deletion mutation affecting the Xp21 region on the short arm of the X chromosome. Dystrophin, the large cytoskeletal protein normally encoded by this gene locus, is absent from the muscle fibers of patients with Duchenne muscular dystrophy. The precise function of dystrophin in maintaining the integrity of muscle and the mechanism by which dystrophin deficiency produces progressive muscle destruction remain to be determined. Becker muscular dystrophy, an allelic disorder affecting 1 in 30,000 male births, is distinguished clinically by later age of onset, slower rate of progression, and longer survival and biochemically by the presence of dystrophin of abnormal molecular weight.

Clinical manifestations of Duchenne muscular dystrophy do not usually appear until the second year of life. Early developmental milestones are normally attained, although the first attempts at walking may be delayed. Gait is often clumsy and awkward from the start, and the ability to run is never normally attained. Difficulty in climbing stairs, frequent falls, and progressive difficulty in rising from the floor are early features. To rise from the floor, the child may at first need only to push with one hand on a knee (Fig. 15-54). However, as weakness of the extensors of the hips becomes more pronounced, rising from the floor becomes increasingly difficult and requires the use of the hands to "climb up the legs" (the Gower maneuver) (Fig. 15-55).

Progressive gluteal weakness leads to the assumption of a compensatory posture characterized by a broadened base, accentuated lumbar lordosis, and forward thrusting of the abdomen (Fig. 15-56). Although weakness of the arms is not a common early symptom, proximal upper extremity weakness is easily detected on clinical examination when the child is lifted with the examiner's hands placed beneath the arms. There is marked laxity of the shoulder girdle musculature associated with upward displacement of the shoulders and abnormal rotation of the scapulae (Fig. 15-57, *A*). In addition, spontaneous winging of the scapulae may be prominent (Fig. 15-57, *B*).

Weakness of the neck flexors, as evidenced by marked head lag when pulled to sit from the supine position (Fig. 15-58), is an early finding. Enlargement of muscles, particularly in the calves (Fig. 15-59), is a common feature by 5 or 6 years of age. The abnormally enlarged muscles have an unusually firm, rubbery consistency on palpation. Early in the clinical course, this increase in muscle volume may result from true hypertrophy, with muscle strength proportional to bulk. Later, infiltration by fat and connective tissue sometimes maintains this bulk in spite of loss of muscle fibers. This is called *pseudohypertrophy*.

Charcot-Marie-Tooth Disease

Charcot-Marie-Tooth disease, also known as *hereditary motor-sensory neuropathy, type 1 (HMSN-1)*, is an autosomal dominant demyelinating form of peroneal muscular atrophy. Deoxyribonucleic acid studies have distinguished two genetic disorders, HMSN-1A, associated with a gene mutation of chromosome 17, and HMSN-1B, caused by a mutation on chromosome 1. Both share similar clinical features. The onset of symptoms is usually in the second decade, the presenting complaints being foot deformities and gait abnormalities. Often, pes cavus or hammertoe deformities develop in early childhood long before more overt symptoms appear (see Fig. 21-104). The clinical picture is quite variable, and because most affected persons do not consult a physician for their neurologic problems, the majority of cases remain undiagnosed. The astute physician considers the diagnosis when a patient who presents with unrelated symptoms is found to have pes cavus or hammertoes and symmetric distal weakness.

Muscle weakness and atrophy begin insidiously in the foot and leg muscles. The intrinsic muscles of the foot are often affected first, followed by involvement of the peronei, anterior tibial, long toe extensor, intrinsic hand, and gastrocnemius muscles. Weakness and atrophy may spread to the more proximal muscles of the leg and forearm. The degree of muscle wasting is often mild; however, in some cases the loss of muscle mass in the distal lower extremities is severe, giving rise to a striking "stork-leg" appearance (Fig. 15-60). With involvement of the

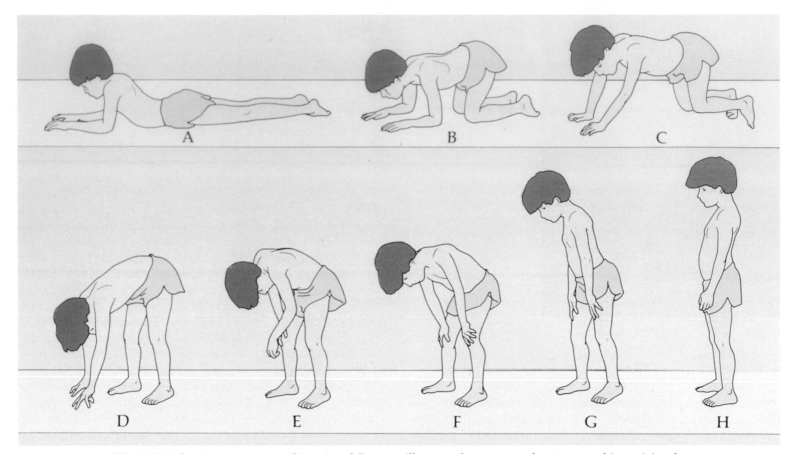

FIG. 15-55 The Gower maneuver. This series of diagrams illustrates the sequence of postures used in attaining the upright position. *A* to *C,* First, the legs are pulled up under the body, and the weight is shifted to rest on the hands and feet. *D,* The hips are then thrust in the air as the knees are straightened and the hands are brought close to the legs. *E* to *G,* Finally, the trunk is slowly extended by the hands walking up the thigh. *H,* The erect position is attained.

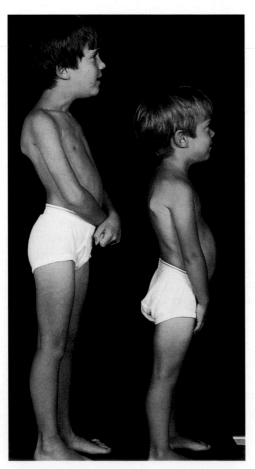

FIG. 15-56 Duchenne muscular dystrophy. These brothers, ages 5 and 8, show progressive compensatory postural adjustments with broadening of stance, accentuated lumbar lordosis, and forward thrusting of the abdomen.

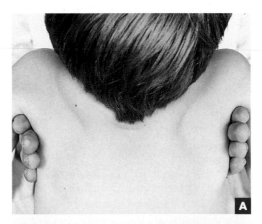

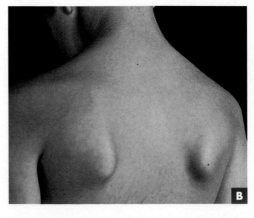

FIG. 15-57 Duchenne muscular dystrophy. *A,* This child, age 5, demonstrates weakness and hypotonia of the shoulder girdle musculature. Upward displacement of the shoulders and abnormal rotation of the scapulae are seen when the child is lifted with the examiner's hands under his arms. *B,* Spontaneous winging of the scapulae can be noted in this 8-year-old child.

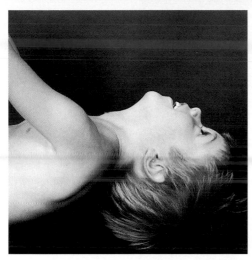

FIG. 15-58 Duchenne muscular dystrophy. This 5-year-old child has neck flexor weakness. Note the marked head lag when the patient is pulled to sit from the supine position.

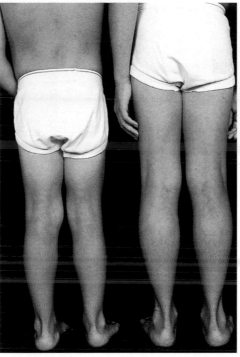

FIG. 15-59 Duchenne muscular dystrophy. Enlargement of the calves in brothers, ages 5 and 8.

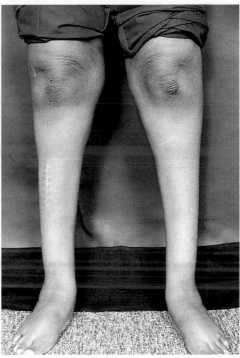

FIG. 15-60 Charcot-Marie-Tooth disease. Patient, age 15, with distal muscular atrophy of the lower extremities ("stork-leg" appearance).

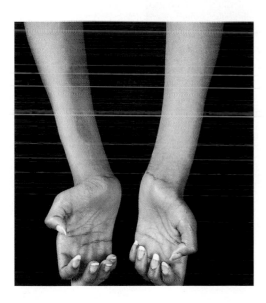

FIG. 15-61 Charcot-Marie-Tooth disease. This 15-year-old has atrophy of the forearm and intrinsic hand muscles and "claw-hand" deformity.

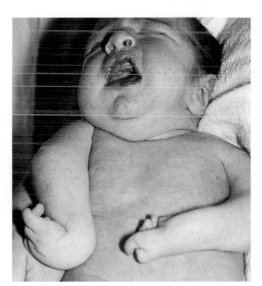

FIG. 15-62 Congenital cervical spinal atrophy. This 2-day-old infant has flaccid paresis limited to the upper extremities and associated congenital flexion contractures.

distal upper extremities there may be obvious wasting of the intrinsic hand muscles and development of secondary "claw deformities" (Fig. 15-61). Deep tendon reflexes are first lost in the gastrocnemius and soleus muscles, and subsequently in the quadriceps femoris muscle and upper limbs. Sensation may be mildly impaired in the distal lower extremities.

Congenital Cervical Spinal Atrophy

Congenital cervical spinal atrophy, a rare disorder, presents at birth with dramatic flaccid paresis of the upper extremities (Fig. 15-62). The presence of congenital flexion contractures suggests chronic denervation that must have occurred in utero and allows this syndrome to be

distinguished from injury to the cervical spine or brachial plexuses during delivery (see Chapter 2). Abnormalities in the formation of the transverse palmar creases are present in all cases (Fig. 15-63), suggesting an antenatal insult during the first trimester. The disorder is nonprogressive.

Myotonia Congenita

Myotonia congenita is an inherited disorder of skeletal muscle in which muscle stiffness is the only complaint. There are autosomal dominant and autosomal recessive forms related to different mutations of the skeletal muscle chloride channel gene on chromosome 7. The clinical symptoms are rather stereotypic. After a period of inactivity, the mus-

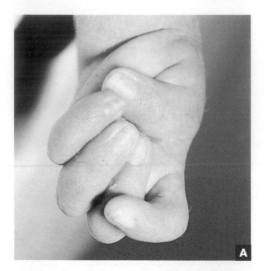

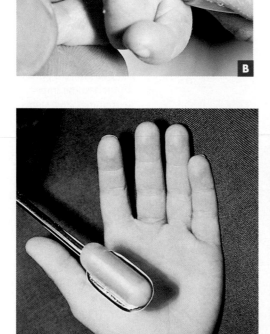

FIG. 15-63 Congenital cervical spinal atrophy. Wasting and atrophy of the intrinsic hand muscles with flexion contractures of the fingers *(A)* and poorly developed transverse palmar creases *(B)* can be seen in this 2-day-old infant.

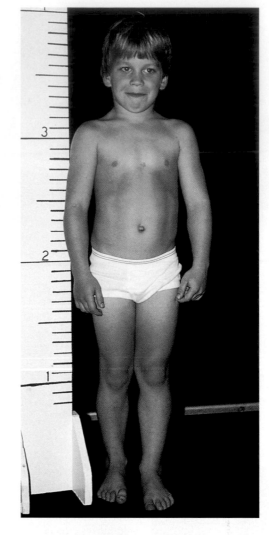

FIG. 15-64 Myotonia congenita. Patient, age 8, demonstrates generalized muscular hypertrophy, giving a well-developed, athletic appearance.

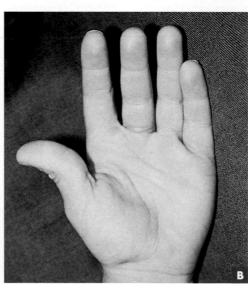

FIG. 15-65 Myotonia congenita. Percussion of the thenar eminence *(A)* is followed by involuntary opposition of the thumb and visible contraction of the muscles of the thenar eminence *(B),* which lasts for several seconds.

cles stiffen and are difficult to maneuver; however, with continued activity, the stiffness diminishes, and movement becomes almost normal. Typically, the child moves clumsily with a stiff awkward gait and falls often. However, as activity continues, the child begins to walk freely and with adequate "warm-up" is able to run without difficulty.

Generalized muscular hypertrophy is a frequent finding on examination, with affected children often having an unusually well-developed, athletic appearance (Fig. 15-64). This belies their sedentary habits and physical ineptitude resulting from muscle stiffness. Clinically, myotonia may be demonstrated by observing delayed relaxation of the muscles

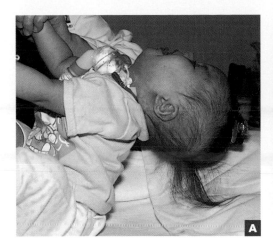
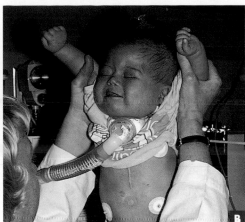

FIG. 15-66 Hypotonic infant. *A,* Abnormal traction response. The head falls into extreme extention. The limbs fail to flex to counter the traction applied by the examiner. *B,* When held under the arms, the infant tends to slip through the examiner's hands.

TABLE 15-7

Differential Diagnosis of Hypotonia

Disorders of the CNS	Disorders of the PNS
Chromosome disorders	Spinal muscular atrophies
Trisomy	Congenital polyneuropathies
Prader-Willi syndrome	Transient neonatal myasthenia
Other	Congenital myasthenic
Other genetic defects	syndromes
Static encephalopathies	Congenital muscular dystrophy
Congenital malformation	Myotonic dystrophy
Perinatal acquired	Fukuyama type dystrophy
encephalopathy	Other
Postnatal acquired	Congenital myopathies
encephalopathy	Metabolic myopathies
Inborn errors of metabolism	Systemic illness
Amino acid disorders	Benign congenital hypotonia
Organic acid disorders	
Urea cycle disorders	
Peroxisomal disorders	
Lysosomal disorders	
Neonatal spinal cord injury	

after sustained voluntary contraction such as clenching of the hand. Myotonia may also be elicited by percussion of the thenar eminence (Fig. 15-65).

Hypotonic Infant

Since depression of muscle tone is manifested by paucity of movement, unusual postures, diminished resistance to passive movement, and increased range of movement of joints, the hypotonic infant has been likened to a rag doll. The legs lie externally rotated and abducted, with their lateral surface in contact with the bed while the arms are extended at the sides or flexed so that the hands lie beside the head. When the infant is pulled by the hands from the supine position (traction response), the head falls into extreme extension, and the limbs fail to flex to counter the traction (Fig. 15-66, *A*). In horizontal suspension with the chest and abdomen supported by the examiner's hand, the infant with hypotonia drapes limply like an inverted U. When held under the arms, the hypotomic infant tends to slip through the examiner's hands

(Fig. 15-66, *B*). Because maintenance of normal postural tone requires functional integrity of both the CNS and PNS, hypotonia is a common symptom of many disorders affecting the brain, spinal cord, peripheral nerves, and muscle (Table 15-7). Hypotonia also occurs as a nonspecific manifestation of systemic illness. The term *benign congenital hypotonia* is reserved for infants with isolated depression of the postural tone that resolves with growth and maturation, usually by 1 year of age.

BIBLIOGRAPHY

Bell WE, McCormick WF: *Increased intracranial pressure in children,* ed 2, Philadelphia, 1978, WB Saunders.

Brooke MH: *A clinician's view of neuromuscular diseases,* ed 2, Baltimore, 1987, Williams & Wilkins.

Chao DH: Congenital neurocutaneous syndromes of childhood. III. Sturge-Weber disease, *J Pediatr* 55:635-649, 1959.

Dubozitz V: *The floppy infant,* ed 2, Philadelphia, 1980, JB Lippincott.

Emery AEH: *Duchenne muscular dystrophy,* ed 2, Oxford, England, 1993, Oxford University Press.

Enjolras O, Riche MC, Merland JJ: Facial port-wine stains and Sturge-Weber syndrome, *Pediatrics* 76:48-52, 1985.

Fenichel GM: *Clinical pediatric neurology: a signs and symptoms approach,* ed 2, Philadelphia, 1993, WB Saunders.

Goldstein SM, Curless RG, Post JD, Quencer RM: A new sign of neurofibromatosis on magnetic resonance imaging of children, *Arch Neurol* 46:1222-1224, 1989.

Gomez MR, ed: *Tuberous sclerosis,* ed 2, New York, 1988, Raven Press.

Hoffman EP, Fishbeck KH, Brown RH, et al: Characterization of dystrophin in muscle-biopsy specimens from patients with Duchenne's or Becker's muscular dystrophy, *N Engl J Med* 318:1363-1368, 1988.

Martuza RL, Eldridge R: Neurofibromatosis 2, *N Engl J Med* 318:684-688, 1988.

Menkes JH: *Textbook of child neurology,* ed 4, Philadelphia, 1990, Lea & Febiger.

Osborne JP: Diagnosis of tuberous sclerosis, *Arch Dis Child* 63:1423-1425, 1988.

Paller AS: The Sturge-Weber syndrome, *Pediatr Dermatol* 4:300-304, 1987.

Riccardi VM: Von Recklinghausen neurofibromatosis, *N Engl J Med* 305:1617-1627, 1981.

Roach ES, William DP, Laster DW: Magnetic resonance imaging in tuberous sclerosis, *Arch Neurol* 44:301-303, 1987.

Swaiman KF: *Pediatric neurology: principles and practice,* ed 2, St Louis, 1994, Mosby.

Warkany J, Lemire RJ, Cohen MM: *Mental retardation and congenital malformations of the central nervous system,* St Louis, 1981, Mosby.

16

Pulmonary Disorders

JONATHAN D. FINDER ❦ BLAKESLEE E. NOYES

DAVID M. ORENSTEIN

The respiratory system can be thought of as having six compartments: airway, airspace, interstitium, vascular space, pleural space, and chest wall/diaphragm. Diseases of the chest often overlap, but it is useful to think of respiratory disease as affecting one of these compartments primarily. A careful history and physical examination go a long way in directing the evaluation toward one or another of these compartments. Airway diseases frequently manifest as cough and/or wheeze. Interstitial diseases often are insidious in onset and associated with a dry cough and resting tachypnea; fine crackles are common on examination. Most airspace diseases in the pediatric patient are infectious and associated with fever; auscultatory abnormalities can be minimal, although absent breath sounds are common. Vascular diseases in children tend to be chronic and often result in chronic hypoxemia; vascular rings are often mistaken for asthma.

Diseases of the pediatric chest are acquired or congenital. Some congenital structural processes are symptomatic at all times rather than episodically. A child who has chronic noisy breathing from a vascular ring (congenital), for example, is not as likely as the youngster with reactive airway disease to have intermittent periods of wheezing with long intervals of normal breathing. Many congenital malformations of the chest are not apparent until an infection occurs or they are discovered as incidental findings on a routine chest radiograph.

History

Every pediatric history should begin with the obstetric history. A history of respiratory distress at birth or of intubation, however brief, is important. Noisy breathing starting early in the first month of life suggests congenital airway obstruction and should be evaluated. Although failure to thrive is a worrisome finding, excellent weight gain in a child with noisy breathing is reassuring to the pediatric pulmonologist.

Distinguishing between constant and intermittent symptoms can be one of the most important means of diagnosing diseases of the pediatric chest. A good "cough history" and "wheeze history" are important and have similar elements. The clinician should inquire about the chronicity of the symptoms, association with feeding, colds, exposures (pets, dust, and especially cigarette smoking are important), and fevers. The effect of previous medications may give important diagnostic information. The nature of the cough is extremely important: wet or dry, parox-

ysmal or continuous, or staccato (as seen in neonatal chlamydial pneumonia); posttussive emesis is a "red flag" to the clinician. Another worrisome finding is that the cough awakens the child at night or keeps the child up much of the night. Conversely, disappearance of a persistent cough in sleep strongly suggests the diagnosis of psychogenic, or habit, cough. In pursuing a history of wheeze, it is important to ask the parents or historians what they mean by the term; it may mean "noisy breathing" and may even be applied to stridor.

In evaluating the infant with frequent episodes of cough and/or wheeze the clinician should inquire about symptoms and signs of gastroesophageal reflux (GER): food refusal, arching, frequent spitting, and milk or formula on the bed next to the infant's head in the morning. Recurrent croup occurs in some patients with pathologic GER.

A family history of atopy, including eczema and environmental allergies, should be investigated. In inquiring about cystic fibrosis, an autosomal recessive trait, an extended family medical history, which extends to the grandparents and cousins, should be taken. Frequent infections, particularly those requiring hospitalization, suggest immunodeficiency.

Immunization history is essential in identifying patients at risk for pertussis. Often, parents state that the immunizations are "up to date" although the child has not had any pertussis vaccinations.

Intolerance of exercise is one of the chief ways in which airflow limitation presents. The neonate's main output of energy is in feeding, and thus difficulties with feedings should be monitored; toddlers are expected to keep up with peers and/or siblings in play; the school-age child's gym performance should be scrutinized. Wheezing or coughing fits after vigorous exercise can occur in reactive airway disease.

Physical Examination

The chest examination of the uncooperative youngster is notoriously difficult, but with patience and a few tricks this need not be the case. Sir William Osler's four steps in the physical examination—inspection, palpation, percussion, and auscultation—are well applied to the examination of the chest.

Inspection should include evaluation for digital clubbing (Fig. 16-16). Decreased subcutaneous adipose tissue as seen in a newly diagnosed cystic fibrosis patient should be noted. The pattern of breathing should always be evaluated while the child is disrobed. Any use of expiratory musculature is abnormal. Suprasternal and intercostal retractions reflect ex-

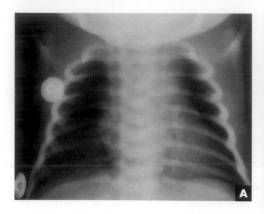

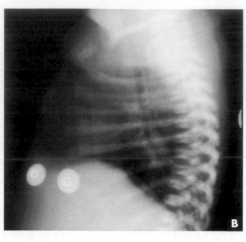

FIG. 16-1 Normal posteroanterior (*A*) and lateral (*B*) chest radiographs in a 1-month-old infant. (Courtesy Dr. Beverly Newman, Pittsburgh.)

cessive negative pleural pressure and can be seen in normal children with thin chest walls after vigorous exercise. Subcostal retractions are always pathologic and are the result of a flattened diaphragm pulling inward on the chest wall. In advanced lung disease the use of accessory muscles of inspiration can be noted; the sternocleidomastoid muscle, for example, helps lift the chest and increase its AP diameter, thereby increasing intrathoracic volume. In respiratory muscle fatigue, including impending respiratory failure, a pattern of breathing can be observed in which the diaphragm alternates with the intercostal muscles to inflate the lungs. This is known as *respiratory alternans* and is seen as alternating abdominal and chest expansion instead of the usual pattern of simultaneous chest and abdominal expansion. Chest wall deformities, such as pectus excavatum or pectus carinatum (see Figs. 17-99 and 17-100), should be noted.

Palpation of the chest can reveal significant findings. The patient takes a deep breath while the examiner's hands are on either side of the chest. The chest should expand symmetrically; asymmetry is seen in pulmonary hypoplasia, mainstem bronchial obstruction, and diaphragmatic paresis. Laying a hand on the upper abdomen just over the insertion of the rectus muscles into the lower ribcage reveals subtle use of expiratory muscles in children with obstructive lower airway disease. With the patient's head in midline position the trachea should be palpated at the sternal notch to evaluate for tracheal deviation as seen with mediastinal shift. Vocal fremitus should be assessed in patients with suspected pleural fluid accumulation; the vibrations transmitted from the larynx are diminished when there is an accumulation of air or fluid in the pleural space. The standard phrase patients say is "ninety-nine."

Percussion of the chest can reveal much more than hyperresonance and dullness over an area of consolidation. Air trapping is the hallmark of small airway disease and results in a depressed position of the diaphragm in midposition. Ordinarily the diaphragm is found just at or slightly below the tip of the scapula when the patient's arm is at his or her side. In the patient with hyperinflation the diaphragm is found several fingerbreadths below the scapular tips. This finding, even in the absence of wheezing on auscultation, suggests a lesion of the small airways. An area of consolidation or pleural effusion results in dullness to percussion. Another disease that results in asymmetry of percussion of the two hemithoraces is diaphragmatic eventration (a congenital lesion of the diaphragm in which the diaphragm is replaced with a fibrous membrane without contractile properties). Postoperative diaphragmatic paralysis (rarely found after cardiac surgery) is diagnosed by percussion of the cooperative patient holding his or her breath at maximal inspiration and at end-expiration.

Auscultation of the pediatric chest requires patience and experience. The infant or toddler is best examined with his or her shirt off while being held upright in the arms of a parent. The patient should face the parent; this maximizes contact with the parent and allows the patient to feel safe. The room temperature should be comfortable. The stethoscope head should be warmed in the clinician's hand or pocket for several minutes before use. Abnormal (or adventitial) breath sounds are defined as coarse or fine crackles and low- or high-pitched wheezes. A wheeze is a continuous noise, whereas a crackle is a discontinuous sound. Wheezes and crackles can be inspiratory or expiratory, although crackles are more commonly heard on inspiration and wheezes are more commonly heard on expiration. Wheezes probably arise from the vibration of partially obstructed large- and medium-sized airway walls. In a patient experiencing an acute exacerbation of asthma the lungs have wheezes in a range of pitches (polyphonic) with substantial regional differences in auscultation. Patients with central airway obstruction, such as tracheomalacia, on the other hand, have a lower-pitched wheeze that sounds the same in all lung fields (monophonic) and is heard loudest over the sternum. Foreign bodies can cause a monophonic wheeze that can vary in pitch depending on the degree of obstruction. Some crackles are believed to arise from the popping open of fluid menisci in medium-sized airways. The crackles heard in the lungs of patients with interstitial lung disease have yet to be explained adequately, but they may arise from the popping open of small airways. Coarse crackles are often audible at the mouth and are late findings in cystic fibrosis patients with advanced bronchiectasis. Other sounds that can be heard are friction rubs, which are creaking sounds heard during both phases of respiration as inflamed pleural surfaces rub over one another. One of the most important abnormal findings in children is the absence of breath sounds over an area of collapse or consolidation. Phase delay in air entry (such as in unilateral bronchial obstruction) can be detected only by using the differential stethoscope and is found in unilateral bronchial obstruction.

Radiology

The pediatric chest radiograph is unique in that normal findings may vary with age. In the chest x-ray examination of a normal infant (Fig. 16-1) the width of the chest on the lateral projection is about the same as the transverse dimension on a frontal projection and the lungs may appear relatively radiolucent. Further, in contrast to the older child (more than 2 years of age) the cardiothoracic ratio in the infant may be as high as 0.65. The width of the superior mediastinum at this age also may be striking because the thymic shadow is particularly prominent during the first few months of life before the normal process of involution occurs. The normal chest x-ray examination of an older child (Fig. 16-2) shows the diaphragm on an inspiratory film at the eighth or ninth rib posteriorly (sixth rib ante-

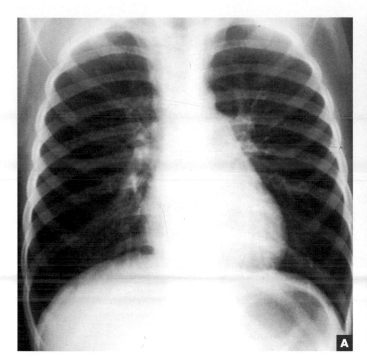
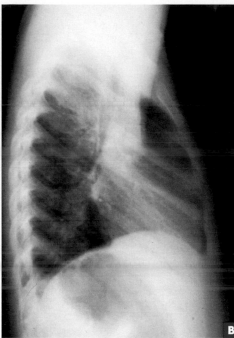

FIG. 16-2 Normal posteroanterior *(A)* and lateral *(B)* chest radiographs in a 6-year-old child.

TABLE 16-1

Causes of Cough According to Age

Infancy (Under 1 Year)
Congenital and neonatal infections
Chlamydia
Viral (e.g., RSV, CMV, rubella)
Bacterial (e.g., pertussis)
Pneumocystis carinii

Congenital malformations
Tracheoesophageal fistula
Vascular ring
Airway malformations
  (e.g., laryngeal cleft)
Pulmonary sequestration

Other
Cystic fibrosis
Reactive airway disease
Recurrent viral bronchiolitis/
  bronchitis
Gastroesophageal reflux
Interstitial pneumonitides
  Lymphoid interstitial
    pneumonitis
  Diffuse interstitial
    pneumonitis

Preschool
Inhaled foreign body
Reactive airway disease
Suppurative lung disease
  Cystic fibrosis
  Bronchiectasis

Right middle lobe syndrome
Ciliary dyskinesia syndromes
Upper respiratory tract
  disease
Recurrent viral
  infection/bronchitis
Passive smoke inhalation
Gastroesophageal reflux
Interstitial pneumonitides
Pulmonary hemosiderosis

School Age to Adolescence
Reactive airway disease
Cystic fibrosis
Mycoplasma pneumoniae
  infection
Psychogenic or habit cough
Cigarette smoking
Pulmonary hemosiderosis
Interstitial pneumonitides
Ciliary dyskinesia syndromes

All Ages
Recurrent viral illness
Asthma
Cystic fibrosis
Granulomatous lung disease
Foreign body aspiration
Pertussis infection

riorly), a cardiothoracic ratio of 0.5, and pulmonary vessels extending two thirds of the way to the periphery. In most situations a lateral radiograph should accompany the posteroanterior (PA) view because some pathologic findings may be missed on a single projection. For example, a lateral x-ray examination yields the best information about the anterior mediastinum and the tracheal air column and also may reveal a small pleural effusion that is unsuspected on the basis of a PA radiograph alone. In combination with the PA view, the lateral projection may help localize an abnormal finding to a particular lobe or segment. In most situations the chest x-ray film taken at full inspiration is most helpful. In the evaluation for bronchial foreign bodies a comparison of inspiratory and expiratory views can help if one lung is unable to empty. In looking for a small pneumothorax, the expiratory film is more helpful because the smaller lung volume allows extrapulmonary air to expand and be more evident.

Cough

Persistent or chronic cough is one of the most common and vexing problems in pediatrics. In most circumstances the tracheobronchial tree is kept clean by airway macrophages and the mucociliary escalator, but cough becomes an important component of this defense system when excessive or abnormal materials are present or when mucociliary clearance is reduced, such as during a viral respiratory illness. A cough clears airway secretions and inhaled particulate matter through a combination of the high airflow velocities generated during the expiratory phase of the cough and the compression of smaller airways, which "milks" the secretions into larger bronchi where they can then be eliminated by a subsequent cough. Cough is generally produced by a reflex response arising from cough receptors located in ciliated epithelia in the lower respiratory tract but can be suppressed or initiated at higher cortical centers. One of the most common causes of cough in pediatric patients is the self-limited cough of an acute viral lower respiratory illness or bronchitis that lasts 1 to 2 weeks. The cough that persists longer than 2 weeks is potentially more worrisome. A diagnostic approach to chronic cough is best served by considering the age of the child (Table 16-1).

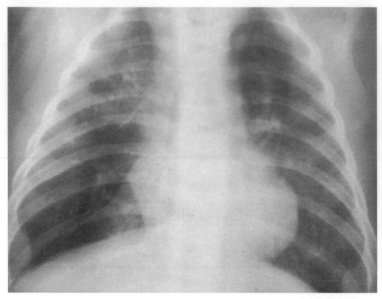

FIG. 16-3   Pneumonia caused by cytomegalovirus in an infant.

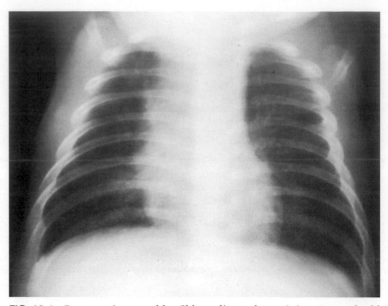

FIG. 16-4   Pneumonia caused by *Chlamydia trachomatis* in a 3-month-old infant with inclusion conjunctivitis.

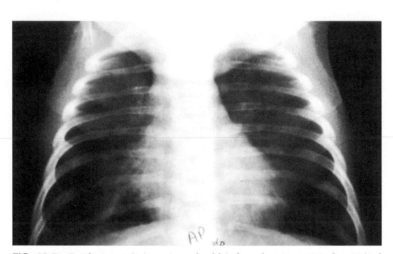

FIG. 16-5   Fatal pertussis in a 6-week-old infant demonstrates the typical radiographic pattern of perihilar involvement.

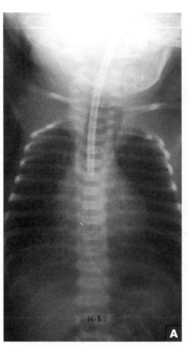
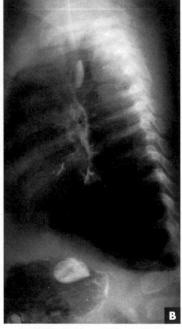

FIG. 16-6   Tracheoesophageal fistula. *A,* Frontal projection shows feeding tube passing no further than proximal esophagus. *B,* Barium swallow in same infant reveals aspiration of barium into the tracheobronchial tree.

There are several causes of persistent cough, however, that are common to all pediatric age groups, such as recurrent viral bronchitis, hyperactive airway disease, cystic fibrosis, granulomatous lung disease (e.g., tuberculosis), foreign body aspiration, and pertussis.

Age and Cause

Infancy (Under 1 Year)

Cough starting at birth or shortly afterward may be a sign of serious respiratory disease and must be evaluated assiduously. Cough beginning at this time raises the possibility of congenital infections, such as cytomegalovirus (Fig. 16-3) or rubella, which are often associated with other findings, such as hepatosplenomegaly, thrombocytopenia, or cen-

tral nervous system involvement. Pneumonia caused by *Chlamydia trachomatis* (Fig. 16-4) generally develops after the first month of life and presents as an afebrile pneumonitis with congestion, wheezing, fine diffuse crackles, a paroxysmal cough, and in approximately 50% of cases a prior or concomitant inclusion conjunctivitis. Pneumonia caused by *Bordetella pertussis* is a possibly life-threatening illness characterized by severe paroxysmal coughing episodes followed by cyanosis and apnea and often associated with an inspiratory "whoop." The latter finding may be missing in very young infants or those weakened by the recurrent coughing spasms. Newborns and young infants may have apnea as the primary sign of a *Bordetella pertussis* infection. The chest radiograph (Fig. 16-5) may show perihilar infiltrates, atelectasis, hyperinflation and in some cases interstitial or subcutaneous emphysema,

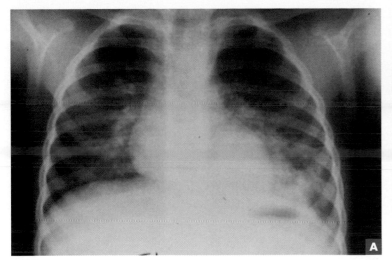

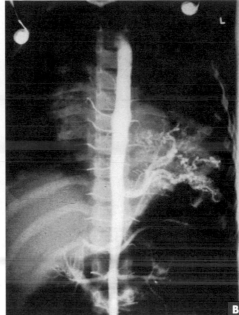

FIG. 16-7 Pulmonary sequestration. Aortic angiogram demonstrates anomalous origin of pulmonary blood supply from abdominal aorta to the left lower lobe in a 7-year-old girl with extralobar sequestration. (Courtesy Dr. Geoffrey Kurland, Pittsburgh.)

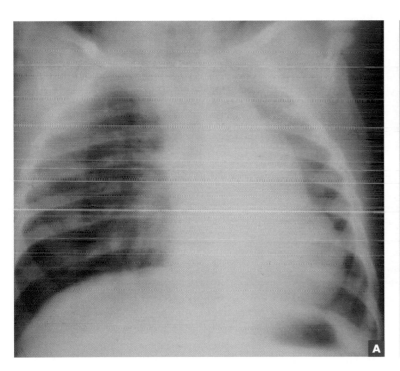

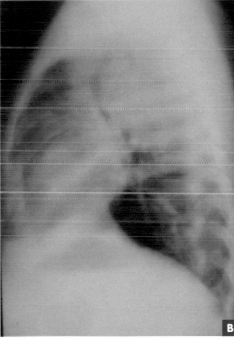

FIG. 16-8 Bronchogenic cyst. *A,* The posteroanterior radiograph has a hyperinflated right lung and a mediastinal shift to the left. *B,* The lateral film has ventral bowing of the tracheal air column. (Courtesy Dr. Beverly Newman, Pittsburgh.)

or it can be normal. A high white blood cell count with a predominance of lymphocytes supports the diagnosis, but unfortunately once the patient has passed through the usually innocent-appearing catarrhal stage into the paroxysmal stage, all diagnostic tests have a lower yield. More recently, *Ureaplasma urealyticum* and *Pneumocystis carinii* have been recognized as causes of pneumonia, and hence persistent cough, in this age group.

Congenital malformations, such as tracheoesophageal fistula (Fig. 16-6) and laryngeal cleft or web, can produce cough via chronic aspiration of gastric contents, milk, or saliva. These anomalies are associated with feeding-related coughing, choking, and occasional cyanosis. Infants with neurologic disorders may have incoordinated swallowing and sucking reflexes that lead to inhalation of milk or gastric contents

into the lung. Pulmonary sequestration (Fig. 16-7) and bronchogenic cysts (Fig. 16-8) are rare congenital anomalies that may compress the pulmonary tree or become infected, thereby producing a cough. Aberrant major blood vessels generally cause inspiratory stridor and expiratory wheezing from tracheal compression (Fig. 16-9), but a brassy cough also may be observed, as may dysphagia from the associated esophageal compression.

The triad of poor weight gain, steatorrhea, and chronic cough at this age makes cystic fibrosis a strong consideration, and a sweat test is therefore mandatory. Reactive airway disease or bronchial hyperresponsiveness is a common and probably underdiagnosed cause of cough in infancy. Cough or persistent wheezing can be found in these infants, who may have a history of viral lower respiratory tract illness or a fam-

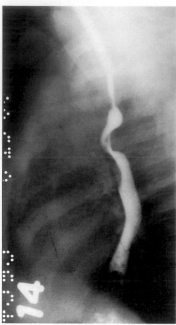

FIG. 16-9 Vascular ring. Barium swallow in a toddler with posterior compression of esophagus and trachea from a vascular ring. (Courtesy Department of Radiology, Children's Hospital of Pittsburgh.)

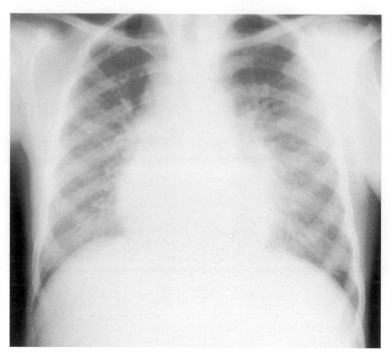

FIG. 16-10 Lymphocytic interstitial pneumonitis in a 10-year-old boy shows a diffuse increase in interstitial markings.

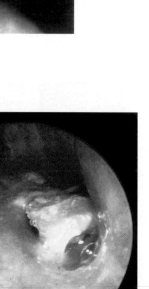

FIG. 16-11 Portion of a carrot lodged in the right mainstem bronchus, as seen through a rigid bronchoscope. (Courtesy Dr. S. Stool, Children's Hospital of Pittsburgh.)

Preschool

The two most common reasons for a persistent cough in this age group are recurrent viral infections with bronchitis and reactive airway disease. The child with reactive airway disease may not manifest the common finding of audible wheezing or dyspnea but rather has cough during and especially after vigorous activity or exposure to noxious inhalants, such as cigarette smoke.

Upper respiratory tract disease and sinusitis have been implicated in the pathogenesis of chronic cough, presumably through the stimulation of pharyngeal cough receptors by upper airway secretions. Parental smoking without evidence of reactive airway disease may be a cause of cough in a small population of preschool children. GER more commonly causes cough at a younger age but may appear at any age. The interstitial pneumonitides may also produce a chronic cough in this age group.

An inhaled foreign body in the esophagus or tracheobronchial tree is an important cause of chronic cough, especially in toddlers. A history of gagging or choking may be absent at this age, physical examination may be unrevealing, and the plain chest radiograph may be normal. Subtle differences in air entry into homologous lung segments detected by the differential (two-headed) stethoscope may be the only indication of a foreign body in the airway. Cough is present in more than 90% of cases; it is usually of abrupt onset, but a quiescent period may occur after inhalation and cough may disappear as irritant receptors adjust to the object's presence. A mobile foreign body may result in the recurrence of cough as new receptors are stimulated by the object. Although inspiratory and expiratory radiography and fluoroscopy are essential in the evaluation of a child who may have inhaled a foreign body, they may be normal and a bronchoscopy may be necessary to confirm or disprove the presence of a foreign object (Fig. 16-11). Unilateral air trapping demonstrated by inspiratory and expiratory radiographs (Fig. 16-12) strongly suggests an inhaled foreign body.

Suppurative lung diseases, such as cystic fibrosis or bronchiectasis (Fig. 16-13), from any other causes (e.g., tuberculosis) characteristically result in a chronic cough, producing purulent sputum. Right middle lobe syndrome, commonly associated with enlarged lymph nodes surrounding the right middle lobe bronchus in tuberculosis, has also been described in asthma and a number of other illnesses and may

ily history of wheezing and/or asthma. Babies with GER may have a combination of wheezing and coughing and in some cases poor weight gain. The absence of a history of "spitting" does not eliminate GER as a diagnostic consideration in infants with persistent coughing because occult reflux may stimulate bronchospasm via vagal reflexes. Lymphocytic interstitial pneumonia (LIP) and the diffuse interstital pneumonitides are rare causes of cough in children and are of unknown etiology. Usual interstitial pneumonitis (UIP) and desquamative interstitial pneumonitis (DIP) present with an insidious onset of cough, dyspnea, anorexia, weight loss, tachypnea, and scattered bibasilar crackles. Later, cyanosis and clubbing are noted on physical examination. LIP may present in a similar fashion but must also be suspected in those patients at risk for human immunodeficiency virus (HIV) infection. The diagnosis of interstitial pneumonitis depends on tissue obtained at lung biopsy. An interstitial pattern on chest radiograph (Fig. 16-10) is seen with varying degrees of hyperinflation or patchy atelectasis. Computed tomography (CT) is a much more sensitive tool for the diagnosis of interstitial lung disease than is the routine chest radiograph.

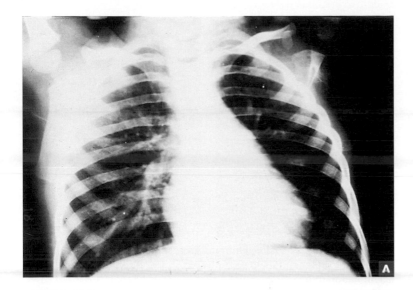

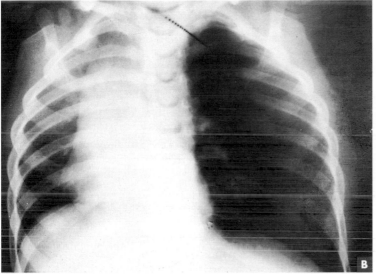

FIG. 16-12 Inspiratory *(A)* and expiratory *(B)* radiograph in a child with an inhaled foreign body lodged in the left mainstem bronchus reveals hyperlucency of the left hemithorax and compensatory shift of the mediastinal structures to the right because the left lung does not empty in expiration.

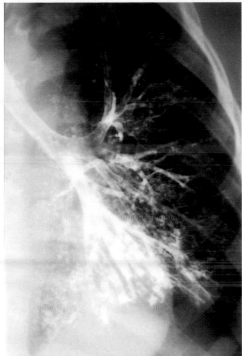

FIG. 16-13 Bronchogram shows cylindrical bronchiectasis of the left lower lobe in a 5-year-old girl with recurrent pneumonia and chronic cough.

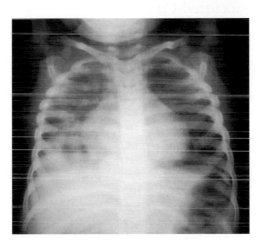

FIG. 16-14 Idiopathic pulmonary hemosiderosis in a youngster with hemoptysis and wheezing and mostly right-sided radiographic involvement.

cause chronic cough. Recurrent infection of the middle lobe can lead to the development of bronchiectasis or fibrosis.

Disorders of ciliary motility may produce insidious symptoms of productive cough, nasal drainage, recurrent middle ear infections, and fever. Clinical findings include basilar crackles and, later, radiographic changes of recurrent lower lobe infections and eventually bronchiectasis. Repetitive infections occur unless measures such as chest physical therapy, postural drainage, and liberal use of antibiotics are employed. The classic triad described by Kartagener of situs inversus, sinusitis, and bronchiectasis fits only a limited number of patients because situs inversus occurs in only about half of all patients with dysmotile-cilia syndrome.

Pulmonary hemosiderosis is a potentially fatal disorder that has been described in association with cardiac or panorganic disease, glomerulonephritis (Goodpasture syndrome), infantile hypersensitivity to cow's milk protein (Heiner syndrome), and collagen-vascular diseases and as an idiopathic form. Idiopathic pulmonary hemosiderosis (IPH) is a disease of unknown etiology characterized by episodes of

dyspnea, cough and/or hemoptysis, wheezing, cyanosis, fever, and iron deficiency anemia. Hematemesis or melena may be the only complaint in some patients without symptoms referable to the respiratory tract. As a result of recurrent bleeding episodes, jaundice may be observed, and clubbing develops over time in some patients. Laboratory findings include iron deficiency anemia and, in a small number of patients, peripheral eosinophilia. Radiographic findings (Fig. 16-14) are quite variable, with some patients demonstrating scant transient infiltrates and others showing widespread parenchymal infiltrates that resemble miliary tuberculosis. Hemosiderin-laden macrophages obtained from sputum, gastric washings, or bronchoalveolar lavage suggest the diagnosis, but a lung biopsy may be necessary. A percutaneous renal biopsy may help in cases of hemosiderosis associated with Goodpasture syndrome.

School Age to Adolescence

Because children are exposed to numerous respiratory viruses during the first several years of school, recurrent viral infection remains an important cause of chronic cough in this age group. Reactive airway

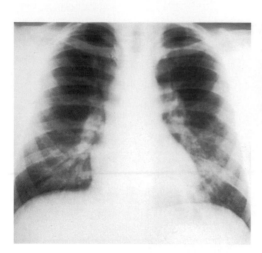

FIG. 16-15 Mycoplasma pneumonia in an adolescent shows typical lower-lobe involvement by chest x-ray examination. (Courtesy Dr. A. Urbach, Pittsburgh.)

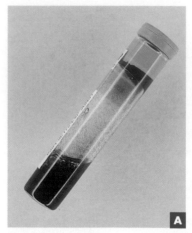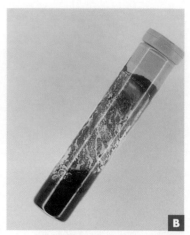

FIG. 16-16 Bedside cold agglutinins (see text for explanation of technique). *A,* Purple-top tube before placing on ice. *B,* Positive result shows agglutination of heparinized blood after exposure to cold. (Courtesy Dr. H. Davis, Pittsburgh.)

TABLE 16-2

Characteristics of Chronic Coughs and Associated Conditions

Characteristic	Associated condition
Loose, productive	Cystic fibrosis, bronchiectasis, ciliary dyskinesia
Croupy	Laryngotracheobronchitis
Paroxysmal	Cystic fibrosis, pertussis syndrome, foreign body inhalation, *Mycoplasma, Chlamydia*
Brassy	Tracheitis, upper airway drainage, psychogenic cough
After feedings	Pharyngeal incoordination, pharyngeal mass, tracheoesophageal fistula, gastroesophageal reflux
Nocturnal	Upper respiratory tract disease, sinusitis, asthma, cystic fibrosis, gastroesophageal reflux
Most severe in morning	Cystic fibrosis, bronchiectasis
With exercise	Asthma (including exercise-induced), cystic fibrosis, bronchiectasis
Loud, honking, or bizarre	Psychogenic cough
Disappears with sleep	Psychogenic cough

---

disease continues to be a consideration in the patient with a chronic cough. Patients in this age group can perform pulmonary function tests, including bronchodilator responsiveness or bronchial provocation studies, to confirm the diagnosis. Other disorders may present with chronic cough at this age, including cystic fibrosis, pulmonary hemosiderosis, interstitial pneumonitis, and ciliary dyskinesia syndromes.

Mycoplasma pneumoniae infection is an important cause of chronic cough among school-age children. Although the lung is the primary site of infection and cough is a striking feature of the disease, the gradual onset of extrapulmonary symptoms, such as malaise, headache, fever, and sore throat, may be the initial clues to the diagnosis. Cough generally produces mucoid sputum, and hemoptysis may develop later. The

cough can persist for 3 to 4 months. Physical findings tend to be minimal, although crackles are the most common sign, with wheezing often noted in younger children. The chest radiograph is not diagnostic, and the findings may be either interstitial or bronchopneumonic in character, with predilection for the lower lobes (Fig. 16-15). Bedside cold agglutinins are a simple means of confirming the suspected diagnosis and may be positive in about one half of cases but are not specific. About 1 ml of blood is collected in an sodium ethylene diamine tetra-acetic acid (NaEDTA or "purple-top") tube and placed on ice for 30 to 60 seconds. The presence of agglutination that disappears upon rewarming to 37°C suggests a positive result (Fig. 16-16). A positive result correlates with a serum cold agglutinin titer of at least 1:64. During the acute stage of the illness the presence of specific IgM antibody to mycoplasma or a rise in the level of specific IgG antibody may confirm the diagnostic impression.

A psychogenic or habit cough may be observed after a lower respiratory tract illness. Habit cough may persist for weeks or months after the acute process has subsided. A psychogenic cough tends to be very loud and bizarre in nature and timing and is often described as "honking" or "barking." This type of cough is short, nonproductive, and nonparoxysmal; it is quite disturbing to family members and classmates, to the point that the child may be excluded from school and other activities. It always disappears with sleep. The cough becomes more obvious in stressful situations or when parents (or physicians) express undue interest or anxiety regarding the cough. For this reason, extensive evaluations by medical personnel may merely exacerbate the problem when the diagnosis can be made on the basis of the characteristic quality of the cough and its disappearance in sleep.

Cigarette smoking in this group also should be a consideration and, unless the rapport between physician and adolescent is particularly strong, it is likely that the history will be unrevealing. Staining of the teeth or fingers or the presence of conjunctivitis may be indirect clues to the underlying cause of the cough.

Evaluation

The history may suggest the underlying cause of the cough (Table 16-2) and, perhaps more importantly, eliciting the cough during the physical examination can help. A loose or productive cough suggests suppurative lung disease such as cystic fibrosis, other forms of bronchiectasis, or ciliary dyskinesia syndromes. The cough in these patients tends to be most

TABLE 16-3

Diagnostic Approach to Cough

Complete history and physical examination
Chest and sinus radiographs
CBC with differential
Pulmonary function tests (including bronchoprovocation tests)
Sweat test (pilocarpine iontophoresis method)
Trial of bronchodilators
Sputum for Gram stain, AFB, bacterial, viral, and fungal cultures
Quantitative immunoglobulins
Tuberculin skin test/anergy panel
Serologic tests for *Mycoplasma pneumoniae*
Bronchoscopy
Barium swallow
pH probe or Bernstein test

AFB, Acid fast bacillus.

severe in the morning because excessive and inadequately cleared secretions pool in the tracheobronchial tree during sleep. A croupy cough may be observed in patients with acute laryngotracheobronchitis, and there may be associated wheezing. A dry or brassy cough generally is seen in patients with larger airway pathology, as in tracheitis or drainage from upper respiratory tract disease; a psychogenic cough may produce similar findings but may be distinguished from the others by its disappearance with sleep. As noted previously, a psychogenic cough is often (but not always) very loud, honking, bizarre, and disruptive. A paroxysmal cough is seen in patients with pertussis syndrome, *Mycoplasma*, *Chlamydia*, foreign body inhalation, or cystic fibrosis. A coughing episode associated with feedings suggests pharyngeal incoordination or mass, tracheoesophageal fistula, or GER. Nighttime coughing is noted in cystic fibrosis, asthma, GER, sinusitis, and upper respiratory tract disease. Cough occurring during or shortly after activities suggests asthma, cystic fibrosis, or bronchiectasis.

Examination of the sputum also may help suggest the diagnosis. Clear, mucoid sputum containing eosinophils is likely to represent asthma, whereas purulent green sputum suggests suppurative lung disease, such as cystic fibrosis. A yellow color can be imparted to the sputum by breakdown products of white blood cells; therefore yellow sputum can be seen with infection (polymorphonuclear leukocytes breaking down) or asthma (eosinophils breaking down). Bloody sputum can occur in cystic fibrosis, retained foreign body, idiopathic pulmonary hemosiderosis, tuberculosis, bronchiectasis, or some infections. Upper respiratory tract irritation may lead to the mistaken notion that hemoptysis is occurring. Hematemesis also may be mistaken for hemoptysis.

Clinical findings associated with a cough also may point to the nature of the problem. A cough occurring in the presence of poor weight gain and malabsorption makes cystic fibrosis a concern. A cough occurring with wheezing suggests asthma, and if evidence of rhinitis, conjunctivitis, or "allergic shiners" is present, allergic disease also is a consideration (see Chapter 4). A cough that is worse in spring and summer months or occurs only after exercise suggests asthma. A worsening of the cough in the winter is consistent with cold-induced bronchospasm or recurrent viral illnesses.

Diagnostic Approach

The approach to diagnosing a patient with persistent cough begins with a complete history in which some of the factors alluded to earlier (Table

16-3) are targeted. On physical examination, close attention to nutritional status, presence of associated upper respiratory tract disease, or clubbing of the digits is as important as the examination of the chest. Clubbing of the fingers raises the possibility of cystic fibrosis; any patient with this finding requires a sweat test performed by quantitative pilocarpine iontophoresis. On auscultation of the chest a localized wheeze, particularly if associated with delayed air entry, suggests a foreign body or focal airway lesion leading to narrowing. Inspiratory crackles may be noted in cystic fibrosis, bronchiectasis from other causes, interstitial lung disease, or pneumonia. Crackles also are present during one third to one half of untreated asthma attacks, even in the absence of infection.

Most patients with prolonged cough should have a chest x-ray examination and, if historical or physical findings are suggestive, sinus x-ray films as well. Inspiratory and expiratory radiographs and fluoroscopy are indicated if inhalation of a foreign body is suspected. A complete blood cell count with differential may suggest the diagnosis in some patients, with eosinophilia seen in allergic disease, lymphocytosis in pertussis and other viral diseases, and an increased proportion of neutrophils in bacterial infections. In a child old enough to cooperate, pulmonary function tests may detect lower airway obstruction and determine its reversibility with bronchodilator administration. Abnormalities of the shape of the inspiratory or expiratory loops during spirometry suggests upper airway pathology (discussed later). In some cases an outpatient trial of bronchodilators for several weeks may confirm the suspicion of cough-variant asthma. Failure to respond to this regimen suggests that asthma is not the problem but also could be the result of noncompliance with the prescribed medications. Examination of sputum produced by the patient with Wright or Gram stain or by cultures may lead to a diagnosis. The presence of eosinophils suggests allergic disease, and polymorphonuclear leukocytes with organisms suggest a bacterial infection. Quantitative immunoglobulins and immunoglobulin subclasses may help detect some immunodeficiencies, and an elevated IgE suggests allergic disease. A purified protein derivative (PPD) intradermal skin test placed in conjunction with other antigens of known immunogenicity (e.g., candida or mumps) may be important in some patients. In the appropriate clinical setting, serologic studies for *Mycoplasma pneumoniae* are occasionally fruitful. Bronchoscopy may exclude the diagnosis of foreign body or airway malformation as the cause of chronic cough. If foreign body inhalation is likely (based on history and/or physical examination), bronchoscopy is essential and should be performed under general anesthesia with the rigid bronchoscope to provide adequate airway control.

Chest CT may confirm the diagnosis of bronchiectasis and should be performed if surgical removal of the affected segment is contemplated. A barium swallow is useful in patients with suspected tracheoesophageal fistula or various pharyngeal disorders. Prolonged monitoring of the pH in the distal esophagus may confirm the suspicion of GER. The appearance of symptoms with acid infusion into the distal esophagus (Bernstein test) can confirm the causal relationship between acid reflux and cough. Finally, on rare occasions a nasal ciliary biopsy for examination by light and electron microscopy or a nuclear medicine scan measuring the movement of inhaled radiolabeled particles may be indicated in patients with suspected ciliary dysmotility.

Stridor

A number of clinical entities can produce persistent or recurrent stridor (Table 16-4), and some of these also may be associated with a chronic cough, as described earlier. Stridor is characteristically a harsh inspiratory noise created by obstruction of the larynx or the extrathoracic tra-

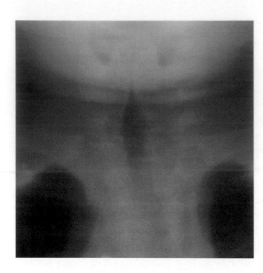

FIG. 16-17 The "steeple sign" shows subglottic narrowing of the trachea caused by croup (laryngotracheobronchitis). (Courtesy Dr. Beverly Newman, Pittsburgh.)

TABLE 16-4

Causes of Recurrent or Chronic Stridor

Croup	Pharyngeal or laryngeal masses
Infectious	Papilloma
Allergic/angioneurotic	Hemangioma
edema	Laryngocele
Laryngomalacia	Web
Tracheomalacia	Foreign body
Subglottic stenosis	Tracheoesophageal fistula
Extrinsic airway compression	Vocal cord paralysis
Vascular ring	Hysterical or psychogenic
Mediastinal mass	
Lobar emphysema	
Bronchogenic cyst	
Foreign body in esophagus	
Thyromegaly	

TABLE 16-5

Causes of Chronic or Recurrent Wheezing

Reactive airway disease	Ciliary dyskinesia
Asthma	syndromes
Exercise-induced asthma	Tracheomalacia and/or
Gastroesophageal reflux	bronchomalacia
Hypersensitivity reactions	Congestive heart failure
(e.g., ABPA)	Bronchopulmonary he-
Cystic fibrosis	mosiderosis or Heiner
Aspiration	syndrome
Tracheoesophageal fistula	Endobronchial lesions,
Foreign body	including localized
Gastroesophageal reflux	stenosis
Laryngeal cleft	Interstitial pneumonitides
Pharyngeal dysmotility	Bronchiolitis obliterans
Extrinsic masses	
Vascular ring	
Cystic adenomatoid	
malformation	
Lymph nodes	
Tumors	

ABPA, Allergic bronchopulmonary aspergillosis.

---

chea. With a mild degree of airway narrowing, breath sounds may be normal when the infant or child is at rest, but with any activity that increases tidal breathing, for example, crying, feeding, or agitation, inspiratory stridor may become noticeable.

The most common cause of inspiratory stridor in the pediatric population is infectious croup or acute laryngotracheobronchitis. The disease generally is caused by a respiratory virus (parainfluenza, respiratory syncytial, influenza, or rhinovirus), and the patient typically has coryza for 24 to 48 hours before the appearance of croupy cough, hoarseness, and stridor. Occasionally the inflammatory process may spread to the smaller airways and produce wheezing in addition to these symptoms. The "steeple sign" is a characteristic radiographic sign on anteroposterior projections (Fig. 16-17) that may be accompanied by marked dilation of supraglottic structures, particularly on lateral films. In the majority of patients, serious airway obstruction does not occur and the disease is self-limited. Acute angioneurotic edema is a less common cause of stridor. In most cases it results from an allergic reaction and is potentially fatal. Some children suffer recurrent bouts of stridor, usually in the middle of the night. This entity is often termed *spasmodic croup* and is poorly understood, with various causes having been postulated but not proved. GER appears to play a role in some of these cases.

The stridor associated with laryngomalacia (Fig. 16-18) generally begins within the first month of life, varies with activity, may be expiratory, and is more noticeable when the child is in the supine position. Clinical symptoms may suggest the diagnosis, but bronchoscopic visualization of airway dynamics by flexible bronchoscopy is a safe and reliable method of confirming laryngomalacia. Tracheomalacia can produce stridor or wheezing as the compliant posterior tracheal wall collapses anteriorly with increased respiratory effort. Parents can be reassured that these entities are self-limited, become less marked after 6 to 10 months of age, and rarely cause serious problems.

Narrowing of the subglottic region can be congenital or acquired, as in subglottic stenosis associated with endotracheal intubation. Congenital subglottic stenosis improves as the child grows older, but narrowing associated with tracheal intubation may require a tracheostomy, particularly if the infant remains dependent on ventilatory support.

Congenital laryngeal or pharyngeal masses also can produce stridor by obstructing airflow. Laryngeal papillomatosis (Fig. 16-19) is a rare and life-threatening illness that generally presents in the first decade of life. Papillomas can involve the vocal cords as in the aforementioned figure, but there also may be widespread involvement of the remainder of the tracheobronchial tree. Although inspiratory stridor may be observed, hoarseness is a more common feature. Hemangiomas of the larynx or trachea also may produce stridor or a brassy or dry cough. Cutaneous or mucosal hemangiomas noted during the physical examination suggest the diagnosis. Laryngeal webs (Fig. 16-20), cysts, and laryngoceles are uncommon, are all accompanied by respiratory distress and stridor, and are occasionally accompanied by feeding difficulties and cyanosis. Diagnosis is made by bronchoscopy. A foreign body in the pharynx or larynx also may cause stridor.

Vocal cord paralysis, either unilateral or bilateral, may present in the neonatal period, although in the case of unilateral paralysis several weeks may pass before the diagnosis is suspected. A weak or absent cry, hoarseness, inspiratory stridor with or without respiratory distress, and feeding difficulties are usual signs of vocal cord paralysis. Bilateral vocal cord paralysis may be seen with hydrocephalus, myelomeningocele, Arnold-Chiari malformation, or other malformations of the brain. Unilateral and bilateral cord paralyses are observed in patients with abnormalities of the cardiovascular system that are accompanied by cardiomegaly (ventricular septal defect or tetralogy of Fallot) or that cause abnormalities of the great vessels (e.g., vascular ring, transposition, patent ductus arteriosus). The diagnosis is best made by flexible bron-

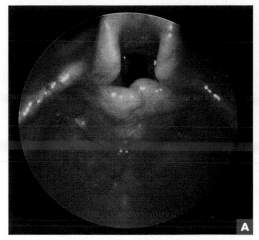

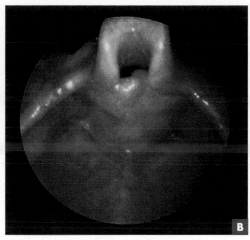

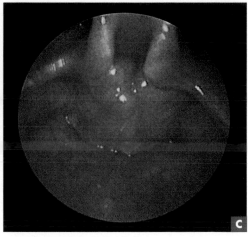

FIG. 16-18 A sequence of photographs demonstrates the degree of airway compromise occurring during inspiration in laryngomalacia. The epiglottis is supported by a laryngoscope blade, but the progressive collapse of the other laryngeal structures during inspiration, especially the arytenoid cartilages, is shown clearly. (From Benjamin B: *Atlas of paediatric endoscopy,* London, 1981, Oxford University Press.)

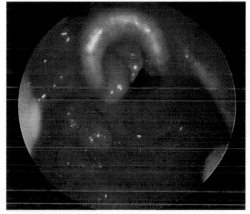

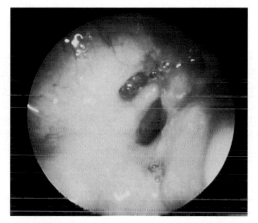

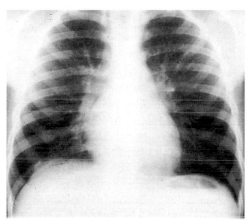

FIG. 16-19 Multiple papillomas involving the larynx. (From Benjamin B: *Atlas of paediatric endoscopy,* London, 1981, Oxford University Press.)

FIG. 16-20 Expiratory view of a laryngeal web in an infant with inspiratory stridor that was exaggerated by crying noted at birth. The web is seen traversing the area of the glottis. (From Boehringer Ingelheim International GmbH.)

FIG. 16-21 The chest x-ray film of an adolescent with asthma and allergic bronchopulmonary aspergillosis shows hyperinflation and patchy atelectasis.

choscopy under minimal sedation so that vocal cord movement can be examined adequately.

A bronchogenic cyst (Fig. 16-18) in the newborn can cause stridor because the cyst fills with air after birth and compresses large airways. It also can cause tachypnea, dyspnea, cyanosis, and diminished breath sounds on the affected side. Later the cyst may become infected, leading to recurrent bouts of fever, cough, and hemoptysis. Finally an esophageal foreign body may compress the compliant posterior wall of the trachea and produce stridor, cough, and dysphagia.

The diagnosis of hysterical or psychogenic stridor is generally made during adolescence and is more common in girls. As in psychogenic cough, psychogenic stridor disappears with sleep and is more noticeable with anxiety or when excessive attention is given to the patient.

Wheezing

Many of the diseases that produce chronic wheezing in pediatric patients (Table 16-5) overlap with entities that cause coughing or stridor.

Wheezing results from obstruction of airflow in intrathoracic airways. This obstruction can be at the lower trachea "downstream" to the small bronchi and in the large bronchioles. Wheezes can be heard on expiration or, less commonly, during both phases of respiration. The pitch of the wheeze, the variation in its pitch throughout the lung fields, and an association with hyperinflation as defined by percussion (described previously) can help differentiate wheezing resulting from obstruction in the small airways from that in the large airways. Response to bronchodilator medication and/or steroids is useful in differentiating true reactive airway disease (which should improve with these treatments) from wheezing resulting from tracheomalacia or bronchomalacia (which does not improve and may even worsen with bronchodilators). Reactive airway disease (with obstruction of the lower intrathoracic airways) is the most common cause of wheezing in pediatric patients. It invariably is associated with some degree of hyperinflation in the untreated patient. Reactive airway disease may take many different forms, including typical asthma, cough-variant asthma, exercise-induced asthma, and wheezing associated with GER.

The development of increased wheezing in a previously well-

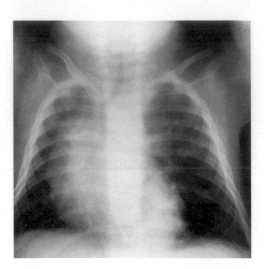

FIG. 16-22 Cystic areas in the left lower lobe caused by congenital cystadenomatoid malformation in an infant with respiratory distress and wheezing.

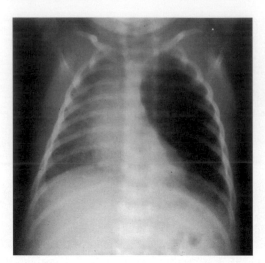

FIG. 16-23 Congenital lobar emphysema of the left upper lobe shows hyperlucency of the affected globe, atelectasis of the lower lobe, and mediastinal shift.

controlled asthmatic patient raises the possibility of allergic bronchopulmonary aspergillosis (ABPA). These patients often have an insidious onset of low-grade fever, fatigue, weight loss, and productive cough. Physical findings include expiratory wheezes and bibasilar crackles and, later in the course, clubbing of the digits. Radiographic features of ABPA (Fig. 16-21) include areas of consolidation, atelectasis, and evidence of dilated bronchi radiating from the hila. Diagnosis can be made by positive skin test results with *Aspergillus fumigatus* antigens, elevated total serum IgE levels, elevation of specific IgE, presence of serum precipitins to aspergillus organisms, and isolation of *A. fumigatus* from the sputum culture. Pulmonary function study results may worsen considerably during episodes of ABPA with evidence of increased airway obstruction. A host of other hypersensitivity reactions produce extrinsic allergic alveolitis with wheezing (see any of the standard pulmonary texts listed in the bibliography for a further discussion of these entities).

Other disorders that can provoke wheezing include cystic fibrosis, aspiration events from any cause, and extrinsic masses that compress the airways.

Congenital cystic adenomatoid malformation is a rare cause of extrinsic airway compression in which symptoms generally begin at birth or shortly afterward as a normal lung is compressed by the lesion with the onset of tachypnea, respiratory distress, and cyanosis. Hydramnios is often noted at birth. Rarely, smaller cysts may be an incidental finding on chest x-ray examination, or symptoms may develop after infection of the cysts occurs. The radiographic appearance (Fig. 16-22) is that of multiple cystlike areas compressing the normal lung with mediastinal displacement. It is usually confined to a single lobe, and there is no apparent predilection for a particular lobe.

Airway compression from extrinsic factors may produce wheezing or stridor, depending on the site of obstruction. A vascular ring (Fig. 16-9) is much more likely to cause expiratory wheezing than inspiratory stridor (see Chapter 5). Diagnosis can be made by barium swallow, echocardiography, magnetic resonance imaging, or bronchoscopy; the last may demonstrate a pulsatile lesion compressing the trachea. Mediastinal masses or occasionally enlargement of the thyroid gland may produce tracheal compression and stridor. Congenital or acquired lobar emphysema usually produces tachypnea and other respiratory symptoms, such as cough, wheeze, intermittent cyanosis, and occasionally stridor. The

chest radiograph in lobar emphysema (Fig. 16-23) demonstrates a large, hyperlucent area with few bronchovascular markings and usually compression atelectasis of adjacent lobes. Left upper lobe involvement is most common, but right middle lobe emphysema also is seen. For the infant who is growing well and in whom tachypnea is the primary symptom or in lobar emphysema associated with a mucous plug, conservative management is indicated. In the symptomatic infant with compression atelectasis and wheezing and/or chronic respiratory distress, resection of the affected lobe is indicated.

Bronchopulmonary dysplasia (BPD), one of the sequelae of hyaline membrane disease and its treatment, is associated with recurrent episodes of wheezing, respiratory distress, and tachypnea (see Chapter 2). Otherwise mild respiratory illnesses in these infants may progress to lower respiratory tract disease necessitating frequent hospitalization. Patients with BPD may develop chronic respiratory insufficiency, pulmonary hypertension, and cor pulmonale. The frequency of wheezing episodes may diminish with age, although it appears that these patients continue to have airway hyperreactivity that is triggered by any number of insults.

Miscellaneous causes of wheezing include idiopathic pulmonary hemosiderosis, endobronchial lesions associated with localized stenosis, interstitial lung disease, and bronchiolitis obliterans. The last has been described in an idiopathic form, following adenoviral infections or inhalation of toxic agents, and in conjunction with other diseases (including rheumatoid arthritis) in adults. Its most common clinical setting in pediatrics in the 1990s is the organ transplant recipient. Patients initially may have fever, cough, or tachypnea and subsequently develop dyspnea and wheezing. Physical findings include both wheezing and crackles. The radiographic pattern (Fig. 16-24) is that of diffusely increased interstitial markings with areas of atelectasis and consolidation. Complications of adenovirus-induced bronchiolitis obliterans include bronchiectasis, overinflation, recurrent atelectasis, and pneumonia. In many patients the prognosis is poor.

Cystic Fibrosis

Cystic fibrosis (CF) is the most common life-shortening genetic disease among white North Americans, afflicting 1 in 2500 newborns in this

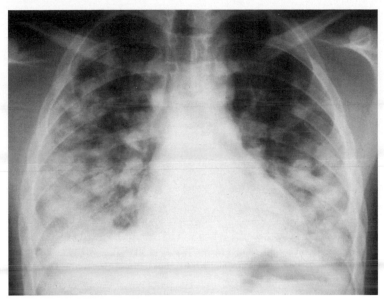

FIG. 16-24 Bronchiolitis obliterans of unknown cause in a 12-year-old boy demonstrates extensive pulmonary involvement.

TABLE 16-6

Presentations of Cystic Fibrosis

General
    Failure to thrive
    Salty taste to skin
GI/Nutritional
    Meconium ileus
    Foul-smelling stools, bloating, abdominal pain
    Rectal prolapse
    Intestinal impaction and obstruction
    Pancreatitis, acute and chronic
    Hypoproteinemia and edema
    Neonatal hyperbilirubinemia
    Cholelithiasis, cholecystitis
    Cirrhosis or portal hypertension
    Fat-soluble vitamin deficiency (A, D, E, K)
Metabolic
    Hyponatremic hypochloremic dehydration
    Heat stroke
    Metabolic alkalosis
    Diabetes mellitus
Respiratory
    Clubbing
    Asthma
    Chronic obstructive pulmonary disease
    Recurrent pulmonary infiltrates
    Chronic cough or sputum production
    Barrel chest
    Hemoptysis
    Pneumothorax
    Cor pulmonale
    Nasal polyps
Other
    Infertility (males)

group. The incidence in African-Americans is about 1 in 17,000, and in people of Asian background, 1 in 90,000. It is estimated that the carrier rate in whites is 1 in 25. CF is a generalized exocrinopathy characterized by the inspissation of abnormally thick and tenacious secretions, principally involving the pancreas and lungs. In the lungs the secretions obstruct the airways, resulting in recurrent infections and an inflammatory process that leads to bronchiolitis, bronchitis, bronchiectasis, and bronchiolectasis. Eventually, pulmonary function declines and respiratory disease accounts for the majority of CF deaths. In the pancreas, ducts are obstructed by the abnormal secretions, preventing pancreatic enzymes from entering the duodenum and therefore preventing breakdown of dietary fat and protein. The pancreas undergoes autodigestion and is replaced by scar tissue; lifetime deficiency of pancreatic exocrine function results. In 40% to 50% of newborns with CF, pancreatic enzyme secretion is largely intact. This condition has recently been labeled *pancreatic sufficiency.* By age 4 to 8 years, the proportion of patients with pancreatic sufficiency has fallen to 10% to 15%, where it remains. The prognosis for patients with CF has improved dramatically over the last several decades. By 1994 the median survival for patients had risen to age 29 years.

The disease is inherited as an autosomal recessive trait. The protein product of the CF gene, the cystic fibrosis transmembrane chloride conductance regulator (CFTR), functions as an epithelial chloride channel. Inhibition of chloride transport and overactive sodium pumping across various epithelia result in abnormally viscid and poorly hydrated secretions. The most common defect found in North America is referred to as delta-F508. This mutation is the result of the deletion of three base pairs in the gene and results in a protein missing a phenylalanine residue at position 508. When genetic testing for CF became available, there was optimism that a handful of mutations at the CF locus (located on the long arm of chromosome 7) would account for the majority of the patients with the disease and lead the way to population-wide screening. This, unfortunately, is not the case. There are, at last count, more than 550 reported mutations in this gene. The majority of these mutations, however, are isolated to a single patient or family; only 32 mutations account for 92% of CF alleles in North America. In approximately 70% of CF genes delta-F508 is found. This means that half of CF patients in North America are homozygous for delta-F508. Half of the remaining patients are compound heterozygotes with delta-F508

coupled with another CF allele; the remaining patients have other non–delta F508 mutations. A number of investigators have tried to discover genotype-phenotype correlations. The most reliable phenotypic correlate of genotype has been the pancreatic status. Respiratory disease severity has not been well correlated to genotype. Although genetic testing is not needed in patients with elevated sweat chloride and typical clinical features of CF, it is somewhat useful in the evaluation of the occasional infant who produces too little sweat for analysis, the patient with borderline sweat chloride, or the patient with normal sweat chloride but clinical features characteristic of CF.

Presentations

CF can present in any number of fashions (Table 16-6), but most symptoms are referable to respiratory or gastrointestinal involvement. The presenting sign in 5% to 10% of patients with CF is meconium ileus, which is noted at or shortly after birth. Meconium ileus is a common cause of intestinal obstruction in the newborn; these infants present with abdominal distension, bilious vomiting, and failure to pass meconium stools. Abdominal radiographs show dilated loops of small bowel and a ground-grass appearance in the cecal region, signifying pockets of air within the thick meconium. A barium or Gastrografin contrast enema

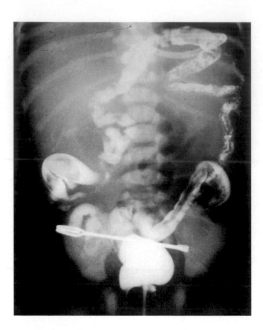

FIG. 16-25 Barium enema in a newborn with meconium peritonitis and evidence of a small, unused distal colon (note small extraluminal calcifications).

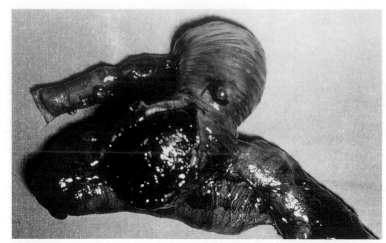

FIG. 16-26 Gross appearance of the thick, tarlike meconium found at laparotomy in meconium ileus.

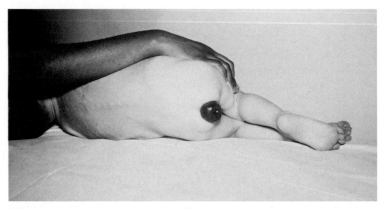

FIG. 16-27 Rectal prolapse in a toddler not previously recognized as having CF.

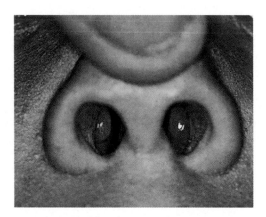

FIG. 16-28 Nasal polyps in a patient with CF.

may show a very small distal colon (Fig. 16-25). In cases of meconium ileus associated with prenatal rupture and meconium peritonitis, abdominal calcification may be noted on plain radiographs, and at laparotomy thick, tarlike meconium is found in the terminal ileum (Fig. 16-26). Prolonged neonatal jaundice, generalized edema in a breast-fed or soy formula–fed infant, and hypoelectrolytemia with heat prostration are less common presentations of CF in early infancy.

A combination of poor weight gain; loose, foul-smelling, bulky stools; and a voracious appetite are signs and symptoms that most clinicians associate with CF and rarely present a diagnostic problem. Rectal prolapse (Fig. 16-27) may be the presenting feature of CF in about 5% of cases and may recur multiple times. Rarely the patient may undergo a surgical procedure for the rectal prolapse before the underlying diagnosis is suspected. Rectal prolapse is thought to result from chronic malnutrition, reduced abdominal musculature, and voluminous stools. It does not generally pose problems once the diagnosis has been made and the patient has been started on supplemental pancreatic enzymes. Acute or chronic pancreatitis occurs occasionally, almost exclusively in patients with pancreatic sufficiency. These patients present with the acute onset of abdominal pain and vomiting and may have recurrent bouts of pancreatitis before the pancreas "burns itself out." Diagnostic laboratory evaluations include elevations of serum lipase and amylase. The differential diagnosis in CF patients with acute abdominal pain and

vomiting includes cholecystitis, appendicitis, and distal intestinal obstruction syndrome. The last is characterized by crampy abdominal pain, constipation, vomiting, and occasionally a palpable mass in the right lower quadrant. There may be a history of missed pancreatic enzyme supplements, especially in adolescents. Other possible signs of CF with respect to the gastrointestinal system include cirrhosis, portal hypertension, esophageal varices, and clinical evidence of fat-soluble vitamin deficiency.

A chronic productive cough or wheezing in a patient with digital clubbing suggests the diagnosis of CF until proved otherwise. Patients may present with a history of recurrent pneumonia or sinus disease; it is worth noting that the majority of patients with CF demonstrate pansinusitis radiographically. Nasal polyps (Fig. 16-28) may be a manifestation of CF and are seen in about 20% of patients during the course of the disease. Other initial respiratory symptoms are listed in Table 16-6.

The clinical course and severity of the disease vary remarkably. Many patients do not develop signs or symptoms of respiratory disease other than an intermittent, loose cough for years. Other patients have persistent symptoms from early infancy and are rarely without a cough. These patients require frequent visits to the physician, frequent hospitalization, and are more likely to have poor weight gain. Virtually all patients develop a loose, productive cough; the sputum may be blood-tinged during acute respiratory illnesses. Hemoptysis occurs in more

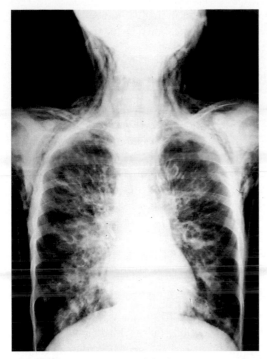

FIG. 16-29 A teenager with CF, severe respiratory disease, pneumomediastinum, and massive subcutaneous emphysema.

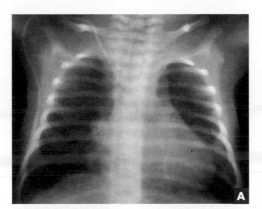

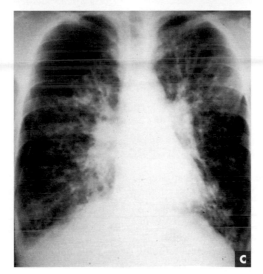

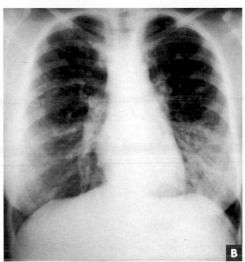

FIG. 16-30 Typical progression of radiographic changes in cystic fibrosis. *A*, A 2-month old child with hyperinflation and right middle lobe atelectasis. *B*, A 15-year-old girl with peribronchial cuffing, hyperinflation, and bronchiectatic changes, particularly of the lower lobes. *C*, A 21-year-old man with severe respiratory involvement and an unsuspected right pneumothorax.

than half of adult patients with CF and a considerable proportion of adolescents as well. Tachypnea, dyspnea, diffuse crackles, and digital clubbing develop in most patients. Later, diffuse bronchiectasis, hyperinflation, and barrel-chest deformity are noted. The usual cause of death in patients with CF is respiratory failure, often in conjunction with cor pulmonale.

Complications

The complications of CF include hemoptysis, pneumothorax, pneumomediastinum, hypertrophic pulmonary osteoarthropathy, distal intestinal obstructive syndrome (meconium ileus equivalent), liver disease, pancreatitis, and cor pulmonale. Among the respiratory complications, massive hemoptysis and pneumothorax with or without pneumomediastinum are potentially life-threatening. Blood streaking of sputum is not uncommon, and massive hemoptysis from rupture of large blood vessels during chronic suppurative infections may occur in a small percentage of patients. Pneumothorax (Fig. 16-30, *C*) generally occurs from rupture of bullous lesions created from chronic airway obstruction and presents with acute onset of chest pain and shortness of breath with or without cyanosis. Pneumomediastinum and massive subcutaneous emphysema may result (Fig. 16-29). Hypertrophic pulmonary osteoarthropathy involving the knees and other major joints occurs in about

5% of patients with severe lung disease and is characterized by pain, swelling, and limited mobility in the affected joint. Right ventricular hypertrophy and cor pulmonale are findings in the terminal stages of many CF patients with severe pulmonary disease.

Radiographic Findings

The radiographic findings in CF vary from early hyperinflation and patchy areas of atelectasis to a generalized increase in peribronchial markings with bronchiectasis, parenchymal densities, and large cystic areas noted in severe disease (Fig. 16-30). The Brasfield scoring system is widely used to classify chest radiographs of these patients. It is based on a point system for findings such as hyperinflation, linear densities, cystic lesions, atelectasis, and right-sided cardiac enlargement or pneumothorax.

Diagnosis

The sweat test performed by pilocarpine iontophoresis with quantitative analysis of chloride and/or sodium remains the laboratory evaluation of choice, even in the era of molecular diagnostics. The sweat test must be performed in an experienced laboratory, such as those associated with one of the Cystic Fibrosis Foundation–approved CF centers.

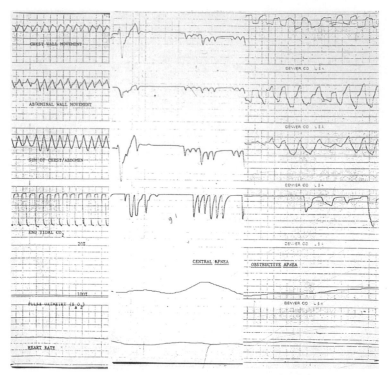

FIG. 16-31 Representative set of tracings from a 6-channel sleep study recording. The first panel shows a normal tracing. In the center panel, the cessation of both respiratory efforts and airflow at the nose is shown in a patient with central apnea. The right panel depicts obstructive apnea with continued chest and abdominal wall motion despite a lack of airflow. The last two tracings also demonstrate a significant fall in oxygen saturation during and after the apneic episode.

False negative and false positive results are common in inexperienced hands. In the appropriate clinical setting of chronic lung disease, malabsorption, or a family history of CF, a sweat chloride or sodium level greater than 60 mEq/l based on a collection of at least 100 mg of sweat is diagnostic of the disorder. Values below 40 mEq/l are normal, and those between 40 and 60 mEq/l are suspicious for CF and should be repeated. In competent laboratories, false negative values are rare and the sweat test should be repeated in those cases where the suspicion is high. False positive values occasionally occur, but disorders that cause this are readily distinguished clinically from CF. Other entities that elevate sweat chloride levels include adrenal insufficiency, ectodermal dysplasia, nephrogenic diabetes insipidus, hypothyroidism, mucopolysaccharidoses, glucose-6-phosphatase deficiency, hypoproteinemia, and anemia associated with malnutrition. Patients with CF who suffer severe malnutrition and edema may have false negative values on initial sweat tests until their nutritional status improves. Newborn screening, recently adopted at many hospitals throughout the country, is based on the demonstration of elevated levels of immunoreactive serum trypsin by blood spot analysis. It is recommended that a single blood spot with elevation of serum immunoreactive trypsin (IRT) be repeated, and if this value remains high, a sweat chloride test should be performed. The false positive rate after two positive IRTs is quite high, at 20%, and the false negative rate may be as high as 10%. In the patient with insufficient sweat for analysis or with a sweat test result at variance with the clinical picture, DNA analysis for CF mutations may give additional information. At present, commercial laboratories test for approximately 30 of the over 550 known mutations that account for roughly 90% of CF genes. It is not considered sensitive enough for population-wide carrier

screening; defining the genotype of an individual patient adds nothing to pilocarpine iontophoresis in the clinical management of CF.

Apnea and Sudden Infant Death Syndrome

Sudden infant death syndrome (SIDS) is the unexpected death of an infant who has been otherwise healthy and in whom there is no demonstrable pathologic basis for the death as determined by a thorough postmortem examination. The incidence of SIDS in the United States is 2 deaths per 1000 live births, resulting in approximately 10,000 deaths annually. SIDS is the leading cause of death after the neonatal period, with a peak incidence at 2 to 4 months postnatally and rarely occurring after 10 months of age. Most of these infants die soundlessly during sleep, without any obvious sign of agitation. Occasionally a history of the recent onset of a viral illness may be elicited.

Clinically meaningful apnea is the absence of airflow for at least 20 seconds or apnea accompanied by cyanosis or bradycardia. Infants who experience these apparently life-threatening events are at increased risk for SIDS, but the precise cause of SIDS remains elusive. Other infants at high risk for sudden death include those with a family history of SIDS (particularly in a sibling); premature infants with prolonged apnea and bradycardia; infants with significant illness, such as bronchopulmonary dysplasia or congenital heart disease; infants with viral bronchiolitis (especially caused by respiratory syncytial virus); and infants born to mothers of lower socioeconomic class; or those whose mothers abused alcohol, drugs, or tobacco during or after pregnancy. Several different forms of apnea are recognized in pediatric patients: obstructive, central, and mixed (Fig. 16-31). Obstructive apnea is characterized by the lack of airflow at the nose or mouth despite continued respiratory efforts, whereas absence of airflow accompanied by the cessation of chest and abdominal wall movement distinguishes central apnea.

The number of hospital evaluations for infants with apneic episodes has increased dramatically in recent years, as has the number of infants who receive months of home apnea monitoring. No specific test can accurately predict the infant at risk for SIDS, and the assessment of an infant with clinically significant apnea varies depending on findings uncovered during the initial history and physical examination. Factors that may be indicative in an otherwise healthy infant include infection (sepsis, central nervous system infection, infantile botulism), cardiac disease (congenital or cardiac dysrhythmias), metabolic disease (including electrolyte abnormalities), neurologic disease (seizures, intraventricular hemorrhage, increased intracranial pressure), and GER. Studies that may be helpful include a sleep study that measures respiratory and abdominal wall movement, airflow at the mouth or nose, pulse oximetry, and heart rate and in some cases pH monitoring of the distal esophagus. Episodes of obstructive, mixed, and/or central apnea may be observed during a sleep study (Fig. 16-31). Obstructive apnea can occur in cases of extreme obesity, in infants with GER, in patients with severe laxity of the supraglottic structures, or in older patients with marked adenoidal or tonsillar enlargement. Central apnea may occur in infants with seizure disorders or central nervous system pathology, such as intraventricular hemorrhage; in premature infants with immature respiratory control mechanisms; and in congenital central hypoventilation syndrome (formerly known as *Ondine's curse*). Mixed apnea generally occurs when an obstructive apneic episode is followed by a central pattern of apnea. Other useful studies include ventilatory responses to hypercapnea or hypoxia, chest x-ray examination, an electroencephalogram, Holter monitoring, and bronchoscopic evaluation of the airway, particularly in those patients with evidence of obstructive apnea. Laboratory evaluation may include the following: CBC, arterial or venous blood gases, chest radiography, and electrocardiogram. Unfortunately,

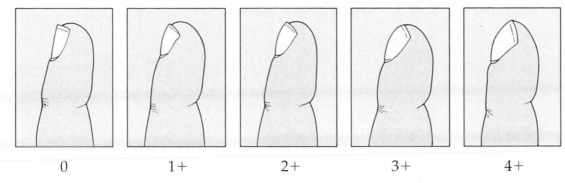

| 0 | 1+ | 2+ | 3+ | 4+ |

FIG. 16-32 Degrees of clubbing.

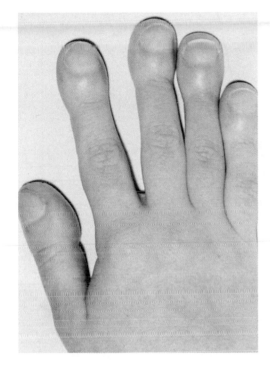

FIG. 16-33 Patient with CF and finger clubbing.

TABLE 16-7

Causes of Clubbing

Pulmonary	Cardiac
Cystic fibrosis	Cyanotic congenital heart
Other bronchiectasis	disease
Pulmonary abscess	Subacute bacterial endocarditis
Empyema	Gastrointestinal or hepatic
Neoplasms	Ulcerative colitis
Interstitial fibrosis	Crohn disease
Pulmonary alveolar	Polyposis
proteinosis	Biliary cirrhosis/atresia
Interstitial pneumonitis	Familial
Chronic pneumonia	Thyrotoxicosis

despite the battery of sophisticated tests available to the clinician, none can predict the subsequent risk for SIDS or determine which patients are appropriate candidates for home monitoring. As a result, a clinical judgment weighing the results of testing, the assessment of the home situation, and the seriousness of the original event is required for decisions regarding therapeutic intervention. Complicating this decision is the fact that there is no convincing evidence that home apnea monitoring prevents SIDS.

An area of controversy within the SIDS literature has been the issue of sleep positioning. In 1992 the National Institute of Child Health and Human Development released a study showing a weak but statistically significant association between the prone position in sleep and SIDS. These data supported previous studies conducted in Australia, England, and New Zealand in which national educational measures were undertaken to discourage parents from placing their infants in the prone position for sleep and found that the rate of SIDS decreased. In May 1992 the American Academy of Pediatrics (AAP) Task Force on Infant Positioning and SIDS recommended that for healthy full-term infants, the prone sleep position should be discouraged in favor of the side or supine position. This recommendation has been challenged on the basis that the risks of the supine position have not been fully studied, that the studies conducted were insufficiently rigorous in the

definition of SIDS and investigation of the death scene, and that the application of data obtained in countries with substantially different sleep practices may not be appropriate to children in the United States. Although the AAP has excluded those infants with known GER from the supine or lateral recommendation because the supine position is provocative for GER, the risk of aspiration and other reflux complications in those infants with unrecognized GER is unknown. Because the AAP policy is in place and data are being collected, we will probably have a clearer idea of the impact of supine or lateral positioning in the coming years.

Diagnostic Techniques

The notion that the examination of the lungs begins at the fingertips is an important one because digital clubbing may indicate severe lung disease. Various stages of clubbing, from mild to severe, are depicted in Figs. 16-32 and 16-33. Not all digital clubbing is associated with pulmonary disease (Table 16-7); nonpulmonary causes include cardiac, gastrointestinal, hepatic, and familial, as well as clubbing observed with thyrotoxicosis. Bronchiectasis from CF or from other infectious causes is the major cause of clubbing among all pulmonary diseases.

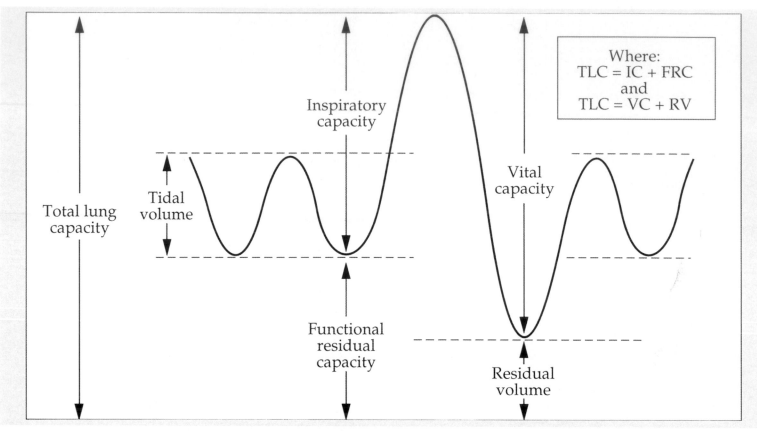

FIG. 16-34 Schematic representation of lung volumes.

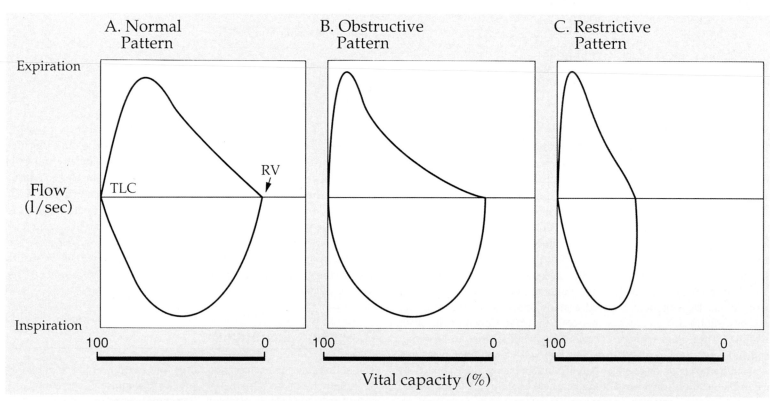

FIG. 16-35 Flow-volume curves obtained by spirometry. *A,* Normal configuration of expiratory flow curve. *B,* Reduced expiratory flow rates suggest obstructive airway disease. *C,* Preservation of flow rates with a diminished vital capacity consistent with restrictive lung disease.

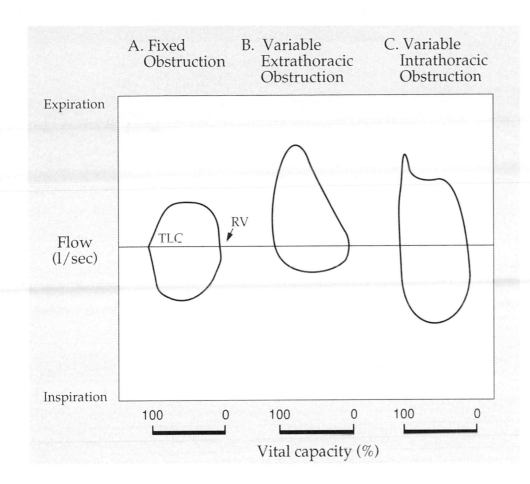

A. Fixed
Obstruction

B. Variable
Extrathoracic
Obstruction

C. Variable
Intrathoracic
Obstruction

Expiration

Flow
(l/sec)

TLC

RV

Inspiration

100   0   100   0   100   0

Vital capacity (%)

FIG. 16-36 *A*, Fixed obstruction of upper airways with reduction in inspiratory and expiratory flow loops. *B*, Reduction in peak inspiratory flow observed in variable extrathoracic airway obstruction. *C*, Reduction and flattening of the expiratory limb in variable intrathoracic obstruction.

Digital clubbing in any child with a chronic cough or wheezing warrants thorough evaluation and investigation to determine the underlying disorder.

Diagnosis and treatment of children with respiratory complaints may be facilitated by the use of pulmonary function tests (PFTs). With appropriate training and with the technician's patience and encouragement, most children 5 or 6 years of age or older cooperate with simple spirometry and measurements of lung volumes (Fig. 16-34). Interpretation of PFT results in children must take into account variability in performance and differences in age, height, weight, sex, and race. In children, PFTs may be useful in establishing the severity of respiratory disease, in guiding the choice of therapy, and in some cases in measuring the response to a therapeutic regimen. In some diseases, such as cystic fibrosis or asthma, evidence of increasing airway obstruction may indicate the need to initiate or increase the aggressiveness of therapeutic intervention.

The inspection of the shape of flow-volume curves generated during forced expiratory maneuvers is critical for the appropriate interpretation of PFT results (Fig. 16-35). The initial portion of the flow-volume curve is effort dependent, but the terminal 75% of the expiratory maneuver is dependent on elastic recoil and airway resistance and is relatively independent of patient effort. A normal-appearing flow-volume curve is shown in Fig. 16-35, *A*. With increased airway resistance distal to the central, large airways, the curve becomes concave to the abscissa. This type of concavity therefore suggests obstruction to airflow (Fig. 16-35, *B*). Patients with suspected reactive airway disease may develop this type of flow-volume curve after bronchoprovocation tests, such as inhaled histamine, methacholine, or cold air, or after exercise testing.

The restrictive pattern shown in Fig. 16-35, *C*, demonstrates preservation of expiratory flow function but a reduction in total lung volume.

Neuromuscular disorders, such as Duchenne muscular dystrophy, scoliosis, and interstitial lung disease, are among the entities that typically produce this pattern on PFTs.

The shape of the flow-volume curve may also help evaluate upper or central airway pathology (Fig. 16-36). Fixed obstruction of the upper airways, as in tracheal stenosis, produces a limitation and plateau of both the inspiratory and expiratory loops of the flow volume curve. A reduced inspiratory flow and a plateau of the inspiratory loop suggest variable extrathoracic obstruction seen in disorders such as laryngomalacia. Chondromalacia of the intrathoracic trachea or major bronchi results in variable intrathoracic obstruction with reduction and flattening of the expiratory limb because pleural pressures exceed pressure within the lumen.

Exercise tests can be a valuable tool to assess the cardiorespiratory fitness of a subject and may provide further information regarding a patient's respiratory reserve in addition to that found during routine PFTs. A progressive exercise study by bicycle ergometry can give important information regarding ventilatory effort, heart-rate responses, oxygen delivery and uptake, and carbon dioxide production. Evaluation of these parameters may provide information regarding exercise fitness and, if limited, identify whether the limiting factor is ventilatory or cardiac. Like PFTs, exercise tests can be used to assess the severity or progress of disease, evaluate effects of changes in treatment, and provide information about the safety or appropriateness of an exercise program in children with chronic lung disease.

Flexible fiberoptic bronchoscopy (Fig. 16-37) is a relatively new procedure available to the pediatric pulmonologist. It can be extremely useful in the diagnosis of lesions of the pulmonary tree and in isolating organisms from patients with pneumonia. Compared with traditional open-tube ("rigid") bronchoscopy, flexible bronchoscopy offers the advantages of avoiding general anesthesia and allowing the study of air-

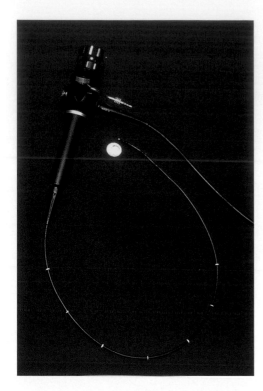

FIG. 16-37 Flexible fiberoptic broncho-scope (Olympus BF3C10, 3.5-mm OD) shown next to a dime, for size comparison.

TABLE 16-8			
Range of Normal Arterial Blood Gas Values by Age			
	pH	pCO$_2$	pO$_2$
Newborn	7.33-7.49	27-41	>60
Infant (<1 year)	7.34-7.46	26-41	>75
Older child	7.35-7.45	35-45	>75

artifact can lead to serious errors in assessment. Venous or capillary blood gases can accurately estimate pH and CO$_2$, but may significantly underestimate real pO$_2$. Normal arterial pH, pO$_2$, and pCO$_2$ values are provided in Table 16-8.

ACKNOWLEDGMENT

The authors thank Dr. Geoffrey Kurland for his assistance with photographs and clinical material.

way dynamics during regular tidal breathing. Indications for pediatric flexible bronchoscopy include evaluation of stridor, unexplained or chronic cough or wheeze, suspected airway malformations or compression, atelectasis, or recurrent pneumonia. To obviate the need for open lung biopsy, flexible bronchoscopy and bronchoalveolar lavage may be particularly useful in immunosuppressed patients with unexplained pneumonia. Flexible bronchoscopy should not be attempted when there is a strong clinical or radiographic suggestion of inhaled foreign body. In these cases rigid bronchoscopy is the procedure of choice to remove the object.

Arterial blood gas measurements are the standard for assessing gas exchange. Pulse oximetry and analysis of the CO$_2$ in exhaled air are useful noninvasive tools appropriate for a select number of patients with respiratory compromise, but technical difficulties in interpretation and

BIBLIOGRAPHY

Benjamin B: *Atlas of paediatric endoscopy*, London, 1981, Oxford University Press.

Chernick V, Kendig EL: *Disorders of the respiratory tract in children*, ed 5, Philadelphia, 1990, WB Saunders.

Eigen HE: The clinical evaluation of chronic cough, *Pediatr Clin North Am* 29:67-78, 1982.

Fishman AP: *Pulmonary diseases and disorders*, ed 2, New York, 1988, McGraw-Hill.

Lloyd-Still JD: *Textbook of cystic fibrosis*, Boston, 1983, John Wright.

Phelan PD, Landau LI, Olinsky A: *Respiratory illness in children*, ed 3, London, 1990, Blackwell Scientific Publications.

Singleton EB, Wagner MI, Dutton RV: *Radiologic atlas of pulmonary abnormalities in children*, Philadelphia, 1988, WB Saunders.

Taussig LM: *Cystic fibrosis*, New York, 1984, Thieme-Stratton.

17

Surgery

DON K. NAKAYAMA

This chapter encompasses many common general pediatric surgical disorders but is not intended to be an exhaustive survey. The emphasis is on surgical conditions likely to be encountered in general pediatric practice, amplified by the inclusion of some rare disorders.

Respiratory Distress

Surgical causes of respiratory distress are uncommon but demand immediate attention and should be considered in the evaluation of newborns who demonstrate signs of dyspnea or stridor.

On rare occasions the cause is obvious, such as a neck mass compressing the airway or abdominal distension elevating the diaphragm. Often the presence of a surgical condition causing respiratory symptoms is obscure, and its detection is difficult because medical causes of dyspnea are so common. Two broad situations suggest a surgical cause for respiratory distress. First, an apparently healthy baby develops signs of stridor or severe respiratory distress. A clinician does not expect a vigorous, full-term infant to have respiratory distress syndrome or atelectasis, and routine studies exclude pneumothorax and sepsis. An example is the baby with diaphragmatic hernia. Another example is an otherwise healthy infant who has noisy breathing resulting from a constricting vascular ring. Second, an infant being treated for a common cause of respiratory distress fails to respond to therapy as expected. Because prematurity and respiratory distress syndrome are common, a coexisting surgical condition may not be suspected. Examples include a premature newborn with tracheoesophageal fistula and esophageal atresia and an infant with group B streptococcal sepsis who later develops a right diaphragmatic hernia.

Plain film evaluation should include both anteroposterior and lateral views of the chest, with special attention to the airway contour and lateral soft-tissue views of the upper airway. Examination under fluoroscopy gives valuable information regarding changes in airway contour and diaphragmatic motion during the respiratory cycle. Barium swallow helps to locate masses within the mediastinum and establish the presence of a vascular ring anomaly (Fig. 17-1). Laryngoscopy and endoscopic examinations of the upper airway, the tracheobronchial tree, and the esophagus become necessary when the procedures previously mentioned fail to yield a clear-cut diagnosis. The different surgical causes of respiratory distress are grouped most conveniently by anatomic site: upper airway, thoracic, and extrathoracic.

Upper Airway

Newborns are unable to breathe through the mouth until several days after birth. Thus an obstructive lesion of the upper airway must be considered in any infant who demonstrates cyclic dyspnea (recurring episodes of asphyxia followed by crying, mouth breathing, quiet, and then asphyxia again) or inability to nurse. An obstructive airway within the extrathoracic area forces the infant to gasp to breathe because the upper airway tends to collapse onto the lesion at inspiration. The airway enlarges during expiration, which is relatively unlabored. The voice is normal unless the larynx itself is occluded. The differential diagnosis should include choanal atresia, tracheoesophageal fistula, esophageal atresia, vocal chord paralysis, presence of a foreign body, and tumors or other lesions in the nasopharynx or oropharynx.

Passage of a nasogastric tube is a basic procedure during the initial evaluation of the newborn with possible airway obstruction. Inability to reach the pharynx suggests choanal atresia. The obstruction is bony in 90% of patients and is membranous in 10%. About half of all cases are associated with other anomalies, including craniofacial, cardiovascular, and abdominal. Endoscopic examination or contrast roentgenography of the nasopharynx confirms the diagnosis. Maintenance of an oral airway and gavage feeding are necessary until transpalatal repair is performed.

Macroglossia may obstruct the oropharynx and cause respiratory distress. Diffuse enlargement of the tongue from lymphangioma is the most common cause. Hypertrophy of the tongue is characteristic of Beckwith-Wiedemann syndrome. In contrast, a hypoplastic and recessed mandible causes a normal-sized tongue to fall posteriorly and obstruct the airway in Pierre Robin sequence (Fig. 17-2). Cleft palate and cardiac anomalies frequently complicate the latter condition. Placing the baby in the prone position may open the airway; this allows many infants to be managed without tracheostomy. The infant eventually learns to keep the tongue away from the larynx, and sufficient mandibular growth occurs. Some infants, however, still require tracheotomy.

Lesions of the larynx are characterized by a husky, hoarse, or whispered cry or complete aphonia in association with dyspnea. Laryngeal atresia, webs, cysts, laryngomalacia, subglottic stenosis, and vocal cord paralysis are included in the differential diagnosis. The need for tracheotomy becomes urgent when a severe obstruction prevents placement of an orotracheal tube, as in cases of laryngeal atresia. Laryngeal cleft allows feedings in the pharynx to enter the airway directly through a defect between the arytenoids in the posterior larynx.

487

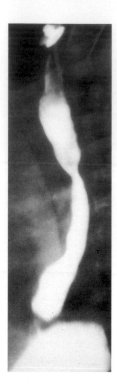

FIG. 17-1 Midthoracic compressions into the esophageal barium column identify the presence of vascular ring anomalies (in this case, pulmonary artery sling).

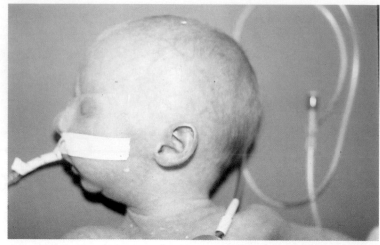

FIG. 17-2 In Pierre Robin sequence, the hypoplastic mandible positions the tongue posteriorly, potentially obstructing the upper airway.

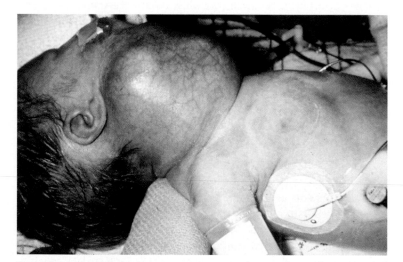

FIG. 17-3 Cervical teratoma may compress the esophagus in utero, and produce polyhydramnios. After delivery, compression of the upper airway from the mass may create a surgical emergency.

TABLE 17-1

Mediastinal Masses in Childhood

Anterior and superior	Middle	Posterior
Teratoma, including dermoid cyst	Bronchogenic cyst	Neurogenic tumor Enterogenous cyst
Normal thymus	Pericardial	Pulmonary
Lymphoma	cyst	sequestration
Vascular malformation		
Thymic cyst		
Cystic hygroma		
Intrathoracic goiter		

Cysts and other tumors that lie within the pharynx may cause upper airway obstruction. Examples include dermoids, branchial cleft remnants, lingual thyroid, intraoral thyroglossal duct cysts, hemangioma, duplications, and palatal teratoma (epulis). Large masses in the neck may compress the airway and cause dyspnea, such as cervical teratoma (Fig. 17-3).

Thoracic

Mediastinum and Diaphragm

Mediastinal lesions cause respiratory distress through compression of the airway and produce other clinical effects (dyspnea, plethora of the head and upper extremities) by compressing other nearby structures (esophagus, superior vena cava) (Table 17-1). Location of the mass within the mediastinum and the age of the patient give the most important clues to the identification of mediastinal masses. Abnormalities of the superior and anterior mediastinum include cystic hygroma, lymphoma, teratoma, and dermoid cysts. Here the thymus is normally prominent in infants (Fig. 17-4). Pericardial and bronchogenic cysts arise in the middle mediastinum. Foregut duplications (Fig. 17-5), neurenteric cysts, extralobar sequestration, anterior myelomeningocele, and neuroblastoma arise in the posterior mediastinum.

Inability to pass a nasogastric tube into the stomach (the same tube to exclude choanal atresia) results in the diagnosis of esophageal atre-

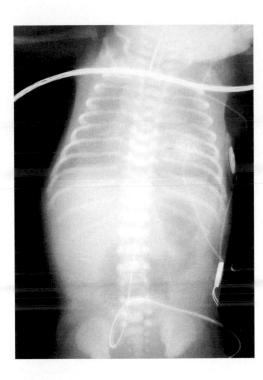

FIG. 17-4 The large thymus of newborns should not be confused with an upper mediastinal mass on chest film.

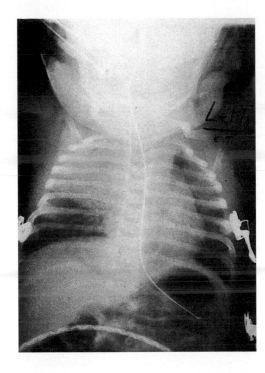

FIG. 17-5 Posterior mediastinal masses include esophageal duplication (illustrated here), neurenteric cysts, extralobar sequestration, anterior myelomeningocele, and neural tumors. Vertebral anomalies coexist frequently.

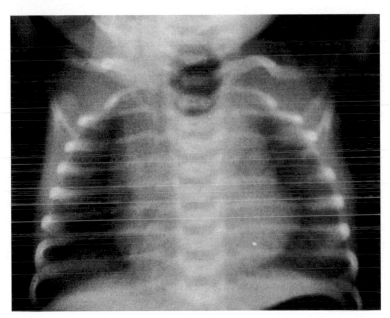

FIG. 17-6 A distended esophageal pouch identifies esophageal atresia; air within the gastrointestinal tract indicates that a distal tracheoesophageal fistula is also present.

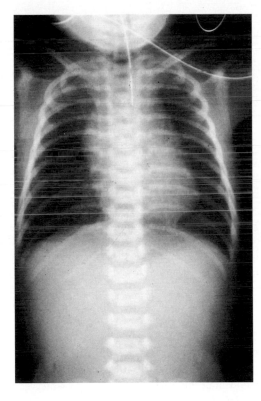

FIG. 17-7 In contrast with Fig. 17-6, the absence of air in the abdomen means that no tracheoesophageal fistula is present, and the esophageal atresia (identified by a coiled nasogastric tube in the upper mediastinum) is isolated.

sia. A fistula from the carina to the distal esophageal remnant (distal tracheoesophageal fistula) completes the most common combination of tracheoesophageal anomalies (present in 85% of cases). The fistula allows air to fill the stomach, a feature on plain film that distinguishes cases of esophageal atresia associated with a distal tracheoesophageal fistula (Fig. 17-6) from those without a tracheoesophageal communication (pure esophageal atresia, Fig. 17-7). The third most common pattern of tracheoesophageal anomalies, tracheoesophageal fistula without esophageal atresia, has no esophageal obstruction, so a nasogastric tube passes freely into the stomach. The fistula arises from the trachea and passes distally into the esophagus, creating an N rather than a horizontal H-shaped communication between the two structures. This an-

gle may impede reflux of material from the esophagus into the trachea, including contrast. To keep the lungs free from foreign material, barium swallow to opacify the fistula is not recommended. Its diagnosis requires confirmation by bronchoscopy (Fig. 17-8).

Respiratory distress results from the esophageal obstruction and the communication between the airway and esophagus. Babies with esophageal atresia salivate excessively and are unable to swallow feedings. The baby may aspirate formula and saliva pooled in the obstructed upper esophageal pouch. Gastric juice refluxes into the distal esophageal segment and enters the tracheobronchial tree through the fistula. While awaiting surgical repair, the baby is kept in a flat, head-up position to minimize gastroesophageal reflux. An infant sump tube

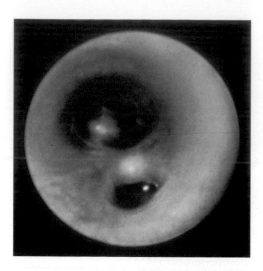

FIG. 17-8 Broncho-scopy visualizes tra-cheoesophageal fis-tula, seen as a posteri-orly positioned orifice (*bottom*) in the upper trachea. The carina, seen toward the top of the picture, lies distally.

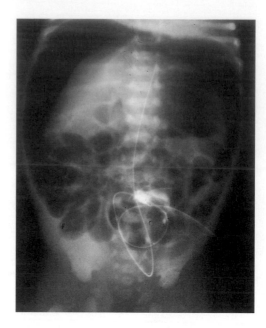

FIG. 17-9 Tracheoe-sophageal fistula al-lows air to be forced into the stomach dur-ing positive pressure ventilation by bag and mask or through an en-dotracheal tube. The stomach may perforate or ventilation may be-come suddenly ineffec-tive if a gastrotomy is placed initially during surgical repair.

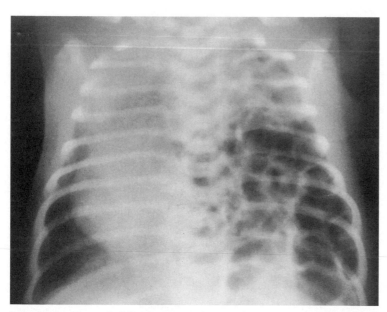

FIG. 17-10 Congenital diaphragmatic hernia allows the intestines to enter the chest in utero and pushes the mediastinum to the contralateral side.

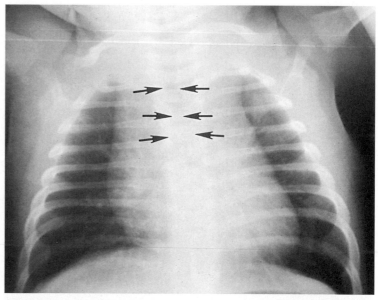

FIG. 17-11 Narrowing (*arrows*) or disappearance of the tracheal air con-tour suggests tracheal compression by a vascular ring, an often subtle sign that should be followed by a barium swallow in the evaluation.

(Replogle tube) keeps the upper esophageal pouch decompressed. A problem arises when respiratory distress is severe, either from aspira-tion or from pulmonary immaturity. The gastrointestinal tract may of-fer less resistance to inflation than the lungs, so positive pressure ven-tilation by mask or endotracheal tube may force air into the stomach. Respiratory insufficiency may worsen, and perforation of the stom-ach may occur (Fig. 17-9).

Congenital diaphragmatic hernia results from persistence of the fora-men of Bochdalek (Fig. 17-10). Most (85%) are left-sided. Intestines en-ter the thorax during early gestation, inhibiting pulmonary develop-ment and leading to hypoplasia of the lung. Once placental circulation is interrupted at birth, respiratory distress develops rapidly. Because the intestines are in the chest, the abdomen appears scaphoid. The left hemithorax is dull to percussion, and breath sounds may be poor or ab-sent. Heart sounds are heard best on the side opposite the hernia be-cause of displacement of the mediastinum. Chest film reveals air-filled loops within the hemithorax that appear to push the mediastinum into the contralateral lung, which is collapsed. Cystic adenomatoid malfor-mation may mimic the roentgenographic appearance of diaphragmatic hernia; the location of the stomach bubble is the abdomen in the for-mer and the chest in the latter. Respiratory insufficiency is severe, the result of pulmonary hypoplasia and pulmonary hypertension. Despite early operative repair and aggressive management with advanced modalities of critical care, including extracorporeal membrane oxy-genation, mortality remains high.

The persistence of the embryonic aortic arches creates complete vas-cular rings around the trachea and the esophagus. Symptoms arise from compression of the trachea (dyspnea) and the esophagus (dysphagia). Narrowing of the tracheal air contour within the mediastinum on chest film (Fig. 17-11) suggests the presence of a vascular ring. Barium swal-low shows compression on the esophagus (Fig. 17-1) and confirms the diagnosis. Bronchoscopy (Fig. 17-12), a necessary part of the preoper-ative assessment, must be performed by the attending surgeon in the operating room, if the procedure induces closure of a critically nar-rowed airway. Aortography provides the necessary anatomic detail for surgery.

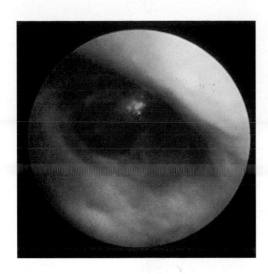

FIG. 17-12 Anterior compression of the trachea by an innominate artery with an anomalous leftward origin, as viewed at bronchoscopy.

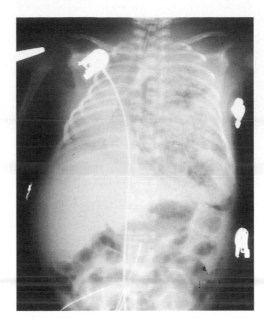

FIG. 17-13 Microcystic adenomatoid malformation of the left lung. Large cystic lesions can be mistaken for bowel loops herniating through a diaphragmatic hernia (Fig. 17-10).

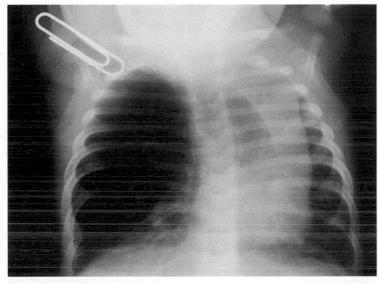

FIG. 17-14 Lobar emphysema, usually involving the upper lobes, may become hugely distended and may cause life-threatening respiratory distress.

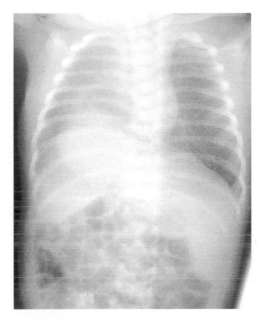

FIG. 17-15 Persistent infiltration of the lung parenchyma may indicate an intralobar sequestration, shown here involving the right lower lobe. Also shown is a right diaphragmatic hernia, a frequently associated malformation.

Although an important cause of respiratory insufficiency, congenital heart disease is beyond the scope of this discussion (see Chapter 5).

Lung

Anomalies of lung bud development lead to cystic diseases of the lung and pulmonary sequestration, the most common surgical causes of respiratory distress that arise within the lung itself. Growth of these lesions within the thorax compresses normal lung parenchyma, causing dyspnea early in life. Large or rapidly expanding lesions may require emergency surgical excision. Rupture of an expanding cyst is rare, except as a complication of diagnostic aspiration, which is recommended only as a temporizing procedure before surgery in patients with severe symptoms. Some patients are relatively free of dyspnea, and later in infancy or childhood they develop cough, fever, and recurrent pulmonary infections.

There are three varieties of cystic adenomatoid malformation of the lung, based on the size of the cysts: large (1 to 4 cm, the type mistaken for diaphragmatic hernia on plain film), small (less than 1 cm, Fig. 17-13),

and solid (noncystic). Like diaphragmatic hernia, cystic adenomatoid malformation can produce life-threatening symptoms soon after birth and may be complicated by pulmonary hypertension. Overexpansion of a segment or lobe of a lung leads to congenital lobar emphysema (Fig. 17-14). About half of all cases become symptomatic within the first week of life, but symptoms may not develop until 1 to 4 or more months later. Chest films show a hyperlucent, overexpanded area of the lung, usually either upper lobes or the right middle lobe. Infants and children who develop dyspnea require resection. Asymptomatic lesions that do not cause significant compressive effects do not require removal. In patients with congenital lobar emphysema, positive pressure ventilation (upon anesthetic induction or during resuscitation) may cause acute cardiorespiratory decompensation by overdistending the affected lobe.

Pulmonary sequestrations are accessory lobes of lung tissue that reside separately from the architecture of the normal lung, within a normal lobe (intralobar type, Fig. 17-15) or lying separately from the normal lobes of the lung, invested in its own pleura (extralobar type, Fig. 17-16). Most frequently found in the lower left posterior chest, many sequestra-

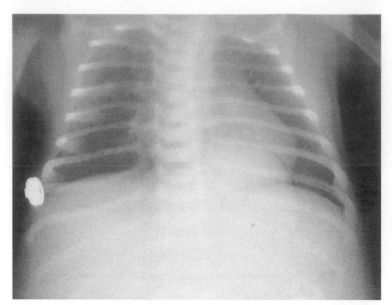

FIG. 17-16   Extralobar sequestration appears typically as a nonaerated intrathoracic mass in the lower posterior thorax, shown here on the left.

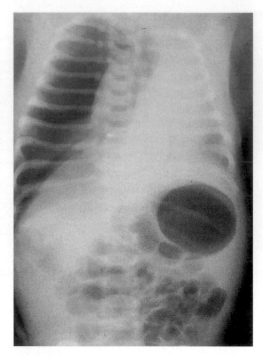

FIG. 17-17   This chest film shows typical radiologic signs of tension pneumothorax: mediastinal shift, flattening of the diaphragm, and widening of the intercostal spaces.

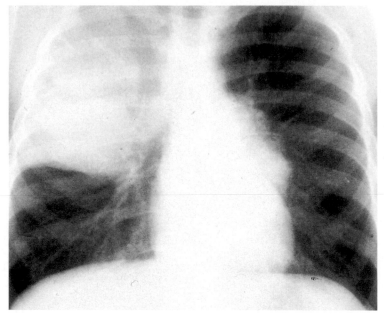

FIG. 17-18   Chest film in a child with allergic bronchopulmonary aspergillosis of the right upper lobe, which ultimately required resection.

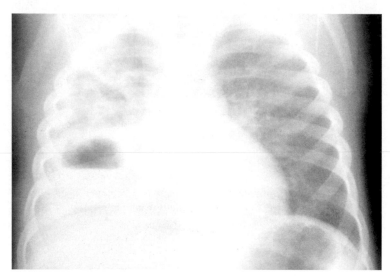

FIG. 17-19   Chest film in a child with a cavitary lung abscess.

tions derive a systemic blood supply from the thoracic or the abdominal aorta. A few cases retain a bronchial communication with the foregut. Most cases are asymptomatic and are found as an airless posterior mediastinal mass during repair of a diaphragmatic hernia or in a chest film taken for other indications. Recurring localized infection in a fluid-filled cyst is the most common presentation. Aortography or high-resolution Doppler ultrasound establishes the diagnosis by demonstration of a systemic arterial supply.

Pneumothorax may result from blunt and penetrating trauma to the chest. It complicates positive pressure ventilation in critical care units and spontaneously breathing children with advanced cystic fibrosis. The ipsilateral thorax is expanded, is tympanic to percussion, and has decreased breath sounds. Breath sounds, however, may be transmitted from the opposite, unaffected side, particularly in infants. Tension pneumothorax causes the diaphragm to flatten and forces the mediastinum to shift to the opposite side (Fig. 17-17). The heart shifts as well, disturbing its relationship to systemic and pulmonary veins, thus embarrassing venous return. Hypotension results and may preclude x-ray confirmation of the diagnosis. Needle decompression may be lifesaving.

Resection may be necessary in pulmonary infections that persist despite antibiotic therapy or in cases in which the diagnosis remains in doubt. Failure of an infiltrate to resolve suggests the presence of a resistant organism (Fig. 17-18); development of a lung abscess, a diag-

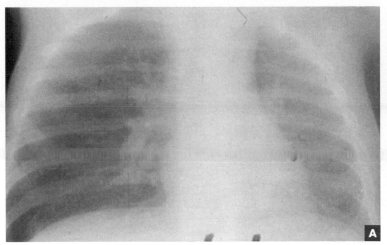
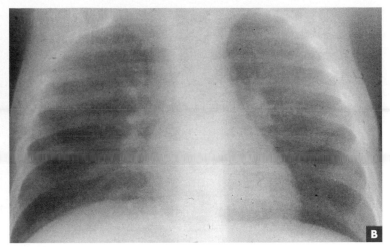

FIG. 17-20 Signs of a radiolucent foreign body are often subtle. Persistent overdistension of the right lung during expiration *(A)* was due to right mainstem bronchial occlusion. Less marked changes are seen during inhalation *(B)*.

nosis that becomes obvious when cavitation occurs (Fig. 17-19); or the presence of a pulmonary malignancy. A foreign body that occludes a bronchus (Fig. 17-20) may produce pulmonary consolidation.

Extrathoracic Causes

Abdominal distension of any cause elevates the diaphragm, decreases intrathoracic volume, and may lead to respiratory insufficiency. In infants, common causes include tumors, ascites, and intestinal obstruction. On pediatric surgical services, the use of narcotics for postoperative pain control may lead to respiratory depression, apnea, and, on occasion, arrest.

Vomiting

The major surgical causes of vomiting are obstruction of the gastrointestinal tract and inflammatory processes that involve the intestine, such as appendicitis. The clinical challenge is to distinguish the relatively few cases that require surgery from the many children with self-limited conditions and medical illnesses that cause vomiting but do not demand operation or even plain films, contrast studies, or medical and surgical consultation. Certain clinical signs direct attention to a surgical etiology. Bilious vomiting and abdominal distension are signs of intestinal obstruction. It is unusual for patients with medical illnesses to vomit bile. Lesions that obstruct the intestine distend the abdomen and reflux bile into the stomach, where it appears in the vomitus. Fever, abdominal pain, and abdominal tenderness suggest an inflammatory process and peritonitis. Vomiting is a reflex reaction to irritation of the visceral peritoneum and ileus. Conditions that cause abdominal pain are discussed more completely in a later section of this chapter.

Bilious vomiting is a key finding in newborns. When it occurs in an infant without abdominal distension, malrotation and volvulus become the paramount concerns; when the abdomen is distended, distal small bowel obstruction must be considered. Blood in the stool may indicate the presence of intestinal ischemia resulting from, for example, intussusception or malrotation. Failure to pass meconium in the first day of life in full-term infants should increase suspicions that a congenital obstruction is present. An abdominal surgical scar identifies the child at risk for postoperative adhesion obstruction. A vomiting child must always be checked for a fixed, tender groin bulge.

Plain film evaluation should include both anteroposterior and left lateral recumbent views (patient on his or her side, left side down, film taken "cross-table") of the abdomen. These views easily demonstrate air-fluid loops and free intraabdominal air, if present.

Newborns have unique radiologic requirements. No radiographic contrast is needed to make the diagnosis of esophageal atresia and duodenal atresia. A small amount of air injected into the stomach through the gastric tube may help demonstrate the characteristic "double bubble" in the latter diagnosis. If air is present distal to the duodenal bulb, an upper gastrointestinal series is the examination of choice to establish the presence of normal intestinal rotation. Intraabdominal calcification identifies perforation and meconium peritonitis. Digital rectal examination and the use of suppositories and enemas may decompress the distended colon above the transitional aganglionic zone in Hirschsprung disease, causing a valuable radiographic sign to disappear. Therefore a contrast enema study of the infant with distended abdomen and bilious vomiting should precede other manipulations of the anorectum. Barium provides excellent opacification of the transition zone, if present. If no transition zone is demonstrated, water-soluble contrast is used. Encountering a microcolon suggests meconium ileus, particularly if mucus concretions ("rabbit pellets") are present, or small bowel atresia. A transition zone from a small left colon to a distended transverse colon identifies small left colon syndrome. Water-soluble contrast may relieve obstruction in both meconium ileus and small left colon syndrome. In cases in which no radiographic diagnosis can be made, abdominal films obtained 1 to several days later may reveal delayed passage of administered contrast, a sign of Hirschsprung disease.

The different surgical causes of vomiting are grouped most conveniently into two age groups: (1) newborns and (2) older infants and children.

Newborns

A practical way to divide causes of vomiting in newborns distinguishes those cases associated with bilious versus nonbilious vomiting and those cases that cause abdominal distension versus those that do not.

Nonbilious Vomiting
Nearly all infants have gastroesophageal reflux, the most common cause of nonbilious vomiting during the first year of life. The condition

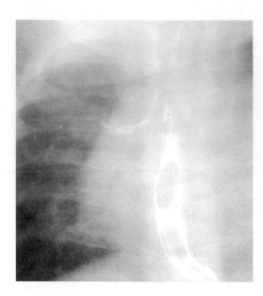

FIG. 17-21 Fluoroscopic examination of the infant during barium swallow must be of sufficient duration to allow the identification of episodes of reflux (here associated with aspiration into the tracheobronchial tree).

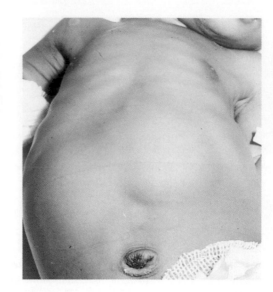

FIG. 17-22 Pyloric stenosis may cause epigastric distension by the obstructed stomach. This patient also demonstrates a visible wave of peristalsis, which moves from left to right.

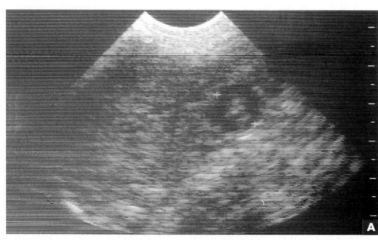

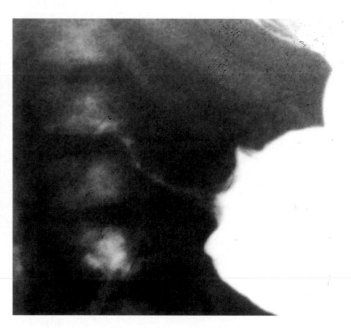

FIG. 17-23 Hypertrophic pyloric stenosis. *A,* Ultrasonographic scan of the upper abdomen demonstrates the thickened pyloric muscle, indicated by the cursors. *B,* Barium study of the stomach *(right)* shows thin streaks of barium in the pyloric canal. The hypertrophic pyloric muscle bulged into the gastric antrum produces a "reversed 3" configuration.

is self-limited, and three fourths of infants are reflux-free by 9 months of age. The tendency to vomit is worsened by overfeeding, failure to burp the baby, and overstimulating the baby after feeding, so a careful feeding history may indicate the cause of vomiting.

A number of tests confirm the diagnosis and establish the need for surgery. In addition to demonstrating episodes of reflux, barium swallow (Fig. 17-21) rules out pyloric stenosis and malrotation and gives roentgenographic evidence of esophageal stricture and motility disturbances. Radionuclide milk scan detects episodes of reflux, quantifies esophageal and gastric clearance, and detects aspiration when radioactivity is present over lung fields. A pH probe placed in the distal esophagus gives the duration and number of reflux episodes, usually during an overnight period, and is the most sensitive test. The presence of esophagitis on biopsy of the distal esophageal mucosa confirms a complication of reflux that may require corrective surgery.

Even in severe cases, conservative management successfully controls vomiting. Surgical procedures to strengthen the lower esophageal antireflux mechanism (fundoplication procedures) are applied to those cases associated with the following complications: esophageal stricture, aspiration, failure to gain weight, and documentation of life-threatening

episodes of apnea associated with reflux. Hiatal hernia is usually absent; in rare cases the stomach may slip through the hiatus into the chest, a situation that risks gastric volvulus. Reflux in children with neurologic handicaps is particularly severe and often requires fundoplication. Fundoplication may render the child unable to vomit. Should adhesions from surgery form and obstruct the intestine distally, a closed loop obstruction results and may lead rapidly to intestinal ischemia. Immediate placement of a nasogastric tube is required for the child with a fundoplication who develops abdominal distension.

Pyloric stenosis is the most common surgical condition of the newborn period, present in 1 in 700 live births. The etiology is unknown, but heredity has some influence: it is more common in boys, develops in 7% of children with affected parents, and is four times more likely when the mother was affected. Vomiting begins at 1 to 6 weeks of age, generally about 3 weeks, and is frequently projectile. Peristalsis of a distended stomach may become visible (Fig. 17-22). The lesion itself is palpable in the epigastrium, between the midline and the right midclavicular line, having the consistency of a small, firm olive. The child must be relaxed, and the stomach must be empty to allow adequate examination. Maneuvers that are sometimes helpful include raising the

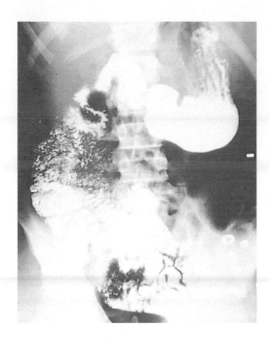

FIG. 17-24 The ligament of Treitz in malrotation is either absent or abnormally located, and the duodenum and small intestine lie on the right side of the abdomen. Duodenal obstruction may be partial (caused by Ladd's bands, as seen here) or complete (caused by volvulus).

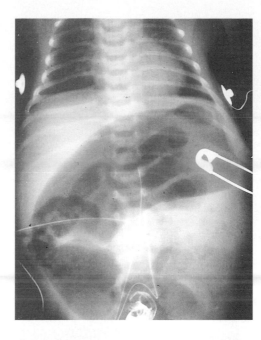

FIG. 17-25 Complete duodenal obstruction from midgut volvulus. Air in the distal gastrointestinal tract fails to rule out complete obstruction from volvulus and distinguishes the diagnosis from duodenal atresia.

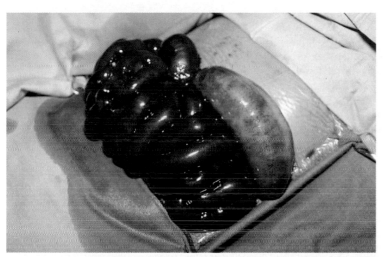

FIG. 17-26 Malrotation predisposes to volvulus and infarction of the entire midgut.

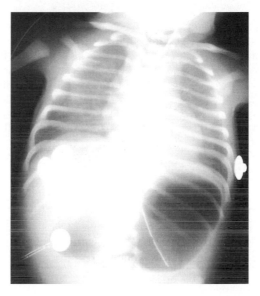

FIG. 17-27 Swallowed air distends the stomach and the first portion of the duodenum in duodenal atresia, producing the characteristic "double bubble" on plain film and making other contrast studies unnecessary.

baby into a semirecumbent position to allow the pylorus to fall inferiorly and flexing the legs to relax abdominal muscles. When the mass is not palpable, the most productive alternative is a second physical examination in about an hour, when the child is sleeping, and other examiners are gone. An affected pylorus is palpable in 70% to 90% of cases. Once felt, no further tests are necessary before pyloromyotomy. If the diagnosis remains in doubt, an upper gastrointestinal series is preferred because other causes of vomiting can be diagnosed if pyloric stenosis is not present (Fig. 17-23). Ultrasound examination is a reliable alternative when an experienced sonographer is present.

Bilious Vomiting, No Abdominal Distension

Malrotation is the failure of the midgut (small intestine and right colon) to achieve its normal anatomic position during development. The cecum and colon lie in the left abdomen; the duodenum and small intestine lie on the right side. Retroperitoneal attachment is inadequate and the mesenteric pedicle is narrow, factors that easily lead to volvulus. Volvulus leads to high intestinal obstruction and vomiting (Fig. 17-24 and 17-25). Twisting of the mesenteric vessels causes intestinal ischemia and midgut infarction (Fig. 17-26). Bloody stool or nasogastric drainage,

the development of abdominal distension, guarding, abdominal wall erythema, and edema indicate intestinal gangrene. The result is death or extreme short-gut syndrome if ischemia of the midgut is irreversible.

Although only a fraction of infants with bilious vomiting have malrotation, the consequences of undiagnosed cases are so grave that many surgeons strongly recommend that all newborns with bilious vomiting undergo urgent evaluation by upper gastrointestinal series. The key finding on contrast study is the location of the ligament of Treitz, which should be to the left of the vertebral column and behind the stomach bubble. An inadequately configured duodenal C-loop that fails to cross to the left of midline and the proximal jejunal loops lying in the right side of the abdomen are diagnostic of malrotation (Fig. 17-24). The cecum on barium enema examination lies in the right upper quadrant or left side of the abdomen. Barium enema detects malrotation less reliably because the cecum in the infant is mobile. A dilated duodenal loop (Fig. 17-25) suggests that obstruction has occurred, resulting from volvulus (Fig. 17-26) or peritoneal bands overlying the duodenum (Ladd bands). Plain films are not diagnostic. The obstructed midgut may fill with fluid and produce a "gasless" abdomen.

Duodenal atresia produces the characteristic double bubble on plain film (Fig. 17-27). Vomiting typically occurs soon after birth. Duodenal

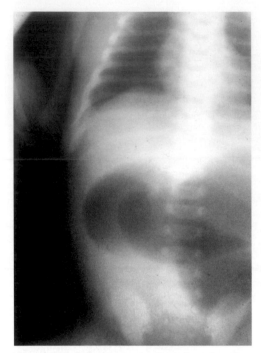

FIG. 17-28 Jejunal atresia distends only a few bowel loops proximally, distinguishing it from duodenal and ileal atresia.

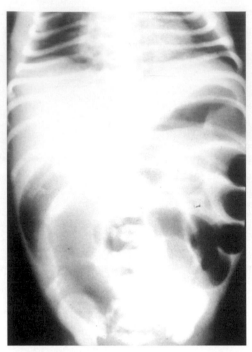

FIG. 17-29 Many intestinal loops become distended in patients with ileal atresia (pictured here), making the distinction between this diagnosis and other causes of distal bowel obstruction difficult. Other signs (such as intraperitoneal calcification, indicating meconium peritonitis) and contrast enema are necessary to identify the cause of obstruction.

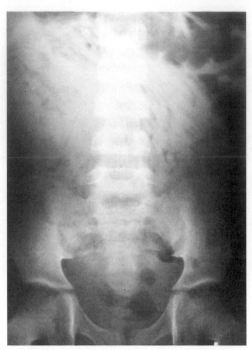

FIG. 17-30 This plain film shows two signs indicative of meconium ileus: a "soap bubble" mass in the right iliac fossa, produced by the impacted meconium, and distended loops of different diameters, reflecting the gradual distension of the small bowel to the area of obstruction.

atresia frequently accompanies Down syndrome and congenital heart defects. Congenital stenosis of the duodenum, duodenal web, and annular pancreas causes partial duodenal obstruction distinguished by the presence of air distal to the dilated duodenal bubble. Because malrotation may also cause partial duodenal obstruction by Ladd bands or volvulus, urgent contrast examination of the duodenal anatomy is required.

Bilious Vomiting, Distended Abdomen

Small bowel atresias arise from intrauterine vascular insults. They may form relatively late in gestation, and meconium may have formed and passed distally by that time. Alone, passage of meconium after birth does not rule out the presence of an atresia. Proximal jejunal atresia results in upper abdominal distension, with only a few distended loops on abdominal plain film, which is diagnostic (Fig. 17-28). No contrast studies are needed. More generalized distension results from atresias located more distally, and contrast studies may be required to distinguish ileal atresia from other causes of distal bowel obstruction, such as Hirschsprung disease and meconium ileus (Fig. 17-29). Distension develops 12 to 24 hours after birth. Distension present at birth suggests meconium ileus or meconium peritonitis. Jejunoileal atresia may coexist with malrotation, meconium peritonitis, meconium ileus, and rarely Hirschsprung disease. The different anatomic variants are classified based on whether the bowel and mesentery are intact. Two rare variants, "apple peel" atresia (the distal small bowel spirals around the ileocecal artery in a retrograde direction, a consequence of a major mesenteric arterial occlusion) and multiple atresia ("string of sausages"), are likely to leave the baby with short-gut syndrome.

Meconium ileus is the first manifestation of cystic fibrosis in about 10% to 15% of affected children. A family history of cystic fibrosis is present in one third of all cases. The meconium in cystic fibrosis is abnormally thick and tenacious and impacts in the ileum, causing intestinal

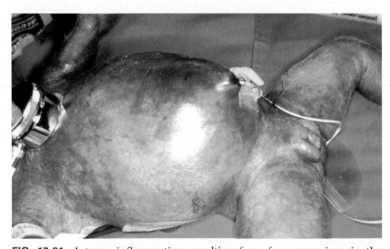

FIG. 17-31 Intense inflammation resulting from free meconium in the peritoneal cavity (meconium peritonitis) may produce visible erythema and edema over the abdominal wall.

obstruction. Distally the ileum and colon are tiny and contain concretions of mucus ("rabbit pellets"). The site of impact becomes hugely distended with meconium, seen as a "soap bubble" mass in the right iliac fossa on plain film (Fig. 17-30). No air-fluid levels are visible, because the meconium cannot easily form layers. The gradual distension of small bowel along its length causes loops of bowel of different sizes to be seen on abdominal film. Contrast enema demonstrates the microcolon and rabbit pellets of inspissated mucus. Water-soluble contrast refluxed into the impacted ileum may result in passage of the meconium and relief of the obstruction in about half of patients with uncomplicated meconium ileus. Meconium ileus can be complicated by small bowel atresia, gangrene, volvulus of the impacted area, and perforation with meconium

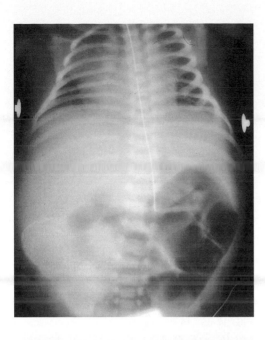

FIG. 17-32 Calcification in an area of meconium peritonitis in the right iliac fossa.

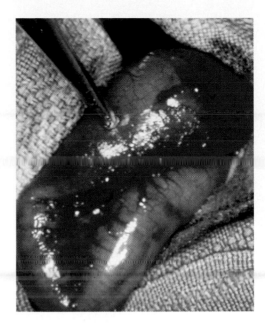

FIG. 17-33 The absence of intramural ganglion cells prevents intestinal peristalsis through segments affected by Hirschsprung disease, causing a functional bowel obstruction. The involved segment appears narrow when compared with the distended, obstructed proximal bowel, which possesses normal ganglion cells.

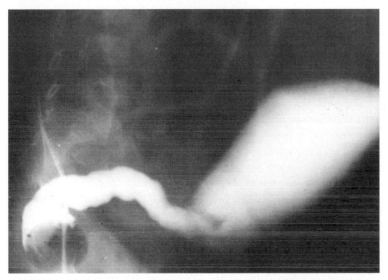

FIG. 17-34 Barium enema outlines the transition zone between the contracted (aganglionic) rectosigmoid lying distal to the obstructed, but normally innervated, colon. To demonstrate this sign, the examination must be conducted in an unprepped patient who has undergone neither enemas nor digital rectal examination.

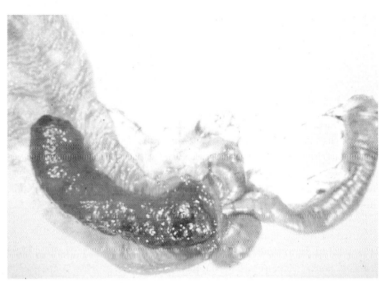

FIG. 17-35 The intestine invaginates into itself in intussusception. The ileum is pulled through the ileocecal valve into the colon, the most common pattern seen in infancy, pictured here.

peritonitis. Presence of an atretic segment prevents further passage of a contrast enema, a point that must be kept in mind during attempts at enema reduction in what is thought to be an uncomplicated case. Meconium peritonitis may cause an intense peritoneal reaction with erythema and edema of the abdominal wall (Fig. 17-31). Free meconium in the peritoneum calcifies, which is visible on plain film (Fig. 17-32).

In Hirschsprung disease, intramural ganglion cells are absent in the distal rectum and for a variable distance proximally. No peristalsis occurs in the affected segment, causing a functional distal bowel obstruction. Symptoms in the newborn are failure to pass meconium, abdominal distension, and, later, bilious vomiting (Fig. 17-33). Gas-filled bowel loops fill the abdomen on plain film. Barium enema examination demonstrates the distended bowel (which has normal ganglion cells) tapering over a transition zone to the narrowed, aganglionic distal segment (Fig. 17-34). Barium enema should precede rectal examination or attempts at decompression. A suppository or saline enema may decompress the bowel proximal to the aganglionic zone, causing the di-

agnostic transition zone to disappear. The diagnosis is confirmed by suction rectal biopsy, a procedure that does not require anesthesia.

Symptoms from Hirschsprung disease may not develop until later in infancy or childhood. Older children may have chronic constipation, abdominal distension, and failure to thrive. A potentially lethal complication of uncorrected Hirschsprung disease is acute enterocolitis, which may be the presenting manifestation. The child has the acute onset of abdominal distension, fulminant diarrhea, and diarrhea. Urgent rectal biopsy to make the diagnosis and colostomy to decompress the bowel are necessary.

Older Infants and Children

Invagination of a portion of the intestine into itself, intussusception, causes both vomiting and abdominal pain (Fig. 17-35). Intussusception occurs most frequently between the ages of 3 and 18 months; in this age group its cause is usually unknown. In contrast, the small number

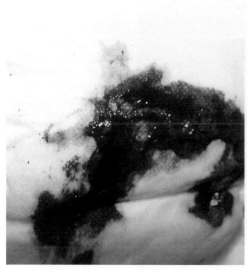

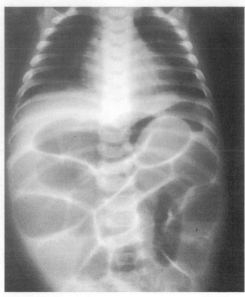

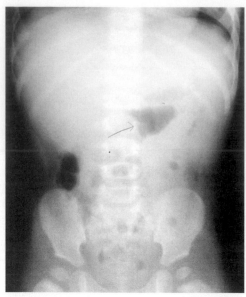

FIG. 17-36 The intussusception—the invaginated portion of bowel—becomes congested and ischemic, leading to the passage of bloody stool mixed with mucus.

FIG. 17-37 Small bowel obstruction occurs late in intussusception.

FIG. 17-38 In some cases the intussusceptum can be seen as a meniscus-shaped mass outlined by air in the colon.

of cases occurring in older children generally has an anatomic abnormality that acts as a lead point for the intussusception. Examples include children with Meckel diverticulum, intestinal lymphoma, polyps, cysts, areas of hemorrhage from Henoch-Schönlein purpura and hemophilia, and, for obscure reasons, children with cystic fibrosis and normal children who are recovering from operation (postoperative intussusception). Among cases of idiopathic intussusception, the majority originate at or near the ileocecal valve. The classic clinical picture is of a well infant who suddenly appears to have violent abdominal pain and vomits. Soon thereafter he or she passes a normal stool and appears to recover, being relaxed, even playful and hungry. However, bouts of colic recur, causing the child to draw up his or her thighs and cry or alternatively become pale, sweaty, and apathetic. Vomiting returns, and the baby begins to pass bloody stools. The vomiting at first is nonbilious, arising as a reflex response from traction on the involved mesentery. As obstruction becomes complete, vomiting later becomes bilious and the abdomen becomes distended. The intussusceptum (the segment of invaginated bowel) becomes engorged with blood and with time becomes ischemic. "Currant jelly" describes the bloody mucus from the intussusceptum that appears in the diaper (Fig. 17-36). On occasion the intussusceptum reaches the anus, where it can be felt on rectal examination. A sausage-shaped mass can be palpated in the majority of cases; because the process pulls the ileocecal area distally, the right iliac fossa may be scaphoid (Dance sign).

Plain film examination of the abdomen may reveal obstruction (Fig. 17-37), an intussusceptum seen as a soft-tissue density meniscus outlined by the air-filled distal colon (Fig. 17-38), or no abnormalities. Barium enema (Fig. 17-39) confirms the diagnosis and offers an opportunity to reduce the intussusception with a low rate of recurrence (less than 5%). Barium must be administered by gravity, without external manipulation of the bowel. Contrast must reflux freely into the small bowel to assure complete reduction and the absence of another intussusception in a more proximal location. A failed attempt requires immediate operation; thus a surgeon must be involved directly in the management of the child. Intussusception that recurs after barium en-

ema reduction or in older children requires operative reduction and exploration for a possible lead point. Contrast enemas usually cannot reach intussusceptions that are restricted to the small bowel, which renders them useless in diagnosis and management. Upper gastrointestinal series with follow-through into the small bowel may help diagnose small bowel intussusceptions (Fig. 17-40). Those that occur after operations cause small bowel obstruction and require reexploration, making contrast studies unnecessary. Small bowel intussusceptions require surgical reduction.

Volvulus around intraperitoneal bands and hernia can produce intestinal obstruction. Internal hernia from omphalomesenteric remnants may cause intestinal obstruction. Omphalomesenteric duct remnants may persist as a band that extends from the small bowel mesentery to the umbilicus. The omphalomesenteric artery originates the end artery of the superior mesenteric artery and extends to the tip of a Meckel diverticulum, but it remains suspended like a bowstring away from the mesentery and bowel. Inadequate retroperitoneal fixation of the bowel, considered a form of malrotation, leaves retroperitoneal pockets (paraduodenal hernia) into which small bowel can become entrapped. The most common source of intraabdominal bands remains postoperative adhesions from prior surgery or abdominal trauma.

Incarcerated hernia, a common cause of intestinal obstruction, is discussed with inguinal-scrotal abnormalities (p. 520).

Gastrointestinal Bleeding

The evaluation of an infant or child bleeding from the gastrointestinal tract involves obtaining answers to a few basic questions.

1. Is it blood? Red dyes in sodas and food, such as beets, produce red stool, and ingested iron gives stool the appearance of melena.
2. In infants, is it maternal blood? The Apt test distinguishes maternal, adult hemoglobin from fetal hemoglobin, thus identifying blood in the newborn as either swallowed during delivery or from the baby itself.

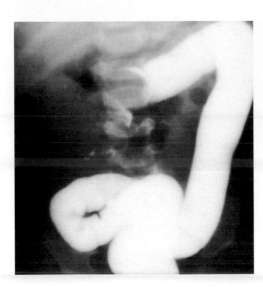

FIG. 17-39 Barium enema confirms the diagnosis by outlining the intussusceptum. The column of contrast can then be used to push the invaginated bowel proximally. Free reflux of contrast into the bowel proximally signals complete reduction of the intussusception.

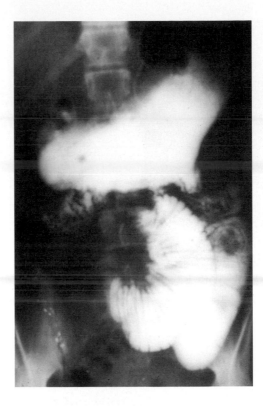

FIG. 17-40 Proximal small bowel intussusceptions require upper gastrointestinal series for diagnosis because enema studies cannot reliably reach the lesions. In contrast to those intussusceptions that occur after operations in infants and small children, those that occur *de novo* have a lead point; a small bowel polyp in a patient with Peutz-Jegher syndrome is shown.

3. Does the bleeding come from an upper or lower source? Bilious fluid free of blood sampled from a gastric tube shows that the bleeding source is distal to the ligament of Treitz. Bright red blood passed from the rectum may be from an upper source with rapid transit to the rectum. A closely related question is whether the bleeding source is the gastrointestinal tract at all. Nosebleeds and hemoptysis may mimic upper tract bleeding; bleeding from the urinary tract or vagina may be interpreted as coming from the rectum.

4. Does the child have a coagulopathy? Gastrointestinal bleeding may be the initial manifestation of congenital or acquired coagulopathies or a hematologic malignancy, or it may be a complication of liver disease or medications.

5. How much blood has been lost? The volume of blood loss is often overestimated, but children in shock must be recognized and treated aggressively. Postural vital signs, appearance of the skin, and hematocrit reflect the amount of blood that has been lost. Bright red blood issuing in large amounts from the gastric tube or anus demands large-bore intravenous catheters and arrangements for prompt blood replacement to coincide with diagnostic workup.

The age of the patient, his or her appearance (how sick he or she appears), and the bleeding site (upper versus lower) give clues to the diagnosis. The discussion in the next section follows this format (Tables 17-2 and 17-3).

TABLE 17-2

Common Causes of Gastrointestinal Hemorrhage

	Patients <1 year	Patients >1 year
Upper	Gastritis	Peptic ulcer
	Swallowed maternal blood	Varices
	Peptic ulcer (duodenal and gastric)	
	Malrotation and volvulus	
Lower	Anal fissure	Colonic polyps
	Intussusception	Intussusception
	Necrotizing enterocolitis	Meckel diverticulum
	Meckel diverticulum	Infectious diarrhea
	Malrotation and volvulus	Inflammatory bowel disease

Infants

The infant who has swallowed maternal blood looks well and has normal vital signs and hematocrit. The Apt test identifies the blood as having adult hemoglobin, establishing its source. (The mixture of one volume of the gastric aspirate and four parts of water is centrifuged. The supernatant is in turn mixed in a 4:1 ratio with 1% sodium hydroxide. If the liquid remains pink, the blood has fetal hemoglobin; if it turns brown, the blood had a maternal source.) Nasogastric tube suction causes trauma to the gastric mucosa, a common cause of small amounts of bleeding in hospitalized patients. This bleeding easily clears with lavage, and as a rule it resolves when suction is discontinued. Although hemorrhagic disease of the newborn is now extremely rare because all babies receive intramuscular injections of vitamin K shortly after birth, it may arise in extremely ill babies who are transferred to other hospitals and in whom this injection has been overlooked. Healthy infants who pass large, hard stools may bleed small amounts

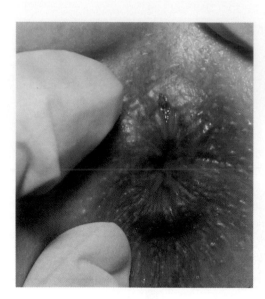

FIG. 17-41 Small tears in the anoderm may bleed, producing small amounts of blood on the stool of healthy infants.

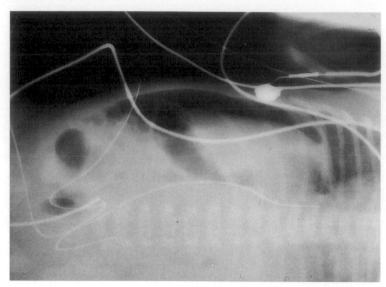

FIG. 17-42 The large quantity of free air within the abdomen resulting from a gastric perforation (shown here outlining the edge of the liver) suggests its source.

TABLE 17-3

Causes of Gastrointestinal Bleeding

Location	Appearance	Newborn	Infant	Child
			Age	
Upper				
	Well	Maternal blood	Nosebleeds	Nosebleeds
		Nasogastric tube	Nasogastric tube	Nasogastric tube
		Pyloric stenosis	Esophagitis	
		Esophagitis		
	Ill	Peptic ulcer disease	Varices	Varices
		Necrotizing enterocolitis	Peptic ulcer disease	Peptic ulcer disease
		Volvulus	Medications	Medications
Lower				
	Well	Anal fissure	Anal fissure	Anal fissure
		Maternal blood	Meckel diverticulum	Juvenile polyp
		Hemangioma	Duplication	Meckel diverticulum
		Duplication		Rectal prolapse
	Ill	Necrotizing enterocolitis	Intussusception	Infectious diarrhea
		Volvulus	Infectious diarrhea	Intussusception
		Infectious diarrhea	Medications	Trauma
			Henoch-Schönlein purpura	Medications
			Hemolytic-uremic syndrome	Hemolytic-uremic syndrome
				Henoch-Schönlein purpura
				Inflammatory bowel disease

of red blood from anal fissures (Fig. 17-41). These fissures are easily seen by spreading the intergluteal cleft; trying to see a fissure through a test tube in the anus is futile.

Acute gastric ulcer during the newborn period may cause a large amount of upper tract bleeding and may produce shock. Typically located in the lesser curve of the stomach, the ulcer may also perforate and cause free air in the abdomen (Fig. 17-42). Newborns in the first week of life are at the highest risk. Malrotation and volvulus may produce gastrointestinal bleeding from ischemic bowel or from coagulopa-

thy induced by midgut infarction and septicemia (discussed as a cause of vomiting on p. 495).

Necrotizing enterocolitis is the most common abdominal surgical emergency in newborns. Intestinal necrosis is variable, ranging from mucosal to transmural in extent. The terminal ileum is involved most commonly, followed in frequency by the colon and the jejunum. The disease can affect only a single segment, multiple segments with areas of relatively normal bowel, or the entire gut. It primarily affects premature infants, generally between 2 and 8 weeks of life. When full-term

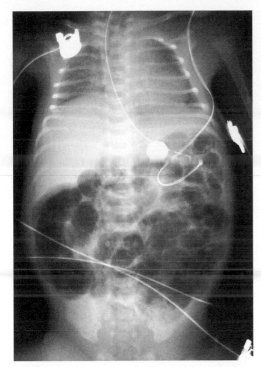

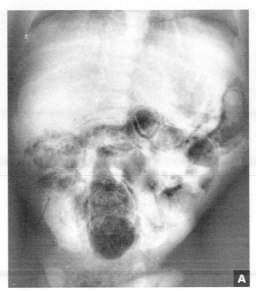

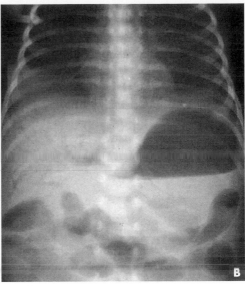

FIG. 17-44 Pneumatosis intestinalis is seen most easily as linear streaks of air outlining the bowel and producing concentric rings when viewed on end. More common, however, is the bubbly pattern seen in the right iliac fossa in this patient, appearing like stool within the lumen (*A*). In severely affected infants, gas may fill the portal system and produce visible streaks of air on abdominal plain film (*B*).

FIG. 17-43 Ileus is the earliest sign of necrotizing enterocolitis, seen as distended bowel loops on abdominal plain film. A careful search should be made for pneumatosis intestinalis, an often subtle and transient sign that establishes the diagnosis, here seen best in the area of the splenic flexure in the left upper quadrant.

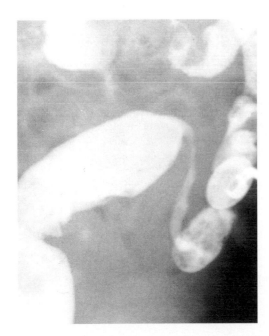

FIG. 17-45 In a patient who develops intestinal obstruction during recovery from necrotizing enterocolitis a colonic stricture must be suspected.

testinal disease. The white blood cell count may be elevated or depressed. Immature forms may predominate on differential count. Severely ill babies develop thrombocytopenia and metabolic acidosis. Bowel distension on abdominal plain film examination may precede clinical illness by several hours (Fig. 17-43). Pneumatosis intestinalis, the radiologic hallmark of the disease (Fig. 17-44), arises from cysts of gas that collect within the intestinal wall and beneath the serosa. Its appearance may be transient. Gas within the portal vein is seen in a branching pattern in the area of the liver (Fig. 17-44), and its appearance also may be fleeting. Perforation of the intestine leads to pneumoperitoneum, best seen on the left lateral decubitus view of the abdomen. Unless there is evidence of intestinal necrosis or perforation, the initial treatment of necrotizing enterocolitis is nonoperative: gastric decompression, intravenous hydration, and broad spectrum antibiotic coverage. Deterioration or perforation is an indication for surgery. Many babies successfully managed without operation may develop late strictures, most frequently in the colon (Fig. 17-45). Those who develop symptoms require resection of the involved segment.

Intussusception, a common cause of rectal bleeding in infancy, is discussed as a cause of vomiting (p. 497).

Toddlers (1 to 4 Years)

Bleeding from a Meckel diverticulum is usually painless and is most often seen in children under 5 years of age, the majority occurring in children under 2 years (Fig. 17-46). Its source arises from peptic ulceration of the ileum adjacent to ectopic gastric mucosa within the diverticulum. The volume of bleeding varies, but typically large amounts of blood are lost and are passed from the rectum as bright red blood. Bleeding is episodic; stools may return to normal color after an episode

infants are affected, the onset of symptoms tends to be earlier, frequently in the first week. The etiology of necrotizing enterocolitis remains obscure, but it probably involves a number of factors that include host defense, feeding routines, influences that reduce intestinal blood flow, and infectious agents.

Abdominal distension from ileus, gastric retention, or vomiting and rectal bleeding are common physical findings. Lethargy, temperature instability, apnea, and bradycardia reflect the severity of illness. Abdominal wall erythema and edema reflect peritonitis and severe in-

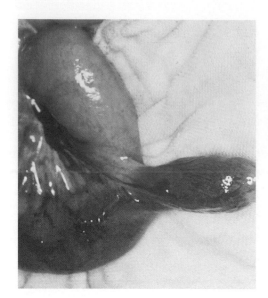

FIG. 17-46 A Meckel diverticulum emerges from the antimesenteric border of the ileum. The mesodiverticular artery courses along the axis of the diverticulum. Erosion of an ulcer into the artery produces massive hemorrhage. When the artery is incompletely attached to the bowel (mesodiverticular band), internal herniation beneath it causes intestinal obstruction.

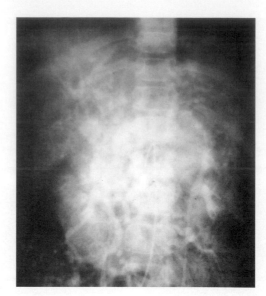

FIG. 17-47 Venous phase of mesenteric angiography demonstrates the abrupt cutoff of the portal vein and ropy, distended varices throughout the mesenteric system. The most significant varices lie in the stomach and esophagus because of the risk of exsanguinating gastrointestinal hemorrhage.

but continue to test positive for blood. Technetium 99m pertechnetate localizes in gastric mucosa, including that found ectopically in a Meckel diverticulum. Helpful when positive, nuclear studies have occasional false positive and relatively frequent false negative results. Contrast studies of the distal small bowel (enteroclysis) may opacify the diverticulum but are not reliable as routine studies. The child therefore may have to undergo exploratory laparotomy on the basis of clinical findings alone. Because bleeding generally ceases spontaneously, resection can be performed electively during the same hospitalization when the child is stable. Other manifestations of Meckel diverticulum that are unrelated to bleeding include obstruction (discussed previously as a cause of vomiting), diverticulitis (clinically indistinguishable from appendicitis and rare), and persistent omphalomesenteric fistula.

Bleeding from esophageal varices arises from portal hypertension. Portal hypertension in childhood has two major causes: extrahepatic portal vein occlusion and cirrhosis. Omphalitis in the newborn, one of the complications of umbilical vessel catheterization, may cause thrombosis of the portal vein. Despite a successful portoenterostomy that clears jaundice, cirrhosis still may develop in cases of biliary atresia. Other causes of cirrhosis in childhood include congenital hepatic fibrosis, cystic fibrosis, alpha$_1$-antitripsin deficiency, and end-stage liver disease following viral hepatitis. Endoscopy gives the most direct and reliable means of diagnosis of bleeding varices. Contrast opacification of the portal vein and its tributaries is necessary if surgical portal decompression becomes necessary (Fig. 17-47). However, most bleeding episodes are self-limited. Persistent bleeding is controlled effectively in nearly all cases by endoscopic injection of a sclerosant into the bleeding varix, and surgery is seldom necessary.

Vasculitis from Henoch-Schönlein purpura may cause lower tract bleeding in this age group. A viral or streptococcal infection may precede the development of arthralgias and confluent purpura primarily over the lower extremities. The diagnosis is made difficult when bleeding or abdominal pain precedes the appearance of the rash. Bloody diarrhea and abdominal pain may accompany hemolytic-uremic syndrome. Hemolytic anemia on blood count and smear, azotemia, and thrombocytopenia establish the diagnosis. Infectious diarrhea may produce bloody bowel motions. The diagnosis is suggested by fever and

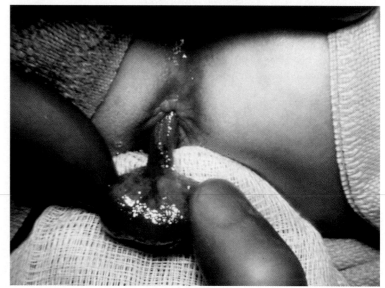

FIG. 17-48 Juvenile polyps are found most often in the rectosigmoid colon. On occasion they may prolapse through the anus.

the presence of white blood cells in the stool, and it is confirmed by culture.

Older Children

Juvenile polyps of the colon are benign hamartomas covered with flattened epithelium and granulation tissue (Fig. 17-48). Children aged 2 to 8 years are affected most frequently. Most occur singly; when multiple, usually they number less than 12. Two thirds of symptomatic polyps occur in the rectum, and 90% occur distal to the sigmoid. Bleeding is painless, small in amount, and found on the surface of the stool. The polyp may prolapse out the anus. Surgical resection of those that prolapse out the anus, or endoscopic resection, is curative. Diffuse gas-

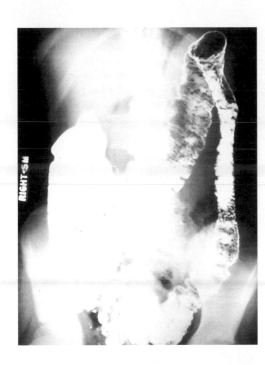

FIG. 17-49 Familial adenomatous polyposis. A barium enema study demonstrates multiple small polyps throughout the colon.

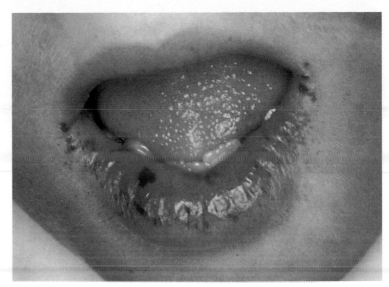

FIG. 17-50 The characteristic melanotic spots of Peutz-Jegher syndrome are seen on the lips, buccal mucosa, and anus.

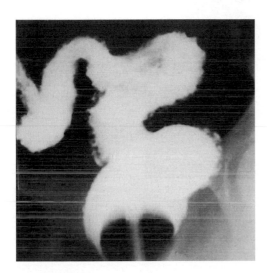

FIG. 17-51 Linear ulcerations and crypt abscesses fill and leave islands of mucosa, which appear as pseudopolyps on barium enema.

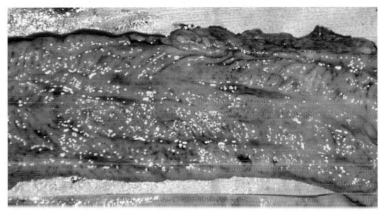

FIG. 17-52 This opened colectomy specimen demonstrates the linear ulcerations in the mucosa of a patient with ulcerative colitis.

trointestinal juvenile polyposis is a rare entity that causes bleeding, diarrhea, rectal prolapse, intussusception, and protein-losing enteropathy. A life-threatening condition, diffuse juvenile polyposis requires total colectomy.

Adenomatous polyps are extremely rare as solitary colonic polyps in children. Children of families with familial adenomatous polyposis usually develop symptoms at puberty or late adolescence. Innumerable adenomatous polyps carpet the colon and cause bloody diarrhea, tenesmus, and abdominal pain (Fig. 17-49). Polyps associated with Peutz-Jegher syndrome are also adenomatous, but they are fewer in number and are located at all levels of the gastrointestinal tract from stomach to rectum. Mucocutaneous melanin spots are present on the lips and face, buccal mucosa, and fingers and may precede the development of abdominal symptoms by years (Fig. 17-50). Gastrointestinal bleeding is usually occult. Colic is the major abdominal symptom, caused by transient intussusception with a polyp as the lead point (Fig. 17-40).

The common causes of bleeding among children as they get older are those common among adults, such as peptic ulcer disease, gastritis, Mallory-Weiss tear, and inflammatory bowel disease (Fig. 17-51 and 17-52). Endoscopy provides the most direct means to diagnosis.

Abdominal Pain

Acute appendicitis is the most common surgical emergency of the abdomen during childhood and adolescence. Obstruction of the appen-

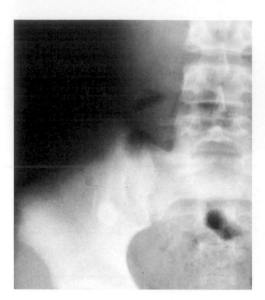

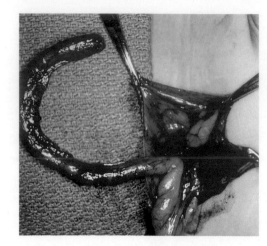

FIG. 17-53 A fecalith, the round calcification in the iliac fossa, obstructs the appendiceal lumen and initiates inflammatory processes that produce appendicitis.

FIG. 17-54 The purple color of the appendix in this case of appendicitis contrasts with the pink color of the healthy serosa of the cecum at its base.

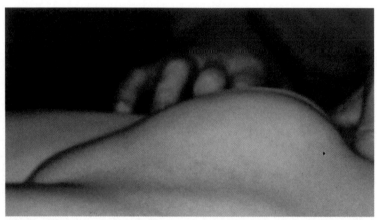

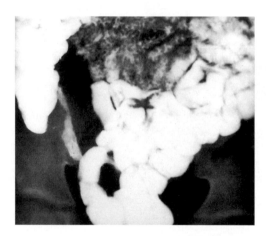

FIG. 17-56 Stricture of the terminal ileum and segmental involvement of the small bowel and colon are characteristic findings on barium enema examination of a child with Crohn disease.

FIG. 17-55 A large ovarian cyst in a prepubertal girl can be demonstrated easily on abdominal examination.

diceal lumen, commonly by a fecalith visible on abdominal plain film (Fig. 17-53), leads to appendiceal edema, ischemia, and ultimately necrosis and gangrene (Fig. 17-54). The classic progression of symptoms begins with vague periumbilical pain. Transmural inflammation follows and produces fever and leukocytosis. As the appendix distends, the child loses his or her appetite and begins to vomit. When the inflamed appendix comes in contact with the abdominal wall, the child perceives the localization of pain in the right lower quadrant. Any sudden movement, such as coughing, walking, jumping, or palpation by a physician, causes pain at that point, so the child lies still on his or her side, draws up the legs at the hips, and resists examination. Involuntary guarding develops, detected on palpation as muscular spasm in the area where the child is most tender. Mild sedation, administered to facilitate examination, never masks true involuntary guarding. Tenderness may be mild in cases in which a retrocecal appendix fails to impinge the anterior abdominal wall but may produce instead a positive psoas or obturator sign. When the appendix perforates, pain at first decreases as the appendix decompresses. Perforation soils the peritoneum, and generalized peritonitis produces diffuse abdominal pain, distension, and rigidity. The omentum and adjacent loops of bowel may limit the perforation to the right lower quadrant, forming an abscess and creating a mass in the right lower quadrant.

Appendicitis occurring in children and adolescent boys seldom presents problems in diagnosis, and the rate of normal appendices removed (negative appendectomy) is less than 5%. The prevalence of acute salpingitis and other uterine tubo-ovarian pathology leads to a high negative appendectomy rate in adolescent girls. The fever and symptoms closely related to the onset of menses, tenderness upon movement of the cervix, and the absence of gastrointestinal complaints suggest acute salpingitis. A twisted ovarian cyst produces a mobile mass in the lower abdomen and causes severe pain without gastrointestinal symptoms or abdominal tenderness (Fig. 17-55). Abdominal ultrasound helps to delineate the presence of ovarian cysts or tubo-ovarian abscess. Appendicitis in preschool children is difficult to diagnose at an early, nonperforated stage because of problems in obtaining precise details of clinical history and adequate physical examinations. Because diagnosis is often delayed, the rate of perforation among young children exceeds 50%. A number of extraabdominal and systemic inflammatory conditions, including otitis media, pneumonia, urinary tract infections, diabetes mellitus, Henoch-Schönlein purpura, rheumatic fever, and sickle cell disease, can cause abdominal pain. In all ages, other acute intestinal conditions can closely mimic acute appendicitis. Viral and bacterial enteritis are most common. Inflammatory bowel disease becomes more common in older children (Figs. 17-56

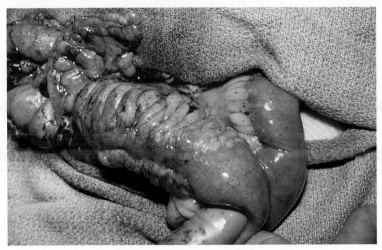

FIG. 17-57 Findings at laparotomy in Crohn disease reveal petechiae over the serosa of thickened small bowel, which has mesenteric fat "creeping" over its surface.

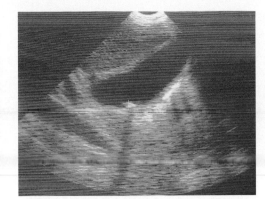

FIG. 17-58 Ultrasound examination of the right upper quadrant easily demonstrates stones within the gallbladder. An acoustic shadow extends beneath the stone.

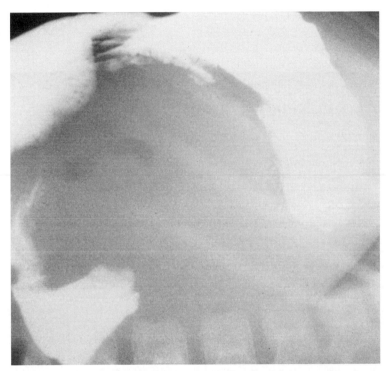

FIG. 17-59 Pancreatic pseudocyst, a complication of pancreatitis of any cause, may grow large enough to displace the stomach anteriorly.

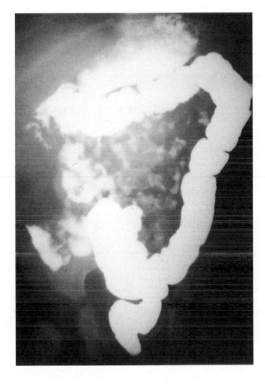

FIG. 17-60 An omental cyst has displaced the right colon.

and 17-57). Intussusception becomes more prevalent among the younger age group and should be considered, rather than appendicitis, in infants who exhibit abdominal pain and vomiting. Meckel diverticulitis, clinically indistinguishable from acute appendicitis, results from peptic perforation of the diverticulum. It is the least common clinical manifestation of Meckel diverticulum.

Other surgical causes of abdominal pain are rare in childhood. Right upper quadrant pain suggests a biliary tract pathology, particularly when jaundice coexists. Acute cholecystitis occurs in children with hemoglobinopathy or hematologic conditions that cause unusual degrees of hemolysis and in adolescent girls who develop "adult" cholesterol gallstones. Ultrasound examination reveals gallstones, distended gallbladder (Fig. 17-58), and biliary tract dilation, if present. Right upper quadrant pain, jaundice, and mass represent the classic triad of choledochal cyst. Pancreatitis produces epigastric pain and the serum amylase becomes elevated. A child with pancreatitis who develops an epigastric mass requires an ultrasound examination to rule out pancreatic pseudocyst (Fig. 17-59). Urinalysis and renal ultrasound identify the urinary tract as the source of abdominal pain, usually located in the flank but sometimes the source of confusion when pain occurs more anteriorly.

Abdominal Masses

The presence of an abdominal mass in an infant or child is always abnormal and requires evaluation. The etiology of abdominal masses includes congenital and neoplastic lesions, as well as complications of in-

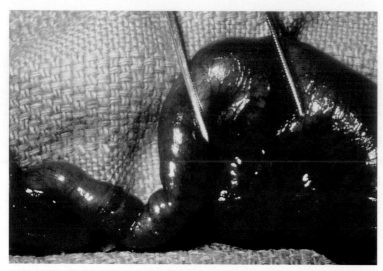

FIG. 17-61 Duplications typically lie within the mesentery and involve the terminal ileum. They may be spherical (pictured here) or tubular. An obstructed duplication may become palpable as an abdominal mass; one with ectopic gastric mucosa may produce gastrointestinal bleeding; another may act as a lead point for intussusception.

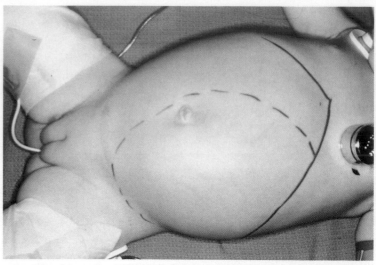

FIG. 17-62 The dashed line indicates the extent of a flank mass in an infant with ureteropelvic junction obstruction.

TABLE 17-4

Possible Diagnoses of Abdominal Masses in Infancy and Childhood

Region	Organ	Diagnosis
Epigastrium	Stomach	Distended stomach from pyloric stenosis, duplication
	Pancreas	Pseudocyst
Flank	Kidney	Hydronephrosis, Wilms tumor, dysplastic kidney ureteral duplication
	Adrenal	Neuroblastoma, ganglioneuroblastoma, ganglioneuroma
	Retroperitoneal	Neuroblastoma, ganglioneuroblastoma, ganglioneuroma, teratoma
Lower abdomen	Ovary	Dermoid, teratoma, ovarian tumors, torsion of ovary
	Kidney	Pelvic kidney
	Urachus	Urachal cyst
	Omentum, mesentery	Omental, mesenteric, peritoneal cysts
Pelvic	Bladder, prostate	Obstructed bladder, rhabdomyoscarcoma
	Uterus, vagina	Hydrometrocolpos, hydrocolpos, rhabdomyosarcoma
Right upper quadrant	Biliary tract	Cholecystitis, choledochal cyst
	Liver	Hematomegaly resulting from congestion, hepatitis, or tumor; mesenchymal hamartoma; hemangioendothelioma; hepatoblastoma; hepatocellular carcinoma; hepatic abscess; hydatid cyst
	Intestine	Intussusception, duplication
Left upper quadrant	Spleen	Splenomegaly resulting from congestion, infectious mononucleosis, leukemic infiltration or lymphoma; splenic abscess; cyst
Right lower quadrant	Appendix	Appendiceal abscess
	Ileum	Meconium ileus, inflammatory mass (complicated Crohn's disease), intestinal duplication
	Lymphatic	Lymphoma, lymphangioma
Left lower quadrant	Colon	Fecal impaction
	Lymphatic	Lymphoma, lymphangioma

flammatory conditions. Discovery of a mass requires early surgical consultation because nearly half (45%) are surgical lesions. Of this group, neoplasm represents about 45% of lesions and hydronephrosis causes about one third (32%). Less common causes of abdominal masses include multicystic kidney, hydrocolpos, omental and mesenteric cysts (Fig. 17-60), and duplications (Fig. 17-61).

The etiology of abdominal masses changes with the age of the child and the location of the mass. A mass in a newborn is a benign obstructive renal lesion in 75% to 80% of cases. Unusual congenital intraabdominal masses, such as ovarian and omental cysts and duplications, are frequently found during early infancy. In older age groups, the majority of masses are malignant tumors. Table

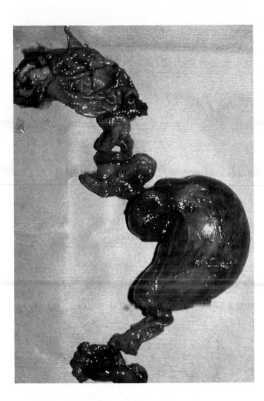

FIG. 17-63 Irregular dilations along the course of an obstructed duplicated ureter may become palpable as flank masses.

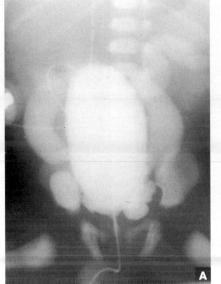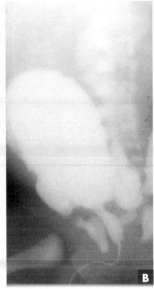

FIG. 17-64 Posterior urethral valves cause dilation of the bladder and both upper tracts, shown here on a retrograde contrast study.

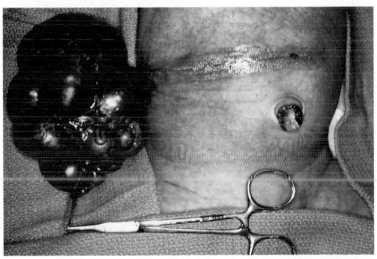

FIG. 17-65 A multicystic kidney produces a knobby flank mass.

17-4 summarizes the causes of abdominal masses by age and location.

Signs of inflammation, such as tenderness, fever, leukocytosis, and overlying tenderness, suggest an inflammatory cause, such as abscess from appendicitis, Crohn disease, or an infected peritoneal cyst associated with a ventriculoperitoneal shunt.

Abdominal plain films provide basic information regarding the location of the mass. The mass may be intraluminal, as in an infant with meconium ileus (see Fig. 17-30), intussusception (see Fig. 17-38), or an older child with constipation. An extraluminal mass generally displaces intestinal loops, giving an indication of its location. If plain films reveal intestinal obstruction from a particularly large mass or one that involves the stomach or intestine, emergency surgery becomes necessary. Calcifications within the mass on plain film suggest the presence of a neuroblastoma. Contrast study of the stomach and the intestine helps to identify inflammatory bowel disease and the anatomic relationships between the mass and the gastrointestinal tract, but it should be de-

ferred if ultrasound, computed tomography, magnetic resonance imaging, or other special imaging studies are planned.

Ultrasonography is useful early in the evaluation to distinguish between solid tumors from obstructive uropathy and other fluid-filled masses. Ultrasound identifies the lesion as arising from the kidney (such as Wilms tumor) or outside the kidney (adrenal neuroblastoma). Abdominal plain film, seldom diagnostic, may demonstrate calcifications from a neuroblastoma. Computed tomography gives more precise anatomic information than ultrasonography, demonstrating enlarged lymph nodes and other masses within the chest or abdomen that might represent metastases.

Oral and intravenous contrast are essential in computed tomography examinations so that gastrointestinal and urinary structures can be identified. Particularly important is to establish whether both kidneys excrete dye and are thus functional, a point of obvious surgical importance if nephrectomy is necessary. Magnetic resonance imaging has been used increasingly in the evaluation of abdominal neoplasms.

Genitourinary Obstructions

Hydronephrosis is the most common cause of an abdominal mass in the newborn and is usually painless. In contrast, hydronephrosis in older children is rarely palpable and causes pain and urinary tract infection. Ureteropelvic junction obstruction results in a large, smooth flank mass that is treated by pyeloplasty (Fig. 17-62). Ureteral duplication causes ureteral dilation of the upper pole ureter from obstruction and the lower pole ureter from reflux. The ureters may become palpable as a knobby flank mass (Fig. 17-63). Stasis within the ureters may cause urinary tract infection. Ureterocele associated with a duplicated system may obstruct the bladder. Posterior urethral valves are the most common cause of lower urinary tract obstruction in boys (Fig. 17-64). The distended bladder drains inadequately and is palpable in the lower abdomen. Hydroureteronephrosis may be present and may produce bilateral flank masses. Multicystic kidney produces a large, knobby mass in infants (Fig. 17-65), a diagnosis easily confirmed on ultrasonography.

An obstructed female genital tract may cause hydrometrocolpos in infancy, usually palpated as a smooth mass placed centrally in the

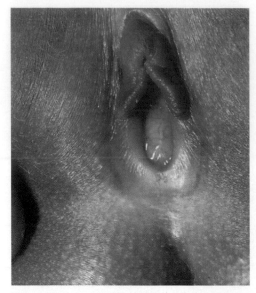

FIG. 17-66 Imperforate hymen. Accumulated secretions in the vagina and uterus caused bulging of the hymen and a pelvic mass in this newborn.

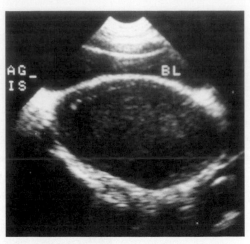

FIG. 17-67 A pelvic mass arising at the expected time of menarche suggests the presence of an obstructed uterine anomaly, here demonstrated by pelvic ultrasound as an oval mass compressing the bladder anteriorly. Urinary anomalies commonly coexist.

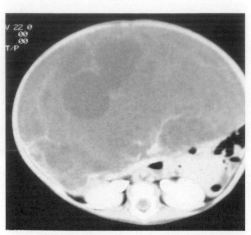

FIG. 17-68 Computed tomography of a mesenchymal hamartoma of the liver. In contrast to the neovascularization within a hepatic tumor, a hamartoma fails to show contrast enhancement.

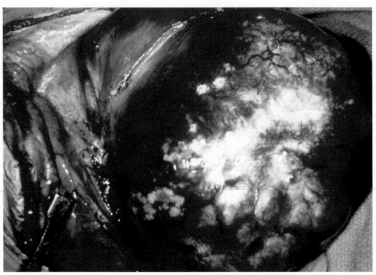

FIG. 17-69 A large hepatoblastoma of the right lobe of the liver. Intravenous urography, computed tomography, and ultrasonography all identify it as a hepatic tumor instead of one arising from the kidney or an adrenal gland.

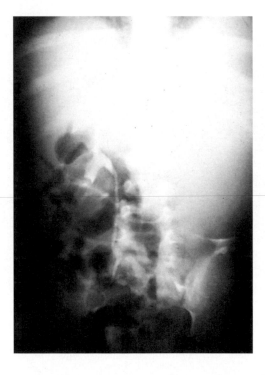

FIG. 17-70 A large Wilms tumor has splayed the collecting system of the left kidney on intravenous urogram so that calyces are visible deep in the left iliac fossa. This distortion of the collecting system identifies a mass as arising from the kidney, one of the radiologic signs of Wilms tumor.

lower abdomen but occasionally as a huge mass that fills the abdomen. Symptoms may not arise until menarche, when the obstructed genital tract fills with blood, creating a hematocolpos (Figs. 17-66 and 17-67). Menstrual bleeding that is unable to drain externally creates a slowly expanding lower abdominal mass with pain that becomes worse every 3 to 4 weeks. Urinary anomalies are common and should be sought out during evaluation.

Abdominal Neoplasms

Hepatic enlargement shortly after birth may represent a subcapsular hematoma from birth trauma. Diffuse enlargement of the liver that develops in early infancy may be due to hemangioendothelioma; enlargement may be so severe that respiratory insufficiency results. Blood flow through the liver may create an audible bruit. Platelet trapping may result in thrombocytopenia. Hemangioendothelioma usually regresses with time without treatment; severe symptoms may require treatment with steroids, radiation, or chemotherapy. Similarly, hepatic metastases from stage IV-S neuroblastoma regress completely without treatment in most cases. However, abdominal distension from hepatic enlargement may cause respiratory insufficiency severe enough to require radiation therapy or chemotherapy. Mesenchymal hamartoma is the most common benign hepatic tumor in infancy, creating homogeneous cystic areas on ultrasound and computed tomography (Fig. 17-68). Hepatoblastoma, primarily affecting infants under 2 years of age (Fig. 17-69), and hepatocellular carcinoma, primarily seen in preadolescents, represent the primary malignant hepatic tumors of childhood. Serum alpha-fetoprotein levels are elevated in most cases, and this elevation is use-

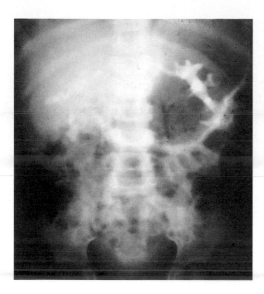

FIG. 17-71 Wilms tumor arising in the lower poles of both kidneys. When possible, the surgical goal is conservative excision of the tumor, leaving as much functioning kidney as possible.

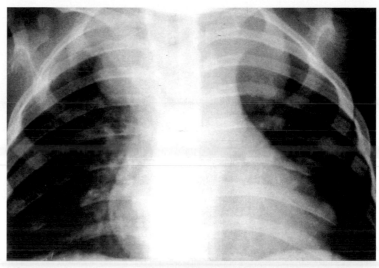

FIG. 17-72 An upper thoracic neuroblastoma shown here in the right superior sulcus of the thorax, may produce unilateral Horner syndrome.

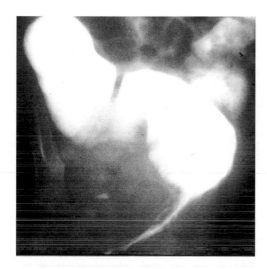

FIG. 17-73 A pelvic neuroblastoma causes compression of the rectum on barium enema study.

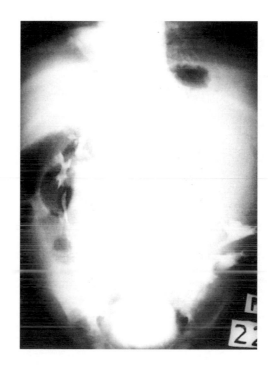

FIG. 17-74 Downward displacement of the entire kidney by a left adrenal neuroblastoma leaves the intrarenal collecting system anatomically intact but gives it a "drooping lily" appearance.

ful as a tumor marker to detect recurrence after resection. Hepatocellular carcinoma occurs more frequently in cases of preexisting liver disease, such as biliary atresia.

Wilms tumor is the most common intraabdominal malignancy in childhood. Nearly all cases occur by the age of 6 years. In addition to a flank mass, hematuria and hypertension may be present. Children with aniridia and hemihypertrophy are considered to be at increased risk for the development of Wilms tumor and should be monitored with semiannual ultrasound examinations. Intravenous urography (Fig. 17-70) and ultrasonography verify the presence of an intrarenal solid mass within the kidney. Ultrasound identifies the presence of tumor lying within the renal vein and inferior vena cava, points of surgical significance. Wilms tumor may arise in both kidneys (Fig. 17-71); in such cases it is a therapeutic challenge to excise the tumor yet leave the child with as much functioning renal mass as possible. Computed tomography also may identify nodal enlargement and liver nodules that may represent metastasis. Chest film and chest computed tomography help to identify metastases to the lung, the most common site. Children with clear cell

sarcoma, previously considered to be a variant of Wilms tumor but now considered a distinct neoplasm, frequently have bone metastasis and should receive a bone scan. Mesoblastic nephroma is an uncommon, relatively benign variant of Wilms tumor and is present most frequently in infants.

Neuroblastoma is the second most common solid tumor in childhood, exceeded only by brain tumors (Fig. 17-72). Tumors may arise in the adrenal glands, sympathetic ganglia, and organs of Zuckerkandl and so may be found in the neck, chest, abdomen, and pelvis (Fig. 17-73). Young children under 5 years of age are most commonly affected. Systemic symptoms, such as fever and failure to thrive, and remote effects of tumor, such as proptosis, opsomyoclonus, and ataxia, may predominate the clinical picture, and the tumor may be relatively small or nonpalpable. More than 70% of children have metastases when first seen, accounting for the poor prognosis of neuroblastoma in general. Radiologic studies of an adrenal neuroblastoma reveal an extrarenal mass; inferior displacement of opacified calyces on intravenous pyelography gives a characteristic "drooping lily" sign (Fig. 17-74). Because of the

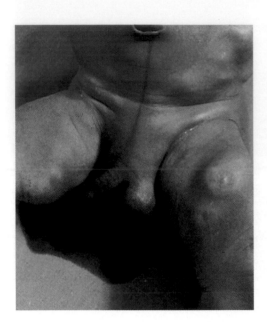

FIG. 17-75 Subcutaneous metastasis in IV-S neuroblastoma gives infants a "blueberry muffin" appearance. The lesions generally regress without chemotherapy or radiation therapy, and the survival rate exceeds 70%.

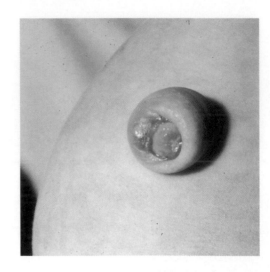

FIG. 17-76 A urachal cyst abscess produces a tender mass beneath the umbilicus, which also may become enlarged and tender.

TABLE 17-5

Common Lesions of the Head and Neck in Infancy and Childhood

Region	Location	Common Lesions
Head	Scalp	Hemangioma, dermoid cyst
	Ear	Preauricular sinus, tag
	Eyebrow	Dermoid cyst
	Base of nose	Meningocele, encephalocele
	Parotid gland	Hemangioma, lymphangioma, rhabdomyoscarcoma, lymphoma, mixed tumor, parotitis
Mouth	Tongue	Tongue tie, macroglossia, lingual thyroid
	Floor of mouth	Ranula
	Cheek and lip	Papilloma, mucocele
	Alveolar ridge	Tooth bud, epignathus
Neck	Midline	Thyroglossal duct cyst, dermoid cyst, submental lymph node, goiter
	Lateral	Branchial cleft cyst or sinus, lymphadenitis, lymphoma, lymphangioma, torticollis

frequency of metastases, workup should include computed tomography of the chest and abdomen and bone scan. Laboratory findings have prognostic significance; survival is higher when serum ferritin is less than 150 ng/ml, neuron-specific enolase is less than 100 ng/ml, and the ratio of vanillylmandelic acid to homovanilic acid in the urine is greater than 1 Stage IV-S neuroblastoma, a variant of metastatic disease that often regresses completely without therapy, is characterized by a localized primary tumor with metastases to the liver, bone marrow, or skin (Fig. 17-75).

Non-Hodgkin lymphoma involves abdominal sites in one fourth to one half of all cases. It has a peak incidence of 5 to 8 years and afflicts boys more often than girls. Pain is frequently the earliest symptom, and a mass may become palpable. The tumor is located in the small bowel in the majority of cases and may lead to intussusception. Tumors may arise in other segments of the bowel, other organs, and retroperitoneum. Non-Hodgkin lymphoma grows rapidly but generally responds promptly to chemotherapy, so aggressive workup including biopsy is warranted.

In contrast to rhabdomyosarcoma of the trunk and extremities, those that involve the bladder, inguinal canal, and vagina commonly have a nonalveolar histology and carry a good prognosis. Ovarian tumors are varied in histology, including both benign (cystic teratoma, follicular cyst) and malignant (teratocarcinoma, germ cell tumors, dysgerminoma). Germ cell tumors may be presacral in location and palpable only on rectal examination, causing no visible mass either in the perineum or in the lower abdomen.

Inflammatory Masses

Adjacent loops of bowel and the omentum may localize perforated appendicitis in the right iliac fossa; appendicitis was discussed previously as a cause of abdominal pain. An infected urachal cyst causes a tender midline mass below the umbilicus (Fig. 17-76). Cellulitis may involve the overlying skin and the umbilicus. Sonography shows a fluid collection anterior to the bladder. Children with ventriculoperitoneal shunts may develop infected collections of fluid in the abdomen associated with shunt infections. Fever and abdominal discomfort usually resolve promptly after exteriorization of the shunt and administration of intravenous antibiotics. Persistence of fever or symptoms suggests that an abscess has formed, from inadequate resolution of an infected fluid collection or from intestinal perforation.

Crohn disease may produce a tender right lower abdominal mass. Effective medical management leads to resolution of the mass. Persistence or enlargement of the mass may indicate fistula formation and abscess development. Ultrasound detects a fluid collection that identifies an abscess and may show abnormal dilation of the urinary tract from involvement of the ureter in the inflammatory process. Contrast enema and follow through of barium into the small bowel define the extent of Crohn disease and may help define the presence of fistulae.

Head and Neck

The locations of head and neck lesions provide the most information regarding the probable diagnosis. Table 17-5 summarizes some of the more common lesions grouped by location. Most are benign. Physical

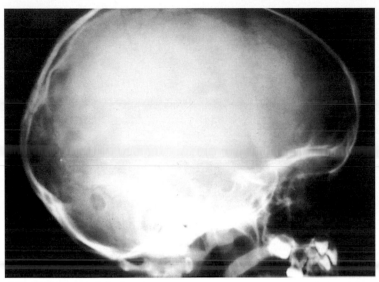

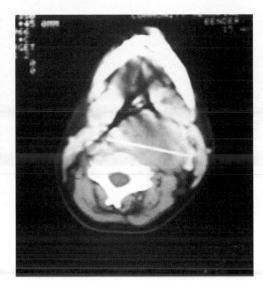

FIG. 17-78 Computed tomography of the neck shows a ganglioneuroma lying below the mandible, distorting the airway toward the contralateral side.

FIG. 17-77 Lateral skull radiograph shows a circular defect in the occipital region of a patient who presented with a superficial dermoid cyst over the occiput. The cyst extended through the defect into the intracranial cavity.

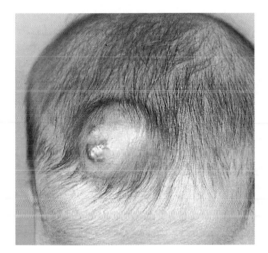

FIG. 17-79 Cavernous hemangioma of the scalp, with overlying skin involvement.

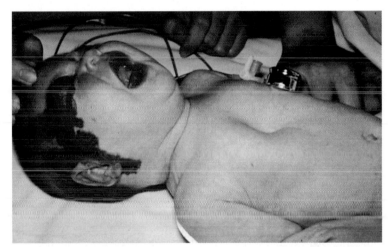

FIG. 17-80 Facial hemangioma covering the eye requires intervention with prednisone to hasten resolution and avoid loss of sight from amblyopia.

examination should note the consistency and mobility of the mass, signs of inflammation, and any abnormal drainage. Masses that impinge upon the airway or compromise vision require immediate attention.

Skull, facial, and mandible films identify bone tumors and superficial lesions that cause bony erosion (Fig. 17-77). Children with lesions causing respiratory distress or dysphagia require x-ray views that show details of the airway and soft tissue and endoscopic examination of the larynx, tracheobronchial tree, and esophagus. Other tests, such as computed tomography and barium swallow, may provide valuable information (Fig. 17-78).

Most head and neck lesions require surgery: drainage of abscesses, evaluation and relief of obstructive lesions, diagnostic biopsy of lesions to exclude malignancy, and removal of benign lesions for cosmetic reasons. However, many cases do not require surgical intervention, including most cases of cervical adenitis, torticollis, and hemangioma.

Scalp

Hemangiomas are common lesions in infancy that are soft or firm in consistency, bright red, and elevated (Fig. 17-79). They blanch when compressed and reexpand when released. A capillary hemangioma frequently involves the overlying skin. Large lesions may cover extensive regions of the scalp and face (Fig. 17-80). However, most lesions involute spontaneously over a period of 4 to 6 years, and expectant management has surprisingly good cosmetic results. Lesions that cover the eyes or occlude the airway require immediate intervention with prednisone, radiation therapy, or tracheotomy to bypass an obstruction.

Dermoid (or epidermal) cysts occur in regions of embryologic fusion. Hence they are frequently found at the corners of the eye, along the sternocleidomastoid, or in the midline of the face and neck (Fig. 17-81). They may be freely movable in the subcutaneous tissue or fixed to the skin or underlying skull. Those found in the preauricular area almost al-

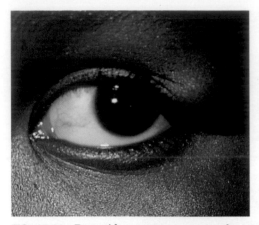

FIG. 17-81 Dermoid cyst occurs commonly at the lateral corner of the eye, pictured here, in the eyebrow, anterior to the ear, and in the midline of the neck.

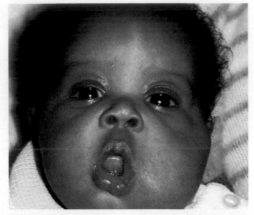

FIG. 17-82 A nontender mass over the parotid in an infant identifies a parotid hemangioma. This lesion will involute over the next few years and does not require excision.

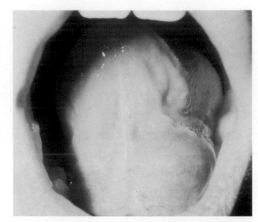

FIG. 17-83 A ranula arises in the floor of the mouth, created by congenital obstruction of the sublingual duct.

ways have a deep attachment to the origin of the helix cartilage. They have a thin wall that contains keratin and occasionally hair. Treatment is excision.

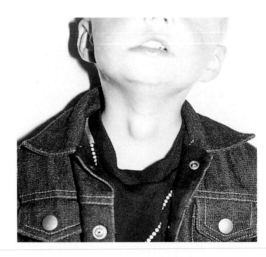

FIG. 17-84 Thyroglossal duct cyst produces a firm swelling in the midline of the neck. Its initial manifestation is sometimes a midline cervical abscess.

Face

Preauricular tags, cartilaginous remnants anterior to the ear, are common minor anomalies that are thought not to have a branchial cleft origin. Most are asymptomatic. Indications for removal are cosmetic. Preauricular sinus tracts end blindly beneath the skin, with hair or other epidermal elements at the base, and are probably closely related to preauricular dermoid cysts. Both tend to become infected, and complete removal of any subcutaneous portion is necessary to prevent recurrence.

Surgical lesions of the salivary glands are uncommon in infancy and childhood. Hemangioma of the parotid, the most common benign lesion, produces a unilateral swelling of the parotid within the first month of life (Fig. 17-82). It may increase in size over several months but involutes over 4 to 6 years (like most hemangiomas of the face and neck). A cutaneous sentinel hemangioma provides positive identification, and biopsy is usually unnecessary. Parotid swelling from inflammatory causes, such as mumps, bacteria (usually staphylococci or gram-negative rods), and different causes of chronic parotitis (chronic sialadenitis, sarcoidosis, and tuberculosis), cause tenderness and redness over the involved gland. The duct orifice may appear red or "pouting" when an inflammatory cause is present.

Mouth

Tongue-tie (ankyloglossia inferior), common in infancy, usually disappears spontaneously or with sucking. A thick, stout frenulum may interfere with speech development. Division of the frenulum is a simple cure.

A ranula forms from obstruction of the sublingual duct, forming a pseudocyst in the floor of the mouth (Fig. 17-83). A large ranula may cause upper airway obstruction in infancy. Marsupialization of the pseudocyst is an effective treatment.

Oral lymphangioma presents difficult problems in both short- and long-term management. It is the most common cause of macroglossia in infancy, although other causes, such as Beckwith syndrome and hypothyroidism, must be considered. An oral lymphangioma appears as a

raised, firm mass in the tongue and floor of the mouth, with tiny cysts over its surface. When extensive, the cysts may obstruct the upper airway. Suppurative glossitis, a common complication, is treated by intravenous antibiotics. Subtotal glossectomy is recommended to prevent prognathism and facilitate speech.

Lingual thyroid appears as a hill-like mass at the foramen cecum. An unusually large lingual thyroid may obstruct the airway in infants, but most present later in childhood as a "lump in the throat" when swallowing. The lingual thyroid, generally the only thyroid tissue present, produces insufficient thyroid hormone. Hypothyroidism may be present. Thyroid replacement is necessary after transoral excision, which is the treatment of choice.

Neck-Midline

Thyroglossal duct remnants, dermoid cysts, and enlarged lymph nodes are the common midline masses in the neck. During embryologic development, the thyroglossal duct arises from the foramen cecum, descends in the midline close to the hyoid, and gives rise to the thyroid gland upon reaching the neck. Incomplete regression of the duct may cause a cyst to form anywhere along its course from foramen cecum to sternal notch, most commonly just below the hyoid (Fig. 17-84). The cyst moves with swallowing and movement of the tongue, but these maneuvers do not distinguish a thyroglossal duct cyst with certainty.

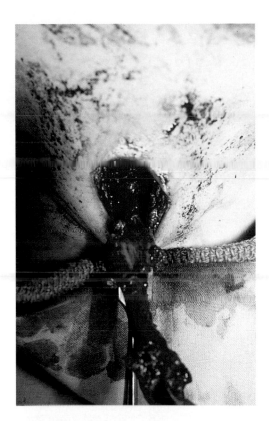

FIG. 17-85 The surgical specimen shows the thyroglossal duct as it courses from the lesion (pulled by the clamp), to the hyoid bone (swelling at the margin of the incision), and to the base of the tongue (in the depth of the incision).

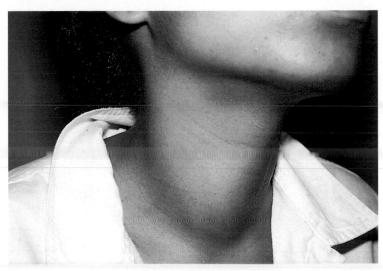

FIG. 17-86 Goiter in a 15-year-old girl, resulting from Hashimoto thyroiditis.

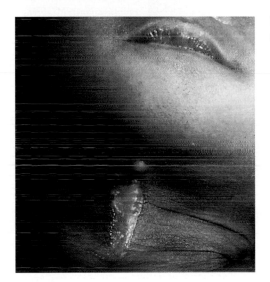

FIG. 17-87 Midline cervical cleft.

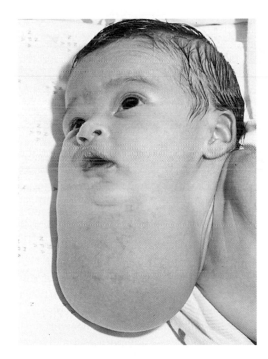

FIG. 17-88 Cystic hygroma involving the anterior triangle of the neck and the floor of the mouth. The cysts, which are large over the neck, are tiny and infiltrate the tongue and floor of the mouth, causing diffuse swelling that may compromise the upper airway.

Infection may result from its communication with the oropharynx. To reduce the risk of recurrence after surgical excision, the entire cyst and duct must be removed to the level of the foramen cecum, including the midportion of the hyoid (Fig. 17-85).

Thyroid nodules occur in children as in adults (Fig. 17-86). However, benign nodules are much less common, and the possibility that a palpable nodule is malignant is considerably greater in a child than in an adult. More than half of solitary nodules in children are malignant, and nearly all are papillary carcinomas. Nodular Hashimoto disease is the most common benign lesion. Thyroid scans are useful only in the identification of hyperfunctioning nodules, all of which are benign and are rarely seen in pediatrics. Fine-needle aspiration generally yields a

diagnosis in solid lesions and "cures" cystic ones, making ultrasound examination unnecessary. Total thyroidectomy is recommended for malignant thyroid lesions; lobectomy and isthmusectomy are recommended for benign lesions in which cancer cannot be ruled out.

Midline cervical cleft is a vertical streak of thinly epithelialized tissue in the anterior midline of the neck, probably the result of defective midline fusion of the branchial arches (Fig. 17-87).

Neck-Lateral

Cystic hygromas occur most commonly in the neck and axilla (Figs. 17-88 and 17-89). Most are discovered at birth; smaller lesions may be found

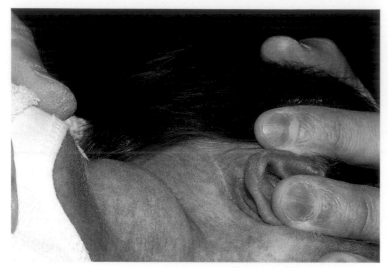

FIG. 17-89 Cystic hygroma extending from the posterior triangle.

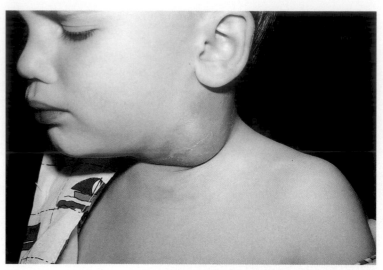

FIG. 17-90 Erythema and fluctuance identify the presence of an abscess. An abscess may be present without fluctuance, however, the result of induration from surrounding inflammation.

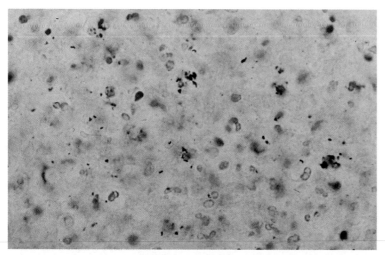

FIG. 17-91 Warthin-Starry silver stain identifies the black-staining organisms associated with cat-scratch disease, seen on examination of an enlarged lymph node.

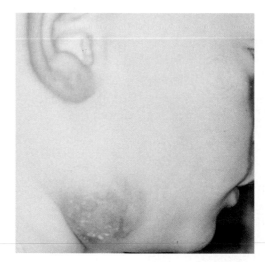

FIG. 17-92 The skin overlying a tuberculous lymph node is often discolored and may break down into a chronically draining sinus.

later in infancy. Composed of fluid-filled, thin-walled cysts, they are soft and transilluminate brightly. Those in the neck may compress the trachea or spread into the floor of the mouth or tongue, thus causing upper airway obstruction. Complications include hemorrhage and infection.

Benign lymphadenopathy of one of the anterior cervical lymph nodes is by far the most common neck mass. Nearly all cases result from nonspecific reactive hyperplasia to an infection in the ears, nose, mouth, throat, face, or scalp. Enlarged reactive nodes are generally small (less than 2 cm in diameter), minimally tender, and high in the anterior cervical chain (most commonly the so-called tonsillar node near the angle of the jaw), and they regress with resolution of the primary infection. Infection of the node itself makes the node more tender and enlarged, and the overlying skin becomes red. Early antibiotic therapy against staphylococci and streptococci may clear the infection. The development of fluctuance means suppuration has occurred, and incision and drainage are required for cure (Fig. 17-90). Needle aspiration may indicate the presence of pus within an involved node that is firm and free from areas of fluctuance.

Causes of chronic cervical adenopathy include cat-scratch disease, atypical mycobacteria (mycobacterium avium-intracellulare scrofulum,

or MAIS), and tuberculosis. Lymphadenopathy in cat-scratch disease arises 2 to 4 weeks after the animal scratch, which is usually healed and forgotten. Regression of node enlargement usually takes 2 to 4 weeks, but some cases may require months. When excised, silver stains reveal the cat-scratch organism (Fig. 17-91). Skin tests depend upon the availability of a reliable preparation of cat-scratch antigen.

Skin tests and chest films help to distinguish different causes of mycobacterial cervical adenitis. The most common cause is one of the MAIS complex. This form of mycobacterial infection is free from pulmonary involvement. Submandibular and preauricular lymph nodes typically are involved and are remarkably free from pain or tenderness. The nodes are fixed to surrounding tissues by perinodal inflammation. The overlying skin has a blue discoloration and may break down to form a draining sinus. Excision of the node and sinus is curative, and no antituberculous chemotherapy is required. In contrast, adenitis from *M. tuberculosis* (Fig. 17-92) is commonly complicated by coexisting chest disease, and antituberculous chemotherapy for active disease is necessary.

Painless cervical adenopathy is the most common presentation of Hodgkin disease, and on occasion it is the first manifestation of non-

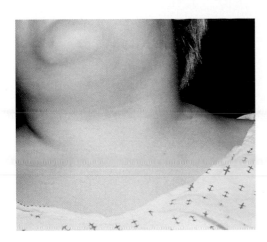

FIG. 17-93 Enlarged lymph nodes in unusual locations, such as in this patient with supraclavicular lymphadenopathy from non Hodgkin lymphoma, require excisional biopsy to rule out malignancy.

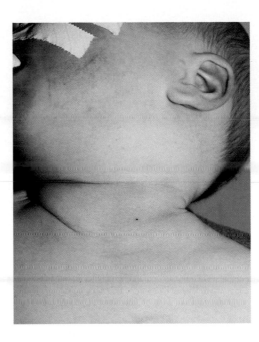

FIG. 17-94 Mucus may drain from a small punctum at the anterior border of the sternocleidomastoid, identifying it as the secondary opening of a second branchial cleft fistula. The primary opening lies in the tonsillar fossa.

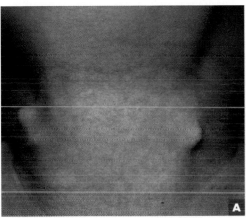

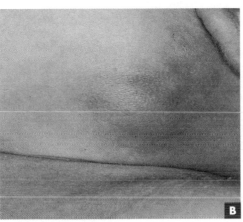

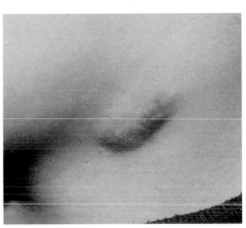

FIG. 17-95 Cartilaginous remnants from the second branchial cleft present as a mobile cyst beneath the anterior border of the sternocleidomastoid *(A)*. In another patient *(B)* the cyst was infected, producing redness of the overlying skin.

FIG. 17-96 First branchial arch fistula, previously diagnosed as an infected lymph node. The location of the secondary opening is near the angle of the mandible.

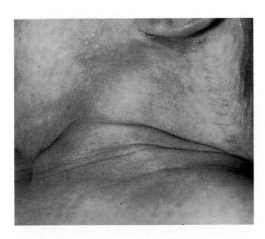

FIG. 17-97 The sternocleidomastoid in a newborn with torticollis may exist as a tight tendonlike cord or may swell and appear as a discrete tumor in the midportion of the muscle, pictured here.

Hodgkin lymphoma. Nodes involved with malignant lymphoma are enlarged, nontender, firm, and rubbery. Malignancy should be considered when large, painless nodes without signs of inflammation are discovered, particularly low in the neck and in the supraclavicular regions (Fig. 17-93). Incisional biopsy is necessary when studies fail to confirm

a definite diagnosis or enlargement continues despite treatment for a presumed infectious cause.

Branchial cleft remnants lead to the formation of cysts and fistulas in the lateral neck. A remnant of the second branchial cleft, the most common form, has an opening in the tonsillar fossa in the pharynx that runs along the anterior border of the sternocleidomastoid. A complete fistula drains mucus from a punctum located along this border (Fig. 17-94). When no cutaneous opening is present, a firm, mobile cyst forms. A neck abscess forms from superinfection (Fig. 17-95). Removal of the entire tract to the level of the primary opening in the tonsillar fossa prevents recurrence. First branchial cleft remnants, which are very rare, usually cannot be distinguished from an enlarged cervical node (Fig. 17-96). First branchial cleft fistulas lead from the external auditory canal to a point high in the neck at the angle of the mandible, very near branches of the facial nerve, a feature of obvious surgical importance.

Fibrous dysplasia of the sternocleidomastoid is the most common cause of torticollis in childhood. Two thirds of children have a firm, painless tumor within the muscle (Figs. 17-97 and 17-98), whereas the remainder have torticollis without the tumor. Daily exercises that force full rotation of the head upon the neck from side to side correct torti-

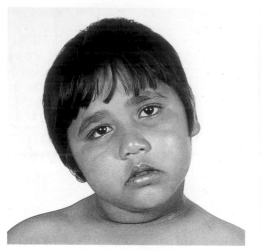

FIG. 17-98 Long-standing torticollis may cause permanent "wry-neck," facial shortening of the affected side of the face, and plagiocephaly.

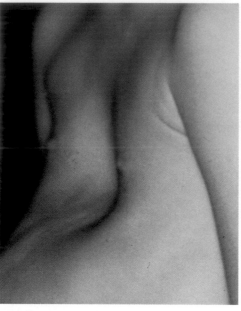

FIG. 17-99 Pectus excavatum (funnel chest) seldom creates cardiorespiratory symptoms, but psychologic consequences may be severe.

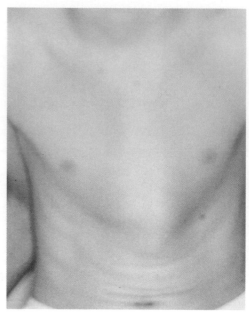

FIG. 17-100 The sternum projects like a keel in front of the anterior chest wall in pectus carinatum (pigeon chest). Like pectus excavatum, pectus carinatum produces no symptoms.

collis in most children, with surgical division of the muscle reserved for those who fail to respond. Neglected cases may lead to facial asymmetry and plagiocephaly.

Chest Wall

The sternum is concave downward, as well as side to side, in pectus excavatum (funnel chest), the most common congenital deformity of the chest wall (Fig. 17-99). The concavity also involves the costal cartilages and rotates to the right. Although infants with dyspnea exhibit sternal retractions and ultimately may develop a fixed deformity, the pectus excavatum frequently arises in children free from respiratory problems. The deformity arises gradually in infancy and becomes more pronounced as the child grows. It fails to significantly compromise cardiorespiratory function in nearly all cases. Its appearance produces psychologic effects that may lead to withdrawal from activities that expose the chest (such as swimming).

The sternum pushes forward like a keel in pectus carinatum (pigeon chest), with depression of the costal cartilages on either side (Fig. 17-100). A second form, "pouter pigeon chest," appears as a Z in profile: prominence of the manubrium, depression of the upper sternum, and protrusion of the lower sternum. The deformity first becomes obvious at age 3 to 4 years and becomes increasingly apparent. There are no functional side effects.

Poland syndrome is a rare chest anomaly that includes unilateral absence of the second, third, and fourth costal cartilages and ribs, with hypoplasia or absence of the overlying pectoralis muscles, subcutaneous tissue, breast, and nipple (Fig. 17-101). The ipsilateral fingers may be short and webbed. Ectopia cordis may complicate sternal cleft, one of the features of pentalogy of Cantrell, discussed later as an abdominal wall anomaly. Complex congenital heart defects complicate ectopia cordis frequently; tetralogy of Fallot and ventricular diverticulum are common.

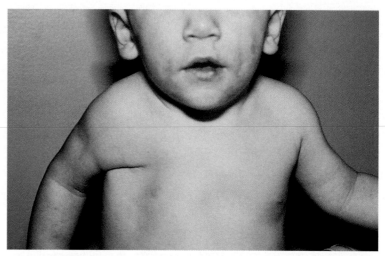

FIG. 17-101 Congenital unilateral absence of the anterior ribs, muscle, and soft tissues characterize Poland syndrome, producing its typical appearance pictured here.

Along with the neck, the axilla is the most common site of cystic hygroma, which may communicate between the two regions. A chest film is necessary because the lesion may extend into the mediastinum.

Mastitis and abscess are the most common breast lesions in newborns. Nearly all cases of mastitis respond to warm compresses and antibiotics; failure of inflammation to resolve indicates an abscess that requires drainage. Localized breast masses in children are nearly always benign. Fibroadenomas, accounting for up to 90% of reported cases, form a mobile, smooth mass within the breast. Growth may produce lesions that replace a large portion of the breast, making a cosmetically pleasing excision difficult. Fibrocystic disease, another common disorder, affects primarily older adolescents. One to several firm, fixed masses gradually become prominent in a breast that has diffuse areas of cordlike thickening, which represent overgrowth of fibrous tissue.

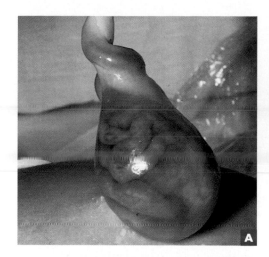

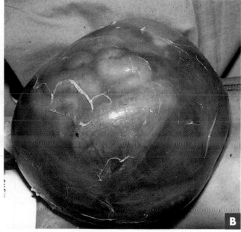

FIG. 17-102 *A,* A small omphalocele with the umbilical cord attached to the apex of the sac. In the absence of chromosomal anomalies, other anomalies are rare and the ultimate prognosis is good. *B,* A giant omphalocele containing liver, stomach, and intestines. Other anomalies, particularly cardiac, that affect prognosis are common.

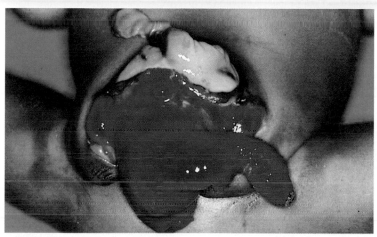

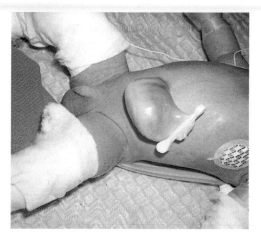

FIG. 17-104 A small omphalocele is easily reduced into the abdomen.

FIG. 17-103 Cloacal exstrophy consists of an omphalocele superiorly, below which the bladder is separated into halves by the exposed intestine. Both the proximal and distal bowel loops have prolapsed, producing the "elephant trunk" appearance.

Size, consistency, and tenderness of the masses change with different phases of the menstrual cycle, a characteristic of the disease. Because the condition increases the patient's risk for breast cancer, breast self-examination should begin at an early age. Nipple discharge, unusual in childhood and adolescence, indicates the presence of intraductal papilloma, fibrocystic disease, or ductal ectasia. Cytologic examination of fine-needle aspiration from the mass provides a reliable means of diagnosis. Excisional biopsy should be avoided in prepubertal girls because surgical damage to the small, immature breast magnifies as the breast increases in size at maturity, with potential disfigurement. Rapidly enlarging breast masses should be removed to avoid distortion of the architecture of the remaining breast tissue. Small lesions can be safely monitored after confirmation of a benign diagnosis clinically or by fine-needle aspiration. Breast enlargement in boys is common in the first 2 years after the onset of puberty; thereafter resolution is gradual and complete. Psychologic problems and social pressures justify subcutaneous mastectomies in boys with persistent enlargement or prominent breasts.

Abdominal Wall

Gastroschisis and Omphalocele

Omphalocele and gastroschisis are the two major congenital abdominal wall defects of the newborn. In omphalocele the viscera herniates through the umbilical region of the abdomen, covered by peritoneum and amniotic membrane. The umbilical cord emerges from the sac that covers the herniated organs. In the most common form of omphalocele, the defect is placed centrally in the abdomen and contains the liver, stomach, and intestine (Fig. 17-102). Failure of the upper abdominal fold to form causes a defect in the epigastrium and lower chest; ectopia cordis with intracardiac malformation, sternal cleft, and diaphragmatic hernia may be present in addition to omphalocele (pentalogy of Cantrell). Failure of the lower abdominal fold to form creates an omphalocele inferior to the umbilicus, which is associated with a number of lower body structures: spina bifida with myelomeningocele, imperforate anus, and cloacal exstrophy (caudal regression syndrome, Fig. 17-103). Chromosomal anomalies, cardiac defects, and other extraabdominal anomalies occur commonly in large omphaloceles and are the primary limitations of survival. The volume of herniated viscera may preclude primary closure of the abdomen, making a staged closure using a silastic abdominal prosthesis necessary. With either approach, reduction of the viscera may lead to respiratory insufficiency.

An umbilical defect less than 4 cm in diameter and containing only loops of intestine represents a small omphalocele or hernia of the umbilical cord (Fig. 17-104). Those not associated with chromosomal anomalies are frequently free from any other anomalies. Repair is simple and gives a good cosmetic result.

The defect in gastroschisis is a hole to the right of the umbilical cord, which lies intact and separate from the defect (Fig. 17-105). Often

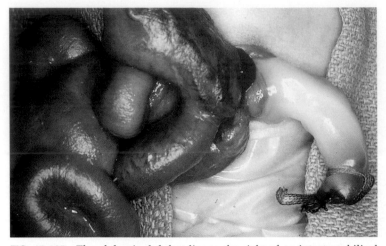

FIG. 17-105   The abdominal defect lies to the right of an intact umbilical cord, and the intestines lie exposed without a covering sac, free in the amniotic fluid. Both distinguish gastroschisis, pictured here, from omphalocele.

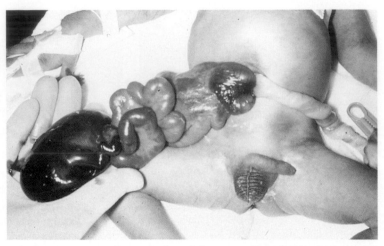

FIG. 17-106   Intrauterine volvulus of the cecum (purple in color) complicates this case of gastroschisis. Occurrence earlier in gestation may have led to absorption of the involved loop of bowel and may have resulted in an atresia. Extraintestinal anomalies are rare in gastrochisis.

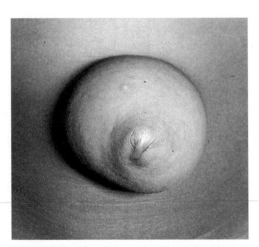

FIG. 17-107   Most infants with umbilical hernia undergo spontaneous closure by age 3 to 4 years. Those that persist require repair.

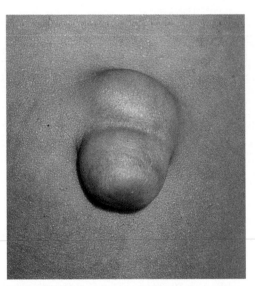

FIG. 17-108   Supraumbilical hernia, shown here as a crescent-shaped defect above an umbilical hernia, does not close spontaneously and requires repair.

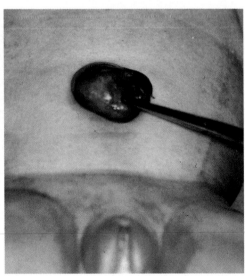

FIG. 17-109   Intestinal contents drain from the umbilicus through an omphalomesenteric fistula.

a thick inflammatory membrane ("peel") covers the extruded intestine, which lies outside the abdomen without covering. The stomach and bladder, but not the liver, may also lie outside the body. The identification of organs that lie outside the body contour and the presence of a sac represent important differentiating signs on antenatal diagnosis. Intestinal atresias complicate gastroschisis in some cases, probably a result of inflammation induced by exposure to amniotic fluid in utero or volvulus (Fig. 17-106). Extraintestinal anomalies are uncommon. Some authors suggest that gastroschisis may represent hernias of the cord that ruptured in utero; these are similar in that both are largely free from associated anomalies. The right-sided location is a consequence of the absence of the right umbilical vein in humans, leaving a relatively weak area at the base of the cord on the right side. Primary closure of gastroschisis is the preferred mode of management, but some may require a staged repair. Parenteral nutritional support is a frequent necessity because slow recovery of intestinal function is characteristic.

Umbilicus

The most common minor umbilical anomaly is umbilical hernia (Fig. 17-107). It is six to ten times more prevalent in black children than in whites. Most close spontaneously, the majority within the first 3 years of life. They rarely incarcerate, and so repair is reserved for cases that do not close by 3 to 4 years of age. Resembling an umbilical hernia but actually situated superior to the umbilicus, a supraumbilical hernia does not resolve spontaneously and requires repair (Fig. 17-108). An umbilical granuloma forms after separation of the cord remnant in infants. Easily recognized as a friable polypoid mass emerging from a short stalk, it is treated by simple ligation. Drainage of intestinal contents signifies the presence of an omphalomesenteric fistula (Fig. 17-109), which represents a persistence of the communication between the embryonic midgut and the yolk sac. Division of the fistula is necessary to stop the drainage and prevent volvulus. Drainage of urine indicates the presence of a patent urachus, which represents a remnant of the connection between the embryonic

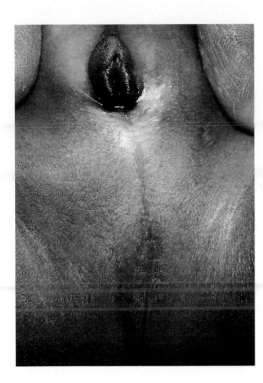

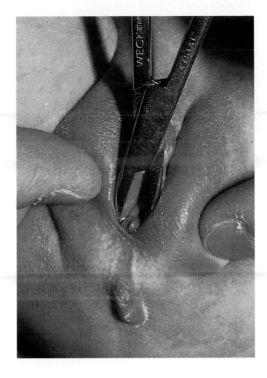

FIG. 17-123 Cloacal anomaly is the most complete expression of imperforate anus in girls, with urinary, genital, and intestinal tracts converging into a single cloacal channel that exists as the sole perineal opening.

FIG. 17-124 An intermediate lesion passes partially through the levator ani but fails to approach the perineum as closely as low lesions.

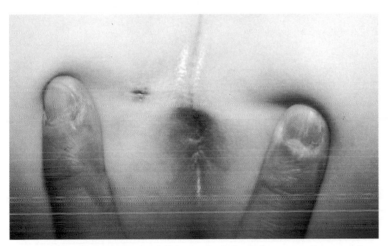

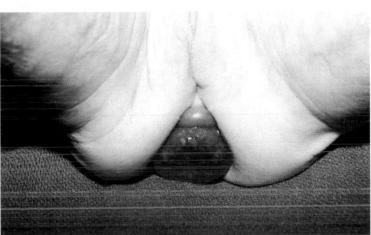

FIG. 17-125 A punctum is visible to the left of the anus, the secondary opening of a fistula arising from an anal crypt within the anal canal. Recurrent abscesses arise from a well-formed fistula like this one, an indication of fistulectomy.

FIG. 17-126 Although the cause of rectal prolapse is unknown in the majority of cases, all infants should be evaluated for cystic fibrosis.

granulomatous disease, nearly all cases that occur in infancy are idiopathic.

The cause of rectal prolapse is unknown in the majority of cases (Fig. 17-126). Inadequate perineal innervation and atrophy of the supporting musculature of the perineum explains rectal prolapse in children with spina bifida. Prolapse also occurs in children with cystic fibrosis, where the cause is less clear. Hookworm infestation can cause tenesmus and straining that can result in prolapse. Idiopathic rectal prolapse has a peak incidence in the second year of life, often brought on by an acute diarrheal illness or a severe episode of constipation. Incarceration is extremely rare, and the parents should be instructed how to reduce the prolapsed rectum. The condition resolves with resolution of diarrhea or effective dietary changes that address constipation. All such patients should undergo a sweat test to rule out cystic fibrosis. Refractory cases should undergo stool examination for ova and parasites, as well as sigmoidoscopy and contrast study of the colon to check for the possible presence of polyps and worm infestation. Circumferential

injection of a sclerosing solution, such as 20% dextrose solution, into the submucosa is simple and effective treatment.

Anal fissure, another common problem among infants, was discussed previously as a cause of gastrointestinal bleeding.

BIBLIOGRAPHY

Ashcraft KW, Holder TM: *Pediatric surgery,* ed 2 Philadelphia, 1992, WB Saunders.

Knight PJ, Reiner CB: Superficial lumps in children: what, when and why? *Pediatrics* 72:147-153, 1983.

Rowe MI, O'Neill JA Jr, Grosfeld JL, et al: *Essentials of pediatric surgery,* St Louis, 1995, Mosby-Year Book.

Sheldon CA, Martin LW: Pediatric surgery, *Surg Clin North Am* 65:1059-1687, 1985.

Welch KJ, Randolph JG, Ravitch MM, et al: *Pediatric surgery,* ed 4, Chicago, 1986, Year Book.

18

Pediatric and Adolescent Gynecology

PAMELA J. MURRAY ❦ HOLLY W. DAVIS
MELISSA HAMP

Pediatricians and other primary care physicians who treat children and adolescents are increasingly confronted with patients with gynecologic complaints. This trend stems in part from earlier onset of sexual activity and consequent concerns about pregnancy prevention and sexually transmitted diseases (STDs). In addition, there is increased media, public, and family discussion of sexual and gynecologic subjects. Today, young women and their mothers are more inclined to seek medical attention for reproductive system problems, including dysmenorrhea, abnormal uterine bleeding, and vaginal discharges. The increased survival of children with chronic illnesses creates another patient group in need of skilled and sensitive attention to the psychologic and physiologic aspects of their sexual development.

Among primary care physicians there is a growing interest in gynecologic pediatrics and adolescent medicine. Many are increasing their understanding of the gynecologic conditions affecting children and adolescents, including vulvovaginitis, STDs, menstrual disorders, and sexual abuse. In the current practice environment there are pressures and incentives to evaluate and treat problems without referral, incorporating women's gynecologic health concerns into primary care. Hence, an adolescent's first pelvic examination may no longer require transferring "well-child care" to a gynecologist. Accordingly this chapter emphasizes normal anatomy, techniques of examination, and the pathologic conditions most commonly encountered: inflammation, infections, gynecologic trauma, and obstructive anatomic abnormalities.

See Chapter 6 for a more detailed description of the approach to sexual abuse and an outline of specimen collection in the prepubertal girl. Chapter 9 illustrates Tanner staging and discusses normal, delayed, and precocious puberty.

Normal Female Genitalia

Newborn and Prepubertal Periods

In the newborn girl the physical appearance of the genitalia reflects stimulation by maternal hormones. The labia majora appear puffy, and the thickened labia minora protrude between them (Fig. 18-1). Separa-

tion of the labia minora reveals thick, redundant hymenal folds that often hide the small central vaginal opening and urethral meatus. The mucosa is pink and moist, vaginal pH is acidic, and a milky discharge (physiologic leukorrhea) is seen often. Vaginal bleeding during the first week of life is common. It is caused by the withdrawal of maternal estrogen, and parents can be reassured that this is normal. Breast development with palpable breast tissue, engorgement, and less commonly a clear or cloudy discharge is observed in full-term neonates of both genders (see Chapter 2). Without ongoing estrogen stimulation, these findings gradually subside over several months as maternal estrogen levels fall. During this period, infants are at increased risk for developing breast inflammation and infection (see Chapter 12). Local trauma, including squeezing, may increase the likelihood of infection.

Similarly, over the first 6 to 8 weeks of life the effect of maternal hormones on the female genitalia abates; the labia majora lose their fullness, and the labia minora and hymen gradually become thinner and flatter. Separation of the labia minora usually exposes the vaginal opening (Fig. 18-2). As the young infant matures, the labia cover less of the vaginal vestibule, particularly when the infant or child is sitting, and thus offer incomplete protection from external sources of irritation. The mucosa is thin, relatively atrophic, and has a glistening, reddish hue. On first inspection this normal red vascular appearance sometimes is mistaken for inflammation by observers unaccustomed to examining prepubertal genitalia. Vaginal pH is now neutral or alkaline, and secretions are minimal.

Physiologic changes also cause variations in the appearance of the hymenal tissues during childhood. During infancy the tissues remain relatively thick and often are redundant (Fig. 18-3, A), but by about 18 to 24 months of age the hymen is thin and translucent, with smooth edges (Figs. 18-2 and 18-3, B to D). When the child enters puberty, the hymen thickens under the influence of estradiol.

The shape of the vaginal orifice also varies. Annular (Fig. 18-3, B), crescentic (Fig. 18-3, C and D), and fimbriated hymens are all normal variations. Fimbriated hymens become less common as girls approach school age. Other irregular shapes occur, such as a teardrop with the narrow portion formed by a notch to one side of the clitoris (Fig. 18-6,

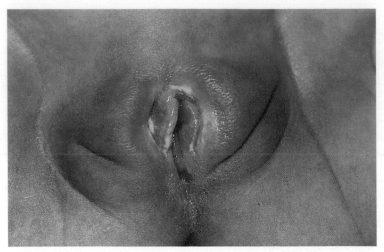

FIG. 18-1 Normal appearance of the genitalia in a newborn girl. The labia majora are full, and the thickened labia minora protrude between them. The mucosa is pink, and a milky white discharge is seen, reflecting stimulation by maternal hormones. (Courtesy Dr. Ian Holzman, New York.)

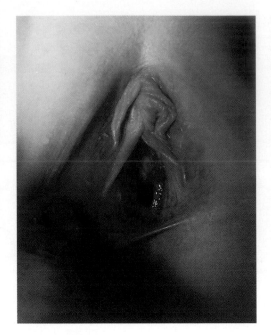

FIG. 18-2 Normal appearance of the genitalia of a 2-year-old girl. The labia majora are flattened, and the labia minora and hymen are thin and flat. The vaginal orifice is easily seen, and the mucosa is thin, relatively atrophic, and red in color. Visualization was facilitated by use of the labial traction technique with the patient in the semisupine lithotomy position.

A and *D*). On rare occasions a complete septum (Fig. 18-3, *E*) or a fenestrated hymen is seen.

The normal transverse diameter of the hymenal orifice is approximately 1 mm per year of age, although deviations of 2 to 3 mm in either direction can be within normal limits. The appearance of the hymen is probably of greater significance in the diagnosis of sexual abuse than is the transverse diameter alone (see Chapter 6).

From about 6 to 8 weeks of age until puberty the perineum, perivaginal tissues, and pelvic supporting structures are relatively rigid and inelastic. This factor increases the likelihood of tearing as a result of trauma. In addition, before the onset of puberty, the ovaries are positioned above the pelvic brim. This intraabdominal location accounts for the fact that ovarian disorders in childhood more frequently present with abdominal than pelvic signs and symptoms.

Peripubertal Period

With the onset of puberty the mons pubis begins to thicken and midline hair begins to form. Fat deposition fills out the labia majora. The labia minora thicken, become softer, and are more rounded. The clitoris enlarges slightly, and the urethra becomes more prominent. The hymen also thickens as its central orifice enlarges. The vaginal mucosa thickens and softens and becomes moist and pink because secretions increase and pH levels drop. Perineal and pelvic tissues become more elastic, and the ovaries gradually descend into the pelvis. In the months preceding menarche, physiologic leukorrhea increases and becomes noticeable. It consists of a white discharge containing mature epithelial cells and vaginal secretions stimulated by estrogen (Fig. 18-4). The developmental aspects of gynecologic anatomy and physiology are summarized in Table 18-1. The Tanner stages of pubertal development are presented in Chapter 9.

Gynecologic Evaluation

Examination of the Prepubertal Patient

Indications

Inspection of the external genitalia should be a part of every general physical examination. Careful perineal inspection of girls at the new-

born, 2-week, and 8-week visits enables early identification of congenital anomalies of the labia and hymen. Anomalies of these structures are relatively uncommon and, with the exception of vaginal agenesis, are not associated with malformations of the upper genital or urinary tract.

Evidence of virilization noted in the newborn, especially when accompanied by hyperpigmentation, should prompt immediate laboratory investigation for evidence of salt-losing adrenal hyperplasia.

The uterus, cervix, and fallopian tubes are derived from the müllerian, or paramesonephric, ducts and develop concurrently with the urinary tract. Thus girls with renal and/or urinary tract abnormalities are at greater risk for having associated anomalies of internal genital structures. During puberty, if menarche is delayed or unusually problematic (e.g., excessive pain, unusually irregular flow patterns) ultrasound evaluation should be considered for these patients. Before puberty, ultrasound examination of the internal pelvic structure is unreliable.

Routine inspection of the external genitalia at each subsequent well-child care visit is recommended because it facilitates early diagnosis of any problems that may arise. This practice also creates an opportunity to discuss normal anatomy and behaviors, including masturbation; to distinguish acceptable from unacceptable (abusive) forms of touching; and to help overcome the reluctance of some parents to express concerns about the genitalia. Ultimately, making assessment and counseling a routine part of well-child care may help reduce anxiety and embarrassment for the child when pelvic examinations are necessary after puberty.

Patients who have certain complaints at acute care visits warrant inspection of the genitalia and on occasion internal examination. These complaints include abdominal pain; dysuria, urinary frequency, urgency, incontinence, or enuresis; constipation or encopresis; perineal pruritus and/or pain; vaginal discharge or bleeding before menarche; and suspected or acknowledged sexual abuse. Maternal diethylstilbestrol (DES) exposure during pregnancy is an indication for earlier and special gynecologic evaluation. There should be no in utero DES exposure among young people born after 1972.

Technique

Whether the patient is being seen for a routine checkup or for a specific problem, the gynecologic portion of the assessment should occur after establishing rapport to avoid frightening the child. Parental and

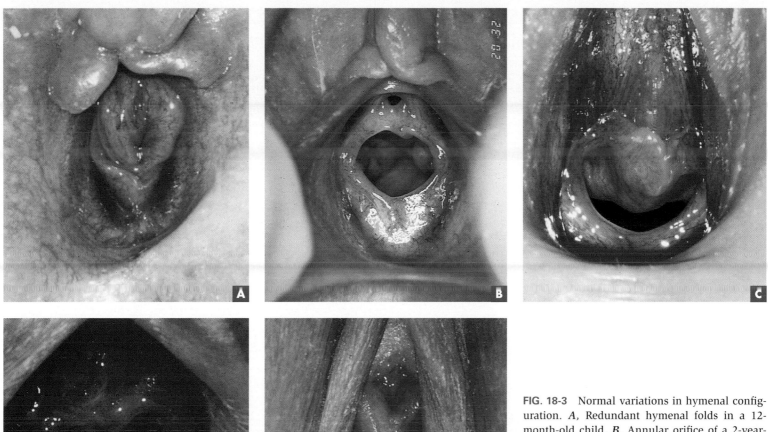

FIG. 18-3 Normal variations in hymenal configuration. *A,* Redundant hymenal folds in a 12-month-old child. *B,* Annular orifice of a 2-year-old. Note the thin sharp edges of the membrane. *C,* Crescentic hymenal orifice. *D,* Crescentic orifice with septal remnants at 1 and 5 o'clock. *E,* Septate hymen. See also Fig. 18-6 (*A, C, D,* and *E* courtesy Dr. Pat Bruno, Sunbury Community Hospital Center for Child Protection, Sunbury, Penn; *B* courtesy Dr. John McCann, University of California at Davis.)

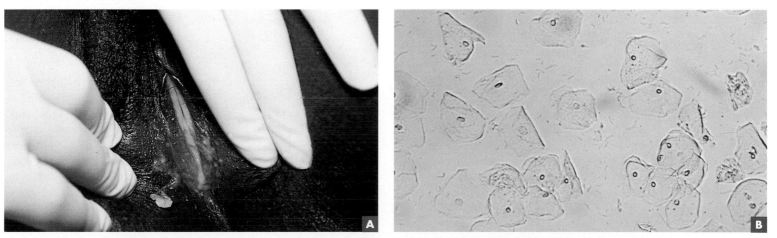

FIG. 18-4 Physiologic leukorrhea. *A,* The clinical appearance of this milky discharge is seen on the perineum of this normal adolescent. It consists of cervical and vaginal secretions produced in response to estrogen stimulation and is evident in the newborn, peripubertal, and postpubertal periods. *B,* On microscopy the discharge is found to contain sheets of estrogenized vaginal epithelial cells. Leukocytes are not increased and lactobacilli are the predominant flora.

TABLE 18-1

Developmental Gynecologic Anatomy and Physiology

	Newborn	Early childhood	Peripuberty (8–13 yrs)	Postmenarche (>13 yrs)
Ovary	Not palpable 0.1–0.2 cc	Pelvic brim 0.7–0.9 cc	Within pelvis 2–10 cc	1.5 × 2.5 × 4 cm 15 cc
Uterine length (cm)	2.5–4.0	2.0–3.0	3.2–5.4	8.0 (nulliparous) (8 × 5 × 2.5)
Corpus-cervix ratio	3:1	2:1	1:1	2–3:1
Vaginal length (cm)	4	4–5	7–8.5	10–12
Hymen				
Orifice diameter (mm)	1–4	1–6	5–10	10
Thickness	Thick	Thin	Thickening	—
Clitoris				
Width (mm)	5	2–5	2–5	≤10
Length (mm)	10–15			15–20
Labia minora	Smooth	Smooth, flat	Progressive increase in size and texture	Tanner stages IV-V completed
Labia majora	Hairless, prominent	Hairless, thin	Hair growth, vulval growth	Separation and differentiation of labia minora and majora
Vaginal secretions	Whitish-clear, copious	Minimal	Physiologic leukorrhea	Physiologic leukorrhea may decrease
pH	5.5–7.0	6.5–7.5	4.5–5.5	3.5–5.0
Normal flora	Maternal enteric	Nonpathogenic flora including Staph and coliforms	Mixed vaginal flora	Lactobacilli dominant
Hormonal influence	Maternal hormones	Minimal sex steroids	Low and variable levels of endogenous estrogen and androgens	High levels of endogenous cyclic hormones
Maturation index of vaginal epithelium				Proliferative phase* / Secretory phase†
Parabasal (%)	0	90-100	20-70	0 / 0
Intermediate (%)	95	0-10	25-50	70 / 95
Superficial (%)	5	10	10-20	30 / 5

*First half of cycle.
†Second half of cycle.

physician comfort levels are communicated to the child. A discussion of any parental anxieties and the clinician's self-awareness of his or her own attitudes may facilitate a more successful examination. Careful evaluation of physical growth and secondary sex characteristics is important for patients in the peripubertal and pubertal periods. All children with potential gynecologic problems deserve a thorough abdominal and inguinal examination.

Adequate preparation is important before the gynecologic assessment. Using terms or language familiar to the child may facilitate cooperation, and interspersing anatomically correct vocabulary may be educational and can enhance understanding. For routine checkups the task is simple external inspection. In such instances, after abdominal and inguinal examination, the clinician generally can say to patients old enough to understand, "Now, I need to take a look at your bottom, and you can help me." The desired position for examination can be ex-

plained or demonstrated and the patient shown how to maneuver into it. Drapes generally are unnecessary because they are isolating and often perceived as threatening by prepubertal and peripubertal patients.

Young infants can be assessed easily on an examination table after being positioned by the examiner. Older infants, toddlers, and preschool children tend to be more relaxed when examined on their mother's lap, with the mother assisting by gently holding the child in either the frog-leg or lithotomy position (Fig. 18-5). School-age children usually are able to be examined on the table in the frog-leg, lithotomy, or knee-chest position (see Chapter 6). The latter enables the best visualization of the vagina and may even permit inspection of the cervix because on deep breathing the vaginal orifice tends to open widely (Fig. 18-6, A). This phenomenon also facilitates specimen collection. Although the knee-chest position is unacceptable to some patients who feel threatened by examination from behind, it can be very useful for selected school-age patients.

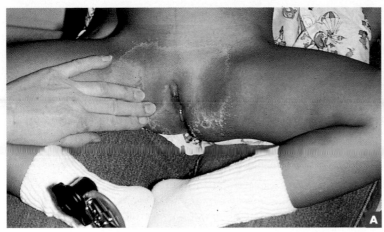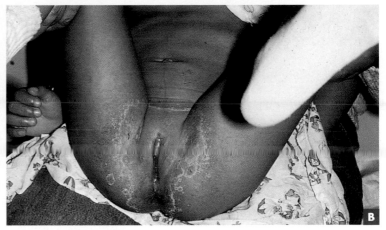

FIG. 18-5 Optimal positions for perineal inspection of the young prepubertal girl. *A,* Frog leg position on the mother's lap. *B,* Lithotomy position on the mother's lap.

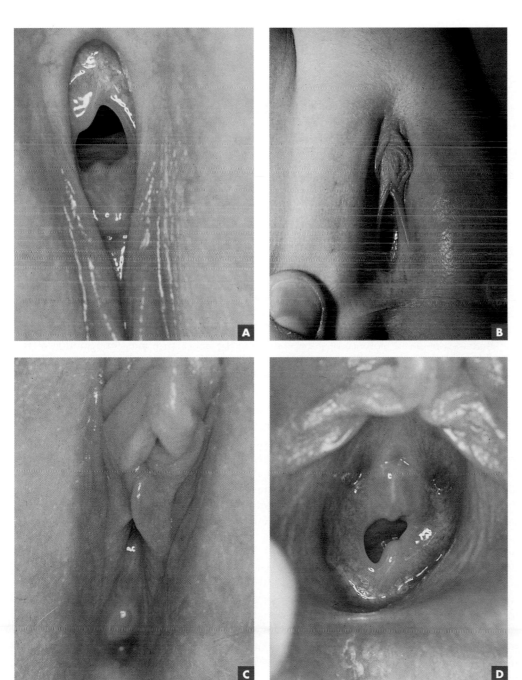

FIG. 18-6 Perineal visualization in various positions and with different techniques of parting the labia. *A,* Knee-chest position. *B,* Semisupine lithotomy position with labial separation. To facilitate visualization of the introitus and lower third of the vagina, the examiner can either press down and laterally on the labia majora with the index and middle fingers of both hands as shown here or gently grasp the labia majora between thumbs and index fingers and pull down and laterally. *C,* Supine frog-leg position with labial separation *D,* Supine frog-leg position with labial traction. *A, C,* and *D* are views of the same child, taken on the same day and clearly show the variations in appearance using different positions and different techniques. *B* and Fig. 18-2 are two views of another child. (*A, C,* and *D* courtesy Dr. Mary Carrasco, Children's Hospital of Pittsburgh.)

TABLE 18-2

Laboratory Investigations Contributing to the Diagnosis of Vulvovaginitis with Vaginal Discharge

Laboratory study	Indication
Saline wet mount	Yeast, *Trichomonas* organisms, clue cells, inflammatory cells, pinworms, sperm
Gram stain	Inflammatory cells, gram-negative intracellular diplococci (gonorrhea), other bacteria, clue cells
KOH	Yeast, "whiff test" for bacterial vaginosis (also can be positive for *Trichomonas* organisms)
Vaginal pH	Bacterial vaginosis, *Trichomonas* organisms, (lateral or anterior wall, not pooled secretions)
Cervical/vaginal cultures	Routine culture for normal flora, nonvenereal pathogens; gonorrhea culture; culture in stool transport media for enteric bacteria, especially *Shigella* organisms; anaerobic cultures; viral culture for herpes simplex virus (HSV); chlamydia culture (for prepubertal patients and forensic evidence); *Mycoplasma* and *Ureaplasma* organism cultures; *Trichomonas* organism culture
Urethral cultures	Chlamydia, gonorrhea, *Trichomonas* organisms
Pap smear	Squamous intraepithelial lesions; precancerous and cancerous cervical lesions: nonspecific inflammation or evidence suggestive of HPV (koilocytes), HSV, fungi*, *Trichomonas* organisms*, chlamydia; cell maturation index (estrogenization)
Tzanck smear (Giemsa stain)	HSV (multinucleated giant cells)
Perianal Scotch tape test	Pinworms and eggs
Blood test	Rapid plasma reagin (RPR) for syphilis, HIV titers, hepatitis serology
Urine test	Urinalysis, and urine culture, *Trichomonas* organisms
DNA-PCR	Chlamydia
Antigen-detection assays	Chlamydia, (chlamydiazyme, Micro-tek)
Biopsy	Dysplastic, atrophic, and unusual lesions of vulva, vagina, and cervix
DNA probes (without amplification)	GC, chlamydia, *Trichomonas* organisms, yeast, and bacterial vaginosis

*See text, do not treat based on Pap results alone.

Inspection is facilitated by use of good, focused lighting. In the office setting the otoscope provides light and magnification. However, many young children associate it with discomfort and restraint because of prior painful experiences during otoscopy. Hence, before its use, the patient must be reassured that no speculum is attached and that she will not be forcibly restrained. Colposcopes and hand-held lenses also provide good magnification when available.

Once the patient is in position, visualization of the introitus, hymen, and lower portion of the vagina is facilitated by maneuvers that separate the labia. These maneuvers should be explained first and the child reassured that the examiner is just going to look. If the patient desires or is mildly anxious, she may place her hands beneath the examiner's, or the mother may be enlisted to perform the maneuver. Some girls prefer to separate their labia themselves. The maneuvers include labial separation, which is achieved by pressing down and laterally with the index and middle fingers of both hands on the lower portion of the labia majora (Fig. 18-6, *B* and *C*), and labial traction, which involves grasping the labia majora between the thumbs and index fingers and gently pulling them down laterally and slightly toward the examiner (Figs. 18-6, *D* and 18-2). Care must be taken to ensure that excess traction is not applied during these maneuvers because it can result in painful tearing of labial adhesions, if present.

If the patient is unusually anxious about the procedure and cannot be reassured, the examination should be deferred to a later date. At no time should an anxious, struggling child be physically restrained and forced to undergo examination; the yield is minimal and the experience physically and emotionally traumatic.

On inspection the physician can readily ascertain the presence or absence of pubic hair; note the appearance and configuration of the labia majora, labia minora, clitoris, urethra, hymen, and vaginal orifice; observe the color of the mucosa and the presence or absence of rash or discharge; and visualize the distal vagina. Vaginoscopy is required only occasionally in the prepubertal child and then only in those with specific problems. These problems include vaginal bleeding with or without evidence of trauma, discharges resistant to routine therapy, a suspected vaginal foreign body, and suspected vaginal tumors. Because of the high potential for inflicting pain, especially if the patient moves suddenly, vaginoscopy generally is best performed under anesthesia. Older school-age children may tolerate internal examination by a skilled examiner without sedation if preparation is careful. Again, a traumatic experience should be avoided.

If a child with vaginal discharge or perineal or urinary complaints is to be evaluated, it is advisable to ask the family not to bathe the patient or apply any creams for at least 12 hours before the examination. Similarly, adolescents should be advised never to douche or use tampons or intravaginal creams before an examination. The patient should always be prepared for the procedure with simple and truthful explanations. It is often helpful to let her handle a swab or catheter and touch herself with it.

TABLE 18-3

Indications for Pelvic Examination of Adolescent Patients

Abnormal vaginal discharge
Pain
  Pelvic
  Perineal
  Dysuria
  Abdominal (unexplained)
Sexual activity
  Routine sexual health care (i.e., routine health care for sexually active individual)
  Sexual contact with partner with a suspected or confirmed STD or related genital symptoms
Suspected sexual abuse (see Chapter 6)
Concerns with pubertal development (see Chapter 9)
  No secondary sexual development by age 14
  No menarche by age 16, earlier if start of puberty >2 years and no menarche
  Abnormal sequence or plateau of pubertal development
  Anatomic abnormalities on genital inspection
  Increased body hair, severe acne, or masculinization
Menstrual disturbances
  Severe dysmenorrhea
  Amenorrhea or oligomenorrhea
  Abnormal uterine bleeding or polymenorrhea
Patient request (with support from history)
DES exposure (little use after 1971)

When specimens of vaginal secretions are required for cultures, wet mounts, cytology, or maturation index, they can be collected easily and with little or no discomfort by use of Dacron wire swabs premoistened with sterile nonbacteriostatic saline. However, if collection is likely to be difficult because of pain or anxiety or because the orifice is very small, application of 2% lidocaine ointment to the perineal and hymenal area 5 minutes beforehand is often beneficial.

Routine bacterial cultures, including those for gonococci can be collected from any visible discharge on the perineum; chlamydia cultures however, must contain superficial cells from the vaginal wall. Herpes cultures should be obtained from the base of fresh vesicles or ulcers. If no discharge is visible on the perineum, having the patient perform a Valsalva maneuver may bring discharge down to the introitus. If this fails and specimens must be collected because of history of discharge or suspicion of sexual abuse, a small, premoistened swab or soft 18- to 19-gauge catheter is inserted gently through the vaginal opening with care taken to avoid contact with the hymen, which is exquisitely sensitive. Dry cotton-tipped swabs should be avoided because they tend to abrade the thin vaginal mucosa of the prepubertal child. When a discharge is present, it can be gently aspirated through a catheter. In the absence of discharge, 1 to 2 cc of prewarmed sterile nonbacteriostatic saline can be instilled slowly and then aspirated back. Because single chambered catheters can adhere to the vaginal wall when suction is applied, a double catheter described by Pokorny is preferable. By using a soft catheter, enough material can be obtained via aspiration for multi-ple culture swabs and smears. Chlamydia cultures, however, must include cellular material obtained directly from the mucosal surface, necessitating use of a Dacron swab moistened with nonbacteriostatic saline. Table 18-2 lists the specimens that may be considered in evaluating patients with symptoms of vulvitis, vaginitis, or vaginal discharge.

Patients with precocious puberty, suspected abdominal masses, suspected vaginal foreign body, and/or abdominal pain should undergo rectal bimanual examination (vaginal bimanual is rarely if ever necessary) in which adequate lubricant and a gentle slow technique are used. In most cases this can be accomplished readily in the office with good preparation of the patient as described previously. If the patient is unable to cooperate, the procedure should be deferred and an examination under anesthesia considered, if warranted based on clinical circumstances or the results of ancillary studies such as sonography or CT scan.

Examination of the Adolescent or Pubertal Patient

Indications

A pelvic examination is part of the evaluation of any postmenarchal adolescent with numerous complaints and concerns (Table 18-3). These include abnormal vaginal discharge; pelvic, abdominal, or perineal pain or dysuria; severe dysmenorrhea, amenorrhea, oligomenorrhea, polymenorrhea, or abnormal uterine bleeding; sexual contact with a partner with a suspected or confirmed STD; suspected sexual abuse; concerns with pubertal development, including absence of secondary sex characteristics by age 14, no menarche by age 16, no menarche with mature secondary sex characteristics within 2 years after the onset of puberty, hirsutism and/or masculinization, abnormal sequence of pubertal development or anatomic genital anomalies; and history of DES exposure. A pelvic examination should also be a part of routine health care for sexually active adolescent girls (Table 18-4), and should be given serious consideration when requested by the patient. In the absence of the above complaints and sexual activity, the first pelvic examination should occur at age 18.

The nature of the initial experience with pelvic examination may greatly affect a young woman's comfort with her body and the ease with which she experiences routine gynecologic care throughout her adult life. The examiner's approach should be sympathetic, unhurried, and sensitive to the modesty of the patient. A thorough and directed history precedes the examination. A comprehensive outline is suggested in Table 18-5. When patients have had pelvic examinations in the past, it is helpful to ask them about their experience to avoid repeating any previous emotional or physical trauma.

Before the examination, adequate time should be devoted to interviewing the patient alone, which provides an opportunity to ask questions about voluntary and involuntary sexual activity and explore other concerns that may be difficult to discuss in the presence of a parent. A similar opportunity should be given to the parent to express any particular concerns or worries that they have been reluctant to share in their daughter's presence.

Young women should be given the choice to be examined with or without an accompanying adult in the room. The older teenager generally prefers not to have her mother present during the pelvic examination; but if she wishes her mother to remain, this wish should be respected. Early adolescents may be conflicted between their desire for support and their extreme modesty. On occasion an accompanying friend or partner provides additional history or support, if the patient permits involvement of a non-family member. Setting a guideline that the support person must stay at the head of the table and using drapes without creating a total visual barrier is often the most comfortable

TABLE 18-4

Sexual Health Care Guidelines for Sexually Active Adolescent Girls

Procedure	Examination				
	Initial	6-month	Annual	3-month* pill-check	STD follow-up
Complete H&P	X				
Update H&P			X		
Problem-focused H&P		X		X	X
Pelvic examination	X	X	X		X
Weight	X	X	X	X	
Blood pressure	X	X	X	X	
Breast examination & SBE education	X		X		
Pap smear	X	H/C†	X		
GC culture	X	X‡	X		H/C§
Chlamydia determination	X	X‡	X		H/C§
Oral & rectal STD specimens	H/C	H/C	H/C	H/C	H/C§
Wet mount (saline/KOH)	X	X‡,‖	X	H/C	H/C‖
RPR	X		H/C‡		
Rubella titer or 2nd MMR	X				
Pregnancy prevention	X	X	X	X	X
STD/AIDS prevention	X	X	X	X	X
HIV risk assessment	X	X	X	X	X
HIV counseling and titer#	H/C	H/C	H/C		
CBC	X (and then every 2 yrs)				
UA or dipstick	X	H/C	X		
Cholesterol	H/C				
Pregnancy test	X	H/C	H/C	X	H/C
Hepatitis B immunization	X¶				

SBE, Self-breast examination; *H/C*, if indicated by history or clinical findings; *H&P*, history and physical; *GC*, gonorrhea; *MMR*, measles, mumps, rubella shot; *UA*, urinalysis.

*Patients starting oral contraceptives should be seen after 3 cycles, then at 6 months from the initial visit, then every 6 months for routine care.

†If previously abnormal or clinical HPV infection is present.

‡The frequency of these studies is related to the STD prevalence in a given patient population. Cultures at 6-month intervals are routine in high-risk populations, as are more frequent RPR and HIV titers.

§STD tests of cure are not current CDC recommendations. Because of the high rate of inadequate treatment of patients and partners, and reinfection, a test of cure provides prudent follow-up.

‖At times a wet mount of a deep vaginal specimen may provide indication for a more extensive exam at non-routine exam visits.

¶Hepatitis series may require additional visits, or accommodated to fit sexual health care schedule.

#HIV determinations should be done in the context of documented pre- and post-test counseling protocols.

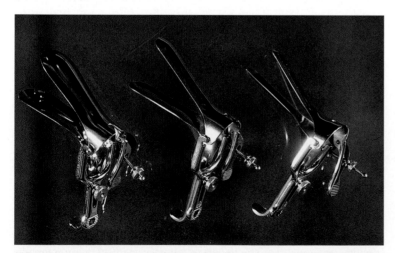

FIG. 18-7 Equipment needed for pelvic examination of adolescent patients. From left to right, a Graves speculum, a Pedersen speculum, and a narrow-bladed Huffman speculum are shown. The Graves and Pedersen speculums are useful for examining sexually active patients, and the Huffman is ideal for virginal adolescents.

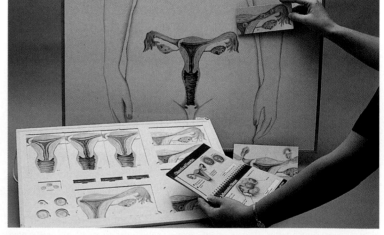

FIG. 18-8 Anatomic drawings are useful in preparation of the adolescent patient for examination and in gynecologic education.

TABLE 18-5

Complete History of an Adolescent with Gynecologic Concerns

Home	Who lives there and quality of relationships; sources of conflict and support
Education/Employment	School, grades, curriculum, repeated grades, goals, behavioral or learning difficulties; if working—type, occupational hazards, hours
Activities	Exercise, nutritional content (specifically calcium, iron, fat), body image, eating patterns, peer activities, friends, hobbies
Drugs	Caffeine, tobacco, alcohol, marijuana, crack, cocaine, pills, injectable drugs; rehabilitation or treatment history
Suicide	Depression, anxiety, psychiatric treatment, medications, major losses or disruptions
Abuse	Physical, sexual, or emotional; family, peer and community violence
Obstetric and Gynecologic History	
Menstrual	Menarche (age), cycles (length, duration, quantity of flow, use of pads or tampons); last menstrual period (LMP)—first day of; dysmenorrhea, associated disability; premenstrual symptoms (PMS); abnormal bleeding and other irregularities; mittelschmerz, midcycle spotting; douching; feminine hygiene product use (including scented products and deodorants);
STD	Herpes, GC, Chlamydia, syphilis, PID, pubic lice ("crabs"), HIV, HPV (venereal warts), Trichomonas, etc.
Pap	Abnormal smears, colposcopy, biopsies, treatments, follow-up
Vaginitis	Yeast, bacterial vaginosis, Trichomoniasis
Urologic	Urinary tract infection or kidney problems, enuresis, incontinence, dysuria, urgency, frequency
Vaginal discharge	Color, odor, quantity, duration, abnormal bleeding, pelvic pain, pruritis
Obstetric	Previous pregnancies and outcomes, future plans, fertility, concerns
Sexual	Last and other recent intercourse and protection; specific HIV risk of self and partners; sexual experience and age of onset; sexual practices, condom use; gender of partners, sexual orientation; number of partners, lifetime and recent; satisfaction with sexual experience; sexual problems with self or partner
Contraceptive	Current and past methods, satisfaction, consistency of use, problems
Past Medical History	Prior sources of care (routine, episodic, and emergency); hepatitis B immunization; rubella and varicella status
Family History	Disease or death caused by alcohol, drugs, tobacco; gynecologic or obstetric problems; age of childbearing; endocrine problems (especially thyroid); bleeding problems (especially ob-gyn–related); congenital malformations, mental retardation, reproductive loss

compromise for younger adolescents. In general, and particularly if the examiner is a man, the presence of a chaperone (such as a nurse or an aide) is recommended for propriety and to facilitate handling of specimens.

Because of patient anxiety, at times it is impossible to do a full pelvic examination. In such cases a partial, less invasive examination still provides valuable information. This may include inspection of the external genitalia, obtaining vaginal specimens with swabs for a wet preparation and cultures, and performing a rectal-bimanual examination. Though vaginal cultures for gonorrhea and chlamydia polymerase chain reaction (PCR) may not match the cervical gold standard, they contribute useful diagnostic information. Some girls who initially refuse an "internal examination" are persuaded by the finding of visible discharge or an abnormal microscopic wet preparation. A pelvic ultrasound is an expensive alternative, and its costs and benefits should be weighed carefully, assessing each patient individually.

Technique

Successful examination depends on adequate patient preparation and use of appropriate instruments. For virginal adolescents, the narrow-bladed Huffman speculum ($\frac{1}{2}" \times 4\frac{1}{2}"$) is recommended. Although it's long enough to expose the cervix, its narrow blades are inserted easily through the virginal introitus. Most sexually active adolescents can be examined with the straight-sided Pedersen speculum ($1" \times 4\frac{1}{2}"$); however, the Huffman speculum should be considered as an alternative for a first pelvic examination or for particularly anxious patients. The duck-billed Graves speculum ($1\frac{3}{8}" \times 3\frac{3}{4}"$) is useful in parous patients (Fig. 18-7). Gloves should be available in the examining room and worn by the practitioner for external and internal examinations.

Before beginning, the examiner should carefully explain the various parts of the examination: inspection of the external genitalia, speculum examination of the vagina and cervix, and bimanual palpation. Use of anatomic drawings and/or models can be helpful and educational (Fig. 18-8).

The patient should be shown the speculum and allowed to touch it if she so desires. Patients experiencing their first pelvic examination should be reassured that only the blades of the speculum will be inserted. Comparing the size of an open speculum to a finger or tampon often is reassuring. Both plastic and metal speculums can be moistened

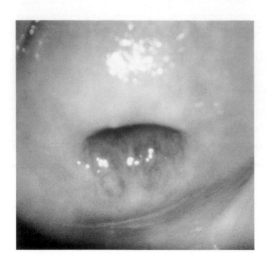

FIG. 18-9 Normal nulliparous cervix. The surface is covered with pink squamous epithelium that is uniform in consistency. The os is small and round. A small area of ectropion is visible inferior to the os. (Courtesy C. Stevens.)

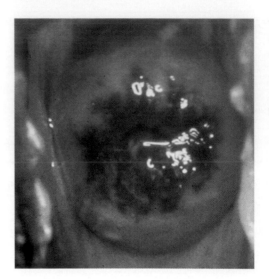

FIG. 18-10 Ectropion. Columnar mucosal cells usually found in the endocervical canal have extended out into the surface of the cervix, creating a circular raised erythematous appearance. Note the normal nonpurulent cervical mucus. This normal variant is not to be confused with cervicitis. (Courtesy Dr. E. Jerome.)

with warm water (but not lubricant) to increase comfort and ease of insertion. This does not compromise specimen collection. If only a single size of disposable plastic specula is routinely used at a facility, it is important to have a back-up supply of smaller metal speculums.

Before and during the examination, the examiner should talk to the patient to explain what she or he is seeing and to provide reassurance and education. Maintaining a dialogue throughout the procedure also usually helps the patient relax. Conversation can confirm normal anatomic findings and provide the patient with examples of a correct and comfortable vocabulary describing her reproductive anatomy and function. A hand mirror held by the patient is often useful for similar reasons. The patient should be told that she will feel "a sense of pressure," not pain, during speculum insertion and should be reminded to breathe at a regular rate because tensing abdominal or pelvic muscles can produce discomfort and make the examination more difficult to perform.

The pelvic examination is usually done after other components of the physical examination. The patient should empty her bladder beforehand, and a urine specimen can be collected at this time. Raising the head of the examination table 20 to 45 degrees helps relax abdominal muscles and facilitates maintenance of visual contact with the patient. She is then assisted into the lithotomy position at the end of the examination table. Her comfort with being touched may be increased by identifying then touching distal areas first and moving proximally (e.g., knees, thighs, groin, labia, introitus). Next the external genitalia are inspected. Pubic hair pattern and clitoral size are assessed. The presence of vulvar lesions or vaginal discharge on the perineum should be noted. The introital opening is examined and its edges palpated for any swellings in the regions of the Bartholin glands. The urethral opening is then inspected, and if erythema or discharge is noted, the urethra is gently stripped with a gloved finger along the vaginal roof. Any purulent material obtained should be cultured. Swabs used to obtain chlamydia cultures from the urethra and any other sites must have direct contact with the mucosal surface, rather than the discharge itself.

The examiner then should gently insert the index finger into the vagina to assess the size of the introital opening and to locate the cervix. Vaginal muscle tone can be assessed by asking the patient to "tighten her muscles" around the examiner's finger. Conscious relaxation can be practiced by asking the patient to relax those same muscles and to push her buttocks onto the examining table. With the index finger partially withdrawn but gently pressing on the vaginal floor, the

speculum (premoistened with warm water, not lubricant) is inserted over the finger into the vagina. This is done at an oblique angle to accommodate the vertical introitus and avoid traumatizing the urethra, which lies above the anterior vaginal wall. Another technique that effectively assists insertion involves using the thumb and index fingers to stretch the posterior labial folds down and out before inserting the speculum. Care must be taken to avoid catching pubic hairs or the labia in the mechanism of the speculum.

With the speculum in place the vaginal walls are inspected for erythema, lesions, and quality of discharge. The vaginal pH level is measured by holding pH paper (with an appropriate range of 3.6 to 6.1) against the lateral vaginal wall, away from pooled secretions. This is useful because vaginal pH levels are elevated in bacterial vaginosis and tend to be increased with trichomonal and decreased with candidal infections, respectively. Visible vaginal secretions from the posterior vaginal pool should be sampled with a cotton or Dacron swab and placed in a small amount of nonbacteriostatic normal saline for wet mount and KOH examination. The cervix is then examined. Cervical mucus should be gently removed from the cervical surface with cotton swabs before inspection of the cervix or sampling of cervical secretions. Purulent secretions (mucopus) typically turn the swab yellow and may be saved for microscopic examination. The normal nulliparous cervix usually has a small round os and is covered with squamous epithelium that is pink and uniform in consistency (Fig. 18-9). Cervical lesions (cysts, warts, polyps, vesicles) should be noted. An ectropion (or eversion) of the endocervical columnar epithelium onto the cervical surface is common and normal in adolescents (Fig. 18-10). Ectropion should be distinguished from cervicitis, the latter being suggested by erythema, friability, or mucopurulent cervical discharge (Fig. 18-36, *B*). If the endocervical epithelium extends onto the vaginal walls or the cervical shape is abnormal or hypoplastic, this raises the possibility of in utero DES exposure and gynecologic referral is warranted.

Cervical specimens are then collected. First, a Pap smear is obtained by rotating a wooden Ayre spatula circumferentially around the cervical os. The entire squamocolumnar junction should be gently scraped. A sample from the endocervical canal is collected with a cytobrush (or a cotton swab if the patient is pregnant). Each sample is smeared onto a labeled glass slide according to laboratory protocol and treated immediately with fixative. Pap smear results may be uninterpretable in the presence of inflammation, bleeding, or inadequate fixation. Ideally, Pap smears collected to screen for cervical dysplasia should be deferred

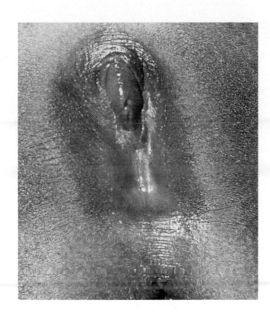

FIG. 18-11 Labial adhesions. Agglutination and adhesion of the labia minora, as a result of healing after inflammation, produce the appearance of a smooth flat surface overlying the introitus, divided centrally by a thin lucent line. (Courtesy Dr. D Lloyd.)

examiner can review the wet mount and KOH preparations. A drop of the saline solution of vaginal secretions is examined under low ($\times$ 10) and high ($\times$ 40) power for distribution of epithelial cells, leukocytes, yeast forms, *Trichomonas* organisms, and clue cells. A drop of 10% KOH is added to a second drop of the saline solution. This preparation is immediately "whiffed" for the presence of the acrid odor associated with amines. Microscopic scanning of a KOH preparation facilitates identification of yeast forms that may be obscured by epithelial cells on the wet mount.

With this additional information, the practitioner can review the presenting problems and subsequent findings with the patient. Use of printed pictures or line drawings enhances the patient's understanding of the discussion (Fig. 18-8). This is also an opportunity to encourage communication between the young woman and her parent, as appropriate to the circumstance.

Genital Tract Obstruction

Labial Adhesions

until infections are treated and menstrual bleeding has finished. Concerns about patient compliance and follow-up or urgent clinical needs may justify collection of Pap specimens at less optimal times. Sometimes Pap smear results contribute to the diagnosis of abnormal bleeding or chronic cervicitis when problems are caused by infection with human papilloma virus (HPV), herpes simplex virus (HSV), or *Trichomonas* organisms.

For routine sexual health care or evaluation of pain, bleeding, or discharge from the cervix, specimens should be obtained to determine the presence of infection. A saline wet mount for microscopic evaluation in the office can be prepared by placing a sample of cervical discharge into a small amount (1 ml) of saline or by placement directly onto a slide with a drop of saline. Gonorrhea cultures are obtained from the endocervical canal. A sterile swab is inserted into the canal and rotated for at least 10 seconds. The swab is placed immediately into a selective transport or culture medium. Either medium must be at room temperature before inoculation. It is possible but less than ideal to grow gonorrhea from routine culture specimens. Gonorrhea-specific media prevent bacterial overgrowth by other species and allow a longer transport time. Chlamydia cultures, DNA-PCR or DNA probes, or ELISA assays (e.g., Chlamydiazyme) require mucosal surface cells because the pathogen is an obligate intracellular organism. Dacron swabs are placed in the endocervical canal and thoroughly rotated to obtain the necessary cellular material. Wooden swabs are not acceptable for chlamydia tests. Nonamplified DNA techniques have lower sensitivities and specificities than other methods. After these routine specimens are obtained, the examination may continue, using acetic acid if genital warts are suspected.

The speculum is then removed, and the bimanual (vaginal-abdominal) examination is performed. Water-based lubricant is placed on the two gloved fingers to be used before inserting them carefully through the introitus into the vagina. The examiner should note the size, consistency, position, and mobility of the uterus and check for tenderness on cervical or fundal motion. The adnexa should be palpated for enlargement or tenderness. After changing the glove on the examining hand, a rectovaginal examination using the index and middle finger is then performed to confirm the vaginal-abdominal examination, palpate the cul-de-sac, and examine a retroflexed uterus.

Once the examination is completed, the patient should be helped out of the lithotomy position, given tissues to wipe away any lubricant or discharge, and allowed privacy to get dressed. During this time the

The most common form of vaginal obstruction in prepubertal patients is a partial obstruction produced by "fusion" of the labia minora as a result of labial adhesions. On inspection the clinician finds a smooth, flat membrane with a thin lucent central line overlying the introitus. It is postulated that inflammation and erosion of the superficial layers of the mucosa—whether caused by infection, dermatitis, or mechanical trauma—result in agglutination of the apposed labia minora by fibrous tissue upon healing. The process typically begins posteriorly and extends forward. In most cases the fused portion is less than 1 cm in length, but on occasion it can extend to cover the vaginal vestibule and rarely the urethra (Fig. 18-11). Even when fusion is extensive, urine flow and vaginal secretions are able to exit through the opening anteriorly. Although most patients with labial fusion are asymptomatic, some have symptoms of lower urinary tract and vulval inflammation.

If resolution of the fused labia is desired, the condition readily responds to application of estrogen cream along the line of fusion twice daily for 2 weeks followed by nightly application for an additional week. After the labia have separated, lubricant should be applied nightly for several months to prevent recurrence. The patient's parent should be informed that topical estrogen may cause transient hyperpigmentation of the labia and the areolae and an increase in breast tissue, but that these changes regress once therapy is completed. An estrogen-withdrawal bleed (similar to that seen in the neonate) occasionally occurs. Removal of irritants, treatment of infections, and instructions on good perineal hygiene tend to prevent recurrence. Nonetheless, recurrence is common, but repeated treatment is not necessary if the child is asymptomatic.

Manual separation of fused labia is painful, traumatic, and frequently followed by a recurrence. Hence this practice should be abandoned. True fusion—adhesions present in the first months of life or adhesions that do not respond to the prescribed therapy—requires further evaluation for abnormalities in gender differentiation or androgen production.

Imperforate Hymen

The anomaly referred to as *imperforate hymen* consists of an imperforate membrane located just inside the hymenal ring. This is the most common truly obstructive abnormality. It is frequently missed on the newborn examination because of the redundancy of hymenal folds. However, it may become evident by 8 to 12 weeks of age on careful per-

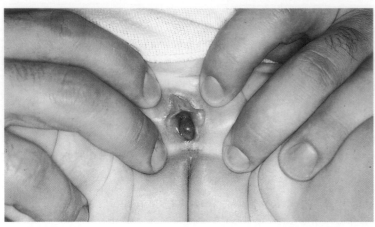

FIG. 18-12   Imperforate hymen with neonatal hematocolpos. A dark purplish bulge at the introitus was noted by the mother during a diaper change.

TABLE 18-6

Causes of Genital Tract Obstruction

Labial fusion (underlying endocrine pathology)
Imperforate hymen
Vaginal atresia (failure to canalize the vaginal plate)
Vaginal (with or without uterine) agenesis, including Mayer-Rokitansky-Kuster-Hauser syndrome (müllerian aplasia); congenital absence of the vagina and uterus
Transverse vaginal septum at the junction of the upper one third and lower two thirds of the vagina
Longitudinal vaginal septum
Androgen insensitivity (testicular feminization syndrome)
Absence of the cervix and/or uterus
Obstructing müllerian malformations, with elements of duplication, agenesis, and/or incomplete fusion
Tumors of the upper and lower genital tracts; other pelvic masses
Labial adhesions (cause only partial obstruction)

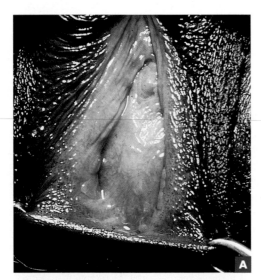

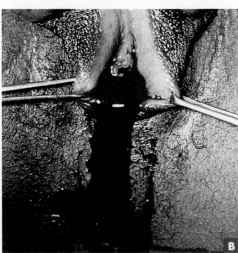

FIG. 18-13   Imperforate hymen with hematocolpos. This adolescent presented with a 2-month history of intermittent crampy lower abdominal pain, which had acutely worsened. She had well-developed secondary sex characteristics but was premenarchal by history. *A,* Examination revealed midline fullness and tenderness of the lower abdomen and a smooth bulging mass at the introitus. *B,* Incision of the imperforate membrane just inside the hymenal ring allowed the accumulated menstrual blood and vaginal secretions to drain. (Courtesy Dr. D. Lloyd.)

ineal inspection, appearing as a thin, white transparent hymenal membrane that bulges when the infant cries or strains. Occasionally, young infants with this anomaly have copious vaginal secretions secondary to stimulation by maternal hormones, and as a result they develop hydrocolpos. In such cases the infant may have midline swelling of the lower abdomen (especially noticeable when the bladder is full) that feels cystic on palpation. Perineal inspection reveals a whitish, bulging membrane at the introitus. The cystic mass also may be palpable on rectal examination. In the presence of a neonatal withdrawal bleed or trauma, a hematocolpos may develop. This presents as a red or purplish bulge (Fig. 18-12). Treatment consists of incision of the membrane to allow drainage, followed by excision of redundant portions.

If her condition goes undetected in infancy, the patient with an imperforate hymen usually develops hematocolpos in late puberty. The major complaints are intermittent lower abdominal and low back pain, which rapidly progress in severity and duration. Over time difficulty in urination and defecation may develop, and a lower abdominal swelling may become noticeable. The patient has well-developed secondary sex characteristics but has had no menstrual periods. Perineal inspection reveals a thick, tense, bulging membrane, often bluish in color, at the introitus (Fig. 18-13, *A*). A low cystic swelling is palpable anteriorly on rectal examination. Operative excision allows drainage of the accumulated blood and vaginal secretions (Fig. 18-13, *B*). Other partially obstructive hymenal abnormalities may allow menstrual blood to flow but later cause difficulty inserting tampons or initiating intercourse. Because hymens are not of müllerian origin, imperforate hymens are not associated with other genitourinary abnormalities.

Other forms of genital tract obstruction (Table 18-6) are rare. In most cases early routine genital inspection reveals the absence of a vaginal orifice, enabling early delineation of the anomaly and thus facilitating treatment. If missed in infancy or childhood, partial or complete obstruction can present with a wide range of signs and symptoms (Table 18-7). These may include cyclic or persistent vaginal, pelvic, or abdominal pain; primary amenorrhea or irregular vaginal bleeding; urinary tract symptoms; and difficulty inserting tampons and initiating intercourse, or dyspareunia. Clinically a vaginal, pelvic, or abdominal mass may be found, reflecting hydrocolpos, hematocolpos, pyohematocolpos, or hematometra.

TABLE 18-7
Symptoms and Signs Associated With Genital Tract Obstructions

Symptoms
Vaginal, pelvic, or abdominal pain (especially cyclic)
Dysmenorrhea
Urinary tract symptoms
Primary amenorrhea
Irregular vaginal bleeding
Purulent vaginal discharge
Difficulty initiating intercourse
Dyspareunia

Signs
Vaginal, pelvic, or abdominal mass
Hydrocolpos (mucus in vagina)
Hematocolpos (blood in vagina)
Pyohematocolpos (pus and blood in vagina)
Hematometria (blood within the uterus)

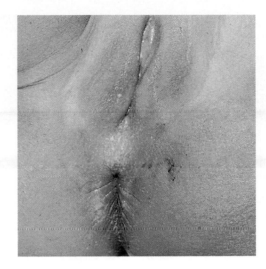

FIG. 18-14 Superficial blunt trauma. Healing abrasions are seen in this patient who was a victim of sexual abuse. Note their posterior location.

Over the past several years an increased use of ultrasound to investigate lower abdominal complaints in prepubertal girls has resulted in numerous mistaken diagnoses of uterine and ovarian agenesis. This is because current ultrasound technology is not sensitive enough to reliably detect the presence of these organs before puberty. Recognition of this fact is important because overinterpretation of ultrasound findings has caused parents and children great concern and unnecessary worry.

Genital Trauma

As mentioned earlier, the genital structures and pelvic supporting tissues of the prepubescent girl are smaller and considerably more rigid than those of the adolescent or adult woman. This inelasticity significantly increases the risks of tearing with either blunt or penetrating trauma, and of internal extension of injury, especially in cases of penetrating trauma. Appropriate assessment and management necessitate appreciation of these differences because serious internal injuries of the vagina, rectum, urethra, bladder, and peritoneal structures may underlie deceptively mild external abnormalities. Careful attention must be given to vital signs; abdominal examination; and evaluation of the urethra, hymen, lower vagina, perineal body, and rectum.

Clues to internal extension of injury include hymenal tears, vaginal bleeding and/or vaginal hematoma, tears of the perineal body, inability to urinate or gross hematuria, and abnormal sphincter tone or rectal bleeding. When injuries have extended to involve peritoneal structures, lower abdominal tenderness is seen and at times is associated with signs of hypovolemia. Direct tenderness may range from mild to marked and may or may not be accompanied by rebound tenderness. Occasionally a palpable mass is present.

Adolescents, in contrast, are more likely to have contusions than tears and are much less likely to have internal extension of injury unless the applied force is very great.

The role of the primary care or emergency physician is to assess the patient's general status and determine the likely extent and cause of the injury. This can be accomplished largely with a good general examination, careful perineal inspection, rectal examination, and urinalysis. The physician must be sensitive to the patient's physical discomfort and emotional distress at all times, providing emotional support and appropriate pain control whenever possible. Patients should also be protected from having to undergo multiple examinations, a particular risk in teaching hospitals.

When external inspection suggests that the prepubertal patient's injury is more than superficial, internal examination under anesthesia (by a pediatric surgeon or gynecologist) should be arranged. This enables meticulous inspection, wound exploration, and repair under optimal conditions without further traumatizing the child.

Some adolescents may be able to tolerate inspection and internal examination as outpatients. However, if injuries are severe or if the postmenarchal patient is too anxious to undergo pelvic examination when indicated, examination under anesthesia is the better course.

Superficial Perineal Injuries

The majority of superficial perineal trauma cases are the result of mild, blunt force incurred via straddle injury, minor falls, or sexual abuse. Patients with accidental injuries that result in pain, swelling, or bleeding are rapidly brought to medical attention. A clear history of the preceding incident (often witnessed) is usually given, and findings fit the reported mechanism of injury. However, accidentally incurred superficial abrasions may not be noticed by parents until the child cries on urination, complains of dysuria, or a small amount of blood is noticed on the child's underwear or toilet paper. As noted in Chapter 6, victims of sexual abuse may complain of abuse but more often complain of unexplained bleeding or pain with no history of trauma.

Typical lesions include superficial abrasions, mild contusions, and occasionally superficial lacerations (Fig. 18-14). The latter are found most frequently at the junction of the labia majora and minora and usually are only 1 to 3 mm deep. Accidental straddle injuries result in the

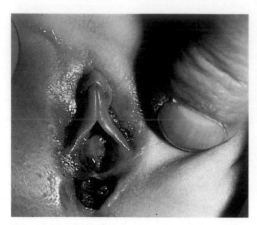

FIG. 18-15 Superficial penetrating injury. This infant had a chief complaint of blood spotting on the diaper. Inspection revealed a perineal tear just posterior to the hymenal ring. There was no evidence of internal extension on vaginoscopy under anesthesia. Sexual abuse was suspected.

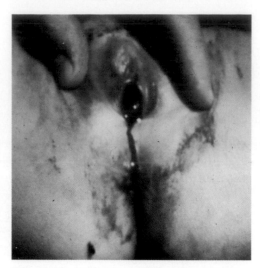

FIG. 18-16 Moderate genital trauma. After a straddle injury on a diving board, this 9-year-old girl had vaginal bleeding. Inspection disclosed a hematoma of the anterior portion of the right labium majora, contusions of the introitus, and a hematoma protruding through the vaginal opening. A small superficial laceration is present on the left, between the labia majora and minora, and another on the right between the superior portion of the anterior portion of introitus and the labium minora. At vaginoscopy under anesthesia a vaginal tear involving the right lateral wall was found. (Courtesy Dr. K. Sukarochana.)

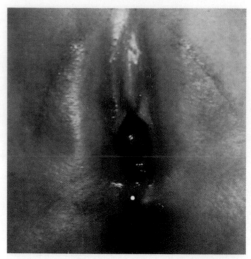

FIG. 18-17 Moderate blunt trauma. This 6-year-old girl had painless vaginal bleeding, which had soaked three sanitary pads in 2 hours. External inspection revealed a superficial tear of the anterior portion of the perineal body, a small hematoma to the right of the introitus, and blood trickling through the vaginal orifice. Examination under anesthesia disclosed a tear of the lateral vaginal wall. Sexual abuse was strongly suspected. (Courtesy Dr. K. Sukarochana.)

crushing of the perineal soft tissues between the pubis and the object on which the patient falls or bumps herself. Hence these tend to produce contusions or tears in and around the area of the clitoris and the anterior portions of the labia majora and minora (Fig. 18-16). In contrast to accidental injuries, those that result from sexual abuse tend to be more posteriorly located and typically involve tears of the posterior portion of the hymen (see Chapter 6). Minor falls onto or scrapes against sharp objects tend to produce simple perineal and vulval lacerations. As in cases of mild blunt trauma, the junction of the labia minora and majora is the site most frequently involved; however, tears of the labia majora or perineal body are not uncommon (Fig. 18-15).

Whether blunt or penetrating, when injuries are truly superficial, bleeding if present at all tends to be scant. The exception to this is a penetrating injury involving the corpus cavernosum of the labia majora, in which case hemorrhage may be profuse. Patients may experience mild perineal discomfort and pain on urination but otherwise are asymptomatic. Most of these injuries can be managed supportively with analgesia, topical bacteriostatic and/or anesthetic ointments, sitz baths, and careful perineal cleansing. Application of the ointment before urinating relieves dysuria as does urinating in a tub of water. If urinary retention continues to be a problem, use of a topical anesthetic ointment may be necessary for the first day or two. Deeper tears of the labia majora necessitate control of bleeding vessels and suturing under anesthesia.

Urethral prolapse and lichen sclerosus et atrophicus may cause bleeding that mimics superficial perineal injury, and the edematous friable appearance of the prolapsed urethra often has been mistakenly attributed to trauma. Knowledge of the clinical appearance of these conditions is important to avoid misdiagnosis (Figs. 18-25 and 18-26).

Moderate Genital Trauma

Moderately forceful blunt trauma often results in perineal tears and in venous disruption and hematoma formation. Hematomas of the perineum appear as tense round swellings with purplish discoloration, which are tender on palpation (Fig. 18-16). When large, these may cause intense perineal pain. Those located in the periurethral area may interfere with urination. Moderate blunt force also can produce submucosal tears and vaginal mucosal separation with resultant vaginal bleeding or vaginal hematoma formation (Figs. 18-16 and 18-17). In some cases the associated external injuries can be deceptively mild (Fig. 18-17). Vaginal hematomas are the source of significant pain that usually is perceived as perineal and/or vaginal but at times is referred to the rectum or buttocks. Inspection through the vaginal orifice reveals a bluish swelling involving one of the lateral walls. This also may be evident as a tender swelling anterolaterally on rectal examination.

Moderate penetrating injuries result primarily from falls onto sharp objects ("picket fence injury"), rape, sexual molestation with phallic-shaped objects, and occasionally auto accidents. Lesions include perineal tears that extend into the vagina, rectum, or bladder but do not breach the peritoneum. Although many patients have external lacerations that obviously are extensive on inspection (Fig. 18-18; see Chapter 6), a significant proportion have deceptively minor external injuries. In the absence of associated hematomas, extensive tears may produce little pain. Furthermore, although most such injuries result in moderate bleeding, some patients have remarkably little blood loss.

Whether the mechanism of injury involves blunt force or penetration, when physical findings include bleeding through the vaginal orifice; a vaginal hematoma; rectal bleeding, rectal tenderness, or abnormal sphincter tone; gross hematuria or inability to urinate; internal ex-

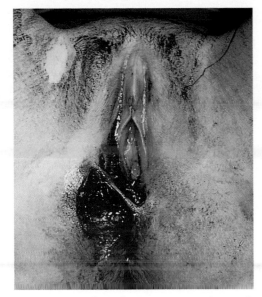

FIG. 18-18 Moderately severe penetrating genital trauma. This youngster fell while roller skating and slid on her bottom for several feet, tearing her perineum on an object projecting up from the ground. A laceration involving the right labia majora and minora, extending through the perineal body to the anus is evident on inspection. The patient complained of only minor discomfort. Examination under anesthesia revealed vaginal and rectal extension of the tear with complete transection of the external anal sphincter. The peritoneum was intact.

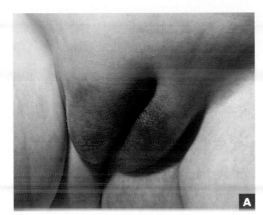
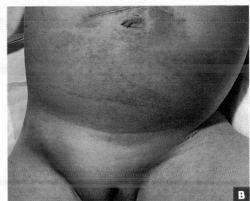

FIG. 18-19 Severe blunt perineal trauma. Following a fall from a height in which she had landed on her bottom, this young child had (*A*), labial contusions and hematomas, lower abdominal tenderness, and signs of hypovolemia. The force of the fall ruptured pelvic vessels, resulting in retroperitoneal bleeding that (*B*) ultimately extended along the anterior abdominal wall. These photographs were taken several days after the injury. (Courtesy Dr. Marc Rowe, Children's Hospital of Pittsburgh.)

tension of injury is probable. All such patients warrant exploration and repair in the operating room. This obviates the need for extensive examination in the office or emergency department.

Severe Genital Trauma

Severe falls from heights onto flat surfaces can produce major perineal lacerations simulating penetrating injury. In addition, they occasionally disrupt the pelvic vessels, mesentery, and intestine, with or without pelvic fracture (Fig. 18-19). Similarly, severe penetrating injury may produce tears that extend through the cul-de-sac, rupturing pelvic vessels and tearing intraabdominal structures. Although external injuries in these cases usually are extensive and associated with significant bleeding, they can be incredibly minor in appearance, particularly when penetration is the source. These children complain of lower abdominal and perineal pain, which may radiate down one leg. Abdominal examination should reveal at least mild direct tenderness early on. Later, guarding and rebound tenderness may be noted. Patients with pelvic bleeding ultimately have signs of hypovolemia, although these signs may not be evident immediately after the injury. Any patient with clinical signs of peritoneal extension of genital trauma warrants prompt hemodynamic stabilization followed by appropriate imaging, surgical exploration, and repair.

Nontraumatic Vulvovaginal Disorders

Prepubertal "Vulvovaginitis"

Strictly defined, the term *vulvovaginitis* denotes an inflammatory process involving both the vulva and the vagina. In practice, however, the term is used less precisely to refer to patients who describe symptoms of dysuria, vulvar pain or itching, or vaginal discharge but who often lack signs of inflammation or who have evidence of vulvar inflammation without vaginal involvement.

Vulvovaginitis is relatively common in prepubertal girls and accounts for a majority of genital complaints before menarche. Its frequent occurrence is explained in part by the fact that the labia do not fully cover and thus do not completely protect the vaginal vestibule from friction and external irritants, especially when the child is sitting or squatting. Additionally the unestrogenized vaginal epithelium is thin, relatively friable, and more easily traumatized. Transient irritation without discharge is common in the young child because of exposure to chemical irritants, inconsistent hygiene, and poor aeration. Finally, young children are less careful than older children and adults about cleansing their perineum and avoiding contamination with stool.

Causes of vulvovaginitis are most easily classified into noninfectious and infectious subgroups, with the latter subclassified into nonsexually and sexually transmitted infections. Table 18-8 presents the most common causes of noninfectious vulvovaginitis with specific historic clues suggestive of each condition. Table 18-9 presents the infectious causes. Nonsexually transmitted bacterial pathogens and the herpes simplex viruses often are spread to the vulvovaginal area from another site (e.g., nose, mouth, throat, skin, or GI tract) by the patient's hands, whereas involvement with viral organisms is more often a part of systemic infection. Although a common cause of diaper dermatitis, *Candida* organisms rarely cause vulvovaginitis in the prepubertal child. Occasionally they are seen in children who are receiving systemic antibiotics or steroids, are using topical steroid hormone creams, or have underlying diabetes mellitus. Vulvovaginitis caused by sexually trans-

---

TABLE 18-8

Causes of Noninfectious Vulvovaginitis and Dysuria

Condition	Historic clues
Poor hygiene	Infrequent bathing, hand washing, and clothing changes; soiled underwear, toilet independence
Poor perineal aeration	Tight clothing, nylon underwear, tights and leotards; wearing wet bathing suits for long periods; hot tubs; obesity
Frictional trauma	Tight clothing, sports, sand from sandbox or beach play, excessive masturbation or sexual abuse, obesity
Chemical irritants	Bubble bath, harsh or perfumed soaps or detergents, powder, water softeners, perfumed and dyed toilet paper; ammonia; douches and feminine hygiene products in adolescents
Contact dermatitis	Poison ivy, topical creams or ointments
Vaginal foreign bodies	Wiping habits, excessive masturbation or self-exploration, sexual abuse
Parasites, insect bites, infestations	Home environment, pets, sandboxes, travel, camping, exposure to woods or beach
Medication-related	Topical steroid or hormone creams, antibiotics, chemotherapy
Generalized skin disorders	History of pruritis, chronic skin lesions, prior diagnosis
Anatomic anomalies	Vesicovaginal fistulas, rectovaginal fistulas, ectopic ureters, spina bifida
Long-term effect of DES	Maternal history
Neoplasms	Discharge, bleeding, bulging abdomen, change in bowel or bladder function, premature puberty
Systemic illness (Steven-Johnson syndrome, Crohn disease with perineal fistulas, toxic shock syndrome)	Prior infection or medication use; tampon use; evidence from other physical findings, including rash, failure to gain weight or height, abdominal pain, diarrhea
Pelvic appendiceal abscess	History of fever, anorexia, vomiting, progression of periumbilical to right lower quadrant pain

---

mitted pathogens is almost always acquired through sexual contact. Specific conditions are discussed in the ensuing sections.

In contrast to adolescents and adults, prepubertal girls are at less risk for internal extension of vulvovaginal infections (cervicitis and pelvic inflammatory disease) because the unestrogenized genital tract does not support the ascent of infection through the uterus and fallopian tubes.

The evaluation of these patients must include questions related to symptoms and duration of problems; recent respiratory, gastrointestinal, and urinary tract infections; exposure to irritants such as bath additives, laundry detergents, fabric softeners, bubble bath, and harsh soaps; hygenic practices; bowel and bladder habits; type of clothing worn; recent activities; medications and topical agents; concurrent abdominal pain; the child's caretakers; and possible sexual contact. Developmental, behavioral, environmental, and medical histories may contribute to a diagnosis and aid in the formulation of a therapeutic plan.

Physical assessment must include determination of the degree of pubertal development; inguinal, abdominal, and often rectal examination; along with careful perineal and vaginal inspection. The degree and extent of inflammation and excoriation should be documented. Parents should be encouraged to bring in samples of soiled or discolored underwear, which should be checked for fit, cleanliness, and signs of blood, discharge, stool, and urine. When patients are seen by appointment for vulvovaginal complaints, the parents should be asked to neither bathe nor apply creams to the child for 12 to 24 hours before the

evaluation; otherwise, many children with a history of discharge have none when examined.

The presence of a vaginal discharge necessitates specimen collection (Table 18-2; see section on Examination of the Prepubertal Patient). Urine should be collected for urinalysis and culture. If a vaginal foreign body is suspected, rectal examination and vaginoscopy are indicated in consultation with a practitioner experienced in such procedures.

Vulvovaginal Complaints in Adolescents

Among sexually active adolescent girls, infectious processes are the major source of vulvovaginal inflammation and sexually transmitted pathogens are the predominant offending organisms. Estrogenization and maturation of the genital tract alter its pathophysiologic response, favoring upward spread of some infectious processes, particularly those of gonorrhea and chlamydiae. As a result asymptomatic subclinical infection, cervicitis, and pelvic inflammatory disease are significant concerns, in addition to vulvovaginitis after menarche.

Vulvar lesions, vaginal discharge, odor, pruritus, and dysuria are common problems in adolescents; but irregular or postcoital bleeding dyspareunia, pelvic pain, and fever may be prominent complaints as well. These symptoms are relatively nonspecific and may represent the final common pathway of different causes of irritation, infection, or infestation.

In addition to identification of specific etiologic agents, a major goal of evaluation is to differentiate vulvovaginal or cervical processes from

TABLE 18-9

Infectious Causes of Prepubertal and Pubertal Vulvovaginitis

Nonsexually transmitted pathogens	Sexually transmitted pathogens
Bacterial Respiratory and/or Skin Pathogens	**Bacterial Pathogens**
Group A beta-hemolytic streptococci*	*Chlamydia trachomatis**
*Streptococcus pneumoniae**	*Neisseria gonorrhoeae**
*Haemophilus influenzae**	*Treponema pallidum*
Neisseria meningitidis	*Mycoplasma species**
Staphylococci	*Ureaplasma species**
	Protozoa
Viral Pathogens	*Trichomonas vaginalis**
Varicella-zoster virus	
Herpes simplex viruses types 1 and 2*	**Viral Pathogens**
Adenoviruses*	Herpes simplex viruses types and 1 and 2*
Echoviruses*	Human papilloma virus
Measles virus	Human immunodeficiency virus
Gastrointestinal Pathogens	**Parasites**
Candida species*	*Phthirius pubis* (lice)
Shigella species*	*Sarcoptes scabiei*
Enterobius vermicularis	
Yersinia species	
*Escherichia coli**	

*Conditions in which vaginal discharge is prominent.

pregnancy (normal or ectopic), from upper tract disease (e.g., pelvic inflammatory disease, adnexal torsion or cysts), and from intraabdominal processes (e.g., appendicitis, endometriosis, or tumors). Hence a complete pelvic examination is necessary when evaluating adolescents with vulvovaginal complaints. Systemic signs and symptoms and abnormalities on bimanual pelvic examination suggest processes involving the uterus and adnexal and/or peritoneal structures. In contrast, isolated vulvovaginal disorders rarely are accompanied by such findings. In the majority of cases, careful history, inspection, "bench" lab tests (such as wet mount, KOH preparation, Gram stain, pregnancy test, urine dipstick, and vaginal pH), and selected cultures provide a specific diagnosis on which to base treatment decisions. Some of the clinical and laboratory features of various etiologic agents of vaginal discharge are presented in Table 18-10.

Physiologic Leukorrhea

Physiologic leukorrhea, though often perceived as a vaginal discharge, is in actuality a normal phenomenon and not a form of vulvovaginitis. These normal secretions are produced in response to estrogen stimulation and thus are seen in the newborn period and return in the 6 to 12 months preceding the onset of menses. Physiologic leukorrhea is clear or milky, relatively thin, odorless, and nonirritating (Fig. 18-4, *A*). When dried on underwear, it may appear yellow or brown. Perimenarchal patients often complain of discharge because they and their mothers are not aware that the secretions are normal. These children are otherwise asymptomatic.

Examination reveals normal pubertal development including findings of breast development, presence of pubic hair, and evidence of estrogenization of the labia and distal vaginal mucosa along with the typical discharge. Diagnosis is confirmed by findings on wet preparation microscopy, which disclose estrogenized epithelial cells with no increase in leukocytes (Fig. 18-4, *B*). As a general guide, there should be no more than one polymorphonuclear leukocyte for every vaginal epithelial cell. Neither bimanual nor speculum examinations are necessary, unless other symptoms or findings suggest other etiologies. Treatment consists of reassurance and education.

Noninfectious Vulvovaginitis

Clinical findings of noninfectious vulvovaginitis vary considerably depending on cause. Although the physical examination often is unimpressive, patient and parental concern with the symptoms may be great. In some patients the vulva and vagina appear normal, whereas in others varying degrees of inflammation or irritation are present, at times accompanied by signs of excoriation. Vaginal discharge is unusual, however, and vaginal cultures grow normal or nonspecific flora (Table 18-11). These disorders are common in prepubertal children but are relatively infrequent after menarche. Individuals with underlying dermatologic disorders may be more susceptible to noninfectious causes of vulvovaginitis. Symptoms are similar for most etiologies: perineal itching, external or contact dysuria, pain, and occasionally vaginal discharge. Treatment consists of removal of the offending agent or causative circumstance along with symptomatic measures. Recommended hygienic practices include providing a sufficient number of opportunities to urinate, use of a front-to-back wiping technique, and regular washing with mild soap without excessive scrubbing. Products to avoid include skin and vaginal cosmetics, bubble bath and other bath additives, and douches. Patients with vulvovaginal inflammation are encouraged to wear loose-fitting clothes and white cotton underwear that is well rinsed after regular washing. Failure to improve should lead to consideration of other etiologies, the possibility of noncompliance with treatment, or sexual abuse.

Noninfectious Vulvovaginitis Secondary to Environmental Conditions

Irritation Secondary to Poor Hygiene

Poor perineal hygiene is one of the most common causes of irritation. Examination typically reveals mild nonspecific vulvar inflammation. Pieces of stool and toilet paper may be seen adhering to the perineum and perianal areas, and smegma may be found around the clitoris and labia (Fig. 18-20). Underwear is often soiled. Coliforms tend to predominate on vaginal culture when there is associated vaginal inflammation. In the majority of cases the search for other causes is unrewarding, and symptoms resolve with a regimen of sitz baths and careful cleansing after urination and defecation. Finding a frankly feculent vaginal discharge should lead to the consideration of a rectovaginal fistula.

Maceration Secondary to Poor Perineal Aeration

Moisture, whether from normal secretions, perspiration, or swimming, when unable to evaporate, promotes maceration and inflammation of perineal tissues. Obesity, wearing tight clothing or tights over nylon underwear, and sitting for long periods in a wet bathing suit or leotard are common predisposing factors to this form of vulvar irritation. Nonspecific inflammation, often with frank maceration, is the predominant physical finding (Fig. 18-21). Patients with urinary incontinence, a vesicovaginal fistula, or ectopic ureter can also have these findings. A history of a chronically wet perineum and the smell of urine on the child's underclothes should lead the clinician to consider these possibilities.

TABLE 18-10

Clinical and Laboratory Features of Disorders Causing Vaginal Discharge in Adolescents

	Physiologic	Candida	Chlamydia	Gonorrhea	Trichomonas	Bacterial vaginosis	HPV
Appearance of discharge	White, gray, or clear, flocculent	White, curdlike, with adherent plaques	Mucopus at cervix, +friable cervix with bloody discharge	Mucopus at cervix; white, yellow, or greenish discharge	Gray, yellow, or green; sometimes frothy; malodorous	Gray, white; homogeneous	White or clear, generalized or localized inflammation
Amount	Variable	Variable	Scant to variable	Scant to variable	Large	Large	Scant
Vulvar and vaginal inflammation	None	Usual	Not usual, with or without Bartholin gland abscess	Variable, with or without Bartholin gland abscess	Occasional	Rare	Common, evidence of HPV with acetic acid wash or overt condylomata
pH of discharge	≤4.5	≤4.5	≤4.5	≤4.5	≥4.5	≥4.5	≤4.5
Microscopy	Epithelial cells, few WBCs, lactobacilli	↑WBCs, +KOH with pseudohyphae and budding yeast in 50% of symptomatic patients	↑WBCs	↑↑WBCs	↑WBCs, motile trichomonads (in saline prep) in 40%-60% of symptomatic patients; trichomonads in urine	Few WBCs, +clue cells in saline prep	Moderate ↑WBCs
Predisposing or concurrent factors	Secretion of estrogen	Menstruation, broad spectrum antibiotics, diabetes, local heat and moisture, pregnancy, OCPs, AIDS, topical steroid or hormone creams, immune deficiencies	Bacterial vaginosis, gonorrhea	Often accompanied by Chlamydia, symptoms often develop toward the end of a menstrual period	Other STDs	Previous BV, sexual activity, douching	Abnormal Pap smear, other STDs; history of genital warts or recurrent unexplained vulvovaginitis
Other clinical signs and symptoms	None	Itching prominent, may have dysuria or dyspareunia	Urethritis, PID, perihepatitis Negative	Pharyngitis, with or without PID, proctitis, urethritis, systemic illness, arthritis, tenosinovitis, perihepatitis, skin lesions	Vulvar itching and burning prominent, dysuria, pelvic discomfort	Fishy odor, odor ↑ after unprotected intercourse	Visible external or flat warts, chronic low-grade vulvovaginitis, fissures, failure of other therapies
Whiff test (+ amine odor on addition of 10% KOH)	Negative	Negative		Negative	Sometimes positive	Positive	Negative

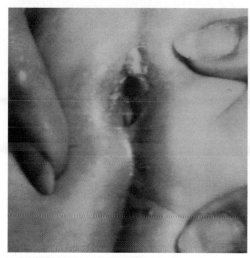

FIG. 18-20 Poor perineal hygiene. Despite prior cleansing by a nurse for a "clean-catch" urine the initial specimen contained numerous white cells and debris. When the perineum was rechecked, the infant was found to have copious amounts of smegma adhering to the clitoris and labia minora. Urine obtained after thorough re-cleansing was normal.

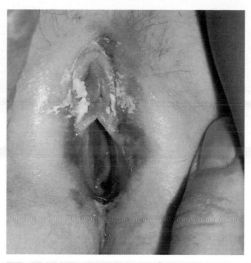

FIG. 18-21 Maceration secondary to poor perineal aeration. This child's chief complaint was one of dysuria. On examination the inner surfaces of the labia were found to be macerated and mildly inflamed. Adherent smegma is also visible. The child had been wearing tights over nylon underwear.

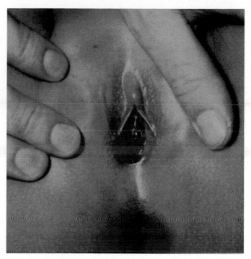

FIG. 18-22 Nonspecific inflammation characteristic of chemical irritant vulvovaginitis.

TABLE 18-11

Organisms Thought to Constitute Normal or Nonpathogenic Vaginal Flora

Aerobes and Facultative Anaerobes

Branhamella catarrhalis	*Pseudomonas* species
Candida albicans and other yeasts*	*Staphylococcus* species
Corynebacterium species	*Streptococcus* species
Diphtheroids	
Enterococcus species	**Anaerobes**
Escherichia coli	*Bacteroides* species
Haemophilus species	*Clostridium* species
Lactobacillus species	*Peptococcus* species
Klebsiella species	*Peptostreptococcus*
Mycoplasma species*	species
Neisseria sicca	
Proteus species	

*Mycoplasma hominis, Ureaplasma urealyticum, and *Candida* species can constitute normal flora in asymptomatic women; however, they may be responsible for genital tract infections as well.*

When maceration occurs, secondary infection is common, and some patients have associated intertrigo. Attention to perineal hygiene and drying, weight loss (when appropriate), avoidance of tight clothing, and treatment of secondary infection are the mainstays of management.

Contact Dermatitis, Allergic Vulvitis

Allergic vulvitis should be considered in patients whose most prominent symptom is pruritis, although scratching and excoriation may result in secondary burning and dysuria. When patients are seen in the acute phase, inspection of the labia and vestibule reveals a microvesicular papular eruption that tends to be intensely erythematous and somewhat edematous. Excoriated scratch marks are common. When the process has become chronic, the vulvar skin has an eczematoid appearance with cracks, fissures, and lichenification. Topical ointments, creams, and lotions; perfumed soaps and toilet paper; and poison ivy are common causative factors in prepubertal children. In adolescents, feminine hygiene products, cosmetics, spermicides, douches, and perfumed sanitary pads or tampons may be responsible.

Chemical Irritant Vulvovaginitis

Many of the agents capable of causing allergic vulvitis can also act as chemical irritants. Bubble bath, harsh soaps, laundry detergents, fabric and water softeners, feminine hygiene products, and perfumed or dyed toilet paper are common offenders. Furthermore, before toilet training, children whose diapers are changed infrequently may develop irritation caused by ammonia produced when the organisms in stool split the urea in urine. Itching and dysuria are prominent symptoms, and examination usually discloses mild nonspecific inflammation (Fig. 18-22), at times associated with signs of scratching. On occasion, findings are normal. Diagnosis is dependent on history (Table 18-8).

Frictional Trauma

Frictional trauma may be the source of superficial abrasive changes and, when chronic, may result in lichenification or even atrophic skin changes (Fig. 18-23). Wearing tight clothing, certain sporting activities (especially long-distance bicycle riding and running), sand from sandboxes, and excessive masturbation are the major predisposing factors.

Other Noninfectious Inflammatory Conditions

Sympathetic Inflammation and Fistulas

APPENDICITIS WITH PELVIC APPENDICEAL ABSCESS. Preschool and young school-age children with appendicitis often do not come to medical attention until after appendiceal rupture has occurred. Girls with a pelvic

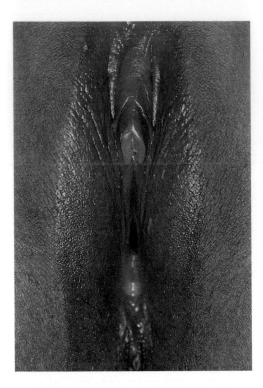

FIG. 18-23 Frictional trauma (nonspecific thickening of the vulvar skin). This patient's labial skin is thickened and mildly irritated. She had a history of recurrent vaginal foreign bodies and was strongly suspected to be a victim of chronic sexual abuse. (Courtesy Dr. K. Sukarochana.)

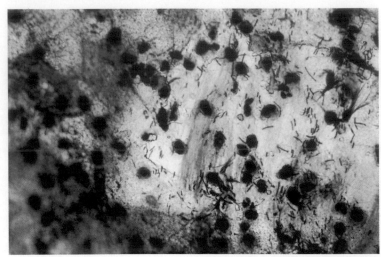

FIG. 18-24 Sympathetic purulent vaginal discharge. This photomicrograph shows numerous leukocytes and epithelial cells, with mixed flora. The patient had vomiting, anorexia, lower abdominal pain, and a purulent vaginal discharge and was found to have a pelvic appendiceal abscess. The vaginal discharge was the result of sympathetic inflammation.

appendix who wall off the rupture in a periappendiceal abscess may develop a copious purulent vaginal discharge caused by sympathetic inflammation of the vaginal wall. On microscopy the discharge contains numerous leukocytes, epithelial cells, and mixed flora (Fig. 18-24). The antecedent clinical course consisting of anorexia, nausea and vomiting, and abdominal pain along with findings on examination suggest the diagnosis. The latter may include abdominal distension, direct and percussion tenderness (especially in the right lower quadrant), and a tender cystic mass palpable on rectal examination. The fact that the unestrogenized genital tract of the prepubertal girl does not promote the ascent of sexually transmitted infections eliminates pelvic inflammatory disease from the differential diagnosis.

FISTULAS. Patients with vesicovaginal fistulas and ectopic ureters can have symptoms of vulvovaginitis. They have a history of a constantly wet perineum. Nonspecific inflammation and maceration are the predominant physical findings (Fig. 18-21; see Chapter 14).

Rectovaginal fistulas also can cause vulvovaginal inflammation, but the presence of a grossly feculent vaginal discharge usually makes diagnosis relatively easy. When rectovaginal fistulas are neither congenital nor posttraumatic in origin or when a perianal fistula is found, inflammatory bowel disease should be considered (see Chapter 10).

Vaginal Foreign Body

The hallmark of a vaginal foreign body is the presence of a profuse, foul-smelling, brownish or blood-streaked vaginal discharge. However, some children have a less dramatic presentation with a yellow, mildly purulent discharge. The majority of patients are in the 3- to 8-year-old age group. Some have developmental delay or other psychobehavioral problems. Although wads of toilet tissue, paper, cotton, crayons, and small toys are the materials found most often, all types of small objects have been retrieved. There may be a long noninflammatory latency period for inert materials. The objects most commonly found in adolescents are forgotten tampons or retained condoms. Nondissolved vaginal suppositories, substances inserted for therapeutic purposes, or objects used in sexual activity may also cause problems. Objects made of hard materials may be palpable on rectal examination.

Radiographs are rarely necessary because direct vaginoscopy is almost always required. Results of wet preparation, Gram stain and culture are nonspecific. Vaginoscopy is diagnostic and, when tolerated, it provides access for extraction, which is curative, once secondary infections are treated. In the prepubertal age group, it is best accomplished under general anesthesia.

When a prepubertal patient is found to have a vaginal foreign body, it is important to obtain a detailed behavioral history of the child in addition to a family psychosocial history because the problem often is recurrent and may be the result of disturbed behavior by the patient or of chronic sexual abuse.

Major differential diagnostic considerations are *Shigella vaginitis*, seen in prepubertal patients, and necrotic tumors, which can produce a discharge that is clinically indistinguishable from that of a vaginal foreign body.

Conditions That Can Be Mistaken for Vulvovaginitis

Urethral Prolapse

Urethral prolapse is often mistaken for vulvovaginitis or perineal trauma. Dysuria, perineal pain, and bleeding are the most frequent symptoms. The phenomenon occurs most frequently among obese prepubertal school-age girls. Increased intraabdominal pressure often precipitates the prolapse of the urethra through the urethral meatus. Constipation, coughing, and crying may all contribute. The classic physical finding is a red, swollen, and friable piece of tissue lying over the anterior introitus (Fig. 18-25). It often has a doughnut shape and is tender. With optimal positioning and careful visualization, the clinician can see that it encircles the urethral meatus. Because the urethral mucosa is responsive to estrogen, application of estrogen cream twice daily usually results in resolution. Oral analgesics and topical antibacterial and/or anesthetic creams provide symptomatic relief. Treatment of underlying causes reduces the risk of recurrence.

Lichen Sclerosus et Atrophicus

Lichen sclerosus et atrophicus is a chronic dermatologic disorder of unknown etiology that primarily involves the perineum and perianal area in prepubertal girls. It begins insidiously with perineal itching; later chronic itching may be accompanied by dysuria and skin break-

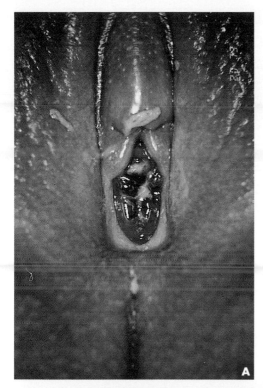

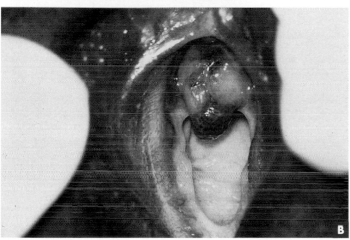

FIG. 18-25 Urethral prolapse. *A,* This child had acute complaints of bleeding and dysuria. The prolapsed urethral mucosa is red, friable, and has a doughnut shape encircling the urethra. *B,* In another patient the prolapsed mucosal tissue is thickened and erythema is less prominent. (*A* courtesy Dr. John McCann, University of California at Davis; *B* courtesy Dr. Carole Jenny, The Children's Hospital, Denver.)

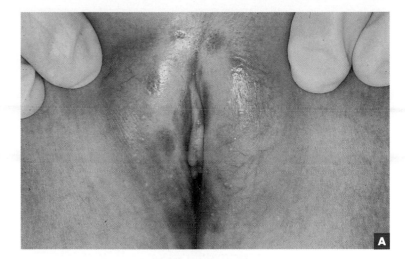

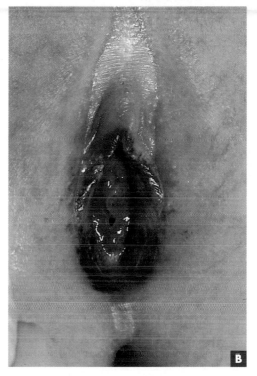

FIG. 18-26 Lichen sclerosis et atrophicus. *A,* The skin overlying the labia majora has become atrophic and appears pale and thin. It is dotted with small, superficial ulcerations. *B,* In this child with complaints of bleeding and pruritus, skin breakdown is evident along with petechial hemorrhage.

down with bleeding. Initially there may be no readily visible signs, and symptomatic treatment is often prescribed to no effect. Eventually, skin changes occur with intermittent breakdown. Clinical findings include patchy areas of atrophy in which the skin appears pale and thinned, ulceration and bleeding, and lichenification (Fig. 18-26, *A* and *B*). A definitive diagnosis is made by biopsy. The problem often responds to treatment with high-potency topical steroids.

Infectious Vulvovaginitis

In contrast to most of the primarily noninfectious forms of vulvovaginitis, vaginal discharge is usually a prominent part of the clinical picture of infectious vulvovaginitis in all age groups. Although a few pathogens produce a fairly characteristic clinical picture, most do not, the symptoms and discharge seen with many pathogens being relatively nonspecific. Furthermore, in the case of sexually transmitted infections, more than one pathogen may be present. For these reasons, careful attention to smear and culture techniques is important.

There are two major subgroups of vulvovaginal infection. In the first subgroup genital involvement is secondary, being part of a systemic infection or the result of transfer of the pathogen from another primary site such as the skin or the respiratory, gastrointestinal, or urinary tracts via contaminated fingers or proximity (Table 18-9). Infection at the primary site may precede or coexist with the genital infection, and in some cases colonization of another site, without overt infection, appears to predispose. This nonvenereal infectious vulvovaginitis is common in prepubertal patients, but is rare in adolescents because the mature female genital tract does not support growth of most of these pathogens.

The second subgroup of infectious vulvovaginitis consists of those infections caused by venereal pathogens (Tables 18-9 and 18-10). Both prepubertal and postmenarchal patients can have vulvovaginitis when infected with these organisms. After puberty, however, patients can have other clinical pictures as well, including cervicitis (with or without vulvovaginal inflammation) and salpingitis. Table 18-12 enumerates the possible clinical features seen in adolescent girls with sexually

TABLE 18-12

Major Characteristics of the Most Common Sexually Transmitted Diseases and Diagnostic Measures

	HSV	HPV	HIV	Trichomonas	Gonorrhea	Chlamydia	Syphilis
Possible clinical findings	Vulvar skin lesions, vulvitis, vaginitis, cervicitis; may be normal	Nonspecific vulvovaginal inflammation; subclinical lesions revealed by acid wash; vulvar, vaginal, and/or cervical condylomata	Unusually severe presentation of candida, HSV, or molluscum contagiosum, often resistant to treatment	Vaginitis, vulvitis, vaginal and/or cervical petechiae	May be normal, cervicitis, salpingitis, vaginitis, vulvitis, occasionally proctitis, pharyngitis, or urethritis	Often normal, cervicitis, salpingitis, occasionally vaginitis and vulvitis, occasionally urethritis	Primary—vulvar, vaginal, or cervical chancre; secondary—condylomata lata involving vulva with or without generalized exanthem
Incubation period	3–14 days	1–3 months (up to 9 months)	Acute flulike viral illness (several weeks); AIDS (variable—up to 10 years)	3—30 days	2–7 days	7–21 days	Primary (15–90 days); secondary (6 wks–6 mo); tertiary (2–20 yrs)
Infectivity	75%–80% (with active infection)	60%–70%	Varies with infecting behavior	70%–90% for male-to-female transmission, less for female-to-male	100% male-to-female; 25% female-to-male	45% male-to-female	10% single encounter; 30% after 1 month of sexual activity
Duration	Primary (2–3 wks); Secondary (7–12 days)	Variable	Acute infection (2–3 weeks); asymptomatic phase (months); symptomatic, not AIDS (months—years); AIDS (months—several years, fatal)	Self-limiting in many males; persistent in most females until treated	Until treated	Until treated	Primary (2–6 wks); secondary (2–6 wks) may recur; teritiary persists until treated
Recurrence	60% (HSV-1); 90% (HSV-2) (within 1 yr)	Variable	Persistence	With reinfection	With reinfection	With reinfection	With reinfection
Routine diagnostic techniques	Culture, Tzanck prep, Pap smear	Inspection, Pap smear, acetic acid wash, colposcopy	ELISA, Western blot, viral culture	Wet prep, urinalysis, Pap smear	Cervical culture, pharyngeal or rectal culture, Gram stain, DNA probe	PCR, antigen detection by ELISA-Chlamydiazyme or direct immunofluoroescence, tissue culture, DNA probe	Dark-field microscopy, serologic tests including VDRL, RPR, and FTA
Antenatal or perinatal transmission	Yes—can cause skin, CNS, and disseminated infection	Yes—can cause laryngeal papillomas and perineal lesions	Yes, and postpartum via breast milk	Yes—may have neonatal vaginal discharge or asymptomatic colonization	Yes—can cause conjunctivitis, septicemia, meningitis	Yes—can cause conjunctivitis and/or pneumonia	Yes, and postpartum via breast milk
Partner evaluation	Inspection	Inspection and acetic acid wash	Antibody test	Antimicrobial Rx	Cultures and antimicrobial Rx	Specimen collection and antimicrobial Rx	Serologic and clinical, antimicrobial Rx

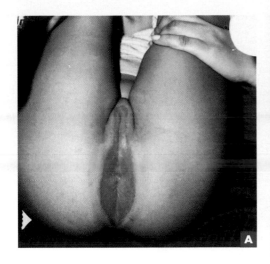

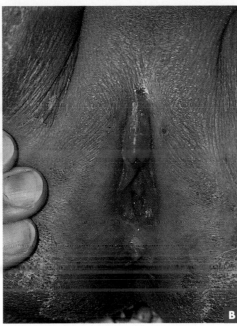

FIG. 18-27 Streptococcal vulvovaginitis. *A,* In this child, who had acute vulvar pain, dysuria, and discharge, the area of inflammation is sharply circumscribed and extends from the vulva to the perianal area. *B,* In this patient, who presented late in the course of a case of scarlet fever, vulvar inflammation is still evident and desquamation has begun.

transmitted infections and summarizes other major epidemiologic characteristics and appropriate diagnostic measures.

Regardless of age, the most frequent mode of transmission of venereal infection is sexual contact. The majority of these infections in prepubertal patients are the result of sexual abuse, although in a minority of cases transmission occurs perinatally or as a result of sex play with other children who have been abused (see Chapter 6). Hence, when venereal disease is found in the prepubertal child, the possibility of sexual abuse *must* be investigated. In adolescence, consensual sexual activity is the major mode of infection by sexually transmitted pathogens, although sexual exploitation and abuse remain significant possibilities. These factors necessitate obtaining a confidential history of sexual activity and case finding of sexual partners. *The presence of one venereal pathogen in any child or adolescent should prompt investigation for others because multiple infections are common* (see section on Genital Infections Caused by Sexually Transmitted Pathogens).

Infectious Vulvovaginitis Caused by Nonsexually Transmitted Pathogens
Vulvovaginitis caused by Respiratory and/or Skin Pathogens

Bacterial respiratory pathogens can cause vulvovaginitis in prepubertal patients, presumably as a result of orodigital transmission. *Streptococcus pneumoniae* and *Haemophilus influenzae* cause purulent vaginal discharge, with associated vulvitis and vaginitis, after or concurrent with upper respiratory tract infection. The most dramatic form of bacterial vulvovaginitis caused by a primary respiratory pathogen is that caused by group-A beta-hemolytic streptococci. This infection may be associated with streptococcal nasopharyngitis or scarlet fever; it may occur in apparent isolation, although a throat culture is often positive for strep even in the absence of pharyngeal or upper respiratory symptoms. The onset of vulvovaginal symptoms is abrupt, with severe perineal burning and dysuria. Inspection reveals a sharply circumscribed area of intense erythema involving the vulva, distal vagina, and perianal area (Fig. 18-27, *A*). The involved skin may weep serous fluid. Most patients have a serosanguineous or grayish-white vaginal discharge, and about one third have vaginal petechiae. Culture of perineal skin and/or discharge is positive. Desquamation ensues with recovery (Fig. 18-27, *B*).

Viral pathogens also are linked to vulvovaginitis in young children. Varicella is perhaps the most common, with pruritus and dysuria as its most prominent symptoms. Inspection reveals typical lesions involving the perineum and/or vagina (see Chapter 12). Adenovirus is reported to cause vulvovaginitis with a serous discharge in association with pharyngitis, conjunctivitis, and an exanthem, whereas echovirus causes a thick, clear vaginal discharge concurrent with gastroenteritis.

Impetigo and folliculitis may occur in the vulvar area of patients of any age and generally is secondary to poor hygiene, excessive sweating, shaving, or mechanical irritation. Simultaneous involvement of the buttocks or other skin sites is common (see Chapter 12). Some young women with increased androgens as a result of congenital adrenal hyperplasia or polycystic ovarian syndrome, children with a familial predisposition to keratosis pilaris, and patients with Down syndrome may be especially prone to developing folliculitis or impetigo.

Vulvovaginitis Caused by Gastrointestinal Pathogens

SHIGELLA. A distinct form of vulvovaginitis caused by *Shigella* species has been recognized in prepubertal patients. The majority have no overt gastrointestinal symptoms, although approximately one third have had associated diarrhea.

The predominant complaint is one of an acute or chronic vaginal discharge. Most patients are otherwise asymptomatic although some have dysuria. A greenish-brown, often blood-streaked, purulent, and foul-smelling vaginal discharge is seen on inspection, along with vulvar and vaginal erythema. The clinical appearance of the discharge may be indistinguishable from that seen with a vaginal foreign body. Gram stain reveals polymorphonuclear leukocytes and a predominance of gram-negative rods. A positive culture is diagnostic, but enteric-specific bacteriologic methods must be used. Antibiotic sensitivities may demonstrate broad resistance. Without proper treatment the discharge may persist for months. A high rate of coinfection with pinworms has been reported.

PINWORMS. Intestinal infestation with pinworms (*Enterobius vermicularis*) is primarily associated with perianal pruritus. However, the worms may crawl forward into the vagina, bringing enteric flora with them and depositing eggs. In some cases vaginal infection and discharge may result. Scratching may produce excoriation and secondary dysuria. A history of preceding perianal pruritus generally is elicited.

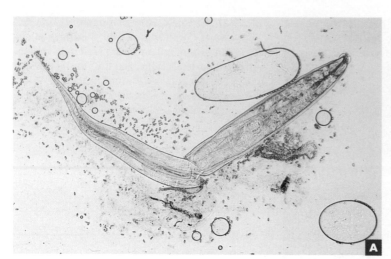

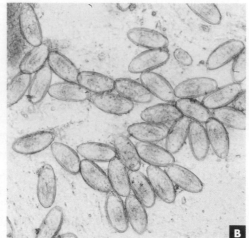

FIG. 18-28 Pinworms (*Enterobius vermicularis*). On this wet mount (*A*) a mature worm is shown surrounded by eggs, which are shown more clearly at higher power (*B*). Patients with intestinal infestation may have vulvovaginal symptoms as a result of scratching and excoriation or migration of the worms into the vagina.

Inflammatory changes are nonspecific. Pinworm ova and/or adult worms may be found on wet mount examination of vaginal secretions (Fig. 18-28). In the occasional patient with associated vaginal discharge, culture is positive for enteric pathogens. When pinworm infestation is suspected despite negative vaginal smears, the perianal Scotch tape test should be obtained by the mother during the night to increase the likelihood of detection.

Candida Vulvovaginitis

Candida species are one of the more common sources of nonvenereal infectious vulvovaginitis after puberty. This is rare in the healthy prepubertal child. Predisposing factors include recent antibiotic intake, poor perineal ventilation, diabetes mellitus, immunodeficiency, pregnancy, and the use of oral contraceptives. Pruritus, contact dysuria, and dyspareunia are the most prominent complaints. Symptoms are most likely to develop in the perimenstrual phase of the patient's cycle. Examination usually discloses diffuse erythema of the vulva associated with a thick cheesy vaginal discharge (Fig. 18-29, *A*). With chronic involvement, white or pink cobblestoned plaques on an erythematous base may be seen over the vulva. Excoriations from scratching also may be noted, and satellite lesions on the perineum are common. In some cases, signs of perianal dermatitis and intertrigo are found in association with vulvovaginal involvement.

Inspection of the lower third of the vagina in young patients and speculum examination in adolescents may reveal a thick white discharge of creamy or cheesy consistency. Whitish plaques may adhere to the vaginal mucosa or to the cervix in adolescents (Fig. 18-29, *B*). A KOH or wet prep confirms the presence of budding yeast and pseudohyphae in 50% to 80% of cases and may demonstrate an increase in inflammatory cells (Fig. 18-29, *C* and *D*). Vaginal pH is low (3.5 to 5).

Topical application of antifungal cream into the lower vagina is the treatment of choice. Single dose oral regimens are less efficacious but are simple and may be more reliable when problems with compliance are an issue. In sexually active adolescents, careful consideration must be given to the possibility of pregnancy before prescribing antimicrobials or any other medication. In patients with recurrences, predisposing factors, such as medications and HIV infection, should be considered. An infected male partner with subacute or chronic monilial balanitis rarely may be the source of recurrences in sexually active patients. This infection generally is not transmitted sexually, and treatment of the partner does not decrease recurrence rates.

Genital Infections Caused by Sexually Transmitted Pathogens

The number of pathogens identified as being transmitted by intimate sexual contact has mushroomed in the past two decades (Table 18-9). The rise in prevalence of venereal disease and the recognition of an increasing array of pathogens have prompted research that has produced a better understanding of their pathophysiology and the clinical pictures they produce (Table 18-12). It also has made the evaluation of patients with STDs considerably more complex. The majority of infections are manifested by external lesions and/or vulvovaginal inflammation with vaginal discharge. Although some infections produce relatively specific clinical findings, many are characterized by nonspecific signs and symptoms that appear to represent a final common pathway of a number of different etiologic agents of irritation, infection, or infestation. Several pathogens can induce two or three different clinical pictures (or a mixed picture) in adolescents. Furthermore the high frequency of multiple simultaneous infections adds to the complexity and necessitates more extensive laboratory evaluation. The clinical approach to these patients must be sensitive and individualized but also must differ considerably depending on whether or not the patient is premenarchal or postmenarchal.

Approach to STDs in Prepubertal Patients

Before menarche, lack of estrogenization inhibits ascent of infection and subclinical infection is probably unusual if not rare. Hence manifestations of venereal infection are primarily confined to the vulva and lower vagina. As a result, external inspection of the perineum and lower vagina and laboratory evaluation of vaginal discharge samples are sufficient for identification of most pathogens and for institution of therapy. This does not complete the assessment, however, because whenever venereal disease is identified in a prepubertal patient, *sexual abuse must be considered as the probable source*. This necessitates obtaining an extensive psychosocial history and initiating a thorough investigation to find the person responsible for transmitting the infection to the child (see Chapter 6).

Approach to STDs in Pubertal Patients

Complaints of pubertal patients with vulvovaginitis include vulvar lesions, vaginal discharge, odor, pruritus or perineal discomfort, and dysuria. These symptoms also may be associated with pelvic pain, dyspareunia, fever, and irregular bleeding. A number of pathogens cause inflammation of not only the vulva and vagina but may involve the cervix as well. Herpes simplex, *Trichomonas vaginalis*, and human papilloma viruses are

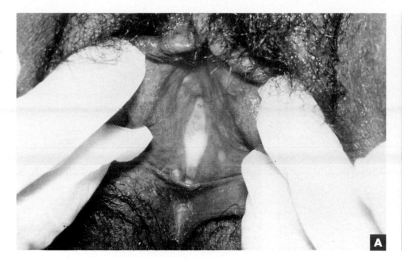

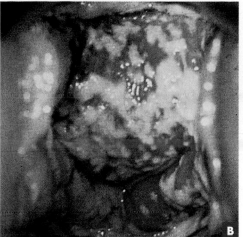

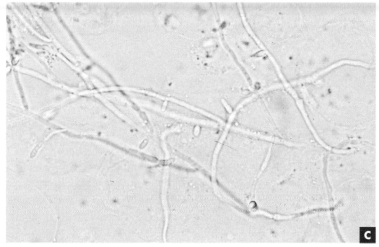

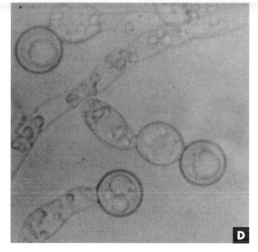

FIG. 18-29 Candida vulvovaginitis and cervicitis. *A,* The vulva is intensely hyperemic, and a thick, cheesy, white discharge covers the urethra, introitus, and hymenal area. *B,* Whitish plaques may be seen on the perineum and vaginal mucosa and occasionally on the cervix in adolescents. A whitish cheesy or creamy vaginal discharge may be noted as well. *C* and *D,* These low- and high-power wet mount specimens contain pseudohyphae and budding yeast. (*A* courtesy Dr. B. Cohen, Johns Hopkins Hospital, Baltimore; *B* and *D* courtesy Dr. Ellen Wald, Children's Hospital of Pittsburgh.)

prime examples. Patients infected with *Neisseria gonorrhoeae* or *Chlamydia trachomatis* may be asymptomatic even in the presence of cervicitis. When symptomatic, they may have vulvovaginitis; vaginal discharge; or, with ascent of infection to the upper tract, signs of salpingitis, although this too can be clinically silent (Tables 18-10 and 18-12). *N. gonorrhoeae* and *C. trachomatis* also infect the columnar epithelium of other genital sites, including the Bartholin glands, Skene ducts, urethra, and rectum.

Hence, a complete pelvic examination is necessary when evaluating adolescents for vulvovaginal complaints and possible STDs. After inspection of the perineum, the vaginal mucosa and the cervix must be visualized and their appearance assessed for signs of erythema, friability, focal lesions, and mucopurulent discharge. To differentiate a true cervical discharge from normal pooled vaginal secretions adhering to the cervix, visible discharge should be removed gently with cotton swabs before inspection. Cervical secretions should be sampled (for wet prep and cultures) by insertion of a swab into the os. The finding of cervicitis with a mucopurulent cervical discharge suggests gonorrheal and/or chlamydial infection and necessitates an attempt to identify or rule out upper tract involvement via bimanual examination. Cervical motion and uterine tenderness and/or a tender, palpable adnexal mass with or without systemic signs and symptoms suggest this possibility (see section on Pelvic Inflammatory Disease).

A number of additional considerations are important in evaluating postpubertal patients suspected of having an STD. A sexual history obtained in confidence is essential, and although consensual activity is common in adolescence, these patients may be victims of sexual abuse, including incest, sexual exploitation, and date rape. Sexual partners

should be evaluated and treated whenever an STD is identified; otherwise reinfection is probable.

Adolescent girls with asymptomatic cervical infections may serve as silent reservoirs of venereal pathogens. This phenomenon is quite significant in the epidemiology of STDs. Hence, women partners of men known to have gonorrhea or nongonococcal urethritis should be cultured and treated appropriately. The patient and partner must be advised to abstain from sexual intercourse until the course of treatment is completed. They also should be seen in follow-up for test of cure, and once cured, they should be seen at least every 6 months for STD surveillance because of the significant incidence of recurrent (often subclinical) infection.

The importance of aggressive case finding, diagnosis, and treatment cannot be overemphasized because of the potential for spread to others and major sequelae that include ectopic pregnancy and infertility as a result of smoldering or recurrent acute upper genital tract disease. Finally, it is the clinician's responsibility to provide education regarding STDs. Patients should understand how the disease was contracted and how to prevent recurrence. Use of condoms and spermicides should be encouraged. Education includes discussion of responsible sexuality, including use of contraceptives and safer sex practices, as appropriate to the patient.

Surface Infestations and Perineal Lesions

PARASITIC INFESTATIONS. Two parasitic infestations—scabies and pubic lice—may be transmitted via sexual contact. Both produce symptoms of vulvar and inguinal pruritus and irritation often accompanied by finding blood on underwear caused by excoriation from scratching.

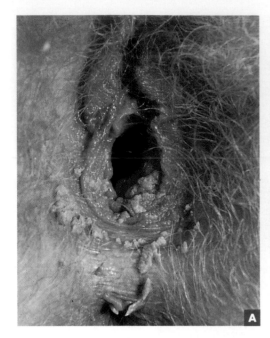

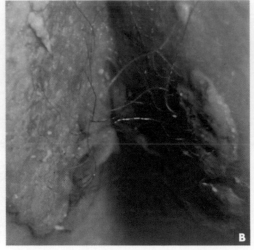

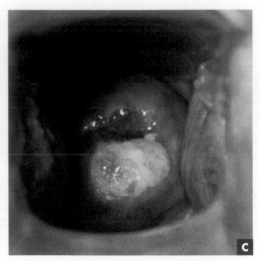

FIG. 18-30 *Condylomata acuminata.* These sexually transmitted viral warts (*A*) tend to be discrete early on, but (*B*) with evolution become confluent. Adolescents have a significant risk of developing vaginal and cervical lesions (*C*) (*A* and *C* courtesy Dr. E. Jerome; *B* courtesy Dr. M. Sherlock.)

Sexual transmission is more likely in adolescents than in young children, who may acquire the parasites by close nonsexual contact. Development of pubic hair is necessary for acquisition of pubic lice. Meticulous inspection of the pubic area for nits and adult lice ("crabs") may be necessary to discover early infestations. The clinical findings of both disorders are presented in Chapter 8.

HUMAN PAPILLOMA VIRUS. HPV has emerged as the most prevalent sexually transmitted pathogen found in adolescent girls. Genital or venereal warts, also called *condylomata acuminata,* are no longer an isolated nuisance, being but one manifestation of a spectrum of lower genital tract diseases caused by HPV. The virus recently has been implicated in playing a critical role in the development of cervical intraepithelial neoplasia (CIN) or dysplasia and is believed to be a cofactor or precursor of invasive carcinoma of the cervix and similarly carcinoma of other genital tissues in both men and women.

Transmission is usually via sexual contact in adolescents. Passage to neonates during delivery also has been documented and can result in subsequent development of laryngeal papillomata and perineal lesions. Vaginal involvement is uncommon in the prepubertal child, but when present, it is often accompanied by a vaginal discharge. The incubation period is variable and ranges from 1 to 9 months (Table 18-12).

Condylomata may emerge after subclinical, acute, or chronic nonspecific vulvovaginal inflammation incited by the virus. In mose cases the lesions are asymptomatic, although pruritis is reported by some patients. However, when the warts are traumatized or become secondarily infected, pain may be a complaint. A rapid increase in warty tissue may be associated with pregnancy or HIV infection.

Generally the warts appear as fleshy, rounded or ragged papules often located at the posterior edge of the introitus and/or in the perianal region. Lesions may be discrete early on (Fig. 18-30, *A*), but with evolution, they tend to become confluent (Fig. 18-30, *B*). The warts can also be flat or even clinically inapparent to the naked eye. Although most lesions involve the perineum and perianal areas, vaginal and cervical involvement also are common in adolescents (Fig. 18-30, *C*). Hence, when vulvar condylomata are found in postmenarchal patients, inspection of the vagina and cervix should be undertaken and a cervical Pap smear obtained. The virus also can infect other mucous membranes, including the anus, urethra, mouth, larynx, and conjunctiva.

Clinical diagnosis is made by careful inspection of the external genitalia, vagina, cervix (in adolescents), and perianal areas for visible warts. Examination of genital tissue after washing or soaking with 5% acetic acid (household vinegar) for up to 5 minutes reveals subclinical lesions. Acetic acid causes proliferating and immature epithelium to turn white because of disordered orientation of intracellular fibers. Most normal tissues retain a pink color. Other causes of aceto-white changes include injury, contact dermatitis, candidiasis, folliculitis, and allergic excoriation.

HPV infection is identified cytologically on the Pap smear by characteristic changes, including koilocytosis, which is pathognomonic for HPV infection. DNA hybridization has identified more than 60 subtypes of the virus, many of which are site- and pattern-specific in their disease expression. Viral Paps and DNA probes are used for identification of subtypes, but the clinical utility of these tests is not yet known. A negative VDRL or RPR helps differentiate HPV disease from the condylomata lata of secondary syphilis. Patients with cervical lesions merit gynecologic referral for colposcopy, biopsy, and definitive treatment, because of the potential of these lesions to undergo malignant transformation.

MOLLUSCUM CONTAGIOSUM. These sharply circumscribed, waxy, papular, umbilicated lesions caused by a pox virus can be spread as a result of sexual contact, in which case lesions are found predominantly on the labia, mons pubis, buttocks, and lower abdomen. This mode of spread is much more likely in the adolescent than in the young child. The clinical characteristics of molluscum lesions are presented in Chapter 8.

SYPHILIS

SYPHILITIC CHANCRE. Primary syphilis should be considered in any patient with a genital ulcer. The typical syphilitic chancre is painless and indurated with rolled margins and a smooth base (Fig. 18-31). It begins as an erythematous papule that erodes centrally. Most involve the genitalia, and in women they tend to be found more often on the cervix or vaginal walls than on the labia. Although a single lesion is typical, multiple chancres are seen in some cases. The chancre usually appears 3 to 4 weeks (up to 3 months) after inoculation with *Treponema pallidum* and is accompanied by inguinal adenopathy. Involved nodes are firm, mobile, and nontender. Because atypical lesions are common, all suspicious ulcers should prompt investigation by darkfield examination of

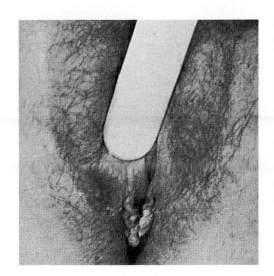

FIG. 18-31 Primary syphilis. This syphylitic chancre was painless and indurated on palpation. The base is smooth, and the margins are rolled. This patient also has condylomata acuminata. (Courtesy Dr. Ellen Wald, Children's Hospital of Pittsburgh.)

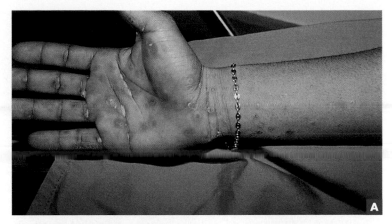

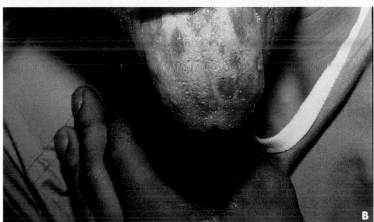

FIG. 18-32 Secondary syphilis. *A,* This adolescent had flulike symptoms and a generalized papulosquamous eruption involving the palms and soles. *B,* Mucosal lesions were also prominent. The systemic symptoms, mucosal lesions, and involvement of palms and soles helped distinguish the eruption from that of pityriasis rosea, with which it is commonly confused. (Courtesy Dr. Robert Hickey, Children's Hospital of Pittsburgh.)

scrapings from the base of the ulcer or of material aspirated from an enlarged regional node. Prior application of topical antibiotic ointment to a chancre can give false-negative results with ulcer scrapings. Reagin serologic tests (VDRL or RPR) usually become positive within 1 to 2 weeks after the appearance of the chancre and are uniformly elevated after a month. Positive reagin tests should always be confirmed by a fluorescent treponemal antibody test.

SECONDARY SYPHILIS. After an incubation period of about 6 to 9 weeks (sometimes months), hematogenous spread occurs and the lesions of secondary syphilis appear. These lesions are accompanied by generalized adenopathy and often are associated with flulike symptoms of headache, malaise, arthralgia, sore throat, and rhinorrhea. The rash generalizes rapidly, has a symmetric distribution, and involves the palms and soles. The lesions usually are reddish-brown maculopapules, although papulosquamous lesions are common (Fig. 18-32, *A*), and follicular and even pustular lesions may be seen, making secondary syphilis the "great mimicker." They range in size from a few millimeters to 1 cm and can be round or oval. Occasionally they clear centrally, becoming annular. As in pityriasis rosea for which the rash is often mistaken, they are frequently oriented along lines of skin cleavage. Moist papules, called *condylomata lata,* are found in the genital folds, gluteal cleft, and over the medial surfaces of the upper thighs. These papules often resemble small mushroom caps or have a warty appearance with a pinkish-gray color and range in size from 1 to 3 cm. Many patients develop an associated patchy alopecia.

Mucosal lesions, termed *mucous patches,* (Fig. 18-32, *B*) appear as centrally eroded, grayish-white plaques ½ to 1 cm in diameter and can be found on all mucosal surfaces. Condylomata lata and mucosal lesions teem with organisms and are thus highly infectious and are ideal sites for obtaining specimens for darkfield examination. Serologic tests are positive at this stage.

BARTHOLIN GLAND ABSCESS. This problem presents as a unilateral red, hot, tender mass at the posterior margin of the introitus at the base of a labia majorum (Fig. 18-36, *A*). It is generally seen in adolescents with gonorrhea, but it can occur in younger patients infected with gonococci, and it is increasingly associated with chlamydiae. When such a mass is encountered, material expressed from the abscess should be cultured because other agents such as streptococci and vaginal anaer-

obes also have been documented as pathogens. A full evaluation for STDs, including cervical swabs, may be necessary for organism identification. Treatment is based on Gram stain and culture results. Occasionally incision and drainage are required.

Lower Tract Disease

A number of sexually transmitted infections that are manifest as vulvovaginitis in the prepubertal patient produce findings limited to the lower genital tract (e.g., vaginitis and cervicitis) in the adolescent. A discussion of these infections follows. Upper tract manifestations are discussed later in the section on Pelvic Inflammatory Disease.

GENITAL HERPES. Herpes simplex viruses (HSV) type 2 and less commonly type 1 have been confirmed as genital pathogens in both pubertal and prepubertal girls. In adolescents, genital infection is acquired almost exclusively by sexual or intimate contact with infected mucosal surfaces. In prepubertal children, vulvar involvement can also result from sexual contact but more often results from spread from another infected site, such as the lip, mouth, or an herpetic whitlow. It has also been acquired from parents with herpes labialis who fail to wash their hands properly before changing diapers or before assisting young children with toileting. After exposure to the virus, 75% to 80% of individuals develop signs of infection after an incubation period of 3 to 14 days. Most infections are symptomatic, but occasionally individuals have no symptoms. An antibody response, with or without symptoms, can be produced within a few days.

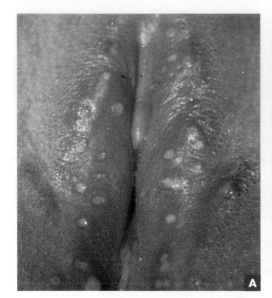
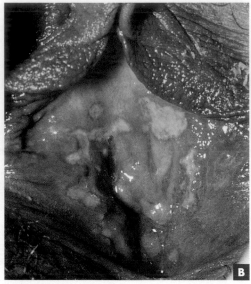
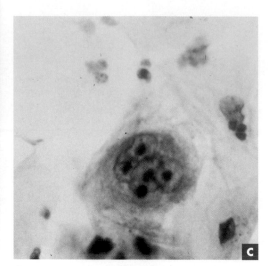

FIG. 18-33 Herpes simplex. *A,* This prepubertal child had intense dysuria, perineal pain, and numerous thick-walled vesicular lesions over her perineum. *B,* The ulcerative phase of herpetic vulvitis is seen in this adolescent patient. *C,* Wright-Giemsa stain of scrapings from the base of an herpetic ulcer demonstrates a typical multinucleated giant cell, with viral inclusions. (*C* courtesy Dr. Ellen Wald, Children's Hospital of Pittsburgh.)

Patients with primary infection frequently have systemic symptoms of fever, malaise, and myalgia, in addition to severe perineal pain and dysuria. Tender inguinal adenopathy usually is prominent but may not develop for several days. Perineal inspection reveals single or clustered vesicular lesions and/or ulcers on erythematous and edematous bases (Fig. 18-33, *A*). Acute ulcerations are typically covered by yellow exudate and may be quite extensive (Fig. 18-33, *B*). A copious, foul-smelling, watery, yellow vaginal discharge may be seen as well. Associated sterile pyuria may be a feature. Dysuria may be so severe as to cause acute urinary retention. The ulcerative phase gradually resolves as the lesions heal within a period of 14 to 21 days. Following primary infection, a persistent subclinical infection is established in the lumbosacral ganglia.

Diagnosis usually can be made on the basis of clinical appearance but can be confirmed in the laboratory by finding multinucleated giant cells on cytologic smears obtained by scraping the base of a lesion, smearing the specimen on a glass slide, and staining it with Wright-Giemsa stain (Fig. 18-33, *C*). Viral culture of a fresh and ideally vesicular lesion usually is confirmatory within a few days and is the diagnostic test of choice. Antiviral treatment is most effective when initiated early. Strong clinical suspicion is the usual indication for initiating antiviral therapy.

Recurrences are common and generally are milder, of shorter duration, and only locally symptomatic. Possible triggers of recurrence include fever, menstruation, emotional stress, and friction. Occasionally, prodromal tingling, pain, burning, or hyperesthesia is noticed in the area where vesicles ultimately recur. The interval between episodes varies widely.

Postmenarchal patients with vulvar herpetic lesions require speculum examination to look for the presence of herpes cervicitis, which is characterized by ulceration, friability, and a serosanguineous discharge. Herpetic ulcers are often found on the vaginal mucosa as well. Additionally, because of the risk of transmitting the virus to the newborn during vaginal delivery, pregnant young women with a history of genital herpes should have careful obstetric follow-up and serial cultures during the last trimester. If evidence of active infection is present, elective cesarean section is recommended.

TRICHOMONAS ORGANISMS. *T. vaginalis* is a flagellated protozoan. It has been found in the vaginal discharge of neonates delivered of mothers infected at the time of delivery, but thereafter it tends to be an unusual finding until the peripubertal period. This is thought to be due to the alkaline environment of the unestrogenized vaginal mucosa, which is unfavorable for growth of the organism. Beyond the neonatal period it is acquired almost exclusively by sexual contact, often in concert with other sexually transmitted pathogens. However, trichomonads can live on warm, moist surfaces outside a living host for up to 3 hours. Hence, transmission via fomites is possible. Although infection is occasionally asymptomatic in adolescents, the majority of patients have vulvar pruritus, burning, and dysuria, in association with a profuse vaginal discharge. The latter may be watery, yellowish-gray, or green. In some cases it is bubbly; in others it is homogeneous. Frequently the discharge has a foul, acrid odor. Some affected adolescents may complain of pelvic pain or heaviness.

On inspection the vulva may be hyperemic and edematous, but the degree of inflammation is highly variable. Because the discharge is profuse, it tends to be present on the perineum (Fig. 18-34, *A*). It pools in dependent portions of the vagina and coats the vaginal walls. The vaginal mucosa is erythematous, and punctate petechial lesions may be noted. In the adolescent these hemorrhagic areas may involve the cervical mucosa, producing the so-called strawberry cervix (Fig. 18-34, *B*). This organism does not routinely ascend to infect the upper genital tract.

Diagnosis is made by finding mobile trichomonads on microscopic examination of a saline wet mount (Fig. 18-34, *C*), but this is positive in only 50% to 60% of infections. On close observation, whiplike flagellar movements are noted. Leukocytes are usually seen in increased numbers and may surround the organisms, making detection more difficult. Warming the saline solution to body temperature and diluting a densely cellular discharge may make it easier to see the organisms moving. The slide must be examined soon after preparation because drying makes it uninterpretable. A positive whiff test (release of amine odor on addition of 10% KOH to a drop of discharge) is also common. Trichomonads may also be found in urine specimens. Reports of trichomonads on Pap smears have a high rate false positives and false

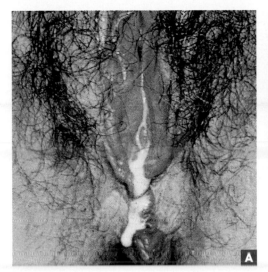
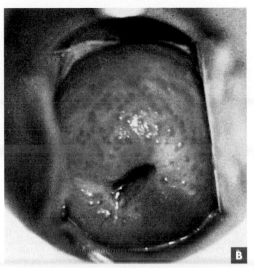
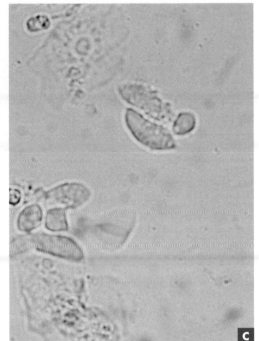

FIG. 18-34 Trichomonas. *A, T. vaginalis* produces a profuse acrid-smelling thin discharge that often is visible on perineal inspection. In some cases it is homogeneous, and in others it is bubbly. Vulvar pruritus often is intense. *B,* The vaginal mucosa is inflamed and often speckled with petechial lesions. In adolescents, petechial hemorrhages may also be found on the cervix, resulting in the so-called strawberry cervix. *C,* Microscopic examination of a wet mount reveals multiple motile trichomonads. A sperm is seen in the upper portion of the picture. (*A* and *B* courtesy Dr. Ellen Wald, Children's Hospital of Pittsburgh.)

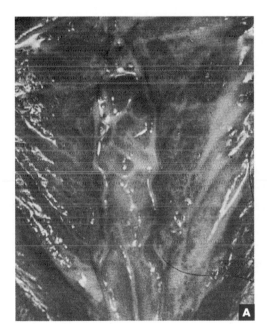
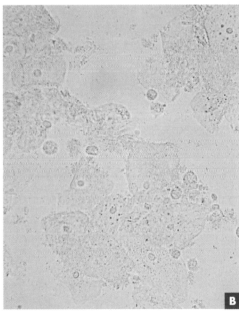

FIG. 18-35 Bacterial vaginosis (previously called *Gardnerella vaginalis*). This surface pathogen acts in concert with vaginal anaerobes to produce this form of vaginosis. *A,* The major symptom is one of a malodorous homogeneous vaginal discharge. *B,* Characteristic "clue cells" are seen on wet mount and consist of vaginal epithelial cells covered with adherent refractile bacteria. Since the organism is noninvasive, leukocytes are not increased and mucosal changes are not present. (*A* courtesy Dr. Ellen Wald, Children's Hospital of Pittsburgh.)

negatives. Positive reports in a symptomatic patient warrant treatment. Finding an elevated vaginal pH also may support a diagnosis. Latex-agglutination and DNA-probe office-based tests are now available, with variable specificity and sensitivity. *Trichomonas* organism cultures, the gold standard of diagnosis, generally are not available in clinical settings.

Oral metronidazole is effective for treatment, but should be avoided in pregnant patients because of its teratogenic potential. Intravaginal metronidazole does not have sufficient absorption to reach the multiple sites of trichomonal infection, including the urethra and skene glands. Sexual partners usually are asymptomatic carriers of small numbers of organisms, but occasionally they have symptoms of urethritis. They should be treated whether or not they have symptoms.

BACTERIAL VAGINOSIS. BV is a noninflammatory condition that represents a disturbance in the vaginal ecosystem. Women with BV have an overgrowth of *Gardnerella vaginalis* and other anaerobic bacteria and a corresponding decrease in their population of lactobacilli. The overall concentration of bacteria increases 100-fold. BV is associated with increased frequency of preterm labor, and data suggest an association with increased incidence of pelvic inflammatory disease. The major symptom in all age groups is a vaginal discharge with a noticeable fishy odor. Adolescents with BV have little vulvovaginal irritation, and the cervix and upper genital tract are spared.

On inspection, discharge is frequently present on the perineum (Fig. 18-35, *A*) and may be seen adhering to the vaginal walls, which do not appear to be inflamed. Generally the discharge is thin and ho-

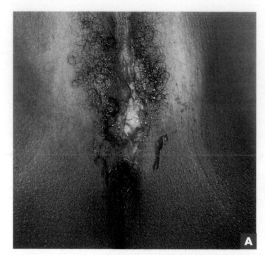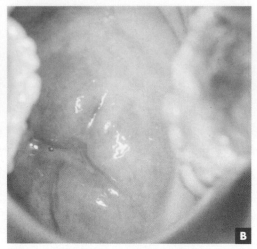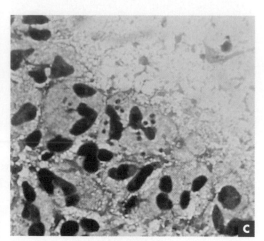

FIG. 18-36 Gonorrhea. *A,* Vulvar inflammation, edema, and a purulent vaginal discharge are seen in this peripubertal child who was a victim of sexual abuse. She also has a unilateral Bartholin gland abscess. *B,* Adolescents are vulnerable to ascent of infection and usually have findings of cervical inflammation with mucopurulent discharge. *C,* On Gram stain the vaginal discharge from the patient in *A* is found to contain sheets of leukocytes, many of which contain gram-negative intracellular diplococci. This test is highly reliable for prepubertal girls and for boys with a urethral discharge, but adolescent girls have a significant incidence of false negatives. (*B* courtesy Dr. L. Vontver.)

mogeneous in consistency, grayish-white in color, and malodorous. Addition of 10% KOH to a sample of the discharge produces a noticeable amine odor (positive whiff test). A saline wet prep usually reveals characteristic "clue cells," vaginal epithelial cells with a stippled cell membrane that is covered with adherent refractile bacteria (Fig. 18-35, *B*). On Gram stain the cells appear studded with gram-negative or gram-variable rods.

The diagnosis is made clinically by meeting three out of the following four criteria: homogeneous white discharge, a positive whiff test, clue cells representing more than 20% of the epithelial cells on a saline wet mount preparation, and vaginal secretions with a pH greater than 4.5. Because BV alone is rarely associated with evidence of tissue invasion, leukocytes should not be seen in increased numbers. If they are, additional pathogens should be sought and are often found. Both oral and intravaginal metronidazole and intravaginal clindamycin are acceptable forms of treatment in the nonpregnant patient.

GONORRHEA ORGANISMS. Gonococci are still a common cause of treatable bacterial cervicitis in the adolescent and vulvovaginitis in the prepubertal child. The major complaint is of a purulent vaginal discharge. Before menarche the child may be otherwise asymptomatic, but most experience some degree of vulvar discomfort, pruritus, or dysuria. Symptomatic adolescents without upper genital tract extension can have a similar picture. Inspection reveals a profuse purulent discharge that usually is greenish-yellow but also can be creamy, yellow, green, or white (Fig. 18-36, *A*). Inspection of the distal vaginal mucosa in younger children reveals prominent inflammation. In adolescents the vaginal mucosa can appear normal, but the cervix usually is erythematous and friable, with purulent material seen draining through the os (Fig. 18-36, *B*). Patients in this age group also may have evidence of urethritis manifested by erythema, edema, and tenderness of the urethra. When the latter findings are present, purulent material can be expressed by pressing along the length of the urethra through the anterior vaginal wall. A sample of this material should be sent for culture. Other sites with columnar epithelium are similarly vulnerable to infection. These include the Bartholin and Skene glands and the rectum.

Laboratory studies are essential for accurate diagnosis. In prepubertal patients a Gram-stained smear of the vaginal discharge is reliably

positive for large numbers of leukocytes and gram-negative intracellular diplococci and is adequate for initiation of treatment (Fig. 18-36, *C*). Culture is important to detect the few cases with a false-negative Gram stain, to determine antimicrobial sensitivity, and for medicolegal confirmation. Since simultaneous throat and anal cultures commonly are positive (despite the absence of anorectal or pharyngeal symptoms), these sites should also be cultured when gonorrhea is suspected or confirmed. They may be positive when the vaginal culture is negative. Both tonsils and the posterior pharyngeal wall should be swabbed in obtaining the throat specimen, and the rectal swab should be inserted no more than 1 to 2 cm past the anal orifice to avoid fecal contamination. Culture swabs should be placed immediately in appropriate transport medium or plated promptly on Thayer-Martin culture plates and incubated under appropriate exacting conditions to maximize the chance for positive results.

In adolescents with symptomatic gonorrhea, Gram stain of the mucopurulent cervical discharge reveals a predominance of leukocytes that may contain gram-negative intracellular diplococci. When results are positive, this is specific and treatment may be instituted. The incidence of false-negative Gram stains is significant, however. False positives also may be encountered in asymptomatic women colonized by other *Neisseria* species. Cultures are thus essential. Recent studies of women with culture-proven gonococcal cervicitis have shown concurrent chlamydial infection in about one third of these patients. Thus when purulent cervicitis is found, specific specimens for detection of *Chlamydia* organisms should also be obtained and treatment for both pathogens begun empirically.

Knowledge of local patterns of bacterial resistance dictates antibiotic choices. Several single-dose oral therapies are usually acceptable for cervicitis. Pharyngeal and anal infection with *N. gonorrhoeae* and the risk of acquiring concomitant syphilis may also influence antibiotic choice, and current Centers for Disease Control (CDC) guidelines should be consulted.

On occasion, patients with gonorrhea may develop disseminated gonococcal infection via hematogenous spread. This phenomenon may occur at any age. It is more common in adolescent girls with asymptomatic (and therefore, untreated) endocervical infection, in men with

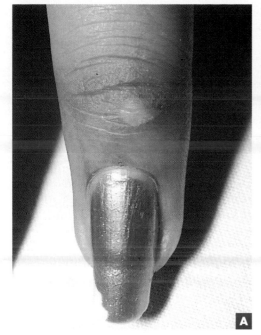
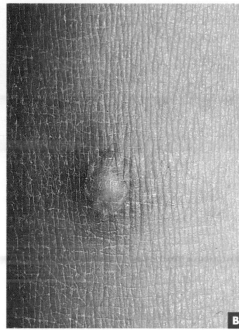
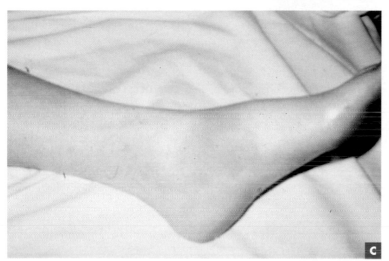
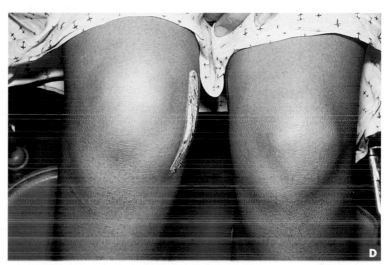

FIG. 18-37 Disseminated gonococcal infection. *A* and *B,* These pustular skin lesions with red halos are characteristic of disseminated gonorrhea, which can occur at any age. *C* and *D,* Tenosynovitis and monoarticular arthritis are commonly seen in association with skin lesions in disseminated disease. Note the signs of effusion in this girl's knee, which was aspirated for culture. (*D* courtesy Dr. Robert Hickey, Children's Hospital of Pittsburgh.)

asymptomatic urethral infection, and in patients of both genders and all ages with silent anal or pharyngeal infections. Yet it also can be seen in patients with symptomatic vulvovaginitis, cervicitis, or urethritis. In postmenarchal women, symptoms are more likely to develop during a menstrual period or during pregnancy.

The clinical picture often has two stages. Initially fever and chills are prominent, and the patient is intermittently bacteremic. During this stage, which lasts 2 to 5 days, polyarthralgias are experienced (involving the knees, wrists, ankles, elbows, and hands) and characteristic skin lesions often appear. The latter begin as small erythematous papules or petechiae that usually evolve to form pustules surrounded by red halos (Fig. 18-37, *A* and *B*). Later, these may necrose centrally. Lesions often contain gram-negative diplococci, which can be seen on a gram stain, but usually fail to grow on culture. If not diagnosed and treated promptly, patients progress to a second phase, characterized by monoarticular arthritis with effusion or tenosynovitis (Fig. 18-37, *C* and *D*). In up to 50% of these cases, culture of joint aspirates is positive. Specialized techniques to isolate cell-wall–deficient organisms further increase culture yield. Myocarditis, pericarditis, endocarditis, and meningitis are other complications of hematogenous seeding.

CHLAMYDIA TRACHOMATIS. Chlamydia is the most prevalent treatable STD and has replaced gonorrhea as the most common sexually trans-

mitted pathogen causing cervicitis and upper genital tract disease. Its high prevalence (up to 25%) in adolescent populations and its serious sequelae make its proper diagnosis and treatment an important aspect of adolescent sexual health care. When compared with gonococcal infection, its transmission rate for a single episode of intercourse is lower, but its prevalence is greater and infection persists longer. Of women whose male partners are infected with chlamydia, 45% are infected.

Chlamydiae are unique microorganisms. They are obligate intracellular parasites that cannot be cultivated on artificial media and depend on their cellular hosts for high-energy ATP and other nutrients. Identification has become more accessible with PCR-DNA probes, ELISA (Chlamydiazyme), tissue culture, and monoclonal antibody techniques, but all are still relatively expensive laboratory procedures. Specimens must be appropriately collected and transported. Chlamydia cultures are the gold standard and must be used for prepubertal, medicolegal, and rectal specimens. For all collections, cell scrapings are necessary rather than secretions or discharge because of the intracellular nature of the organism. Swabs or cytologic brushes are acceptable for specimen collection. External mucus and debris should be removed first. A Dacron swab with a plastic shaft should be used for culture because cotton swabs may interfere with recovery of the organism from tissue culture. Calcium alginate-tipped swabs may produce false-positive

Chlamydiazyme results when specimens are not processed shortly after collection. Serologic tests are not useful, except for confirmation of lymphogranuloma venereum caused by specific immunotypes. Tests of cure are not reliable for several weeks after treatment and are not recommended by the CDC. Reinfection is common.

Although some are asymptomatic, most prepubertal girls infected with chlamydia tend to have vaginal discharge and/or bleeding, vulvar pruritis or pain, and vulvar erythema. Symptoms may be intermittent or persistent and coinfection with *N. gonorrhoeae* is common.

Adolescent girls have symptoms of both cervical and urethral infection. Pelvic or abdominal pain, spotting or irregular-vaginal bleeding, dysuria, or vaginal discharge may accompany infection. A picture indistinguishable from that of symptomatic gonorrhea, with purulent vaginal discharge, perineal irritation, and findings of cervicitis with mucopurulent discharge, also can be seen (Fig. 18-36, *B*). Endometritis is common with cervicitis, even in the absence of classic symptoms of pelvic inflammatory disease, and Bartholin duct infections also occur. Asymptomatic chlamydial infection in both females and males is common.

On examination of the cervix, the presence of yellowish-green mucopus, cervical ectopy, and erythema are all associated with chlamydial infection. Often the cervix is friable, bleeding during the minimal manipulation necessary to obtain specimens. When seen as an isolated infection, the cervical discharge contains increased numbers of leukocytes without intracellular organisms. Microscopic evidence of other infections does not decrease the likelihood of chlamydia coinfection and should not deter the practitioner from treating for chlamydia if its presence is suggested by the history or physical findings. Patients commonly have simultaneous infection with gonococci and chlamydia—hence the rationale for culturing for both organisms and covering for both with treatment, when purulent cervicitis is found on examination.

Chlamydia can also produce an acute urethral syndrome in postpubertal patients. Dysuria, urgency, and frequency may be accompanied by physical signs of urethral discharge, meatal redness, and swelling. Pyuria may exist in the absence of bacteriuria. Urethral specimens for Chlamydia must be collected by inserting a thin Dacron swab 2 cm into the urethra and rotating it 360 degrees before withdrawal. First void urine specimens from males can be used for Chlamydiazyme and DNA-PCR testing, but urine is not an acceptable specimen from females. Rectal infection exists in both heterosexual and homosexual populations. Pharyngeal infection is rarely detected. A careful sexual history may reveal possible extragenital sites of infection, but treatment at other sites is not known to differ, as it does with extragenital gonorrhea.

Genital Mycoplasmas

Mycoplasma hominis, M. genitalium, and *Ureaplasma urealyticum* are the three species of mycoplasma implicated in genital infections. The organisms may be cultured from vaginal specimens of neonates and sexually active women in the absence of disease, but colonization in the prepubertal girl is rare. Mycoplasmas also have been cultured from polymicrobial upper genital tract infections, but it remains unclear whether they are initiators of ascending infections or they behave as normal bacterial flora accompanying the primary ascending infection of gonorrhea or chlamydia organisms, becoming pathogenic once relocated in the fallopian tubes. Mycoplasmas have also been found causative in some cases of acute urethral syndrome.

The currently widespread practice of broad spectrum antimicrobial treatment of STDs to include chlamydia and the general unavailability of laboratory confirmation of *Mycoplasma* organism involvement in infection have made it difficult to further understand the role of these organisms. This broad-spectrum therapy, however, has provided treatment for problems that might have persisted because of an inability to establish a precise diagnosis. Although routine cultures for mycoplasmas are not justified, they should be considered for infections resistant to documented therapy in the absence of reinfection by an untreated partner.

HUMAN IMMUNODEFICIENCY VIRUS (HIV). Acquired immunodeficiency syndrome (AIDS) and other manifestations of HIV infection are discussed in Chapter 4. The adolescent history outlined previously (Table 18-5) should identify teenagers at risk of acquiring HIV infection. In an attempt to reduce subsequent transmission and treat infection early, confidential HIV testing is encouraged for teens at risk of exposure to the virus. The definition of moderate to high risk has been regularly changing as our understanding of the disease, its epidemiology, and treatment opportunities evolve. Reliable sources of such information (e.g., the CDC) should be consulted regularly.

From the gynecologic perspective, a number of infections may present differently in the HIV-infected individual. These include infections with *Candida* organisms, human papilloma viruses, herpes simplex viruses, and molluscum contagiosum. In such cases the disease may be unusually severe, may present atypically, or may be resistant to treatment.

Pelvic Inflammatory Disease

An important complication of lower genital tract infection in the postmenarchal female is pelvic inflammatory disease (PID). PID results from ascending spread of a cervical infection that may or may not have been symptomatic. Though classically attributed to gonorrhea, PID is being increasingly recognized as a polymicrobial infection. Initiating pathogens implicated include *N. gonorrhoeae, C. trachomatis,* and *M. hominis.* Other organisms, usually considered normal vaginal or enteric flora, are potentially pathogenic when introduced into the upper genital tract. Among these are *Bacteroides* species; other anaerobic gram-positive bacilli and cocci; and aerobes, including streptococcal species, *E. coli,* and *Klebsiella* and *Proteus* species (Table 18-11). The majority of cases of salpingitis are due to mixed anaerobic and aerobic infection, although the classically recognized venereal pathogens play a critical initiating role.

Risk factors for developing upper genital tract infection include being an adolescent, having multiple sexual partners, use of an IUD, and previous PID. Because menstruation facilitates ascent of pathogenic organisms from the cervix to the uterus and fallopian tubes, the onset of symptoms is often during or shortly after a menstrual period. Long-term morbidity includes an increased incidence of ectopic pregnancy, decreased fertility, and chronic pelvic pain. These sequelae are secondary to tubal occlusion and scarring of pelvic structures. It is estimated that for each episode of PID there is an additional 15% chance of subsequent fertility problems.

The "textbook" picture of acute PID is one of a sexually active female who abruptly develops a high fever and shaking chills in association with intense lower abdominal pain. Nausea and vomiting are common. The patient appears acutely ill and uncomfortable and may have pain on walking with an antalgic gait. On abdominal examination there is prominent lower abdominal tenderness and guarding. Cervical visualization discloses signs of cervicitis with mucopurulent discharge. Bimanual palpation elicits extreme pain on cervical motion and reveals marked tenderness of the fundus and adnexa. Adnexal enlargement, if present, suggests abscess formation. The sedimentation rate is markedly elevated, and there is a pronounced leukocytosis with a left shift on CBC and differential. This "classic" picture has the highest likelihood of being associated with positive cultures for *N. gonorrhoeae.* It is not the most typical scenario, however. More commonly the onset of symptoms is insidious and the clinical picture more subtle. This is particularly likely with nongonococcal PID. Fever may be absent or low grade; the abdomen and pelvis may be only mildly tender; and blood work frequently is normal. In such cases diagnosis can be particularly difficult, requiring considerable suspicion and a readiness for obtaining cultures on the part of the clinician. Lower abdominal or pelvic pain, cervical motion tenderness, and some evidence of lower genital tract inflammation usually are present. However, some cases of chronic PID may not fit even this milder picture. A low-grade tubal infection may produce more in the way of adnexal findings and few, if any, uterine signs.

Diagnosis is complicated by the fact that, not only is there a wide range in severity of the clinical picture but also a lack of clear, quantifiable diagnostic guidelines for PID. Furthermore acute salpingitis may mimic a number of other disorders, including ectopic or intrauterine pregnancy and appendicitis or appendiceal abscess (in cases with right-lower-quadrant abdominal pain and tenderness). Torsion or hemorrhage of an ovarian cyst, septic abortion, endometriosis, pyelonephritis, cholecystitis, pelvic tumors, inflammatory and irritable bowel disease, and severe dysmenorrhea are other differential diagnostic possibilities (Table 18-13).

The adolescent with right-lower-quadrant abdominal pain is particularly challenging diagnostically. Table 18-14 summarizes clinical findings that may aid in distinguishing among the many potential causes. Fig. 18-38 illustrates some of the ultrasound findings in disorders that may cause pelvic or right-lower-quadrant abdominal pain.

Because of the potentially devastating long-term sequelae of PID, aggressive and largely empiric antimicrobial therapy is warranted. Treatment should include antibiotics that cover the common organisms in accordance with current CDC recommendations. Polymicrobial coverage is prescribed at the time of presumptive diagnosis.

According to the CDC and generally subscribed to clinical practice guidelines, all adolescents with PID should be admitted to the hospital for parenteral antibiotic treatment and serial reexaminations to assess response. Hospitalization and parenteral therapy are also recommended for patients suspected of having an abscess, patients in whom the diagnosis is uncertain, patients with manifestations of toxicity, and those who are pregnant or unable to comply with outpatient treatment. If a patient with suspected PID is treated as an outpatient, it is mandatory that she be reexamined within 24 to 48 hours to document improvement. If no such improvement has occurred she should be admitted and treated parenterally. In addition to antibiotic resistance, failure to improve promptly on therapy raises the possibility of complications such as abscess formation; development of a tuboovarian complex; or a missed diagnosis of ectopic pregnancy, miscarriage, or appendicitis. Sonography is useful in evaluating masses and suspected tuboovarian complexes. Additional procedures such as culdocentesis or laparoscopy may be necessary in unusual cases in which surgical conditions are suspected or medical treatment fails. The risks of complicated PID and tuboovarian abscess increase with each subsequent episode of PID.

PERIHEPATITIS (FITZ-HUGH-CURTIS SYNDROME). One of the more acute complications of PID, seen in 5% to 20% of cases, presents as right-upper-quadrant pain caused by perihepatitis. The inflammatory process probably ascends from the fallopian tubes along the paracolic gutters to the right upper quadrant, resulting in inflammation of the liver capsule and adjacent peritoneum.

The clinical picture is one of sudden onset of severe pleuritic right-upper-quadrant pain, which may be referred to the right shoulder, and is associated with chills, fever, nausea, and vomiting. Although in the majority of cases the pain develops simultaneously with pelvic symptoms of PID, it may present in the course of an asymptomatic ascending lower genital tract infection before genital tract signs emerge or later in the course of a partially treated infection. Upper abdominal pain may be so severe that the patient is relatively unconcerned about lower abdominal and pelvic complaints.

TABLE 18-13

Medical Conditions Presenting With Acute Right-Sided Abdominal Pain in Adolescent Girls

Pulmonary
Pneumonia, pleuritis, pleurodynia

Hepatic
Fitz-Hugh-Curtis syndrome
Viral hepatitis (A, B, C, etc.)
Drug-induced hepatitis
Autoimmune hepatitis
Alcoholic hepatitis
Hepatitis secondary to bacteremia
Epstein-Barr virus hepatitis

Biliary
Acute cholecystitis
Gallstones
Cholelithiasis

Intestinal
Inflammatory bowel disease
Irritable bowel syndrome
Constipation
Lactose intolerance

Pancreatic
Drug induced
Alcohol related
Traumatic
Viral
Autoimmune

Other Gastrointestinal
Subdiaphragmatic abscess
Appendicitis
Perforated gastric or duodenal ulcer

Renal
Acute pyelonephritis or perinephric abscess

Gynecologic
PID
Ovarian cyst, torsion, rupture, hemorrhage
Dysmenorrhea
Ectopic pregnancy

Right-upper-quadrant tenderness and guarding are the major physical findings; peritoneal signs may be present. Gynecologic examination in most instances discloses findings of purulent cervicitis and PID. *N. gonorrhoeae* and *C. trachomatis* are the major pathogens associated with this syndrome. When nongonococcal in origin, the predisposing salpringitis may be silent.

The sedimentation rate may be elevated, but there are minimal if any abnormalities of liver function tests. Although usually not necessary, ultrasound examination of the right upper quadrant should demonstrate a normal liver, biliary tree and gallbladder. Laparoscopic findings of purulent and fibrinous inflammation of the capsule and hemorrhagic areas of adjacent parietal peritoneum are diagnostic, but laparoscopy is rarely indicated for this condition.

Major differential diagnostic considerations include viral and drug-induced hepatitis; hepatitis secondary to bacteremia; pneumonia, pleuritis, and pleurodynia; subphrenic abscess; and acute cholecystitis. Perforated gastric or duodenal ulcers and pancreatitis may cause right-upper-quadrant pain but are more likely to cause burning epigastric pain or boring epigastric pain, respectively (Tables 18-13 and 18-14).

Although psychosomatic factors may be the most common cause of recurrent abdominal pain and should be carefully addressed in history taking, many such cases are of organic origin and a diagnosis of functional abdominal pain is a diagnosis of exclusion. Furthermore patients with sudden onset of severe abdominal pain are highly likely to have a significant underlying organic cause.

TABLE 18-14

Pertinent Clinical Characteristics of Disorders Causing Right-Sided Abdominal Pain in Adolescent Girls

	PID	Ovarian torsion	Ovarian cyst	Ectopic pregnancy
Location and quality of pain	Mid and lateral pelvis, usually bilateral; can be vague, dull, crampy, or sharp	Unilateral RLQ or LLQ (R:L,3:2), colicky	RLQ or LLQ, colicky, but usually asymptomatic	Lateral pain, colicky, +/− uterine cramping
Onset	GC—immediately post-menstrual and rapid Chlamydia—gradual over days to months	Sudden	Gradual, though rupture or hemorrhage associated with acutely increased pain	Gradual with sudden exacerbation
History	Unprotected sexual intercourse, previous PID or STDs, multiple partners	+/− history of similar pain with resolution, increased ovarian size (anatomic variation predisposes)	Midcycle or luteal phase, physiologic rupture causes Mittelschmerz of 24 to 48 hours' duration	Amenorrhea (75%), +/− pregnancy signs and symptoms
GI symptoms (vomiting/diarrhea)	Nausea, vomiting, anorexia (not necessarily present)	Vomiting with onset of pain (25%)	Rare	GI symptoms secondary to pregnancy or severe vomiting secondary to rupture and peritonitis
Masses	Occasional; if present, consider tuboovarian complex or ectopic pregnancy	Usually present, increased size secondary to edema	Often palpable if not physiologic cyst	Adnexal mass palpable in 50% of cases
Physical examination and lab findings	Cervical motion and adnexal tenderness, clinical and lab evidence of cervicitis; vaginal bleeding; +/− discharge; +/− RUQ pain; perihepatitis; + cervical cultures for gonorrhea or Chlamydia	Tender adnexa, +/− guarding or peritoneal signs	Unilateral cystic adnexal mass, x-ray rules out dermoid	Normal uterus; unilateral or bilateral adnexal tenderness; +pregnancy test in most, but inadequate β-HCG Rise/48 hr; drop in Hct with rupture
Ultrasound findings	Usually normal, tuboovarian complex in 10%–15%	Usually solid ovarian mass, +/− compromised blood supply on Doppler	Cyst >3 cm, +/− fluid in cul-de-sac—frequent incidental finding on U/S	Tubal mass, vaginal probe enhances detection

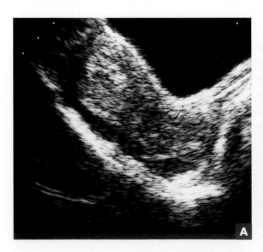
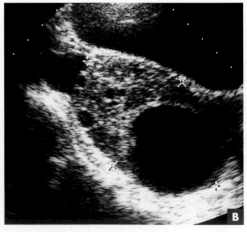

FIG. 18-38 Ultrasound findings in the diagnosis of pelvic or abdominal pain. *A,* This image shows an abnormal amount of fluid in the cul-de-sac released from a ruptured ovarian cyst in a 15-year-old with left-lower-quadrant and midline pelvic pain. *B,* In a 12-year-old girl with a 4-day history of colicky right-lower-quadrant pain, ultrasound demonstrates a single large abnormal cyst and multiple small physiologic cysts. Operative diagnosis was right ovarian torsion.

TABLE 18-14

Pertinent Clinical Characteristics of Disorders Causing Right-Sided Abdominal Pain in Adolescent Girls—cont'd

	Inflammatory bowel disease	Appendicitis	Irritable bowel/constipation	Dysmenorrhea	Intrauterine pregnancy
Location and quality of pain	LLQ, crampy	Periumbilical cramping changing to RLQ cramping or sharp pain	LLQ, crampy or colicky	Suprapubic, mid-abdominal, lower back, dull cramping	Midline fullness
Onset	Gradual, weeks to months with exacerbations	Gradual over hours to days	Long history of GI problems, months to years	Periodic, evolving over hours	Gradual over weeks or months
History	Weight loss or growth failure, fatigue, rashes, arthritis, fever	Usually no prior pain	+/− constipation or diarrhea, distension common, + family Hx, symptoms increase with stress	If unusual pattern or severity, consider congenital abnormalities or obstruction, threatened abortion or ectopic pregnancy	Amenorrhea, pregnancy signs and symptoms
GI symptoms (vomiting/diarrhea)	Increased stool frequency, nocturnal stools, sometimes bloody diarrhea	Vomiting may follow onset of pain, anorexia	Long intermittent history of constipation, +/− diarrhea	Diarrhea, flatulence, or vomiting not uncommon	Nausea with vomiting, worse in morning
Masses	Unusual, except with chronic complicated disease	Rare	Feces	None	Smooth midline pelvic or abdominal mass palpable above symphys pubis
Physical examination and lab findings	Rectoabdominal tenderness, hematologic abnormalities, stool heme +	↑WBCs, fever, evolving peritoneal signs	Ocasional tender colon, usually normal	Normal	+Serum pregnancy test 8-10 days after conception, + urine test 10-14 days
Ultrasound findings	Normal	Appendix frequently visible	Normal	Normal	Gestational sac after 4 weeks or with β-HCG >1500 MIU/ml

Pregnancy

Sexual activity among teenagers has dramatically increased since the early 1970s, with a greater percentage of young women of all ages reporting having had sexual intercourse. The pregnancy rate for adolescents in the U.S. is approximately 110 per 1000 for 15- to 19-year-old girls per year. It remains one of the highest among industrialized countries. Although the birth rate of 15- to 19-year-olds has declined slightly since 1974, the rate of pregnancies and births among younger adolescents (below age 15) has increased. As a result, the total number of teenage pregnancies has stayed about the same. These pregnancies are usually unintended and unplanned, and many occur within 6 months after first intercourse. A number of factors contribute to this problem, including social and cultural factors and values and misconceptions

about reproductive functioning and contraceptive use and its risks and effectiveness. The misconceptions stem in part from lack of access to early comprehensive sex education and counseling and in part from reluctance to seek and use professional services. This explains to some extent the fact that the average adolescent seeks contraceptive counseling almost 1 year after initiating sexual activity.

Some of the forces that delay education, counseling, and medical care needed to effectively prevent pregnancy also contribute to delayed pregnancy diagnosis and failure to get good antenatal care. Furthermore, in many instances of unplanned pregnancy, adolescents deny their condition for extended periods to themselves, their parents, and others. This delay is associated with increases in complications of pregnancy and neonatal morbidity. Vaginal bleeding or spotting in early pregnancy may falsely reassure a young woman that she is not preg-

TABLE 18-15

Signs and Symptoms of Pregnancy

First trimester (6-12 weeks)	Second trimester (12+ weeks)
Amenorrhea	Increased size of breasts, abdomen, waist
Light, irregular vaginal bleeding	Increased weight and clothing size
Syncope or fainting	Increased vaginal discharge
Fatigue	Increased skin pigmentation
Urinary frequency	Congestion of vaginal mucosa
Mood swings	
"Morning" sickness	
Nausea and vomiting	
Food cravings	
Increased facial oil gland activity ("glow")	
Elevated body temperature	
Chloasma (dark facial pigmentation)	
Nasal stuffiness or mucous membrane congestion	

TABLE 18-17

Causes of False-Positive and False-Negative Pregnancy Tests

False-negative	False-positive
Too early (commonly) or too late (rarely)	Hydatidiform mole
Adulterated urine	Malignancies
Ectopic pregnancy (occasionally negative, most are positive)	Postabortion (up to 4 weeks)
	Midcycle LH surge
	Perimenopausal (LH elevation)
Impending or missed abortion	Premature ovarian failure (LH elevation)
Dilute urine	

TABLE 18-16

Clinical and Laboratory Correlations of Pregnancy

Gestation (wks)	Pregnancy detection by lab test	Fundal height	Urine HCG (MIU/ml)	Signs, symptoms, and significant events
1				LMP
2			5	Conception
3	Serum ELISA		(24 hrs after implantation)	Implantation
4	Urine ELISA assay		70–100	Missed period, vaginal ultrasound detects pregnancy
5	Urine β-HCG assay, other methods		>250	Pelvic ultrasound detects pregnancy; breast changes—tender, swollen; nipples—sensitive, dark
6			>1000	Nausea, morning sickness; **Hegar sign**—softening of lower corpus;
7				**Chadwick sign**—bluish color of
8			>10,000	cervix; **Goodell sign**—softening of cervix
10			100,000 (peak)	
12		Pelvic brim		Uterine enlargement; fetal heart tones detectable with Doppler
14				Decrease in early signs and symptoms
16		Midway between pelvic brim and umbilicus	10,000; false negatives may occur in 2nd and 3rd trimesters	Fetus visualized by x-ray; perception of fetal movement
20		Umbilicus		

HCG, Human chorionic gonadotrophin; *LMP,* last menstrual period; *MIU,* mili international units.

nant, and minimal weight gain (whether voluntary or involuntary) may further facilitate denial. Patients may have substitute chief complaints. Amongst these are pelvic, abdominal, or back pain; vomiting and dehydration; constipation; urinary complaints; and urinary tract infection. Phlebitis, rupture of membranes, symptoms of gestational diabetes, or secondary problems of insomnia or headache may bring the patient to medical attention.

At the time of presentation the teenager or the parent may suspect pregnancy. Interviewing the patient and parent separately and sensitively addressing underlying concerns is usually the best way to get a complete and honest history.

Considering the frequency of teenage pregnancy and the tendency of individuals to have alternate chief complaints, practitioners who care for adolescents should be familiar with the signs, symptoms, and methods of diagnosing pregnancy.

In the first trimester, patients often experience fatigue and mood swings. At about 5 weeks gestation, breast tenderness, swelling, and darkening and increased sensitivity of the nipples develop. Nausea and vomiting, especially in the morning, tend to begin at about 6 weeks gestation. Weight changes, food cravings, and increased facial oil gland activity and chloasma (darkening of facial pigmentation) may be noted. If a pregnant adolescent is examined between the sixth and eighth weeks, the Hegar sign (softening of the lower corpus), Chadwick sign (bluish discoloration of the cervix), and Goodell sign (softening of the cervix) may be noted. Ultrasonography can detect the fetus after the sixth week of pregnancy.

In the second and third trimesters, breast enlargement increases as do abdominal girth and weight. Normal vaginal discharge increases as well. On examination, congestion of the vaginal mucosa is seen. The uterus is palpable as a midline mass, with its dome at the pelvic brim at about 12 weeks; midway between the pelvic brim and the umbilicus at 16 weeks; and at the level of the umbilicus at 20 weeks. Fetal heart tones become detectable with Doppler between 12 and 14 weeks, and fetal movements are perceptible between 16 and 20 weeks gestation. Signs and symptoms of pregnancy are outlined in Table 18-15.

Current laboratory pregnancy tests give us the opportunity to diagnose pregnancy earlier and with greater reliability. Serum radioimmune assay for beta-HCG is positive 24 to 48 hours after implantation (about 7 days after conception). A urine specimen gives a positive result on a sensitive urine ELISA assay for an intrauterine pregnancy 10 days after conception. A chronology of laboratory and clinical findings during pregnancy is presented in Table 18-16.

Home pregnancy tests are variable in sensitivity. Some are identical to and as sensitive as office laboratory ELISA assays, and others may not give a positive result on a first-morning specimen until 14 to 21 days after conception. False-positive and false-negative results are encountered less frequently and are most often caused by errors of timing and dilution. In particular, false positives are not caused by foods, drugs, and other medical conditions (Table 18-17). They can occur in adolescents with hydatidiform moles or malignancies, after abortion, or during a midcycle lutenizing hormone surge. Causes of false-negative findings include testing too early (mentioned earlier) or too late (after 16 to 20 weeks), very dilute urine (specific gravity <1.010), adulterated urine, ectopic pregnancy, or an impending or missed abortion (Table 18-17).

Pregnancies are dated from the last normal menstrual period and not from conception, which occurs 2 weeks later. This is not well known by the public and should be explained to minimize confusion, facilitate decision making, and clarify paternity.

BIBLIOGRAPHY

Bacon JL: Pediatric vulvovaginitis, *Adolesc Pediatr Gynecol* 2:86-93, 1989.

Berenson AB, et al: Appearance of the hymen in prepubertal girls, *Pediatrics* 89(3):387-394, 1992.

Berenson AB: Appearance of the hymen at birth and one year of age: a longitudinal study, *Pediatrics* 91(4):820-825, 1993.

Centers for Disease Control: 1993 Sexually transmitted diseases treatment guidelines, *MMWR* 42:1-102, 1993.

Emans SJ, Goldstein DP: *Pediatric and adolescent gynecology*, ed 3, Boston, 1990, Little, Brown.

Emans SJ, Woods ER, Flagg NT, Freeman A: Genital findings in sexually abused, symptomatic and asymptomatic girls, *Pediatrics* 79:778-785, 1987.

Hammerschlag MR, Rosner AS, et al: Microbiology of the vagina in children: normal and potentially pathogenic oraganisms, *Pediatrics* 62:57-62, 1978.

Hatcher RA, et al: *Contraceptive technology*, ed 16, New York, 1994, Irvington.

Holmes KK, et al: *Sexually transmitted diseases*, ed 2, New York, 1990, McGraw-Hill.

Huffman JW: *The gynecology of childhood and adolescence*, ed 2, Philadelphia, 1981, WB Saunders.

McCann J, Wells R, Simon M, Voris J: Genital findings in prepubertal girls selected for nonabuse: a descriptive study, *Pediatrics* 86:428-439, 1990.

McCann J, Voris J, Simon M, Wells R: Comparison of genital examination techniques in prepubertal girls, *Pediatrics* 85:182-187, 1990.

Murray P: Vulvitis, vaginitis, urethritis. In Burg FD, Ingelfinger JR, Wald ER, eds: *Gellis and Kagan's current pediatric therapy*, ed 15, Philadelphia, 1995, WB Saunders.

Paradise JE, Campos JM, Friedman HM, Frishmuth G: Vulvovaginitis in premenarchal girls: clinical features and diagnostic evaluation, *Pediatrics* 70:193-198, 1982.

Pokorny SF, Kozinetz CA: Configuration and other anatomic details of the prepubertal hymen, *Adolesc Pediatr Gynecol* 1:97-103, 1988.

Pokorny SF, Pokorny WJ, Kramer W: Acute genital injury in the prepubertal girl, *Am J Obstet Gynecol* 166:5:1461-1466, 1992.

Pokorny SF, Stormer J: Atraumatic removal of secretions from the prepubertal vagina, *Am J Obstet Gynecol* 156:3:581-582, 1987.

Sanfilippo JS, et al: *Pediatric and adolescent gynecology*, Philadelphia, 1994, WB Saunders.

Treatment of sexually transmitted diseases, *The Medical Letter* 32(810):5-9, 1995.

19

Ophthalmology

KENNETH P. CHENG ❦ ALBERT W. BIGLAN

DAVID A. HILES

*O*ver the past three decades pediatric ophthalmology has become established as a distinct subspecialty of ophthalmology.

Common problems include refractive errors, strabismus, amblyopia, and infections or trauma that involve the eye or its surrounding tissues. Other problems encountered include ocular complications of systemic disease, developmental and genetic conditions, and neoplasms affecting the globe and orbits.

Anatomy of the Visual System

The visual system is conveniently separated into three principal parts: the globe and surrounding structures (Fig. 19-1), the visual pathways, and the visual or calcarine cortex.

The eyelids provide protection for the globe and assist in even distribution of the tear film over the cornea to provide a clear, undistorted optical system for focusing light. The crystalline lens complements the cornea's refracting power with its ability to adjust the focal length of the optical system so that incoming light from objects at any distance may be clearly imaged on the retina. During the first 2 to 3 months of life, children develop the ability to focus images at any range (accommodation). Light is focused on the macula, the portion of the retina responsible for the central field of vision (Fig. 19-2). The retina contains the sensory receptors: the rods and cones. The fovea centralis is the center of the macula; it has the greatest concentration of cones and therefore has the greatest potential for visual acuity.

Light falling on the fovea and peripheral retina is converted into nerve impulses by the rods and cones. Nerve fibers emanate from the ganglion cell layer of the retina, coalesce to form the optic nerve, and synapse in the lateral geniculate body. Fibers from the temporal retina travel without crossing at the chiasm to the ipsilateral visual cortex (Fig. 19-3). Nerve fibers from the nasal retina decussate at the chiasm and are directed toward the contralateral visual cortex. This decussation of nerve fibers causes portions of each retina to image a different part of the visual field. For example, if an object is seen off to the person's left, the image is received by the nasal retina of the left eye and the temporal retina of the right eye. Similarly, if the object is off to the person's right, the image will fall on the nasal retina of the right eye and the temporal retina of the left eye. The temporal retina images objects in the contralateral visual field, and the nasal retina images ob-

jects in the ipsilateral visual field. Because of the decussation of nasal retinal fibers, the right visual cortex will therefore receive images from the left visual field and the left visual cortex will receive images from the right visual field.

Lesions of the visual pathways produce predictable patterns of visual field loss; for example, a left homonymous hemianopsia is produced by a lesion of the right occipital cortex. Visual field defects that respect or do not extend across the vertical midline suggest pathology involving the intracranial portion of the visual system.

The visual field can be arbitrarily divided into the central field of vision and the peripheral field. The macula is responsible for the central field. A physiologic blind spot is found about 10 to 15 degrees temporal to central fixation (the fovea) and represents the area of the field that corresponds to the optic nerve head (optic disc). Precise measurement of the visual field of each eye can be obtained in a cooperative child or adult using a visual field perimeter. This test requires steady fixation and concentration for roughly 30 minutes. In young children, it is impractical to attempt this tedious measurement. A young patient's visual fields are grossly assessed by observation of the child's eyes fixating on small targets brought into the peripheral field of vision in each quadrant of the visual field. Visual fields may be also assessed using a confrontation method where the child fixates on the examiner's nose and is asked to count the examiner's fingers as they are presented in each quadrant of the visual field.

Evaluation of Vision

The most valuable assessment of visual function is measurement of visual acuity. Selection of a test to measure it will depend on the patient's age, cooperation, and level of development.

The evaluation of vision in a young infant requires the use of the fixation reflex. This reflex develops during the first month or two of life. By 3 months, an infant should be able to steadily fixate on and begin to follow a face, toy, or penlight. By age 5 to 6 months a child should be able to follow a fixation target into all fields of gaze. The level of vision can be estimated by the quality and intensity of the fixation response. If the visual acuity is normal, central fixation will be steady and maintained (CSM) on objects. If visual acuity is profoundly decreased, the quality of fixation may be wandering in nature, poorly maintained, or eccentric. Central, steady, maintained fixation equates to visual acu-

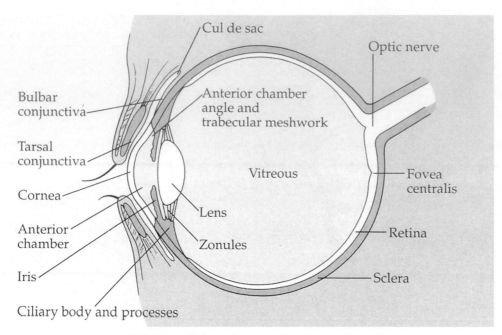

FIG. 19-1   Globe and surrounding structures.

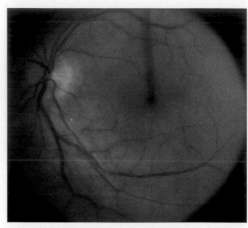

FIG. 19-2   Normal fundus. Posterior pole of fundus with normal optic disc and retinal vasculature. The macula is visualized as an area of increased pigmentation surrounded by retinal vessels. The fovea centralis or center of the macula is maintaining fixation on the end of a vertical fixation target.

FIG. 19-3   Visual field and visual pathways.

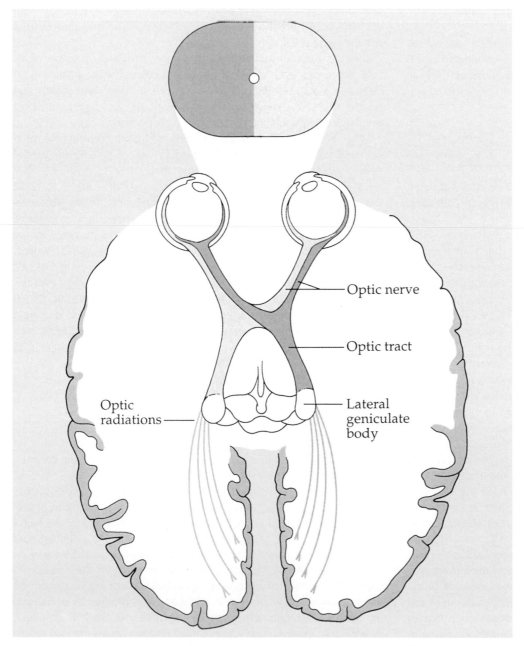

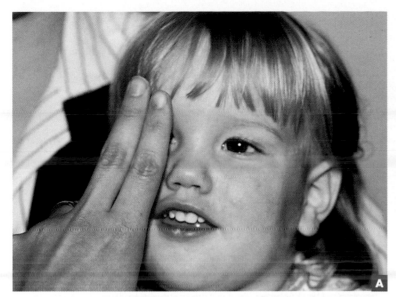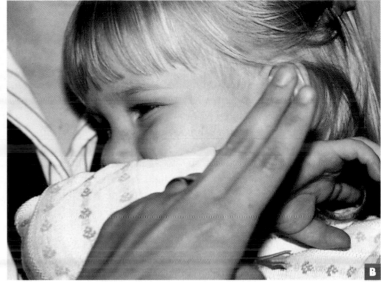

FIG. 19-4 Test for central fixation. *A,* An alert child seated on her mother's lap with one eye covered. The child is content to fix and follow with the normal left eye. *B,* The cover (in this case, fingers) is then transferred to the normal eye. The child becomes disturbed, pushes the hand away, and moves her head to see. This suggests that the visual acuity in the right eye is not as good as the acuity in the left eye.

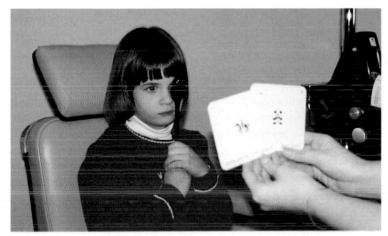

FIG. 19-5 Visual acuity testing with the Allen object recognition cards. Recognition of each figure at a distance of 20 feet is equivalent to a visual acuity of 20/30. The visual acuity is quantitated as the number of feet at which each figure may be recognized over 30 (e.g., 5/30, 15/30, 20/30).

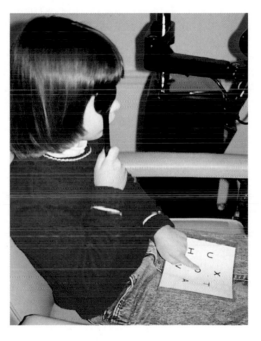

FIG. 19-6 The Sheridan-Gardiner visual acuity test presents letters of decreasing size to a child who matches the figure presented to one on a card held on his or her lap. This test provides an accurate assessment of visual acuity for children who have not yet mastered reading the alphabet.

ity of 20/200 or better. Eyes with unsteady or wandering fixation usually have visual acuity decreased to the 20/800 range (Fig. 19-4).

The Allen object recognition cards, simple pictures of common objects, are useful for assessing visual acuity in a 2- to 3½-year-old child who cannot comprehend the E game or recognize Snellen letters. To perform this test the child is taught what the pictures are, and then one eye is occluded and picture cards are individually presented at increasing distances until the patient recognizes the cards at 20 feet or fails to recognize the cards (Fig. 19-5). The visual acuity is quantitated as the number of feet at which a picture equal to 20/30 visual acuity can be recognized (e.g., 5/30, 15/30, 20/30). This is a measurement of recognition visual acuity. Although use of isolated targets is not ideal for detection of amblyopia, comparison of vision between the eyes will detect most cases of amblyopia and other defects in visual acuity.

The Sheridan-Gardiner or HOTV visual acuity tests are easy-to-administer tests that more accurately measure visual acuity in young children. In the HOTV test the letters H, O, T, and V are individually presented on cards and the child matches the letter with a corresponding letter on a card that is held on the lap (Fig. 19-6).

Another commonly used test to measure the visual acuity in 3½-year-old children is the "E game." The letter E in decreasing size is presented to the child rotated in an up, down, right, or left orientation, and the child indicates the direction of the crossbars of the E by pointing.

The "gold standard" for measurement of visual acuity is the presentation of a full line of Snellen letters. This presentation is best achieved with a wall chart or by projection of the letters onto a standardized reflective surface. Because dim illumination increases measured visual acuity in eyes that have amblyopia, testing should be performed in a well-illuminated, glare-free room.

Normal values for visual acuity will depend on the patient's age. A child at 6 months of age should have a visual acuity of 20/60 to 20/100. A child who is 3 years old can be expected to have an acuity in the range of 20/25 or 20/30 using the E game or a recognition target test. With further maturation, a 5- to 7-year-old child will have visual acuity of 20/20 to 20/25 as tested with a full line presentation of Snellen letters. All children over age 8 should be able to achieve 20/20 visual acuity with their best possible eyeglass correction in place. Those who cannot should be referred for evaluation to explain the reason for the defective vision.

The visual pathways coalesce in the visual cortex. Electrical impulses in the visual cortex produced by light stimulation of the retina can be measured by placement of sensitive electrodes on the overlying scalp. This is termed *the visual evoked response* (VER). The pattern visual evoked potential (PVEP) is generated with a CRT monitor that produces an alternating checkerboard stimulus, which can be controlled to produce a pattern of checks that may be increased or decreased in size. This test can be used to estimate visual acuity. Caution must be used in interpreting this test, however, since children and adults with known 20/20 vision can suppress the VER. Additionally, children who have significant decreases in their visual acuity may give a VER that overestimates the visual acuity.

It is recommended that vision screening be conducted as part of well-child care at regularly scheduled intervals in the pediatrician's or family practitioner's office. In infancy, the response of each eye to a fixation target should be recorded. Beginning at age 3, quantitation of the visual acuity using Allen cards, the E game, or an HOTV chart should be completed. Later, a Snellen visual acuity test should be performed by the office staff or physician, and the results should be recorded as part of the patient's medical record. If the physician has special concerns, referral to an ophthalmologist for examination may be appropriate.

Once children enter school, some state laws require that visual acuity be measured at 1- to 2-year intervals. Children who fail these examinations (visual acuity <20/40 in either eye) are referred to eye-care specialists for further evaluation.

Refractive Errors

Subnormal visual acuity may be the result of an error in the refractive power of the eye. This may be due to variation in the curvature of the cornea or lens or variation in the axial length of the eye. If visual acuity is improved by looking through a pinhole held in front of an eye, a refractive error is the cause of the decrease in visual acuity. The pinhole eliminates the off-central rays of light that require refraction. Patients demonstrate the pinhole effect by squinting to compensate for refractive errors. Those patients who do not have an improvement in visual acuity with a pinhole usually have ocular pathology.

Determination of the refractive state of the eye is part of a comprehensive ophthalmic evaluation. In children, an objective measurement of the refractive error may be obtained by using drugs that temporarily inhibit accommodation and cause pupillary dilation. Only 30 minutes after cycloplegic-mydriatic agents such as cyclopentolate or tropicamide are instilled, accommodation is paralyzed and the pupil is dilated. A retinoscope is used to project a beam of light into the eye and illuminate the retina. The light is then reflected back through the pupil. The focus of the reflected light is neutralized by placement of appropriate lenses in front of the eye, and the refractive error is accurately and objectively measured (Fig. 19-7).

Low levels of hyperopia (farsightedness) in the range of +1.50 to +2.00 diopters are normal during childhood and are easily compensated for by the focusing mechanism of the lens, accommodation, so that

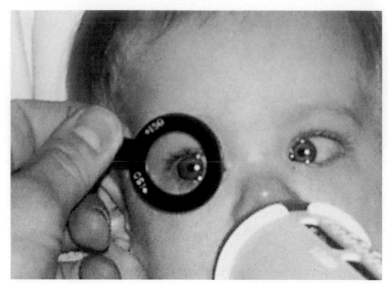

FIG. 19-7 The examiner is viewing light emanating from the retina through the retinoscope. A lens is held in front of the patient's eye to neutralize refractive errors.

glasses are not necessary. The amount of hyperopia normally increases until age 6 years and then decreases. Under normal circumstances, emmetropia, or no refractive error, is achieved around adolescence. If excessive axial growth of the eye occurs, myopia (nearsightedness) develops. A patient's refractive error is for the most part genetically predetermined. The effect that environment has on refractive error remains unclear.

The optical image formed by a hyperopic eye is in focus behind the retina (Fig. 19-8, *C*). By changing the shape of the lens with accommodation, the image can be brought into focus on the retina and glasses may not be required. If a large amount of hyperopia is present (+4.00 diopters or more), fatigue, headaches, asthenopia, and blurring of vision, especially at near, may occur. Hyperopia greater than +5.00 or +6.00 diopters may cause ametropic amblyopia. When this occurs, glasses are prescribed to correct the child's refractive error and stimulate the development of normal vision. If large hyperopic refractive errors are not treated by the age of 6 to 8 years, the resultant amblyopia may be irreversible. The optic discs in eyes with large degrees of hyperopia may have an appearance simulating papilledema (Fig. 19-9).

Myopia is frequently caused by an increase in axial length of the eye with respect to the optical power of the eye (Fig. 19-8, *B*). Children who are myopic can see near objects clearly; objects at distance are blurred and cannot be brought into focus without the aid of glasses or a contact lens. High degrees of myopia ranging from −8.00 to −20.00 diopters may be associated with systemic conditions, such as Stickler syndrome, a condition associated with increased axial length of the eye. Myopia is inherited as a multifactorial trait.

High myopia with extreme lengthening of the globe may be associated with retinal thinning, peripapillary pigment crescents, staphylomas (a focal area of bulging of the posterior globe wall), and decreased macular function with poor visual acuity. The optic nerve may appear to enter the eye at an angle (Fig. 19-10).

Myopia may be present at birth but usually develops with growth spurts that occur between 8 and 10 years of age. The amount of myopia present usually increases until growth is completed.

In astigmatism the refractive power of the eye is different in different meridians (Fig. 19-8, *D*). This produces a blurred retinal image for objects at any distance, which requires optical correction with glasses.

REFRACTIVE ERRORS

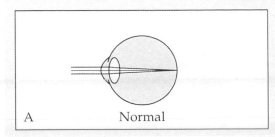

A   Normal

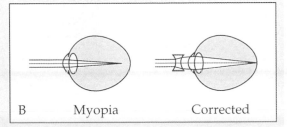

B   Myopia   Corrected

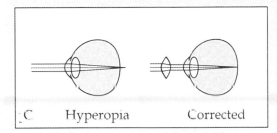

C   Hyperopia   Corrected

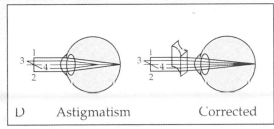

D   Astigmatism   Corrected

FIG. 19-8 In the normal or emmetropic eye, light from a distant object is focused on the retina. In a myopic eye, it is focused in front of the retina; in a hyperopic eye, it is focused behind the retina; and in an astigmatic eye, light in different meridians is brought to focus either in front of or behind the retina.

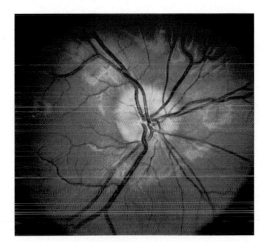

FIG. 19-9 Funduscopic view of pseudopapilledema in a hyperopic child. Vessels are normal sized; small vessels are continuously visible at the disc margins. There are no hemorrhages or exudates.

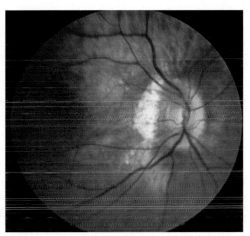

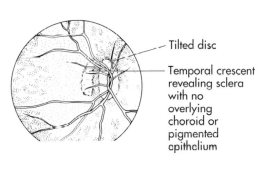

Tilted disc

Temporal crescent revealing sclera with no overlying choroid or pigmented epithelium

FIG. 19-10 Ophthalmoscopic view of an eye with high myopia. Thinning of the retinal pigment epithelium produces a tessellated fundus appearance. A temporal crescent adjacent to the optic disc is present.

Astigmatism occurs when the cornea, lens, or retinal surface has a toric shape rather than a spherical one. This may be likened to the two different curves that give a football its characteristic shape. Bulky masses in the lids, such as chalazions or hemangiomas, may compress the cornea and induce astigmatic refractive errors.

Anisometropia refers to the condition in which one eye has a different refractive error than the other. Usually the eye with the least amount of hyperopia or refractive error is the dominant or preferred eye. The fellow eye may be suppressed and frequently will develop amblyopia. Anisometropia may occur with hyperopia, myopia, astigmatism, aphakia (absence of the lens), or a combination of these refractive errors. If the degree of anisometropia is large, the optical properties of the required correcting lenses produce a difference in image size between the two eyes. This is called *aniseikonia.*

Strabismus

Misalignment of the visual axes is referred to as *strabismus.* Strabismus may be congenital or acquired. It occurs in 1% to 4% of the population. It may occur on a hereditary basis. Strabismus may be caused by cranial nerve paralysis or neuromuscular disorders (myasthenia gravis).

Voluntary and reflex movement of the eyes is mediated via the extraocular muscles. These muscles are coordinated in their saccadic and pursuit movements by centers in the frontal and occipital areas of the cerebral cortex with modification by the cerebellum. Saccades are voluntary movements used to move the eyes to the object of regard. These are rapid eye movements. Pursuit or following movements are used to track or follow moving objects. These are slow eye movements.

The third, fourth, and sixth cranial nerve nuclei, located in the brainstem, are the centers responsible for innervating the extraocular

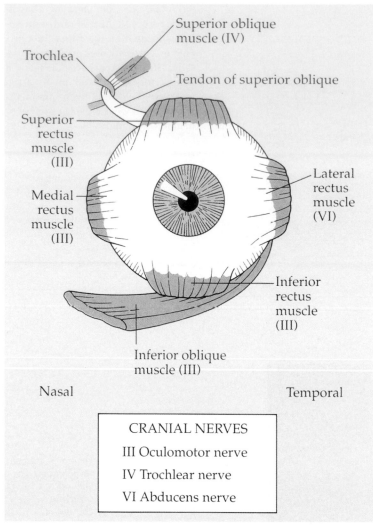

FIG. 19-11 Innervation of extraocular muscles.

CRANIAL NERVES

III Oculomotor nerve

IV Trochlear nerve

VI Abducens nerve

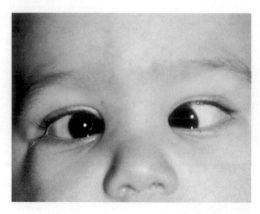

FIG. 19-12 Infantile esotropia with asymmetric corneal light reflexes.

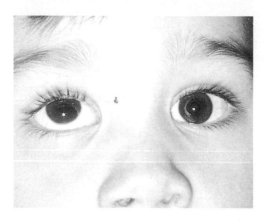

FIG. 19-13 Dissociative vertical deviation, an upward and outward drifting of the right eye. Covering the fixating left eye in the cover-uncover test causes the deviating right eye to move into alignment with the left eye.

muscles. In addition to innervation of the inferior oblique, medial, inferior, and superior recti, the third cranial nerve is responsible for innervation of the levator muscle, pupillary constriction, and accommodation of the lens. The fourth cranial nerve provides innervation to the superior oblique muscle, and the sixth cranial nerve supplies the lateral rectus muscle (Fig. 19-11).

Simultaneous fixation with the use of both eyes eliminates problems of diplopia or the need to suppress the vision from one eye and produces stereoacuity or an enhancement of the perception of depth. To achieve this, the eyes must be aligned and their movement coordinated. Control of conjugate movement of the eyes is a complex reflex arc that involves the visual images projected on each retina and the controlling centers located in the brainstem and higher cortical centers. Information is relayed to the muscles that move the eyes through the third, fourth, and sixth cranial nerve nuclei and their efferent pathways.

An abnormal head posture may be a sign of strabismus. These postures are usually observed in children who have good binocular function. Head postures are used to compensate for double vision caused by horizontal, vertical, or cyclovertical muscle palsies. In a patient with nystagmus, a head posture may be used to place the eyes in the null point or direction of gaze where the amplitude of nystagmus is the least.

Versions

Eye movements are tested by moving the eyes right, left, up, down, up and right, down and right, up and left, and down and left. This tests the function of each of the extraocular muscles and its counterpart or yoke muscle in the fellow eye. A duction is the movement of a single eye. Versions refer to movement of both eyes together in conjugate gaze. Normal version movements should be present by 4 months of age.

Vergence movements consist of convergence or divergence of the eyes. Vergences are well established by 6 months of age. Convergence of the eyes, coupled with accommodation and miosis of the pupil, is referred to as the *near response*. Convergence facilitates alignment of the eyes at near.

Phorias and Tropias

If strabismus is present, it may be manifest, a tropia, or it may be held latent by sensory fusion, a phoria. When the fusion of a patient with a phoria is interrupted by placing an occluder in front of one eye, the eye seeks a position of rest and deviates from the visual axis of the fellow eye. When the eye is uncovered and binocular vision is reestablished, the fusion response assists in the realignment of the eyes on the object of regard. A phoria may produce symptoms of intermittent double vision, fatigue, blurring, or movement of objects. Phorias become symptomatic at times of fatigue, stress, or illness.

A tropia is a constant or intermittently present ocular deviation. The fusion mechanism is unable to maintain alignment of the eyes on an object of fixation. The deviation may occur in one or all positions of gaze.

Phorias and tropias are classified according to the pattern of the eye deviation. The prefixes *eso-* and *exo-* classify horizontal strabismus, *hyper-* and *hypo-* are used for vertical deviations, and *incyclo-* and *excyclo-* for torsional deviations.

Esodeviations

An esodeviation is a convergent deviation of the eyes. The deviation may be latent, a phoria (esophoria), or it may occur as a manifest de-

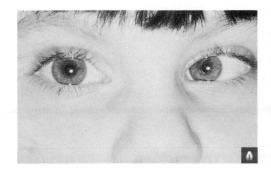

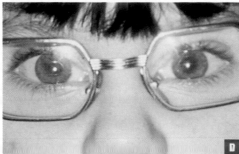

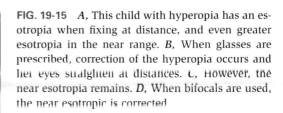

FIG. 19-14 The child in *A* has esotropia with a high degree of hyperopia. In *B*, we see that corrective glasses have reduced the hypertropia, and her esotropic eye has returned to orthophoria.

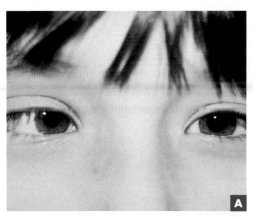

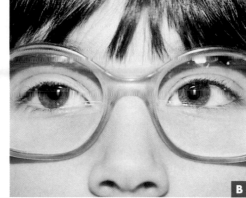

FIG. 19-15 *A*, This child with hyperopia has an esotropia when fixing at distance, and even greater esotropia in the near range. *B*, When glasses are prescribed, correction of the hyperopia occurs and her eyes straighten at distances. *C*, However, the near esotropia remains. *D*, When bifocals are used, the near esotropic is corrected

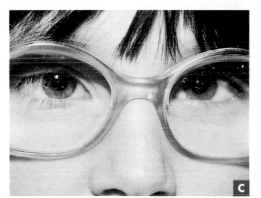

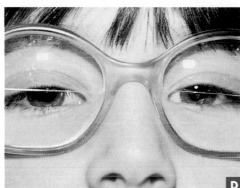

viation, a tropia (esotropia). Common esodeviations seen in children are infantile esotropia, accommodative esotropia, esotropia resulting from sixth cranial nerve palsy, and Duane syndrome.

Infantile Esotropia

The most common esodeviation in children is infantile, or congenital esotropia (Fig. 19-12). There is frequently a family history of infantile esotropia, and the eyes will be crossed at birth or shortly thereafter. The angle of esodeviation is large and constant. Defects in abduction may appear to be present, and differentiation from sixth cranial nerve palsy may be difficult. Cross-fixation is usually present, with the adducted right eye used for vision to the left and the adducted left eye used for vision to the right. Children with this condition usually maintain good visual acuity and are otherwise systemically normal.

Infantile esotropia requires surgical correction. After correction, the ocular alignment remains unstable, and inferior oblique overaction or dissociated vertical deviations frequently develop later in childhood or adolesence. Inferior oblique overaction is seen as an elevation of one or both eyes in adduction. Dissociated vertical deviation (DVD) (Fig. 19-13) is an upward and outward "floating" movement of one or both eyes that becomes prominent with fatigue or inattention. These patients do not experience diplopia.

Accommodative Esotropia

Accommodative esotropia most commonly presents as an acquired strabismus at $2\frac{1}{2}$ to 5 years of age. Family histories of esotropia and amblyopia are common. Uncorrected hyperopia stimulates accommodation to obtain clear vision. With accommodation, the synkinetic near response, which includes miosis, accommodation, and convergence of the eyes, occurs. If the fusion mechanism is unable to diverge the eyes to compensate for the convergence, esotropia results.

If an esodeviation is associated with a modest degree of farsightedness, treatment of the hyperopia is indicated. In patients with pure accommodative esotropia, this measure alone may completely correct the deviation (Fig. 19-14). More often than not, a residual esodeviation will remain, and if this is large, surgical correction may be recommended.

In another form of accommodative esotropia, the ratio between accommodative convergence and accommodation (AC/A ratio) may be abnormally high, producing excessive convergence when focusing on near objects. In high AC/A ratio accommodative esotropia, the esodeviation with near vision is greater in magnitude than it is with distance vision (Fig. 19-15).

Nonaccommodative Esotropia

Children may develop an esodeviation that is not associated with a hyperopic refractive error (Fig. 19-16). These nonaccommodative eso-

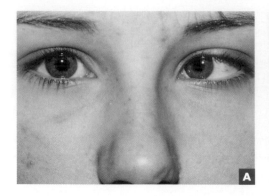

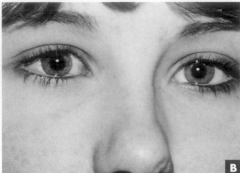

FIG. 19-16 The girl in *A* shows nonaccommodative esotropia, an esotropia that could not be corrected with glasses or miotics. Surgery was performed, and the 1-week postoperative photograph in *B* shows reduced esotropia with normal alignment.

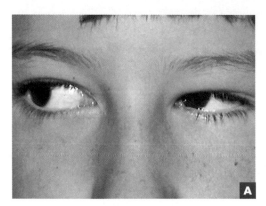

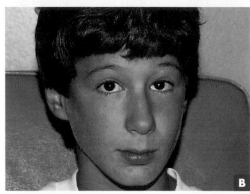

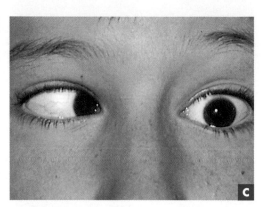

FIG. 19-17 Left Duane syndrome. *A,* Right gaze. While the left eye is noted to move into adduction, retraction of the globe is noted along with narrowing of the palpebral fissure. The globe retraction and lid changes are due to cocontraction of the medial rectus and lateral rectus muscles on the involved side. *B,* Fixation target directly in front of patient. The patient is noted to maintain a slight left head turn to maintain normal alignment of the eyes with the affected left eye held slightly in adduction. If the patient's head is forced out of the slight left head turn, the left eye would become slightly esotropic. *C,* Left gaze. The affected left eye is seen to have an absence of abduction resulting from aberrant innervation of the lateral rectus muscle.

deviations may be associated with poor vision, trauma, prematurity, aphakia, or high myopia. Nonaccommodative esotropia may also develop if accommodative esotropias are left untreated for too long.

Other Causes of Esotropia

Unilateral or bilateral sixth cranial nerve palsy causes deficient abduction and an esodeviation. In sixth nerve palsy the esotropia increases with gaze directed toward the side of the palsy. Patients may display a head turn toward the side of the palsy to hold the involved eye in adduction and maintain binocular vision. Sixth cranial nerve palsies in children may be associated with increased intracranial pressure, trauma, tumor, or antecedent viral illness. In benign or "postviral" and traumatic cases the lateral rectus function may return fully over a 6-month period. In idiopathic cases if improvement does not occur, if the deviation increases, or if a gaze palsy develops, suspicion should be raised that a pontine glioma is the cause for the sixth nerve paralysis.

Duane syndrome is a congenital unilateral or bilateral defect characterized by inability to abduct an eye. This may be accompanied by an up or down shoot of the eye and narrowing of the lid fissure on attempted adduction. In attempted abduction the palpebral fissure widens. Duane syndrome is caused by a malformation of the cranial nerve nuclei producing coinnervation of the medial and lateral rectus muscles. The lateral rectus muscle does not contract with abduction and paradoxically cocontracts along with the medial rectus on adduc-

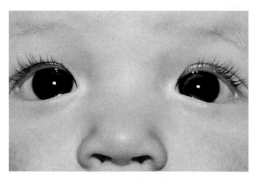

FIG. 19-18 This infant has pseudostrabismus, caused by a flat nasal bridge, wide epicanthal folds, and closely placed eyes.

tion. Patients with Duane syndrome may be esotropic and have a head turn toward the involved side analogous to those seen with a sixth cranial nerve palsy. The changes in lid position and vertical deviations help to differentiate the two conditions (Fig. 19-17).

Pseudostrabismus

Pseudostrabismus is seen in infants with prominent epicanthal folds, closely placed eyes, and flat nasal bridges. Asymmetry of the lids or nasal bridge may also produce pseudostrabismus. When these facial features are present, the white of the sclera between the cornea and inner canthus frequently may be obscured, giving the optical illusion that the eyes are esotropic (Fig. 19-18 and 19-19). Parents and caretakers frequently report esodeviations that worsen with gaze to the right or

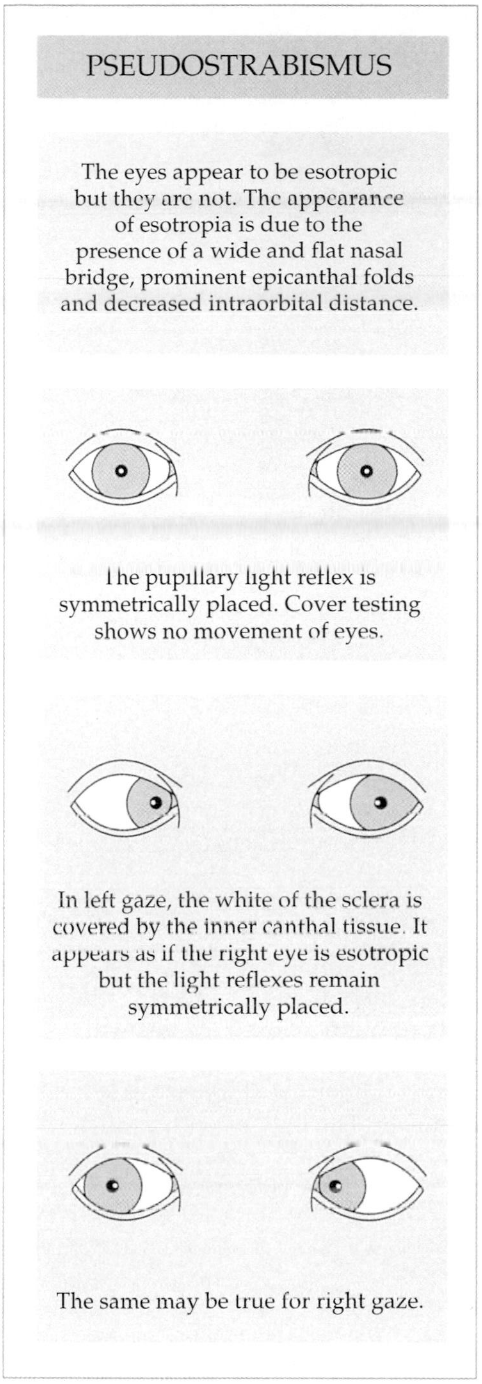

FIG. 19-19 The characteristics of pseudostrabismus are illustrated.

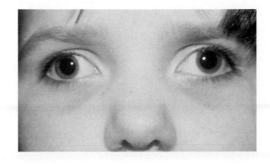

FIG. 19-20 Exotropia, a divergent deviation of the eyes.

left. Observation of symmetric corneal light reflexes or cover testing confirms or excludes the presence of a true deviation.

Exodeviations

When the visual axes are divergent, an exodeviation is present (Fig. 19-20). Many children with exodeviations will have family histories of strabismus. Exodeviations may also occur with vision loss in one eye (sensory exotropia) and cranial nerve paralysis. An exodeviation may be controlled by fusion (exophoria), be manifest intermittently (intermittent exotropia), or be constant (exotropia). Intermittent exodeviations become manifest with fatigue, daydreaming, or illness. Patients with exodeviations frequently squint one eye

in bright light and may complain of discomfort at night or when tired.

If there is a defect in visual acuity, the decreased visual stimulation may produce a sensory deviation. Generally speaking, if the onset of decreased vision occurs after the age of 4 years, an exodeviation will occur; however, if sensory input to the eye is decreased before the age of 2 years, an esodeviation usually occurs.

Exodeviations may be simulated in patients with widely spaced eyes (hypertelorism) or in those whose maculae are temporally displaced, as may occur in retinopathy of prematurity. When the macula is displaced temporally, the eye rotates outward to align its visual axis on the fixation target. This simulates an exodeviation. The term *positive angle kappa* is used to describe this condition (Fig. 19-21).

Convergence Insufficiency

Convergence insufficiency describes an exodeviation in which the size of the deviation is greater in the near range than at distance. This may cause symptoms of discomfort while reading and possibly intermittent double vision at near. To test for convergence insufficiency, the child is asked to fixate on a target with detail as the target is brought progressively closer. Normally the child should be able to converge to a point 10 cm from the nose. If the eyes converge, then break their alignment and diverge at a distance greater than 10 cm from the eyes, the patient should be evaluated for convergence insufficiency.

Third (Oculomotor) Cranial Nerve Palsy

The third cranial nerve innervates the medial rectus muscle. In third nerve paralysis the action of the lateral rectus muscle, innervated by the sixth cranial nerve, is unopposed and produces an exodeviation. The third nerve also innervates the superior and inferior recti; the inferior oblique muscles; the levator palpebrae superioris, which elevates the lid; the ciliary muscle, which is responsible for accommodation of the lens; and the iris sphincter muscle, which produces miosis of the pupil. In the presence of a complete third cranial nerve palsy, the eye assumes a down and outward position, the eyelid is ptotic, and the pupil is enlarged (Fig. 19-22). Elevation of the eye with forced eyelid closure (Bell phenomenon) is typically absent in patients with a third cranial nerve palsy (Fig. 19-23). The most common causes for third cranial nerve palsy in children are trauma and tumor.

Vertical Deviations

Isolated vertical misalignment of the eyes is uncommon. Vertical deviations may occur in only one field of gaze, or they may be concomitant and equal in all fields of gaze. Vertical deviations may have a cyclotorsional component and be associated with a head tilt or head posture to eliminate double vision. All patients with torticollis should be evaluated for cyclovertical muscle palsies.

The most common cyclovertical deviation is due to a palsy of the fourth cranial (trochlear) nerve (Fig. 19-24). Fourth nerve palsies in

ANGLE KAPPA

Positive angle kappa produces an appearance of exotropia. This appearance is caused by a temporal displacement of the fovea, usually due to cicatricial changes of the retina after retinopathy of prematurity.

The left eye appears exotropic; however, cover testing shows no movement of the eyes.

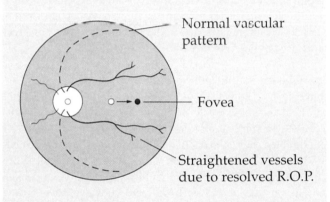

Normal vascular pattern

Fovea

Straightened vessels due to resolved R.O.P.

Retinal cicatricial changes after resolution of stage 3 R.O.P. have caused the fovea to be displaced temporally.

Angle Kappa

The fovea has been displaced and retains fixation. The eye therefore rotates outward to focus light on the fovea. The eye appears exotropic but is not.

FIG. 19-21 Angle kappa.

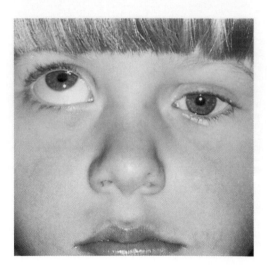

FIG. 19-22 Left third nerve palsy with ptosis and an inability to elevate and adduct the eye.

THIRD CRANIAL NERVE PALSY

A patient with left third cranial nerve palsy will not have a Bell's phenomenon on the affected side. The forced opening of tightly closed eyelids will normally reveal an upward, slightly outward movement of the eye under the closed eyelids (normal Bell's response). The patient with a third cranial nerve palsy cannot elevate or adduct the eye. The affected eye will not be elevated.

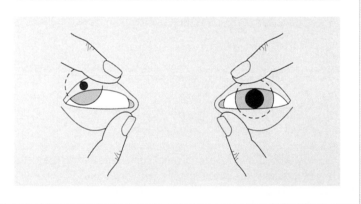

FIG. 19-23 Third cranial nerve palsy.

children occur congenitally and secondary to trauma. The eye is excyclorotated, and the head is tilted to the shoulder opposite the side of the paretic superior oblique muscle. Other features are elevation of the eye and difficulty depressing the eye in adduction (Fig. 19-25). Patients with fourth nerve palsies have diplopia in the affected field of gaze. Patients with congenital palsies may not always recognize this diplopia, however.

Brown syndrome describes an isolated motility disorder in which there is an inability to elevate the eye when it is adducted (Fig. 19-26). This may be due to a defect in the superior oblique tendon as it passes through the trochlea or to a congenital anomaly of the superior oblique tendon.

Abnormalities of extraocular muscle innervation rarely cause vertical deviations. Double elevator palsy is an inherited unilateral or

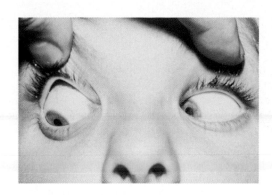

FIG. 19-24 Left fourth nerve palsy with an inability to depress the involved eye in adduction. Abnormal head posture is common, as is overaction of the direct antagonistic inferior oblique muscle.

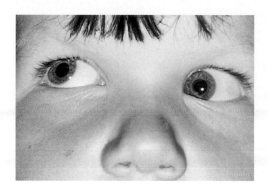

FIG. 19-26 Brown syndrome, an inability to elevate an eye in adduction resulting from a tight superior oblique tendon.

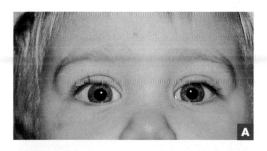

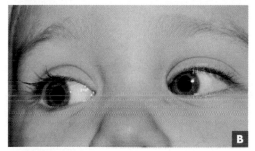

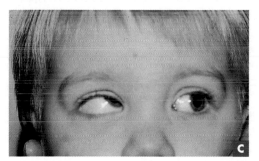

FIG. 19-25 Right inferior oblique overaction. In primary (straight ahead) *(A)* and right gaze *(B)* the eyes are well aligned. In left gaze *(C)* the right eye is elevated or hypertropic because of overaction of the right inferior oblique.

HIRSCHBERG TEST FOR OCULAR ALIGNMENT

A penlight is held 1 meter from and directly in front of the eyes. The pupillary light reflex is observed and its relationship to the center of the pupil is noted.

Normal Corneal Light Reflex
The reflexes are symmetrical and slightly displaced nasal to the center of the pupils.

Left Estropia
The reflex is displaced temporal to the center of the pupil.

Left Exotropia
The corneal light reflex is displaced nasal to the center of the pupil.

FIG. 19-27 Hirschberg test for ocular alignment.

bilateral condition in which there is hypotropia and limitation of elevation of the involved eye. To achieve binocularity, patients tilt their chins up and position their heads back. Ptosis is frequently present.

Additional causes of vertical deviations include myasthenia gravis, thyroid ophthalmopathy, external ophthalmoplegia, orbital fractures with muscle entrapment, and orbital disease with intraorbital masses.

Tests for Strabismus

The type and degree of ocular misalignment may be estimated using the corneal light reflex test or Hirschberg method. The patient fixates on a penlight held at 1 m. Using the pupil as a point of reference, if the light reflex is displaced temporally, an esotropia is present. If the light reflex is displaced nasally in comparison with the other eye, an exodeviation is present (Fig. 19-27). This test only estimates ocular align-

HETEROPHORIAS

Normally, both eyes appear to be aligned and centrally fixed

Exophoria

Cover one eye—that eye deviates away from the other eye

The cover is then removed—the now uncovered eye returns to a central position

The same procedure is then performed on the other eye

Esophoria

Cover one eye—that eye deviates toward the other eye

The cover is then removed—the now uncovered eye returns to a central position

The same procedure is then performed on the other eye

Hyperphoria

Cover one eye—that eye deviates superiorly

The cover is then removed—the now uncovered eye returns to a central position

The same procedure is then performed on the other eye

FIG. 19-28 The cover-uncover test for heterophorias.

HETEROTROPIAS

In esotropia, one eye is deviated inward. Note that the corneal light reflex is not centrally placed.

Cover the esotropic eye—there is no movement of either eye and the preferred fixating eye maintains fixation.

The cover is then removed—again, there is no movement of either eye.

The other eye is now covered—the previously esotropic eye moves to take up fixation and the covered eye turns in under the cover.

If the cover is removed and no eye movement occurs, this indicates an absence of a strong fixation preference or that the eyes have equal visual acuity. This indicates a relative absence of amblyopia.

If the cover is removed and both eyes move so that the original fixating eye is again centrally fixed, and the originally esotropic eye is again esotropic, this indicates a fixation preference and that amblyopia is present.

The same maneuvers can be used to determine the presence of exotropia (outward deviation), hyper- and hypotropia (upward and downward deviation), and cyclotropia (rotary displacement).

FIG. 19-29 The cover-uncover test for heterotropias.

ment. The most accurate test to measure defects in alignment of the eyes is the prism and alternate cover test.

The cover test requires vision in each eye and use of a target that stimulates accommodation. Cover testing is performed while the patient maintains fixation on targets at 20 feet and at 13 to 14 inches. The cover-uncover test is used to detect phorias. This test is performed by placing a cover over one eye and disrupting fusion or binocularity. As

AMBLYOPIA

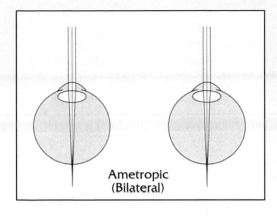

Ametropic
(Bilateral)

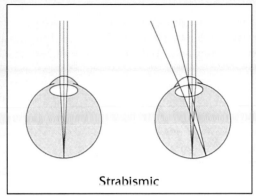

Strabismic

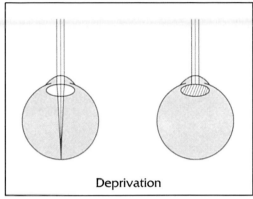

Deprivation

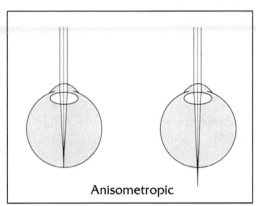

Anisometropic

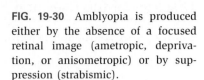

FIG. 19-30 Amblyopia is produced either by the absence of a focused retinal image (ametropic, deprivation, or anisometropic) or by suppression (strabismic).

the cover is removed, the previously covered eye is observed. If the eye does not move, both eyes are aligned on the object at that distance; orthophoria is present. If the eye deviates while covered and then moves to regain fusion and assumes fixation as the cover is removed, a phoria exists. The test is then repeated, covering and uncovering the other eye (Fig. 19-28).

The second component of the cover test is performed by covering one eye and observing the movement of the other. If neither eye moves as the eyes are alternately covered, the eyes are both aligned on the fixation target and the term *orthophoria* is used. No deviation is present in this case. If a tropia and a fixation preference are present, a fixation movement occurs when the preferred fixating eye is covered and the deviating eye is uncovered; when the cover is transferred back, the previously deviating eye again deviates behind the cover (Fig. 19-29). If a deviation is well controlled by fusion (a phoria) and is small in size, it may be safely observed if there are no symptoms and the fundus is normal. When a tropia is present, either constantly or intermittently, after 3 months of age, the patient should be referred to an ophthalmologist.

Amblyopia

Amblyopia is a decrease in vision in one or both eyes for which no organic cause can be detected. Amblyopia is caused by form depriva-

tion, the absence of stimulation of the immature visual system by a focused retinal image, or strabismus resulting from abnormal binocular interaction. Visual deprivation amblyopia may be caused by a corneal opacity, a dense cataract, high hyperopia, or anisometropia (Fig. 19-30).

In anisometropic amblyopia an image is clearly focused on the fovea of one eye, but in the other eye the image is out of focus. The blurred retinal image is suppressed by the child's immature visual system. In high hyperopia, ametropic amblyopia may occur if the child does not or cannot accommodate to produce a focused retinal image to stimulate the visual system. Patients with strabismic amblyopia have suppression of the second image produced by the deviating eye so that diplopia is not recognized.

The severity of the visual loss produced by amblyopia is determined by the nature of the visual deprivation, the age of onset, its consistency, severity, and duration. If a patient is suspected of having amblyopia, careful measurement of visual acuity is performed in a well-illuminated room. Suspicion is heightened if there is a coexistent strabismus or if there is evidence of an opacity that interferes with visualization of the fundus. Patients who are suspected of having amblyopia should be promptly referred to an ophthalmologist. Amblyopia responds best to treatment begun early in life. Treatment is rarely effective after 8 years of age.

Diseases of the Eyes and Surrounding Structures

Eyelids and Adnexae—Anatomy of the Eyelid

The eyelid is composed of skin and its related appendages, glands that contribute to the tear film and muscular structures that permit the eyelid to open and close (Fig. 19-31). Conditions affecting the eyelid are related to these anatomic structures.

Telecanthus refers to an increase in the distance between the inner canthus of each eye (Fig. 19-32). Telecanthus can be due to the hereditary transmission of facial features, midline embryonic defects, or related to a syndrome such as the blepharophimosis or Komoto syndrome (Fig. 19-33). This inherited syndrome consists of telecanthus, epicanthus inversus (a skinfold projecting over the inner angle of the eye and covering part of the canthus, arising from the lower lid skin), blepharophimosis (horizontal shortening of the lid fissure), and ptosis. *Hypertelorism* refers to an increase in the distance between the nasal walls of the orbits. This is usually associated with telecanthus.

Blepharoptosis, or ptosis, is a unilateral or bilateral decrease in the vertical distance between the upper and lower eyelids (palpebral fissure) because of dysfunction of the levator muscle (Fig. 19-34). Congenital blepharoptosis is frequently transmitted as an autosomal dominant trait with variable penetrance. Other causes for blepharoptosis include ocular inflammation, chronic irritation of the anterior segment of the eye, chronic use of topical steroid eyedrops, third nerve palsy, and trauma. Ptosis may be severe enough to cause visual deprivation and amblyopia.

The Marcus Gunn, or jaw-winking, phenomenon is caused by a misdirection of the motor division of the fifth cranial nerve to the ipsilateral levator muscle of the eyelid (Fig. 19-35). With jaw movement to the ipsilateral side the eyelid droops, and when the jaw is moved to the contralateral side, the eyelid elevates. The eyelid "winks" with chewing or feeding. Marcus Gunn phenomenon is not associated with other neurologic abnormalities.

Trichiasis is the term used to describe misdirected eyelashes that irritate the cornea or conjunctiva. It can be caused by chronic inflammation of the eyelids, entropion (inturning of the eyelid), eyelid trauma, or inflammatory conditions with scarring of the conjunctiva, such as Stevens-Johnson syndrome.

Districhiasis describes a condition where there is an accessory row of eyelashes (cilia) along the posterior border of the eyelid (Fig. 19-36). Eyelid eversion or ectropion frequently coexists because of defects in the tarsal plate. This condition is inherited as an autosomal dominant condition, but it may also be a sequela of severe ocular inflammation.

Ectropion is an outward rotation of the eyelid margin. If severe, ectropion can lead to problems of corneal exposure. Ectropion may be congenital or caused by any condition (trauma, scleroderma) causing the eyelid skin to contract and evert the eyelid (Fig. 19-37). Ectropion may occur after seventh cranial nerve palsy with paralysis of the facial musculature.

Entropion is an inverted eyelid with the lashes rubbing against the conjunctiva or cornea. This may be present at birth, associated with a horizontal kink in the tarsus, or occur with severe blepharospasm, inflammation, or trauma. If severe, the abrasion of the cornea by the lashes can cause permanent corneal scarring (Fig. 19-38).

In epiblepharon a skinfold extends over the lid margin and presses the lashes against the globe. It is commonly observed during the first year of life (Fig. 19-39). The lower lid is more commonly affected in whites, and the upper lid is occasionally affected in Asian infants. This defect usually corrects itself spontaneously by 1 year of age. Corneal abrasion usually does not occur because of the soft texture of the infant's eyelashes.

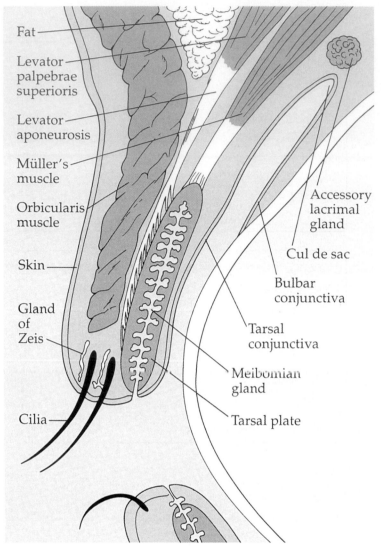

FIG. 19-31 Eyelids and adnexae. Cross-section of the eyelid.

Congenital eyelid colobomas are defects or notches in the eyelid margin caused by failed fusion of embryonic fissures early in development. These may be isolated defects or associated with conditions such as Goldenhar syndrome (Fig. 19-40). Goldenhar syndrome consists of eyelid colobomas, vertebral anomalies, corneal limbal dermoids, and preauricular skin tags.

Ankyloblepharon is a fusion of the upper and lower eyelid margins. This may range from a few thin strands of tissue to complete fusion of the lids.

Children frequently have a low-grade inflammation of the eyelid margin, chronic blepharitis, caused by staphylococcus infection. Blepharitis may be associated with seborrhea or allergies and occurs commonly in children with Down syndrome. Symptoms include itching, light sensitivity, and irritation of the lids. The lashes may be matted and adherent in the morning. This chronic problem causes thickening of the eyelid and misdirection of the eyelashes to the point where they may invert and irritate the cornea or conjunctiva (Fig. 19-41). Complications include ulceration of the lid margin, abscess or hordeolum formation, chronic conjunctivitis, and keratitis (corneal irritation and inflammation).

A hordeolum is a staphylococcal infection involving the glands of Zeis at the base of the cilia (Fig. 19-42). This produces painful swelling and erythema of the eyelid. A purulent discharge may be seen, and spontaneous resolution frequently occurs. Preseptal cellulitis may occur as a complication.

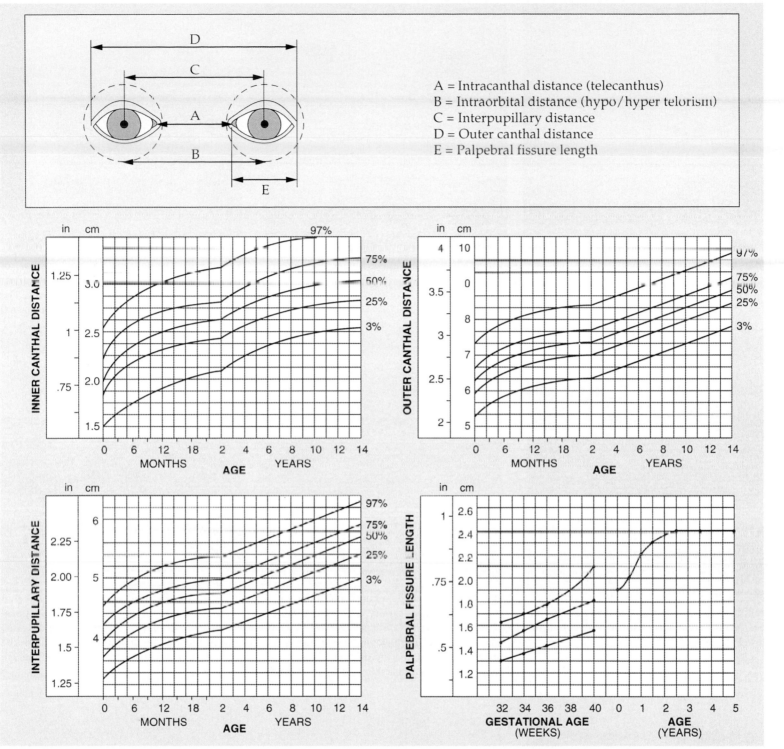

A = Intracanthal distance (telecanthus)
B = Intraorbital distance (hypo/hyper telorism)
C = Interpupillary distance
D = Outer canthal distance
E = Palpebral fissure length

FIG. 19-32 Normal adnexal measurements.

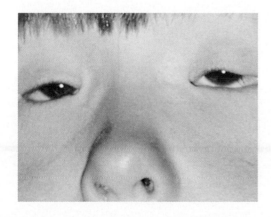

FIG. 19-33 Komoto syndrome, a combination of blepharophimosis, ptosis, epicanthus inversus, and telecanthus.

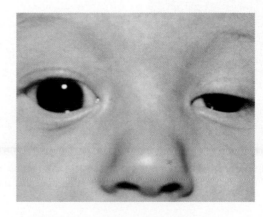

FIG. 19-34 Unilateral congenital ptosis with lid covering pupil.

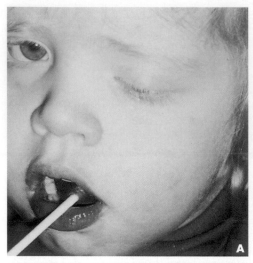

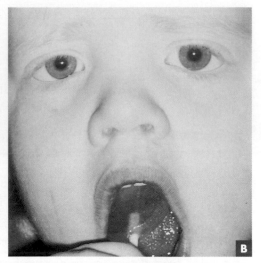

FIG. 19-35 *A,* The toddler exhibits the Marcus Gunn jaw-winking phenomenon with ptosis, whereas in *B,* he shows a wide-open lid with movements of the jaw.

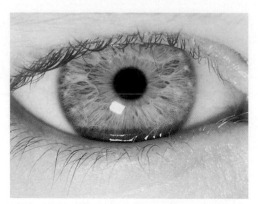

FIG. 19-36 Districhiasis, a double row of lashes. One row, directed toward the cornea, arises from the meibomian gland orifices. The second row is directed outward in the normal position.

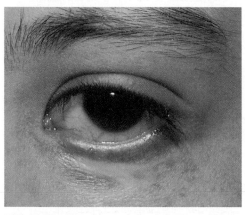

FIG. 19-37 Ectropion of the left lower lid resulting from scleroderma. The lower eyelid skin has become contracted, causing eversion of the lower eyelid.

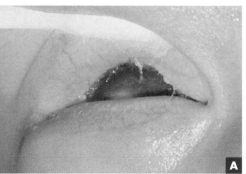

FIG. 19-38 Congenital entropion of the right upper lid. The lid is inverted, and the lashes and skin rest on the corneal surface. This case is caused by a congenital horizontal kink in the upper tarsal plate. *A,* The eyelid is propped up with a cotton-tipped applicator displaying the area of skin inverted against the eye. The Betadine prep solution has not coated the affected area of the lid. *B,* With the upper lid everted and the lids held widely open, extensive corneal scarring caused by the abrasion caused by the inverted skin and lashes is seen.

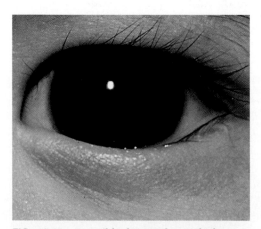

FIG. 19-39 In epiblepharon the eyelashes are rotated upward against the globe in the medial third of the eyelid.

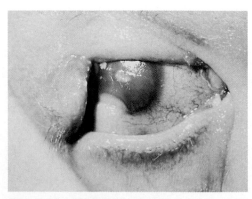

FIG. 19-40 Goldenhar syndrome with eyelid coloboma and corneal limbal dermoid.

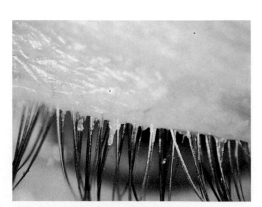

FIG. 19-41 Thickened lids with crusts around lashes in a patient with blepharitis.

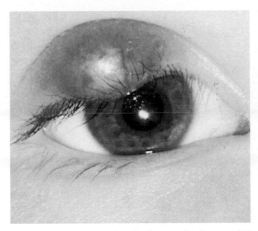

FIG. 19-42 Acute hordeolum of the eyelid (pointing externally) with swelling, induration, and purulent contents.

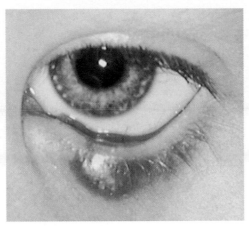

FIG. 19-43 Chalazion, a painless lid mass pointing externally or internally.

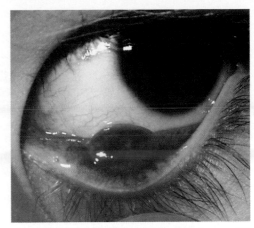

FIG. 19-44 Chalazion of the left lower lid pointed internally. A pyogenic granuloma consisting of a vascularized mound of conjunctival tissue has developed over the chalazion because of spontaneous rupture of the chalazion under the palpebral conjunctiva.

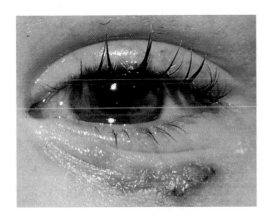

FIG. 19-45 Primary herpes simplex infection involving the periocular area. Primary infection is frequently associated with a mild diffuse keratoconjunctivitis; dendritic corneal lesions are uncommon in primary infections.

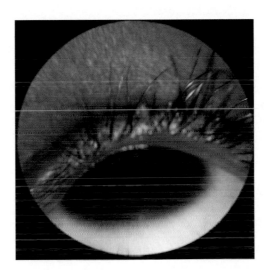

FIG. 19-46 Infestation of the eyelashes with the crab louse *Phthirus pubis.* The lid margin has a crusty appearance because of the presence of adult organisms and eggs adherent to the eyelashes. The salivary material of the parasites results in toxic and immunologic reactions that cause itching and burning of the eyes.

A chalazion is a chronic granulomatous inflammation of the meibomian glands within the tarsal plate. There is painful swelling and redness of the eyelid resulting from distension of the gland and the inflammatory response caused by the retained glandular secretions. The gland may spontaneously rupture either to the conjunctival surface or externally to the skin (Figs. 19-43 and 19-44). Spontaneous resolution may occur; however, tissue reaction may persist and leave a firm mass within the lid.

Primary herpes simplex infection may affect the periocular skin (Fig. 19-45). This is characterized by small skin vesicles, frequently unilateral, with an associated mild conjunctivitis and punctate keratitis. Varicella produces eyelid swelling and vesicular skin eruptions, usually without scarring. Conjunctival vesicles and keratitis may also occur. Herpes zoster is uncommon in children. A lesion on the tip of the nose indicates involvement of the ophthalmic division of the maxillary nerve and possible involvement of the eye with keratitis, uveitis, and glaucoma. Another common eyelid lesion found in children is caused by *molluscum contagiosum.* Molluscum is characterized by elevated, 1- to 2-mm umbilicated lesions of the eyelid skin. If the lesions involve the eyelid margin, they may cause an associated keratoconjunctivitis (see

Chapter 8). Molluscum is included in the differential diagnosis of chronic conjunctivitis.

Phthiriasis, or infestation of the lashes with the crab louse *Phthirus pubis,* is manifested as a crusty appearance of the lid margin. Closer inspection reveals egg cases and the adult louse (Fig. 19-46). Phthiriasis may also produce chronic conjunctivitis.

Lacrimal Gland and Nasolacrimal Drainage System

Reflex tears are produced by the lacrimal gland, whereas the basal secretion of tears comes from the accessory lacrimal glands (Fig. 19-47). The secretions from the glands of Zeis and the meibomian glands contribute to the tear film. During the first month of life the eye remains moist, but reflex tearing or tearing resulting from emotion does not occur until the second month of life.

Disorders of the lacrimal gland are rare in children. Acute dacryoadenitis may occur with viral infections, most frequently mumps (Fig. 19-48). Chronic diseases, such as sarcoid, Hodgkin disease, leukemia, and mononucleosis, may produce lacrimal gland swelling with a palpable mass in the upper outer portion of the orbit.

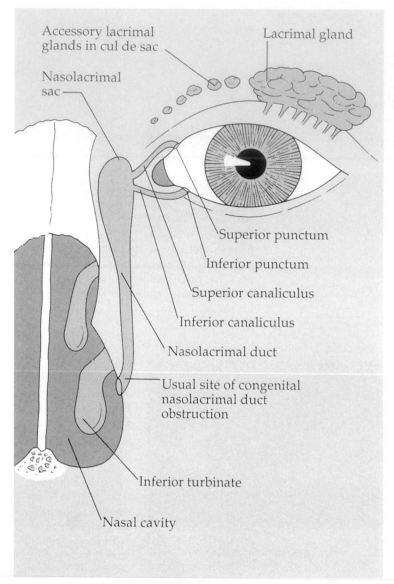

FIG. 19-47   Lacrimal secretory and collecting system.

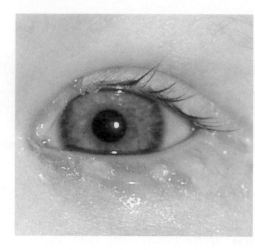

FIG. 19-49   Obstruction of the left nasolacrimal duct has led to the development of mucopurulent discharge and tearing.

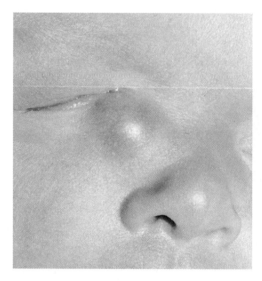

FIG. 19-50   Congenital nasolacrimal sac mucocele presents shortly after birth as a bluish mass below the medial canthal tendon.

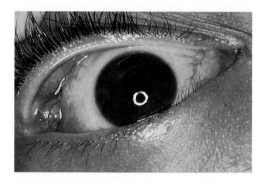

FIG. 19-48   Dacryoadenitis. The lacrimal gland has become swollen and inflamed and is visible beneath the lateral aspect of the upper eyelid. The swelling is frequently accompanied by symptoms of pain and tenderness.

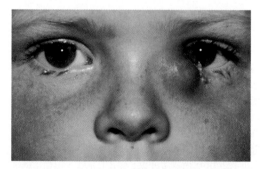

FIG. 19-51   Acute dacryocystitis caused by bacterial infection of the nasolacrimal sac associated with nasolacrimal duct obstruction. The infection of the nasolacrimal sac has spread to the surrounding tissues, producing a cellulitis.

The tears are drained from the eye by the superior and inferior puncta, which connect to the superior and inferior canaliculi (Fig. 19-47). The canaliculi may unite before they enter the nasolacrimal sac, or they may enter the sac separately. The medial canthal tendon is anterior to the nasolacrimal sac. The sac is connected to the nasolacrimal duct, which is located in the nasal bone. The distal portion of the nasolacrimal duct enters the nasal antrum beneath the inferior turbinate.

Stenosis or obstruction of the nasolacrimal duct is present in 30% of newborns (Fig. 19-49). Signs include tearing and mucopurulent discharge, which usually begin 3 to 5 weeks after birth. A helpful diagnostic technique is to apply gentle pressure over the nasolacrimal sac to cause reflux of tears and mucopurulent material from the sac. Spontaneous resolution of the obstruction is common before 6 months of age. If the obstruction has not cleared by this age, spontaneous resolution is much less likely and the patient should be referred for probing of the nasolacrimal duct.

If both the nasolacrimal duct and the canaliculi entering the sac are obstructed at birth, a bluish swelling will occur over the nasolacrimal sac (congenital nasolacrimal sac mucocele or dacryocele) (Fig. 19-50). Other congenital defects of the nasolacrimal collecting system include

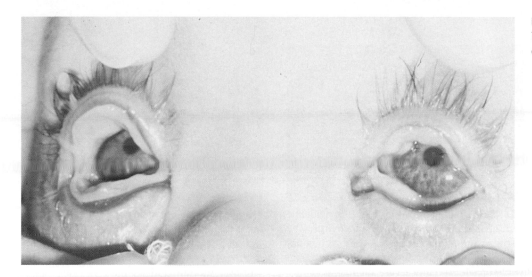

FIG. 19-52 Ophthalmia neonatorum, a hyperacute bacterial conjunctivitis, with thick purulent discharge and red swollen lids.

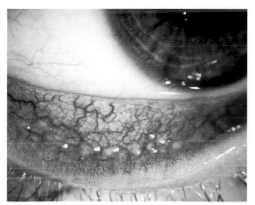

FIG. 19-53 Follicular conjunctivitis of viral origin.

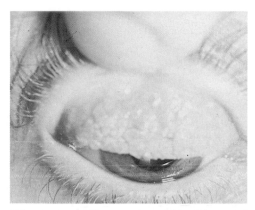

FIG. 19-54 Papillary conjunctivitis of bacterial or allergic origin.

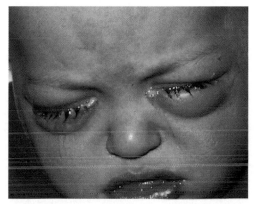

FIG. 19-55 Acute bacterial conjunctivitis. Copious amounts of mucopurulent discharge have made the upper and lower eyelids adherent to each other. Chemosis of the upper and lower lids may also make opening of the eyelids difficult.

absence of the puncta and fistulae from the nasolacrimal sac to the overlying skin.

Obstruction of the nasolacrimal system may also occur secondary to infections such as viral conjunctivitis, trachoma, tuberculosis, or fungal infections. Dacryocystitis, infection and inflammation of the lacrimal sac and passages, may spread to the surrounding tissues producing a periorbital cellulitis. Acute dacryocystitis is usually due to bacterial infection (Fig. 19-51).

Conjunctiva

The conjunctiva is a mucous membrane that covers the posterior aspect of the eyelids. It is reflected into the cul-de-sac and extends onto the globe, where it fuses to the sclera at the corneal scleral limbus. The conjunctiva has goblet cells that contribute mucin to the tear film. When the eyelids are closed, the oxygen supplied by the blood vessels of the conjunctiva is responsible for maintaining oxygenation of the cornea. *Conjunctivitis* refers to inflammation of the conjunctiva. Infections of the conjunctiva may be bacterial or viral.

The etiology of neonatal conjunctivitis is related to the time of onset. Neonatal conjunctivitis occurring within the first day or two of life usually is due to the use of Credé prophylaxis. One percent silver nitrate solution may cause a mild chemical conjunctivitis that spontaneously resolves within 1 or 2 days. Neonatal conjunctivitis occurring 2 to 4 days after birth and accompanied by a copious purulent dis-

charge, either with or without corneal involvement, usually is due to gonococci (Fig. 19-52). Infectious neonatal conjunctivitis occurring after 8 days (but before 2 weeks) and accompanied by a watery discharge is often due to chlamydiae. Conjunctivitis is usually contracted after early rupture of membranes or during passage through the birth canal.

Conjunctiva has a limited variety of responses to infection or inflammation. Inflammation of the conjunctiva results in the formation of follicles or papillae. A follicle is an aggregate of lymphocytes with an avascular center and a peripheral vascular network (Fig. 19-53). Newborns seldom develop follicles because lymphoid tissues have not yet developed. Viral infections frequently lead to follicular reaction.

Papillae are small, raised nodules with a central vascular core (Fig. 19-54). They may be located on the tarsal surface of the upper and lower eyelids. Papillae may become large, measuring 1 to 2 mm in diameter if inflammation is chronic. Papillae are the conjunctiva's response to bacterial or allergic conjunctivitis. Giant papillae may be produced by the continuous irritation caused by a contact lens.

Bacterial conjunctivitis may be acute or chronic. Acute conjunctivitis is painful with lid edema and keratitis. The bulbar conjunctiva will swell (chemosis) and become hyperemic (injection). Corneal ulceration may occur as a complication. Acute bacterial conjunctivitis is usually due to staphylococcal, pneumococcal, or *Haemophilus* infections. Mucopurulent discharge is associated with tearing, and the eyelids may be stuck together on awakening (Fig. 19-55).

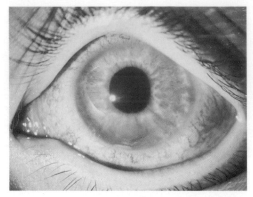

FIG. 19-56   Viral conjunctivitis with hyperemia and a watery discharge.

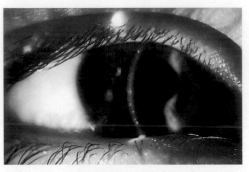

FIG. 19-57   Subepithelial infiltrates of epidemic keratoconjunctivitis caused by adenovirus. The beam of the slit-lamp light is used to demonstrate corneal subepithelial infiltrates (small white opacities). Only severe adenoviral keratoconjunctivitis produces subepithelial infiltrates. These may persist for months, causing symptoms of glare and blurring of vision.

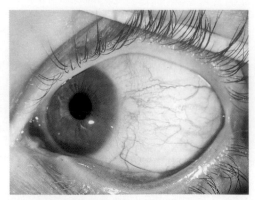

FIG. 19-58   Conjunctival phlyctenule. A raised area of conjunctival infiltration and localized injection is commonly seen at the corneal-scleral limbus. The center of the lesion is clear or white and may ulcerate. Phlyctenules may also occur elsewhere on the bulbar or tarsal conjunctiva or on the cornea. (Courtesy Dr. Robert Arffa, Pittsburgh, Penn.)

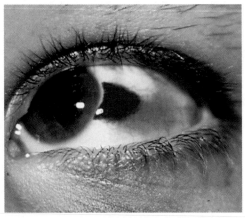

FIG. 19-59   Subconjunctival hemorrhage secondary to blunt ocular trauma.

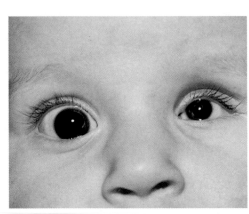

FIG. 19-60   Unilateral microcornea and microphthalmos.

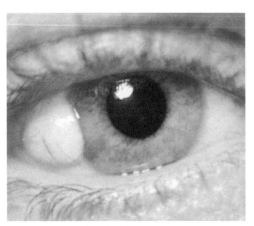

FIG. 19-61   Corneal-limbal dermoid, often associated with Goldenhar syndrome.

Chronic bacterial conjunctivitis results from bacterial toxins of *Staphylococcus aureus*, *Proteus* organisms, *Moraxella* organisms, or, in third world countries, trachomata. A foreign body sensation may be experienced, and the eyes may be hyperemic with a chronic, mucopurulent, or watery discharge. Papillary hyperplasia and thickening of the conjunctiva may also occur.

Viral conjunctivitis usually is caused by various strains of adenovirus (Fig. 19-56). The eyes are extremely light sensitive because of subepithelial infiltrates of the cornea (Fig. 19-57). Signs include copious tearing with a watery or thin mucopurulent discharge, conjunctival redness, and preauricular lymph node enlargement. Viral conjunctivitis is self-limited and usually resolves in 7 to 10 days depending on the viral strain. Viral conjunctivitis is highly contagious.

Allergic conjunctivitis occurs as a hypersensitivity response to dust, pollen, animal dander, or other airborne allergens. The eyes exhibit copious tearing, itching, and photophobia. The eyelids and palpebral conjunctiva are hyperemic and edemetous (see Chapter 4). Acute chemosis may cause a startling collection of serous discharge under the conjunctiva so that the conjunctiva may protrude between the eyelids to the extent of obscuring the cornea. This is usually self-limited

and resolves within several hours. Allergic conjunctivitis may become chronic with repeated exposure to the allergen. In cases of chronic allergic conjunctivitis, the conjunctiva becomes pale and boggy and demonstrates a papillary reaction. Complications include keratitis and, rarely, iritis.

Phlyctenular conjunctivitis is the result of a cell-mediated hypersensitivity reaction (Fig. 19-58). Phlyctenular lesions are small, pinkish-white vesicles or pustules in the center of hyperemic areas of conjunctiva. These lesions may occur at the limbus, on the conjunctiva, or more rarely, on the cornea. Phlyctenulosis most commonly occurs in association with chronic staphylococcal infection. Symptoms consist of itching, tearing, and irritation. A mucopurulent discharge may occur if secondary infection is present. Patients with corneal phlyctenulosis have more severe symptoms of pain, light sensitivity, and tearing.

Subconjunctival hemorrhages may occur spontaneously, or they may be secondary to trauma (Fig. 19-59). Such a hemorrhage presents as a striking bright red discoloration underneath the bulbar conjunctiva. The size and configuration of the hemorrhage depends on the amount and location of the blood between the conjunctiva and the globe. Spontaneous resolution occurs within 1 to 2 weeks.

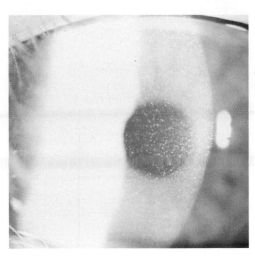

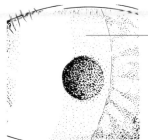

Cystine crystal
in cornea

FIG. 19-62 Cystinosis of the cornea with deposition of L-cystine crystals in the corneal stroma.

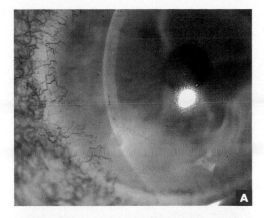

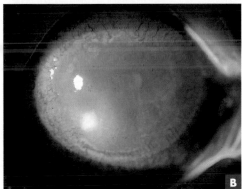

FIG. 19-63 Bacterial corneal ulcer. *A,* The conjunctiva displays a marked inflammatory response with injection, most prominent in the quadrant nearest the corneal ulcer. The ulcer is visualized in the slit beam as a small white infiltrate of the corneal stroma. There is an overlying epithelial defect. *B,* The epithelial defect is easier to visualize after the application of fluorescein dye. The dye is taken up by the corneal stroma in the area of the epithelial defect. The areas fluoresce with cobalt blue light illumination.

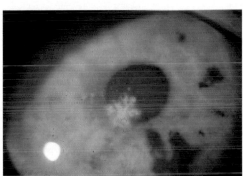

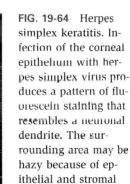

FIG. 19-64 Herpes simplex keratitis. Infection of the corneal epithelium with herpes simplex virus produces a pattern of fluorescein staining that resembles a neuronal dendrite. The surrounding area may be hazy because of epithelial and stromal edema and infiltration. Conjunctival injection is typically present.

Cornea

Developmental anomalies of the cornea include sclerocornea, Rieger syndrome, microcornea, and corneal dermoid.

Sclerocornea, present at birth, is a rare condition in which the cornea is white and resembles sclera. Rieger syndrome, a variant of anterior segment dysgenesis, is a dominant hereditary disorder that affects development of the anterior segment of the eye. Features include hyperplasia of the iris stroma, pupillary anomalies, anomalies of the trabecular meshwork, and early-onset glaucoma. Microcornea, whether an isolated anomaly or associated with glaucoma, cataracts, iris abnormalities, or anterior segment dysgenesis, is present when the corneal diameter is 9 mm or less (Fig. 19-60).

The developmental abnormalities mentioned necessitate further tests to exclude glaucoma. If the anterior segment of the eye is severely disorganized, the cornea is opaque, or glaucoma exists, surgical reconstruction and repair are indicated. The prognosis for vision is guarded for severe cases.

Corneal dermoids occur at the limbus (junction between the cornea and sclera), grow slowly, and may encroach upon the visual axis or cause high degrees of astigmatism (Fig. 19-61). They are composed of fibrolipoid tissue containing hair follicles and sebaceous glands.

The cornea is also the site of many systemic diseases. Hurler syndrome, a mucopolysaccharidosis, produces clouding of the cornea. The cornea, clear at birth, develops an opacification by 2 to 3 years of age. Pigmentary retinopathy and optic atrophy coexist.

Cystinosis, seen in the early months of life, involves the deposition of L-cystine in the cornea. This may be seen as a very subtle haze of the cornea. Slit-lamp examination is necessary to clearly visualize the corneal deposits (Fig. 19-62).

Corneal inflammations are associated with bacterial, viral, mycotic, and allergic diseases. Corneal ulcers are caused by the invasion of bacterial organisms into the corneal stroma, leading to abscess formation (Fig. 19-63). The infection may involve the entire cornea and result in visual impairment, corneal perforation, and loss of the globe. Bacteria commonly involved include staphylococci, pneumococci, *Moraxella organisms, Pseudomonas aeruginosa, Escherichia coli,* and *Klebsiella pneumoniae.* Appropriate smears and cultures are obtained and treatment started as soon as the diagnosis is suspected.

Herpes simplex, a severe viral infection of the cornea, may be transmitted from active herpes in the maternal birth canal, or it may result from direct contact with infected individuals. Primary herpes is a unilateral lesion associated with regional lymphadenopathy. A few weeks after infection, half of all patients develop a punctate or typical dendritic keratitis (Fig. 19-64). This is best seen using a fluorescein stain and a cobalt blue filter over a penlight.

Recurrent herpes keratitis occurs in 25% of infected individuals. The lesions may have a typical appearance of branching dendrites. Recur-

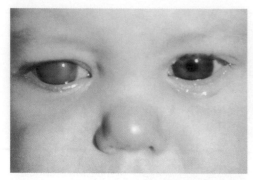

FIG. 19-65 Congenital glaucoma. The right cornea is hazy and opaque resulting from corneal edema. Breakdown of the corneal epithelium has caused ocular irritation, and the conjunctiva is slightly injected. Epiphora is present because of reflex tearing caused by the pain of epithelial breakdown and increased intraocular pressure.

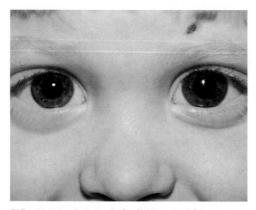

FIG. 19-67 Congenital glaucoma. This patient has corneal asymmetry resulting from glaucoma in the left eye. The horizontal corneal diameter is 11.0 mm in the right eye and 13.5 mm in the left eye. The entire left eye has become enlarged, and the axial length is greater than normal. The increase in axial length of the left eye has produced a myopic refractive error.

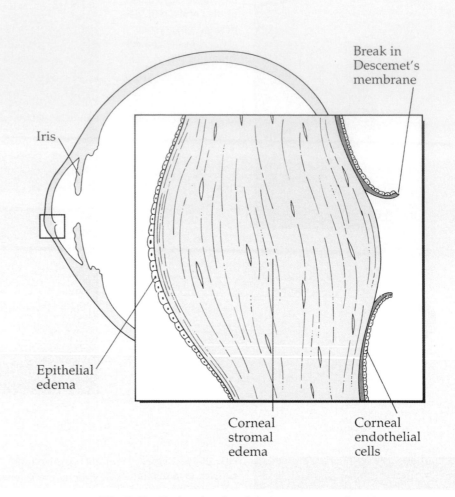

FIG. 19-66   Haab striae (break in Descemet membrane).

rences may be complicated by stromal keratitis, keratouveitis, and anesthesia of the cornea. Stromal disease is a serious complication that reduces visual recovery because of corneal vascularization and scarring. Patients with a history of herpes keratitis must be evaluated by an ophthalmologist for any episode of conjunctivitis.

Anterior Chamber

The term *anterior chamber* refers to the fluid-filled space between the cornea and the iris diaphragm. The aqueous fluid is optically clear, and it provides nutrition for the corneal endothelial surface. The aqueous fluid is secreted by the ciliary processes, reaches the anterior chamber by passing through the pupillary space, and leaves via the trabecular meshwork in the periphery of the anterior chamber angle.

Glaucoma

The incidence of infantile or congenital glaucoma is approximately 1 in 12,500 births. The inheritance of congenital glaucoma is multifactorial; parents of an affected child have a 5% chance of having another child with glaucoma, and an affected parent has a 5% chance of having an affected child. Two thirds of all patients are male. Glaucoma can present at birth, but more commonly, clinical signs develop during the first several weeks or months of life. An embryonic defect in the development of the trabecular meshwork or filtration area of the eye has been hypothesized as the cause.

Infants with glaucoma have corneal edema, which gives the cornea a hazy or cloudy appearance. Corneal edema may produce an irregular corneal light reflex or dull the red reflex. Initially, the edema may be limited to the epithelium, but stromal edema may follow (Fig. 19-65). As this increases, Descemet membrane may rupture and produce Haab striae (Fig. 19-66).

A break in Descemet membrane may produce a corneal opacity, or if edema is not present, it may be visualized against the red reflex when viewed with a slit lamp or direct ophthalmoscope. Breaks in Descemet membrane can produce irregular astigmatism. Glare from the scatter of light produced by the epithelial and stromal edema is responsible for photophobia and blinking. Breakdown of the corneal epithelium may produce pain, squinting, and blepharospasm.

In children less than 2 years of age, an increase in corneal diameter frequently indicates increased intraocular pressure (Fig. 19-67). An in-

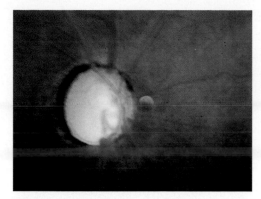

FIG. 19-68 Glaucomatous optic atrophy. In glaucoma, excavation extends to the disc edge in contrast to the cupped disc seen in myopia where a normal rim of tissue exists. Retinal vessels emerge from under the disc edge.

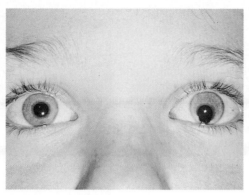

FIG. 19-69 Typical unilateral iris coloboma in an otherwise normal left eye.

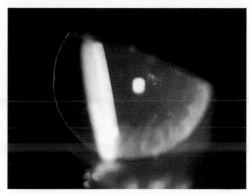

FIG. 19-70 Aniridia. Iris structures are present only as rudimentary findings and the red reflex fills the entire corneal diameter. The edge of the lens is visible peripherally, and early cataractous lens changes are present centrally.

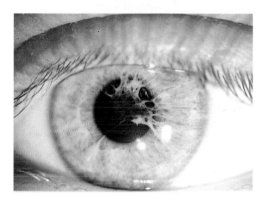

FIG. 19-71 Persistent pupillary membranes. Hyperplasia of the mesoderm of the anterior layer of the iris has caused iris strands to become adherent to the anterior lens surface. The lens is clear, and these are visually insignificant.

fant's horizontal corneal diameter is normally 9.5 mm; this increases over the first 2 years of life to a normal corneal diameter of 11.5 mm. In addition to enlargement of the corneal diameter, chronic elevated intraocular pressure may also enlarge the entire eye. This produces an increase in axial length and a myopic refractive error. A rapid increase in myopia may be a sign of glaucoma. The anterior chamber in infancy is shallow when compared with older children. An anterior chamber that is deeper than normal is a sign of congenital glaucoma.

Epiphora, or tearing, is a sign of glaucoma and is differentiated from nasolacrimal duct obstruction by the presence of rhinorrhea. When the nasolacrimal duct is obstructed, rhinorrhea is absent.

The optic nerve damage caused by elevated intraocular pressure is reflected in the degree of enlargement of the optic cup (Fig. 19-68). Asymmetry of the cup/disc ratio between the eyes or an increase in cup/disc ratio to greater than 0.5 indicates glaucoma. Enlargement of the optic cup is reversible in infants and young children but is usually permanent in adults. Enlargement of the optic cups without glaucoma may be inherited; examination of family members may be of value.

Elevation of intraocular pressure is the hallmark of congenital glaucoma. Normal intraocular pressure (IOP) in infants and young children is less than 20 mm Hg. Pressures greater than 25 mm Hg strongly suggest glaucoma.

Precise measurement of pressure is difficult in children. An estimate of the IOP may be obtained by palpating the globes with the fingertips over closed eyelids. More precise measurements are obtained with a handheld Schiotz tonometer or an applanation tonometer. These pro-

cedures and decisions regarding the management of the pressure may require an examination that is conducted under general anesthesia. Unfortunately, some anesthetic agents alter IOP.

Glaucoma may occur with congenital ocular malformations such as aniridia or mesodermal (iridocorneal) dysgenesis, in systemic syndromes, or after trauma. Sturge-Weber syndrome, neurofibromatosis, Lowe syndrome, Rubinstein-Taybi syndrome, and congenital rubella syndrome are associated with congenital glaucoma. Patients with chronic uveitis frequently develop glaucoma and 8% to 25% and of children with congenital cataracts develop glaucoma at some point in life.

Iris

A coloboma results from failed fusion of the embryonic fissure of the optic cup anywhere from the optic disc to the iris (Fig. 19-69). The defect is usually inferior and nasal in location, and it may involve any ocular structure.

Colobomas occur either as isolated defects or in association with systemic syndromes. Iris colobomas occur in the CHARGE association, cat-eye syndrome, Rieger syndrome, and the facioauriculovertebral anomalies. Isolated colobomas may be inherited as a dominant trait.

Aniridia, an apparent absence of the iris, is due to failure of the mesoderm to grow outward from the iris root during the fourth month of gestation. The pupil appears the same size as the cornea, and iris structures are present as only rudimentary findings (Fig. 19-70). A fibrovascular membrane can form between the rudimentary iris and the trabecular meshwork and cause glaucoma.

Hypoplasia of the macula occurs in patients with aniridia, and visual acuity is decreased to the 20/400 level. Associated defects include corneal opacities, lens dislocations, and cataracts. Affected patients have photophobia and nystagmus.

An autosomal-dominant inheritance pattern is present in two thirds of all patients. It is estimated that 1 to 70 patients with sporadic aniridia will have Wilms tumor, and 90% of these will occur before age 3. Other genitourinary defects and mental retardation may occur, and many of these patients have abnormalities of the 11 p chromosome.

Persistent pupillary membranes are caused by hyperplasia of the mesoderm of the anterior layer of the iris and are a frequent finding in children born prematurely (Fig. 19-71). Instead of terminating at the pupillary margin, iris strands with accompanying blood vessels en-

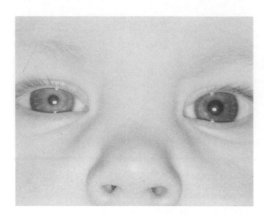

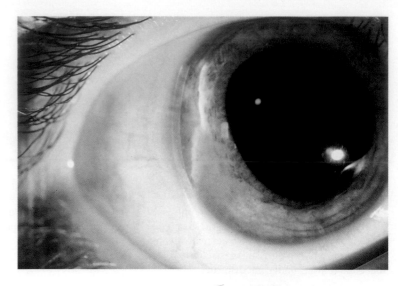

FIG. 19-72 Horner syndrome (right side) with iris heterochromia. The right upper lid is slightly ptotic, and the right lower lid is slightly higher than its mate. Anisocoria is present. The right pupil is smaller than the left. The iris on the side affected by Horner syndrome is lighter in color than the iris of the fellow eye.

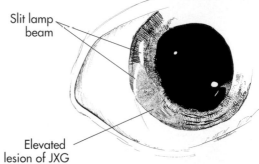

FIG. 19-73 Juvenile xanthogranuloma (JXG). The ocular lesion of JXG is visualized as a fleshy, yellowish-brown tumor on the surface of the iris. The lesions are vascular, bleed easily, and can cause spontaneous hyphemas.

TABLE 19-1

Differential Diagnosis of Leukocoria

Angiomatosis retinae
Cataracts
Coats disease
Colobomas
Congenital retinal fold
High myopia
Incontinentia pigmenti
Medulloepithelioma
Myelinated nerve fibers
Persistent hyperplastic primary vitreous
Retinal detachment
Retinal dysplasia
Retinoblastoma
Retinopathy of prematurity
Toxocariasis
Uveitis
Vitreous hemorrhage

croach on the pupillary space or adhere to the anterior lens surface. They are rarely visually significant.

Heterochromia iridis, or asymmetry in the color of the iris, if isolated, is visually insignificant. Heterochromia may occur in congenital Horner syndrome, the eye with Horner syndrome being lighter in color. Heterochromia may also occur secondary to inflammation or after intraocular surgery or ocular trauma. Trauma may cause the affected iris to become darker than the fellow iris as late as many years after the incident (Fig. 19-72).

The iris may provide signs that aid in the diagnosis of systemic conditions. Patients with neurofibromatosis may have multiple small melanocytic iris nevi, Lisch nodules, on the surface of the iris (see Chapter 15). These may be identified with magnification provided by the direct ophthalmoscope, or by slit-lamp examination. Other ocular findings associated with neurofibromatosis include plexiform neurofibromas of the lids, thickened corneal nerves, congenital glaucoma, and optic nerve gliomas.

Patients, usually less than 1 year of age, with juvenile xanthogranuloma (JXG) may develop unilateral asymptomatic fleshy, yellowish-brown tumors on the surface of the iris (Fig. 19-73). These vascular lesions bleed easily and may produce a spontaneous hyphema.

Brushfield spots are found in patients with Down syndrome. The spots consist of tiny areas of normal iris stroma that are surrounded by rings of mild iris hypoplasia. Brushfield spots give the iris a speckled appearance.

Lens

The lens may be affected by developmental, hereditary, syndrome-related, inflammatory, metabolic, or traumatic conditions. This can result in the development of a cataract, an opacification of the crystalline lens, which may be either partial or complete. The lens may also be dislocated from its supporting zonulae or subluxated.

Cataracts

Leukocoria refers to the white pupillary reflex produced by reflection of light from a light-colored intraocular mass or structure. Several conditions of variable severity and prognosis produce leukocoria (Table 19-1).

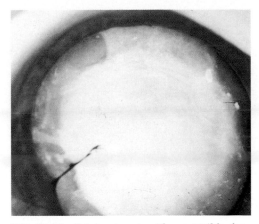

FIG. 19-74 Total cataract with no visible fundus details.

FIG. 19-75 Spokelike cortical cataract of Down syndrome. The lens opacification does not affect the visual axis and is visually insignificant. Lens opacification such as this may rapidly progress and produce visual loss, or they may remain unchanged for years.

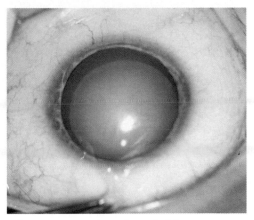

FIG. 19-76 A microspherophakic cataractous lens in rubella syndrome.

TABLE 19-2

Syndromes Associated with Cataracts

Albright hereditary osteodystrophy	Lantieri syndrome
Alport syndrome	Laurence-Moon-Bardet-Biedel syndrome
Cat-eye syndrome	Lowe syndrome
Cerebrooculofacial-skeletal syndrome	Marinesco-Sjögren syndrome
Chondrodysplasia punctata (Conradi-Hünermann syndrome)	Marshall syndrome
	Myotonic dystrophy
	Osteogensis imperfecta
Cockayne syndrome	Patau syndrome
Congenital ichthyosis	(trisomy 13-15)
Conradi syndrome	Progeria
Craniofacial syndromes (Apert and Crouzon syndromes)	Roberts syndrome
	Rothman-Thomson syndrome
Down syndrome (trisomy 21)	Rubinstein-Taybi syndrome
Edward syndrome (trisomy 18)	Smith-Lemli-Opitz syndrome
Hallgren syndrome	
Hallmann-Streiff syndrome	Stickler syndrome
Ichthyosis	Turner syndrome
Incontinentia pigmenti	Zellweger syndrome
Kniest syndrome	

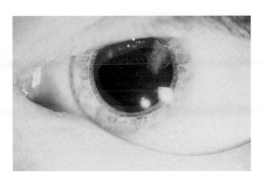

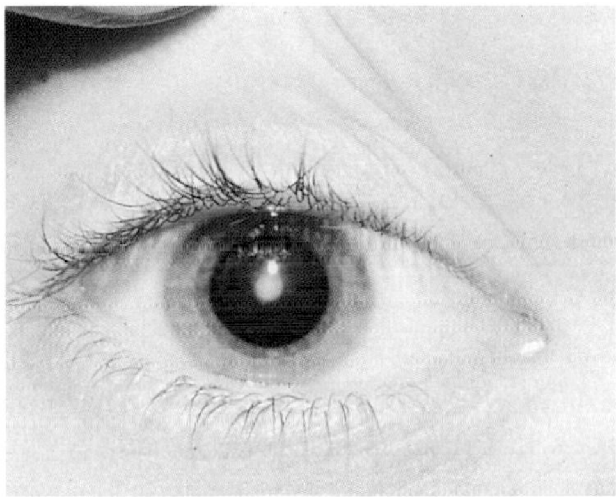

FIG. 19-77 Anterior polar cataract. This type of lens opacity is a developmental abnormality that in most cases remains stable and rarely affects vision.

Examination with a penlight, the plus lens of a direct ophthalmoscope, or slit-lamp biomicroscopy will help to differentiate lens opacification (cataract) from other forms of leukocoria.

Congenital or infantile cataracts may be unilateral or bilateral, and the extent of opacification may be complete or partial (Fig. 19-74). Bilateral cataracts usually arise early in infancy and, if not treated early, may produce severe visual deprivation accompanied by poor fixation and nystagmus. Visually significant unilateral cataracts are associated with severe deprivation amblyopia and strabismus.

Opacification of a child's lens may be due to heredity (autosomal dominant), chromosomal disorders (trisomy, 13, 18, and 21) (Fig. 19-75), inflammation (iritis and uveitis), infection (TORCH), metabolic disorders (galactosemia and disorders of calcium and phosphorous metabolism),

exposure to toxins, vitamin deficiencies (vitamins A and D), systemic syndromes with cataracts (Table 19-2), ocular conditions producing retinal detachment, radiation exposure, and trauma. Roughly one third of pediatric cataracts are hereditary, one third are syndrome or disease related, and one third are attributed to undetermined causes.

The presence of ocular anomalies frequently identifies a developmental defect as being the cause for the cataract. Microphthalmia, the globe being smaller than normal, may be caused by ocular disease or inflammation, or it may be present as a developmental defect (Fig. 19-60). Eyes with persistent hyperplastic primary vitreous (PHPV) are usually microphthalmic and frequently have cataracts.

The morphology of the lens opacification may provide a clue to the cause of a congenital cataract if opacification is not complete. During development, the lens cells lay down fibers that grow out from the peripheral lens to the anterior and posterior lens surfaces. These will form sutures. Because of this the gestational age at the time of cataract development determines the location of the opacity. For example, the nuclear cataracts of rubella syndrome (Fig. 19-76) indicate infection early in gestation, whereas a zonular or lamellar cataract represents an insult to the lens occurring later in lens development.

Small central opacities on the anterior or posterior poles of the lens, polar cataracts, are developmental abnormalities that remain stable and rarely affect vision (Fig. 19-77). Lamellar or zonular cataracts have a normal, transparent central nucleus, an affected lamellar zone, and a

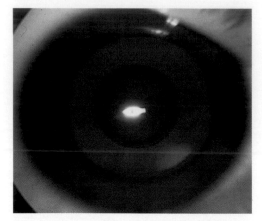

FIG. 19-78 Lamellar cataract with riders, surrounded by a clear cortex.

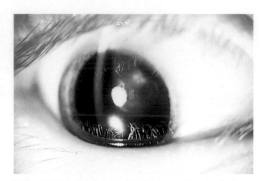

FIG. 19-79 Cataract of galactosemia. Early lens changes cause the nucleus of the lens to have an "oil droplet" configuration resulting from the accumulation of dulcitol, a metabolic product of galactose, within the lens. The resultant osmotic gradient draws water into the lens, producing the opacification. Early lens changes in galactosemia are reversible.

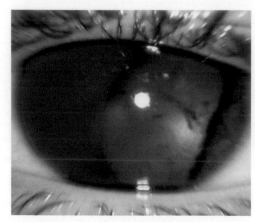

FIG. 19-80 A traumatic, dislocated cataractous lens.

clear outer layer of cortex. Riders or radial extensions frequently are present (Fig. 19-78). Zonular cataracts may be autosomal dominant, associated with vitamin A and D deficiency, or follow hypocalcemia. Multicolored flecks may be seen in hypoparathyroidism or myotonic dystrophy, and an oil droplet configuration is seen in galactosemia (Fig. 19-79).

If a child has no history of trauma, the family history is unremarkable, the general physical examination fails to uncover a systemic syndrome or chromosomal abnormality, and ocular examination does not help to determine the cause of a cataract, then a focused laboratory evaluation to determine the cause of the cataract may be undertaken. The most common metabolic disorders causing congenital cataracts are hypoglycemia and hypocalcemia. Laboratory evaluation for galactosemia and galactokinase deficiency should include blood tests for galactose and galactose-1-phosphate, as well as examination of the urine for reducing substances. Examination of the urine for protein and amino acids will identify patients with Lowe (oculocerebrorenal) syndrome, and a urine nitroprusside test will diagnose homocystinuria. Screening tests for congenital TORCH infections and syphilis also should be performed.

Positional abnormalities of the lens may occur. A partial dislocation of the lens is referred to as *subluxation*. A dislocated lens, ectopia lentis, may cause a profound decrease in vision by producing a large refractive error and amblyopia. Ectopia lentis may be unilateral, bilateral, inherited or sporadic, or it may be due to trauma (Fig. 19-80).

Simple ectopia lentis is a bilateral, symmetric condition with an autosomal dominant inheritance pattern. Bilateral superotemporal lens dislocation is present in 50% to 80% of patients with Marfan syndrome. Of patients with homocystinuria, 90% will have an inferior lens dislocation, and patients with Weill-Marchesani syndrome may have dislocation of their microspherophakic lenses.

Uvea

Inflammation of the uveal tract (iris, ciliary body, and choroid) has many potential causes, including infections (toxoplasmosis, herpes zoster and simplex, and Lyme disease), collagen vascular disease (most frequently juvenile rheumatoid arthritis [JRA] and sarcoidosis), and trauma. In the majority of children the etiologic agent cannot be determined. Advanced retinoblastoma may also present with signs that suggest uveitis.

Involvement of the iris alone (iritis or anterior uveitis) produces pain, ciliary injection (conjunctival redness in the circumlimbal area), tearing, photophobia, and decreased vision. Synechiae, adhesions between the iris and lens or peripheral cornea, may produce corectopia, an abnormally shaped pupil. Inflammatory reaction in the anterior chamber may be viewed with the aid of a slit lamp as inflammatory cells and fibrin or protein (flare) in the aqueous fluid. If marked, this may give the eye a dull or "glassy" appearance (Fig. 19-81). Clumps of inflammatory cells may adhere to the posterior corneal surface, forming keratic precipitates (KP).

Because iritis may be present without signs and symptoms, children with JRA should have periodic screening ophthalmic examinations. Children with polyarticular disease should be examined annually, and those with positive antinuclear antibodies and pauciarticular disease, who are more likely to develop ocular complications, should be examined three to four times a year (see Chapter 8).

Pars planitis, or intermediate uveitis, is an idiopathic, bilateral inflammation of the pars plana or pars ciliaris portions of the ciliary body. Symptoms include light sensitivity, "floaters," and blurring of vision. Inflammatory cells in the anterior vitreous can make visualization of the retina with the direct ophthalmoscope difficult. If the inflammation is severe, it may produce leukocoria. Most cases are self-limited; however, chronic courses with exacerbations and remissions may produce visual loss resulting from cataracts, glaucoma, optic nerve inflammation, and cystoid macular edema. Retinal detachment because of membrane formation and phthisis bulbi may occur in advanced cases (Fig. 19-82).

Posterior uveitis (inflammation of the posterior vitreous, retina, and/or choroid) can be caused by infection, but frequently the precise cause is undetermined. Infection of the retina by protozoa, fungi, and viruses may produce an intense inflammatory response in the vitreous, rendering it hazy or opaque. Leukocoria may be produced if the vitreous is very cloudy or if extensive retinal involvement is present.

Vitreous

Vitreous Hemorrhage

Trauma, be it penetrating, concussive, or the result of shaken baby syndrome, is the most common cause of vitreous hemorrhage. Vitreous hemorrhage may occur with hemorrhagic disease of the newborn (hy-

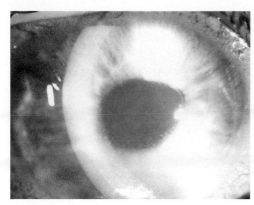

FIG. 19-81 Iritis with circumcorneal ciliary flush.

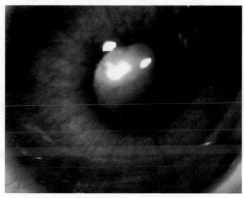

FIG. 19-82 Yellow cyclitic membrane behind a clear lens in a soft phthisic eye.

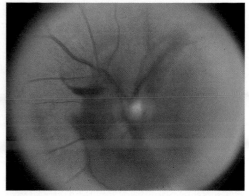

FIG. 19-83 Vitreous hemorrhage. Dispersed red blood cells in the vitreous have made it hazy. The diffraction of light causes blurred vision. Fluid levels often are visible, and collections of blood may appear to "float" within the eye.

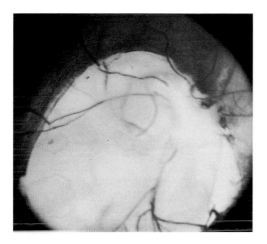

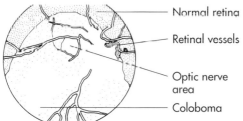

FIG. 19-84 Coloboma of optic nerve, retina, and choroid. Yellowish-white sclera is visible, and retinal vessels can be seen coursing through the coloboma.

- Normal retina
- Retinal vessels
- Optic nerve area
- Coloboma

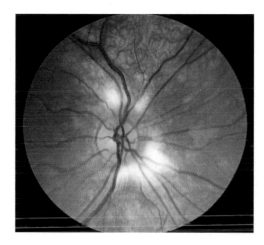

FIG. 19-85 Myelinated nerve fibers. Myelination of the optic nerve fibers may continue beyond the optic disc to include the retinal nerve fibers. This is visible as yellowish-white flame-shaped patches oriented with the retinal nerve fibers. Myelinated nerve fibers may produce the clinical sign of leukocoria.

poprothrombiemia), thrombocytopenia, or in advanced stages of retinopathy of prematurity. Patients with a subarachnoid hemorrhage may develop vitreous hemorrhage (Terson syndrome), and vitreous hemorrhage may also occur in patients with leukemia.

Blood in the vitreous, if located centrally or posteriorly, may be visible with the direct ophthalmoscope. If the vitreous is liquid, the hemorrhage may appear to "float" inside the eye (Fig. 19-83). Blood in the vitreous may produce leukocoria as it organizes and becomes yellow and then gray in color.

Retina

Developmental Abnormalities

Colobomas

Retinal colobomas are caused by a defect in closure of the embryonal fissure of the optic cup. They may occur unilaterally or bilaterally. Large colobomas are manifest as an absence of the retina and choroid with or without marked excavation of the optic disc (Fig. 19-84). There

is usually a ring of pigment around the coloboma. Leukokoria may be produced by the yellowish-white reflection of the underlying sclera. Using a direct ophthalmoscope, an occasional vessel may be seen bridging the area of the coloboma. The coloboma and retina are at a different plane of focus when visualized with the ophthalmoscope.

Colobomas may occur in otherwise normal eyes or in association with microphthalmia or retinal detachment. If the optic disc and macula are not involved, visual acuity may be normal. Colobomas may be inherited as isolated anomalies, or they may be associated with chromosomal defects (trisomy 13) or other syndrome-related entities (CHARGE association).

Myelinated Nerve Fibers

Before birth, myelination of the optic nerve begins in the central nervous system, progresses peripherally, and usually stops at the optic disc before birth. Myelination may continue beyond the optic disc to include the retinal nerve fiber layer. Once completed, the process remains stationary. Myelinated fibers are oriented with the retinal nerve fibers and are easily seen with the direct ophthalmoscope as yellowish-white flame-shaped patches overlying the sensory retina and choroid (Fig. 19-85).

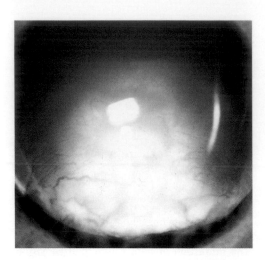

FIG. 19-86 Persistent hyperplastic primary vitreous presenting as a dense fibrovascular retrolental mass with microspherophakia, microphthalmia, and elongated ciliary processes.

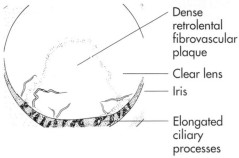

Dense retrolental fibrovascular plaque

Clear lens

Iris

Elongated ciliary processes

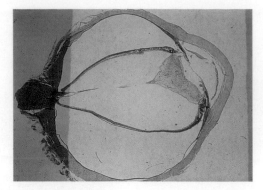

FIG. 19-87 Pathologic section of persistent hypoplastic primary vitreous (PHPV). (Courtesy Dr. BL Johnson.)

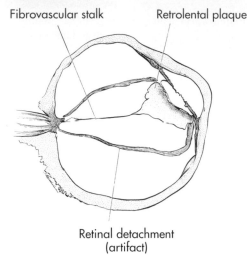

Fibrovascular stalk   Retrolental plaque

Retinal detachment (artifact)

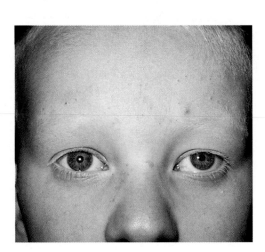

FIG. 19-88 Albinism, characterized by white hair, pale skin, and translucent irides.

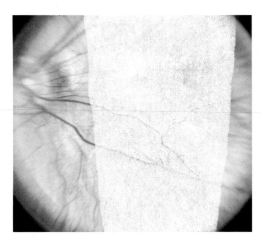

FIG. 19-89 Ophthalmoscopic view of a patient with albinism demonstrates a pale fundus, poor macular development, and prominent choroidal vasculature.

The macula is rarely involved, and normal vision is usually present, although scotomas corresponding to the areas of myelination may be found on visual field examination.

Persistent Hyperplastic Primary Vitreous

PHPV occurs as a unilateral defect in the involution of the primary vitreous during the seventh month of gestation. There are no systemic associations. Eyes with PHPV are usually microphthalmic. PHPV may be associated with cataracts, intraocular hemorrhage, glaucoma, and retinal detachment. Eyes with advanced PHPV can become phthisic (Figs. 19-86 and 19-87).

Albinism

Albinism refers to conditions involving deficiencies of melanin in the skin or eye (Fig. 19-88). The loss of pigmentation may predominantly affect the eye (ocular albinism), be generalized to the skin and

eye (oculocutaneous albinism), or occur in conjunction with a systemic syndrome such as Chédiak-Higashi or Hermansky-Pudlak syndrome.

Ocular albinism occurs as an X-linked or autosomal recessive trait. Photophobia is frequently a symptom. The loss of cutaneous pigmentation may be mild. Patients have iris transillumination defects in which the red reflex is seen through multiple punctate defects in the iris. Absence of pigment in the retinal pigment epithelium layer of the retina makes the fundus appear a lighter yellowish-orange color than usual. The macula and fovea are hypoplastic, and visual acuity is decreased to a degree dependent on the absence of pigment (Fig. 19-89). Ocular albinism must be included in the differential diagnosis of an infant with nystagmus.

Ocular pigmentary abnormalities may also occur in a milder form, albanoidism. Such patients have iris transillumination defects, fundus hy-

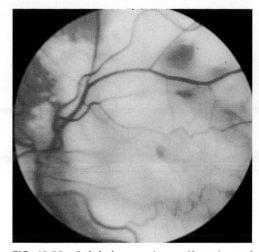

FIG. 19-90 Ophthalmoscopic manifestations of Coats disease. Peripheral telangiectasis along the course of the retinal veins leads to exudation, giving the retina a yellowish-white appearance.

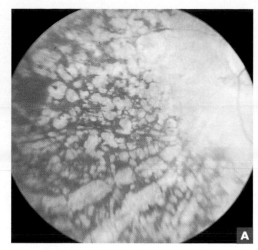

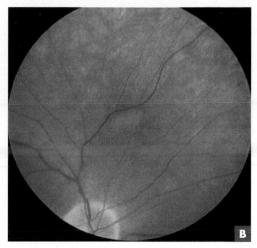

FIG. 19-91 *A*, Retinitis pigmentosa, characterized by retinal pigment disposition, narrow arterioles, and a pale disc. *B*, Early fundus signs of retinitis pigmentosa. The optic disc has a waxy pallor, and the retinal arterial system is sclerotic. In children, pigmentary changes may not be as advanced or as noticeable as in adults.

popigmentation, and photophobia. Their maculae, however, are less severely affected or are normal. Because of this, nystagmus is uncommon and visual acuity is normal or only minimally reduced. Albanoidism is inherited as an autosomal dominant with incomplete penetrance.

Coats Disease (Retinal Telangiectasis)

Coats disease occurs unilaterally in boys younger than 18 years of age. The most common age at diagnosis is between 8 and 10 years. Peripheral retinal vessel telangiectasis and aneurysmal dilation lead to extensive areas of exudation, giving the retina a yellowish-white appearance, which may produce leukokoria (Fig. 19-90). The macula is a common site for exudation to collect; when this occurs, visual loss is profound.

Retinitis Pigmentosa

Retinitis pigmentosa (RP) is a pigmentary retinopathy characterized by visual field loss, night blindness, and a depressed or extinct electroretinogram (ERG). Symptoms of visual loss may be present in childhood but usually do not become apparent until the second or third decade of life. Poor night vision is the earliest symptom, followed by progressive loss of peripheral visual field and, finally, loss of central vision. The rate of progression of visual loss varies for each pedigree and may ultimately be mild or severe.

The retinal pigment epithelial changes include deposition of pigment in a perivascular pattern. Pigment deposition in the midperipheral retina gives a characteristic "bone spicule" pattern late in the course of the disease (Fig. 19-91, *A*). Early in the disease, the optic nerve may have a waxy pallor and the retinal arteries may be attenuated (Fig. 19-91, *B*).

Systemic disease entities are associated with RP. Patients with sensorineural hearing loss should be examined for the associated presence of retinitis pigmentosa (Usher syndrome and Hallgren syndrome). Renal diseases including Fanconi syndrome, cystinuria, cystinosis, and oxalosis may be associated with pigmentary retinal changes, as may the mucopolysaccharidoses, Refsum disease, and syphilis.

Retinal Detachment

Trauma is the most common cause of retinal detachment in children. Leukokoria occurs when the detached retina is in apposition to

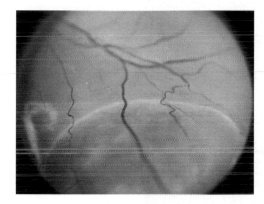

FIG. 19-92 Retinal detachment. The inferior retina is detached, and a demarcation line between the attached and detached retina is visible. Fluid beneath the detached sensory retina shifts with movement of the eye and causes the detached retina to move or undulate.

the lens. Retinal detachments, if located posteriorly, may be viewed with the direct ophthalmoscope as elevations of the retina (Fig. 19-92). The detached retina may move or undulate with eye movement.

Retinopathy of Prematurity

Retinopathy of prematurity (ROP) is characterized by abnormalities in the developing retinal vascular system. Mild forms affect the peripheral retina at the junction between the vascularized and immature avascular retina. These changes can be observed using an indirect ophthalmoscope. Severe forms produce fibrovascular proliferations that extend into the vitreous and cause traction that may lead to poor macular development (temporal macular drag) or detachment of the retina (Fig. 19-93). A white fibrovascular mass may occupy the retrolental space (retrolental fibroplasia) and produce leukokoria.

In 75% of patients, ROP is bilateral and symmetric. Retinopathy of prematurity primarily affects the ill, premature infant whose birthweight is less than 1600 g or who has been exposed to more than 30 days of supplemental oxygen. Because early phases of this disease are treatable, programs to screen neonates at risk for developing this condition are necessary.

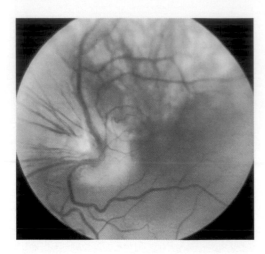

FIG. 19-93 Retrolental fibroplasia with temporal tugging of the disc.

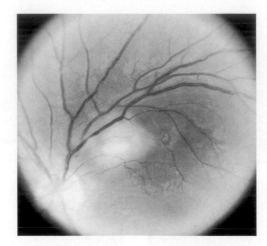

FIG. 19-94 Acute, recurrent, toxoplasmic chorioretinal inflammation adjacent to a healed pigmented lesion.

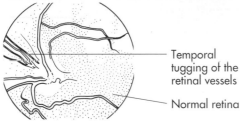

Temporal tugging of the retinal vessels

Normal retina

Area of acute chorioretinitis

Old pigmented lesion

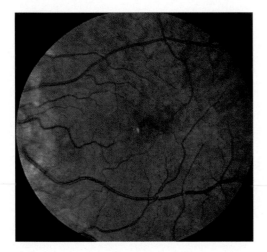

FIG. 19-95 Pigmentary retinopathy in rubella syndrome.

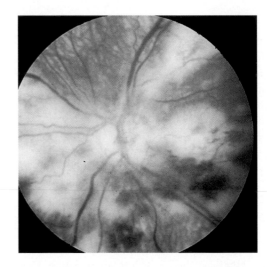

FIG. 19-96 Retinitis, with obvious hemorrhages and perivascular yellowish-white exudates secondary to cytomegalic inclusion disease.

Retinitis and Retinochoroiditis

Inflammation of the retina and choroid is most commonly the result of viral, protozoal, fungal, or bacterial infection. The final common pathway for recovery or resolution of retinal inflammation is the production of a pigmented chorioretinal scar. The characteristics and location of these scars are frequently diagnostic for the infecting agent. In many cases, however, isolated chorioretinal scars do not suggest any particular disease.

A rare cause of retinochoriditis is sympathetic ophthalmia. Sympathetic ophthalmia occurs after an injury of one eye, the "exciting" eye, followed by a latent period and the development of uveitis in the uninjured eye, the "sympathizing" eye. Sympathetic ophthalmia may occur as early as 10 days after the original injury but may also have a delayed onset years after the incident. The etiology of sympathetic ophthalmia is unknown.

Torch Infection

Toxoplasmosis

Toxoplasmosis, a protozoal infection of the retinal cells, is most often considered to be congenital in origin with transplacental transmission. Of neonates severely affected by toxoplasmosis, 80% will have

retinochoroiditis. Involvement is bilateral and often includes the macula. The retinal lesions may develop after birth, and most are inactive when first diagnosed. These lesions characteristically occur as multifocal pigmented chorioretinal scars. Inactive lesions may reactivate anytime throughout life with active inflammation developing adjacent to areas of scarring. This is seen as a white fluffy response that may extend into the vitreous overlying the lesion (Fig. 19-94).

Rubella

Exposure to rubella virus during the first trimester of pregnancy may result in an intrauterine infection manifested as congenital rubella syndrome. Ocular findings include microphthalmia, microcornea, anterior uveitis, iris hypoplasia, nuclear or complete cataracts, corneal opacification, and glaucoma. The retinopathy of rubella syndrome is a diffuse "salt and pepper" retinopathy that develops early in childhood and does not affect vision. The pigmentary changes may be similar in appearance to those of syphilis, retinitis pigmentosa, and Leber congenital amaurosis (Fig. 19-95).

Cytomegalovirus

Cytomegalovirus (CMV) infection produces a bilateral retinochoroiditis manifested as multiple, yellowish-white, fluffy retinal lesions (Fig. 19-96). Hemorrhage is a prominent feature. Other ophthalmic

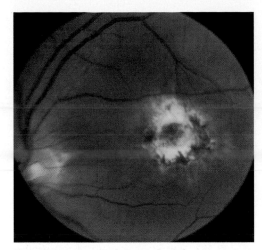

FIG. 19-97 A retinal toxocariasis lesion appears as a white elevated mass with surrounding pigmentation.

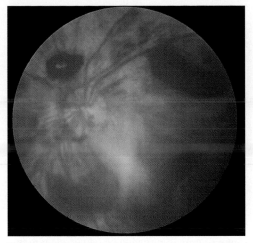

FIG. 19-98 Shaken baby syndrome. Multiple retinal hemorrhages are present in the posterior fundus. There are small flame-shaped hemorrhages within the nerve fiber layer that follow the pattern of the retinal vessels. More extensive areas of hemorrhage have broken through to the preretinal space and are seen as areas of blood that obscure the retina. A Roth spot, a hemorrhage with a white center, is visible just above the optic disc. The white reflection from the camera flash is visible because of dispersed RBCs within the vitreous.

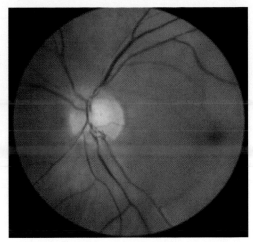

FIG. 19-99 Central retinal artery occlusion. A cherry-red spot is visible in the fovea. This sign is due to edema and opacification of the ganglion cell layer of the retina surrounding the fovea.

manifestations include microphthalmia, uveitis, cataracts, optic disc atrophy, strabismus, and nystagmus.

CMV retinitis may be an opportunistic infection occurring in patients who are immunosuppressed because of immunodeficiency disorders or who are receiving immunosuppressive drugs. Retinal inflammation, edema, and hemorrhage may be extensive and rapidly progressive in these patients.

Herpes Simplex Virus

Herpes simplex virus (HSV) infection may involve the anterior segment of the eye, with conjunctivitis, keratitis, or, when disseminated in the perinatal period, retinochoroiditis. Retinal involvement with disseminated HSV is severe, with extensive inflammatory reaction producing yellowish-white exudates and retinal necrosis.

Syphilis

Congenital syphilis may cause bilateral chorioretinitis, resulting in a "salt and pepper" fundus appearance. Differentiation of the retinopathy of congenital syphilis from retinitis pigmentosa may be difficult. Syphilis may also cause interstitial keratitis, anterior uveitis, glaucoma, and optic nerve atrophy.

Toxocariasis

Toxocara canis larvae infect children from 2 to 9 years of age. When the eye is involved, a white, elevated chorioretinal granuloma develops (Fig. 19-97). Chronic unilateral uveitis with opacification of the vitreous overlying the granuloma may occur. Inflammation in ocular toxocariasis occurs only after the organism dies. Externally, the eye does not appear to be inflamed. With extensive inflammation, fibrotic preretinal membranes may develop and produce retinal detachment. Differentiation from retinoblastoma may be difficult. Calcification of the lesion is rare in toxocariasis as opposed to retinoblastoma. The diagnosis is confirmed by enzyme-linked immunosorbent assay (ELISA) for *T. canis* on blood or intraocular fluid.

Bacterial Endocarditis

"Cotton-wool" spots frequently develop in patients with bacterial endocarditis and septic emboli. These represent infarction of the nerve fiber layer of the retina and appear as white, irregular lesions with indistinct borders. Cotton-wool spots may be seen in any condition that produces retinal ischemia, such as hypertension and diabetes, or in patients with acquired immunodeficiency syndrome (AIDS). Intraretinal hemorrhages occur with septic emboli and are flame shaped or dot-blot in nature. If the hemorrhage has a white center from the accumulation of leukocytes, the term *Roth spot* is used. Roth spots are not specific for bacterial endocarditis. They may occur in leukemia or shaken baby syndrome (Fig. 19-98). Conjunctival petechiae may be present as a sign of septic emboli.

Emboli to the eye may cause a central or branch retinal artery obstruction. Occlusion of the central retinal artery causes a sudden loss in vision, loss of the pupillary direct light reflex, absence of venous pulsations, and the development of a cherry-red spot in the fovea. Edema and opacification of the ganglion cell layer surrounding the fovea produces this sign (Fig. 19-99).

Leukemia

Patients with acute lymphoblastic, myelogenous, or monocytic leukemia may develop flame-shaped intraretinal hemorrhages. These are usually visible with the direct ophthalmoscope. The presence of hemorrhage is not correlated with anemia or thrombocytopenia. Leukemic infiltration may also occur in the retina as a perivascular infiltrate, in the choroid, or in the optic disc, producing disc swelling and a papilledema-like appearance. Leukemic involvement of the orbit may be difficult to distinguish from bacterial cellulitis.

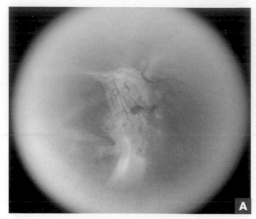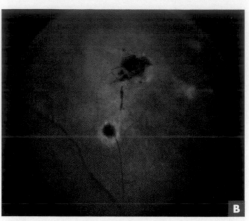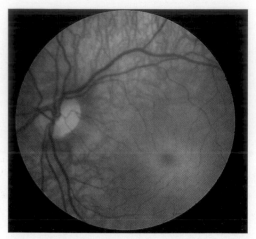

FIG. 19-100   Sickle cell retinopathy. *A,* Neovascularization or growth of fragile blood vessels into the vitreous in the midperipheral retina. The white fibrous tissue present is due to the proliferation of fibroglial elements. This produces traction on the retina, which may subsequently lead to retinal detachment. *B,* The black sunburst lesions are areas of perivascular retinal pigment epithelial hypertrophy with pigment migration. This finding is an example of nonproliferative change.

FIG. 19-101   Tay-Sachs disease. Because the perifoveal area has many retinal ganglion cells and the fovea has none, the fovea retains its orangeish-red color but it is surrounded by retina that is whitish in color. This produces the "cherry-red spot" in the macula.

Diabetes

The most common ocular finding in young diabetic patients is lenticular myopia. This occurs in patients who have had a rapid rise in blood glucose level. Sorbitol accumulates within the lens as a metabolic product, increasing the lens osmolarity, thus causing the lens to swell and produce myopia. After the blood sugar level returns to normal, myopia may continue to persist for several days or even weeks. Children with diabetes rarely develop cataracts.

The earliest sign of background diabetic retinopathy (BDR) is the presence of microaneurysms (tiny discrete red spots). Small retinal hemorrhages, cotton-wool spots, venous dilation, and hard exudates (small, discrete, yellow lesions) may also be seen. The occurrence of background diabetic retinopathy is related to the duration of diabetes; it is rarely seen within 3 years after diagnosis. The prevalence of retinopathy increases to 90% in patients who have had juvenile onset diabetes for greater than 15 years. Proliferative diabetic retinopathy seen in adults essentially does not occur until after puberty.

Sickle Cell Retinopathy

The ocular abnormalities of the hemoglobinopathies are caused by intravascular sickling, hemostasis, and thrombosis. Retinal findings occur in the peripheral fundus and are difficult to visualize with the direct ophthalmoscope. Retinal vascular complications occur most frequently in patients with SC and S-thalassemia disease. Patients with sickle cell disease (Hb SS) are less frequently affected. The decreased hematocrit may provide protection to the retinal vasculature. Rarely, patients with the milder hemoglobinopathies, AS and AC, may have retinal findings.

Retinal findings may be divided into nonproliferative and proliferative changes. Proliferative changes include arteriolar occlusions that lead to arteriovenous anastomosis, causing areas of retinal nonperfusion. Neovascularization occurs at the edge of these areas of nonperfusion, in the form of a gossamer vascular network (a sea fan), and often leads to vitreous hemorrhage, traction, and retinal detachment (Fig. 19-100, *A*). The disease process is similar to that seen in retinopathy of prematurity.

Nonproliferative changes include refractile or iridescent deposits, black sunburst lesions, and salmon patch hemorrhages. Refractile deposits are sequelae of old reabsorbed hemorrhages. Sunburst lesions are areas of perivascular retinal pigment epithelial hypertrophy and pig-

ment migration (Fig. 19-100, *B*). Salmon patch lesions represent areas of intraretinal hemorrhage. Parafoveal capillaries and arterioles may become occluded and produce decreased visual acuity in sickle cell retinopathy. Segmentation of the conjunctival blood vessels produces comma-shaped capillaries ("comma sign").

Metabolic Diseases

The mucopolysaccharidoses (MPS) are syndromes caused by inherited defects in the lysosomal enzymes that degrade acid mucopolysaccharide. All of the mucopolysaccharidoses are transmitted as autosomal recessive traits except type II (Hunter), which is X-linked recessive. A common ocular finding is retinal pigmentary degeneration, which closely resembles retinitis pigmentosa. Optic atrophy also occurs, as does corneal clouding resulting from stromal infiltration.

The sphingolipidoses are caused by a deficiency of the lysosomal enzymes responsible for the degeneration of sphingolipids. Tay-Sachs disease (GM_2 type I gangliosidosis) and Niemann-Pick disease are the two most common sphingolipidoses. Sphingolipids accumulate in the retinal ganglion cells, giving a whitish appearance to the retina. Because the parafoveal area has many retinal ganglion cells and the fovea none, the fovea has its normal orangish-red color, whereas the retina peripheral to the fovea is white. This produces a "cherry-red spot" in the macula (Fig. 19-101).

The mucolipidoses are caused by abnormal glycoprotein metabolism. Mucolipidoses have clinical findings of some of the sphingolipidoses and some of the mucopolysaccharoidoses. The ocular findings include corneal epithelial edema, retinal pigmentary degeneration, macular cherry-red spots, and optic atrophy.

Cystinosis represents a defective transport mechanism for cystine within the lysosomes, which cause intralysosomal accumulation of cystine. Patients develop "salt and pepper" changes of the retinal pigment epithelium and areas of patchy depigmentation with irregularly distributed pigment clumps. These changes do not produce loss of vision. Photophobia is due to the accumulation of corneal crystals.

Retinoblastoma

Retinoblastoma is the most common intraocular malignancy of childhood. It occurs with a frequency of between 1 in 14,000 and 1 in

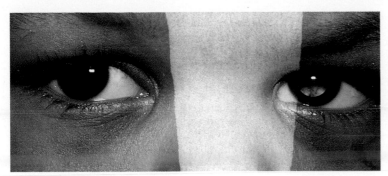

FIG. 19-102 Leukocoria. The patient's left eye has a white pupillary reflex produced by reflection of light from a retinoblastoma. Leukocoria is the most common presenting sign (60%) of retinoblastoma.

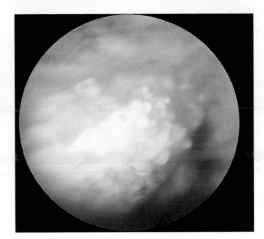

FIG. 19-103 Retinoblastoma. The tumor mass of retinoblastoma usually is elevated and yellow or white in color. Dilated feeding vessels of the tumor may be visible. Seeding into the vitreous from the tumor may produce a cloudy vitreous.

20,000 births. The most common age of diagnosis is between 1 and 1½ years, with 90% of cases presenting before age 3 years. The most common presenting signs of retinoblastoma are leukocoria (60%) and strabismus (22%) (Fig. 19-102). One third of cases are bilateral. The tumor may present as an elevated, round, white or yellow mass (Fig. 19-103). Retinoblastoma may be multicentric, with several tumor masses arising within the same eye. Seeding into the vitreous may occur, producing a cloudy vitreous. A frequent feature of retinoblastoma is the presence of calcification within the mass.

Great advances have occurred in the understanding of the genetics of retinoblastoma. Retinoblastoma may be transmitted in an autosomal dominant inheritance pattern. Of patients with the disease, 60% have a family history of retinoblastoma. Penetrance is high (60% to 90%) but incomplete. Sporadic cases occur as either somatic mutations in 75% of patients or as germinal mutations that may be passed on to offspring. These sporadic cases are almost always unilateral, and the hereditary forms are usually bilateral; however, a patient with a unilateral tumor may have heritable disease. Current research is making it possible to determine which patients with unilateral tumors have the hereditary form of the disease and which patients do not (see Chapter 1).

Optic Nerve

The optic nerve relays information from each eye to the brain. Its function is assessed by measuring visual acuity, visual fields, color vision, and the pupillary response. Visualization and assessment of the morphology of the optic disc with the direct ophthalmoscope provides valuable information regarding the function of the nerve.

Color Vision

Change in color vision, particularly the ability to perceive red, is an early feature seen in disorders that compromise the function of the optic nerve. Patients may complain of subjective changes in color perception, or they may demonstrate defects in color vision on objective tests.

An easy test to assess color vision is to judge color comparison between the two eyes. The patient is asked to look at a red object first with one eye, then with the other, and is asked whether it is more red with one eye or the other. A subjective desaturation of red in one eye is an indication of dyschromatopsia and a potential optic nerve disorder. If the patient reports that the object is only 50% as red to one eye as compared with the other, the results would be recorded as a red desaturation of 50%. In children it is valuable to present the object to the "normal eye" first with the question "If this is $1.00 of red, how much red is it now?" offering a comparison with the fellow eye. A similar comparison may be performed for brightness by shining a light first into one eye and then into the other. The sense of brightness is also decreased in the presence of optic nerve disease. Formal assessment of color vision is performed using color plates such as the Hardy-Rand-Rittler or Ishihara color plates. Patients with heritable congenital color vision defects are equally affected in both eyes. Patients with asymmetric optic nerve disease (optic neuritis, tumor, toxic optic neuropathy) have asymmetrically decreased color vision, especially for the red hues.

Pupils

Assessment of the pupils for size, shape, position, and reactivity is an important part of the neurologic and ophthalmic evaluation. Neurologic abnormalities that effect the pupil include defects of the afferent pathway (the optic nerve and visual system), the parasympathetic pathway (for pupillary constriction), and the sympathetic pathway (for pupillary dilation).

Afferent Pupillary Defects

In a normal patient, shining a penlight in one eye causes both pupils to constrict. Pupillary constriction in the illuminated eye is the direct response, and the constriction in the fellow eye is the consensual response. The pupils are normally equal in size even if one eye is blind; each eye receives equal pupillary innervation.

The swinging flashlight test is used to assess optic nerve function (Fig. 19-104). If an afferent pupillary defect (APD) is present, the term *Marcus Gunn pupil* is used. A penlight is used to illuminate one eye and then the other. The pupil of the illuminated eye is observed. If both eyes have equal afferent input, then illumination of either eye should produce equal constriction of the pupils. Normally, after shining a light in one eye, the response is initial constriction of both pupils followed by a small dilation. If the light is then swung quickly to the fellow eye, the response is the same. When there is a decrease in afferent input for pupillary constriction on one side (e.g., a monocular optic neuritis with one optic nerve acutely affected), constriction is either absent or decreased and the pupils dilate. The critical observation is that when the affected eye is illuminated, a gradual dilation of the pupils occurs as compared with the response of the normal eye. It is important to have the patient maintain fixation on a distant object, since accommodation causes constriction of the pupils and may lead to misinterpretation of the findings.

An APD indicates disease affecting the optic nerve. Unilaterally or bilaterally asymmetric optic nerve disease always causes a relative APD. Mild optic nerve disease producing minimal or no objectively measurable decrease in visual acuity still produces an APD, whereas a retinal defect must be profound to produce an APD. Afferent pupillary defects are not seen with dense cataracts, refractive errors, cortical lesions, or functional visual loss. Amblyopia may produce a subtle APD.

Anisocoria

Lesions of the parasympathetic or sympathetic system cause pupillary constriction or dilation and produce pupils that are unequal in size, anisocoria, if unilateral or asymmetric. Pupillary involvement in third nerve palsy is usually accompanied by ptosis and disturbances in ocular motility. In cases of brainstem herniation and basilar meningitis, however, pupillary dilation may be the only sign of the third nerve palsy. Pharmacologic mydriasis may occur with minimal exposure to atropine, cyclopentolate, or other parasympatholytic agents. Pharmacologic miosis occurs with echothiophate iodide or pilocarpine. Pharmacologic testing with 1% pilocarpine is useful for differentiating pharmacologic mydriasis from third cranial nerve palsy; pupillary constriction occurs in third nerve palsy and does not occur with pharmacologic mydriasis.

A lesion at any point along the sympathetic pathway for pupillary constriction results in Horner syndrome. The classic triad of findings includes ptosis, miosis, and anhidrosis. The anisocoria of Horner syndrome is more apparent in dim illumination, and the affected pupil shows a lag in dilation on dimming of the lights. The light and near pupillary reactions are intact. Paresis of Müller muscle of the lid leads to the mild upper lid ptosis. The lower eyelid on the affected side may rest 1 mm higher than the fellow lid, and the narrowed palpebral fissure gives the appearance of enophthalmos (Fig. 19-72). Anhidrosis of the ipsilateral side of the body, side of the face, or forehead may be present depending on the site of the innervation defect. A characteristic of congenital Horner syndrome is the development of iris heterochromia with the affected iris being lighter in color.

The sympathetic pathway for pupillary constriction involves three neurons. The location of first-order neuron lesions is in the brainstem and spinal cord, examples being cervical trauma or demyelinating disease. Preganglionic or second-order neuron lesions occur within the chest or neck (e.g., neuroblastoma arising in the sympathetic chain). Congenital Horner syndrome caused by birth trauma to the brachial plexus is another cause for a second-order neuron lesion. Third-order neuron lesions, postganglionic in reference to the superior cervical ganglion, are usually benign; however, extracranial or intracranial tumors of the nasopharynx or cavernous sinus may produce such lesions. More common causes for a postganglionic Horner syndrome are migraine variants such as cluster headache.

Physiologic Anisocoria

Approximately 20% of the population has a perceptible anisocoria. The degree of anisocoria may vary from day to day, but usually the difference in pupil size is 1 mm or less. The magnitude of anisocoria remains the same in bright or dim illumination; however, in some cases the anisocoria may be more apparent in dim light than in bright light, thereby simulating Horner syndrome. Differentiating physiologic anisocoria from Horner syndrome may be difficult. In physiologic anisocoria, there is no dilation lag. Pupils with physiologic anisocoria

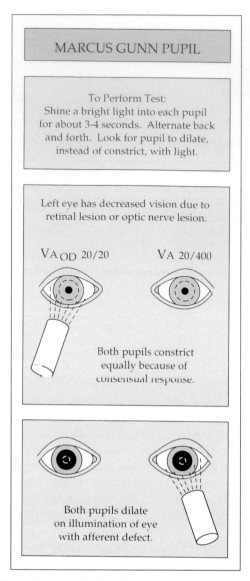

MARCUS GUNN PUPIL

To Perform Test:
Shine a bright light into each pupil for about 3-4 seconds. Alternate back and forth. Look for pupil to dilate, instead of constrict, with light.

Left eye has decreased vision due to retinal lesion or optic nerve lesion.

VA OD 20/20   VA 20/400

Both pupils constrict equally because of consensual response.

Both pupils dilate on illumination of eye with afferent defect.

FIG. 19-104 Swinging flashlight test.

dilate after the instillation of 4% cocaine, whereas a Horner pupil will fail to dilate.

Optic Neuritis

Inflammation of the optic nerve may occur either as a papillitis, referring to the intraocular form in which optic disc swelling is present, or as a retrobulbar neuritis, in which the optic disc appears normal and inflammation of the optic nerve occurs posterior to the globe. Vision loss may be sudden, profound, and accompanied by complaints of pain in or behind the eye, which may be accentuated by movement of the eyes. An afferent pupillary defect is present if the condition is unilateral or if it is bilateral and asymmetric. Visual fields usually show a cecocentral scotoma, an area of vision loss located in the central visual field.

The optic disc, if affected, may show swelling of the peripapillary nerve fiber layer and elevation. Small vessels at the optic disc margin may hemorrhage or become obscured by edema.

Optic neuritis in children is frequently bilateral and usually follows mumps, measles, chicken pox, or meningoencephalitis. Collagen vascular disease, particularly systemic lupus erythematosus (SLE) and sarcoidosis, may be associated with optic neuritis. Syphilis and tuberculosis also cause optic neuritis. Visual acuity gradually improves 1 to 4 weeks after onset and usually returns to normal over several months.

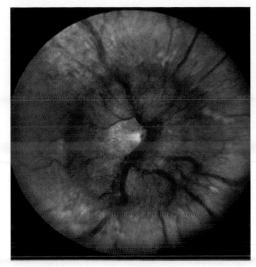

FIG. 19-105 Acute papilledema, characterized by blurred disc edges, an absent physiologic cup, and intraretinal exudates.

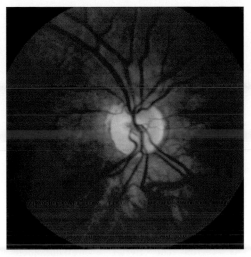

FIG. 19-106 Optic atrophy, characterized by a sharply demarcated, pale yellowish-white disc, with an absence of small vessels and disc substance.

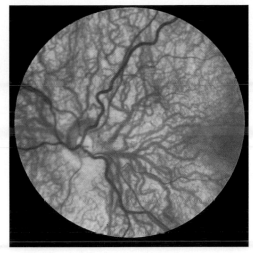

FIG. 19-107 Optic nerve hypoplasia. A pigment crescent surrounds the hypoplastic nerve. This corresponds to the scleral opening for a normal sized optic nerve and is termed the *double ring sign*. In this patient the pattern of the retinal vasculature also is abnormal, as is the retinal pigmentation.

Papilledema

Increased intracranial pressure (ICP) is transmitted to the optic nerves via the cerebrospinal fluid and subarachnoid space and causes papilledema. The axoplasmic flow from the retinal ganglion cells to the cells in the lateral geniculate nucleus is blocked and causes the optic disc to swell. The degree of disc swelling may be asymmetric; however, increased intracranial pressure rarely causes papilledema in only one eye. Ophthalmoscopic signs include blurring of the disc margin and disc edema. The disc may be hyperemic because of telangiectasia of the superficial capillaries on the disc, and small hemorrhages may appear on the disc margin (Fig. 19-105). Visual acuity is normal unless hemorrhage and edema involve the macula. Patients complain of transient obscurations of vision. The visual fields may show an enlarged blind spot, and the pupillary response and color vision are normal.

If papilledema is chronic, elevation of the optic disc may persist but the hemorrhages and exudates seen in the acute phase resolve. When the condition is prolonged, optic nerve atrophy occurs.

Pseudopapilledema

Pseudopapilledema occurs in eyes with high hyperopia or optic disc drusen (Fig. 19-9). The disc is not hyperemic, the vessels of the disc margin remain visible, and there is no nerve fiber layer swelling. There may be anomalous branching and tortuosity of the retinal vessels, and the physiologic cup is usually absent. The disc borders may be irregular. Hemorrhages, exudate, cotton-wool spots, and venous congestion do not occur. Spontaneous venous pulsations are not present in 20% of the normal population. If they are present, they are an indication that the disc swelling is pseudopapilledema and not caused by increased intracranial pressure. Central visual acuity is normal.

Optic Disc Atrophy

Optic nerve atrophy causes the optic disc to lose its reddish-orange color. The lamina cribrosa may become visible with enlargement of the optic cup, leaving a "pinholed" appearance (Fig. 19-106). As the disease process continues, the disc eventually becomes white in color, visual acuity decreases, and visual field defects emerge.

Optic atrophy may occur as a sequela of papilledema, optic neuritis, compressive lesions of the optic nerve or chiasm, trauma, hereditary retinal disease, or glaucoma. Optic atrophy may also be inherited as a recessive or dominant trait. Atrophy may occur as a component of a generalized neurologic condition, such as Behr optic atrophy with cerebellar ataxia, hypotonia, and mental retardation. Leber optic atrophy occurs in late adolescence or early adulthood, with acute disc edema being rapidly followed by progressive bilateral optic atrophy.

Developmental Anomalies of the Optic Nerve

Developmental anomalies of the optic nerve include colobomas, tilted discs, and optic nerve hypoplasia (Figs. 19-9 and 19-84). The level of visual acuity is related to the type and extent of the defect.

Hypoplasia of the optic nerve occurs either unilaterally or bilaterally. The optic disc is smaller than normal and will have a yellowish-white ring that corresponds to the scleral opening for a normal-sized optic nerve. The term *double ring sign* is used to describe the ring with its surrounding pigment crescent. The retinal vessels are normal in size but may appear crowded as they leave the optic disc (Fig. 19-107). Visual acuity is related to the degree of hypoplasia, and an afferent pupillary defect may be present if the degree of involvement is asymmetric. Optic nerve hypoplasia is associated with midline central nervous system abnormalities, including absence of the septum pellucidum (de Morsier syndrome). Children with optic nerve hypoplasia should be examined for abnormalities in pituitary and hypothalamic function.

Orbit

Clinical signs of orbital disease are proptosis and restriction in ocular motility, compression of the optic nerve, optic disc swelling,

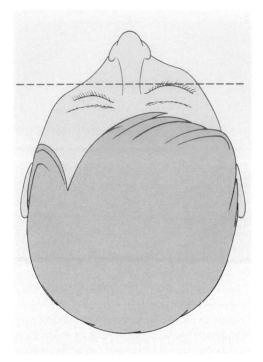

FIG. 19-108 Blowout fracture of inferior orbital wall and dislocation of zygoma (*left side*).

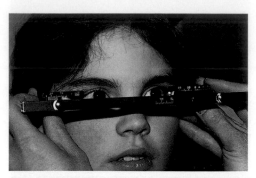

FIG. 19-109 The Hertel exophthalmometer measures the anterior to posterior distance from the corneal surface to the lateral orbital rim. A base measurement, the distance between the two lateral orbital rims, is recorded to ensure repeatable instrument placement. Progression or regression can be determined to ensure reportable instrument placement by comparable serial measurements.

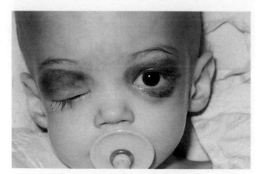

FIG. 19-110 Neuroblastoma. Neuroblastoma metastatic to the orbit may present with an abrupt onset of unilateral or bilateral proptosis and ecchymosis of the eyelids. Neuroblastoma is the most common lesion to metastasize to the orbit in childhood.

changes in refraction, and retinal striae. Retinal striae appear as radial lines on the retinal surface and are caused by compression of the posterior portion of the globe.

Orbital disease or trauma may cause orbital asymmetry with displacement of the globe (Fig. 19-108). Posterior (enophthalmos) or anterior (exophthalmos) displacement of the globe in orbital disease may be subtle. Comparison of the position of the globes in relation to the lateral orbital rims, looking especially for asymmetry, is a valuable clinical test. The Hertel exophthalmometer is an instrument used to compare the position of the globes in relation to the lateral orbital rim (Fig. 19-109). Palpation of the globes over closed eyelids, gently retropulsing the globe into the orbit, may reveal the character of an orbital mass. Ocular rotations are tested looking for restrictions in motility. Other adjuncts to the clinical examination include A and B scan ultrasonography, computed tomography, and magnetic resonance imaging of the orbit.

The most common orbital disease in childhood is cellulitis (see Chapter 22). Capillary hemangioma and lymphangioma are the most common benign primary orbital tumors of childhood. Orbital capillary hemangiomas present shortly after birth, enlarge over the first 6 months of life, and then begin to regress. Lymphangiomas may involve the conjunctiva, lids, or orbit. These tumors may rapidly enlarge during upper respiratory tract infections. Sudden enlargement may occur after hemorrhage within the lesion.

Rhabdomyosarcoma is the most common primary orbital malignancy in childhood. This tumor should be a consideration in any child between the ages of 7 and 8 years who has rapidly progressing unilateral proptosis. The tumor mass may be palpable in the upper eyelid area, or it may be located deeper in the orbit.

The most common metastatic lesion to the orbit in childhood is neuroblastoma. This tumor presents with an abrupt onset of proptosis and ecchymosis that may be bilateral (Fig. 19-110). Metastasis in neuroblastoma typically occurs late in the course of the disease when the primary tumor can easily be detected in the abdomen.

Dermoid and epidermoid cysts are relatively common. These benign masses are usually located anterior to the orbital septum but may extend posteriorly into the orbit. These cysts present as smooth, painless, freely movable round or oval masses and are usually located in the lateral brow area, adjacent to the zygomaticofrontal suture (Fig. 19-111). They may, however, be found near any bony suture. These cysts contain dermal and epidermal elements that have become isolated from the skin during the course of embryonic development. If ruptured by trauma, an intense inflammatory reaction occurs.

Optic nerve gliomas are tumors that occur in children younger than 10 years of age. One third of children have a history of neurofibromatosis. The presenting sign may be loss of vision or painless proptosis. An afferent pupillary defect and optic atrophy are usually present. Papilledema may also occur. Strabismus may be present because of decreased visual acuity (Fig. 19-112).

Plexiform neurofibromas are also seen in association with neurofibromatosis. They occur within the orbit or within the upper lid tissue. This will cause a fullness and ptosis of the lateral portion of the eyelid, causing an "S-shaped" upper lid deformity.

Orbital pseudotumor is a unilateral or bilateral orbital inflammatory process affecting the structures within the orbit. Children with pseudotumor have signs of headache, fever, lethargy, orbital pain, proptosis, lid erythema, conjunctival injection, and restricted ocular motility causing diplopia. The extraocular muscles and their tendons may be thickened. Orbital pseudotumor is a benign condition; however, recurrent tumor with scarring and fibrosis may cause restriction of ocular motility and optic nerve atrophy. Orbital pseudotumor must be differentiated from leukemia. The most common form of leukemia that affects the orbit is acute lymphoblastic leukemia.

Ocular Trauma

In the evaluation of children with orbital or periocular trauma, serious ocular injury must be presumed even if only minimal external signs exist. Before any evaluation or manipulation of the patient, an assessment of visual acuity must be performed. This provides information regarding the severity and nature of the trauma, as well as records data that may be of medicolegal importance.

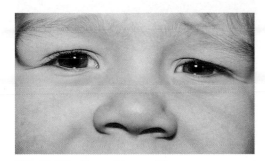

FIG. 19-111 Dermoid cyst. These cysts present as smooth, painless, mobile, subcutaneous, round or oval masses. Dermoid cysts are most frequently located in the lateral brow area adjacent to the zygomaticofrontal suture. Although benign, if they are ruptured by trauma, an intense inflammatory reaction with scarring in the area may occur.

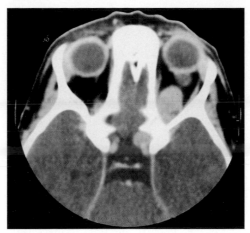

FIG. 19-112 Optic nerve glioma. Its presence may cause a gradual onset of painless proptosis. Children seldom complain of monocular visual loss, and the discovery of a profound loss of vision may be the presenting sign of an optic nerve glioma. In children, optic nerve gliomas are benign lesions that may, however, extend to the optic chiasm or intracranially.

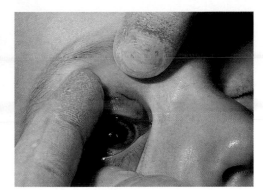

FIG. 19-113 Canalicular laceration. This patient experienced a laceration of the upper canaliculus. Simple apposition of the wound edges in this case will not approximate the cut ends of the canaliculus. Silastic tubes are used to splint the canaliculus during the healing process.

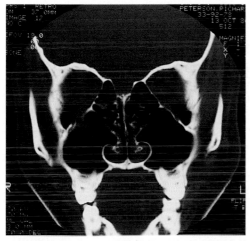

FIG. 19-114 Blowout fracture of the right orbit (coronal CT scan). Protruding through the fracture in the orbital floor into the maxillary sinus is orbital fat. The inferior rectus muscle is potentially entrapped within the fracture site.

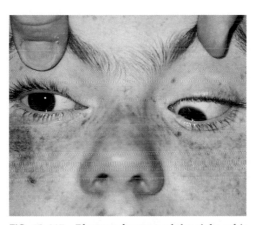

FIG. 19-115 Blowout fracture of the right orbit leading to the inability to depress the right eye.

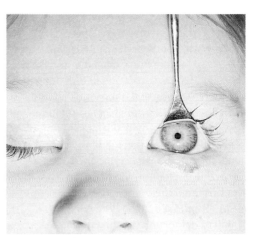

FIG. 19-116 A Desmarres lid retractor may be used to gently open the eyelids of an uncooperative child or in cases of trauma or preseptal cellulitis in which lid swelling makes opening of the lids for globe examination difficult.

The anatomy of a laceration of the eyelid dictates the measures required for repair. The presence of orbital fat indicates penetration of the septum and entrance into the orbit. Additionally, evaluation of the laceration must include the degree of involvement of the lid margin, loss of tissue, injury to the medial and lateral canthal tendons, and injury to the canaliculi of the nasolacrimal drainage system (Fig. 19-113). Each of the above injuries requires a special technique for repair.

Patients who have sustained blunt orbital trauma should be evaluated for a fracture of the orbital floor or the medial wall of the orbit. Signs of a fracture with entrapment of one of the extraocular muscles include enophthalmos, diplopia, restricted gaze, and paresthesias in the distribution of the infraorbital nerve. Fractures may be isolated to the floor, or they may extend to the orbital rim (Fig. 19-114). If subcutaneous air or orbital emphysema is present, the fracture has permitted communication with the sinuses. Intraorbital edema or hemorrhage within extraocular muscle may also restrict ocular motility. The most commonly involved muscles are the inferior and medial rectus muscles (Fig. 19-115).

Conjunctival lacerations may appear greatly disproportionate to their degree of severity. On the other hand, a small penetration of the conjunctiva may be hidden beneath a penetrating injury to the globe.

The use of a topical anesthetic such as tetracaine or proparacaine anesthetizes the cornea and permits a close examination of the cornea and surrounding conjunctiva for foreign bodies. A Desmarres lid retractor may help exert gentle pressure to open the lids of uncooperative children or if swelling of the lids makes examination difficult (Fig. 19-116).

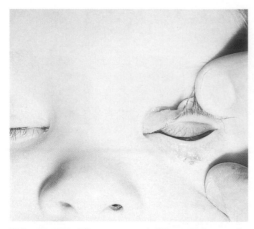

FIG. 19-117 The upper eyelid may be easily everted by placing a cotton swab at the upper edge of the tarsal plate. The lashes are then gently grasped and pulled anteriorly and upward to evert the lid over the cotton swab. The tarsal conjunctiva may be inspected for the presence of a foreign body.

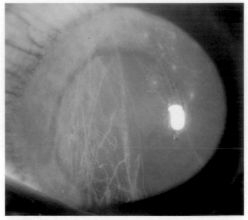

FIG. 19-118 Corneal abrasions stained with fluorescein dye and viewed under blue light. The abrasions appear green in the area of corneal epithelial loss.

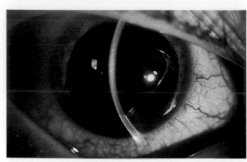

FIG. 19-119 Hyphema. Red blood cells within the anterior chamber have settled into the inferior anterior chamber angle.

The lids may also be everted over a cotton swab to inspect the underside (Fig. 19-117). The presence of a foreign-body under the upper eyelid causes vertical epithelial abrasions on the underlying corneal surface (Fig. 19-118). Corneal abrasions cause extreme pain and photophobia. The use of sodium fluorescein dye applied to the conjunctival cul-de-sac and examination with a cobalt blue filtered light aid in the detection of a superficial epithelial abrasion. The dye stains areas that are missing epithelium. When possible, examination should be conducted with magnification as provided by a slit lamp or magnifying glass.

Blunt trauma to the eye may cause iritis or an anterior uveitis. Patients complain of dull eye pain and light sensitivity. Signs of iritis include miosis of the pupil, tearing, and ciliary injection. With severe blunt trauma, the iris may be avulsed from its insertion (iridodialysis) or the iris and ciliary body may be avulsed (cyclodialysis). Tears of the pupillary sphincter may also occur and are a sign that further evaluation should be conducted. Eyes that receive blunt trauma may develop traumatic angle recession and glaucoma years after the incident.

An injury to the globe may cause bleeding from the small vessels of the peripheral portion of the iris or the ciliary body. Blood, which is heavier than aqueous fluid, usually settles out in the inferior portion of the eye, causing a hyphema (Fig. 19-119). While the red blood cells are dispersed throughout the aqueous fluid, vision may be dramatically decreased. The blood may remain fluid and shift with changes in head position, or it may clot. Complications after a hyphema include rebleeding, glaucoma, and blood staining of the cornea (Fig. 19-120). In the latter case, concurrent increased intraocular pressure increases the risk of developing blood staining. The opacification of the cornea may resolve over several months. In children, this may cause amblyopia.

Immediate or delayed opacification of the lens may occur with penetration of the lens capsule. Blunt trauma may disrupt the lens zonules and dislocate the lens (Fig. 19-80).

All eyes receiving trauma must have an examination of the fundus. Blunt trauma may cause a macular hole or a rupture of the choroid. A choroidal rupture is visualized as a white concentric ring around the optic disc where the underlying sclera has become visible (Fig. 19-121).

Trauma may produce retinal hemorrhages that are limited to the retina or that extend into the vitreous. Crushing injury to the chest may raise intrathoracic pressure with transmission to the retina causing

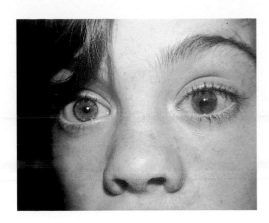

FIG. 19-120 A complication of hyphema is corneal blood staining. This patient's left cornea has an area of brown staining inferiorly because of prolonged presence of blood within the anterior chamber.

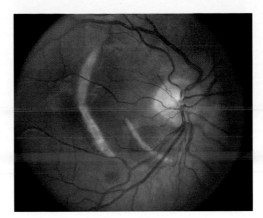

FIG. 19-121 Blunt trauma to the eye has caused a rupture of the choroid. This is visualized as white concentric rings around the optic disc where, beneath the retina, the choroid has separated, making the underlying sclera visible.

hemorrhages. Purtscher retinopathy includes retinal hemorrhages, cotton-wool spots, retinal edema, and fat emboli. Terson syndrome is the transmission of subarachnoid hemorrhage to the optic nerve and disc and results in vitreous and retinal hemorrhages. Infants with shaken baby syndrome may have extensive intraretinal hemorrhages accompanying their intracranial injuries, and the severity of intraocular hemorrhage may correlate with the severity of intracranial injury.

In cases of penetrating injury to the eye, the key to examination is to be brief and gentle so as not to extend the injury by causing expulsion of intraocular contents. Immediately after identifying an ocular injury as penetrating, further examination should be limited and conducted in the operating room under general anesthesia. Topical medications should not be applied to the eye, and the eye should be protected at all times with a shield. Penetrating injuries caused by projectiles or foreign bodies may produce very subtle findings. In cases where the index of suspicion is high, appropriate evaluation may include plain film x-rays or imaging studies including CT or MRI. If the potential intraocular foreign body is metallic, MRI scanning is contraindicated.

BIBLIOGRAPHY

Diamond G, Eggers H: Strabismus and pediatric ophthalmology. In Podos S, Yanoff M, eds: *Textbook of ophthalmology*, vol 5, St Louis, 1994, Mosby.

Fraunfelder FT, Roy FH: *Current ocular therapy*, ed 4, Philadelphia, 1995, WB Saunders.

Helveston EM, Ellis FD: *Pediatric ophthalmology practice*, ed 2, St Louis, 1989, Mosby.

Isenberg SJ: *The eye in infancy*, ed 2, St Louis, 1993, Mosby.

Miller NR: *Clinical neurophthalmology*, ed 4, Baltimore, 1985, Williams & Wilkins.

Nelson LB, Calhoun JH, Harley RD: *Pediatric ophthalmology*, ed 3, Philadelphia, 1991, WB Saunders.

Renie WA: *Goldberg's genetic and metabolic eye disease*, ed 2, Boston, 1986, Little, Brown.

Tasman W, Jaeger EA: *Duane's clinical ophthalmology*, Philadelphia, 1996, JB Lippincott.

Taylor D, ed: *Pediatric ophthalmology*, Boston, 1990, Blackwell Scientific Publications.

von Noorden GK: *Binocular vision and ocular motility: theory and management of strabismus*, ed 5, St Louis, 1996, Mosby.

Yanoff M, Fine BS: *Ocular pathology*, ed 3, Philadelphia, 1989, JB Lippincott.

20

Oral Disorders

MAMOUN M. NAZIF ❦ HOLLY W. DAVIS

DAVID H. MCKIBBEN ❦ MARY ANN READY

Assessment Technique

Because oral and oropharyngeal problems and disorders are common and cause a wide variety of symptoms, a thorough oral examination is an essential component of a complete physical examination, enabling the practitioner to make appropriate diagnoses without undue delay.

Key elements of the oral/dental history include the following:

1. Timing of eruption and exfoliation of primary teeth, timing of eruption of permanent teeth, and any problems encountered
2. Brushing and flossing frequency and technique
3. Dietary habits, including frequency of bottle and breastfeeding in infancy; whether infants and toddlers are put to bed with a bottle; time of weaning; frequency of carbohydrate intake; and possible symptoms of eating disorders in adolescence
4. Current source of dental care and frequency of visits
5. Current history of symptoms: oral pain, redness, swelling, drainage, headaches, abdominal pain, decreased appetite (especially for chewy foods)
6. Problems with bite or occlusion
7. History of dental problems and/or orofacial trauma and their treatment
8. Family history of dental problems or disorders

A systematic approach to the examination of a child's dentition is essential and should include assessment of the following:

1. Facial symmetry and balance
2. Lip seal at rest position
3. Occlusion (bite) and tooth alignment
4. Mandibular excursion in lateral, vertical, and anterior/posterior planes
5. Integrity of enamel, presence of caries
6. Appearance of gingivae from both labial-buccal and lingual sides
7. Condition of the other oral soft tissues: tongue, palate, mucobuccal folds, and sublingual spaces

Successful examination requires close visual inspection of the face; palpation of suspected areas of abnormality, and systematic inspection of the dentition, its supporting structures, and the oral soft tissues. This can be challenging with young children, but patience and a gentle, even playful manner can be of great help. At least initially, young children should be allowed to sit on the parent's lap. Toys, puppets, and a rubber glove blown up into a balloon can serve as useful distractions. Drawing a face

on a tongue depressor and giving it to the child to hold, and letting him look at himself in the dental mirror are good ways to introduce these basic instruments and make them less threatening (Fig. 20-1, A and B). If an otoscope is being used as a light source in a medical office setting, letting the child blow it out is another good introductory game, as is demonstrating the examination on the parent or examiner. Then the examiner can gradually begin the hands-on assessment. If cooperation cannot be achieved despite these measures, immobilization in a papoose board may be necessary. With older children, examination of the patient in the supine or semi-recumbent position with good lighting facilitates visualization and may be more practical.

Use of a tongue depressor is necessary to ensure direct visual access to all intraoral areas, and a dental mirror can be quite helpful, especially in assessing the lingual surfaces of the anterior teeth and gingivae and the buccal surfaces of rear molars (Fig. 20-1, C). Extra effort and patience may be required to ensure that the mucobuccal folds, sublingual space, lingual surface of the anterior teeth, and anterior palate are adequately visualized.

The special aspects of the history and physical assessment of dental and orofacial trauma are detailed in the trauma section of this chapter.

Normal Oral Structures

The oral cavity, including the teeth, gingivae, and periodontal ligaments, is in a constant state of evolution during infancy and childhood. From the early teething stage, through the eruption and exfoliation of the primary dentition, and finally to the eruption of all permanent teeth, the oral cavity provides one of the most visible signs of development.

To facilitate understanding of this chapter and communication when consulting dentists, a review of basic terminology is in order. Each tooth is composed of an outer protective enamel layer; an inner layer of dentin consisting of tubules, which are thought to serve a nutritional function; and a central neurovascular core termed the *pulp*. The roots of the teeth are anchored in the sockets of the alveolar processes of the mandible and maxilla by an encompassing periodontal membrane or ligament. The neurovascular supply to the root apex also passes through this structure. The bony processes between the teeth are referred to as the *interdental septae* (Fig. 20-2).

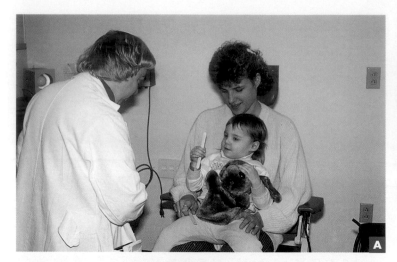

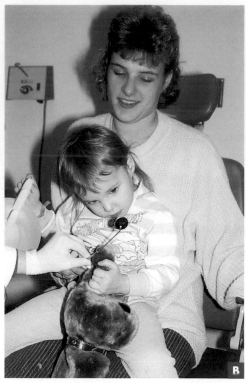

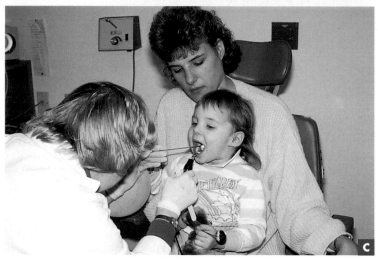

FIG. 20-1   Oral examination of a toddler. *A* and *B,* Use of toys and puppets as distractors, introduction of nonthreatening instruments by drawing a face on the tongue depressor, and letting the child look at herself in the dental mirror facilitate cooperation. *C,* The dental mirror is very useful for visualizing the lingual surfaces of the anterior dentition and gingivae and the buccal surfaces of rear molars.

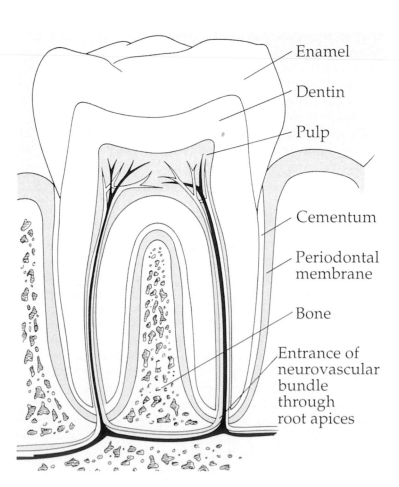

— Enamel

— Dentin

— Pulp

— Cementum

— Periodontal membrane

— Bone

— Entrance of neurovascular bundle through root apices

After eruption, the visible portions of teeth are referred to as the *crowns,* and the interface between them and the gingivae is termed the *gingival crevice.* Finally, the portions of the gingivae located between teeth are called *interdental papillae.*

Oral Cavity in the Newborn

The lips of an infant reveal a prominent line of demarcation at the vermilion border. The mucosa may look wrinkled and slightly purple at birth, but within a few days it exhibits a dryer appearance, with the outer layer forming crusty "sucking calluses." This callus formation affects the central portion of the mucosa and persists for only a few weeks.

The maxillary alveolar arch is separated from the lip by a shallow sulcus. In the midline the labial frenulum extends posteriorly across the alveolar ridge to the palatine incisive papilla. Two lateral miniature frenulae are also evident. The alveolar ridge peaks anteriorly and gradually flattens as the ridge extends posteriorly, forming a pseudoalveolar groove medial to the ridge along its palatal side. This flattened appearance is seen in young infants and gradually disappears with the growth of the alveolar process and the formation and calcification of posterior tooth buds. The mandibular alveolar ridges also peak anteri-

FIG. 20-2   Diagrammatic representation of a molar shows the enamel, dentin, and pulp; the periodontal membrane; the entrance of the neurovascular bundle through the root apices; and the bony supporting structures.

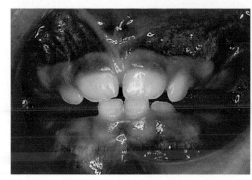

FIG. 20-3 Early primary dentition. The mandibular and maxillary central and lateral incisors are the first to erupt.

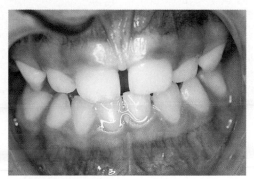

FIG. 20-4 Full primary dentition. By age 3, all 20 primary teeth have erupted.

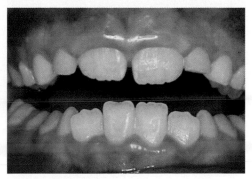

FIG. 20-5 Mixed dentition. This transitional stage from primary to permanent dentition begins at age 6 and lasts for about 6 years.

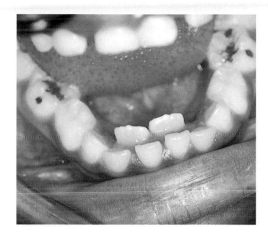

FIG. 20-6 Abnormal eruption patterns frequently occur in the early mixed dentition phase. One example is shown here, with the eruption of the permanent central incisors behind the primary teeth.

orly and flatten posteriorly. The mandibular labial frenulum connects the lower lip to the labial aspect of the alveolar ridge. Careful visual inspection and palpation of the ridges should confirm the presence and location of tooth buds. Anterior tooth buds are located on the labial side of the alveolar ridges, whereas posterior tooth buds are often located closer to the crests of the alveolar ridges. Palatal morphology and color are variable. The tongue and the floor of the mouth differ only slightly from those of older children.

Primary Dentition

Development of the alveolar bone is directly related to the formation and eruption of teeth, and normal patterns of dental development occur symmetrically. At approximately 6 months of age, the mandibular central incisors erupt. This stage is often preceded by a period of increased salivation, local gingival irritation, and irritability. These symptoms may vary in intensity, but they respond well to oral analgesics and usually subside when the last primary tooth erupts into the oral cavity. Other symptoms such as fever or diarrhea have never been proven to be directly related to teething. The lower incisors are soon followed by the maxillary central incisors and the maxillary and mandibular lateral incisors (Fig. 20-3). By the end of the first year, all eight anterior teeth are usually visible. At 2 years, all primary teeth have erupted with the exception of the second primary molars, which erupt shortly thereafter. By the age of 3 years, the primary dentition is fully present and functional (Fig. 20-4).

Any variation in the time and sequence of eruption in an otherwise normal infant may call for early dental referral. In most instances, care-

ful observation is the best course of action. For example, delayed eruption of primary teeth for up to 8 months is occasionally observed and is considered a normal variation. Rarely, retarded eruption is associated with Down syndrome, hypothyroidism, hypopituitarism, achondroplastic dwarfism, osteopetrosis, rickets, or chondroectodermal dysplasia. A significant variation affecting a single tooth or only a few teeth should be carefully investigated as well.

Spacing (extra space between teeth) during this stage is normal and desirable and often indicates that more space is available for the larger permanent teeth. The completed primary dentition establishes a baseline that dictates to a great extent the future alignment of permanent teeth and the future relationship between the maxillary and mandibular arches.

During most of the primary dentition stage, the gingiva appears pink, firm, and not readily retractable. A well-defined zone of firmly attached keratinized gingiva is present, extending from the bottom of the gingival sulcus to the junction of the alveolar mucosa. Rarely, local irritation may develop into acute or subacute pericoronitis, with elevated temperature and associated lymphadenopathy (Fig. 20-50). Topical and/or systemic therapy may be required for treatment; however, lancing the gingiva to relieve such symptoms is not usually indicated.

Mixed Dentition

This stage of development begins with the eruption of the first permanent molars at about 6 years of age and continues for approximately 6 years. During this period, the following teeth erupt from the gums in this sequence: mandibular central incisors, maxillary central incisors, mandibular lateral incisors, maxillary lateral incisors, mandibular cuspids, maxillary and mandibular first premolars, maxillary and mandibular second premolars, maxillary cuspids, and mandibular and maxillary second molars (Fig. 20-5).

The mixed dentition during this stage undergoes certain physiologic changes, including root resorption followed by exfoliation of primary teeth, eruption of their successors, and eruption of the posterior permanent teeth. During the period of root resorption of primary teeth, and for several months after the eruption of permanent teeth, these teeth are relatively loosely imbedded in the alveolar bone and more vulnerable to displacement with trauma. Other minor complications may occur during resorption and exfoliation of primary teeth and eruption of permanent teeth. Gingival irritation can occur as a result of increased mobility of primary teeth but usually disappears spontaneously when the tooth is lost or extracted. Two transient deviations of eruption pattern may occur: the mandibular incisors may erupt in a lingual position behind the primary incisors ("double teeth") (Fig. 20-6), and the max-

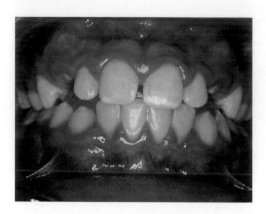

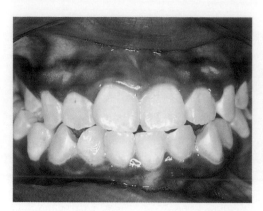

FIG. 20-7 The earliest stage of permanent dentition begins with the eruption of the 6-year molars and central incisors. The cuspids and second molars are the last to erupt.

FIG. 20-8 Gingivitis during puberty. The gingival tissues are mildly erythematous and edematous, and they tend to bleed easily with brushing. Hormonal changes and inattention to careful dental hygiene are thought to be contributory.

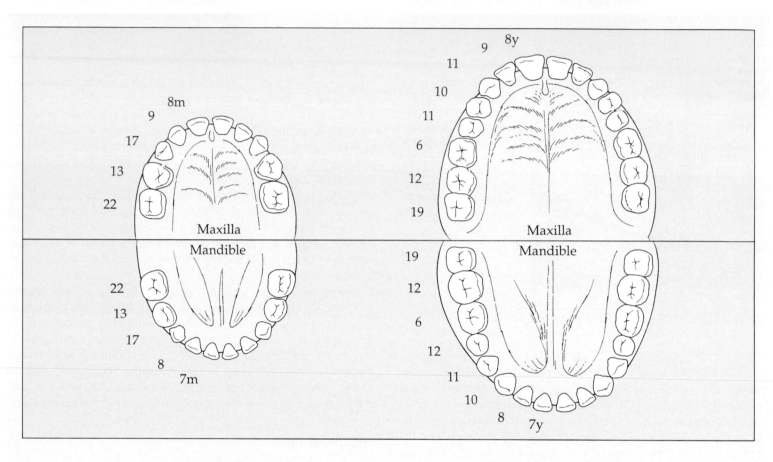

A. Primary Dentition

B. Permanent Dentition

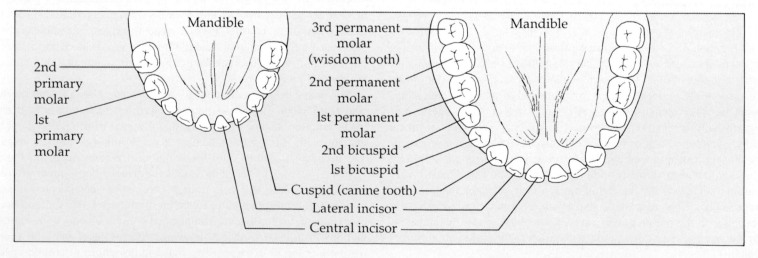

C. Primary Dentition

D. Permanent Dentition

FIG. 20-9 Artist's illustrations of the primary and permanent dentition. *A* and *B,* The numbers represent the average age of eruption for the teeth, indicated in months for the primary teeth and years for the permanent dentition. *C* and *D,* The names of specific teeth in the primary and permanent dentition are shown.

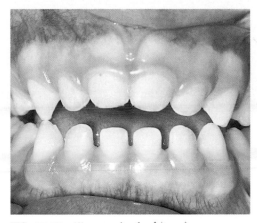

FIG. 20-10 Changes in the bite often occur as the result of prolonged digit sucking. This child's upper arch has been narrowed and an anterior open-bite is developing.

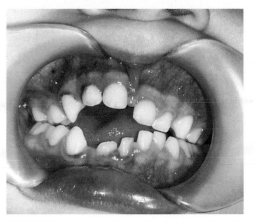

FIG. 20-11 A 2-year-old with a prolonged pacifier-sucking habit has severe deformity of the alveolar arches and teeth caused by the extrinsic force of the pacifier-sucking action.

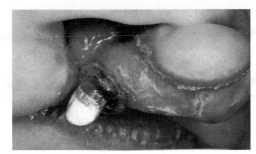

FIG. 20-12 A natal tooth associated with cleft palate. Extraction is necessary only if it is of abnormal morphology or causes feeding difficulties.

illary incisors may assume a widely spaced and labially inclined position ("ugly duckling" stage). Finally, the occlusal surfaces of newly erupted permanent teeth are relatively "rough" (Figs. 20-5 and 20-43), facilitating plaque accumulation that increases the risk of staining, gingivitis, and possibly formation of caries.

Early Permanent Dentition

This stage marks the beginning of a relatively quiescent period in dental development. Activities are limited to root formation of a few permanent teeth and the calcification of the third molars. By this time the length and width of the dental arches are well established (Fig. 20-7); however, the jaws undergo a major growth spurt during puberty that alters their size and relative position. The gingiva begins to assume adult characteristics, becoming firm, pink in color, with an uneven, stippled surface texture and a thin gingival margin. Puberty is occasionally associated with gingivitis, thought secondary in part to hormonal changes (Fig. 20-8). The gingivae become mildly edematous and erythematous and bleed with brushing (the common chief complaint). Inattention to careful dental hygiene also may contribute to development of this disorder, which necessitates good oral hygiene for control.

In Fig. 20-9 the primary and permanent dentition are presented diagrammatically.

Harmful Oral Habits

Children often develop sucking habits, using the thumb, finger(s), or objects. Thumb and finger sucking begins antenatally and is considered a normal behavior pattern. However, if the habit persists beyond the late primary dentition stage of dental arch development (5 years), the extrinsic forces applied by the sucking action can produce pathologic changes in the child's normal arch growth. These deviations range from minor, reversible changes to gross malformations in the dental arches that produce significant anterior open-bites and/or posterior cross bites. The degree of change depends on the duration, frequency, and intensity of the sucking habit (Fig. 20-10).

Bottle and Pacifier Habits

The forces produced by prolonged use of bottles and pacifiers can first cause dental malocclusions and may, if the habit persists, worsen the resulting deformity with the involvement of adjacent jaw structures. Usually, if the child is weaned from the bottle and pacifier by the age of 18 months, no permanent changes in bite development can be expected. The longer any force is applied, the greater the risk that the distortion in the dental arches and adjacent bony structures will not self-correct (Fig. 20-11).

Thus, the use of bottles and pacifiers should be discouraged by the age of 18 months. After this age, changes in the oral structures have been noted and are more likely to be permanent. Counseling parents during the neonatal period not to put their infants to bed with a bottle, but rather to hold them during all feedings, is probably one of the best ways to prevent later difficulties with weaning. Such practices also prevent the development of nursing-bottle caries.

Therapy

Clinical management of harmful oral habits should be customized to the child's age. Obviously, harsh measures to discourage digit sucking in a 2-year-old are not justified and may be counterproductive. Children who receive frequent criticism for thumb sucking are probably more likely to cling to the habit than are those whose families ignore it. However, when the habit persists beyond a reasonable age, calm discussions with the child concerning feelings related to the sucking and the physical damage possible if it continues, often produce the desired results. When a child has expressed a strong will to cease sucking but is unable to accomplish this goal without help, appliance therapy by a dental professional may be indicated. Referral for oral evaluation and consultation is appropriate after the child has passed the appropriate age of the behavior pattern involved, for example, over 5 years of age for digit sucking habits or 18 months for pacifiers.

Natal and Neonatal Abnormalities

Teeth

Teeth present in the oral cavity at birth are called *natal teeth,* whereas those erupting during the neonatal period are called *neonatal teeth.* The incidence of natal teeth has been reported to be approximately 1 in 2000 births. Though seen in normal infants, this anomaly is more frequent in patients with cleft palate (Fig. 20-12), and is often associated with the following syndromes: Ellis-van Creveld, Hallermann-

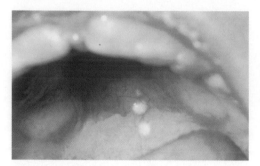

FIG. 20-13 Gingival cysts. The small, whitish cystic lesions along the midpalatine raphe are called *Epstein pearls*.

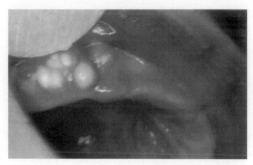

FIG. 20-14 Gingival cysts. The firm, grayish-white mucous gland cysts on the buccal aspect of the alveolar ridges are called *Bohn nodules*.

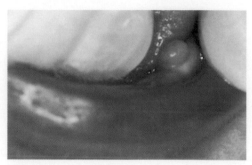

FIG. 20-15 Dental lamina cyst. These cysts are found on the alveolar ridge and usually occur singly.

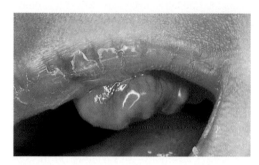

FIG. 20-16 Congenital epulis. This 4-day-old patient has a benign tumor of the anterior maxilla.

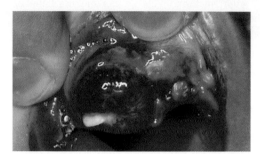

FIG. 20-17 Melanotic neuroectodermal tumor. This benign but locally aggressive tumor of the anterior maxilla has produced elevation of the lip and displaced a primary tooth.

Streiff, and pachyonychia congenita. The majority of such teeth are true primary teeth, but occasionally they are supernumerary. Some are abnormal, with either hypoplastic defects or poor crown or root development. Natal teeth may cause feeding problems for both the infant and mother. Ulceration of the ventral surface of the tongue by sharp tooth edges (Riga-Fede disease) may develop if natal teeth remain in the oral cavity. This condition is usually transient, but in persistent cases symptomatic treatment or extraction of such teeth may be indicated. Most normal-appearing natal teeth can be retained, but those that are supernumerary, abnormal, or very loose may have to be removed.

Gingival Cysts in the Newborn

Gingival cysts of the oral cavity are small, single or multiple superficial lesions that are formed by tissues trapped during embryologic growth and occur in about 80% of newborns. They are asymptomatic, do not enlarge, seldom interfere with feeding, and usually exfoliate within a few weeks.

Three types of cysts exist.

1. Epstein pearls are keratin-filled cystic lesions lined with stratified squamous epithelium. They appear as small, whitish lesions along the midpalatine raphe and contain no mucous glands (Fig. 20-13).
2. Bohn nodules are mucous gland cysts, often found on the buccal or lingual aspects of the alveolar ridges and occasionally on the palate. They are multiple, firm, and grayish-white in appearance. Histologically they show mucous glands and ducts (Fig. 20-14).
3. Dental lamina cysts are found only on the crest of the alveolar mucosa. Histologically these lesions are different because they are formed by remnants of dental lamina epithelium. They may be larger, more lucent, and fluctuant than Epstein pearls or Bohn nodules and are more likely to occur singly (Fig. 20-15).

Congenital Epulis in the Newborn

This benign, soft-tissue tumor is seen on the alveolar mucosa at birth or shortly after. It is usually found on the anterior maxilla as a pedunculated swelling (Fig. 20-16) but may appear on the mandible or occasionally on both jaws. The mass is firm on palpation, and the overlying mucosa appears normal. Histologically, sheets of large granular cells are seen. Differential diagnosis should include rhabdomyoma and melanotic neuroectodermal tumor of infancy. The lesion is amenable to conservative surgical excision, and recurrence is infrequent.

Melanotic Neuroectodermal Tumor of Infancy

This benign yet aggressive tumor occurs during the first year of life and is often found on the anterior maxilla in association with unerupted or erupted teeth. It often bulges and destroys the alveolar bone, thus displacing the associated primary tooth. The tumor mass is grayish-blue, firm on palpation, and spherical in shape (Fig. 20-17). Careful surgical removal is effective, and recurrence is unusual.

Developmental Abnormalities

Soft-Tissue

Geographic Tongue (Benign Migratory Glossitis)

This painless condition is characterized by inflamed, irregularly shaped areas on the dorsum of the tongue that are devoid of filiform papillae. Lesions are red, slightly depressed, and bordered by a whitish band (Fig. 20-18). Spontaneous healing followed by the formation of similar lesions elsewhere on the tongue results in a migrating appearance. Etiology is unknown; however, strong association with stress and allergies is suspected. Although benign, the course of this disorder may be prolonged for months, and it may recur.

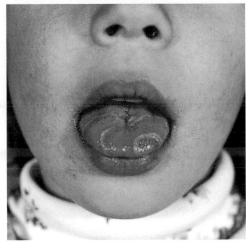

FIG. 20-18 Characteristics of benign migratory glossitis (geographic tongue), which is a chronic and often recurring condition affecting the filiform papillae of the tongue. Lesions are red, slightly depressed, and bordered by a whitish band.

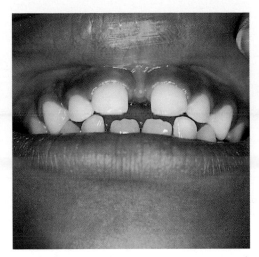

FIG. 20-19 Large diastema (excessive spacing) between the front teeth secondary to an inferiorly positioned maxillary frenum.

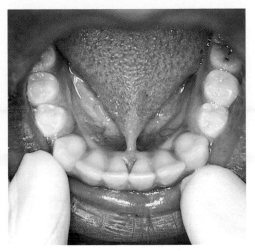

FIG. 20-20 Ankyloglossia. This extremely short lingual frenulum with a high insertion point on the gingival margin is an indication for surgical intervention.

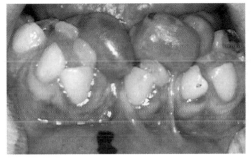

FIG. 20-21 Multiple hyperplastic frenula are seen in this patient with orofaciodigital syndrome. These frenula interfered with the eruption of teeth, causing rotations and crowding.

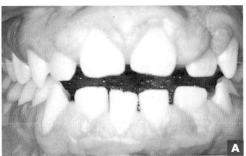
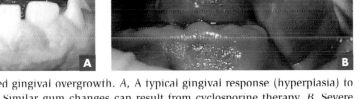

FIG. 20-22 Phenytoin-induced gingival overgrowth. *A,* A typical gingival response (hyperplasia) to chronic phenytoin ingestion. Similar gum changes can result from cyclosporine therapy. *B,* Severe overgrowth. The firm, hyperplastic gingival tissues have completely covered the posterior teeth and are interfering with mastication.

Abnormalities of the Frenula

During embryonic life, the maxillary labial frenulum extends as a band of tissue from the upper lip over and across the alveolar ridge and into the incisive (palatine) papilla. Postnatally, as the alveolar process increases in size, the labial frenulum separates from the incisive papilla and becomes relatively smaller. With the eruption of primary and later permanent teeth, the frenulum attachment moves apically and further atrophies as a result of vertical growth of the alveolar process. The developmental gap (diastema) between the maxillary central incisors tends to close with the full eruption of the maxillary permanent canines. Occasionally the maxillary frenulum fails to atrophy and the diastema persists (Fig. 20-19). The mandibular midline frenulum only rarely maintains a lingual extension and therefore only rarely causes a diastema between the mandibular central incisors.

The lingual frenulum extends almost to the tip of the tongue in early infancy and then gradually recedes. Occasionally, ankyloglossia (tongue tie) is seen (Fig. 20-20), but this is rarely associated with feeding or speech difficulties. Various surgical procedures have been advocated to correct this condition. In general, frenulectomy is seldom indicated and should be recommended only after appropriate justification. Congenital anomalies may include an enlarged frenulum, labiolingual frenulum ex-

tensions, or supernumerary frenula as seen in orofaciodigital syndrome (Fig. 20-21).

Gingival Hyperplasia

Generalized gingival hyperplasia is a fairly common nonspecific pathologic entity. This disorder is frequently a complication of drug therapy as is seen with phenytoin and cyclosporine. Gingival hyperplasia may also be idiopathic or genetically transmitted as in familial fibromatosis. Differentiation of various types of hyperplasia must be based on thorough physical evaluation and appropriate medical history. Histopathologically, it is impossible to differentiate between these various disorders; therefore the final diagnosis and recommendations for therapy should be based on all available clinical data and an appropriate dental consultation.

Phenytoin-Induced Gingival Hyperplasia

The administration of phenytoin over a period of time frequently causes generalized hyperplasia of the gingivae (Fig. 20-22, *A* and *B*). The gingiva may become secondarily inflamed, edematous, and boggy, especially if proper oral hygiene is not practiced. The severity is often related to the degree of local irritation, stemming from poor oral hygiene, mouth breathing, caries, or poor occlusion (alignment). Because

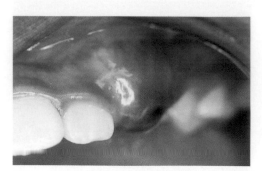

FIG. 20-23 Eruption hematoma. A bluish, fluid-filled, fluctuant swelling can be seen over the crown of an erupting maxillary cuspid. The lesion resolved without treatment when the tooth erupted.

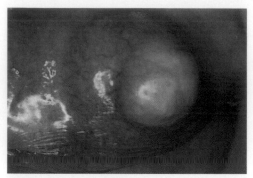

FIG. 20-24 A mucocele on the lower lip with the characteristic translucent coloration secondary to fluid retention.

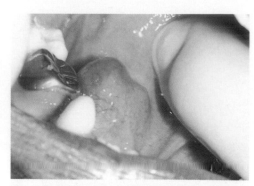

FIG. 20-25 Ranula. The bluish, fluctuant swelling in the floor of the mouth is a retention cyst associated with trauma to a salivary duct.

hyperplasia tends to recur after surgical excision, gingivectomy is usually reserved for those patients whose overgrowth interferes with function and for those whose therapy has been discontinued.

Cyclosporine-Induced Gingival Hyperplasia

Cyclosporine has been used primarily in treating patients after organ transplants. The drug has been demonstrated to directly increase cellular growth of gingival fibroblasts. It also increases the production and retention of collagen. Further, this agent's immunosuppressive action may predispose gingival tissues to invasion by microorganisms, thereby increasing inflammatory changes. Although meticulous oral hygiene reduces inflammation, it has no significant affect on the degree of hyperplasia.

Fibromatosis Gingivae

This rare, genetically determined condition may be clinically evident at birth and in such instances may prevent or slow subsequent dental eruption. The clinical manifestations include the generalized presence of firm fibrous tissue that extends around the crowns of involved teeth. Inflammation, when present, is usually secondary.

Surgical excision of excessive tissues is usually indicated, but recurrence is a distinct possibility.

Idiopathic Gingival Hyperplasia

Different types of patients, often with significant systemic illnesses or syndromes, may manifest generalized gingival enlargements. These may primarily involve the gingival tissues or may sometimes be related to underlying thickening of cortical bone, which causes gingival hyperplasia by impeding dental eruption. Each of these cases must be evaluated individually for possible etiology and appropriate treatment.

Eruption Cysts (Eruption Hematoma)

An eruption cyst is a fluid-filled swelling, nontender in the majority of cases, over the crown of an erupting tooth. When the follicle is dilated with blood, the lesion takes on a bluish color and is termed an *eruption hematoma* (Fig. 20-23). Although the eruption cyst is a superficial form of dentigerous cyst, it rarely impedes eruption, and surgical exposure of the crown is seldom necessary. Very rarely, such a cyst may become secondarily infected. In such cases, patients complain of headache or facial pain, and the cyst is tender on palpation. Incision and drainage are required when infection has developed.

Mucocele and Ranula

A mucocele is a painless, translucent or bluish lesion of traumatic origin, most often involving minor salivary glands of the lower lip (Fig. 20-24). The lesion may alternately enlarge and shrink. The treatment of choice is surgical excision of the lesion and the associated minor salivary gland.

A simple ranula is a retention cyst in the floor of the mouth that is confined to sublingual tissues superior to the mylohyoid muscle. It appears clinically as a bluish, transparent, thin-walled, fluctuant swelling (Fig. 20-25). Herniation of the ranula through the mylohyoid muscle results in a cervical or plunging ranula that becomes more apparent in the oral cavity with the muscle contraction associated with jaw opening. Simple incision and drainage of the ranula is not an acceptable treatment since healing is followed by recurrence. Marsupialization by suturing the edges of the opened cystic wall to the mucous membrane is the recommended treatment. The plunging ranula must be removed in its entirety along with the associated salivary gland to avoid recurrence.

Salivary Calculus (Sialolithiasis)

Formation of a salivary calculus is rare in the pediatric population, but when it does occur it may affect either the Wharton or Stenson duct (Fig. 20-26, *A*). Partial obstruction of the duct results in pain and enlargement of the gland, especially at mealtime. Although palpation of the stone may be possible, dental radiographs confirm the diagnosis and give appropriate information about its size and location (Fig. 20-26, *B*). Larger salivary stones wedged within the ducts may cause localized irritation and secondary infection. If the calculus cannot be manipulated through the duct, surgical intervention may be necessary.

Hard-Tissue

Hyperdontia and Hypodontia

Variations in tooth number include both hyperdontia and hypodontia. Supernumerary teeth occur in about 3% of the normal population, but patients with cleft lip and/or cleft palate and cleidocranial dysostosis have a significantly higher incidence. The most common site is the anterior palate (Fig. 20-27). Supernumerary teeth may have the size and morphology of adjacent teeth or may be small and atypical in shape. They may erupt spontaneously or remain impacted. Early consideration of removal is justified because of complications such as impeded eruption, crowding, or resorption of permanent teeth; cystic changes; or ectopic eruption into the nasal cavity, the maxillary sinus, or other sites (Fig. 20-28).

Congenital absence of teeth is more often seen in the permanent dentition than in the primary. Most frequently missing are third molars,

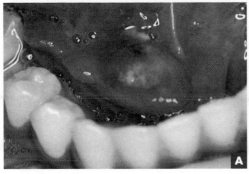

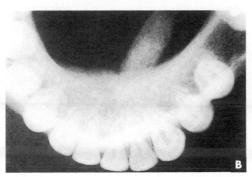

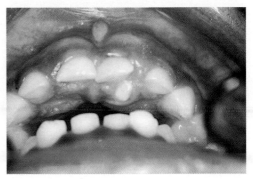

FIG. 20-26 Salivary calculus. *A,* This sialolith obstructing a salivary duct is observed in the floor of the mouth. *B,* A dental radiograph of the sublingual space reveals the size and location of the salivary calculus.

FIG. 20-27 Hyperdontia. Erupted supernumerary tooth lingual to the maxillary central incisor in the deciduous dentition.

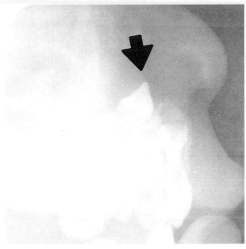

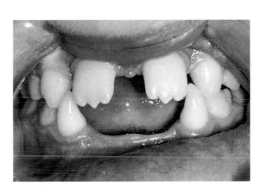

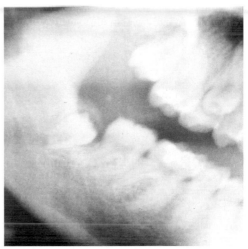

FIG. 20-28 Supernumerary nasal tooth. A lateral radiograph of the maxilla shows a supernumerary tooth erupting through the floor of the nasal cavity in a child with cleft palate who had recurrent epistaxis.

FIG. 20-29 Hypodontia. The congenital absence of teeth is seen in this patient with hereditary ectodermal dysplasia. This phenomenon may be an isolated anomaly or a manifestation of several syndromes.

FIG. 20-30 A microdont can be seen on this panoramic radiograph near the second molar. Microdonts are often seen in the maxillary lateral incisor region.

second premolars, and lateral incisors. Hypodontia is frequently associated with several ectodermal syndromes such as anhidrotic ectodermal dysplasia and chondroectodermal dysplasia (Fig. 20-29).

Alteration in Size and Shape

Teeth that are smaller or larger than normal are termed *microdonts* and *macrodonts,* respectively. These teeth are genetic anomalies. They are clinically significant when a discrepancy in tooth size and dental arch length results in severe crowding or spacing of the teeth. Size abnormalities are often localized to one tooth or to a very small group of teeth (Fig. 20-30).

Variations in shape also result from the joining of teeth or tooth buds. Fusion is the joining of two tooth buds by the dentin. Concrescence is the joining of the roots of two or more teeth by cementum. Gemination (twinning) results from the incomplete division of one tooth bud, resulting in a large crown with a notched incisal edge and a single root (Fig. 20-31).

Hypoplasia and Hypocalcification

Numerous local and systemic insults are capable of causing the enamel defects of hypoplasia and hypocalcification. The most common

etiologic factors are local infections such as an abscessed primary tooth, which, when not diagnosed and treated promptly, may damage the enamel of its developing permanent counterpart. Other causes include systemic infections with associated high fever; trauma such as intrusion of the primary tooth; and chemical injury, of which excessive ingestion of fluoride is an example. Other etiologic factors include nutritional deficiencies, allergies, rubella, cerebral palsy, embryopathy, prematurity, and radiation therapy. Hypoplasia results from an insult during active matrix formation of the enamel and clinically manifests as pitting, furrowing, or thinning of the enamel (Fig. 20-33). Hypocalcification results from an insult during mineralization of the tooth and is seen as opaque, chalky, or white lesions (Fig. 20-32).

Heritable Defects of Enamel and Dentin
Amelogenesis Imperfecta

Amelogenesis imperfecta is the term used to describe a group of genetically determined defects that involve the enamel of primary and permanent teeth without affecting dentin, pulp, or cementum. Although the types of amelogenesis imperfecta are numerous, the major defect in each is hypoplasia, hypomaturation, or hypocalcification. The hypoplastic type results in thin, pitted, or fissured enamel (Fig. 20-33).

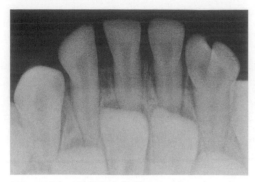

FIG. 20-31 Radiograph demonstrates gemination (twinning), the incomplete division of a tooth bud resulting in a tooth with a large, notched crown and a single root.

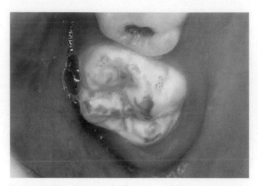

FIG. 20-32 Hypocalcification. This 6-year-old patient exhibits early signs of hypocalcification of his permanent molars. Chalky white spots indicate poor calcification of the enamel.

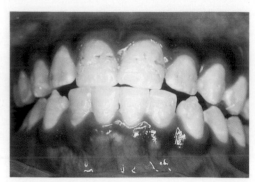

FIG. 20-33 Amelogenesis imperfecta, hypoplastic type. This process results in generalized pitting of the enamel.

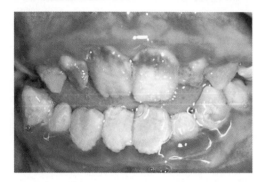

FIG. 20-34 Amelogenesis imperfecta, hypocalcified type. The enamel defects result in discoloration and erosion caused by errors in the mineralization stage of tooth development and secondary staining.

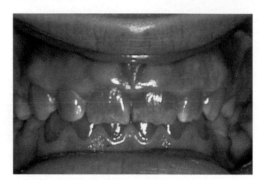

FIG. 20-35 Dentinogenesis imperfecta. The bluish, opalescent sheen on several of these teeth results from genetically defective dentin. This condition may be associated with osteogenesis imperfecta.

Hypomaturation manifests as discolored enamel of full thickness but decreased hardness that tends to chip away slowly, exposing underlying dentin. Radiographic evaluation demonstrates the decreased density of enamel. In the hypocalcified form the enamel is chalky, variable in color, and quickly erodes (Fig. 20-34). Depending on the type of amelogenesis imperfecta, inheritance may be autosomal dominant, autosomal recessive, or X-linked.

Dentinogenesis Imperfecta

Dentinogenesis imperfecta results in dentin defects and is usually inherited as an autosomal dominant trait. The most common manifestation is opalescent dentin, which may be associated with osteogenesis imperfecta. The teeth are blue to pinkish-brown in color and have an opalescent sheen (Fig. 20-35). Despite normal enamel morphology, there is rapid attrition or wearing down of the crowns. The roots are shortened, and the pulp cavities are calcified. Primary teeth are more severely affected than the permanent, although permanent teeth are fracture prone.

Discoloration

Three major types of tooth discoloration are frequently observed: (1) discoloration from stains that adhere externally to the surfaces of the teeth (extrinsic); (2) discoloration from various pigments that are incorporated into the tooth structure during development (intrinsic); and (3) intrinsic discoloration secondary to hereditary defects, which was discussed previously.

Extrinsic

Extrinsic discoloration is primarily limited to patients with poor oral hygiene, those receiving certain medications, those who heavily consume stain-containing foods or drinks, or those who smoke or chew tobacco or other substances. It occurs more often at certain locations, especially on the gingival third of the exposed crown. Diagnosis requires appropriate medical, dental, and dietary histories with emphasis on oral hygiene, food and drug intake, and tobacco habits. Treatment includes scaling, dental prophylaxis and polishing, and the practice of regular oral hygiene. The use of abrasive toothpaste can cause excessive wear of the enamel and should be avoided.

Brownish-black stain on the lingual surfaces of anterior and posterior teeth is most common among young children who are taking liquid oral iron supplements and among adolescents who are smokers and tea drinkers. Green stain on the labial surfaces of the anterior maxillary teeth is common among children with poor oral hygiene. The source is usually chromogenic bacteria and fungi (Fig. 20-36). Orangeish-red stain is unusual, but when it does occur it can be found around the gingival third of the exposed crown. This stain often results from antibiotic intake, which causes a temporary shift in the oral flora.

Intrinsic

Intrinsic discoloration is usually induced during the calcification of dentin and enamel by excessive levels of the body's natural pigments such as hemoglobin and bile or by pigments introduced by the intake of chemicals such as fluorides or tetracyclines. Occasionally, isolated

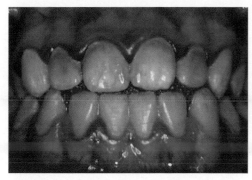

FIG. 20-36 Extrinsic discoloration. The green stain seen on the gingival third of the incisors is associated with poor oral hygiene.

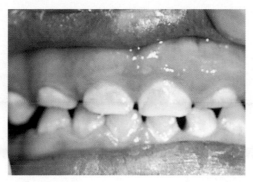

FIG. 20-37 Hepatic discoloration. Generalized intrinsic discoloration of the primary teeth is seen in this patient with biliary atresia.

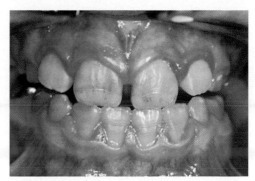

FIG. 20-38 Tetracycline discoloration. The severe discoloration seen in this patient is the result of tetracycline administration during calcification of the permanent teeth.

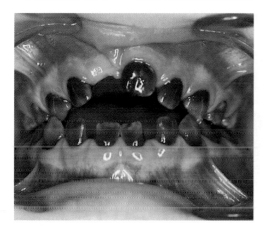

FIG. 20-39 The reddish-brown tooth discoloration associated with prophyria.

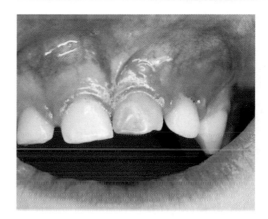

FIG. 20-40 Isolated intrinsic discoloration. The central incisor is discolored secondary to trauma. Often, such a change is a manifestation of pulpal necrosis.

intrinsic discoloration takes place as a result of pulpal necrosis, pulpal calcification, or internal resorption.

Hepatic

Generalized intrinsic discoloration of primary teeth is seen in patients with advanced hepatic disease associated with persistent or recurrent jaundice and hyperbilirubinemia (Fig. 20-37). The intensity of discoloration varies and may be related to the severity of the disease. Color ranges from brown to grayish-brown and usually has no clinical significance unless it is associated with significant hypoplasia of the dentition.

Tetracycline

Teeth stained as a result of tetracycline therapy may vary in color from yellow to brown to dark gray. Staining occurs when the tetracycline is incorporated into calcifying teeth and bone. The enamel and to a greater degree the dentin that are calcifying at the time of intake incorporate tetracycline into their chemical structures. The severity of discoloration depends on the dose, duration, and type of tetracycline administered. The initial yellow or light brown pigmentation tends to darken with age (Fig. 20-38). Tetracyclines readily cross the placenta, so staining of primary teeth is possible if tetracycline is taken during pregnancy. Therefore tetracycline should not be prescribed to pregnant women or to children under 10 years of age.

Erythroblastosis Fetalis

Children born with congenital hemolytic anemia caused by Rh incompatibility may exhibit distinct discoloration of their primary teeth as a result of the deposition of bilirubin in the dentin and enamel during primary tooth development. The color ranges from green to blue to orange. No treatment is indicated unless discoloration is associated with significant hypoplasia or hypocalcification. The permanent dentition is usually not affected.

Porphyria

This hereditary disturbance of porphyrin metabolism may produce a distinct reddish or brownish discoloration of the primary and permanent teeth secondary to deposition of porphyrin in developing teeth (Fig. 20-39).

Isolated Intrinsic

Teeth with necrotic pulps develop an opaque appearance with discoloration ranging from light yellow to gray (Figs. 20-40 and 20-47, *B*). Such teeth may develop abscesses, periapical cystic lesions, or chronic fistulas. Pulpal calcification (Fig. 20-41) is often associated with a localized yellow discoloration. Internal resorption manifests clinically as a pink discoloration secondary to loss of dentin thickness.

Caries

The interaction of microorganisms, especially *Streptococcus mutans*, and fermentable carbohydrates results in acid demineralization of susceptible enamel. Caries are seen as yellowish-brown to gray defects in the enamel surfaces of affected teeth (Fig. 20-42). Untreated carious de-

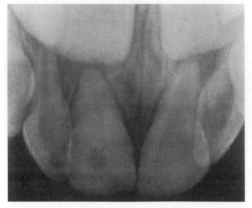

FIG. 20-41 Radiographic evidence of dystrophic calcification of the pulp and root canal of the upper right primary central incisor.

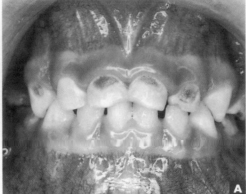

FIG. 20-42 Caries. *A,* The typical pattern of nursing-bottle caries, with the upper incisors being the first involved. *B,* When badly neglected, severe tooth erosion occurs and periapical abscesses may develop.

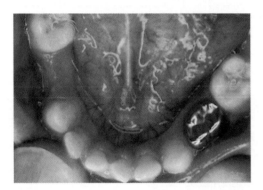

FIG. 20-43 The occlusal surfaces of newly erupted molars exhibit varying degrees of pit and fissure depth. The morphology of these patterns makes these teeth more prone to early decay.

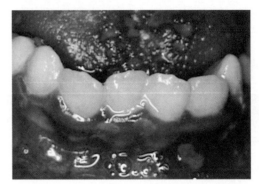

FIG. 20-44 Herpetic gingivostomatitis. The ulcerations seen on the oral mucosa were preceded by fever, headache, and lymphadenopathy. Note the erythematous halos around the ulcerations.

struction progresses through the enamel and dentin and with bacterial contamination of the pulp ultimately renders the pulp necrotic. The deep pits, fissures, and grooves characteristic of the surfaces of newly erupted teeth are at increased risk for developing carious lesions (Fig. 20-43 and Fig. 20-5). Sealing these defects with plastic bonding agents may prevent the initiation of caries. Other preventive methods include brushing and flossing on a daily basis (beginning with eruption of the first tooth) to remove bacteria-containing plaque, implementation of systemic fluoride via the water supply or prescribed supplements, and control of the frequency of intake of fermentable carbohydrates, especially those high in sugar and adhesiveness.

Nursing bottle caries involve the primary dentition of the child who is habitually put to bed with a bottle containing milk or another cariogenic (sugar-containing) liquid. This form of caries was originally associated with bottle-feeding only; however, an association with frequent and prolonged nocturnal breast-feeding has become apparent. Carious lesions initially develop on the maxillary incisors and later on the molars and cuspids (Fig. 20-42, *A* and *B*). The mandibular incisors are spared by the protective position of the tongue during nursing. The deleterious effect of nocturnal nursing is due to the frequency of carbohydrate intake and the decreased rate of swallowing and salivation during sleep. Brushing before bedtime and after any nocturnal feedings is especially important in prevention.

Infections

Viral

Herpetic Gingivostomatitis

Primary herpetic gingivostomatitis, caused by herpes simplex type I, is an extremely painful disease that affects children, especially those between the ages of 6 months and 3 years. The vesicular lesions of the lips, tongue, gingivae, and oral mucosa are preceded by fever, headache, regional lymphadenopathy, and gingival hyperemia and edema. These lesions tend to rupture quickly, leaving shallow ulcerations covered by a gray membrane and surrounded by an erythematous halo (Fig. 20-44). The inflamed gingivae are friable and bleed easily. Lesions heal spontaneously in 1 to 2 weeks without scarring. Since inflammation makes brushing too painful, oral hygiene should be maintained using a preparation such as chlorhexidine or glycerin and peroxide (in very young children) to decrease the incidence of secondary infection. A bland diet and rinsing with viscous lidocaine (in children older than 6 or 7 years) or a solution of equal parts of Benadryl and Maalox, in addition to use of oral analgesics, are indicated to minimize and control pain. In some severe cases, codeine may be required. The use of systemic acyclovir may be indicated in cases with moderate to severe involvement. Topical application of the same drug can be helpful in milder cases.

Recurrent infections caused by reactivation of latent herpes simplex virus are fairly common. Lesions are few in number and more localized; systemic symptoms are absent unless the host is immunocompromised. Lesions are usually located on the lips, with prodromal symptoms of itching and burning preceding the development of thin-walled vesicles that rupture and become crusty in appearance (see Chapter 12). When intraoral lesions occur, they manifest as small vesicles in a localized group on mucosa that is tightly bound to periosteum.

Herpes Zoster (Shingles)

Herpes zoster results from reactivation of the varicella zoster virus and inflammation of the dorsal root or extramedullary cranial nerve ganglion. Although the disease is seen in otherwise healthy children, it is more likely to occur in the severely debilitated or immunosuppressed child. The patient exhibits a prodrome of malaise, fever, headache, and tenderness along the affected dermatome that may last a few to several

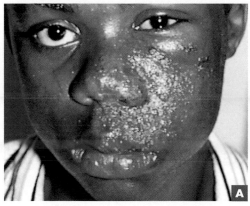
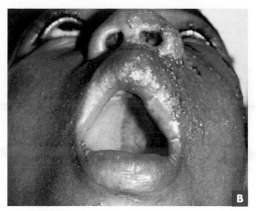

FIG. 20-45　Herpes zoster. This patient's infection involved the trigeminal nerve, including the nasociliary branch. The extraoral *(A)* and the intraoral *(B)* lesions stop at the midline.

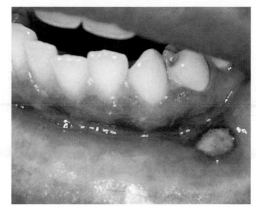

FIG. 20-46　Recurrent aphthous ulcers. The ulceration seen on the labial mucosa is surrounded by a characteristic erythematous halo.

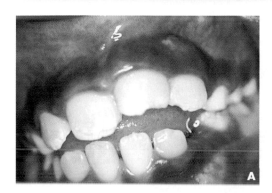
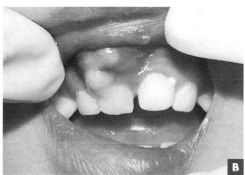

FIG. 20-47　Dental abscesses. *A,* A small abscess above the left upper lateral incisor developed after an injury in which the patient had chipped that tooth and his central incisor. *B,* This abscess above the right central incisor has ruptured through the gingiva and begun to drain. The tooth is discolored as a result of pulp necrosis stemming from an injury 2 years earlier.

days. This is followed by the extraoral formation of painful, grouped vesicular lesions that rupture to form ulcerations. The oral cavity also may be affected with erosions when maxillary and mandibular divisions of the trigeminal nerve are involved (Fig. 20-45).

Recurrent Aphthous Ulcers (Canker Sores)

Aphthous ulcers are similar in appearance to herpetic ulcers but are not of viral origin. Precipitating factors include trauma, stress, sunlight, endocrine disturbances, hematologic disorders, and allergies, alluding to a multifactorial etiology. Onset is usually during adolescence or young adulthood. Unlike herpetic lesions, these ulcerations are not preceded by vesicle formation. They are extremely painful, and have a pseudomembrane and an erythematous halo (Fig. 20-46). They can vary in size, number, and distribution. Small aphthae may coalesce into larger lesions. Although any oral mucosal surface may be involved, freely movable mucosa is more frequently involved than tightly bound. Lesions heal in 1 to 2 weeks without scarring.

Bacterial

Odontogenic infections are caused by both aerobic and anaerobic microorganisms. Streptococci and staphylococci are isolated most frequently; however, any oral flora or opportunistic microorganism may be involved.

Dental Abscesses

Abscesses are most common in children with neglected dental caries as a result of poor dental hygiene and irregular dental care. Once caries extend to the pulp, infection and pulpal necrosis ensue, setting the stage for formation of a periapical abscess. Children with traumatized teeth may go on to develop abscesses, if the resulting pulpal hyperemia is so extreme that it causes pressure necrosis, if the neurovascular bundle is severed, or pulp is exposed by a crown fracture.

Periapical abscesses require endodontic therapy or extraction of the offending tooth. The potential for complications makes early diagnosis important, yet frequently this does not occur because often symptoms are insidious in onset and progression and nonspecific in nature. This is in part because the alveolar processes of the mandible and maxilla in young children are fenestrated anteriorly, facilitating early decompression of the abscess through the alveolus and gingiva. Patients may complain of headaches as the abscess enlarges and pressure builds up, then of abdominal pain after decompression as the draining pus is swallowed, causing gastric irritation. Later in childhood, abscessed maxillary teeth may intermittently decompress through the floor of a maxillary sinus, producing recurrent sinus infections. Other symptoms may include anorexia, avoidance of chewy foods, halitosis, toothaches, a sensitive tooth, or facial swelling. Nonspecific complaints and complaints of referred pain are more common than a toothache in children, some of whom have no overt symptoms but report feeling better after treatment.

On physical examination the examiner may find localized gingival swelling and/or erythema, a gingival abscess, a fistula, or a granuloma (Figs. 20-47 and 20-48, *A*). On occasion there is increased sensitivity to percussion. Left untreated, a periapical abscess of a primary tooth may damage the underlying developing tooth bud. Abscesses may also result in formation of an apical granuloma or a radicular cyst, or they may rupture and spread through the adjacent soft tissues to create a fistula, which drains through the skin (Fig. 20-48, *B*), or cause facial cellulitis (Fig. 20-49). More ominously, the infection may track through lateral pharyngeal, retropharyngeal, or sublingual spaces, threatening the airway and causing sepsis and/or mediastinitis. Rarely, septic thrombosis of the cavernous sinus may result from neglected infections that rupture into the maxillary sinus.

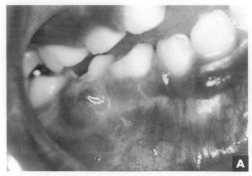
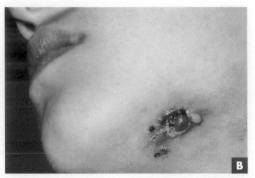
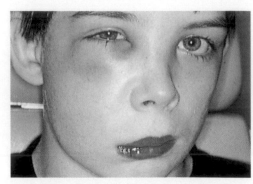

FIG. 20-48 *A,* A deep, neglected cavity in this mandibular molar predisposed to development of a periapical abscess that after rupture, resulted in formation of a gingival granuloma. *B,* Left untreated, such abscesses can be responsible for this type of extraoral lesion in which infection has spread by way of a fistulous tract to the skin. Extraction of the offending tooth is necessary for resolution of the extraoral lesion.

FIG. 20-49 Facial cellulitis associated with an abscessed maxillary tooth. Hospital admission for intravenous antibiotics, incision and drainage, and extraction of the abscessed tooth was necessary.

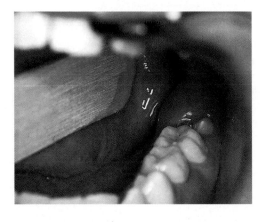
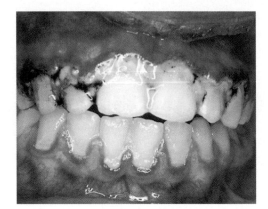

FIG. 20-50 Pericoronitis involving a partially erupted molar. Food particles and bacteria have become trapped under the residual overlying gingiva, resulting in inflammation and abscess formation. This condition can occur with any molar eruption but is most common with partially erupted third molars (wisdom teeth).

FIG. 20-51 Acute necrotizing ulcerative gingivitis. The infected gingiva exhibits localized necrosis and hemorrhage and is covered with pseudomembranes.

Pericoronitis

Pericoronitis is a bacterial infection of the gingival soft tissue surrounding the crown of a partially erupted tooth. This occurs when food particles and plaque become trapped under the residual gingiva, stimulating bacterial growth and abscess formation. The third molars are most commonly involved. Symptoms include localized pain and tenderness and occasionally fever and malaise. Erythema and edema are readily apparent on examination (Fig. 20-50), and an enlarged tender submandibular node is often found.

Acute Necrotizing Ulcerative Gingivitis
(Vincent Infection, Trench Mouth)

This is a fusospirochetal infection caused by fusiform bacilli and *Borrelia vincentii,* which is seldom seen before the age of 10. Patients experience abrupt onset of fever, malaise, severe mouth pain, and anorexia. The gingivae are reddened, edematous, and friable with necrotic punched-out craters in the interdental papillae. Occasionally the palate and tongue are affected as well. Involved areas hemorrhage readily and become covered with a pseudomembrane (Fig. 20-51). The breath is fetid, and cervical and submandibular nodes are enlarged and tender. Treatment generally consists of gentle dental prophylaxis followed by improved oral hygiene measures and topical peroxide appli-

cations. In most cases resolution occurs within several days without the use of antibiotics. Occasionally, secondary infection or severe involvement may necessitate the use of antibiotics; penicillin is then the antibiotic of choice.

Fungal

Candidiasis (Moniliasis, Thrush)

Candidiasis results from the opportunistic pathogen *Candida albicans.* This infection is seen in infants, children with underlying systemic diseases, immunosuppressed children, or those on antibiotic treatment. Common sites of involvement are the buccal mucosa, tongue, palate, and commissures of the lips. The intraoral lesions of acute infection are soft, elevated, creamy white plaques that do not scrape off easily (Fig. 20-52). Chronic candidiasis, usually seen in the immunocompromised host, can result in marked hypertrophy and fissuring of the tongue mucosa. Although culturing is difficult and not reliable, diagnosis may be made on the basis of clinical findings or examination of a KOH preparation. Treatment consists of local application of nystatin (miconazole or ketoconazole for severe or chronic cases), and control of the underlying causes, including sterilization of nipples used for formula feedings.

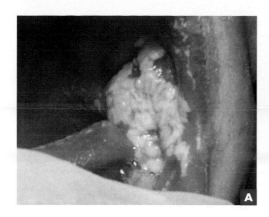
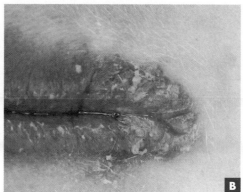

FIG. 20-52 Candidiasis. *A,* Involvement of buccal mucosa with white plaque. *B,* Mucocutaneous infection of the commissures of the lips.

Trauma

Assessment of Patients with Orofacial and Dental Injuries

In evaluating patients with orofacial and dental trauma, key elements of the history include when, where, and how the injury occurred; the child's subsequent behavior; any prior treatment; and general health and tetanus immunization status. In asking about the mechanism of injury, the examiner must determine the forces involved. Did the child trip and fall while walking, or was he or she running; if riding a bike, how fast was he or she going; in the case of falls, from what height, onto what kind of surface? This gives the examiner a better idea of the potential severity of injury and risk of associated injuries.

Physical examination is first directed at determining the adequacy and stability of airway, breathing, and circulation followed by evaluation for associated head and neck injury. When these areas have been cleared and/or stabilized, then the examiner may proceed with the orofacial examination, assessing the extent and nature of injuries. Because the presence of underlying injuries is often belied by the degree and nature of overlying soft tissue trauma, assessment begins with external inspection of facial structures for swelling, deformity, contusions, abrasions, and lacerations. The presence of associated periorbital ecchymoses, or swelling, subconjunctival hemorrhage or edema; diplopia; and nasal bleeding should raise suspicion of frontal skull and midface fractures. Meticulous examination of cranial nerve function is essential. This is followed by observation of occlusion and jaw motion on opening and closing, checking for deviation or trismus. Older patients can be asked if it feels normal when they bite down; parents of young children can report if the child's occlusion looks normal. The temporomandibular joint should be palpated, assessing for tenderness, snap, or pain on opening and closing.

Next, intraoral soft tissues are inspected for evidence of swelling, hematoma, abrasions, and lacerations. Displacement, loosening, and fractures of teeth are noted. Palpation of facial bones and the labial and lingual surfaces of the dental arches and assessment of abnormal maxillary mobility may be best left until last because resulting pain may reduce cooperation. All internal and external lacerations must be carefully inspected to check for injury to underlying neural and ductal structures.

Recommended radiographs include apical and occlusal views for displacement or loosening of a permanent tooth, panoramic and facial bone radiographs for possible mandibular fractures, and a computed tomography (CT) scan for suspected maxillary and midface fractures.

Soft Tissue Injuries

A variety of soft-tissue injuries including lacerations, contusions, abrasions, perforations, avulsions, and burns may occur. Whereas soft tissue injuries may occur in isolation, they often are associated with injuries of teeth and supporting bones. Thus any assessment of a soft-tissue injury must include careful attention to the teeth and underlying structures. The injured area should be cleansed of blood clots, debris, and foreign material, then carefully examined to determine the extent of tissue involvement. Mechanical debridement of any ragged, necrotic, or beveled margins may be necessary. Appropriate tetanus prophylaxis should also be considered. Saline rinses, careful attention to oral hygiene, penicillin prophylaxis, and soft diet are mainstays of management of soft-tissue injuries.

Abrasions

Superficial abrasions usually heal without complications. Extensive abrasions should be covered with a water-soluble, medicated gauze after irrigation. Extensive deep abrasions may require skin grafting.

Contusions

A contusion, or bruise, usually requires no treatment, and healing proceeds favorably in most instances. Contusions are often associated with underlying injuries; therefore a careful examination of adjacent structures is indicated.

Perforations

These small, deep wounds caused by sharp objects are fairly common in children, especially as a result of falls with such an object in the mouth. Careful examination of the wound and the object is essential. Following careful inspection and irrigation, larger wounds should be closed in layers; smaller wounds may not require closure. If doubt exists concerning foreign bodies and/or contamination, a drain should be left in place and proper antibiotics prescribed. The possibility of damage to large vessels should be recognized, especially when the perforation involves the posterolateral palate or a tonsillar pillar (see Chapter 22).

Avulsions (Degloving Injuries)

Avulsions of oral soft tissues are uncommon injuries, yet when they occur they may involve deep and superficial tissues (Fig. 20-53, *A* and *B*). Small avulsions can be treated by undermining and suturing surrounding tissues. Larger avulsions can be treated by reattaching the avulsed tissues or by use of a graft.

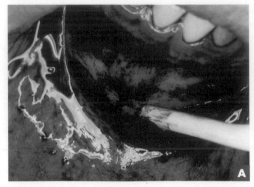 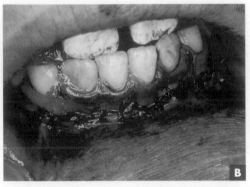 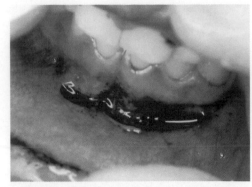

FIG. 20-53 Degloving injury, before *(A)* and after *(B)* repair. Such an injury to the oral mucosa requires immediate inspection, irrigation, approximation, and suturing.

FIG. 20-54 This laceration of the oral mucosa—deep and not well approximated—requires immediate treatment.

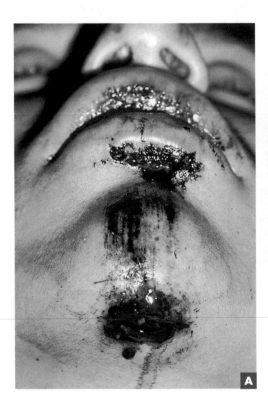 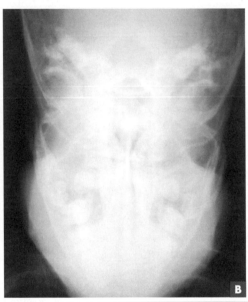

FIG. 20-55 *A,* This boy incurred a forced occlusion injury when hit by a car and thrown from his bike. Note the chin laceration and through-and-through lip laceration. *B,* He also had bilateral condylar neck fractures of the mandible. In this radiograph the condyles bend inward at nearly 90 degrees above the fracture lines.

Lacerations

Lacerations of facial and oral tissues are common in children. Small intraoral lacerations with well-approximated margins do not require suturing. Bleeding usually subsides spontaneously, and healing proceeds satisfactorily. Large lacerations, through-and-through lacerations, and those associated with extensive, recurrent, or uncontrolled bleeding require careful assessment and surgical closure (Fig. 20-54).

Lip lacerations are often caused by penetration of teeth through the labial soft tissues (Fig. 20-55). Thus the adjacent dentition must be carefully inspected for evidence of chipping and for signs of loosening or displacement. If chipping is found, imbedded tooth particles should be suspected. These may be difficult to palpate but are easily detected radiographically. If present, they must be removed to prevent infection.

Because the trauma that results in chin lacerations commonly involves forced occlusion of the dentition with transfer of impact forces to the underlying bone and condyles, these cases warrant assessment of underlying dental and bony structures (Figs. 20-55, 20-65 and 20-66). Forced occlusion injuries can also produce tongue lacerations. Closure is

required for large, gaping wounds with persistent bleeding (Fig. 20-56, *A*), but conservative management is best for smaller lesions (Fig. 20-56, *B*).

Soft-palate lacerations require a thorough pharyngeal inspection. The possibility of foreign body entrapment, immediate or delayed vascular injury (particularly when the laceration involves posterolateral structures), or formation of pharyngeal abscesses should be seriously considered. Lacerations involving the labial frenulum of infants are common and usually require only restriction of lip manipulation and a soft diet.

Burns

Burns involving the oral cavity usually heal rapidly but with contracture and scarring. Burns at the angle of the mouth incurred by chewing on an electrical cord (Fig. 20-57) are particularly problematic. After the injury an eschar forms over the necrotic tissue. This tends to separate approximately 10 days later, at which time profuse bleeding from the labial artery may occur. Splints fabricated from dental materials are important in long-term management to prevent or minimize contracture by maintaining proper anatomic relationships during healing.

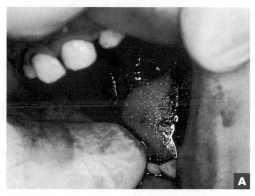

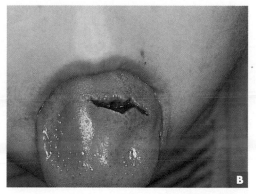

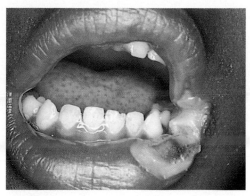

FIG. 20-56 Tongue lacerations. *A,* A large gaping tongue laceration in a toddler produced by the upper front teeth being forced through the tissue by a fall with the tongue protruded. This type of injury usually requires suturing. *B,* This small laceration, though gaping slightly, does not require surgical closure.

FIG. 20-57 This electrical burn was the result of chewing an extension cord. In this site, delayed hemorrhage after separation of the eschar and deformity with scarring are particular problems.

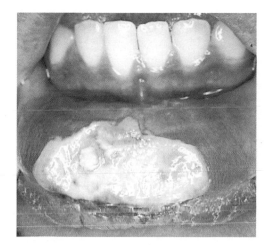

FIG. 20-58 Traumatic lip ulceration caused by lip-biting after administration of local anesthesia.

Traumatic Ulcers

These painful ulcerations result from mechanical, chemical, or thermal trauma. Injury may be secondary to irritation by objects, trauma during mastication, toothbrush trauma, or abnormal habits. Large ulcerations involving the buccal mucosa or lower lip may be associated with cheek or lip biting after inferior alveolar nerve block (Fig. 20-58). Topical peroxide application (Gly-Oxide) is useful in cleansing the area. Lesions usually heal without scarring, but secondarily infected lesions may require antibiotic therapy. Identification and elimination of the habit is necessary for resolution of habit-related lesions.

Trauma to the Dentition

As noted earlier, facial injuries in childhood frequently involve the dentition and supporting bones. One prospective study showed that 50% of children had suffered at least one dental injury by age 14. Although falls are the major source in early childhood, bicycle and skateboard accidents, contact sports, fights, and motor vehicle accidents become more prevalent with advancing age. The risk of such injuries is relatively high in (1) children with neurologic disorders that impair coordination; (2) children with protruding maxillary anterior teeth; and (3) children with a deviant anatomic relationship, such as an anterior open bite or a hypoplastic upper lip. Preventive measures, such as use of helmets, mouthguards, and seat belts, significantly reduce the incidence and severity of such injuries.

Potential Complications

Pulp hemorrhage and/or vasodilation of the pulp vessels are a common response to concussive injury to a tooth and can lead to development of permanent discoloration within 10 to 14 days. Excessive pulpal vasodilation can actually result in pressure necrosis of the pulp. Injuries that produce loosening or displacement of a tooth disrupt the anchoring periodontal ligament. If disruption is mild, there may be no sequelae, although in some cases it stimulates overactive bony repair, ankylosing the tooth in place. When severe, the neurovascular bundle can be torn, resulting in pulp necrosis, which then predisposes to abscess formation. Finally, dental fractures in which dentin and/or pulp are exposed open a pathway for bacteria and predispose to abscess formation. The fracture surface must be sealed and the crown restored emergently.

Several extensive classifications of tooth injuries have been suggested, but for the purpose of this text a more simplified descriptive classification is presented.

Crown Craze or Crack

A significant number of children are discovered during routine physical examination to have "cracks" in the enamel of their teeth. Such cracks are presumably caused by relatively minor trauma or temperature changes. The majority of such teeth are asymptomatic and require no treatment.

Crown Fractures Without Pulpal Exposure

Fractures that traverse only the enamel layer often require no treatment other than smoothing down rough edges and ensuring close follow-up (Fig. 20-47, *A*). However, any fracture of the crown that results in exposure of the dentin requires urgent treatment to prevent infection and subsequent pulp necrosis (Fig. 20-59) because oral flora enter the dentinal tubules and rapidly migrate to the pulp. The treatment of choice is to seal the exposed dentin with calcium hydroxide and to protect it with an acid-etched resin bandage for a minimum of 2 to 3 months to enhance pulpal healing. This procedure should be performed as soon as possible after the

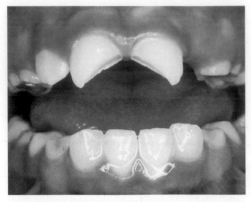

FIG. 20-59 These crown fractures demonstrate involvement of enamel and dentin, without exposure of the pulp. Immediate dental referral is necessary to prevent contamination of the pulp through the dentinal tubules.

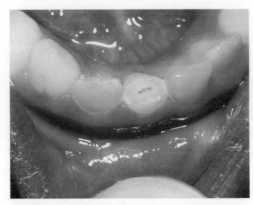

FIG. 20-60 This crown fracture involves enamel, dentin, and the soft tissue of the pulp as well. Immediate dental referral is mandatory to save the tooth.

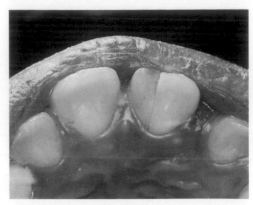

FIG. 20-61 A vertical fracture of the upper central incisor extending below the gum line resulted in pulp exposure.

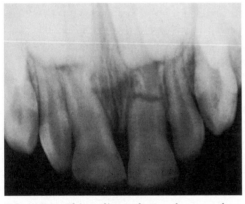

FIG. 20-62 This radiograph reveals a root fracture in the apical third of an upper primary incisor. This was suspected clinically because of tenderness and increased mobility.

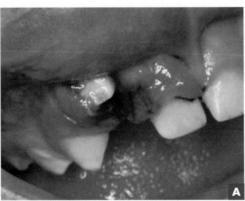

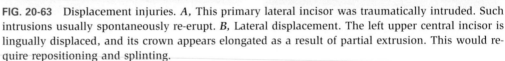

FIG. 20-63 Displacement injuries. *A,* This primary lateral incisor was traumatically intruded. Such intrusions usually spontaneously re-erupt. *B,* Lateral displacement. The left upper central incisor is lingually displaced, and its crown appears elongated as a result of partial extrusion. This would require repositioning and splinting.

injury. As noted earlier, dental fragments are occasionally embedded in the soft tissues of the lip or tongue; therefore appropriate examination and palpation of these areas is indicated. The presence of such fragments may be confirmed by radiographic examination.

Crown Fractures With Pulpal Exposure

Fractures that traverse all three tooth layers to expose the pulp usually involve a significant loss of tooth structure. On physical examination, the fracture surface reveals the pink central pulp surrounded by the brown or beige dentinal layer (Fig. 20-60). Severe vertical or diagonal fractures may also result in pulp exposure and can at times extend to involve the root (Fig. 20-61). Such teeth must be treated urgently with pulp capping, pulpotomy, or root canal therapy, depending on severity.

Root Fractures

Root fractures are less common in the primary dentition, and when they occur they usually require no therapy. Root fractures of permanent teeth may occur with or without loss of crown structure and may be asymptomatic (Fig. 20-62). If a seemingly normal tooth becomes tender

or exhibits increased mobility after trauma, root fracture should be suspected and radiographs obtained. Generally the prognosis is good, and treatment may include splinting the involved segment for 6 to 10 weeks, with or without root canal therapy.

Displacement Injuries

Displacement injuries result in extrusion, intrusion, or lateral displacement (labially or lingually) and are most commonly seen in the primary dentition where the combination of a short root length and a very "pliable" bony structure seem to permit displacement to occur (Fig. 20-63, *A* and *B*). Displacement injuries are often the cause of significant discomfort, bleeding, and possible interference with mastication and occlusion. All result in some degree of disruption of the periodontal ligament. Further, being the result of moderate to severe mechanisms of injury, fractures of underlying bony structures are common associated findings. Because the primary teeth are most vulnerable to these types of injury, there is always a risk of damage to and interference with normal development of permanent tooth buds; therefore immediate care is advised. Treatment may include observation with or without prophylactic antibiotic coverage, immediate correction in cases

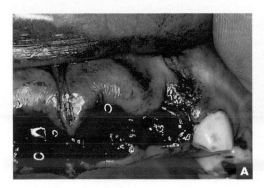
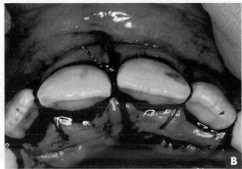

FIG. 20-64 *A,* Four permanent incisors have been avulsed. *B,* The teeth have been reimplanted successfully.

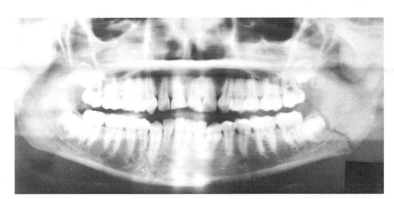

FIG. 20-65 A panoramic radiograph reveals a nondisplaced mandibular fracture extending through the wall of the third molar tooth bud. There is an associated hairline fracture near the midline on the patient's right.

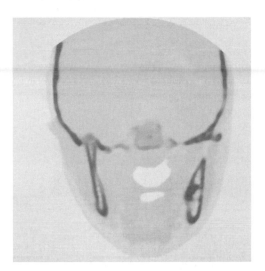

FIG. 20-66 CT scan reveals the intrusion of the mandibular condyle into the middle cranial fossa as a result of an extremely severe forced occlusion injury. Careful "pull back" and splinting is a common treatment for this type of injury.

of lingual displacement caused by interference with mastication, or extraction of the displaced tooth in cases of severe labial or vertical displacement. Most intruded primary teeth reerupt within 6 to 8 weeks with antibiotic coverage, sensible oral hygiene, and an appropriate diet. In general, displaced permanent teeth should be surgically repositioned and splinted, with close follow-up. It is not uncommon for these teeth to require root canal therapy.

Avulsion and Reimplantation

Avulsion is the complete displacement of a tooth from its socket and is seen mostly in preschool and early school-age children. Reimplantation of primary teeth is still experimental and should be done only under selective conditions. However, the prognosis is usually poor, and splinting is not easily carried out.

On the other hand, reimplantation of permanent teeth is an acceptable technique with a relatively good prognosis (Fig. 20-64, *A* and *B*). The major factors in improving prognosis are as follows:

1. A short period between avulsion and reimplantation, preferably less than half an hour.
2. Appropriate storage of the avulsed tooth (the most desirable "media" would be the socket itself, followed by saliva and milk).
3. Appropriate irrigation of the surgical site, replacing the tooth into the socket without pressure, and stabilizing it with the use of a resin-bonded splint.
4. Appropriate removal of the pulp within 2 weeks as a first step in completing root canal treatment, unless the tooth was immature with incomplete root formation.
5. Removal of the splint within 2 weeks.

It is generally accepted that scraping of the root or the socket is contraindicated because preservation of adherent shreds of peridontal membrane appears to improve prognosis.

Trauma to Supporting Structures

The developing facial bones in the young child are small relative to the calvarium and thus somewhat protected by it. They are compact, spongy, and have greater elasticity, which tends to reduce the risk of fractures. However, the relatively thin outer cortices make alveolar process fractures somewhat more likely with dental displacement injuries, and their growth centers and developing tooth buds serve as weak points and thus are major sites of fractures when they do occur (Fig. 20-65). Finally, their thick periosteum has remarkable osteogenic potential, which speeds healing remarkably. Injuries to these bony supporting structures of the dentition may result from birth trauma, bicycle accidents, car accidents, various physical and sporting activities, child abuse, and animal bites. Because major forces are required to produce jaw fractures in children, the examiner must carefully search for evidence of associated head and neck injuries (Fig. 20-66) and be vigilant in observing for evidence of expanding hematomas that may later compromise the airway.

Fractures of the Mandible

Excluding nasal fractures, the most common facial fractures in children involve the mandible. The two major mechanisms are forced occlusion and lateral or frontolateral impact. Forced occlusion can produce hemarthrosis of the temporomandibular joint, a compression fracture of the condylar process, or a greenstick condylar fracture (Fig. 20-55). These injuries are often associated with fractures of the molar crowns. Lateral and frontolateral blows tend to produce fractures of the mandibular body, usually through the wall of a developing tooth bud (Fig. 20-65). Because the mandible is an arch through which the force of the impact is transmitted, these injuries are often associated with a contralateral fracture of the mandibular body or condyle (Fig. 20-65). Important diagnostic clues may include ecchymosis, facial swelling, devia-

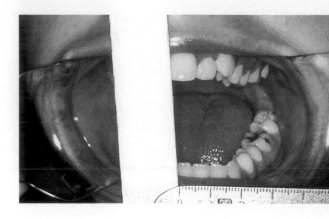

FIG. 20-67 A method of measuring deviation of the mandible on opening is illustrated in this picture showing a shift to the fracture side the width of one lower central incisor.

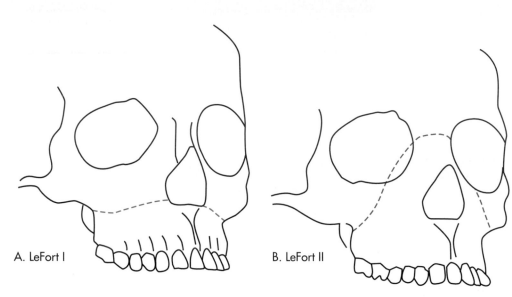

A. LeFort I

B. LeFort II

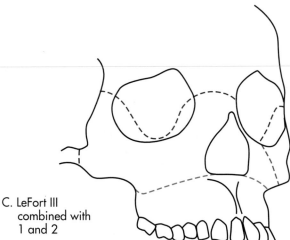

C. LeFort III combined with 1 and 2

FIG. 20-68 Diagrammatic representation of fracture patterns of LeFort fractures. *A,* LeFort I: the fracture separates the maxilla from the pterygoid plates and the nasal complex. *B,* LeFort II: the fracture line separates the maxilla and nasal complex from the orbits and the zygoma. *C,* LeFort III: the fracture line separates the midface from the cranial vault, traversing the zygomaticofrontal sutures and extending through the orbits and the nasoorbital ethmoid complex. Fracture lines of types I and II are shown as well, because they are commonly present with the LeFort III.

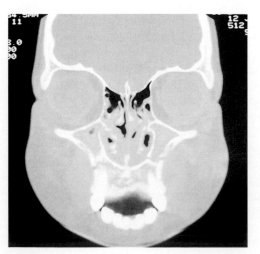

FIG. 20-69 CT scan shows a LeFort I fracture. The maxilla is separated from the midface. The degree is greater on the right.

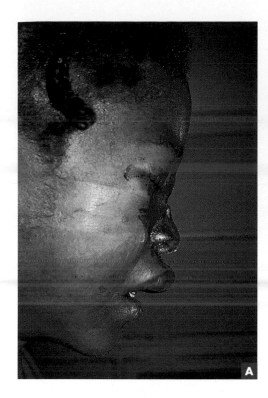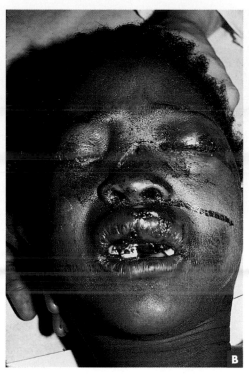

FIG. 20-70 LeFort II fracture. This adolescent boy sustained multiple midfacial and nasoorbital injuries in a motor vehicle accident. A and B, He has a collapsed midface with marked swelling of the upper lip, deviation of the nose and prominent periorbital swelling and ecchymosis. (Courtesy Dr. Joseph Andrews.)

tion on opening or closing (Fig. 20-67), trismus, and malocclusion that may be apparent visibly or only subjectively evident to the patient. Severe bilateral mandibular fractures can result in posterior displacement of the mandible and tongue with secondary airway obstruction. Palpation may reveal localized tenderness and hematoma formation, a step-off, or abnormal mobility with or without gingival tears. Examination of the child with a temporomandibular joint injury may reveal tenderness and decreased motion or a snap when the examiner's fingers are pressed just anterior to the external auditory canal as the child opens and closes the mouth. A panoramic radiograph and a mandibular series should be ordered if there is clinical suspicion of a fracture. If routine views are unrevealing, CT may be called for in certain unusual, difficult, or complex cases.

Management requires careful assessment of the stability and type of erupted dentition, as well as the location of the tooth buds. Nondisplaced fractures with no occlusal abnormalities may require no treatment other than a soft diet. Most displaced fractures can be treated conservatively: first by appropriate reduction, followed by simple intermaxillary fixation or intraoral splints and circumferential wiring (closed reduction). Seldom is open reduction indicated; however, if this technique is used, careful placement of intraosseous holes is essential to avoid damaging the developing tooth buds.

Fractures of the Maxilla and Midface

Other than minor fractures of the alveolar process seen with dental displacement injuries, fractures of the maxilla and midface are very uncommon in infants and young children. This is because the relatively large cranial vault provides protection, with the forehead bearing the brunt of most frontal impacts. The elasticity of the facial bones further reduces the risk of fracture. When such injuries do occur in older children and adolescents, they are generally the result of major impacts and are often associated with injuries to the nose, ethmoid sinuses and orbits, and the frontal portion of the skull. As noted earlier, careful attention must be given to the airway, breathing, and circulation, along with assessment for associated head and neck injuries. Exact diagnosis of the location and extent of maxillary fractures is challenging and ne-

cessitates a thorough and detailed examination and specialized imaging techniques. CT scan of the midface in both sagittal and coronal planes is the most reliable diagnostic tool.

The LeFort classification of midfacial fractures, devised in 1901, divides them into three groups (Fig. 20-68) as follows:

1. The LeFort I primarily involves the maxilla, separating it from the pterygoid plates and the nasal and zygomatic struts (Fig. 20-69)
2. The LeFort II, in which the maxilla and nasal complex are separated from the orbits and the zygoma (Fig. 20-70).
3. The LeFort III, in which there is complete separation of the midface from the cranial vault at the level of the nasoorbital ethmoid complex and the zygomaticofrontal suture area with extension through the orbits (Fig. 20-71).

Often these fractures occur in combination, and the involved maxilla may be further fragmented. It is not unusual to encounter the combination of a LeFort II on one side and a LeFort III on the other. Sagittal splitting of the palate, often accompanied by palatal laceration, is seen in about 10% of patients. Associated mandibular fractures are common.

The diagnosis of LeFort I fracture is often made by finding abnormal mobility of the maxilla when the maxillary dental arch is grasped anteriorly and a vertical "pull-push" maneuver performed, although on occasion the fracture may be impacted or incomplete and malocclusion without mobility is found. Associated findings may include midfacial swelling or ecchymosis (Figs. 20-70 and 20-72), epistaxis, malocclusion, and apparent elongation or shortening of the midface.

LeFort II fractures should be suspected when both the maxilla and nasal complex are mobile. Physical findings are similar to those noted in LeFort I fractures, but wrinkling of the skin above the nose also may be seen.

Beyond these findings, patients with LeFort III fractures tend to have prominent periorbital hematomas and swelling, and may have subconjunctival hemorrhage, disconjugate gaze, and limited extraocular motion, any of which should prompt careful assessment for associated orbital rim and frontal bone fractures. Up to 25% of patients with LeFort II and III fractures have cerebral spinal fluid rhinorrhea and pneumo-

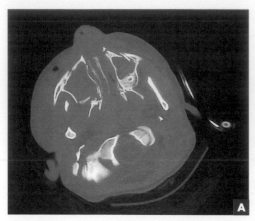

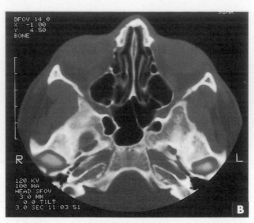

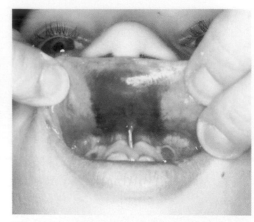

FIG. 20-71   LeFort III fracture. This 10-year-old girl was hit by a car while sled riding. Clinically, she had bilateral raccoon eyes, severe facial edema with a mobile maxilla and bleeding from the nose, mouth, and eyes. She had the constellation of fractures that constitutes a LeFort III fracture and numerous other facial and skull fractures. *A,* In this cut, multiple fractures involving the anterior, posterior, and medial walls of the maxillary sinuses are shown. *B,* Bilateral zygoma fractures are evident in another cut.

FIG. 20-72   Delineated ecchymosis with hematoma formation on the mucosa of the upper lip is a common sign associated with underlying fractures, in this case a fracture of the anterior nasal spine of the maxilla.

cephaly. Injury to the nasoorbital ethmoid complex can also cause detachment of the medial canthal ligaments, with resultant widening of the intercanthal distance.

Progression of edema and often profuse nasopharyngeal bleeding necessitate frequent reassessment of the patient's airway and circulatory status. The airway may need to be stabilized via orotracheal intubation (or rarely tracheotomy) to protect the patient from aspiration of blood or airway narrowing from edema or an expanding hematoma. Total blood loss must be monitored carefully, the patient typed and cross-matched, and blood replacement initiated when necessary.

Once airway, circulatory status, and head and neck injuries have been stabilized or ruled out, appropriate imaging can be performed and treatment initiated. Primary objectives include control of hemorrhage; reestablishing normal occlusion, vertical dimension, and width of the midface; along with immobilization of fractures and restoration of normal frontoorbital architecture. This often necessitates a team approach. It is preferable to plan and carry out the repair as soon as possible after more serious injuries are stabilized because delays increase infection risk and can make repair more difficult as edema worsens and the bones begin to knit over the first 2 to 3 days postinjury.

Temporomandibular Joint Disorders

Temporomandibular Joint Disorders (TMJD) are a heterogenous group of problems with only one common denominator—pain. Their incidence is not specifically known, and the reported signs and symptoms vary considerably, probably because of lack of a scientifically acceptable definition of TMJD.

The origin of TMJD symptoms can be traced to joint dysfunction or inflammation, muscle strain or spasm, trauma, significant malocclusion, and/or stress. In healthy adults, most recent evidence points to stress as a major contributor. Because existing therapeutic modalities seem to have similar results and biofeedback has longer-lasting effects when compared with splints, it is recommended that the most nonin-

vasive and the least expensive modality of treatment be used, with emphasis on stress control.

Specific signs and symptoms, such as clicking or popping of the TMJ, have never been proven reliable indicators of pathology in controlled studies. However, bruxism, clenching of the jaws, or grinding of the teeth should be identified and their diagnostic relevance evaluated.

Examination of the TMJ should include palpation of the immediate area, including the surrounding muscles of mastication, and movement of the condylar heads; assessment of maximum opening; and visual inspection for deviations of the mandible while opening and closing.

Required diagnostic data may include a thorough history, including behavioral assessment and clinical evaluation. Other diagnostic data such as tomography, transcranial radiography, and CT scanning have not been proven reliable under controlled conditions.

In pediatric patients, no good data are yet available, but muscle fatigue and spasm must be first ruled out. History of repetitive habits or activities must be evaluated. Examples include prolonged violin playing, computer games, clenching, grinding, and bruxism. As a general rule, the younger the child, the more likely it is that the pain is muscular in origin. Behavior modification, rest, and changing or modifying repetitive habits usually yield excellent results.

BIBLIOGRAPHY

Bhaskar SN: Oral lesions of infants and newborns, *Dent Clin North Am* July: 421-435, 1966.

Christensen RE Jr: Soft tissue lesions of the head and neck. In Sanders B, ed: *Pediatric oral and maxillofacial surgery,* St. Louis, 1979, Mosby.

Nazif MM, Ruffalo RC: The interaction between dentistry and otolaryngology, *Pediatr Clin North Am* 28(4):977-1010, 1981.

Rapp R: Dental and gingival disorders. In Bluestone CD, Stool SE, eds, *Pediatric otolaryngology,* ed 2, Philadelphia, 1990, Saunders.

Sanders B, et al: Injuries. In Sanders B, ed: *Pediatric oral and maxillofacial surgery,* St. Louis, 1979, Mosby.

Schuit KE, Johnson JT: Infections of the head and neck, *Pediatr Clin North Am* 28(4):965-971, 1981.

21

Orthopedics

W. TIMOTHY WARD & GREG BISIGNANI

HOLLY W. DAVIS & EDWARD N. HANLEY, JR.

hildren with musculoskeletal injuries and afflictions are brought for care because of pain, deformity, or loss of function. Often the clinical challenge lies not so much in recognizing the impaired or injured part, which in most cases is readily accessible to inspection and examination, but in making an accurate diagnosis in order to plan and initiate appropriate treatment. Because of their rapid physical growth and the special properties of their developing bones, children often pose special problems for the clinician.

Musculoskeletal problems in children fall into several general categories.

1. Trauma (discussed here and in Chapter 6).
2. Congenital problems—malformations resulting from genetic factors and from exposure to teratogens during the first trimester, as well as deformations stemming from insults later in pregnancy—many of which are associated with anomalies of other organ systems (discussed here and in Chapters 1, 2, and 15).
3. Infections (see Chapter 12).
4. Inflammatory processes such as the collagen vascular diseases, the vasculitides, rheumatic fever, and inflammatory bowel disease (see Chapters 7 and 10).
5. Metabolic diseases (see Chapters 9, 10, and 13).
6. Neoplastic disorders (see Chapter 11).

This chapter will focus on primary musculoskeletal problems and the discussion is divided into seven sections: (1) development of the skeletal system, (2) physical assessment, (3) musculoskeletal trauma, (4) disorders of the spine, (5) disorders of the upper extremity, (6) disorders of the lower extremity, and (7) generalized musculoskeletal disorders.

Development of the Skeletal System

The assessment, diagnosis, and management of pediatric orthopedic problems necessitate a clear understanding of the physiology of the growing musculoskeletal system and especially of the unique properties of growing bone. The process of growth begins in utero and continues until the end of puberty. Linear growth occurs as the result of multiplication of chondrocytes in the epiphyses, which align themselves vertically, forming a transitional zone of endochondral ossification in the metaphyses. The shafts of long bones widen and flat bones enlarge through the deposition and mineralization of osteoid by the periosteum. Hence, genetic and congenital disorders that affect connective tissue (and thus the skeleton) tend to cause abnormal growth. Most commonly this results in dwarfism, with varying degrees of deformity. However, in some conditions such as Marfan syndrome, excessive linear growth occurs, resulting in an abnormally tall stature and unusually long fingers and toes.

The terminal arterial loops and sinusoidal veins that form the vascular bed of growing metaphyses have sluggish blood flow, which increases the risk of thrombosis and of the deposition of bacteria during periods of bacteremia. As a result, there is a greater risk of developing hematogenous osteomyelitis in pediatric patients than in adults. Furthermore, the epiphyseal plates, which are incompletely formed in infancy, are a less effective barrier to extension of infection into adjacent joints, and the relatively thin diaphyseal cortices tend to permit rupture outward under the overlying periosteum. Similarly, penetration of vascular channels through the vertebral end-plates into the intervertebral discs makes discitis more likely than vertebral osteomyelitis in early childhood (see Chapter 12).

A thorough understanding of musculoskeletal development and of the radiographic findings at differing stages is particularly important in the diagnosis and management of orthopedic injuries. At birth only a few epiphyses have begun to ossify; the remainder are cartilaginous and thus are invisible radiographically. With development, other epiphyses begin to ossify, enlarge, and mature in such an orderly fashion that one can estimate a child's age from the number and configuration of ossification centers (Figs. 21-1 and 21-2). The epiphyseal plates (physes), which are sites of cartilaginous proliferation and growth, do not begin to ossify until puberty (Fig. 21-3). This process starts and ends earlier in girls than in boys. When skeletal injuries involve sites where ossification has not begun or is incomplete, radiographic findings may appear normal or may not reflect the full extent of the injury. This necessitates greater reliance on clinical findings.

Prior to closure of the physis during puberty, the growth plate is actually weaker than nearby ligaments. As a result, injuries that occur near joints are more likely to result in physeal disruption than in ligamentous tearing (i.e., sprains and dislocations are seen less commonly in prepubescent children than in adolescents). Similarly, avulsion fractures at sites where strong muscular attachments join secondary ossification centers are unique to children and adolescents. When there is

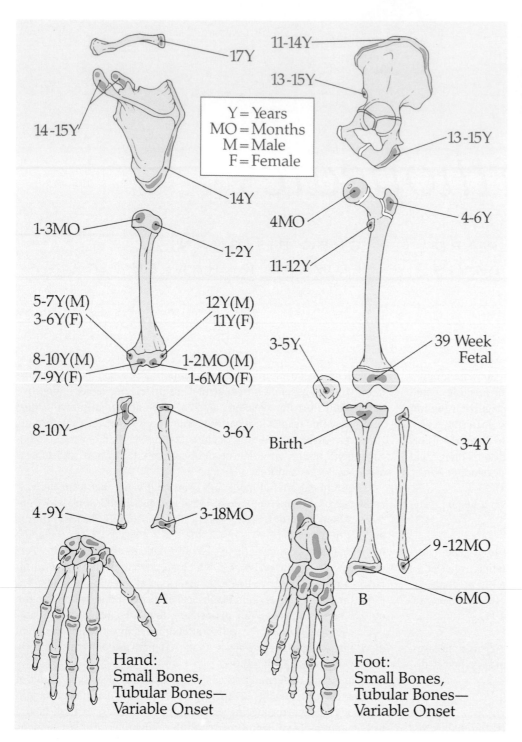

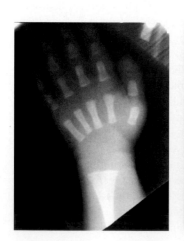
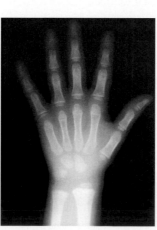
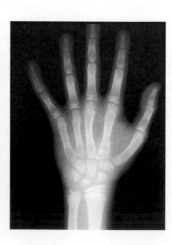

FIG. 21-1 Ages of onset of ossification. At birth only a few epiphyses have begun to ossify. The remainder are cartilaginous and therefore invisible radiographically. With development, other epiphyses begin to ossify, enlarge, and mature in an orderly fashion, making it possible to estimate a child's age from the number and configuration of ossification centers. This forms the basis for the use of bone age as part of the evaluation of children with growth disorders. When evaluating the radiographs of injured children, it is of crucial importance to bear in mind that fractures involving nonossified epiphyses are radiographically invisible until healing begins (see Fig. 21-55).

FIG. 21-2 Increasing numbers of ossification centers become radiographically visible with age. The hands shown are those of a toddler, a young school-age child, and a young adolescent. Injuries affecting unossified bones or growth centers are invisible radiographically.

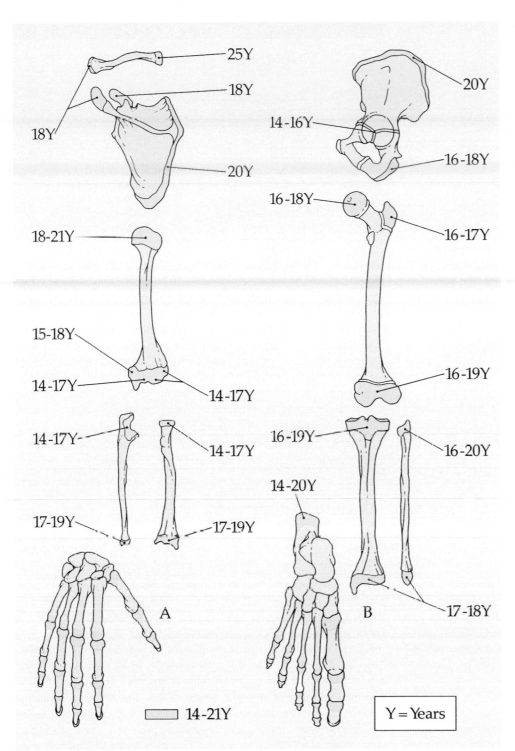

FIG. 21-3 Ages of physeal closure.

displacement of an epiphyseal fracture and the fragments are not anatomically reduced, growth disturbances may occur. Because the epiphysis may not be ossified, radiographs often may fail to reveal the injury, and for this reason, children with injuries at or near joints must be examined with meticulous care so that epiphyseal fractures are not missed.

The periosteum of a child is much thicker than that of an adult, strips more easily from the bone, and rarely is disrupted completely when the underlying bone is fractured. The immature, rapidly growing bone of the child is more porous and pliable than that of the adult and has a greater capacity for plastic deformation but less ability to withstand compressive or tensile forces. Consequently, a given compressive

force that would produce a comminuted fracture in an adult tends to be dissipated in a child in part by the bending that occurs in the more flexible bone of the child. Such a force is thus more likely to result in plastic deformation or to produce an incomplete fracture, such as a torus fracture or a greenstick fracture, in a child.

Thus, fracture patterns in children often differ from those in adults. Their fractures can be considerably harder to detect clinically and radiographically and can result in long-term growth abnormalities. Children do have advantages, however, in that their actively growing bones heal more rapidly and have a remarkable capacity for remodeling.

Finally, numerous genetic, metabolic, endocrine, renal, and inflammatory processes can have an effect not only on growth and ultimate height, but also on skeletal maturation—in some cases delaying it and in others accelerating it. Comparison of the patient's actual bone age, as determined by the number of radiographically visible ossification centers, with his or her chronologic age can help in the diagnosis of these underlying disorders.

Physical Assessment

History

Key historical points in the evaluation of problems not resulting from trauma include:

1. Age of onset of symptoms.
2. Mode of onset.
3. Clinical course, including the manner and rate of progression and associated signs and symptoms.
4. Past medical history with an emphasis on the prenatal and perinatal history in the infant or very young child.
5. Family history, especially of genetic, metabolic, and musculoskeletal problems.

This information helps considerably in narrowing the list of differential diagnostic possibilities.

When the patient's problem is the result of trauma, it is important to obtain the following historical points:

1. The time and place of the accident and whether it was witnessed.
2. The mechanism of injury, including the degree of force applied and the direction of force, if known (e.g., if a fall, from what height, onto what surface?; was the child running or walking [momentum]?; in what position did the child land?; was there any head injury or loss of consciousness?).
3. The child's behavior since the time of injury (e.g., decreased movement, guarding, refusal to walk or limp, any altered level of consciousness).
4. Complaint of pain (if so, how severe, and can it be localized?).
5. Prior treatment or first aid.
6. Past medical history of serious illness and prior injuries.
7. Family history of musculoskeletal problems.

This information helps localize the site or sites of injury and their potential severity, points to the risk of possible associated injuries, gives clues to the possible existence of underlying disorders that may predispose to injury, and may occasionally help raise a suspicion of abuse.

Physical Examination

The orthopedic examination involves a systematic assessment of posture, stance, gait; the symmetry or asymmetry of paired musculoskeletal structures and their motion; muscle strength and tone; and neurovascular status. In pediatrics, the patient's developmental level is a major consideration, not only in terms of the interpretation of findings, but also in terms of the manner in which the examination is conducted. Patience and often some degree of creativity are required on the part of the examiner if the patient is very young. Often, much information can be gleaned from an initial period of observation of the child's demeanor and spontaneous activity. This can be facilitated by providing age-appropriate toys for him or her to play with while the history is being taken and by engaging the patient in play (if circumstances permit) before starting the more formal physical examination. This also helps to alleviate anxiety and gain the child's trust, enhancing his or her cooperation. After spontaneous activity is observed, the relevant parts of the orthopedic examination typically are done by region.

A complete orthopedic examination that assesses every bone, muscle, joint, tendon, and ligament is very lengthy and detailed and rarely

TABLE 21-1

Grading of Muscle Strength

Grade	Physical finding
0/5	No movement seen
1/5	Muscle can move joint with gravity eliminated
2/5	Muscle can move joint against gravity but not against added resistance
3/5	Muscle can move joint against slight resistance
4/5	Muscle can move joint against moderate added resistance
5/5	Normal strength

indicated. Even in multiple-trauma victims and patients whose symptoms point toward an underlying systemic disorder, each region is screened and a full assessment done only of those regions where local musculoskeletal abnormalities are found. Similarly, in patients with focal injuries or deformities, the examination can generally be focused on the *region* involved, with the clinician bearing in mind referral patterns for pain and the maxim that all extremities "begin at the back." Finally, in performing routine physical examinations on healthy children, after a general screening examination of spontaneous movement, posture, gait, station, and stance, the assessment of the musculoskeletal system is focused on areas at risk for the child's age (e.g., the hip for dislocation in the neonate, the spine for scoliosis in the preadolescent and adolescent).

Regional Musculoskeletal Examination

In the regional examination, the area of concern is inspected visually for spontaneous movement, guarding, size, swelling, deformity, and the appearance of overlying skin and the findings compared with those for its paired structure. After this, the normal side, then the affected side, is gently palpated for warmth, induration, and tenderness. Muscle mass, tone, and reflexes on the affected side are compared with those on the normal side, and the presence or absence of spasm is noted. If asymmetry in muscle mass is detected, the circumference is measured bilaterally at a point equidistant from a fixed bony landmark. The child is then asked to move the extremity or handed objects to get him or her to do so, and active motion is observed. If this appears limited, passive range of motion is tested first on the normal then on the affected side, taking care not to cause severe pain. Strength is tested against gravity and then against resistance (Table 21-1), being careful to stay within the limits of pain, and sensation and vascular status are also evaluated.

Joints are further inspected to determine whether there is erythema, obliteration of landmarks that may indicate presence of effusion, evidence of deformity, and position of comfort. Further evaluation to detect joint effusion is done by pressing on one side of a visible joint while feeling for the protrusion of fluid on the other. The joints are palpated to look for evidence of heat and tenderness, range of motion is assessed, and evidence of pain on motion determined.

Assessment of ligamentous stability around joints is discussed under specific sections of the regional examination. However, in cases of acute trauma, especially when deformity or hemarthrosis are evident on initial assessment, tests of ligamentous stability should be deferred, the extremity splinted, and radiographs obtained to check for possible underlying fracture.

Trunk and Neck. With the examiner in front and the patient standing, the sternocleidomastoid muscles, the bony prominences of the

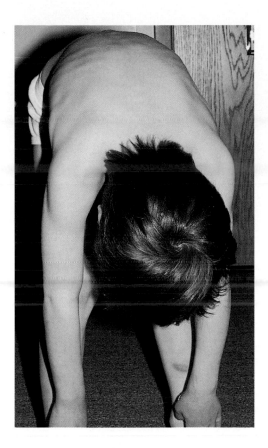

FIG. 21-4 Forward-bending test. Spinal curvature and rotation can be tested by having the patient bend over and touch his or her toes. The trunk should be viewed from behind and in front, observing the alignment of the spinous processes and checking for asymmetry of rib height.

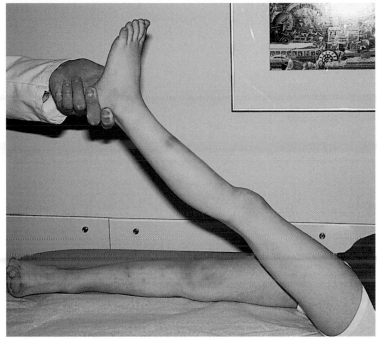

FIG. 21-5 Straight leg–raising test. With the patient supine, the limb to be tested is grasped behind the ankle and elevated into hip flexion with the knee in full extension. If pain is produced well before 90 degrees of flexion is achieved, the test is positive, indicating irritation of a sciatic nerve root.

clavicles, and the respective heights of the acromioclavicular joints, nipples, and anterior iliac crests and sides of the chest wall are inspected for symmetry. The patient is then turned and viewed from behind, and the shoulder and scapular height, the muscle bulk of the trapezius, and the height of the posterior iliac crests and of the depressions over the sacroiliac joints are checked for symmetry. Trapezius strength is determined by having the patient shrug his or her shoulders, first against gravity then against resistance, as the examiner presses down on the shoulders. The muscles supplying the scapula are tested by having the patient press his or her outstretched arms against a wall. Winging of the scapula during this maneuver is suggestive of weakness of the serratus anterior muscle. The line of the spinous processes of the vertebrae is observed for straightness, and the position of the head over the trunk is noted. Normally the head is aligned over the midline of the sacrum.

Next, the sternocleidomastoid and paraspinous muscles of the neck are palpated to assess for bulk, tone, tenderness, and spasm, and the spinous processes of the cervical vertebrae are palpated to assess for tenderness and step-off. In the immobilized trauma patient these observations are made largely with the patient supine on a back board, then log-rolled onto his or her side. It is important to recognize that, in checking for neck injury, the cervical spine can be cleared clinically if the patient is awake and alert and has no complaint of neck pain, no evidence of tenderness or paraspinous muscle spasm, and no extremely painful injury elsewhere. If the patient's level of consciousness is not normal or there is a major distracting injury, the cervical spine cannot be cleared, even if radiographic findings are normal, because spinal cord injury can be present in the absence of bony abnormalities.

Range of neck motion is assessed by having the patient move his or her head. A normal child can touch his or her chin to the chest, extend the neck to look directly above, and bend laterally to 45 degrees, and is capable of symmetrical lateral rotation when turning the head from side to side. Strength is tested by applying pressure to the forehead while the patient flexes his or her neck and to the occiput as the patient extends, and by applying resistance to the opposite side of the head as the patient bends and rotates laterally.

Thoracolumbar Spine. Viewed from the side, the normal child has a lordotic curve in the cervical area with a bony prominence at C7, a mild thoracic kyphosis, a lumbar lordosis, and a sacral kyphosis. Each patient is checked for the presence, absence, or accentuation of these curves. The midline of the back is inspected for evidence of abnormal pigmentation and the presence of hemangiomas, nevi, hairy tufts, dimples, masses, or defects, which may be associated with underlying bony or neural anomalies (see Chapter 15).

Flexion, extension, rotation, and lateral bending of the thoracolumbar spine are primarily motions of the thoracolumbar junction and the lumbar area. Most children can bend forward to touch their toes, bend laterally 20 to 30 degrees (with the pelvis held stable by the examiner's hands on the iliac crests), and rotate 20 to 30 degrees in either direction.

Inspection of the spinous processes with the trunk in forward flexion, the *Adam's forward-bending test,* is particularly useful for demonstrating the spinal curvature and rotation of scoliosis. This can be done from behind while the patient is bent forward with his or her arms hanging freely but should also be done while the examiner is seated in front of the child, thus enabling the examiner to control the forward bending by holding his or her hands together and slowly guiding the forward bend while observing the symmetry of rib height at each level of the spine (Fig. 21-4).

The spinous processes are palpated to evaluate alignment and look for evidence of tenderness or a step-off (suggesting absence of a spinous process with an underlying occult spina bifida). Next, the paraspinous muscles are palpated to detect evidence of any spasm and to locate areas of tenderness.

Any examination of the spine must include a neurologic assessment of strength, tone, reflexes, and sensation. The *straight leg–raising test* (Fig. 21-5) can be helpful in demonstrating nerve root pathology in patients with slipped discs, spinal or paraspinal masses, or inflammatory

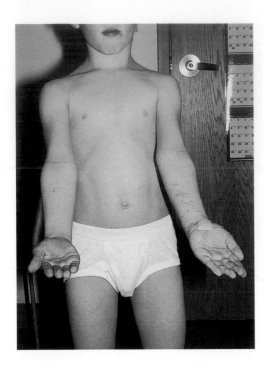

FIG. 21-6 Carrying angle. The normal relationship of the extended supinated forearm to the upper arm is not a straight line but involves 5 to 10 degrees of lateral or valgus angulation.

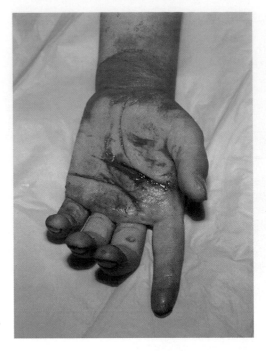

FIG. 21-7 Extensor tendon overpull. This boy's palm laceration involved the flexor tendons to his index finger. With his hand at rest, his index finger lies in extension, in contrast to his other fingers, which are partially flexed. (Courtesy Dr. Robert Hickey, Children's Hospital of Pittsburgh.)

processes. The test is performed with the patient lying supine on the examining table. The limb to be tested is grasped behind the ankle and elevated passively into hip flexion with the knee fully extended. This maneuver stretches the sciatic nerve as it passes behind the hip joint, and if one of its several roots has been irritated by a protruded disc, mass, or inflammatory process, pain will be felt with only 15 to 30 degrees of hip flexion. Normally the straight leg can be brought to 90 degrees of hip flexion without difficulty.

Upper Extremity

SHOULDER. When examining the shoulder, first the position of the upper limbs is observed, at the same time noting whether there is any swelling, asymmetry of height, or visible landmarks and looking for any difference in spontaneous movement. Prominent landmarks that are easily palpable include the acromion process lying laterally and subcutaneously, the clavicle, the spine of the scapula, the coracoid process, and the bicipital groove. Any displacement or tenderness of these structures should be noted. Swelling of the glenohumeral joint capsule and atrophy of the shoulder muscles are best appreciated by viewing from above with the patient seated and by comparison with the normal side.

It is important to assess range of motion because many shoulder problems are manifested by a loss of normal motion. The shoulder is a ball-and-socket joint with six components of movement. Abduction, a function of the deltoid muscle, is tested by having the patient raise the extended, supinated arm up so the hand is directly above the shoulder (180-degree abduction). To test adduction, the patient is asked to flex his or her shoulder to 20 to 30 degrees and then draw the upper arm diagonally across his or her body (75 degrees is normal). Flexion is assessed by having him or her raise the extended pronated arm up and forward until it is parallel to the floor; extension is tested by having him or her return the arm to the neutral position and then lift the arm up and backward (45 to 60 degrees is normal). To check rotation, the upper arm is held to the side with the elbow flexed to 90 degrees and the child is asked to turn the forearm toward the body (medial) and then out to the side (lateral) (60 to 90 degrees is normal).

ELBOW. In the normal relationship of the extended, supinated forearm to the upper arm, there is 5 to 10 degrees of lateral (valgus) angulation, denoted as the *carrying angle* (Fig. 21-6). When this angle is greater than 10 degrees, the deformity is termed *cubitus valgus*, and

when less or reversed, *cubitus varus* (gunstock deformity). The range of motion of the hinge joint of the elbow has four components: extension, a function of the triceps (normally to 0 degree of flexion); flexion, a function of the biceps (normally 145 degrees); supination (normally to 90 degrees); and pronation (80 to 90 degrees). The latter two components are tested by having the patient turn the palm up and down, respectively, with the elbow flexed.

Because of the proximity of the brachial artery and the median, radial, and ulnar nerves to the elbow joint, injuries of the elbow necessitate a careful neurovascular examination.

WRIST AND HAND. During examination of the wrist and hand, one should observe skin color, check capillary refill, and palpate the radial and ulnar pulses to assess circulation. Any swelling or edema should be noted, as well as any abnormal posture or position. The presence of intraarticular fluid in the wrist is manifested by swelling and tenderness, especially evident dorsally, and by restriction of wrist motion. Wrist motion has four components: flexion with the hand held down (normally 70 to 80 degrees), extension with the hand held up (normally 70 degrees), and ulnar and radial deviation (normally 25 degrees and 15 to 20 degrees, respectively).

Examination of hand function can be particularly challenging in young children because of lack of cooperation and developmental limitations. Observation of the position at rest (normally a loose fist with all the fingers pointing in the same direction and with the same degree of flexion) and of use during play is often helpful. Having the parent perform various hand and finger motions while trying to get the child to imitate these can be helpful in some cases. Handing the child a small object such as a key or a thin piece of paper such as a dollar bill may suffice for assessing opposition of thumb to fingers, which in the older child is tested by having him or her touch the tip of the thumb to the tip of the little finger. Normal ranges of motion in the hand are 90 degrees of flexion and 45 degrees of extension for the metacarpophalangeal joints, full extension and 100 degrees of flexion for the proximal interphalangeal joints (PIP), and full extension and 90 degrees of flexion for the distal interphalangeal joints.

Because the bones of the hand are subcutaneous, displaced fractures and dislocations are readily evident on inspection. Laceration or rupture of the tendons is common because of their superficial location. Those involving flexor tendons result in extensor tendon overpull

TABLE 21-2

Signs of Neural Dysfunction With Injury of the Upper Extremity

Nerve	Sign
Radial	↓ strength of wrist and finger extensors ↓ sensation in web space between thumb and index finger, dorsum of hand to proximal interphalangeal joints, and radial aspect of ring finger
Ulnar	↓ strength of wrist flexion and adduction ↓ strength of finger spread ↓ sensation over ulnar aspect of palm and dorsum of hand, little finger, and ulnar aspect of ring finger
Median	↓ strength of wrist flexion and abduction ↓ strength of flexion of proximal interphalangeal joints ↓ strength of opposition of thumb to base of little finger ↓ sensation over radial aspect of palm, thumb, index, and long fingers
Anterior interosseus	↓ strength of flexion of the distal interphalangeal joints of the index finger and thumb

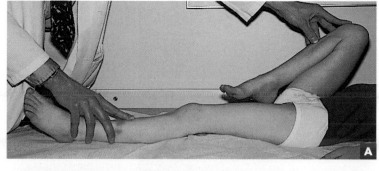
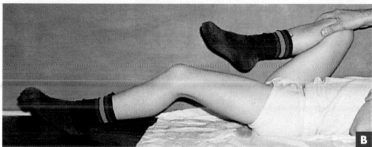

FIG. 21-8   Thomas test. This test of range of hip extension is performed by flexing both hips, then holding one in flexion while the patient is asked to extend the other leg. *A,* Normally full extension is achieved. *B,* Inability to fully extend the hip, seen in this boy with Legg-Calvé-Perthe disease, indicates the presence of a flexion contracture of the hip and constitutes a positive Thomas test.

(Fig. 21-7), with the affected digit lying in greater extension than its neighbors at rest. Conversely, extensor tendon lacerations result in flexor muscle overpull, with the opposite result.

Functional testing of the tendons and intrinsic muscles of the hand is generally possible in older children. They can be asked to extend the fingers at the metacarpophalangeal joints and each interphalangeal joint. Function of the flexor digitorum profundus muscle is tested by holding the PIP joint extended while the patient flexes the tip of the finger. To test the superficialis flexor tendon, adjacent distal interphalangeal joints are held in extension and the patient is asked to flex the finger being tested at the PIP joint. The intrinsic muscles of the hand are evaluated by having the child adduct and abduct the fingers toward and away from the middle finger. Sensation is best tested using two-point discrimination and pinprick in older children and by touch in very young children.

Muscle strength in the upper extremity is largely tested during assessment of range of motion of the joints, with and without resistance. Signs of neural dysfunction with injury of the upper extremity are listed in Table 21-2.

Lower Extremity

HIP. Examination of the hip begins by assessing gait (see later discussion) and stance, checking the latter to see if the anterior superior and posterior superior iliac spines and the greater trochanters are level. If not, a leg-length discrepancy should be suspected and leg length measured. Total length is measured from the bottom of the anterior superior iliac spine to the medial malleolus of the ankle with the patient supine. If inequality is found, the knees are flexed to 90 degrees with the feet flat on the examination table. If as the examiner looks from the foot of the examination table one knee appears higher than the other, the tibias are unequal in length; if one knee is anterior to the other when viewed from the side, the discrepancy involves the femurs. If total leg lengths are equal, the inequality apparent when the patient is standing may be due to pelvic obliquity or flexion contracture of the

hip. The latter may also be associated with a compensatory accentuation of lumbar lordosis.

The thighs are checked next for symmetry and signs of atrophy. If atrophy is found, circumference should be measured and compared at a fixed point below the greater trochanters.

Because the hip lies deep and is surrounded by muscles, direct inspection is impossible and palpation is of limited value (though the femoral triangle, greater trochanter, and posterior aspect should be palpated to check for tenderness). As a result, assessment of the position of comfort (abduction and external rotation are seen with effusion, hemarthrosis, and fracture [see Figs. 21-14, *C,* and 21-87, *B*]), weight-bearing, range of motion, and pain on motion is particularly important (for hip examination in the neonate, see section on Congenital Dislocation of the Hip).

In assessing range of motion of the hip, care must be taken to distinguish true hip motion from that occurring in combination with pelvic rotation or trunk flexion. The range of hip flexion is normally about 120 degrees. It is tested with the child lying supine. The hip to be tested is passively flexed while the contralateral hip and pelvis are observed or stabilized by one hand. The limit of flexion is reached when movement of the contralateral pelvis is noted. Alternatively, both hips can be flexed simultaneously to stabilize the pelvis and eliminate truncal flexion. The *Thomas test* is performed by flexing both hips so that the thighs touch the abdomen. Then one is held in place, thereby eliminating lumbar lordosis and movement of the lumbosacral joint, and the patient is asked to extend the hip to be tested. Normally he or she should be able to extend the hip to 0 degree of flexion (Fig. 21-8, *A*). Failure to do this indicates the presence of a hip flexion contracture, which is a positive Thomas test (Fig. 21-8, *B*). Next the knee and thigh are held with the hip and knee flexed to 90 degrees and internal and external rotation are tested and recorded in degrees. Abduction and adduction are also checked with the hip flexed to 90 degrees. While the examiner places the thumb and index finger of one

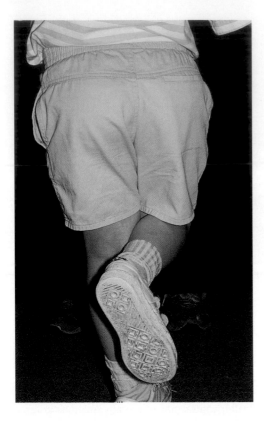

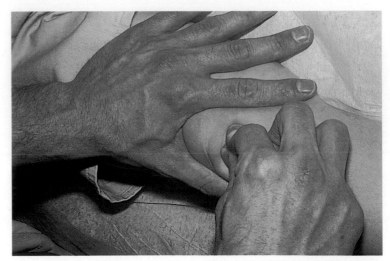

FIG. 21-9 Trendelenburg test. This test is performed to check for weakness of the hip abductors. While lifting his right foot, this patient's left abductor muscles stabilize his pelvis with a slight rise of the pelvis on the right. If left hip abductor weakness were present, the right pelvis would tilt downward when the right leg is lifted.

FIG. 21-10 Test for small knee joint effusions. Moderate pressure is applied over the suprapatellar pouch with the thumb and index finger of one hand, milking any fluid present downward. The other hand simultaneously pushes the patella up toward the femur. When an effusion is present, the patella becomes ballotable and a palpable click is felt as the patella strikes the front of the distal femur.

hand over the patient's pelvis, attempting to span the distance between the anterior superior iliac spines, the hip to be tested is abducted and then adducted. The limit is determined by the point at which the pelvis begins to move (normally 45 degrees of abduction and 30 degrees of adduction). Extension is tested with the patient prone by having him or her lift the leg up from the table (normal, 20 to 30 degrees). Internal and external rotation are also tested with the patient prone and the hip and leg in extension.

When hip abductor weakness is suspected on the basis of the finding of a gait abnormality, the *Trendelenburg test* (Fig. 21-9) is performed. This involves having the child stand and asking him or her to lift one leg up. Normally the pelvis should rise slightly on the side of the leg that is lifted. If instead it drops, abductor weakness is present on the opposite side, and the Trendelenburg test is positive.

Knee. It is important to bear in mind that knee pain is a common reason for seeking orthopedic care and that it is often referred from the hip, thus any patient presenting with knee pain should always be examined for possible limitation of hip motion or pain on motion of the hip.

The knee examination begins with the examiner viewing the joint from the front, side, and back, looking for differences in contour, swelling or masses, and changes in overlying skin. From the front, the knee is inspected for valgus (lower leg points away from the midline) or varus (lower leg deviates toward the midline) deformity and for evidence of effusion, manifested by obliteration of the normal depressions around the patella or by generalized swelling. In viewing the knee from its lateral aspect, the examiner looks for incomplete extension resulting from flexion contracture or excess hyperextension (recurvatum deformity), as well as for symmetry of the tibial tuberosities. From the rear, the popliteal fossae are checked for symmetry and evidence of swelling. The thighs are also observed for comparative size and contour.

The knees are palpated to assess warmth and check for tenderness along the medial and lateral joint lines, the medial and collateral ligaments, the patella and its supporting ligaments, the femoral and tibial condyles, and the tibial tubercles. Palpation is easier with the knee

flexed because the skeletal landmarks are more readily seen and felt, and the muscles, tendons, and ligaments are relaxed in this position.

When there is evidence of a marked effusion, landmarks are obscured and the patella is readily ballotable. This is seen with intraarticular hemorrhage, arthritis, and synovitis, and range of motion is usually significantly limited. If landmarks are only mildly obscured (suggestive of a mild joint effusion or fluid collection in the bursae), pressure should be applied over the suprapatellar pouch with the thumb and index finger of one hand milking down any fluid present while simultaneously pushing the patella up toward the femoral condyles with the other hand (Fig. 21-10). If fluid is present, the patella is ballotable and a palpable click is noted as the patella strikes the front of the femur.

The knee is primarily a hinge joint and is normally capable of 130 to 140 degrees of flexion and 5 degrees of hyperextension. However, it can also rotate approximately 10 degrees internally and externally, and this involves rotation of the tibia on the femur. Flexion is tested with the patient either sitting or lying prone. To test extension, the examiner can either have the patient sit and try to straighten the leg to 0 degree of flexion or try to lift the straightened leg from the examination table while lying supine. Rotation is assessed by turning the foot medially and then laterally with the knee flexed.

With the knees flexed to 80 to 90 degrees, the patellas should face forward when viewed from the front and be located squarely at the ends of the femurs when seen from the side. The *apprehension test* (Fig. 21-11) is performed to check for a subluxating or dislocating patella. With the patient sitting, the examiner supports the lower leg and holds the knee flexed to 30 degrees. The patella is then gently pushed laterally. Any abnormal amount of lateral displacement, pain, or apprehension in response to this maneuver indicates a positive test.

Ligamentous stability of the knee should be assessed in the mediolateral and anteroposterior planes. In patients with acute injuries, especially those involving significant pain and swelling, this should be deferred until x-rays have been obtained to check for associated fractures.

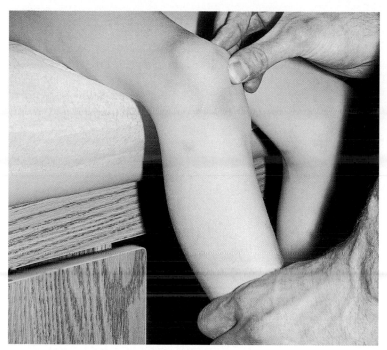

FIG. 21-11 Apprehension test for a subluxing or dislocating patella. With the patient sitting and the knee supported in 30 degrees of flexion, the patella is gently pushed laterally. Any abnormal amount of lateral displacement, pain, or apprehension constitutes a positive test.

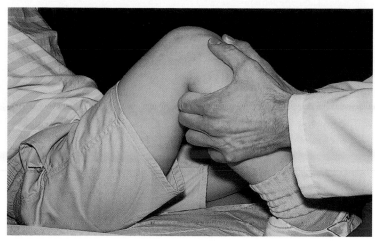

FIG. 21-12 Anterior and posterior draw tests for cruciate ligament stability. With the patient supine, the hips flexed to 45 degrees, and the knees flexed to 90 degrees, the examiner grasps the proximal tibia with his or her fingers behind the knee and thumbs on the anterior joint line and makes a gentle pull-push motion. Forward movement of more than 0.5 to 1 cm indicates anterior cruciate instability, representing a positive anterior draw test. Similar posterior motion on pushing indicates posterior cruciate instability, representing a positive posterior draw test.

The *abduction/adduction stress test* is used to determine the degree of stability of the medial and lateral collateral ligaments. With the supine patient's thigh moved to the side of the examination table and the knee flexed to 30 degrees, the examiner holds the distal thigh in one hand while grasping the inside of the lower leg with the other. To test the medial collaterals, the examiner applies valgus stress by pressing medially against the distal thigh with the upper hand while gently abducting the lower leg. To check the lateral collaterals, the examiner applies varus stress by pressing laterally on the inside of the distal thigh while gently adducting the lower leg. Normally the joint line should open no more than 1 cm on either side.

Anteroposterior ligamentous stability is provided by the anterior and posterior cruciate ligaments of the knee. They are tested by the *anterior and posterior draw* and *Lachman* tests. The former are performed with the patient supine, the hip and knee flexed to 45 and 90 degrees respectively, and the foot planted on the examining table, stabilized by the examiner's thigh or buttock. The examiner then grasps the proximal tibia with his or her fingers behind the knee and the thumbs over the anterior joint line and gently pulls and pushes (Fig. 21-12). In a positive anterior draw test, the tibia moves forward more than 0.5 to 1 cm, indicating instability of the anterior cruciate ligament. Movement backward more than 0.5 to 1 cm indicates instability of the posterior cruciate ligament. In the *Lachman test* (Fig. 21-13) for anterior cruciate tears, the knee is flexed to 15 degrees. The examiner grasps the distal femur with one hand and the proximal tibia with the other. The thumb of the lower hand is placed on the joint line and the femur is pushed backward as the tibia is pulled forward. Abnormal anterior displacement of the tibia on the femur can be seen and felt if instability is present. The amount of excursion is estimated in millimeters, and the endpoint is recorded as soft or firm.

ANKLE. Examination of the ankle begins with inspection for evidence of deformity, swelling, change in color of overlying skin, and abnormal position (especially with weight bearing). Palpation is performed to detect warmth and localize tenderness. In the neutral posi-

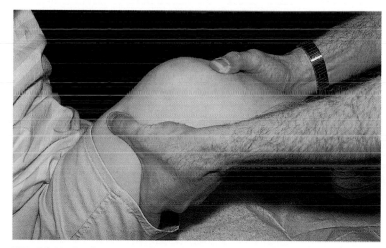

FIG. 21-13 Lachman test for anterior cruciate ligament tear. With the knee flexed to 15 degrees, the distal femur is grasped with one hand and the proximal tibia with the other, with the thumb on the joint line. The tibia is moved forward while the femur is pushed backward. Any abnormal displacement of the tibia on the femur indicates anterior cruciate instability and represents a positive test.

tion, the long axis of the foot should be at 90 degrees to the long axis of the tibia. Normally a child can dorsiflex 20 degrees and plantar flex 30 to 50 degrees from the neutral position, as well as invert and evert approximately 5 degrees. Dorsiflexion and plantar flexion can be checked by observing passive and active motion (with and without resistance) but are perhaps most easily tested by having the ambulating child walk on his or her heels and toes respectively. Similarly, inversion is tested by having him or her walk on the outside of the feet and eversion by having him or her walk on the medial sides.

Tests for ligamentous instability can be important following severe ankle sprains. The *anterior draw test* is used to assess the stability of the anterior talofibular ligament. With the patient's legs dangling over the side of the examination table and the foot in a few degrees of plantar flexion, the examiner grasps the anterior aspect of the distal tibia with one hand while holding the calcaneus cupped in the palm of the other. The calcaneus is then drawn anteriorly while the tibia is pushed posteriorly. Normally there should be no movement, but with instability of the anterior talofibular ligament, the talus slides anteriorly. Lateral instability is seen only with major tears of the anterior talofibular and calcaneofibulare ligaments, occasionally accompanied by tears of the posterior talofibular ligament, and is tested by inverting the calcaneus with one hand while grasping the distal tibia with the other. When present, the talus gaps and rocks in the ankle mortise. Medial instability is exceptionally rare because of the strength of the fan-shaped deltoid ligament. To test for medial instability, the tibia and calcaneus are held in the same manner as they are in testing lateral instability, but the foot is everted instead. Gross gaping of the ankle mortise is felt when there is a major tear.

Gait and Gait Disturbances

Between the onset of walking and 3 years of age, children tend to have a wide-based gait and toddlers often hold their arms out to the side to assist balance. By 3 years of age, children achieve a normal smooth and rhythmic heel-to-toe gait, consisting of two main phases: stance and swing. The stance phase begins when the heel strikes the ground, bears all the weight, and progresses to foot flat, midstance, and push-off as weight is transferred from the heel to the metatarsal heads. The swing phase starts with acceleration after push-off and progresses through midswing to deceleration just before heel strike. During the swing phase, as the leg moves forward, so does the opposite arm. Because stance occupies 60% of the time and weight is borne in this phase, most gait disorders are more evident during the stance phase than during the swing phase. Normally the distance between the two heels (width of the base) is between 5 and 10 cm, the pelvis and trunk shift laterally about 2.5 cm from stance to stance, the center of gravity rises and falls no more than 5 cm, and the pelvis rotates forward about 40 degrees during swing.

Gait is best observed by having the patient walk back and forth in a hall or in a room with a mirror at one end. As the patient walks, the examiner focuses first on overall movement and then on the motion of the pelvis, hips, thighs, knees, lower legs, ankles, and feet in succession, both coming and going. In doing so, he or she looks for the pattern of heel-to-toe motion, for shortening of the stance phase, for evidence of limitation of joint motion or weakness, and for positional changes of the extremities. Checking the patient's shoes for signs of abnormal wear is also helpful.

Most acute and many chronic disturbances of gait in childhood are caused by pain. Others stem from weakness or spasticity caused by neurologic or muscular disorders, from leg-length inequality, or from deformity. Important historical points are the time of onset of the abnormal gait and the circumstances surrounding it; the duration; whether the abnormal gait is constant or intermittent and, if intermittent, the time of tday it is most apparent (A.M., juvenile rheumatoid arthritis; P.M., neuromuscular disorders—symptoms becoming more apparent with fatigue); and its relation to activity or exercise, including its effect on running or climbing stairs. The examiner should note any associated pain and its location, bearing in mind referral patterns (low back to buttocks and lateral thigh; hip to groin, medial thigh, knee and sometimes buttock) and attempting to determine whether the pain is constant (suggestive of tumor or infection) or intermittent.

Gait Disturbances Stemming from Pain, Limb Length Inequality, or Stiffness. An *antalgic gait* is a limp caused by pain on weight-bearing that results in shortening of the stance phase on the affected side. It can be due to pain referred from the back or pain anywhere in the lower ex-

tremity. Causes include trauma, pathologic fracture, infection, inflammatory disorders and other sources of arthritis, malignancy, tight shoes, foreign body in the shoe, and a lesion on the sole of the foot. Careful physical examination combined with a complete history usually enables localization of the problem.

Patients with leg-length inequality manifest depression of the trunk and pelvis during the stance phase on the shorter leg and circumduction of the longer leg during swing. Some try to compensate for the leg-length inequality by toe walking on the shorter extremity.

Patients with limited hip motion compensate by thrusting the pelvis and trunk forward in the swing phase. When knee flexion is limited, children tend to hike up the pelvis on the involved side during the swing phase and circumduct the leg to clear their foot from the floor. A *circumduction gait* can also be related to a painful condition involving the ankle or a limitation of ankle motion. By circumducting the leg laterally during swing phase, the patient reduces the need for ankle motion.

Gait Disturbances Resulting from Weakness or Spasticity. Patients with weakness of the hip abductors (gluteus medius muscle) have a *Trendelenburg gait.* Because they are unable to maintain a level pelvis and linear progression of their center of gravity, their pelvis tilts toward the unsupported side and their shoulder lurches toward the weak side during stance phase to maintain their center of gravity over the foot. Patients with weakness of the gluteus maximus (seen most commonly in children with Duchenne muscular dystrophy) have to hyperextend their trunk and pelvis to maintain their center of gravity posterior to the hip joint. Children with weakness of the quadriceps femoris muscle may have a relatively normal gait on level ground but have difficulty climbing stairs. Weakness of the dorsiflexors of the foot results in foot drop and a *steppage gait.* Because the foot hangs down during swing phase, the patient must lift the knee higher than usual to help the foot clear the floor and the forefoot tends to slap the floor on impact, because smooth deceleration of the foot cannot be controlled. When the plantar flexors are weak, the patient is unable to push off at the end of the stance phase and so the heel and forefoot come off the floor at the same time.

An *equine gait,* characterized by toe walking or a toe-to-heel sequence during the stance phase, is seen in children with heel cord contracture and limited dorsiflexion. It is usually indicative of an underlying neurologic problem with spasticity. Patients with spastic cerebral palsy who are able to ambulate often manifest a stiff-legged *scissors gait,* in which one foot crosses over the other during the swing phase. Vestibular or cerebellar dysfunction or generalized weakness tend to result in a wide-based ataxic gait because of abnormal balance. Absence of the normal arm swing with walking is seen in patients with paresis or cerebellar disease.

Intoeing and Outtoeing. The angular difference between the long axis of the foot and the forward line of progression during walking is called the *foot progression angle.* A minus value is assigned to intoeing, a plus value to outtoeing. The normal range varies from 5 to 10 degrees to 10 to 20 degrees. Femoral anteversion, internal tibial torsion, and metatarsus adductus are common causes of excessive intoeing, or pigeon toe, and femoral eversion and external tibial torsion are common causes of outtoeing, or "slew foot."

Musculoskeletal Trauma

The normal impulsiveness and inquisitiveness of children combined with their lack of caution and love of energetic activities place them at a relatively high risk for accidental injury. The incidence of trauma is further increased by the prevalence of child abuse (see Chapter 6). In fact, beyond infancy, trauma is the leading cause of death in children

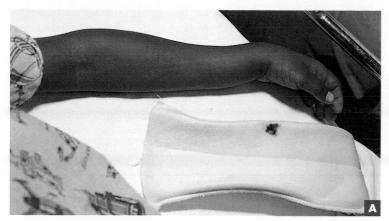

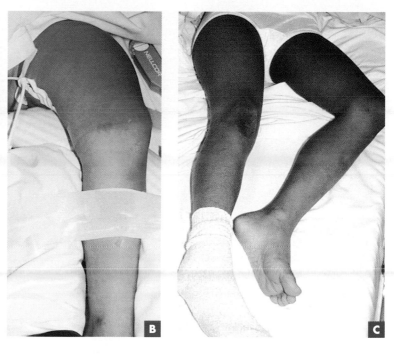

FIG. 21-14 Visible abnormalities seen on inspection in children with fractures. *A,* Distortion and angulation of the distal forearm in a child with fractures of the radius and ulna. *B,* Swelling and angulation of the proximal thigh resulting from a femur fracture. *C,* Longitudinal shortening of the thigh in a child with a proximal femur fracture. Note the characteristic externally rotated position of the injured leg. The child was struck by a car, sustaining a fracture of the femoral neck.

and adolescents and is the source of significant morbidity. Musculoskeletal injuries are very common, whether seen in isolation or as part of multisystem trauma. Although the management of life-threatening injuries to the airway, circulation, and central nervous system (CNS) must take precedence over treatment of accompanying musculoskeletal injuries in cases of multiple trauma, it must be kept in mind that fractures can result in significant blood loss. This is particularly true of pelvic and femoral fractures. Furthermore, prompt attention must be given to assessment of the status of neurovascular structures distal to obvious fractures, because failure to recognize compromise may result in permanent loss of function. Finally, traumatic hip dislocations must be reduced within 6 to 12 hours if the risk of aseptic necrosis and long-term morbidity is to be minimized.

Fractures

Diagnosis

One of the many variables that complicate the diagnosis of the skeletally injured child is that the child, already in pain, is frightened by his or her recent experience and by the strangeness of the hospital or emergency room setting. Many children are too young to give a firsthand history, and the cooperation of toddlers is often limited. The parents are likely to be anxious as well. A calm, empathetic manner is needed to allay their fears. Taking a thorough history before making any attempt to perform a physical assessment will help the examiner establish rapport with the patient and the family. This should include questions concerning the type and direction of the injuring force, the position of the involved extremity at the time of the accident, and the events immediately following the injury, such as measures taken at the scene of the accident. The presence of underlying disorders and the possibility of contamination of an open wound should be determined as well. Physicians also should be alert to signs suggestive of inflicted injury or child abuse.

In cases of suspected fracture, splinting, elevation, and topical application of ice may help reduce discomfort and local swelling. Splinting is particularly important for displaced and unstable fractures because it prevents further soft tissue injuries and reduces the risk of fat embolization. When pain is moderate to severe and there are no car-

diovascular or CNS contraindications, analgesia should be administered promptly. Contrary to the opinion of many physicians, this does not obscure physical findings. Tenderness will not be reduced significantly, swelling will remain, and patient cooperation during the examination may be considerably greater.

Before beginning the physical examination, it is wise for the examiner to talk with the child to further gain his or her trust. Older infants and toddlers are often more comfortable when allowed to sit on a parent's lap, and use of puppets or toys can reduce fear and help gain their cooperation. Because comparison of paired extremities is an integral part of orthopedic assessment, it is best to begin by examining the uninjured side and it is wise to defer palpation of the most likely site of the injury on the affected side until last. If young children are highly anxious, it can be useful to instruct the parent in how to perform passive range of motion and palpation.

The first step in the physical examination is visual inspection of the injured area. The gross position of the extremity should be noted, and attention given to the presence or absence of deformity, distortion or abnormal angulation, and longitudinal shortening (Fig. 21-14). The overlying skin and soft tissues are examined for evidence of swelling, ecchymoses, abrasions, punctures, and lacerations. Comparison with the opposite extremity and measurement of circumference can be very helpful when findings are subtle.

The location of open wounds is important in ascertaining whether an underlying fracture is open or closed and in assessing the risk of joint penetration. Small puncture wounds or lacerations overlying bony structures from which a bloody, fatty exudate is oozing usually reflect communication with the medullary cavity of a fractured bone. Similarly, punctures or tears over joints that weep serous or serosanguineous fluid, especially when drainage is increased on moving the joint, must be assumed to communicate with the joint capsule (Fig. 21-15, *A*). In patients with penetrating joint injuries, radiographs may demonstrate air in the joint, but absence of this does not rule out capsular penetration (Fig. 21-15, *B*). Probing of open wounds that are highly likely to communicate with a fracture or a joint is contraindicated. The wound should be cleaned and covered with a sterile dressing until its extent can be determined under sterile conditions in the operating room.

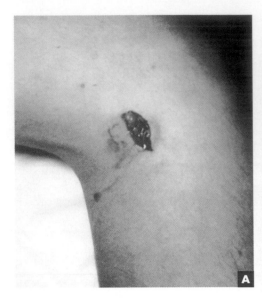

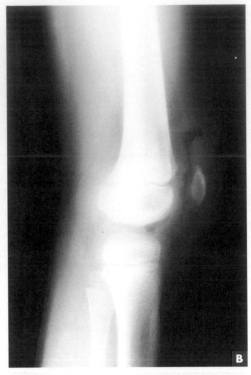

FIG. 21-15 *A,* Penetrating injury of the knee. This child was struck by a stone propelled by the blades of a power lawn mower. Though the laceration appeared to be minor, serosanguinous fluid flowed from it on movement of the knee, suggesting penetration of the joint capsule. This was confirmed on exploration in the operating room. *B,* Air is seen within the knee joint and in the overlying soft tissues in a child who sustained a deep laceration that penetrated the joint capsule. (*A* courtesy Dr. Bruce Watson.)

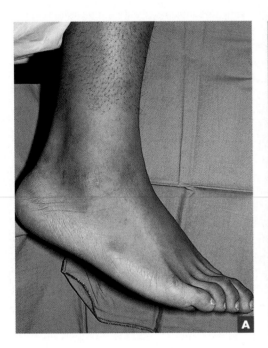

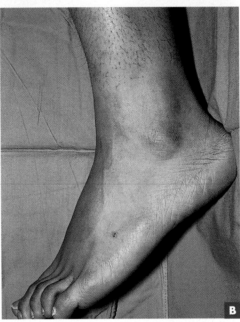

FIG. 21-16 Salter-Harris type I fracture of the distal fibula. *A,* Slight swelling is present over the lateral malleolus. The degree of swelling can only be truly appreciated by comparing the injured ankle to its normal counterpart, shown in *B.* The patient had point tenderness over the affected malleolus. The findings differ from those seen in an ankle sprain, in which tenderness and swelling are greatest over the ligaments inferior to the malleolus (see Fig. 21-63).

After inspection of the most obviously injured area, palpation and assessment of active and passive motion can be performed. It is crucial to remember that in examining an injured limb the entire extremity must be evaluated in order to detect less obvious associated injuries. Localized swelling and tenderness on palpation are significant findings and should alert the examiner to the high likelihood of an underlying fracture. Pain on motion and limitation of motion signal the need for careful scrutiny as well. Assessment of motion involves observation of spontaneous movement, attempts to get the patient to voluntarily move the involved part through its expected range, and passive movement. Particular attention should be paid to the adjacent proximal and distal joints to avoid missing associated injuries. It can be difficult, however, to determine whether motion is limited because of pain, an associated injury, or fear and lack of cooperation.

Clinical findings vary depending on the nature of the fracture. Undisplaced growth plate fractures typically present with mild, localized swelling and point tenderness at the level of the epiphysis (Fig. 21-16). Because ligamentous injury is relatively uncommon in a child, the finding of point tenderness should suffice to prompt treating the injury as a fracture until proven otherwise. Often initial radiographs appear normal and the fracture is confirmed only on follow-up when repeat radiographs disclose evidence of healing. Swelling is typically mild and occasionally imperceptible in cases of torus or buckle fractures and of undisplaced transverse and spiral fractures. Careful palpation should disclose focal tenderness, however. Usually, the patient also experiences some degree of discomfort on motion in some planes or on weight bearing, but it must be remembered that limitation of movement or function can be minimal in patients with such incomplete frac-

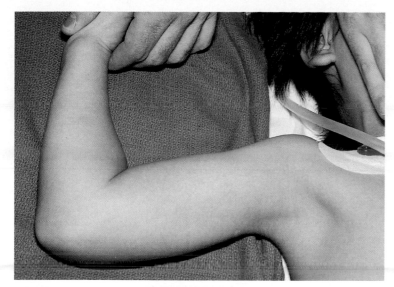

FIG. 21-17 Fracture with overlying soft tissue swelling. This child has a displaced supracondylar fracture of the distal humerus with moderate soft tissue swelling. The degree of swelling becomes evident if the size of the elbow area is compared with the size of the patient's wrist.

tures. In contrast, fractures that completely disrupt the bone and displaced fractures are accompanied by more prominent swelling, more diffuse tenderness, and severe pain, which is markedly increased on motion (Figs. 21-14, *A* and *B*, and 21-17). Crepitus may also be evident on gentle palpation. In examining children with these findings, manipulation must be kept to a minimum to prevent further injury.

Assessment of neurovascular function distal to the injury is essential in evaluating any child with a potential fracture. This includes checking the integrity of pulses and speed of capillary refill as well as testing sensory and motor function. Strength and sensation should be compared to those of the contralateral extremity. Assessment of two-point discrimination is probably the best test of sensory function. Evidence of neurovascular compromise necessitates urgent, often operative, orthopedic treatment. In addition, this assessment is crucial before and after reduction of displaced fractures to determine if the procedure itself has impaired function in any way. Persistence of intense pain following fracture reduction should provoke suspicion of ischemia.

Supracondylar fractures of the humerus, fractures of the distal femoral shaft and proximal tibia, fracture-dislocations of the elbow and knee, and severely displaced ankle fractures are particularly likely to be associated with neurovascular injury.

Even relatively minor fractures of the tibia, forearm bones, metatarsals, and femur can result in *compartment syndrome,* in which bleeding and edema collection within a closed fascial compartment produce increased pressure that causes neurovascular compromise and muscle ischemia. This should be strongly suspected in patients who complain of intense pain that is aggravated by passive stretching of the muscles. On palpation the area is noted to be swollen and tense, at times even hard. The patient may complain of paresthesias and show pallor and decreased pulses. However, it is important to also be aware of the fact that vascular compromise can be present in a patient who has normal distal pulses and good peripheral perfusion (see section on Compartment Syndromes).

In all cases of suspected extremity fractures, the injured part should be properly splinted and elevated and an ice pack applied while the patient awaits transport to the radiography suite. However, to obtain high-quality radiographs, obstructing splints must be removed temporarily.

This presents no major problem in patients with partial or nondisplaced fractures but can create difficulties in patients with severe displaced fractures. To ensure that manipulation is minimal in these patients, splint removal, positioning for radiographs, and splint reapplication should be supervised by a physician and not done merely at the discretion of the x-ray technician.

At a minimum, two radiographs taken at 90-degree angles are obtained, anteroposterior and lateral views being the most common. Oblique views are helpful in fully disclosing the nature and extent of many fracture patterns, especially when the injury involves the ankle, elbow, hand, or foot. They can also prove useful in detecting subtle spiral fractures and in cases in which the anteroposterior (AP) and lateral views are normal, yet a fracture is strongly suspected. Radiographs should include the joints immediately proximal and distal to a fractured long bone, because there may be associated bony or soft tissue injuries in these areas as well. Such associated injuries easily can be missed on clinical examination when assessment of motion is limited by pain or when patient cooperation is limited. It is necessary to obtain comparison views of the opposite side, especially when evaluating patients with suspected physeal injuries who may have very subtle radiographic abnormalities. These views can also prove invaluable in detecting cortical disruptions. In some cases of displaced or angulated fractures, potentially complex intraarticular fractures, and vertebral and pelvic fractures, a computed tomographic (CT) scan can be useful. A bone scan may be necessary to detect subtle stress fractures.

Particular care should be taken in interpreting pediatric radiographs because of the high incidence of subtle or even normal findings in patients with fractures. If the clinical picture strongly suggests a fracture, appropriate treatment should be initiated, even if the radiograph appears normal. Reassessment in 1 to 2 weeks can then clarify the exact nature of the injury.

Fracture Patterns

Fractures should be described in terms of anatomic location, direction of the fracture line, type of fracture, and degree of angulation and of displacement. When the growth plate is involved, use of the Salter-Harris classification system is recommended.

Any specific mechanism of injury results in a readily definable pattern of force application, which tends to produce a typical fracture pattern. Because of this, it is often possible to infer the likely mechanism of injury once the fracture pattern is documented radiographically. If the vector of the direct force is perpendicular to the bone, a transverse fracture is most likely to result, whereas direct force applied at any angle to the bone produces an oblique fracture pattern. Examples of situations resulting in transverse and short oblique fractures include falls in which an extremity strikes the edge of a table, counter, or chair; direct blows with an object such as a stick; and karate chops. These fractures are commonly seen as a result of accidents or fights and in the battered child syndrome. Comminuted fractures generally result from high-velocity, direct forces, such as those characteristic of vehicular accidents, falls from heights, or gunshot wounds. Impacted fractures are produced by forces oriented in a direction parallel to the long axis of the bone. Application of indirect force commonly results in spiral, greenstick, or torus fractures in children.

A common example of a nondisplaced spiral fracture is the *toddler's fracture* (see Fig. 21-42), which results from a fall with a twist. Typically, the child either was running, turned, and then fell; jumped and fell with a twist; or got his foot caught and fell while twisting to extricate himself. If a child's arm or leg is forcibly pulled and twisted, a similar fracture pattern may be seen. Greenstick and torus fractures of the radius or ulna are incurred usually when the child falls on an outstretched arm with the wrist dorsiflexed. Vigorous repetitive shaking

TABLE 21-3

Patterns of Fractures

Fracture pattern	Major feature	Radiographic appearance
Longitudinal	Fracture line is parallel to the axis of a long bone	Fig. 21-18
Transverse	Fracture line is perpendicular to the axis of a long bone	Fig. 21-19
Oblique	Fracture line is at an angle relative to the axis of a bone	Fig. 21-20
Spiral	Fracture line takes a curvilinear course around the axis of a bone	Fig. 21-21
Impacted	Bone ends are crushed together, producing an indistinct fracture line	Fig. 21-22
Comminuted	Fracturing forces produce more than two separate fragments	Fig. 21-23
Bowing	Bone bends to the point of plastic deformation without fracturing	Fig. 21-24
Greenstick	Fracture is complete except for a portion of the cortex on the compression side of the fracture, which is only plastically deformed	Fig. 21-25
Torus	Bone buckles and bends rather than breaks	Fig. 21-26

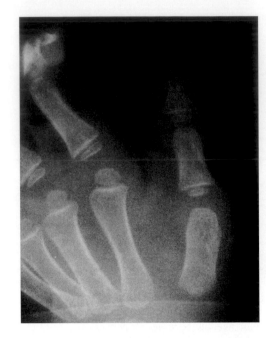

FIG. 21-18 Longitudinal fracture. A direct blow to the thumb from above produced this longitudinal fracture of the distal phalanx.

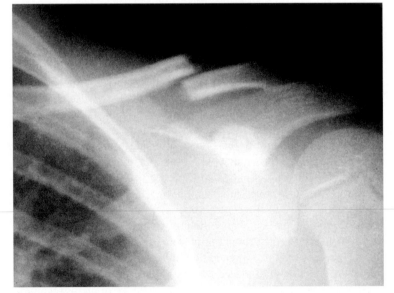

FIG. 21-19 Transverse fracture of the midportion of the clavicle. The fracture line is perpendicular to the long axis of the bone.

while holding a child by the hands, feet, or chest results in small metaphyseal chip or bucket-handle fractures, a major feature of the shaken-baby syndrome (see Chapter 6). Table 21-3 summarizes the major features of these various fracture patterns, which are illustrated in Figures 21-18 through 21-26.

The anatomic location of the fracture line simply refers to that portion of the bone to which the injury force was applied. Table 21-4 presents types of fractures classified by anatomic location. These fractures are illustrated in Figures 21-27 through 21-35. There is some degree of overlap in this method of categorization, however.

Physeal Fractures

An estimated 15% of all fractures in children involve the physis. Because the adjacent epiphyseal plate is not ossified in the young child and therefore is invisible on a radiograph, the fracture may be mistaken for a minor sprain or missed altogether, only to manifest itself at a later date in the appearance of slowed or failed longitudinal limb growth or in the development of an angular deformity. Even if diagnosed and properly treated, physeal injuries may still result in longitudinal or angular abnormalities. This risk is especially high in children with physeal fractures involving the distal femur, proximal tibia, or radial head and neck. Most physeal disruptions occur through the zone of cartilage cell hypertrophy within the physeal plate and thus do not result in permanent damage to the plate. However, a small proportion of disruptions involve the resting or

Text continued on p. 643

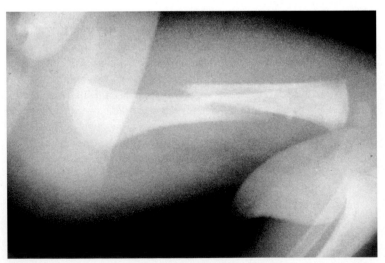

FIG. 21-20 Oblique fracture of the midportion of the femur. The fracture line is angled relative to the axis of the bone.

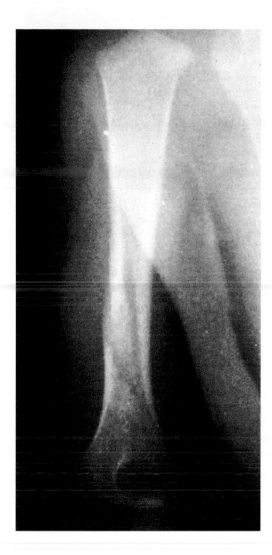

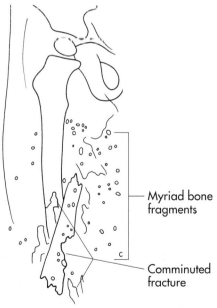

FIG. 21-21 Spiral fracture of the humerus. The fracture line takes a curvilinear course around the axis of the bone.

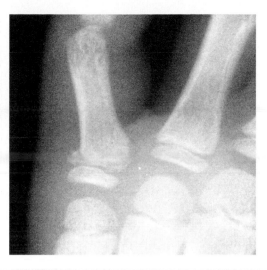

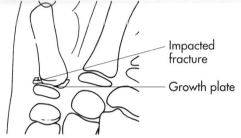

FIG. 21-22 Impacted fracture of the base of the proximal phalanx resulting from axial loading. The fracture line is indistinct, and the fragments appear to be crushed together. The fracture does not actually involve the growth plate but is located just distal to it in the proximal metaphysis.

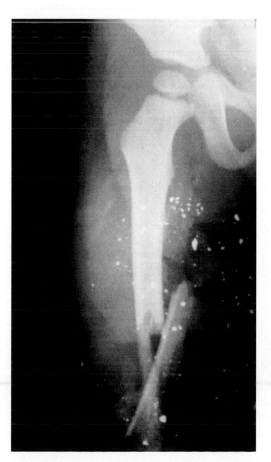

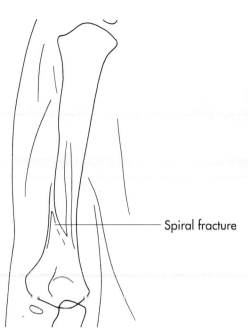

FIG. 21-23 Comminuted fracture of the femur secondary to a gunshot wound. Notice the numerous small fragments of bone in the adjacent soft tissues.

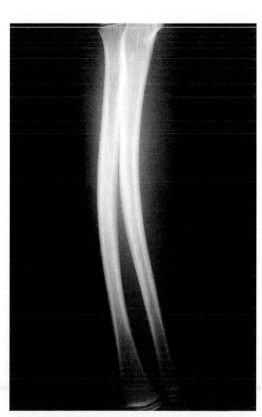

FIG. 21-24 Bowing of the forearm bones in an 8-year-old child. This type of plastic deformation can be expected to remodel with time.

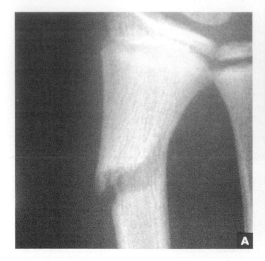

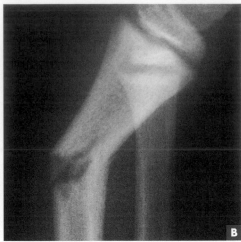

FIG. 21-25 Greenstick fracture of the distal radius. *A,* In this anteroposterior view of the distal radius, a fracture line is seen that is complete, except for a portion of the cortex on the compression side of the fracture. *B,* The lateral radiograph demonstrates more clearly the disrupted and compressed cortices. This resulted from a fall on the outstretched arm with the wrist in dorsiflexion.

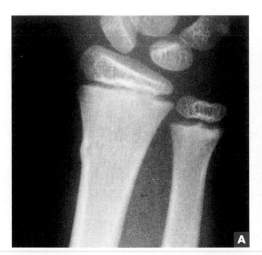

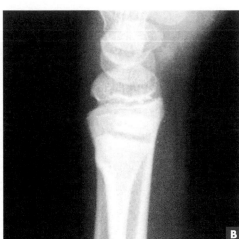

FIG. 21-26 Torus fracture of the distal radius resulting from a fall on an outstretched arm. *A,* An anteroposterior radiograph of the wrist shows a minor torus or buckle fracture of the radius. *B,* The lateral radiograph shows the dorsal location of the deformity. This injury can be expected to completely remodel.

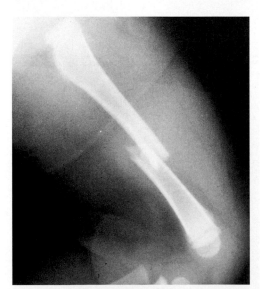

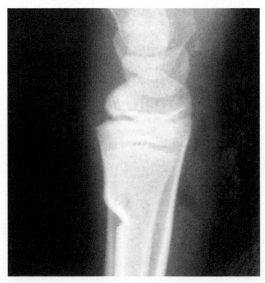

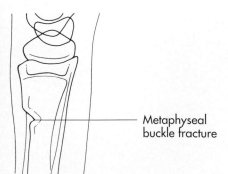

Metaphyseal buckle fracture

FIG. 21-27 Diaphyseal fracture. A transverse fracture line crosses the diaphyseal region of the femur. There is a moderate amount of overlap at the fracture site.

FIG. 21-28 Metaphyseal fracture. This lateral radiograph of the wrist shows a dorsal buckle fracture of the distal radial metaphysis. This fracture resulted from a fall on the outstretched arm with the wrist dorsiflexed and is a common injury in children.

TABLE 21-4

Classification of Fractures by Anatomic Location

Type	Site	Radiographic appearance
Diaphyseal	Fracture involves the central shaft of a long bone	Fig. 21-27
Metaphyseal	Fracture involves the widened end of a long bone	Fig. 21-28
Epiphyseal	Fracture involves the chondro-osseous end of a long bone. Such fractures can also be classified as Salter-Harris fractures.	Fig. 21-29
Articular	Fracture involves the cartilaginous joint surface	Fig. 21-30 (see Figs. 21-39 and 21-40)
Intercondylar	Fracture is located between the condyles of a joint. This is one variant of articular fracture and could also be subclassified as a Salter-Harris fracture.	Fig. 21-30
Physcal	Fracture involves the growth center of long bone. These are subclassified according to the Salter-Harris system.	Fig. 21-31
Transcondylar	Fracture traverses the condyles of a joint	Fig. 21-32
Supracondylar	Fracture line is located just proximal to the condyles of a joint	Fig. 21-33
Epicondylar	Fracture involves an area juxtaposed to thecondylar surface of a joint	Fig. 21-34
Subcapital	Fracture is located just below the epiphyseal head of certain bones	Fig. 21-35

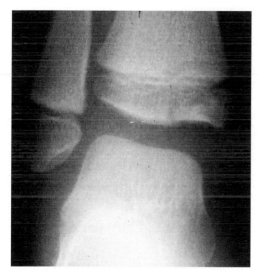

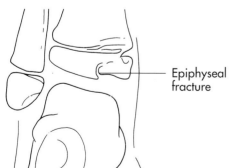

FIG. 21-29 Epiphyseal fracture. A fracture involving the medial aspect of the epiphysis of the distal tibia is seen in this anteroposterior radiograph of the ankle in a 4-year-old girl. A slight step-off is present at the articular surface. This could also be classified as a Salter-Harris type III fracture.

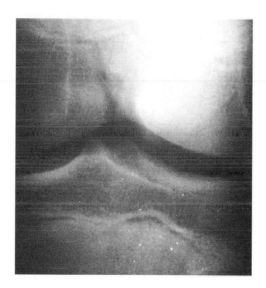

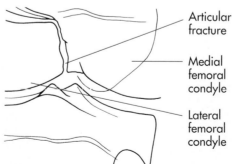

FIG. 21-30 Articular fracture. This anteroposterior view of the knee demonstrates intraarticular extension of a fracture line that exits at the junction of the medial and lateral femoral condyles. The condyles are separated by only a few millimeters. This can also be termed an *intercondylar fracture.*

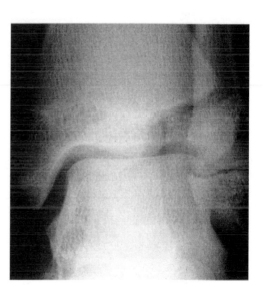

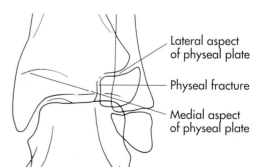

FIG. 21-31 Physeal fracture. A fracture of the lateral aspect of the tibial epiphysis through the lateral aspect of the physeal plate is seen in this anteroposterior view of the ankle of a 13-year-old boy. Also called a *Tillaux fracture,* this pattern is seen in adolescents in whom the medial aspect of the distal tibial physis has closed but not the lateral aspect. Also termed a *Salter-Harris type III fracture.*

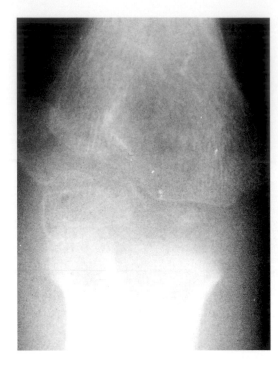

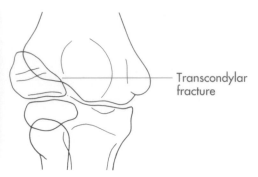

FIG. 21-32   Transcondylar fracture. This anteroposterior radiograph of the elbow shows a fracture of the lateral condyle of the distal humerus. The condyle is displaced proximally and radially. The fragment is always larger than it appears on a radiograph because of the large amount of unossified cartilage present in the distal humerus.

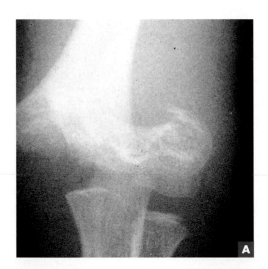

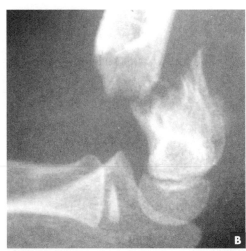

FIG. 21-33   Supracondylar fracture. These radiographs show the most common pattern of a supracondylar humerus fracture seen in children. This injury resulted from a fall backward on the outstretched arm with the elbow in hypertension. This transmitted the force of the impact to the distal humerus, driving the distal fragment posteriorly. *A*, The anteroposterior radiograph shows the distal fragment displaced radially. *B*, In the lateral view, posterior displacement is evident as well.

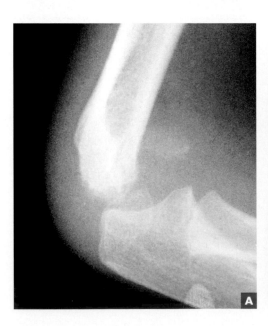

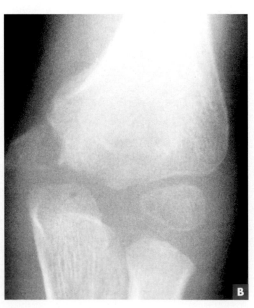

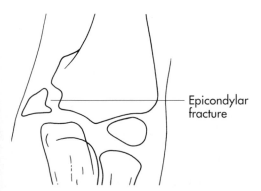

FIG. 21-34   Epicondylar fracture. *A*, This lateral radiograph shows significant proximal migration of the medial epicondyle of the distal humerus. *B*, The anteroposterior view shows slight medial displacement of the medial epicondyle.

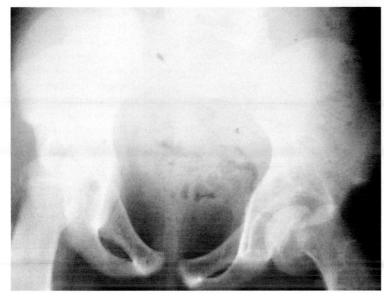

FIG. 21-35 Subcapital fracture. This anteroposterior radiograph of the pelvis shows a displaced subcapital fracture of the right femur. This particular injury may be seen acutely as the result of significant trauma or may develop slowly as a result of gradual slipping at the physeal level.

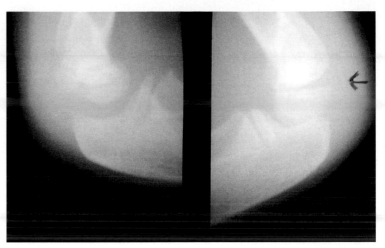

FIG. 21-37 Salter-Harris type I injury. Close inspection shows slight widening of the distal humeral epiphysis. Clinically the patient had pain, tenderness, and decreased range of motion of the elbow. (Courtesy Dr. Jocelyn Ledesma Medina.)

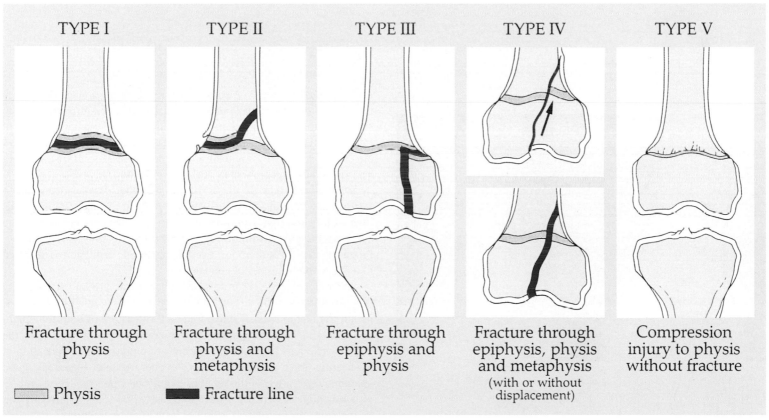

TYPE I	TYPE II	TYPE III	TYPE IV	TYPE V
Fracture through physis	Fracture through physis and metaphysis	Fracture through epiphysis and physis	Fracture through epiphysis, physis and metaphysis (with or without displacement)	Compression injury to physis without fracture

▭ Physis   ▮ Fracture line

FIG. 21-36 Salter-Harris classification of physeal injuries.

germinal layer of the physis and may disrupt the cells permanently, resulting in eventual deformity despite adequate reduction of the fracture fragments.

Because of the potential for long-term morbidity in patients with physeal fractures, great attention has been focused on the classification, diagnosis, treatment, and prognosis of physeal fractures. The Salter-Harris classification scheme is the system most commonly used in North America to classify physeal injuries (Fig. 21-36).

Salter-Harris Type I. This injury consists of a fracture running horizontally through the physis itself, resulting in a variable degree of separation of the epiphysis from the metaphysis. The amount of separation depends on the degree of periosteal disruption. Radiographs are often normal; hence, the diagnosis frequently must be made clinically on the basis of the findings of point tenderness and mild soft tissue swelling over the site of an epiphysis (Fig. 21-37). This injury usually results from a shearing force. Prognosis is usually favorable.

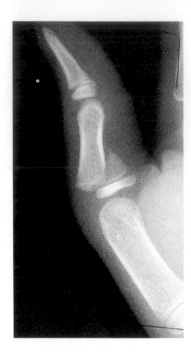

FIG. 21-38 Salter-Harris type II injury. On this lateral radiograph of the thumb, the fracture is seen to involve the proximal phalanx. The fracture line runs through the physis and exits through the metaphysis on the side opposite the site of fracture initiation. A fragment consisting of the entire epiphysis with the attached metaphyseal fragment is produced.

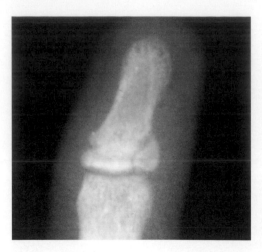

FIG. 21-40 Salter-Harris type IV injury. This patient incurred a fracture of the distal phalanx of the index finger. The fracture line starts at the articular surface, runs through the epiphysis across the physis, and exits through the metaphysis. A single fragment consisting of the epiphysis and the attached metaphysis is thus created.

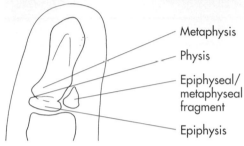

Metaphysis

Physis

Epiphyseal/ metaphyseal fragment

Epiphysis

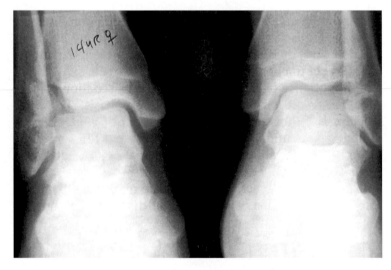

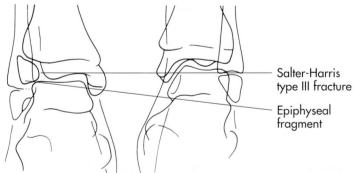

Salter-Harris type III fracture

Epiphyseal fragment

FIG. 21-39 Salter-Harris type III injury. Comparison view of both ankles reveals a fracture involving the lateral aspect of the right, distal tibial epiphysis. This configuration creates a separate fragment without any connection to the metaphysis.

Salter-Harris Type II. Also produced by shearing forces, this injury consists of a fracture line running a variable distance through the physis and exiting through the metaphysis on the side opposite the site of fracture initiation. A fragment consisting of the entire epiphysis with an attached metaphyseal fragment is thus produced (Fig. 21-38). Prognosis is generally favorable with adequate reduction.

Salter-Harris Type III. Intraarticular shearing forces can produce a fracture line running from the articular surface through the epiphysis then exiting through a portion of the physis. This creates a separate epiphyseal fragment with no connection to the metaphysis (Fig. 21-39). Prognosis may be quite poor. Accurate anatomic reduction is required to achieve the best possible outcome.

Salter-Harris Type IV. In this fracture, the fracture line starts at the articular surface, runs through the physis across the epiphysis, and exits out the metaphysis. A single fragment consisting of both the epiphysis and attached metaphysis is thus created (Fig. 21-40). Like the Salter-Harris type III fracture, the injury results from the application of a shearing force. Prognosis may be poor despite seemingly good anatomic restoration of the fracture fragments. Open reduction and internal fixation is virtually always necessary. Both Salter-Harris III and IV fractures also can be classified as intraarticular fractures.

Salter-Harris Type V. This type of fracture is the product of a crushing injury to the physis without physeal fracture or displacement. Radiographic diagnosis is virtually impossible to make at the time of injury; hence, this fracture must be diagnosed on clinical grounds. Distinction between a Salter-Harris type I and a Salter-Harris type V fracture is often possible only when a subsequent growth abnormality has been appreciated. Prognosis is quite poor for normal growth (Fig. 21-41).

Fracture Treatment Principles

The healing and remodeling capacity of the growing bones of a child is considerably greater than that of an adult; the younger the child and

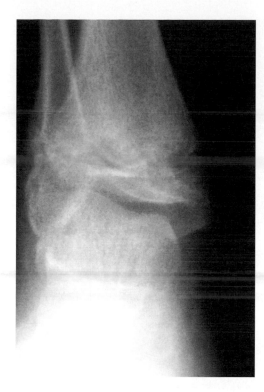

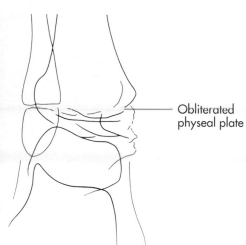

Obliterated
physeal plate

FIG. 21-41 Salter-Harris type V injury. This anteroposterior radiograph of the ankle taken several weeks after a crush injury sustained in an automobile accident reveals obliteration of the distal tibial physeal plate. As is often the case, original radiographs taken at the time of injury looked normal. This fracture must be suspected on clinical grounds and the patient treated and followed accordingly.

the closer the fracture to the epiphysis, the greater is this capacity for regeneration. As a result, healing is rapid, necessitating a shorter period of immobilization; nonunion is rare. Furthermore, in planning fracture reductions, the remodeling capability and the likely addition to bone length as a result of overgrowth must be considered. For example, in managing a toddler with a femur fracture that is displaced in the plane of motion of the adjacent joint, the bone ends must overlap to account for overgrowth and a degree of angulation can be accepted, because this will ultimately be corrected by remodeling. The amount of angulation and the degree of overlap of fracture fragments that can be accepted are difficult to state in numeric terms. Acceptable position is determined in part by the child's age, the nature and position of the fracture, the bone involved, the appearance and condition of the adjacent soft tissues, and the presence or absence of other systemic injuries. Remodeling has its limitations, however. Rotational deformities and angular deformities which are not in the axis of adjacent joint motion are not effectively remodeled. Thus, these must be corrected at the time of initial fracture reduction.

Nondisplaced fractures are simply casted or splinted. Because of the relative rarity of ligamentous injuries prior to epiphyseal closure, patients with an appropriate clinical history and point tenderness over an epiphysis are presumed to have a fracture and should be treated accordingly, even if radiographs are normal. Most displaced fractures not involving the physis can be treated by closed reduction and casting. As a general rule, open reduction and internal fixation are usually reserved for the management of Salter-Harris type III and IV fractures, which have any degree of displacement; for certain open fractures; and for fractures associated with continued neurovascular compromise. Depending on the time of presentation, degree of displacement, and severity of soft tissue swelling, reduction or casting may have to be deferred pending application of traction and subsidence of edema.

The importance of adequate analgesia and sedation before the performance of closed-reduction procedures warrants emphasis. Too often

reduction is performed without the benefit of analgesia and justified by the rationale that "it will only hurt for a minute." This reasoning is callous, and that excruciating "minute" may seem an eternity to the child. After reduction or immobilization in a cast, pain should be markedly alleviated, although some analgesia may be needed for a day or two. Persistence or recurrence of considerable discomfort signifies a complication and warrants prompt reevaluation.

Care must be taken in describing the nature of the injury and its prognosis and in explaining the rationale for proposed treatment measures to the parents. A simpler explanation in terms geared to his or her developmental level should be given to the child. Written instructions regarding home care measures, necessary parent observations, and worrisome signs that signal the need for prompt reevaluation are invaluable.

Special Cases

Clavicular Fractures

Fractures of the clavicle are very common. They are caused by lateral compression forces (as can occur in the process of delivery of the newborn or in falls onto the shoulder), transmission of forces through the glenohumeral joint in a fall to the side on an outstretched arm, or occasionally by a direct blow or impact on the clavicle itself. Most involve the midshaft or distal clavicle. Greenstick fractures are more common in infants and toddlers, whereas through-and-through fractures are more typical of older children and adolescents (see Fig. 21-19). Severe displacement and angulation are usually prevented by the thick periosteum that envelops the clavicle. Clinically, the child complains of pain in the shoulder, is noted to avoid moving the arm on the involved side, and often splints it by holding the arm close against the chest. Tenderness and mild swelling are evident on palpation of the fracture site. Complications are rare and treatment consists in the application of a padded figure-of-eight splint for 2 to 3 weeks. It is advisable to forewarn parents that a hard bump will appear as the fracture heals and that this is due to callus formation because the clavicle's superficial location makes the site of callus formation very prominent.

Rare medial clavicular fractures are caused by high-impact forces and may be accompanied by injuries of mediastinal structures. These warrant meticulous evaluation, including chest CT and often angiography.

Toddler's Fracture

One of the most common orthopedic injuries seen in children between the ages of 1 and 5 years is the toddler's fracture. The child usually has a sudden onset of refusal to bear weight on one leg or of an antalgic limp. Typically this develops after a fall with a twist, to which the unsteady toddler is unusually prone. The child may have gotten his foot caught and fallen while trying to extricate himself, may have fallen while running and making a sudden change of direction, or fallen with a twist upon jumping. Not uncommonly the actual fall is unwitnessed, and the parents are unsure about the nature of the accident. The injury results in a spiral or short oblique fracture of the distal tibia or the junction of the mid and distal tibia (Fig. 21-42). Because the thick periosteum tends to be only partially disrupted, soft tissue swelling is often minimal and tenderness may be subtle. Furthermore, many of these fractures are radiographically invisible or so subtle as to be difficult to detect, although some degree of soft tissue swelling may be evident on the film. Without radiographic evidence of a fracture, the physician must rely on the examination findings to make a clinical diagnosis.

It is generally best to allow the child to remain seated in the parent's lap during the examination. This will help calm the child and ensure a more subdued response to palpation of the uninvolved areas. Attention should first be turned to the normal extremity. The ankle, knee, and hip should be placed through their range of motion. Next, the entire foot, tibia, fibula, and femur should be palpated. The child will cry if upset, but nothing about the examination will otherwise exacerbate the child's baseline irritability. Attention is then directed to the involved extremity, and a similar examination is performed. Palpation over the fracture site usually will be revealed either by a withdrawal reaction or, more commonly, by an increase from baseline irritability, usually manifested by a change in the child's facial expression and in the pattern of crying. In suspected cases in which it is difficult to determine if tenderness is present, a gentle passive twist applied to the tibia may elicit pain. Localized bone tenderness or pain on passive twisting in this setting is clinical proof of a fracture, even if radiographs are normal. In attempting to assess very frightened and highly uncooperative toddlers, it is best to give them time to calm down and then either have the parent perform palpation or introduce puppets and palpate using the puppet's hands.

Treatment consists of either long- or short-leg casting for approximately 4 weeks. Infection must be included in the differential diagnosis of the limping child in this 1- to 5-year age group but usually can be ruled out by lack of fever, absence of local erythema, and normal blood values. If there is no clear history of a fall, only a mild limp, and no evidence of localized tenderness and radiographs are normal, it may be best to defer treatment and observe the child closely.

Fractures Involving the Elbow

Supracondylar, transcondylar, intercondylar, and epicondylar humerus fractures and proximal radius and ulna fractures all involve the elbow, and the major mechanism is a fall onto the arm with the elbow in hyperextension.

Supracondylar fractures account for about 50% of these injuries and usually result from a fall backward onto an outstretched hyperextended arm, which results in posterior displacement of the distal humeral fragment (see Fig. 21-33). More rarely, a direct blow to the posterior aspect of the distal humerus is the cause, in which case the distal fragment is angu-

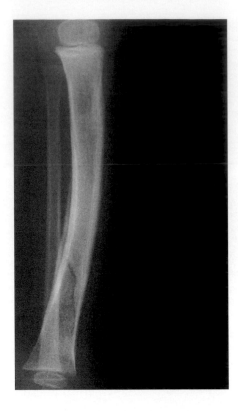

FIG. 21-42 Toddler's fracture. This spiral fracture of the distal tibia was the result of a fall with a twist.

lated anteriorly. Pain, swelling, and tenderness are most prominent over the posterior aspect of the distal humerus. There is a significant risk of associated neurovascular injury in patients with such fractures.

Lateral condylar fractures are transcondylar fractures of the Salter-Harris type IV variety and thus are in part interarticular (see Fig. 21-32). Typically they result from a fall onto an extended and abducted arm. Swelling and tenderness are prominent over the lateral aspect of the elbow. These fractures are generally unstable and often require pinning to ensure optimal reduction.

Medial epicondylar fractures stem from falls in which the hyperextended elbow is subjected to valgus stress (see Fig. 21-34). They are also commonly seen in association with elbow dislocations. These children have swelling and tenderness centered over the medial aspect of the elbow.

Radial head and neck fractures are usually the result of a fall onto an outstretched, supinated arm. Local swelling and tenderness are centered over the proximal radius, although pain is often referred to the wrist. Because they often are accompanied by other fractures, care should be taken to search for associated injuries.

Radiographic findings in patients with fractures about the elbow can be subtle, and oblique and comparison views may be necessary to reveal them. Key signs suggestive of a fracture in the absence of fracture lines are the posterior fat pad sign and displacement of the *anterior humeral line.* The fat pad sign consists of the upward and outward displacement of the posterior fat pad of the distal humerus (Fig. 21-43), which is normally invisible. The finding of a fat pad indicates the presence of a hemarthrosis, and it can be seen in patients with fractures involving the distal humerus, proximal radius, or proximal ulna. The *anterior humeral line* is a line drawn through the anterior cortex of the humerus and normally intersects the middle third of the capitellum. As just noted, hyperextension injuries of the distal humerus resulting in fractures typically displace the distal humeral fragment posteriorly. As a result, the anterior humeral line intersects the anterior third of the capitellum if displacement is slight or misses it entirely if displacement or angulation is marked (Fig. 21-44).

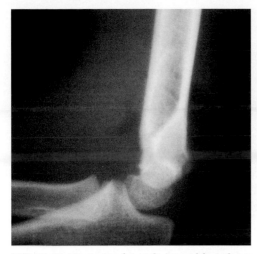

FIG. 21-43 Posterior fat pad sign. Although no clear fracture line is evident in this patient with a supracondylar fracture, the posterior fat pad is readily visible, being displaced upward and outward from the posterior aspect of the distal humerus. (Courtesy Dr. Richard B. Towbin, Children's Hospital of Pittsburgh.)

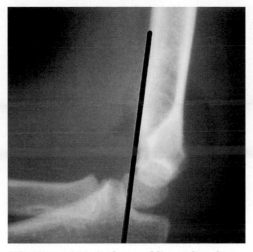

FIG. 21-44 Anterior humeral line. A line drawn through the anterior cortex of the humerus in the patient shown in Fig. 21-43 intersects the anterior third of the capitulum, indicating posterior displacement of the distal humeral fragment. (Courtesy Dr. Richard B. Towbin, Children's Hospital of Pittsburgh.)

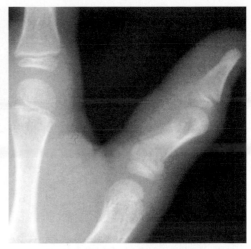

FIG. 21-45 Angulated phalanx fracture. Significant angular deformity is seen in this fracture of the proximal phalanx of the thumb. Such fractures require careful reduction to prevent permanent disability.

Hand and Finger Fractures

Although a complete discussion of the examination of the hand and hand injuries is beyond the scope of this chapter, several key points bear emphasis, as appropriate assessment and management are essential if long-term dysfunction is to be prevented (see Figs. 21-83 and 21-84).

Phalangeal Fractures. The most common mechanism of injury producing phalangeal fractures in young children is a crush injury caused by getting their fingers caught in a door or by the weight of a heavy object falling on them. Crush injuries continue to be common in older children and adolescents, but contact sports and fist fights assume an increasing causative role in this age group.

Meticulous attention must be paid to the assessment of neurovascular and tendon function to detect subtle abnormalities that may reflect significant injury with the potential for long-term complications. This can be difficult in young children. However, much information can be gained from observing the position of the hands at rest and during spontaneous movement and by watching motion as the parents hand objects to the child.

Complete phalangeal fractures typically angulate as a result of the action of the intrinsic muscles of the hand. Any fracture associated with shortening, significant angulation (Fig. 21-45), or rotational deformity, and any intraarticular fracture must be appropriately reduced. Shortening and rotation are best detected by comparison of the injured hand with its normal opposite. Comparison of the plane of the fingernails of both hands with the forearms supinated and the fingers partially flexed is particularly useful in detecting rotational abnormalities (Fig. 21-46).

Determination of the degree of angulation and identification of intraarticular fractures are best done radiographically. X-ray findings can be subtle, necessitating careful comparison with radiographs of the normal hand. It is also important to obtain oblique as well as AP and lateral views.

Chip fractures at the base of the middle or distal phalanges may be associated with avulsion of the flexor or extensor tendons, which may necessitate surgical repair (Fig. 21-47). Clinically, an extensor tendon injury may be manifested by flexor tendon overpull, and conversely,

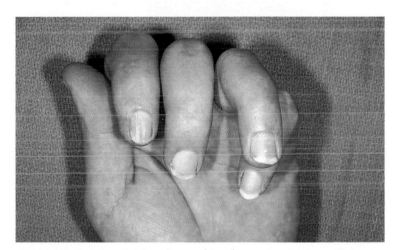

FIG. 21-46 Rotational deformity resulting from a hand injury. With rotational deformity the plane of the nail of the involved finger is seen to deviate from its normal plane of orientation. (Courtesy Dr. Neil Jones, Los Angeles.)

flexor tendon injuries may result in extensor overpull (Fig. 21-7).

Crush injuries of the distal phalanges associated with partial or complete nail avulsions often result in open fractures with laceration of the nail bed (Fig. 21-48). These require careful cleansing, debridement, and nail bed repair and antibiotic prophylaxis.

The volar plate is a cartilaginous plate located at the base of the middle phalanx of each finger. Intraarticular fractures involving the PIP joint may fracture or tear this structure as well. The typical mechanism of injury is usually a blow to the end of the finger in hyperextension. Often a chip of bone avulsed from the middle phalanx is seen radiographically. Clinically, pain and swelling are especially marked over the volar aspect of the PIP joint. A hyperextension deformity of the involved PIP joint may be seen when the fingers are extended, or pain or locking may be noted on attempted flexion. Pain is exacerbated on pas-

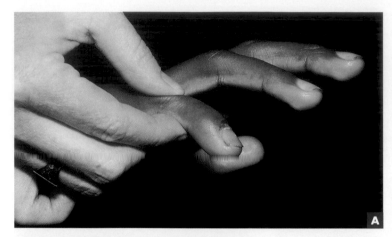

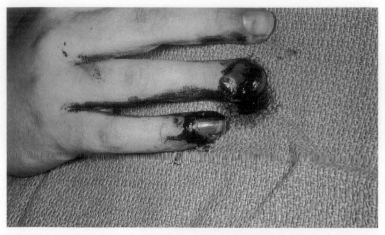

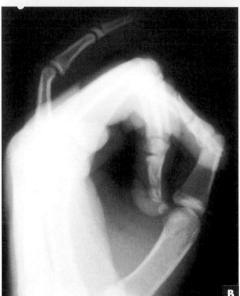

FIG. 21-47 Distal phalanx fracture with extensor tendon injury. *A,* Another player's shoulder landed on this boy's finger. The finger was swollen and painful and maximally tender at the base of the distal phalanx, and the patient was unable to extend the distal interphalangeal joint. *B,* Radiographs revealed separation of the epiphysis at the base of the distal phalanx.

FIG. 21-48 Crush injury of the distal phalanx. This child's finger was slammed in a car door. He incurred a crush fracture of the distal phalanx, partial avulsion of the nail, and a nail bed laceration. By definition, this is an open fracture. (Courtesy Dr. Neil Jones, Los Angeles.)

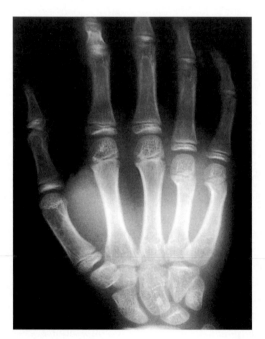

FIG. 21-49 Boxer's fracture. This adolescent presented with pain and swelling of the lateral aspect of his right hand after punching a wall in a fit of temper. Radiographically he has typical boxer's fractures of the necks of the fourth and fifth metacarpals with volar displacement of the distal fragments.

sive hyperextension and reduced on passive flexion. Volar plate injuries may also accompany dislocation of the PIP joint (see section on Ligamentous Injuries).

Metacarpal Fractures. The boxer's fracture, an impacted fracture of the neck of the fifth and often the fourth metacarpal, is among the most common of these injuries (Fig. 21-49). It occurs as a result of direct impact with a partially clenched fist (typically resulting from punching another person or a wall) and is most commonly seen in aggressive adolescents. It can also result from a fall onto a clenched fist. Clinically, depression of the involved knuckle or knuckles may be noted, along with more proximal swelling and discoloration. The involved metacarpals may also appear shortened. An associated rotational deformity, if present, is manifested by rotation of the nails of the corresponding fingers (see Fig. 21-46). If the injury stems from punching another person in the mouth, care must be taken to check for overlying breaks in the skin caused by the opponent's teeth. These are infection-prone wounds and may communicate with metacarpophalangeal joints. Radiographically, volar angulation of the distal segment is typically found. If this exceeds 15 to 20 degrees or a rotational de-

formity is present, the patient should be referred to an orthopedist or hand surgeon for reduction. Nondisplaced, minimally angulated fractures can be treated with an ulnar gutter splint.

Metatarsal Fractures

Most metatarsal fractures are the result of a heavy object dropping onto the foot and thus are crush injuries. Falls in which the patient twists the forefoot can produce transverse fractures at the base of the fifth metatarsal (Fig. 21-50), and injuries of the foot with the ankle inverted and the foot in plantar flexion can avulse the tuberosity from the base of the fifth metatarsal. This must be distinguished from the normal finding of a secondary ossification center, termed the *os vesalianum,* at the base of the fifth metatarsal. The edges of the latter are smooth, rounded, and sclerotic (Fig. 21-51). Mild, localized swelling and point tenderness are noted over the site of a metatarsal fracture; weight-bearing is painful, if not impossible. A short leg cast provides maximal relief.

Adolescents involved in long-distance running or walking may incur stress fractures of the shafts of the second and third metatarsals, which

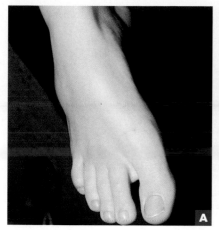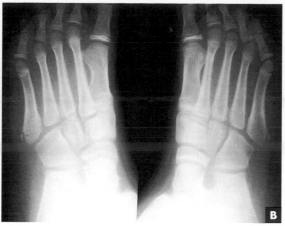

FIG. 21-50 Transverse metatarsal fracture. This adolescent fell forward with her forefoot twisted under her. *A,* Swelling over the proximal portion of the fifth metatarsal was prominent. *B,* The transverse fracture is evident radiographically in these oblique views. Note that she has an os vesalianum, or secondary ossification center, bilaterally.

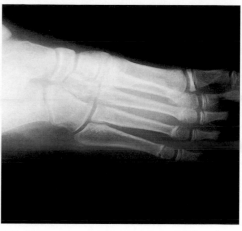

FIG. 21-51 Os vesalianum. Many children have a secondary ossification center at the base of the fifth metatarsal. This can be distinguished from a fracture by the fact that its edges are smooth, rounded, and sclerotic. (Courtesy Dr. Jocelyn Ledesma Medina.)

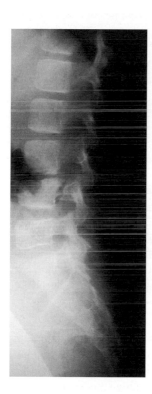

FIG. 21-52 Lap belt fracture. This compression fracture of the L4 vertebral body resulted from hyperflexion against the fulcrum of a backseat lap belt.

sulting in hyperflexion of the lumbar spine over the fulcrum of the lap belt and often causing a compression fracture of the L4 or L5 vertebral body or disruption of the posterior elements of one of these vertebrae. Pain resulting from associated abdominal injuries may overshadow the pain of the vertebral injury; however, localized tenderness or spasm is usually detectable with careful palpation during examination of the back. Radiographic findings may include evidence of vertebral body compression, which is best seen on the lateral view (Fig. 21-52), or displacement of the shadow of the spinous process on the AP view in cases of disruption of the posterior elements. Identification of these fractures and determining whether they are stable or unstable via CT scan is essential before any undue movement is allowed.

Pelvic Avulsion Fractures

Pelvic avulsion fractures are a phenomenon unique to adolescents, with a peak occurrence between 13 and 14 years of age in girls and 15 and 17 years of age in boys. This stems from the fact that the secondary centers of ossification in these young people have not yet fused to the pelvis. They are typically seen in adolescents who are in top physical condition and involved in competitive sports, especially track and field (e.g., sprinting and jumping), soccer, and football. The incidence of these fractures is increasing with the rising participation of adolescents in competitive sports. Most result from a sudden, violent muscular contraction while the ipsilateral extremity is held in a static position or when a muscle is suddenly lengthened during isometric contraction. As the muscle power exceeds the strength of the tendinous unit, it is torn from the apophysis or secondary ossification center. Avulsion fractures of the ischial tuberosity are the most common. They tend to occur during sprinting and are due to the sudden, powerful contraction of the hamstring muscles when the hip is flexed and the knee extended (Fig. 21-53, *A*). Avulsions of the anterior superior and anterior inferior iliac spines (Fig. 21-53, *B*) are caused by strong contractions of the sartorius and rectus femoris muscles respectively. These, too, tend to happen during running, often during an abrupt directional change. In some cases of anterior inferior iliac spine avulsions, they occur with kicking. At the time of injury, the patient experiences sudden pain at the site and difficulty walking. On examination, point tenderness and swelling are noted over the involved apophysis and weakness on active hip motion is seen secondary to pain.

are the site of maximal stress and weight application during the push off phase of walking and running. Pain often increases insidiously and tends to be poorly localized. Swelling may be imperceptible. These are often microfractures and may be radiographically invisible until healing becomes detectable 3 to 4 weeks after onset. Earlier detection is possible with bone scan.

Seat Belt Fractures

Increased awareness of the importance of using seat belts to prevent serious multiple trauma in auto accidents and adherence to recommendations to place children in the back seat of the car have resulted in an increase in the incidence of lap belt fractures in children, because, as yet, most cars to not have three-point belts in the back seat. In a head-on collision, the child's head and torso are thrown forward, re-

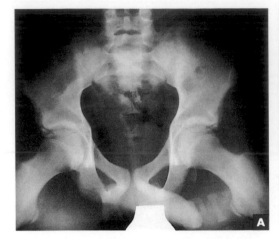

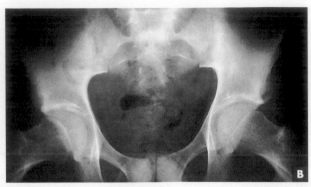

FIG. 21-53 Pelvic avulsion fractures. *A,* Ischial tuberosity avulsion fracture. This 14-year-old football player sprinting for a touchdown fell on his stomach and experienced sharp left hip pain. He could not bear weight after the incident and was found to have tenderness over the left buttock and pain with abduction and flexion of the left hip. The avulsed fragment is best seen on this frog-leg view. *B,* Anterior inferior iliac spine avulsion fracture. While running in gym class, this 15-year-old boy experienced the sudden onset of left hip pain and difficulty walking. He had point tenderness over the anterior inferior iliac spine and full range of hip motion but experienced pain on flexion and internal rotation. If compared with the right, the avulsed apophysis is evident. (Courtesy Dr. Janet Kinnane, Children's Hospital of Pittsburgh.)

In viewing radiographs, it is important to compare the involved side with the normal side to detect displacement of the avulsed fragment and to avoid mistaking a normal apophysis for a fracture.

Treatment is conservative and consists of a few days of bed rest until the pain subsides, followed by 2 to 6 weeks of crutch-walking, with a gradual increase in weight-bearing as pain allows. Thereafter, careful reconditioning allows return to full activity, usually within 6 to 10 weeks.

Pathologic Fractures

Children with severe osteopenia or osteoporosis, whether stemming from an inherited disorder or disuse secondary to neurologic or neuromuscular disease, are at considerably increased risk of incurring fractures as the result of minor falls or even during routine physical therapy exercises. Localized bone lesions, including those caused by osteomyelitis, tumors, or cysts, can cause localized cortical thinning as they expand. Impact on the involved bone can then also result in a pathologic fracture. Examples of these conditions and representative fractures are presented in Chapter 6 (see Figs. 6-39 and 6-40).

Compartment Syndromes

A compartment syndrome arises whenever the interstitial tissue fluid pressure exceeds the capillary perfusion pressure. In clinical practice, the interstitial pressure elevation must reach approximately 35 to 45 mm Hg for this to occur. Because the enclosed fascial boundary of the involved muscle compartment is unyielding, hemorrhage or edema within it can cause interstitial pressure to rise to such levels, resulting in muscle ischemia and neurovascular compromise. Compartment syndromes are not rare in childhood and can be seen after open or closed fractures, crush injuries, or prolonged pressure on an extremity, which can occur in a comatose child who has been lying on an extremity for several hours. A displaced fracture of the proximal tibial metaphysis is the fracture most likely to be complicated by a compartment syndrome. Other fractures that are well documented to predispose to the development of a compartment syndrome include supracondylar humerus fractures and displaced forearm fractures.

Prompt and accurate diagnosis of a compartment syndrome is essential, because if definitive treatment is not implemented within 4 to 6 hours of onset, permanent neuromuscular damage will result. The clinical findings of compartment syndrome are quite classic. The in-

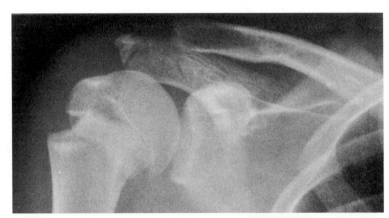

FIG. 21-54 Epiphyseal separation. Because of the elasticity and relatively greater strength of the ligaments, forces that would have resulted in dislocation in an older adolescent have instead caused epiphyseal separation and displacement of the proximal humeral epiphysis in this prepubescent child. (Courtesy Department of Pediatric Radiology, Children's Hospital of Pittsburgh.)

volved extremity is swollen and tense to palpation. The patient complains of severe pain that is unrelieved by elevation, immobilization, and routine doses of narcotics. Passive movement of the terminal digits (fingers or toes) exacerbates the pain, and active motion is avoided. In view of the fact that pulses may never be diminished or absent despite a full-blown, florid compartment syndrome, the diagnosis or decision to treat should never be based solely on the presence or absence of the peripheral pulses. Because the clinical diagnosis of compartment syndrome can be difficult, especially in the uncooperative or comatose child, intracompartmental needle pressure readings are recommended.

Emergent surgical decompression of the fascial covering of all involved compartments is necessary to prevent irreversible muscle and nerve damage. Following fascial decompression, relief of pressure, pain reduction, and return of active muscle power are immediate.

Ligamentous Injuries

Dislocations

The ligaments of a child have great elasticity and are relatively strong compared with bony structures, especially the physis (Fig. 21-54). Consequently, joint dislocations and ligamentous disruptions are rather un-

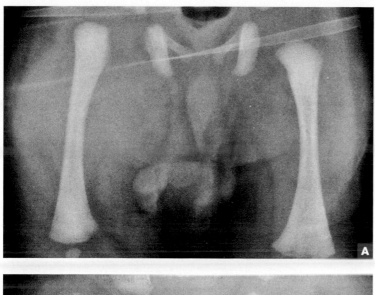

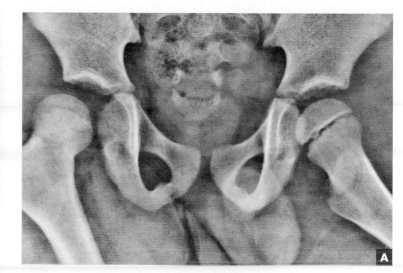

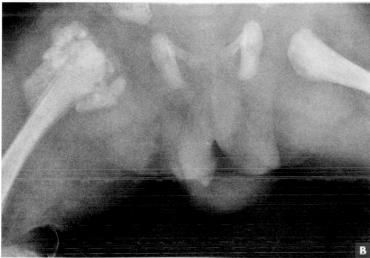

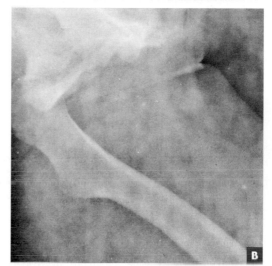

FIG. 21-55 Fracture dislocation, right hip. This young infant presented with what appeared to be a traumatic hip dislocation without an associated fracture. *A*, The right femoral head is displaced laterally and superiorly. *B*, The follow-up film taken 2 weeks later reveals vigorous callus formation around the proximal femur and periosteal new bone formation both proximally and distally, thus confirming the existence of associated femoral fractures. (Courtesy Department of Pediatric Radiology, Children's Hospital of Pittsburgh.)

FIG. 21-56 Traumatic posterior hip dislocation. This child suffered an impaction injury in an automobile accident. *A*, In the anteroposterior view the femoral head appears to be displaced laterally and superiorly. The femur is also adducted and internally rotated. *B*, The frog-leg view discloses the severity of displacement posteriorly.

usual in childhood; when seen, they are usually the result of severe trauma and are commonly associated with fractures. In some instances the dislocation is obvious and the fracture subtle or even invisible radiographically (Fig. 21-55), but often the fracture is the prominent clinical finding and the dislocation less apparent. Hence, the emphasis in pediatric orthopedics is on examining the entire extremity and on including the joints proximal and distal to a suspected fracture site in the radiographic examination. Failure to diagnose the full extent of injury can result in permanent morbidity. It must also be remembered that in infants epiphyseal separations prior to ossification can simulate dislocations. For example, separation of the distal humeral epiphysis presents a radiographic picture suggestive of posterior displacement of the olecranon. The most frequent sites of dislocation in children are the hip, the patellofemoral joint, and the interphalangeal joints.

Hip dislocations in the young are usually the result of falls. In children under 5 years of age, the softness of the acetabulum and relative ligamentous laxity enable dislocation without the application of extreme force, and thus there may be no associated fractures. In older children, violent force is required and dislocation is commonly accom-

panied by fractures of the femur and acetabulum. In most instances the femoral head dislocates posteriorly. The child presents in severe pain with the involved leg held in adduction, internally rotated and flexed (Fig. 21-56). A position of extension, external rotation, and abduction is adopted by patients with the less common anterior dislocation. When the child also has an impressive femoral fracture, his or her pain may be attributed to that and the positional findings missed, unless the clinician specifically looks for them. Even in patients without an obvious associated fracture, epiphyseal separation or avulsion of an acetabular fragment may have occurred. Prompt reduction is important, both to relieve pain and to reduce the risk of secondary avascular necrosis of the femoral head. Postreduction films are important, as these are more likely to disclose the fact that an epiphyseal separation has occurred and will tend to show incomplete reduction if a radiolucent intraarticular fragment is present.

In patellofemoral dislocations the patella usually dislocates laterally (Fig. 21-57). This may occur as the result of laterally directed shearing forces or of a hyperextension injury. Patients with ligamentous laxity appear particularly susceptible. In most instances the patella has relocated

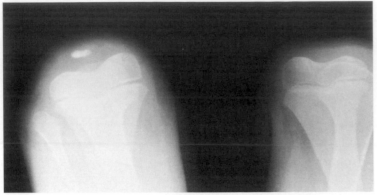

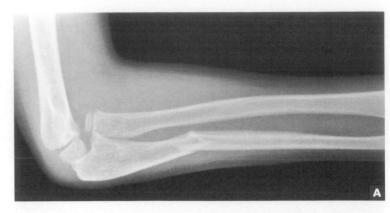

FIG. 21-57   Patellar dislocation. In this flexion view obtained before re-location, the left patella is displaced laterally and there is marked swelling. (Courtesy Department of Pediatric Radiology, Children's Hospital of Pittsburgh.)

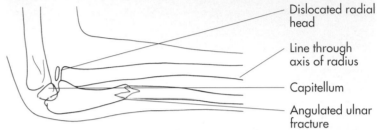

Dislocated radial head

Line through axis of radius

Capitellum

Angulated ulnar fracture

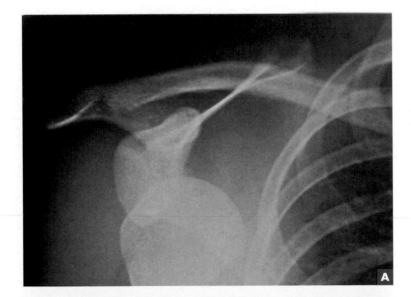

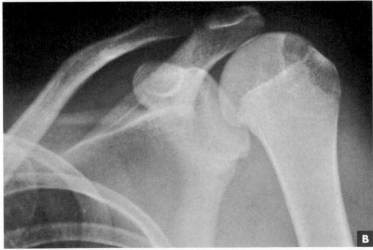

FIG. 21-59   Monteggia fracture. *A,* A displaced fracture of the proximal ulna is accompanied by dislocation of the radial head. A line drawn through the long axis of the radius would intersect the distal humerus above the level of the capitellum. *B,* The comparison view of the normal arm shows the normal position of the radial head. (Courtesy Department of Pediatric Radiology, Children's Hospital of Pittsburgh.)

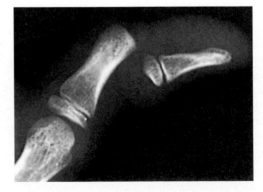

FIG. 21-60   Interphalangeal joint dislocation. The distal phalanx of the thumb is dislocated dorsally. (Courtesy Department of Pediatric Radiology, Children's Hospital of Pittsburgh.)

FIG. 21-58   *A,* Anterior dislocation of the right shoulder. The humeral head is not in the glenoid fossa but is displaced anteriorly. *B,* The normal relationship is seen in this comparison view of the left shoulder. The injury occurred when the patient was taking a back swing for a hockey shot. The patient felt a pop and the immediate onset of severe pain. Note that his epiphyses have fused. (Courtesy Department of Pediatric Radiology, Children's Hospital of Pittsburgh.)

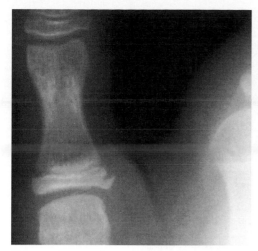

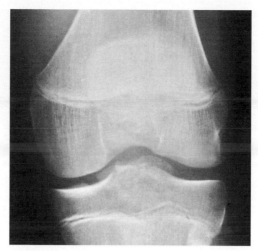

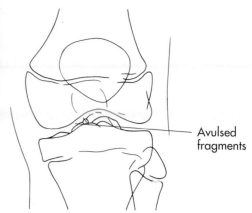

Avulsed fragments

FIG. 21-61 Gamekeeper's thumb. A small avulsion fracture of the epiphysis at the base of the proximal phalanx is associated with rupture of the ulnar collateral ligament. The injury occurred when the patient fell while skiing and the strap of his ski pole forcefully abducted his thumb on impact.

FIG. 21-62 Avulsion fracture of the left tibial spine as the result of a soccer injury (anteroposterior view). Also present were a tear in the cruciate ligament and a lipohemarthrosis. (Courtesy Department of Pediatric Radiology, Children's Hospital of Pittsburgh.)

by the time the patient is seen. If not, the leg should be extended immediately and the patella pushed back into place to alleviate pain. Findings on examination include prominent swelling and hemarthrosis, tenderness along the medial patellar border, a positive apprehension test (see section on knee examination and Fig. 21-11), and increased lateral mobility of the patella. Avulsion fractures of the lateral femoral condyle or medial patella are common associated injuries. Application of ice, rest, and use of a knee immobilizer for 3 weeks are recommended. Currently there is disagreement on whether surgical intervention should be considered after the first episode or deferred until a recurrence.

True shoulder dislocations are seen only in adolescents after epiphyseal fusion. On examination of the shoulder, a loss of the rounded contours lateral and anterior to the acromion is found. When the humeral head dislocates anteriorly, it is displaced medially beneath the coracoid process, where it can be palpated (Fig. 21-58). These patients usually support the affected arm with the opposite hand, with the shoulder in moderate internal rotation. Patients with posterior shoulder dislocations have evidence of a fullness posterior to the glenoid cavity and are unable to externally rotate the involved upper extremity.

Separation of the proximal humeral epiphysis or major fracture dislocations are seen in younger children subjected to forces that would cause shoulder dislocation after puberty (see Fig. 21-54).

Elbow dislocations are rare in the absence of an associated fracture. The fracture may be as subtle as a nonossified fragment avulsed from the medial epicondyle or the ulna or as prominent as a displaced fracture of the ulna or radius. An example of the latter is the Monteggia fracture. In this situation, a displaced fracture of the proximal ulna is accompanied by dislocation of the radial head. A radial dislocation should be suspected if a line drawn through the long axis of the radius fails to pass through the capitellum on any view (Fig. 21-59). Less frequently, fractures of the radius are associated with dislocation of the radioulnar joint, and fractures of the olecranon may be accompanied by dislocation of the radius. A fall onto an extended or partially flexed arm with the forearm supinated can result in posterior dislocation of both the radius and ulna with tearing of the anterior portion of the joint capsule and of the medial collateral ligaments. This injury may be associated with fracture of the medial epicondyle, the coronoid process, the olecranon, or the proximal radius. Clinically the forearm is shortened and there is an obvious deformity and marked swelling of the posterior aspect of the elbow. There is a high risk of neurovascular compromise and compartment syndrome in patients with this injury.

Dislocation of an interphalangeal joint results in an obvious deformity and is an intensely painful injury (Fig. 21-60). Avulsion fractures, volar plate fractures, and tendinous or capsular injury may be associated with it and difficult to detect radiographically. These must be suspected if range of motion is incomplete following relocation. In some cases the associated injury makes closed reduction impossible.

Sprains

A sprain is a ligamentous injury in which some degree of tearing occurs, often as a result of excessive stretching or twisting. As noted in the section on fractures, sprains are less common in children with open epiphyses than they are in older adolescents whose epiphyses are fused. When sprains do occur, they tend to be milder and may be associated with Salter-Harris fractures. This stems from the fact that the growth plate, being weaker than the ligaments, tends to give before significant ligamentous tearing can occur. Thus in children, physeal fractures tend to result from forces that would produce a sprain in older adolescents or adults.

In many other instances, a suspected sprain is actually a small avulsion fracture. If the portion avulsed is ossified, a small fragment may be detectable radiographically, but if the fragment is cartilaginous, it will be radiographically invisible. A particular example of this is the *gamekeeper's thumb*, which is often associated with a small avulsion fracture of the proximal phalanx (Fig. 21-61). In it, an injury causing forceful abduction of the thumb results in rupture of the ulnar collateral ligament at the base of the thumb. Adequate examination necessitates stress testing of the radial and ulnar collateral ligaments by applying varus and valgus stress, respectively, with the thumb in extension. This is often impossible until pain has been reduced by a digital nerve block. If more than 20 degrees of instability is found on stressing the ulnar collaterals, the patient should be referred to an orthopedist or hand surgeon for possible surgical repair. Failure to correct the problem results in a loss of resistance to abduction and a weak pinch.

Before epiphyseal closure, Salter-Harris fractures and avulsion fractures of the distal fibula or tibia should be strongly suspected in children with "sprain-like" injuries of the ankle. Similarly, injuries that rupture the cruciate ligaments of the knee in adults usually avulse the tibial spine in children (Fig. 21-62). Following physeal closure in adolescence, sprains are seen with some frequency.

TABLE 21-5

Classification of Sprains

Grade of sprain	Degree of tearing	Clinical findings
I	A small fragment of ligamentous fibers is disrupted	Pain on motion Local tenderness Mild swelling
II	A moderate percentage of fibers is torn	Pain on motion More diffuse tenderness Moderate swelling, may have joint effusion Mild instability
III	The ligament is completely disrupted	Severe pain on motion Marked swelling, usually with joint effusion Marked tenderness Joint instability

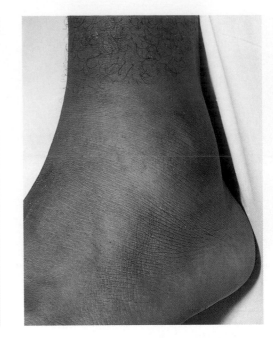

FIG. 21-63 Ankle sprain. Marked tenderness and swelling were maximal inferior to the malleolus of this 17-year-old youth. The anterior talofibular, calcaneofibular, and posterior talofibular ligaments were all tender. This is in contrast to the findings seen with a Salter-Harris type I fracture of the distal tibia (see Fig. 21-16).

Sprains are classified in three grades according to severity (Table 21-5). In contrast to physeal fractures, swelling and tenderness are more likely to be prominent and occur early and are most evident over the involved ligament or ligaments, not over the epiphysis. Pain on motion is often more marked in patients with sprains than in patients with physeal fractures.

Ankle Sprains. An ankle sprain in an adolescent patient is typically caused by a severe inversion stress injury and the presenting findings are diffuse pain and tenderness along with swelling centered below the lateral malleolus, although the superior margin of swelling may cover the malleolus (Fig. 21-63). Areas of maximal tenderness may be found over the anterior talofibular ligament alone or over both it and the calcaneofibular ligament. Rarely the posterior talofibular ligament is also torn in patients with particularly severe sprains, and tenderness and swelling are noted over its course. There is little pain on dorsiflexion or plantar flexion but marked pain on passive inversion. Tests for ligamentous stability are described in the section on ankle examination.

Knee Sprains. Patients with major knee sprains present with marked pain, refusal to bear weight, and swelling resulting from hemarthrosis. Tears of the medial or lateral collateral ligaments of the knee are seen in adolescents and are usually the result of a direct blow that applies valgus or varus stress respectively. A football tackle or being hit by a car from the side are common reported mechanisms. Tenderness is prominent over the involved ligaments. Major tears result in ligamentous instability detected by the *adduction/abduction stress test* (see the section on Knee Examination). Tibial spine avulsion fractures and anterior cruciate ligament tears stem from falls in which the knee is hyperflexed, often a fall from a bicycle or a fall while skiing. Tenderness is marked anteriorly, and instability is demonstrated by the *anterior draw* and *Lachman tests* (see the section on Knee Examination; see also Fig. 21-12).

Because of the frequency of associated fractures in children and adolescents, patients with apparent sprains and hemarthroses should not undergo tests of ligamentous stability until radiographs have been obtained and the possibility of unstable fractures ruled out.

Shoulder Separation. A shoulder separation involves a ligamentous tear at the acromioclavicular joint, usually resulting from a fall onto an outstretched, adducted arm. Clinically the lateral aspect of the clavicle appears to ride higher on the injured side than on the normal side, and with application of pressure it may be forced back into its normal position. If it can also be moved forward and backward, the coracoclavicular ligaments have been torn as well.

In evaluating patients with possible sprains, careful attention must be given not only to assessment of swelling, tenderness, and joint stability, but also to evaluation of adjacent bony structures and to musculotendinous function (see the section on Physical Examination). Complete evaluation may be impossible if initial presentation has been delayed for several hours and secondary effusion, soft tissue swelling, and muscle spasm are pronounced. In such instances, it may be necessary to immobilize the affected joint with a splint and have the patient return for reevaluation in 24 to 72 hours when the swelling has abated.

Rest, the application of ice, use of analgesic anti-inflammatory agents such as ibuprofen, and perhaps use of an Ace wrap or taping, suffice for grade I sprains. Subjective improvement occurs in a few days. Grade II and III sprains necessitate a longer period of immobilization. Splinting or casting for a few to several weeks is generally necessary. Grade III sprains may necessitate surgical intervention.

Subluxation of the Radial Head (Nursemaid's Elbow)

Subluxation of the radial head is the most common elbow injury in childhood and one of the most common ligamentous injuries. The mechanism is one of sudden traction applied to the extended arm. The injury is seen predominantly in children between the ages of 1 and 4 years. The typical history is one of a parent suddenly pulling the child by the arm to prevent a fall, of the child, in a fit of temper, attempting to pull away from the parent, or of a child being swung by the arms. However, in many cases the injury is due to grabbing onto some object in an effort to break a fall. This type of injury can also occur in an infant who is rolled over with an extended arm trapped beneath his or her trunk. After a brief initial period of crying, the child calms down but is unable to use the affected arm, which is held close to the body with the elbow flexed and forearm pronated (Fig. 21-64, *A*). If old enough to talk, the child may complain of elbow, forearm, or even wrist pain. Physical examination reveals no bony tenderness and no evidence of swelling, but on assessment of passive motion, the child resists any attempt at supination and cries in pain. Mild limitation of elbow flexion and extension may also be noted.

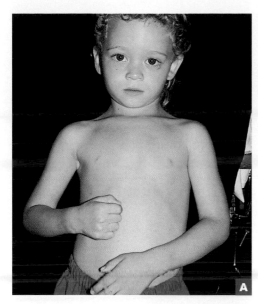

FIG. 21-64 Nursemaid's elbow. *A*, The affected arm is held close to the body with the elbow flexed and the forearm pronated. *B*, Reduction maneuver produces pain, as do attempts at supination during the examination.

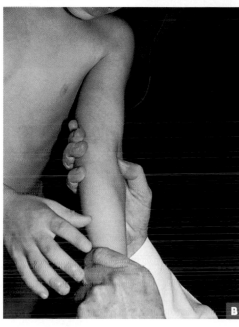

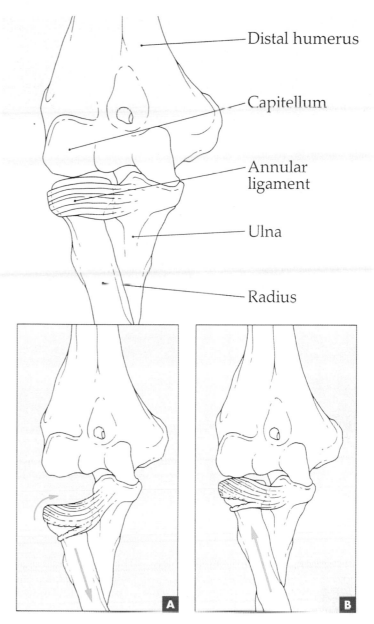

FIG. 21-65 Nursemaid's elbow. *A*, Sudden traction on the outstretched arm pulls the radius distally, causing it to slip partially through the annular ligament and tearing it in the process. *B*, When traction is released, the radial head recoils, trapping the proximal portion of the ligament between it and the capitellum.

Pathologically, when the radial head is subluxated by the sudden pull on the arm, the annular ligament is torn at the site of its attachment to the radius and the radial head slips through the tear. When the traction is released and the radial head recoils, the proximal portion of the annular ligament becomes trapped between the radial head and the capitellum (Fig. 21-65). This limits motion and produces the child's pain. Radiographs are normal because the radial head is not truly subluxed. When a patient presents with a typical history, is found to have no evidence of tenderness, and resists supination, x-ray studies are unnecessary. Reduction, as described later, should be attempted.

Treatment consists of supinating the child's forearm with the elbow in a flexed position while applying pressure over the radial head (see Fig. 21-64, *B*). A click can be perceived as the annular ligament is freed from the joint. Occasionally this maneuver fails, in which case the forearm should be supinated and extended with traction applied distally while pressing down on the radial head. If this fails as well, pronation with the elbow in extension may be attempted. Pain relief is immediate, return of function is evident within 10 to 15 minutes of reduction, and no cast is required. It is often recommended that the child wear a sling for 10 days to reduce use and to allow the annular ligament to heal; compliance is difficult to ensure, however.

If presentation has been delayed for several hours, there may be a longer delay between reduction and resumption of normal use and it may be necessary to administer acetaminophen for 12 to 14 hours to relieve residual aching. Parents should be cautioned to avoid maneuvers that cause excessive traction on the arm, because there is a significant risk of recurrence.

Extremity Pain With Ligamentous Laxity

Children with significant and generalized ligamentous laxity have hypermobile joints and are vulnerable to excessive stretching or stress on ligamentous and musculotendinous structures. They are also some-

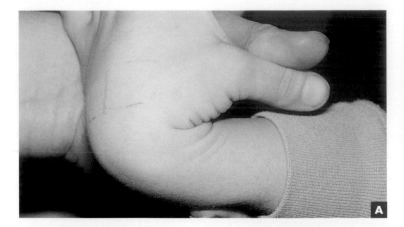

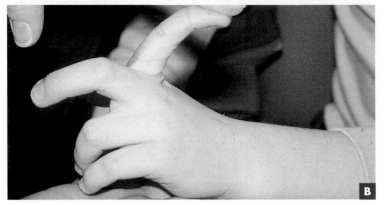

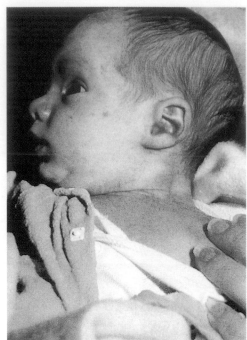

FIG. 21-67 Congenital torticollis. The "tumor" of congenital torticollis is seen as a swelling in the mid-portion of the sternocleidomastoideus muscle. It is firm on palpation, and the muscle itself is shortened. The head tilts toward the affected side, and the chin rotates in the opposite direction. (Courtesy Dr. James Reilly, Children's Hospital of Alabama.)

FIG. 21-66 Ligamentous laxity. This child shows findings typical of the joint hypermobility seen with ligamentous laxity. *A,* He is able to hyperflex the wrist on the forearm. *B,* He also is able to hyperextend the distal interphalangeal joint and the metacarpophalangeal joint.

what more susceptible to joint dislocations. The phenomenon is seen in up to 18% of girls and 6% of boys. After periods of vigorous physical activity, these children often complain of arthralgias or muscular pain and occasionally have evidence of joint swelling. Episodes tend to occur in the evening or at night, are self-limited, lasting 1 to several hours, and respond to rest and acetaminophen or ibuprofen. Many of these children have been accused of attention-getting behavior and hypochondriasis. Others have been dismissed as having "growing pains," and some have undergone extensive testing for rheumatic disorders. A history of greater than average activity on the preceding day and of recurrent short-lived pain usually without objective swelling, combined with findings of ligamentous laxity on examination (Fig. 21-66), should point to this diagnosis. The rarity of joint swelling and the absence of fever and other systemic symptoms help to rule out rheumatic and collagen vascular disorders.

Once the problem is correctly diagnosed, patients can minimize discomfort by avoiding sudden increases in level of activity and by taking a mild analgesic prophylactically after a period of unusually vigorous activity. Graduated strengthening exercises may also be helpful. This is particularly true for children who wish to participate in gymnastics or competitive sports.

Disorders of the Spine

Children with disorders of the axial skeleton most commonly present with some type of deformity. Pain or dysfunction of the associated spinal cord and nerve roots may also prompt evaluation. Because these

conditions often progress with growth, awareness and early recognition are important to facilitate early institution of appropriate treatment and to minimize resultant morbidity.

Congenital Torticollis

Congenital torticollis, or "wry neck," is a positional abnormality of the neck produced by fibrosis and shortening of the sternocleidomastoideus muscle. It is thought to be secondary to abnormal intrauterine positioning or to birth trauma resulting in the formation of a hematoma within the muscle belly. Usually the condition is recognized at or shortly after birth. A palpable swelling or "tumor" is often noted within the muscle. With subsequent fibrosis, the characteristic deformity of torticollis develops, consisting of head tilt toward the affected side with rotation of the chin to the opposite side (Fig. 21-67). Passive rotation is diminished toward the side of the torticollis, and lateral side bending is limited toward the side away from the torticollis. Although the mass usually disappears in the first several weeks of life, contracture of the muscle persists and, if untreated, may result in craniofacial disfigurement with flattening of the face on the affected side. Gentle passive stretching exercises and positioning the child's crib so that external stimuli will cause him or her to turn the head and neck away from the side of deformity may be beneficial. If these measures fail, surgical release of the contracted muscle may be indicated.

Differential diagnoses include Klippel-Feil syndrome; inflammatory or infectious conditions of the head, neck, or nasopharynx; posterior fossa or brainstem neoplasm; traumatic cervical spine injury; and atlantoaxial rotary subluxation. However, with the exception of the

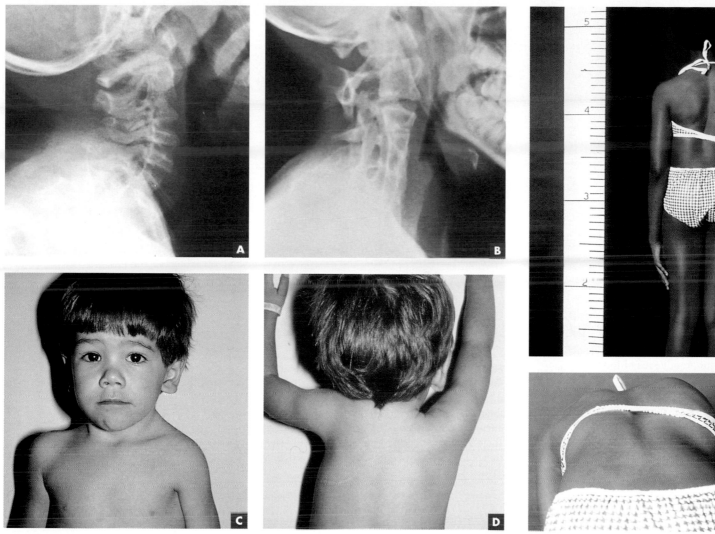

FIG. 21-68 Klippel-Feil syndrome. *A,* This radiograph shows mild osseous involvement with fusion of the upper cervical segments. *B,* Shown in this radiograph is severe osseous involvement in which C3 to C7 are fused and hypoplastic. *C,* The neck appears short and broad in the anterior view of this young child. *D,* In this posterior view, the hairline is low and an associated Sprengel's deformity is present, the left scapula being hypoplastic and high riding. As a result, the patient is unable to fully raise his left arm. Typical webbing is not appreciable in this child.

FIG. 21-69 Moderate thoracic idiopathic adolescent scoliosis. *A,* Scapular asymmetry is easily discernible in the upright position. This results from rotation of the spine and attached rib cage. *B,* Forward flexion reveals a mild rib hump deformity.

Klippel-Feil anomaly, the other conditions tend to occur considerably later in childhood. In addition, a hip examination and an AP pelvis x-ray study should be performed in every child with torticollis, because hip instability or dysplasia is present in approximately 20% of these children.

Klippel-Feil Syndrome

Patients with Klippel-Feil syndrome have a congenital malformation of the neck that results from a failure of segmentation in the developing cervical spine. The condition varies greatly in severity, depending on the number of vertebrae that are fused (Fig. 21-68, *A* and *B*). More severely affected people exhibit a short, broad neck with the appearance of "webbing," a low hairline, and gross restriction of motion (Fig. 21-68, *C* and *D*). The condition may be associated with other congenital malformations, such as Sprengel's deformity (Fig. 21-68, *D;* see Fig. 21-77); rib deformities; scoliosis; CNS defects; and cardiac, pulmonary,

and renal anomalies. Secondary neurologic problems are rare, but accelerated degenerative changes may occur at mobile spinal segments adjacent to the involved vertebrae.

On occasion, range of motion exercises or bracing may be tried to improve mobility or correct the deformity. Surgery, except for cosmesis or the treatment of neurologic dysfunction, is rarely indicated. Mild forms of the malformation may be diagnosed in people only as a result of radiographs taken for other reasons.

Scoliosis

Scoliosis is a curvature of the spine occurring in the lateral plane. It occurs in structural forms, characterized by a fixed curve, and "functional" forms, characterized by a flexible or correctable curve. By anatomic necessity, this lateral deviation is associated with vertebral rotation, such that when this deformity occurs in the thoracic spine, a chest wall deformity, or "rib hump," develops (Fig. 21-69). When it oc-

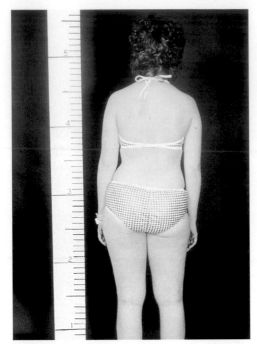

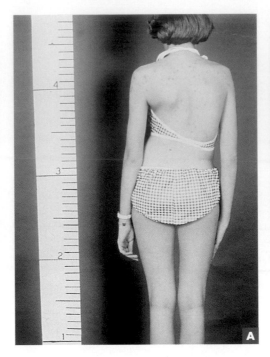

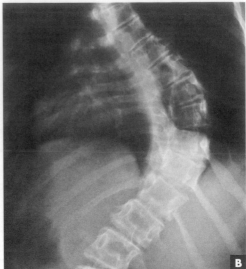

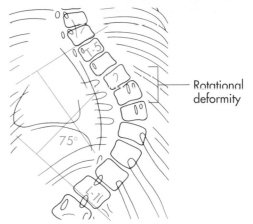

Rotational deformity

FIG. 21-70   Lumbar scoliosis. Pelvic obliquity is present, with prominence of the flank.

FIG. 21-71   Severe thoracic scoliosis secondary to neurofibromatosis. *A,* Note the chest wall deformity and that patient's head is not centered over the pelvis. *B,* The severe curvature is more apparent on this radiograph. The angle of measurement (here 75 degrees) is determined by the intersection of lines drawn perpendicular to the vertebrae at the end of the curve (Cobb's method).

curs in the lumbar spine, a prominence of the flank may be noted (Fig. 21-70). Often there is a primary structural curve with an adjacent secondary compensatory curve. Most cases of structural scoliosis are idiopathic, and their onset occurs in early adolescence. A familial predisposition has been documented, but inheritance of this appears to be multifactorial. Females are affected more often than males, and their curvature is more likely to worsen. Infantile (0 to 3 years) and juvenile (3 to 10 years) forms of idiopathic scoliosis are seen, though much less commonly. Affected infants rapidly develop plagiocephaly with flattening of the head on the concave side of the curve and a corresponding prominence on the opposite side of the head. There is also an increased incidence of associated hip dysplasia, congenital heart disease, inguinal hernias, and mental retardation in these infants. Structural scoliosis can also occur in conjunction with neuromuscular conditions (e.g., cerebral palsy, myelomeningocele, spinocerebellar degeneration, polio, spinal cord tumors); myopathic disorders (arthrogryposis or muscular dystrophy); congenital spinal anomalies (hemivertebrae, trapezoidal vertebrae, unsegmented vertebrae); neurofibromatosis (Fig. 21-71) and mesenchymal disorders; and a variety of other conditions (Table 21-6). These neuromuscular and congenital forms of scoliosis tend to have more rapid progression of curvature than is true of idiopathic scoliosis, and infants with congenital spinal anomalies have a high incidence of associated genitourinary anomalies.

Apparent nonstructural, flexible, or "functional" scoliosis may be seen in association with poor posture, limb-length inequality, or flexion contracture of a hip or knee, in which case the curve disappears when the child is seated. It can also be seen with paraspinous muscle spasm after a back injury; as the result of splinting because of pain in cases of pyelonephritis, appendicitis, or pneumonia; or in patients with a herniated intervertebral disc and secondary nerve root pain (Table 21-6; see Fig. 21-76, *A*). These forms resolve with treatment of the primary disorder.

Except in curvatures resulting from inflammatory or neoplastic processes and from herniation of an intervertebral disc, pain is rarely a complaint in children and adolescents with scoliosis. In fact, patients with pain, signs of nerve root compression, or evidence of new-onset peripheral neurologic deficits should undergo thorough evaluation for a treatable underlying cause.

The clinical signs found during examination in a patient with scoliosis can be separated into true pathognomonic findings and associated stigmata, which may also occur in otherwise normal, nonscoliotic children. The only true pathognomonic sign of scoliosis is the presence of a curve noted on forward bending; this represents a positive Adam's forward-bending test (see the section on Thoracolumbar Spine Examination). An associated convex posterior chest wall prominence (termed *rib hump*) or paralumbar prominence may also be noted on forward bending (see Fig. 21-69, *B*). The rib hump and paralumbar prominence are manifestations of the vertebral rotational deformity seen in scoliosis.

Frequently a diagnosis of scoliosis is not based on a positive forward-bending test, but rather on the presence of so-called stigmata signs. These signs include shoulder asymmetry, unilateral scapular promi-

TABLE 21-6

Causes of Scoliosis

Structural Scoliosis
Idiopathic
Congenital
Neuromuscular
Other conditions that may result in scoliosis:
  Myopathic disorders
  Neurofibromatosis
  Mesenchymal disorders
  Osteochondrodystrophies
  Metabolic disorders
  Trauma, surgery, irradiation, burns

Functional Scoliosis
Herniated lumbar discs
Postural derangements
Limb-length inequality
Irritative or inflammatory disorders
Hysteria

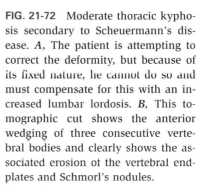

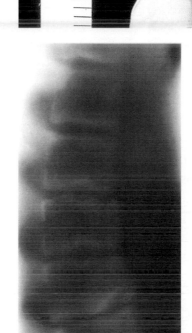

FIG. 21-72 Moderate thoracic kyphosis secondary to Scheuermann's disease. *A,* The patient is attempting to correct the deformity, but because of its fixed nature, he cannot do so and must compensate for this with an increased lumbar lordosis. *B,* This tomographic cut shows the anterior wedging of three consecutive vertebral bodies and clearly shows the associated erosion of the vertebral endplates and Schmorl's nodules.

hence, waist asymmetry, and small chest or paralumbar humps. Any or all of these stigmata signs may be present in a child with true scoliosis, but the mere presence of these stigmata does not always imply the presence of scoliosis. Body asymmetry is a frequent occurrence in the normal nonscoliotic child. A carefully performed Adam's forward-bending test will always determine whether the stigmata signs are associated with true scoliosis or simply evidence of body asymmetry—which does not warrant referral to an orthopedic specialist.

Because screening studies have shown that up to 5% of school-age children and adolescents have lateral curvatures, routine screening by primary care physicians is important. Hence, the forward-bending test should be part of all examinations in children from age 6 to 7 years until the end of puberty (see the section on Thoracolumbar Spine Examination). When true clinical scoliosis is found, the patient should be referred for orthopedic evaluation no matter how small the curve is felt to be. It is probably safer and more cost-effective for the primary care physician to make the referral without obtaining prior radiographs, because typical office radiographs done for scoliosis screening are usually not of high quality. Standing, full-torso x-rays taken on 36-inch (90-cm)–long cassette films with special grids are much more helpful and more readily available in the orthopedic clinic or office. Once a diagnosis of scoliosis has been made, follow-up x-rays are routinely obtained no more frequently than at 6- to 9-month intervals. The goal of close follow-up is to detect progression of curvature early and implement treatment to prevent or reduce it when needed. Idiopathic curves of 20 degrees or more and lesser curves showing rapid progression are treated with spinal bracing and an exercise program. Children with curves exceeding 40 degrees or those with curves that progress rapidly despite bracing require operative intervention.

Patients with untreated curvatures exceeding 60 degrees inevitably suffer significant secondary cardiopulmonary problems, including decreased vital capacity, shunting, decreased oxygen saturation, and cor pulmonale.

Newborns and infants should be screened for congenital and infantile forms of scoliosis. This is often best done by holding the infant prone on the examiner's hand.

Kyphosis

Kyphosis is a curvature of the spine in the sagittal plane. Unlike scoliosis, it is generally not associated with a rotational spinal deformity. It may be purely postural in nature or associated with many pathologic conditions. The latter include congenital vertebral anomalies, spinal growth disturbance (Scheuermann's disease) (Fig. 21-72),

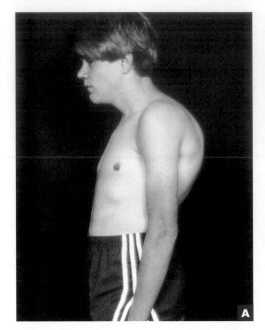

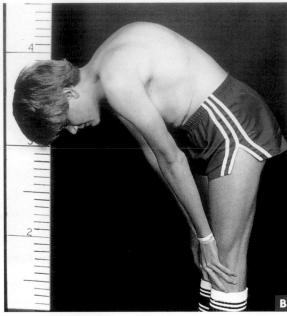

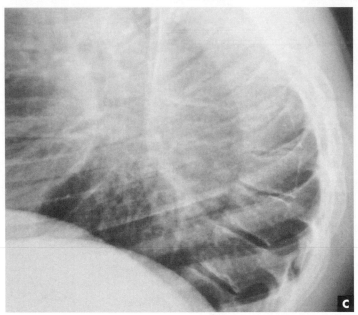

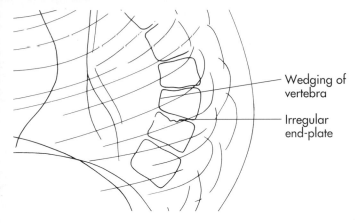

FIG. 21-73 *A,* Severe kyphosis of the thoracic spine secondary to vertebral wedging in a patient with glycogen storage disease. To stand upright, the patient must increase his lumbar lordosis and thrust his head forward to center it above the pelvis. *B,* The kyphotic deformity is accentuated on forward bending. *C,* Radiographically the vertebral wedging that underlies the kyphotic deformity is evident.

Wedging of vertebra

Irregular end-plate

neuromuscular afflictions, skeletal dysplasias, and metabolic diseases (Fig. 21-73). Kyphosis can also develop after spinal trauma or surgery. Patients with a structural deformity may complain of backache aggravated by motion. The deformity is best viewed from the lateral position on forward bending. Evaluation of the effects of posture and of application of pressure over the apex facilitates diagnosis and decisions regarding treatment.

Postural kyphosis is usually seen in preadolescents and consists in a flexible thoracic kyphosis that is correctable on hyperextension. Most affected children have a compensatory increase in lumbar lordosis. Radiographic findings are normal. Treatment consists of an exercise program designed to strengthen trunk and abdominal muscles, which are usually weak in these patients.

Scheuermann's disease, a disorder of unknown etiology, is the most common cause of fixed kyphotic deformity. It can be distinguished clinically from postural kyphosis by its inherent stiffness and the greater magnitude of the deformity. The deformity fails to correct or is only partially correctable on hyperextension or upon the application of pressure over the apex of the curve. Lateral radiographs reveal anterior wedging of three or more consecutive vertebral bodies which are located at the apex of the curve. There is often radiographic evidence of end-plate erosion of the involved vertebrae, and Schmorl's nodules are a common associated finding (see Fig. 21-72).

Exercises and bracing are quite effective in treating mild structural kyphosis in the growing spine. However, when the deformity is severe and fixed, surgical correction and stabilization may be indicated.

Spondylolisthesis

Spondylolisthesis is a condition characterized by the translation or forward displacement of one vertebral body over another and is seen most commonly at the lumbosacral articulation. The problem may develop as a result of insufficiency or fatigue fractures of the pars interarticularis (isthmic), congenital dysplasia of the posterior spinal elements (dysplastic), or degenerative changes of the disc and facets (degenerative), or it may occur secondary to pathologic lesions within the vertebra and its elements (pathologic). Isthmic spondylolisthesis (spondylolysis) is by far the most common type (Fig. 21-74). Patients with a

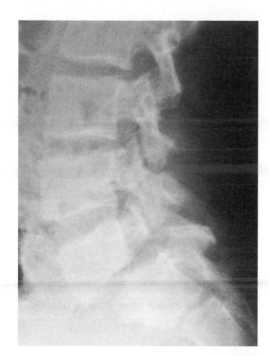

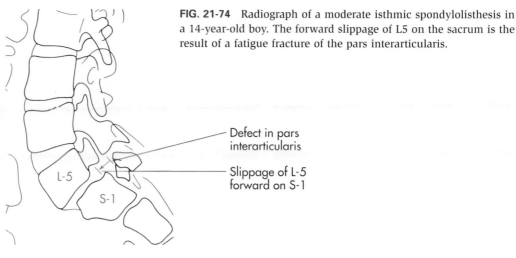

FIG. 21-74 Radiograph of a moderate isthmic spondylolisthesis in a 14-year-old boy. The forward slippage of L5 on the sacrum is the result of a fatigue fracture of the pars interarticularis.

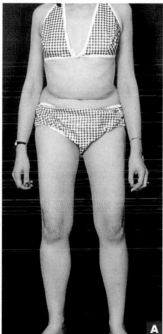

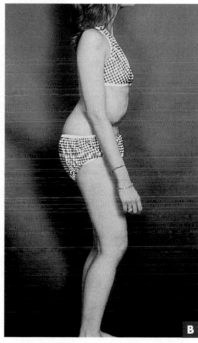

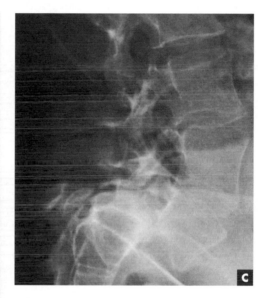

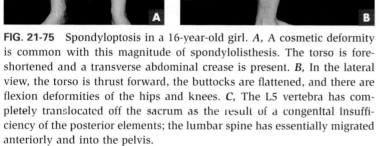

FIG. 21-75 Spondyloptosis in a 16-year-old girl. *A,* A cosmetic deformity is common with this magnitude of spondylolisthesis. The torso is foreshortened and a transverse abdominal crease is present. *B,* In the lateral view, the torso is thrust forward, the buttocks are flattened, and there are flexion deformities of the hips and knees. *C,* The L5 vertebra has completely translocated off the sacrum as the result of a congenital insufficiency of the posterior elements; the lumbar spine has essentially migrated anteriorly and into the pelvis.

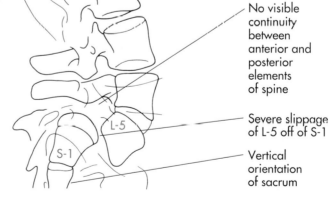

congenital predisposition may show alarming degrees of slippage. The condition is often associated with low back pain that increases with strenuous activities and abates with rest. Some patients have symptoms of nerve root irritation. This necessitates differentiation from inflammatory and neoplastic processes and disc herniation.

Examination often reveals loss of normal lumbar lordosis, tenderness of the involved posterior elements, paravertebral muscle spasm, and secondary tightness of the hamstring muscles. A step-off deformity

may be evident on palpation of the spinous processes. Range of motion is often limited in extension because of pain. Nerve root signs may be present. In its most severe form, spondyloptosis, the L5 vertebral body may completely translate off of the sacrum. These patients characteristically exhibit a waddling gait, a transverse abdominal crease, flattened buttocks, and flexion deformities of the hips and knees and their torso may appear foreshortened (Fig. 21-75, *A* and *B*). Characterization and grading of the process are accomplished with radiographs. The oblique

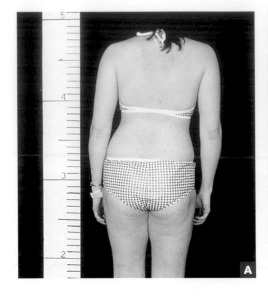
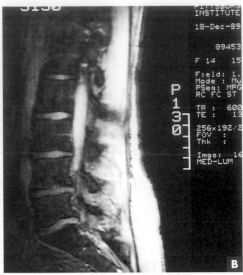

FIG. 21-76 Herniated intervertebral disc. *A,* Discogenic scoliosis in a 16-year-old girl with a herniated disc at L4 to L5. The trunk is shifted away from the affected side. The normal lumbar lordosis is absent, and spinal motion is severely limited. *B,* On this sagittal magnetic resonance image, the L4 to L5 disc bulges posteriorly, compressing the cauda equina. (*B,* Courtesy Department of Pediatric Radiology, Children's Hospital of Pittsburgh.)

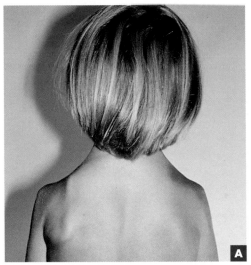
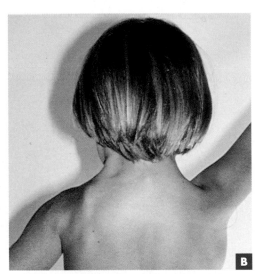
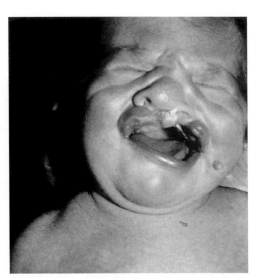

FIG. 21-77 Sprengel's deformity. *A,* The left scapula is high riding and hypoplastic, and its vertebral border is prominent. *B,* Shoulder motion is severely limited, particularly in abduction. (Courtesy Dr. Dana Mears, Shadyside Hospital, Pittsburgh.)

FIG. 21-78 Congenital pseudarthrosis of the clavicle. There is a bulbous, nontender swelling in the region of the midclavicle. The medial aspect of the clavicle is prominent. This patient has associated anomalies.

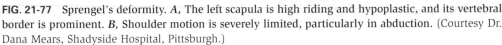

view may reveal a spondylolysis and the lateral view the degree of spondylolisthesis (Figs. 21-74 and 21-75, *C*).

In mild to moderate cases, treatment consists of appropriate exercises and bracing. Patients with progressive slippage require surgical fusion, and those with neural involvement may also require nerve root decompression. In severe spondylolisthesis with cosmetic deformity, functional impairment, and neurologic dysfunction, surgical reduction of the deformity may be attempted, but this is not easy, nor is it without risk to the adjacent neural structures.

Herniated Intervertebral Disc

Although relatively common in adults, herniated discs occur only rarely in children and are almost always limited to the lower two segments of the lumbar spine in adolescents. A history of antecedent trauma is not uncommon. Lower extremity radicular symptoms predominate. Patients often describe a peculiar "pulling" sensation in the lower extremity or liken their pain to a "toothache" in the distribution of the L5 or S1 nerve roots. They may complain of numbness or weakness in the involved limb. Forward flexion, sitting, coughing, or straining aggravate the neurologic symptoms.

On examination, an antalgic scoliosis of the lumbar spine may be apparent, which the patient is unable to reduce (Fig. 21-76, *A*). Inability to reverse the normal lumbar lordosis is present, and symptoms may be aggravated by attempts at flexion. The straight leg–raising test is often positive (radicular symptoms being reproduced when the limb is raised by the examiner [see the section on Thoracolumbar Spine Examination and Fig. 21-5]), and neurologic abnormalities may be found on sensory, motor, and reflex testing. Plain radiographs usually show no abnormality, other than a possible discogenic scoliosis, but the diagnosis may be verified by a myelography, CT, or magnetic resonance imaging (Fig. 21-76, *B*). The differential diagnosis may include hematogenous disc space infection or vertebral osteomyelitis, spinal cord or neural element tumor, and spondylolisthesis with nerve root irritation.

Nonsurgical treatment consisting of rest and antiinflammatory agents may be successful, but if a profound neurologic deficit is present or incapacitating symptoms persist, surgical disc excision may be indicated. Intradiscal chemonucleolysis, as employed for adults, is contraindicated for children. Conservative treatment of radiographically proven disc herniation is not as effective in adolescents as it is in adults.

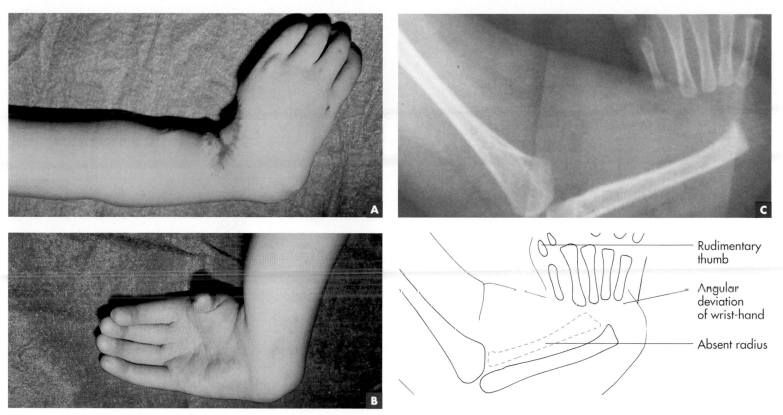

FIG. 21-79 Radial club hand. *A,* The forearm is shortened with radial deviation of the hand and wrist on the ulna. *B,* There is a flexion deformity of the hand and wrist on the forearm and a hypoplastic thumb. *C,* This radiograph shows absence of the radius, dislocation of the carpus, and a rudimentary thumb, all characteristic of radial club hand. (Clinical photographs courtesy Dr. Joseph Imbriglia, Allegheny General Hospital, Pittsburgh.)

Disorders of the Upper Extremity

Because of the importance of prehensile function, disorders affecting any area of the upper limb can result in significant impairment of motor development during childhood. Knowledge of the normal anatomy and actions of the shoulder, arm, elbow, forearm, wrist, and hand is vital for assessment of abnormalities and institution of appropriate treatment.

Sprengel's Deformity

Sprengel's deformity is a congenital malformation characterized by an abnormally small, high-riding scapula. In most cases it is unilateral. The etiology is unknown, but there appears to be a familial predisposition and the condition may be associated with a variety of other congenital anomalies, including Klippel-Feil syndrome (see Fig. 21-68) and rib and vertebral malformations. The small undescended scapula may be attached to the cervical spine by a band of fibrous tissue or bone (omovertebral bone). Scoliosis and torticollis may be associated abnormalities. Cosmetic deformity and limited shoulder motion on the affected side are the usual complaints.

On examination, the scapula is noted to be hypoplastic and high riding in association with asymmetry of the base of the neck and shoulder (Fig. 21-77, *A*). Shoulder motion is usually severely limited, particularly in abduction (Fig. 21-77, *B*). Radiography confirms the abnormal size and position of the scapula.

Nonsurgical treatment consisting of stretching and range-of-motion exercises may be instituted but is rarely successful. Surgery is usually undertaken for cosmetic and functional reasons and may consist of excision of the prominent superior aspect of the scapula or of release and reduction of the scapula accomplished by placing it inferiorly on the chest wall. The latter procedure is not without risk, as brachial plexus palsy may result from the maneuver.

Congenital Pseudarthrosis of the Clavicle

Congenital pseudarthrosis of the clavicle is a rare congenital disorder usually manifested by a painless, nontender bulbous deformity in the region of the midclavicle. It is thought to result from a failure of maturation of the ossification center of the clavicle. It generally involves the right side and on occasion may be associated with other congenital anomalies. In cleidocranial dysostosis the entire clavicle may be absent or may have an appearance similar to that of congenital pseudarthrosis.

On examination, the clavicle appears foreshortened with a prominence evident in its midportion (Fig. 21-78; see Fig. 6-41 for radiographic appearance). Palpation reveals hypermobility of the two ends of the clavicle and crepitance. Range of motion of the shoulder is generally normal. This condition characteristically involves no functional impairment and requires no treatment. Although clavicular fracture as a result of birth trauma may present a similar appearance, it is easily distinguished because of tenderness over the region of deformity.

Radial Club Hand

Radial club hand is the result of congenital absence or hypoplasia of the radial structures of the forearm and hand. Associated muscular structures and the radial nerve are hypoplastic or absent. The anomaly is rare and affects more male than female subjects. Its characteristic clinical presentation is a small, short, bowed forearm and aplasia or hypoplasia of the thumb, and the residual hand is deviated radially (Fig. 21-79, *A* and *B*). Radiographs show absence of bones in the affected area (Fig. 21-79, *C*).

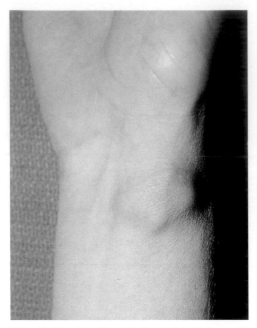

FIG. 21-80 Ganglion of the wrist. This cystic mass overlying the wrist joint and flexor tendons was asymptomatic and nontender.

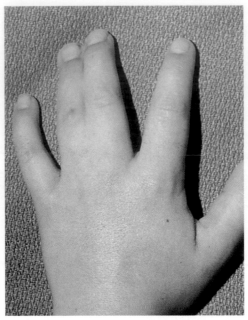

FIG. 21-81 Mild syndactyly involving soft tissues of the middle and ring fingers without bony involvement. (Courtesy Dr. Joseph Imbriglia, Allegheny General Hospital, Pittsburgh.)

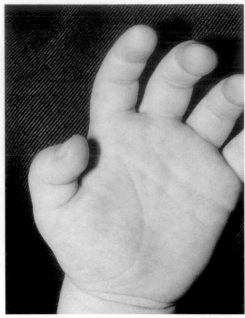

FIG. 21-82 Congenital trigger thumb. There is a fixed flexion deformity at the interphalangeal joint of the thumb resulting from tightness of the tendon sheath of the flexor pollicis longus. The remainder of the hand appears normal.

Treatment is best instituted early with passive stretching exercises and corrective casting. Surgical treatment consists of centralization of the hand on the "one-bone forearm" to maximize function.

Ganglion of the Wrist

A ganglion is a benign cystic mass consisting of an accumulation of synovial fluid or gelatin in an outpouching of a tendon sheath or joint capsule. The exact etiology is unknown, but it is thought to be related to a herniation of synovial tissue with a ball valve effect. Antecedent trauma may be reported. These masses may be present over the dorsal or volar aspects of the wrist and are generally located toward the radial side (Fig. 21-80). They are occasionally seen on the dorsum of the foot or adjacent to one of the malleoli of the ankle (see Fig. 21-103). Their size may fluctuate with time and activity. On examination, they may be either firm or fluctuant and they can be transilluminated. Although most are asymptomatic, an occasional patient may have pain and tenderness.

Treatment is generally unnecessary for patients who are asymptomatic. Occasionally, patients desire removal for cosmetic or psychological reasons. Surgery is not routinely advised for asymptomatic cysts, because the recurrence rate may be as high as 20%. Aspiration, injection, or rupture of these cysts does not eradicate them. Surgical excision with obliteration of the base of the ganglion is the most successful treatment for the occasional patient in whom treatment is indicated.

Syndactyly

Syndactyly is a relatively common congenital affliction involving failure of the digits of the hands or feet to separate. It is more common and disabling in the upper extremity. Bilateral involvement is usual, and a positive family history is not uncommon. It may be associated with other congenital anomalies, particularly Apert's syndrome and Streeter's dys-

plasia. There is great variation in the degree of fusion. In mild cases, only the skin is joined, making reconstructive surgery simple (Fig. 21-81). In more severe cases, the nails, deeper structures, and bones may be conjoined, contributing to deformity and growth abnormalities and making reconstructive treatment more difficult.

Congenital Trigger Thumb

A congenital trigger thumb is characterized by a fixed or intermittent flexion deformity of the interphalangeal joint of the thumb that may be present at birth or may develop shortly thereafter (Fig. 21-82). It is thought to result from tightness of the tendon sheath of the flexor pollicis longus in the region of the metacarpophalangeal joint. The flexion deformity generally cannot be reduced, although in milder cases it may be passively correctable, with a snapping sensation felt as the tendon passes through the stenosed pulley mechanism. If passively correctable, splinting in extension occasionally will result in correction; otherwise, surgery is required.

Boutonnière (Buttonhole) Deformity

A boutonnière deformity of the finger is the end-result of a traumatic avulsion of the central portion of the extensor tendon at its insertion on the middle phalanx of the finger that went unrecognized at the time of initial injury. The mechanism of injury is usually a blow to the tip of the finger that drives it into forced flexion against resistance. A laceration over the dorsum of the finger involving the extensor tendon may produce a similar deformity if tendon involvement is not recognized and repaired at the time. Initially, there may be local tenderness over the dorsal aspect of the PIP joint without deformity. With time, however, the lateral bands of the extensor mechanism migrate volarly, producing a flexion deformity of the PIP joint with a secondary extension deformity of the distal joint (Fig. 21-83). If recognized early, healing

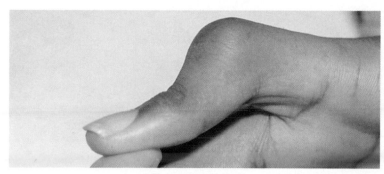

FIG. 21-83 Boutonnière deformity of the finger. There is a fixed flexion contracture of the proximal interphalangeal joint and hyperextension of the distal joint secondary to volar migration of the lateral bands of the extensor mechanism. This is the result of an unrecognized or inadequately treated injury to the extensor tendon at its insertion on the middle phalanx.

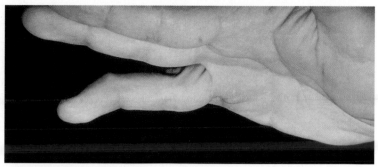

FIG. 21-84 Mallet finger with secondary swan-neck deformity. This is the result of avulsion of the extensor tendon from its insertion at the base of the distal phalanx, which was not recognized at the time of injury. The patient shows a flexion deformity of the distal interphalangeal joint and secondary hyperextension of the proximal interphalangeal joint.

may occur with splinting of the PIP joint in extension. Later, open surgical repair may be necessary to improve function.

Mallet Finger/Swan-Neck Deformity

A mallet finger is the result of avulsion of the extensor tendon from its insertion at the base of the distal phalanx of a finger. It occurs as a result of a blow to the extended finger against resistance. The tendon alone, or a portion of the distal phalanx into which it inserts, may be involved. The clinical appearance is that of a "dropped finger" or flexion deformity of the distal interphalangeal joint with inability to actively extend the joint (see Fig. 21-47). If not recognized and treated at the time of the initial injury, the condition becomes chronic and contracture of the extensor mechanism may occur, with a secondary hyperextension deformity of the proximal interphalangeal joint producing a swan-neck deformity (Fig. 21-84). Treatment consists of splinting the distal joint in an extended position, open reduction if a large fragment of bone is involved, or surgical repair in chronic cases.

Disorders of the Lower Extremity

Normally developed and functional lower extremities permit locomotion with ease and a minimal amount of energy expenditure. A disability resulting from a deformed, shortened, or painful lower limb can be considerable (see the section on Gait and Gait Disturbances).

Many problems of the lower extremities occurring in childhood are congenital and, if they remain unrecognized or are unsuccessfully treated, can result in life-long disability. Knowledge of the normal anatomy and function of the hip, knee, ankle, and foot is necessary to accurately recognize and treat abnormalities in this region (see the section on Lower Extremity Examination).

Congenital Dislocation of the Hip

Congenital dislocation of the hip, or displacement of the femoral head from its normal relationship with the acetabulum, is a relatively frequent problem, with an incidence of 1 to 2 per 1000 births. It is generally detectable at birth or shortly thereafter. Female infants are affected significantly more frequently than male infants, and unilateral dislocation is twice as frequent as bilateral. Congenital dislocation may be divided into idiopathic and teratogenic types. Idiopathic congenital dislocation is more frequent, and patients often have a positive family his-

tory for the defect. Its severity varies from subluxated, to dislocated and reducible, to dislocated and irreducible. This type of congenital dislocation may be related to abnormal intrauterine positioning or restriction of fetal movement in utero, which impedes adequate development and stability of the hip joint complex. The relaxing effect of hormones on soft tissue during pregnancy may also contribute, with affected infants perhaps being more sensitive to the pelvic relaxation effects of maternal estrogen. A history of breech presentation is not uncommon, and these patients often exhibit generalized ligamentous laxity. Teratogenic dislocations of the hip represent a more severe form of the disorder and are probably the result of a germ plasm defect. They occur early in fetal development and result in malformation of both the femoral head and the acetabular socket. Associated congenital anomalies are common in infants whose dislocations are teratogenic. There is a significant association with clubfoot deformity, congenital torticollis, metatarsus adductus, and infantile scoliosis.

The importance of careful hip evaluation in the newborn and at early infant visits cannot be overemphasized. Early diagnosis enables prompt institution of treatment and results in a better outcome. A knowledge of the clinical signs and skill in techniques of examination are necessary.

Typically, the infant with a dislocated hip holds the leg in a position of adduction and external rotation. If the dislocation is unilateral, the skin folds of the thighs and buttocks are often asymmetrical and the involved lower extremity appears shorter than the opposite side (Fig. 21-85, *A*). This foreshortening is accentuated by holding the hips and knees in 90 degrees of flexion (Galeazzi sign). In patients with bilateral dislocations, these asymmetrical findings are not present. In a truly dislocated hip, the most consistent physical finding is that of limited abduction (Fig. 21-85, *B*). Additional diagnostic maneuvers may assist in establishing the diagnosis. In patients with reducible dislocations, Ortolani's sign is positive when a palpable clunk is felt upon abduction and internal rotation (relocation) of the hip. Barlow's test is positive if, with the knees flexed and hips flexed to 90 degrees, the hips are gently adducted with pressure applied on the lesser trochanter by the thumb. A palpable clunk indicating posterior dislocation is appreciated if the hip is unstable or dislocated. When the hip is dislocated and irreducible, only limitation of abduction is apparent.

The radiographic findings of a congenital hip dislocation are characteristic. The femoral head is generally located lateral and superior to its normal position and the acetabulum may be shallow, with lateral deficiency and a characteristic high acetabular index or slope (Fig. 21-85, *C* and *D*). Reduction of the dislocated hip is apparent if,

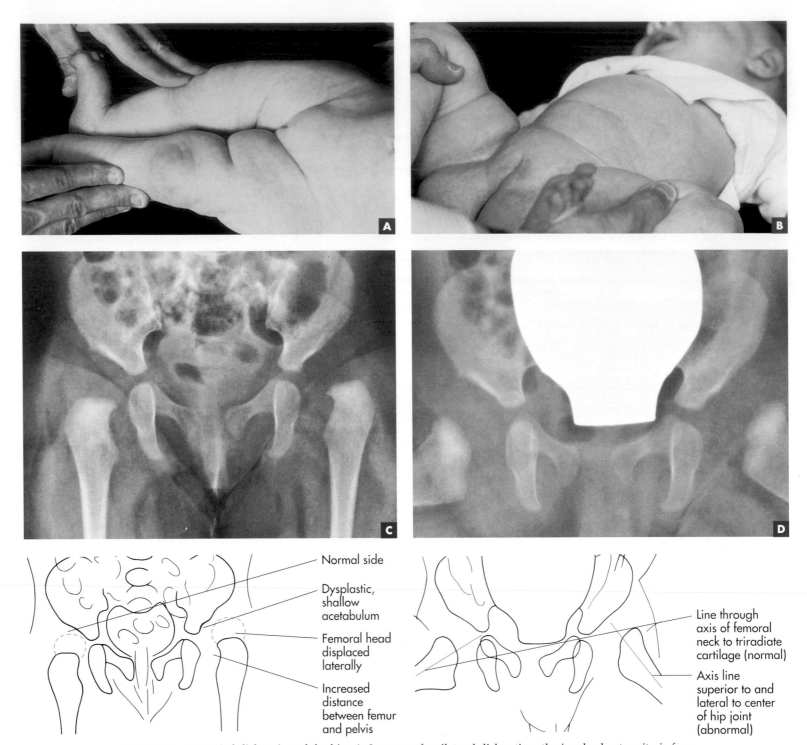

FIG. 21-85   Congenital dislocation of the hip. *A,* In cases of unilateral dislocation, the involved extremity is foreshortened and the thigh and groin creases are asymmetrical. *B,* Limited abduction of the involved hip is seen. This is a consistent finding in infants with a dislocated and irreducible hip. *C,* In this anteroposterior radiograph obtained in a 3-month-old child, the proximal femur is displaced upward and laterally and the acetabulum is shallow. The femoral head is not visible on the radiograph because of the delayed ossification associated with congenital hip dislocation. *D,* In the frog-leg view, the long axis of the affected left femur is directed toward a point superior and lateral to the triradiate cartilage, in contrast to that of the right, which points directly toward this structure.

upon abduction of the hip to 45 degrees, a line drawn through the axis of the metaphysis of the neck crosses the triradiate cartilage (Fig. 21-85). In idiopathic dislocation, ossification of the femoral epiphysis is delayed. Ossification is normally evident radiographically at 3 to 6 months of age but is delayed in congenital dislocation because normal articulation forces are absent. In teratogenic hip dislocation, there may

be hypoplasia of both the acetabular and femoral sides with noncongruent development of one or both of these structures. The early radiographic findings, however, are similar to those already mentioned.

Successful correction depends on the early diagnosis and institution of appropriate treatment. In the first 6 months of life, use of a Pavlik harness, which permits gentle motion of the hip in a flexed and ab-

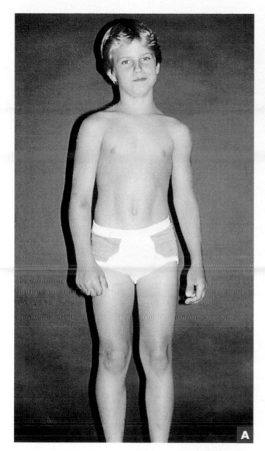

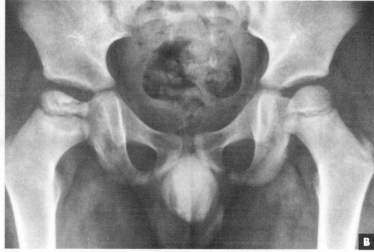

FIG. 21-86 Legg-Calvé-Perthes disease. *A*, This 7-year-old boy is small for his chronologic age. He is bearing less weight on the involved right leg (note the flexed right knee). On examination, a hip flexion contracture, detected by a positive Thomas test (see Fig. 21-8, *B*), and an abductor lurch gait were found. *B*, In this anteroposterior radiograph, the right femoral epiphysis is flattened and fragmented. The proximal femur is also displaced inferiorly and laterally.

ducted position, may achieve and maintain a satisfactory reduction. Between 6 and 18 months of age, gentle closed reduction and immobilization in a spica cast with or without surgical release of the contracted iliopsoas and adductor muscles is indicated. After the age of 18 months, reduction by manipulative measures is difficult owing to contractures of the associated soft tissues. In such instances, open reduction is usually indicated. In cases of teratogenic dislocation, underlying maldevelopment makes the outcome less satisfactory, even with optimal management.

With early recognition and appropriate treatment, a relatively normal hip with satisfactory function can be anticipated. Failure of concentric reduction or complications such as avascular necrosis of the femoral head, resulting from overzealous attempts at closed reduction in long-standing cases, may result in a life-long disability characterized by pain and stiffness in the hip, an antalgic, lurching gait, and shortening of the involved limb.

Legg-Calvé-Perthes Disease

In Legg-Calvé-Perthes disease (coxa plana), impairment of the blood supply to the developing femoral head results in avascular necrosis. The etiology is unknown. Current theories implicate traumatic disruption of the blood supply and recurrent episodes of synovitis during which increased intraarticular pressure compromises blood flow to the developing ossific nucleus as causative. The disorder generally becomes manifest between the ages of 4 and 11 years, with a higher incidence in boys. Affected children often exhibit delayed skeletal maturation and are small for their age. Unilateral involvement is the rule, and if a bilateral case is suspected, some form of epiphyseal dysplasia must be ruled out. The severity of the disease varies greatly, depending on the extent to which the femoral head is affected. Younger children generally have milder involvement, as

a larger portion of the femoral head is still cartilaginous and less dependent on vascular supply.

Onset is often insidious. The child may present with symptoms characteristic of toxic synovitis without radiographic findings. Many children present with a painless limp, and others complain of thigh or knee pain, fatigue on walking, or hip stiffness. Generally, the patient bears less weight on the involved leg when standing and there is a flexion contracture of the involved hip (Figs. 21-8 and 21-86, *A*), with the lower extremity held in a slightly externally rotated position. Pain and limitation of motion are encountered on attempts at internal rotation and abduction. Trendelenburg's sign (failure to maintain a level pelvis when standing on the involved limb) is positive.

Early radiographic findings may include failure of progressive development of the femoral ossific nucleus, a subchondral radiolucent fracture line (Caffey's sign), or evidence of slight subluxation. However, in very early cases, radiographs may be completely normal, though a nuclear bone scan may be useful in verification of impairment of the blood supply to this region. Later, fragmentation of the femoral ossification center may be evident with flattening of the femoral head, extrusion, and frank subluxation (Fig. 21-86, *B*).

The disease is self-limited, typically lasting for 1 to 2 years. Although revascularization and reconstitution of the femoral head always occurs, loss of mechanical integrity of the head with flattening and fragmentation of its surface may result in an irreversible predisposition to degenerative change. Most treatments are based on the principle of "containment" and the maintenance of a normal relationship of the femoral head within the acetabulum so as to minimize permanent joint incongruity. In young children with minimal symptoms and radiographic findings, decreased activity and close observation may be all that is necessary. Antiinflammatory agents and traction are used during episodes of synovitis. In more severe cases, abduction casting, bracing, or surgical treatment with femoral or acetabular osteotomy to reposi-

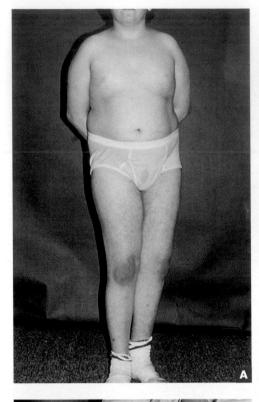

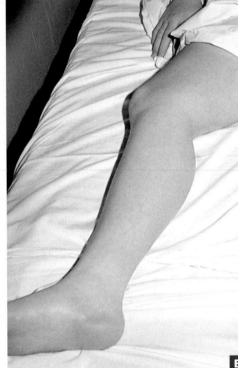

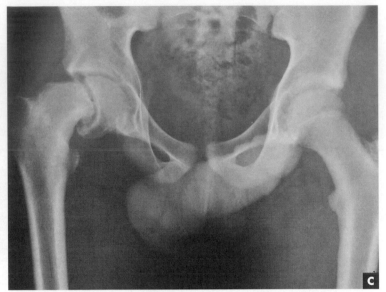

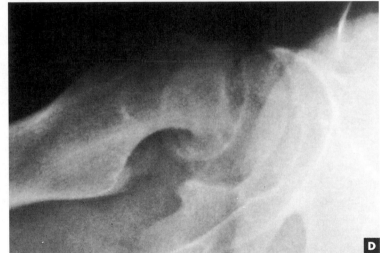

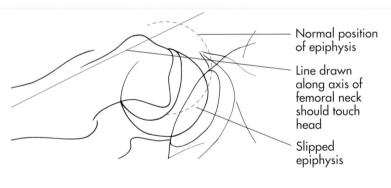

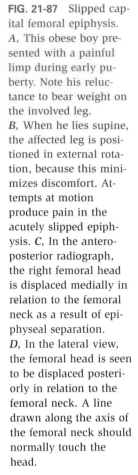

FIG. 21-87 Slipped capital femoral epiphysis. *A,* This obese boy presented with a painful limp during early puberty. Note his reluctance to bear weight on the involved leg. *B,* When he lies supine, the affected leg is positioned in external rotation, because this minimizes discomfort. Attempts at motion produce pain in the acutely slipped epiphysis. *C,* In the anteroposterior radiograph, the right femoral head is displaced medially in relation to the femoral neck as a result of epiphyseal separation. *D,* In the lateral view, the femoral head is seen to be displaced posteriorly in relation to the femoral neck. A line drawn along the axis of the femoral neck should normally touch the head.

Normal position of epiphysis

Line drawn along axis of femoral neck should touch head

Slipped epiphysis

tion the femoral head deeper within the acetabulum may be employed. In patients whose disease is recognized late or who fail to respond to appropriate measures, permanent degenerative change is common and salvage-type surgery may be necessary.

Slipped Capital Femoral Epiphysis

Slipped capital femoral epiphysis, a disorder seen early in puberty, involves displacement of the femoral head from the femoral neck through the epiphyseal plate. It is seen more frequently in males, and occurs bilaterally in approximately 25% of patients. Most commonly, it occurs at the onset of puberty in obese children with delayed sexual maturation.

Although the etiology is unclear, it is generally thought that hormonal changes at the time of puberty may result in loss of mechanical integrity of the growth plate, and that if the epiphysis is then subjected to excessive shear stress, slippage through this area may occur. This condition differs from traumatic epiphyseal fractures because the translational displacement occurs through a different area of the growth plate. In some cases an underlying connective tissue disorder, such as Marfan syndrome, or an endocrinologic problem, such as hypothyroidism, can be identified.

The clinical presentation is quite characteristic, although the duration of symptoms varies. The patient presents with a painful limp and may or may not have a history of recent trauma, which is usually minor, or

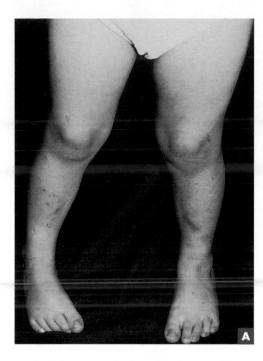

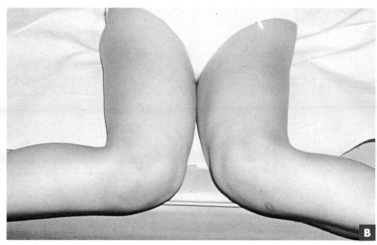

FIG. 21-88 Femoral anteversion. *A,* The condition occurs bilaterally, and in the standing view, both legs appear to turn inward from the hip down. *B,* On assessment of range of motion, the degree of internal rotation of the hips is found to be greater than normal. (Courtesy Dr M. Sherlock.)

pain may have developed after jumping. This injury may have precipitated a slip in the previously weakened epiphysis or may have increased the degree of displacement of a slip that was already in progress. The pain may be perceived as being in the hip or in the thigh or knee. The lower extremity is held in an externally rotated position secondary to deformity at the site of physeal displacement (Fig. 21-87, *A* and *B*). An antalgic and abductor lurch gait is usually apparent. A flexion contracture may be noted, and range of motion tends to be diminished in all planes, particularly internal rotation. Slight shortening of the involved lower extremity is observed in some patients.

Radiographic findings vary from a widened and radiolucent physis (preslip) to a frank deformity with displacement of the femoral head on the proximal femur posteriorly and inferiorly in relation to its normal counterpart (Fig. 21-87, *C* and *D*). The degree of slippage and deformity correlates with the extent of incongruity of the hip joint and the later development of degenerative change and painful symptoms. Prompt intervention to prevent further displacement is an important factor in preventing life-long problems, and awareness, a high index of suspicion, and early recognition are key factors in improving the prognosis.

In patients with undisplaced or mildly displaced slips, cast immobilization or stabilization of the slip with in situ pin fixation is indicated. In patients with acute slipped epiphyses of moderate or severe grade, an attempt at closed reduction followed by surgical pin fixation may be indicated. When the disease is recognized late and deformity is severe, proximal femoral osteotomy may be necessary. Children with unilateral slipped epiphyses must be monitored closely for signs of involvement of the opposite limb.

Femoral Anteversion

Femoral anteversion may be viewed as a normal variation of lower extremity positioning in the developing child. In utero and at birth, the femoral neck sits in an anteverted position relative to that of the adult. During childhood it remodels to a position of slight anteversion and normal alignment of the lower extremities. In certain children, however, delayed rotational correction may result in persistent intoeing. An unsightly gait, kicking of the heels, or tripping on walking or running are frequent related complaints. There may be a history of sitting on the floor with the legs turned outward in a "reversed Tailor position." Generally the condition is bilateral and is not associated with other musculoskeletal problems.

On examination, the child is noted to stand with the entire lower extremities, including the knees and feet, turned inward. An increase in internal rotation over external rotation is apparent on assessment of range of motion of the hip (Fig. 21-88). Radiographic findings are normal. No treatment is indicated, other than reassurance that the condition will correct with growth and instructions to avoid sitting in the predisposing position.

Genu Varum (Physiologic Bowlegs)

Genu varum, or bowlegs, is a normal variation of lower extremity configuration, seen in the 1- to 3-year age-group. It is generally recognized shortly after ambulation begins and may be associated with laxity of other joints and internal tibial torsion. Examination reveals diffuse bowing of the lower extremities with an increased distance between the knees that is accentuated on standing (Fig. 21-89). Varus positioning of the heel with pronation of the feet may be noted on weight-bearing. The child may walk with a waddling gait and kick the heels on running to clear the feet from the ground and avoid hitting the contralateral limb. Laxity of joint capsular structures may be noted with application of a reduction force.

Radiographs show normal osseous and physeal development and may reveal a gentle symmetrical bowing of the femur and tibia. Although there may be slight beaking of the medial metaphyses of the femur and tibia adjacent to the knee joint, there is no fragmentation of the epiphyses or irregularity of the growth plate, as is seen in Blount's disease (see Fig. 21-91). Conditions such as rickets or other metabolic abnormalities, epiphyseal dysplasia, various forms of dwarfism, and pathologic growth disturbances such as Blount's disease also can usually be ruled out on the basis of radiographic findings.

Treatment is rarely indicated, as this condition resolves with growth; in fact, a valgus deformity of the knees may be noted later, at approximately 4 to 5 years of age. Casting, bracing, and corrective shoes are unnecessary, and there is no indication for surgery.

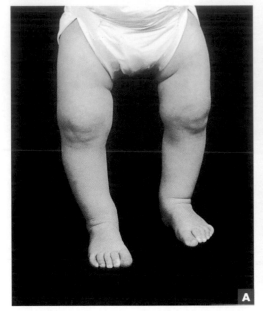

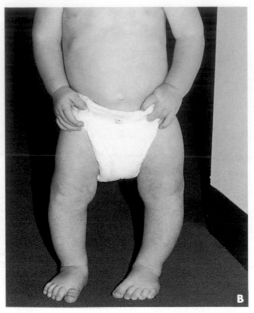

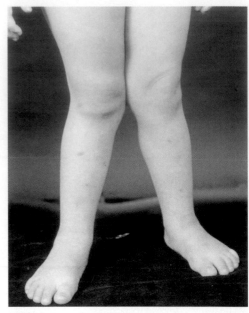

FIG. 21-89   Genu varum. *A,* The mild symmetrical bowing seen in this 1-year-old boy represents a normal variation of lower extremity configuration that occurs in toddlers; correction occurs with growth and remodeling. The bowing is diffuse and involves the upper and lower portions of the legs. *B,* This child has more severe physiologic bowing, which resulted in frequent tripping and a waddling gait. He also had associated ligamentous laxity and intoeing on the left.

FIG. 21-90   Genu valgum. This 3½-year-old girl shows moderate knock-knees. Ligamentous laxity and mild pes planus are associated problems.

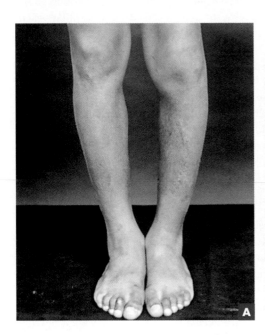

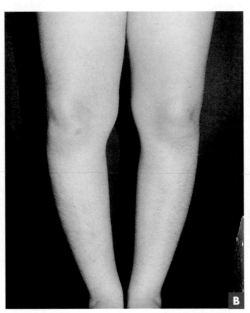

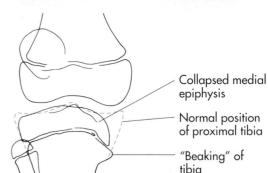

FIG. 21-91   Blount's disease. *A,* This patient has a unilateral angular deformity of the proximal left tibia that gives the appearance of genu varum. *B,* Both proximal tibiae are bowed in another patient as a result of fragmentation and loss of height of the medial epiphyses. In contrast to physiologic bowing, the thighs are straight. *C,* The radiograph shows the typical fragmentation, loss of height, and angular deformity or beaking of the medial portion of the proximal tibia.

Genu Valgum (Physiologic Knock-Knees)

Genu valgum, or knock-knees, is a normal variation of lower extremity configuration, generally noted in children between the ages of 3 and 5 years. The phenomenon is part of the normal process of remodeling of the lower extremities during growth and development. It is more frequently seen in females and may be associated with ligamentous lax-

ity. While standing the child is noted to have an increased distance between the feet when the medial aspects of the knees touch one another (Fig. 21-90). Not uncommonly, the child will place one knee behind the other in an attempt to get the feet together. In some cases, valgus alignment of the feet and a pes planus deformity may be noted. Radiographs reveal no osseous or physeal abnormalities, but accentuation of the an-

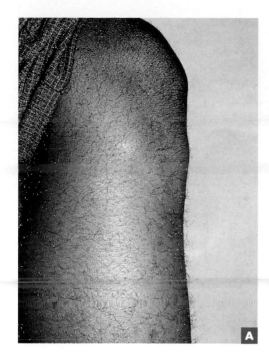 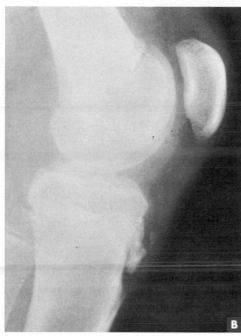

FIG. 21-92 Osgood-Schlatter disease. *A,* Localized swelling is evident in the region of the tibial tubercle. This is generally tender on palpation. The knee is otherwise normal on examination, with the possible exception of mild limitation of flexion. *B,* Irregularity and fragmentation of the tibial tubercle are seen in this radiograph. In less severe cases of shorter duration, soft tissue swelling or irregularity of ossification may be the only findings.

gular deformity of the knee secondary to ligamentous laxity is seen on weight-bearing views. One must rule out the possibility of an underlying metabolic condition such as rickets or renal disease. Treatment is generally not indicated, as the condition gradually corrects with time.

Blount's Disease

Blount's disease is an isolated growth disturbance of the medial tibial epiphysis manifested as an angular varus deformity of the proximal tibia with apparent progressive genu varum. Unilateral and bilateral involvement is seen with nearly equal frequency. The etiology of this condition is unknown, although it appears to be more common in African-Americans. It may represent a compression injury to the medial growth plate of the proximal tibia.

On careful examination, a localized angular deformity of the proximal tibia is apparent (Fig. 21-91, *A* and *B*), in contrast to the diffuse bowing of the lower extremities seen in patients with physiologic bowlegs. Generally there is no evidence of the ligamentous laxity commonly associated with physiologic bowing. Radiographs reveal fragmentation of the medial epiphysis of the tibia associated with beaking and loss of height in this region, as well as the characteristic angular deformity (Fig. 21-91, *C*). A satisfactory response to treatment depends on accurate diagnosis and early recognition, as bracing or surgical osteotomy with realignment of the leg may prevent further progression.

Osgood-Schlatter Disease

Osgood-Schlatter disease is a traction apophysitis of the tibial tubercle which tends to develop during the adolescent growth spurt. It occurs somewhat more frequently in males than females. It is thought that rapid differential growth between the osseous and soft tissue structures and stress on the apophyses produced by vigorous physical activity are contributing factors. Bilateral involvement is usual. Patients have a history of gradually increasing pain and swelling in the region of the tibial tubercle. Discomfort is accentuated by vigorous physical activity, kneeling, or crawling and is relieved by rest.

On examination, a localized tender swelling is noted in the region of the tibial tubercle and patellar tendon (Fig. 21-92, *A*). The knee joint is otherwise normal on examination, with the exception that some patients show limitation of knee flexion with reproduction of their pain. Radiographs may reveal only soft tissue swelling in the region of the proximal tibial apophysis or irregularity of ossification of this structure (Fig. 21-92, *B*). In long-standing cases, frank fragmentation of the apophysis may be seen.

The problem, though self-limited, typically persists for 6 to 24 months. If the condition is only occasionally bothersome and does not limit activities, treatment is unnecessary. If severe pain and a limp are present, a short period of immobilization in a splint or cast may be beneficial. Use of ibuprofen as needed for relieving pain and curtailing activities that produce pain are sufficient treatment for most patients. Steroid injection is contraindicated, because this may cause deterioration of the tendon and provides little in the way of long-term relief.

Popliteal (Baker's) Cyst

Popliteal cysts occurring in childhood are encountered most commonly in children between 5 and 10 years of age and occur significantly more frequently in boys than girls. They are located in the posteromedial aspect of the knee joint in the region of the semimembranosus tendon and medial gastrocnemius muscle belly. Pathologically it is a fibrous tissue or synovial cyst filled with synovial-like fluid. In contrast to those seen in adults, popliteal cysts in childhood generally do not communicate with the joint capsule but originate instead beneath the semimembranosus tendon, presumably as a result of chronic irritation. Occasionally, vague pain is noted, but evaluation is usually sought because of a recently noted painless mass.

On examination, a soft, nontender, cystic mass is found in the described location (Fig. 21-93). Range of motion of the joint is normal unless the cyst is particularly large, limiting flexion. The knee is otherwise normal. Radiographs show no osseous abnormality. Popliteal cysts are benign and may resolve over time, although their surgical excision is reasonable if desired.

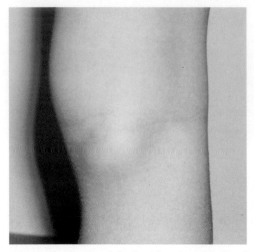

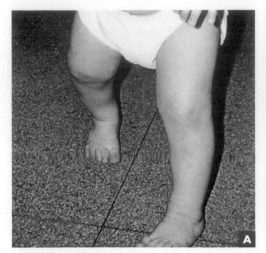

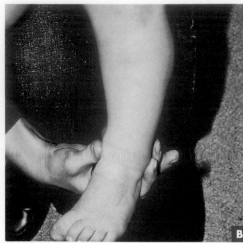

FIG. 21-93 Popliteal (Baker's) cyst. A localized swelling appears in the region of the semimembranosus tendon. This may arise from the synovial lining of the semimembranosus bursa.

FIG. 21-94 Internal tibial torsion. *A,* The hip, thigh, and knee are normally oriented and the patella faces anteriorly, but the lower leg and foot turn inward. The deformity results in prominent intoeing on walking and may cause the child to trip frequently. *B,* The lateral malleolus is positioned anterior to the medial malleolus, thus shifting the ankle mortise and foot to a medially oriented position. (Courtesy Dr. Michael Sherlock.)

Chondromalacia Patella

Chondromalacia patella is a disorder of as yet unclear etiology, although abnormal tracking of the patella is suspected to be causative in part. Patellofemoral incongruity resulting from developmental variations in the shape of the distal femur and patella, malalignment of the quadriceps and patellar tendons, abnormal positioning of the patella in the quadriceps tendon, and weakness of the quadriceps muscle have all been associated with the condition.

Onset of symptoms may be insidious or may abruptly follow trauma. The patient complains of diffuse aching behind the patella that is exacerbated by climbing stairs, pedaling a bicycle, or prolonged sitting. On examination, the patella is found to be tender along its medial border and application of pressure over the patella with the knee slightly flexed elicits pain. When the examiner holds a hand over the patella as the patient flexes and extends the knee, a grating sensation may be felt.

Pathologically, softening and blistering of the articular cartilage are found early on. With progression, the articular cartilage becomes fissured and ultimately eroded.

Treatment consists of quadriceps-strengthening exercises, oral anti-inflammatory agents such as ibuprofen and avoidance of activities such as deep knee bends and weight lifting.

Internal Tibial Torsion

Internal tibial torsion is a nonpathologic variation in the normal development of the lower leg in children under the age of 5 years. It is a rotational deformity that is thought to result from internal molding of the foot and leg in utero. The child is usually brought for evaluation because of concern about prominent intoeing on walking and frequent tripping.

On examination, the hips and knees are found to be normally aligned, with the patellas facing anteriorly, but the lower legs and feet are rotated inwardly. The lateral malleolus, which is normally positioned slightly posterior to the medial malleolus, may be in alignment with it or even anteriorly displaced, thus causing the ankle mortise to shift to a medially directed orientation, resulting in intoeing (Fig. 21-94). The rotational deformity can also be detected by having the patient lie prone on the examining table with the knees flexed. In this position the feet in children with internal tibial torsion turn toward the midline. Radiographs reveal no osseous abnormalities. Treatment is seldom indicated; remodeling gradually corrects the condition as the child grows and develops. Children who have a habit of sitting on their feet on the floor may inhibit the normal remodeling process and should be instructed not to do this. Bracing and special shoes have little effect and are not recommended.

Congenital Clubfoot

Congenital clubfoot (talipes equinovarus) is a teratogenic deformity of the foot that is readily apparent at birth. It is seen more frequently in male than female infants and has an incidence of 1 in 1000 live births. Etiology is probably multifactorial. Findings from familial incidence studies point toward an underlying genetic predisposition. Abnormal intrauterine positioning and pressure at a critical point in development may contribute as well. Neural, muscular, and osseous abnormalities are other proposed predisposing conditions. There is a near equal frequency of unilateral and bilateral involvement. The deformity is characterized by three primary components: (1) the entire foot is positioned in plantar flexion (equinus); (2) the hindfoot is maintained in a position of fixed inversion (varus); and (3) the forefoot exhibits an adductus deformity, often combined with supination (Fig. 21-95, *A* to *C*). In the newborn period the deformity may be passively correctable to some extent. With time, however, deformities become more fixed as a result of contracture of soft tissue structures.

The primary pathologic finding is that of a rotational deformity of the subtalar joint with the os calcis internally rotated beneath the talus, producing the characteristic varus deformity of the heel and mechanically creating a block to dorsiflexion of the foot. The navicular bone is in a medially displaced position on the head or neck of the talus, producing the characteristic adductus deformity of the forefoot (Fig. 21-95, *D* and *E*). Contractures of the Achilles and posterior tibial tendons and of the medial ankle and subtalar joint capsules appear to be secondary factors that contribute to the difficulty of obtaining anatomic reduction. Congenital absence of certain tendinous structures may be found in

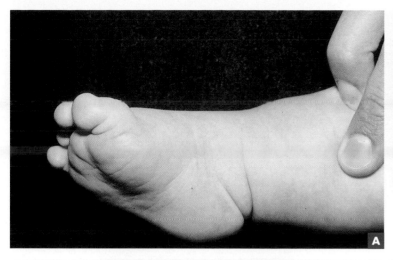

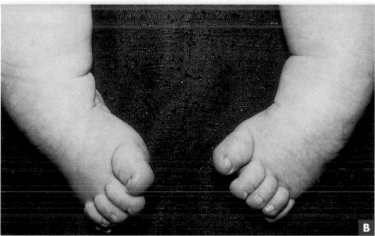

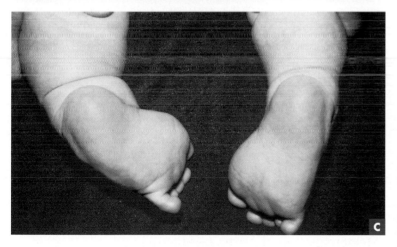

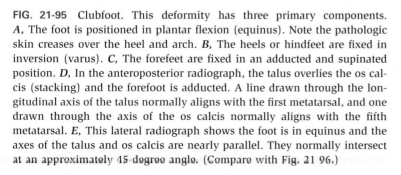

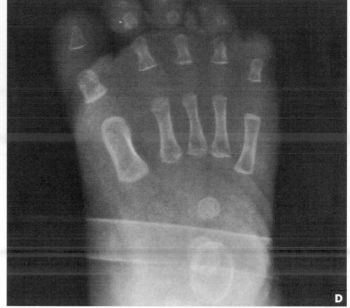

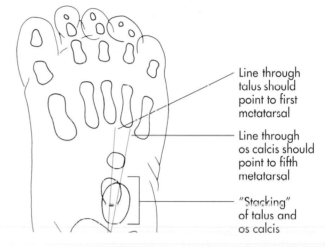

Line through talus should point to first metatarsal

Line through os calcis should point to fifth metatarsal

"Stacking" of talus and os calcis

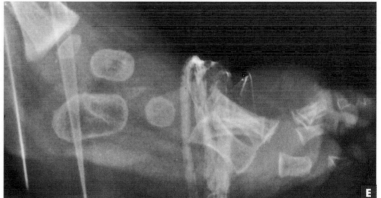

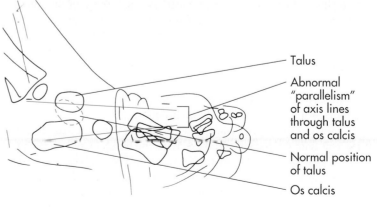

Talus

Abnormal "parallelism" of axis lines through talus and os calcis

Normal position of talus

Os calcis

FIG. 21-95 Clubfoot. This deformity has three primary components. *A,* The foot is positioned in plantar flexion (equinus). Note the pathologic skin creases over the heel and arch. *B,* The heels or hindfeet are fixed in inversion (varus). *C,* The forefeet are fixed in an adducted and supinated position. *D,* In the anteroposterior radiograph, the talus overlies the os calcis (stacking) and the forefoot is adducted. A line drawn through the longitudinal axis of the talus normally aligns with the first metatarsal, and one drawn through the axis of the os calcis normally aligns with the fifth metatarsal. *E,* This lateral radiograph shows the foot is in equinus and the axes of the talus and os calcis are nearly parallel. They normally intersect at an approximately 45-degree angle. (Compare with Fig. 21-96.)

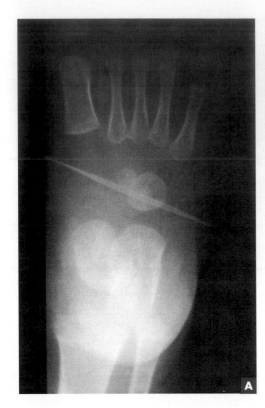

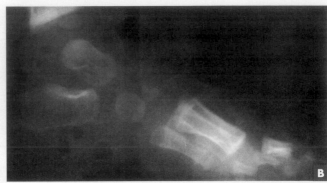

FIG. 21-96 Normal foot. *A,* Anteroposterior and, *B,* lateral views of the foot of a slightly older child show the normal orientation of the tarsal bones, as compared with the findings in congenital clubfoot (shown in Fig. 21-95, *D* and *E*).

rare instances. A small atrophic-appearing calf is frequently noted without pathologic change in its osseous or soft tissue structures. The typical congenital clubfoot deformity must be differentiated from similar foot deformities secondary to neurologic imbalance resulting from myelodysplasia, spinal cord tethering, or degenerative neurologic conditions. Occasionally, tibial hemimelia with deficiency of this bone may present a similar clinical picture. The condition should not be confused with the nonteratogenic occurrence of isolated metatarsus adductus. Its association with arthrogryposis and congenital dislocation of the hips should also be kept in mind.

The roentgenographic difference between a clubfoot and a normal foot can be appreciated by comparing Fig. 21-95, *D* and *F*, with Fig. 21-96.

Early treatment consists of attempts at manipulation and serial casting or cast wedging with progressive correction. When the child is seen late or closed treatment is unsuccessful, open reduction and surgical release of the contracted soft tissues is indicated. Generally these measures should be undertaken before the age at which walking is expected in order to prevent the deformity from impeding the child's motor and social development.

Metatarsus Adductus

Metatarsus adductus (metatarsus varus) is a deformity of the forefoot in which the metatarsals are deviated medially. The condition is probably the result of intrauterine molding and is usually bilateral. Other than the deviation, there are no pathologic changes in the structures of the foot. There is a wide spectrum of severity and resultant intoeing, but otherwise patients are asymptomatic. Clinically it should be distinguished from the more severe and complex deformity of congenital clubfoot, as it carries a more benign prognosis.

Examination is best performed with the foot braced against a flat surface or with the patient standing. With the hindfoot and midfoot positioned straight, the affected forefoot assumes a medially deviated or varus position (Fig. 21-97, *A* and *B*). A skin crease may be located over the medial aspect of the longitudinal arch. When mild, the deviation

may be passively correctable by the physician or actively correctable by the patient. Active correction may be demonstrated by gentle stroking of the foot, stimulating the peroneal muscles to contract. In more severe cases, the deviation may be only partially corrected by these maneuvers. Some patients have an associated internal tibial torsion deformity, but their calf muscle is normal in size. Radiographs demonstrate the abnormal deviation of the metatarsals medially without other osseous abnormalities (Fig. 21-97, *C*).

Treatment depends on the severity of the condition. In very mild cases, passive manipulation of the deformity by the mother several times a day may suffice. In moderate cases, a combination of manipulative stretching and reverse or straight-last shoes may be indicated. More severe cases, which are not passively correctable and which exhibit a prominent deformity and skin crease, necessitate serial manipulation and casting for 6 to 8 weeks. If the deformity persists despite these measures, surgical intervention may be required. Treatment should be undertaken before anticipated ambulation so as to prevent impairment of the patient's motor and social development.

Metatarsus Primus Varus (Adductus)

Metatarsus primus varus is a congenital and often hereditary foot deformity characterized by a broad forefoot with medial deviation of the first metatarsal. It is significantly more frequent in females than males. Examination reveals a wide forefoot with medial deviation of the first metatarsal and normal orientation of the second through fifth metatarsals. There is often an associated varus deviation of the great toe (Fig. 21-98, *A*). Over time, a secondary hallux valgus deformity and bunion may be produced by the abnormal forces exerted on the great toe with weight-bearing and ambulation (Fig. 21-98, *B*). The heel may seem narrow, but this is more apparent than real. Pronation of the forefoot may be present as well. Radiographs confirm the diagnosis by revealing an increased space between the first and second metatarsals and a large first intermetatarsal angle. The first ray through the tarsometatarsal joint may be medially oriented, forming the basis for the deformity.

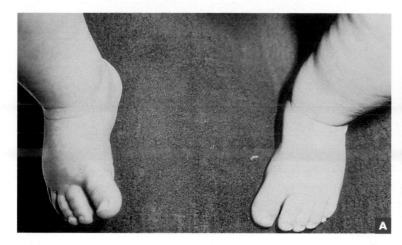

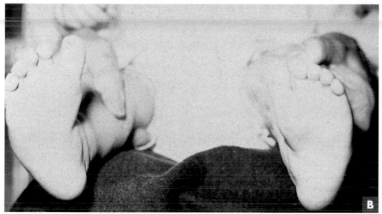

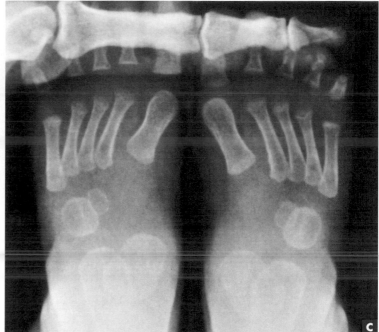

FIG. 21-97 Bilateral metatarsus adductus. *A,* In this view from above, the forefeet are seen to be deviated medially, but otherwise the feet are normal. *B,* When viewed from the plantar aspect, rounding of the lateral border of the feet can be appreciated. *C,* In the anteroposterior radiograph, all five metatarsals can be seen to be deviated medially with respect to the remainder of the foot; otherwise the bony structures are normal. The relationship of the talus and os calcis is normal, unlike the relationship in clubfoot.

Normal metatarsal orientation

Medial deviation of metatarsals

Talus

Os calcis

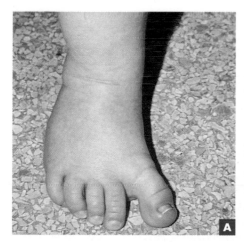

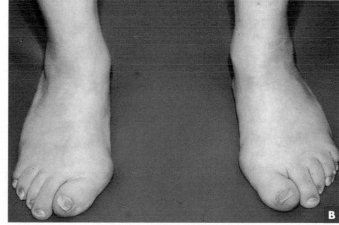

FIG. 21-98 Metatarsus primus varus. *A,* The first metatarsal and great toe are deviated medially; the forefoot is broad. The other metatarsals are normally oriented. *B,* Bilateral metatarsus primus varus with hallux valgus. The forefeet are broad, and the great toes deviate laterally. (*A* courtesy Dr. Michael Sherlock.)

In mild cases, no treatment may be necessary. In moderate or severe cases, foot strain symptoms, bunion pain, and shoe-fitting problems may necessitate treatment. Surgical osteotomy of the medial cuneiform or first metatarsal in conjunction with bunion correction may satisfactorily eliminate the deformity.

Congenital Vertical Talus

Congenital vertical talus is a teratogenic anomaly of the foot noted at birth and characterized by a severe flatfoot deformity. The underlying pathology is a malorientation of the talus, which assumes a more vertical position than normal. The adjacent navicular is dorsally displaced,

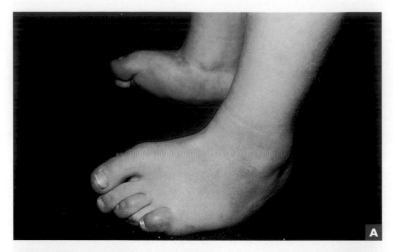

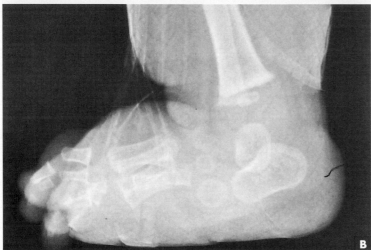

FIG. 21-99 Congenital vertical talus. *A,* The normal longitudinal arch of the foot is absent, a rocker-bottom–type deformity is present and the forefoot is fixed in dorsiflexion. *B,* Note the vertical orientation of the talus in the radiograph. (See Fig. 21-96 for comparison.)

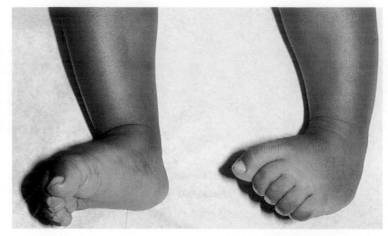

FIG. 21-100 Calcaneovalgus foot deformity. The right foot is held in a position of eversion and dorsiflexion. This deformity is supple, and thus is passively correctable. The contralateral foot exhibits a metatarsus adductus deformity, giving the feet a "windswept" appearance.

Calcaneovalgus Foot Deformity

Physiologic calcaneovalgus is another deformity of the foot thought to result from intrauterine molding. It is normally a supple deformity that is passively correctable, in contrast to the rigid foot characteristic of congenital vertical talus. The condition is evident at birth and at times is associated with a contralateral metatarsus adductus. There are no underlying pathologic changes in the foot and no osseous deformities other than the positional one. On examination, the foot is noted to be held in a dorsiflexed and everted position with some loss of the normal longitudinal arch (Fig. 21-100). Tightness of the anterior tibial tendon and laxity of the Achilles tendon may be noted in association with the positional deformity. Radiographs reveal no pathologic bony changes. Nonoperative treatment is usually successful and consists of serial casting to eliminate the deformity. Later, wearing shoes with inner heel wedges and longitudinal arch supports may help prevent recurrence and improve ambulation.

Pes Planus (Flatfeet)

Pes planus, or physiologic flatfeet, is an extremely common condition for which there is a familial predisposition. It is characterized by laxity of the soft tissues of the foot resulting in loss of the normal longitudinal arch, with pronation or eversion of the forefoot and valgus or lateral orientation of the heel (Fig. 21-101). There may be secondary tightness of the Achilles tendon. The condition is generally asymptomatic in children, and evaluation is sought primarily because of parental concern about the appearance of the foot and the possibility of future problems. Occasionally, affected patients report discomfort after long walks or running.

On examination, the characteristic appearance is easy to recognize and laxity of other joints, particularly the thumb, elbow, and knee may be noted. Weight-bearing radiographs reveal loss of the normal longitudinal arch without osseous abnormality. Treatment is unnecessary if the condition is asymptomatic. Corrective shoes with arch supports are of no use unless symptoms of foot strain are present.

Accessory Tarsal Navicular

An accessory tarsal navicular results from formation of a separate ossification center on the medial aspect of the developing tarsal nav-

articulating with the superior aspect of the neck of the talus and causing the forefoot to assume a dorsiflexed and valgus orientation. In effect, these deformities are the opposite of those seen in congenital clubfoot. The etiology of this condition is unknown, although it may be associated with other musculoskeletal or organ system anomalies. Pathologic analysis reveals normal development of the bones but an abnormal relationship. As in clubfoot, associated soft tissue contractures may occur, particularly of the Achilles tendon, toe extensors, and anterior tibial tendon.

Clinically the deformity is recognizable as a calcaneovalgus foot with loss of the arch, or on some occasions, a rocker-bottom–type foot with a prominent heel (Fig. 21-99, *A*). The head of the talus is often palpable on the medial plantar aspect of the midfoot. The deformity is usually fixed, but passive correction may be obtainable in some instances, particularly if the talus is oriented in a less severe oblique position. Radiographs mirror the clinical appearance, showing a vertical orientation of the talus, a calcaneus deformity of the os calcis, and valgus orientation of the forefoot (Fig. 21-99, *B;* and see Fig. 21-96, *B* for a normal comparison).

Initially, attempts at manipulation and serial casting are indicated. However, if this is unsuccessful, as is often the case, surgery may be necessary.

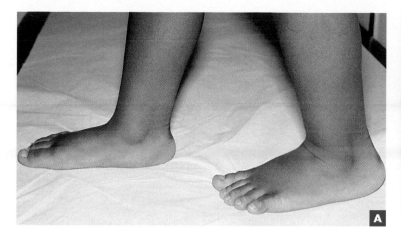

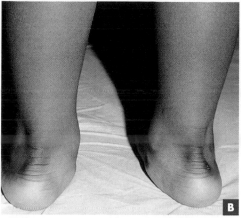

FIG. 21-101 Pes planus. *A,* Laxity of the soft tissue structures of the foot results in a loss of the normal longitudinal arch and pronation or eversion of the forefoot. *B,* Viewed from behind, the characteristic eversion of the heels is appreciated more readily.

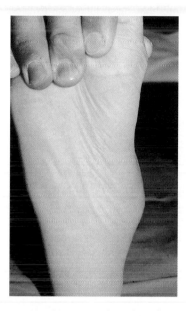

ΓIG. 21-102 Accessory tarsal navicular. A bony prominence produced by the formation of a separate ossification center of the tarsal navicular is present over the medial aspect of the midfoot. It is covered by a painful bursa, produced by chronic rubbing of the prominence against the medial side of the patient's shoes. Patients with this problem usually also have a pes planus deformity as well.

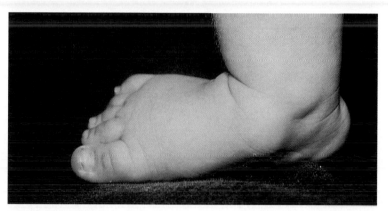

FIG. 21-103 Ganglion of the foot. A prominent soft tissue mass is present over the medial aspect of the midfoot. This represents a ganglion of the posterior tibial tendon sheath.

icular at the insertion site of the posterior tibial tendon. The condition is not uncommon and is usually associated with a pes planus deformity. Clinically, patients exhibit a bony prominence on the medial aspect of the foot that tends to rub on the shoe, thus producing a painful bursa (Fig. 21-102). Radiographs reveal either a separate ossification center or bone medial to the parent navicular, or a medial projection of the navicular when fusion has occurred. Cast immobilization may be helpful in acutely painful cases. Long-term improvement can be obtained by wearing soft supportive shoes with longitudinal arches and a medial heel wedge. Recalcitrant symptoms warrant surgical intervention.

Ganglion of the Foot

A ganglion, or synovial cyst, may occur on the foot. These benign masses are similar to those commonly seen on the wrist. They originate from outpouchings of a joint capsule or tendon sheath. Trauma may be a predisposing factor in their formation. They are most commonly seen on the dorsal or medial aspect of the foot. The mass is soft, nontender, and transilluminates. It does not produce symptoms, other than difficulty in fitting shoes (Fig. 21-103). If this occurs, surgical excision may be indicated.

Cavus Feet and Claw Toes

Cavus feet and claw toes are deformities produced by a muscular imbalance within the foot. Although they may occur for unknown reasons, often they are manifestations of an underlying neurologic disorder such as Charcot-Marie-Tooth disease, Friedreich's ataxia, or spinal cord tethering. These conditions should be considered in each patient presenting with these deformities, particularly if the problem is unilateral. Cavus feet exhibit a high arch with a varus or inversion deformity of the heel. Usually the metatarsal heads appear prominent on the plantar aspect of the foot (Fig. 21-104). This phenomenon is accentuated by overlying callosities that develop as a result of abnormal weight-bearing. With claw toes, the metatarsophalangeal joints are held in extension with the PIP joints in flexion and the distal joint in the neutral or slightly flexed position (Fig. 21-105). Calluses tend to develop over the PIP joints as the result of rubbing against shoes. Neurologic examination may reveal motor weakness, most often involving the anterior tibial, toe extensor, and peroneal muscles.

Logical treatment necessitates identifying and treating the underlying pathologic condition when possible. Nonsurgical measures for managing the deformities and ameliorating the symptoms consist of the wearing of customized shoes and use of a metatarsal bar to relieve pressure on the metatarsal heads and to correct the extension defor-

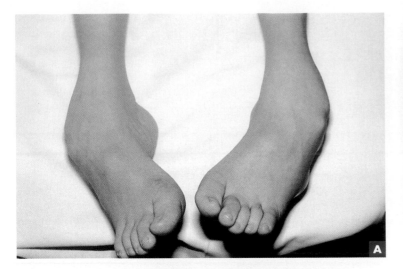

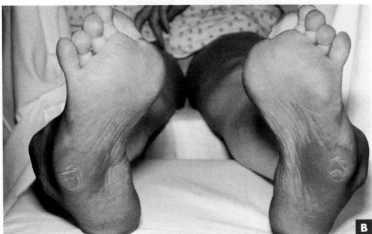

FIG. 21-104   Bilateral cavus feet. *A,* The feet are inverted and have high arches. The deformity is often a feature of neuromuscular disorders; this case is the result of Charcot-Marie-Tooth disease. *B,* In addition to the high arches and varus (inverted) heels seen in the view of the plantar surface, the prominence of the metatarsal head region is apparent. Callosities have developed over the lateral borders of the feet as a result of abnormal weight-bearing in this region.

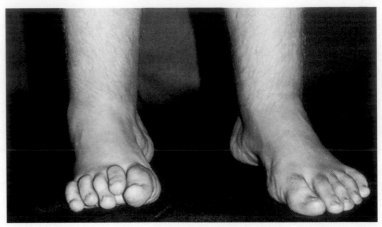

FIG. 21-105   Unilateral claw toes. This child with a tethered spinal cord has unilateral claw toe deformities. The metacarpophalangeal joints are held in extension while the proximal interphalangeal joints are fixed in flexion.

mities at the base of the toes. However, surgical correction is often necessary.

Generalized Musculoskeletal Disorders

Numerous systemic disorders have significant musculoskeletal manifestations. Those relating to genetic, endocrine, collagen-vascular, neurologic, and hematologic problems are discussed in their respective chapters. Three conditions with major musculoskeletal manifestations—cerebral palsy, osteogenesis imperfecta, and arthrogryposis—are discussed in this section.

Cerebral Palsy

Cerebral palsy refers to a group of fixed, nonprogressive neurologic syndromes resulting from static lesions of the developing CNS. Depending on the timing of injury, signs may be present at birth or they may become evident in infancy or early childhood. The primary cerebral insult may be intrauterine or perinatal infection; a prenatal or perinatal vascular accident; anoxia due to placental insufficiency, difficult delivery, or neonatal pulmonary disease; hyperbilirubinemia resulting in kernicterus; or neonatal hypoglycemia. After the newborn period, CNS infections, trauma, and vascular accidents may, when severe, produce the disorder. Abnormal motor function is the most obvious result and may take the form of a spastic neuromuscular disorder (65% of cases), athetosis (25%), or rigidity and/or ataxic neuromuscular dysfunction (10%). Sensory deficits and intellectual impairment are common, and there is a significant incidence of associated seizure disorders.

Because of the number and variety of possible insulting factors, each of which has its own spectrum of severity, there is a broad range in the location and extent of neural damage, and thus in the degree of functional impairment. Patients with severe afflictions generally have early evidence of gross neuromuscular dysfunction. Those with milder involvement may have subtler abnormalities and may be diagnosed only after they fail to achieve normal developmental and motor milestones. Patterns of the affliction include involvement of one or two limbs (monoplegia or hemiplegia), of both lower extremities (diplegia), of all four extremities (quadriplegia) (Fig. 21-106), or of all limbs with poor trunk and head control (pentaplegia). Those patients with a spastic disorder exhibit flexion contractures of the involved limbs, hyperreflexia, and spasticity; those with athetosis exhibit the characteristic movement disorder. Mixed involvement is apparent in some patients. Neurologic examination often reveals the persistence of primitive reflexes. Patients with severe involvement that inhibits sitting and ambulation suffer disuse atrophy of involved muscles and skeletal demineralization that increases their risk of pathologic fractures (see Chapter 6).

In evaluating such patients, one must be careful to rule out a progressive neurologic disorder, such as intracranial or spinal cord neoplasms, degenerative neurologic conditions, and tethering of the spinal cord.

Optimal treatment necessitates a team approach. In addition to general pediatric, neurologic, and orthopedic care, these patients often need the services of a urologist and physical and speech therapists and

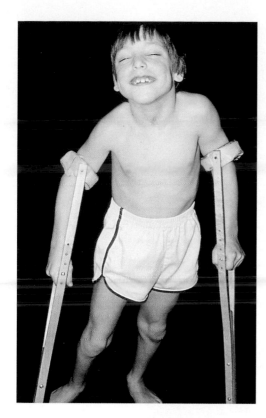

FIG. 21-106 Cerebral palsy. Typical patient with spastic quadriplegia. Note the secondary muscle atrophy especially evident in the lower extremities. He requires crutches to ambulate, seizure medication, and a specialized educational program. His neuromuscular abnormalities are the result of a one-time central nervous system insult and are not progressive.

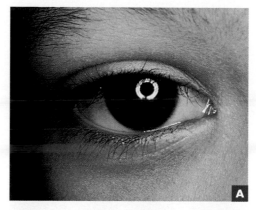

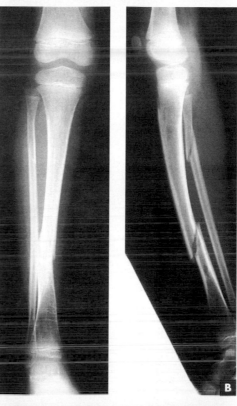

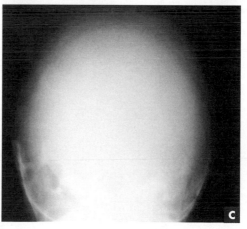

FIG. 21-107 Osteogenesis imperfecta type I. *A*, Blue sclera. *B*, Cortical thinning is evident, especially distal to the spiral fracture of the tibia in this child with OI type I. *C*, Wormian bones. Multiple wormy, irregular lucencies are seen over the occipitoparietal area. This finding is characteristic of all children with OI types I, II, and III and is seen in more than 50% of patients with OI type IV. (*A* and *B* courtesy Dr. Thomas Daley, Bronx-Lebanon Hospital.)

need to be enrolled in individualized educational programs. Family counseling is a necessity. From an orthopedic standpoint, emphasis is placed on optimizing neuromuscular function by attempting to facilitate the achievement of progressive motor milestones, including the ability to sit, stand, walk, and perform activities of daily living. Exercises, bracing, and surgical procedures all have a role, and the institution of specific measures must be timed to fit the pace of growth and development of the individual child. Encouragement and cautious optimism are important. Surgical treatment usually takes the form of soft tissue release to relieve flexion deformities, tendon transfer to optimize functional use of the extremities, osteotomy to correct deformities, and occasionally selective neurectomy to inhibit overactive muscle units.

Osteogenesis Imperfecta

Osteogenesis imperfecta (OI) is a family of inherited disorders in which type I collagen formation is immature and characterized by abnormal cross-linking. Although these disorders affect all connective tissue in the body, their primary clinical manifestations involve the skeleton because of the structural demands placed on the bones. Microscopically, the number of osteoblasts are reduced, osteoid is disorganized and nonossified, and bony trabeculae are sparse. The end-result is osteoporosis with increased susceptibility to fractures.

Formerly divided into two types (congenita and tarda), research using fibroblast culture techniques has now revealed the existence of four major types and several subtypes. Overall, the incidence is thought to be between 1 in 15,000 and 1 in 60,000 births.

Osteogenesis Imperfecta Type I

OI type I accounts for 60% to 80% of cases and is transmitted as an autosomal dominant trait. In subtype A, teeth are normal; in subtype B, dentinogenesis imperfecta is present (see Chapter 20). All affected patients have blue sclerae (Fig. 21-107, *A*), although the degree of blueness varies. Mild to moderate bony fragility is seen in 90% of affected patients but is not present in the remaining 10%. Radiographs

reveal mild to moderate generalized osteoporosis with cortical thinning (Fig. 21-107, *B*). All affected children are seen to have significant wormian bones on skull radiographs (Fig. 21-107, *C*). Although the first fracture usually occurs during the preschool period, 8% to 10% of patients with type IA and 25% of those with type IB have one to a few fractures at birth. Fractures heal normally with normal callus formation, and their frequency decreases after puberty.

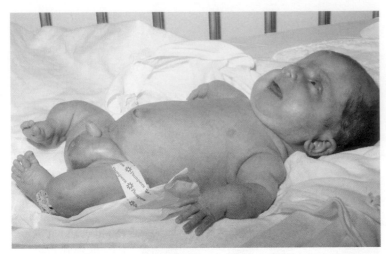

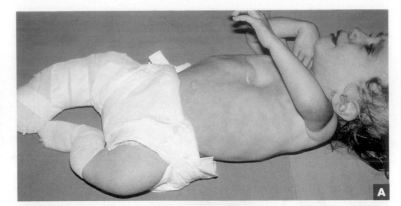

FIG. 21-108 Osteogenesis imperfecta type II. This infant was born with multiple fractures and limb deformities. The thighs are fixed in abduction and external rotation. His sclerae are a dark bluish-gray. He died of respiratory insufficiency in the first month of life as the result of his small thorax.

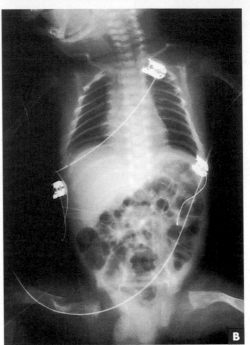

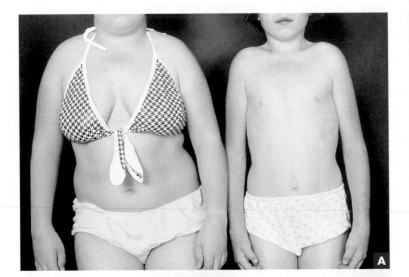

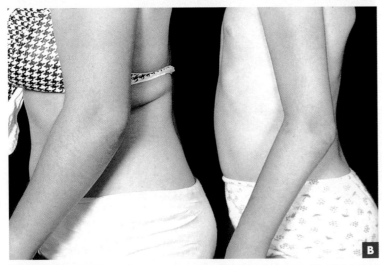

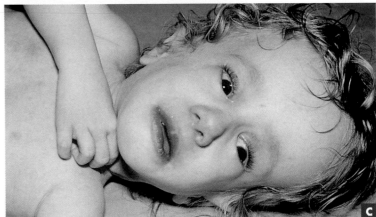

FIG. 21-109 Osteogenesis imperfecta type III. *A,* Note the extremely small stature of this 5-year-old child and the deformities of the rib cage. A recent fracture has been splinted. *B,* Radiograph of an affected infant shows dwarfed, deformed femurs with a new fracture in the midshaft of the right femur. Note also the thin, peculiarly shaped ribs. *C,* In this close-up, the characteristic craniofacial features are seen, consisting of a triangular facies, a broad nose, and frontal and temporal bossing. The sclerae may be normal in color, as in this child, or light blue or gray.

FIG. 21-110 Arthrogryposis. *A,* Two sisters with the generalized form of the disorder. Note the stiff posture and tubular appearance of the limbs. Motion of all joints is limited as a result of failure in the development of or the degeneration of muscular structures. Their stature is short. *B,* The lateral view highlights the flexion contractures of the elbows.

Children with OI type I tend to have generalized ligamentous laxity and joint hypermobility. Anterior and lateral bowing of the femurs and tibias is common, as are valgus knees and pes planus. Ultimate stature is normal or mildly short. Three quarters of these children have easy bruisability, and approximately 35% to 55% suffer conductive hearing loss in early adulthood.

Osteogenesis Imperfecta Type II

OI type II is an extremely severe form of the disease and is lethal in the prenatal or perinatal period. It is usually due to a new autosomal dominant mutation but rarely is inherited as an autosomal recessive trait. It accounts for less than 10% of all cases of OI. Intrauterine growth is severely retarded, and affected infants are born with multiple fractures and severe deformities stemming from extreme osteoporosis (Fig. 21-108). The extremities are short, bowed, and bent, and the thighs are fixed in abduction and external rotation. The calvarium is large and soft with palpable bony islands, and poor mineralization and wormian bones are evident radiographically (see Fig. 21-107, *C*). The face is triangular with a beaked nose and the sclerae are blue-black. The chest is so small that those who are liveborn die of respiratory insufficiency in the first few weeks. Three subtypes have been identified on the basis of the radiographic appearance of the ribs and long bones.

Osteogenesis Imperfecta Type III

OI type III, the severe progressive form accounting for approximately 15% of cases of OI, also is usually the result of a new autosomal dominant mutation, although on rare occasion it is transmitted as an autosomal recessive trait. Osteoporosis is severe, resulting in moderately severe to severe fragility. Most affected children are born with multiple fractures and deformities. Those who are not have multiple fractures by 1 to 2 years of age. The osteopenia and fractures produce progressive shortening, bowing, and angulation of the long bones (Fig. 21-109, *A* and *B*) and severe progressive kyphoscoliosis, which results in marked dwarfism and ultimately causes cardiopulmonary compromise. The calvarium is large and thin and radiographically is seen to be poorly ossified with multiple wormian bones (see Fig. 21-107, *C*). Frontal and temporal bossing are common, and the facies is triangular (Fig. 21-109, *C*). The sclerae can be normal or light blue or gray, changing to white by puberty. Approximately half of these patients have associated ligamentous laxity and half have dentinogenesis imperfecta. Easy bruising is seen in about 25% of patients.

Osteogenesis Imperfecta Type IV

This mild form is rare, accounting for less than 5% of all cases of OI, with an estimated incidence of 1 in 1 to 3 million live births. It is inherited as an autosomal dominant trait. There are two subtypes: IVA with normal teeth and IVB with dentinogenesis imperfecta. Bony fragility varies from mild to moderately severe, and osteoporosis is gradually progressive, although it may be minimal or absent at the time of the first fracture. About one third of patients have one to a few fractures at birth, and most experience their first fracture by 5 years of age. More than 50% have wormian bones on skull radiographs (see Fig. 21-107, *C*). Bowing of the lower extremities is common, with or without fractures, and most affected individuals have short stature. The sclerae may be normal in color or light blue at birth, gradually changing to white later in childhood. Easy bruisability is unusual in this group.

Treatment

Patients with OI types I and IV may require only routine orthopedic care for their fractures and counseling regarding accident prevention and safety. Palliative supportive care and minimal handling are the only measures available for infants with OI type II. Treatment of infants and children with OI type III is geared toward minimizing the frequency of fractures and preventing deformities. In infancy this may mean limited handling of the child and use of a padded carrying device. Later, bracing and surgical treatment in the form of osteotomy and internal stabilization of long bones with intermedullary rod fixation may be necessary. Maintenance of activity and the avoidance of repeated prolonged periods of immobilization help prevent disuse atrophy.

Arthrogryposis

Arthrogryposis is a nonprogressive muscular disorder of unknown etiology, which appears to be related either to failure of development in or degeneration of muscular structures. Neural factors have been implicated in its pathogenesis, because in some instances the spinal cord has been found to be reduced in size, with a decreased number of anterior horn cells. Generally all limbs are involved. On occasion the disease may be confined to one or a few limbs only. Primary manifestations consist of joint contractures with secondary deformities and limited motion. Deformities include clubfeet, dislocated hips, and contractures of the knees, elbows, wrists, and hands (Fig. 21-110). Motion of the involved joints is severely limited, but patients generally are able to compensate for this functional limitation. Radiographs show relatively normal appearing bones and joints, but fat density is noted in the areas where muscles are normally seen. On pathologic analysis, there is a striking absence of muscle tissue with strands of fat permeating the area.

Orthopedic treatment is aimed at providing optimal motor function. Range of motion exercises may maintain what motion is present but rarely result in an increase. Surgery rarely results in improved range of motion but is indicated to restore functional position in those patients with clubfeet and/or hip dislocation. Gradual recurrence of the deformity after surgery is not uncommon, however.

BIBLIOGRAPHY

Ablin DS, Greenspan A, Reinhart M, Grix A. Differentiation of child abuse from osteogenesis imperfecta, *Am J Radiol* 154:1035-1046, 1990.

Aegerter E, Kirkpatrick JA Jr: *Orthopedic diseases, physiology, pathology, radiology,* ed 4, Philadelphia, 1975, WB Saunders.

American Orthopaedic Association: *Manual of orthopaedic surgery,* ed 6, Philadelphia, 1985, The Association.

American Society for Surgery of the Hand: *The hand: examination and diagnosis,* Edinburgh, 1983, Churchill Livingstone.

American Society for Surgery of the Hand: *The hand: primary care of common problems,* Aurora, CO, 1985, Churchill Livingstone.

Bachman D, Santora S: Orthopedic trauma. In Fleisher GR, Ludwig S, eds: *Textbook of pediatric emergency medicine,* ed 3, Baltimore, 1993, Williams & Wilkins.

Edmonson AS, Crenshaw AH: *Campbell's operative orthopaedics,* ed 8, St Louis, 1992, Mosby.

Ferguson AB Jr: *Orthopedic surgery in infancy and childhood,* ed 5, Baltimore, 1981, Williams & Wilkins.

Hoppenfeld S: *Physical examination of the spine and extremities,* New York, 1976, Appleton-Century-Crofts.

Lovell WW, Winter RB: *Pediatric orthopedics,* ed 4, Philadelphia, 1996, JB Lippincott.

Moe JH, Winter RB, Bradford DS, Lonstein JE: *Scoliosis and other spinal deformities,* Philadelphia, 1978, WB Saunders.

Ogden JA: *Skeletal injury in the child,* ed 2, Philadelphia, 1989, Lea & Febiger.

Rang M: *Children's fractures,* ed 2, Philadelphia, 1983, JB Lippincott.

Rockwood CA Jr, Wilkins KE, King RE: *Fractures in children,* vol 3, ed 3, Philadelphia, 1991, JB Lippincott.

Salter RB: *Textbook of disorders and injuries of the musculoskeletal system,* ed 2, Baltimore, 1983, Williams & Wilkins.

Scoles PV: *Pediatric orthopedics in clinical practice,* Chicago, 1982, Year Book.

Simon RR, Koenigsknecht SJ: *Orthopedics in emergency medicine: the extremities,* New York, 1982, Appleton.

Staheli LT: *Fundamentals of pediatric orthopedics,* New York, 1992, Raven Press.

Tachidjian MO: *Pediatric orthopedics,* ed 2, Philadelphia, 1990, WB Saunders.

22

Otolaryngology

TIMOTHY P. McBRIDE   HOLLY W. DAVIS

JAMES S. REILLY

The importance of pediatricians and family physicians having an understanding of and experience with otolaryngologic problems and being skilled in techniques of examination of the head and neck region cannot be overemphasized. A recent study revealed that more than one third of all visits to pediatricians' offices were prompted by ear symptoms. When nasal and oral symptoms are included, ear, nose, and throat pathology accounts for more than 50% of all visits. With patience and proper equipment, pediatricians can complete a thorough examination on almost all children. Then, if a disorder fails to respond to therapy or becomes chronic or recurrent or if an unusual problem is encountered, consultation with a pediatric otolaryngologist should be sought.

Successful examination of the ears, nose, and oropharynx of a young child can present some challenges, especially with older infants and toddlers who fail to appreciate the need for (and thus often vigorously resist) examination. This can be a particular problem in children who have had previous bad experiences. Patience, warmth, and careful explanation on the part of the examiner help reduce fear and enhance cooperation.

Whenever possible, the child should be allowed to sit on the parent's lap. Pacifiers, puppets, other toys, and tongue blades with faces drawn on them can all serve to reduce anxiety, enlist the child's trust, and distract attention. Gradual introduction of the equipment also can be helpful, especially if done in a playful way. The child can be asked to blow out the otoscope light while the examiner turns it off, urged to catch the light spot as the examiner moves it around, and even allowed to look in the parent's or examiner's ears (Fig. 22-1, A to D). Parents also can help demonstrate maneuvers for opening the mouth, panting to depress the tongue, and holding the head back. Although this may take a little additional time at the outset, it often saves considerable time in the long run and makes future follow-up examinations far easier.

Ear Disorders

Ear pain (otalgia), discharge from the ear (otorrhea), and suspected hearing loss are three of the more common and specific otic symptoms for which parents seek medical attention for their children. Less specific symptoms such as pulling or tugging at the ears, fussiness, and fever are also frequently encountered, particularly in children less than 2 years of age.

History should center on the nature and duration of symptoms, character of the clinical course, and possible antecedent treatment. Because many infections of the ear are recurrent and/or chronic, the parent should be asked about previous medical or surgical therapy (e.g., antibiotics, myringotomy and tubes).

A brief review of the anatomy of the ear is helpful in developing a logical approach to any clinical abnormalities that may be encountered. The ear is conveniently divided into the following three regions (Fig. 22-2):

1. The **external ear** includes the pinna, or auricle, and the external auditory canal, up to and including the tympanic membrane.
2. The **middle ear** is made up of the middle-ear space, the inner surface of the eardrum, the ossicles, and the mastoid.
3. The **inner ear** comprises the cochlea (hearing), the semicircular canals (balance), and the main nerve trunks of the seventh and eighth cranial nerves.

The examination should include inspection of the auricle, periauricular tissues, and external auditory canal and visualization of the entire tympanic membrane, including assessment of its mobility in response to positive and negative pressure. This often necessitates clearing the canal of cerumen or discharge by using a curette, cotton wick, lavage, or suction (Fig. 22-3, A and B). Use of a surgical otoscope head or an examining microscope facilitate visualization during the cleaning process. These procedures should be performed carefully and gently and attempted only after the child has been carefully immobilized to avoid trauma (Fig. 22-4). It is extraordinarily easy to injure the canal during the process of cleaning the external ear. Hence great care must be taken; otherwise bleeding from the ensuing trauma obscures the examination and upsets the patient and parent. Both the patient and parent should be given a clear explanation of the procedure beforehand. Allowing older children to handle and look through the equipment beforehand reduces anxiety and enhances cooperation (Fig. 22-3, C).

Because the external auditory canal is often slightly angulated in infants and young children, gentle lateral traction on the pinna is frequently necessary to facilitate visualization of the eardrum itself (Fig. 22-5). In infancy the tympanic membrane also tends to be oriented at an angle (Fig. 22-6), the landmarks are less prominent, and the

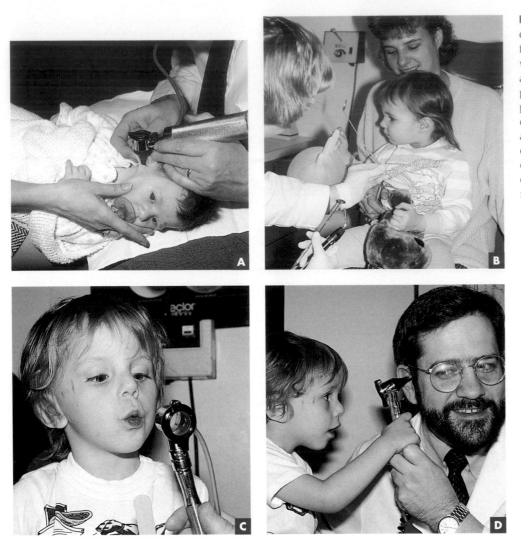

FIG. 22-1 Techniques to facilitate examination of a child's ears, nose, and oropharynx. *A,* Young infants often can be examined on their mother's lap, with gentle immobilization provided by the parent and the examiner's hand. *B,* Having a toddler or preschooler sit on the mother's lap and using puppets, other toys, and tongue blades with faces drawn on them while gradually introducing the examining instruments reduces anxiety and enlists cooperation. *C* and *D,* Making a game of blowing out the otoscope light and allowing the patient to check the examiner first convey that otoscopy does not have to hurt.

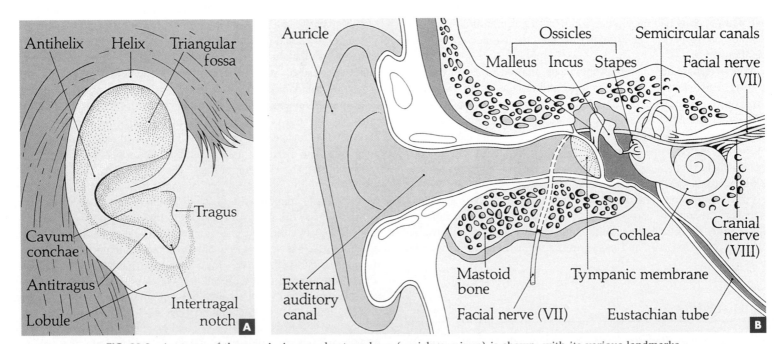

FIG. 22-2 Anatomy of the ear. *A,* A normal external ear (auricle or pinna) is shown, with its various landmarks labeled. It is helpful to refer to such a diagram in assessing congenital anomalies. *B,* This coronal section shows the various structures of the hearing and vestibular apparatus. The three main regions are the external ear, middle ear, and inner ear. The eustachian tube connects the middle ear and the pharynx and serves to vent the middle ear.

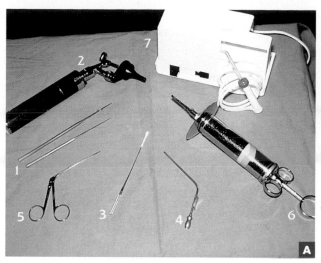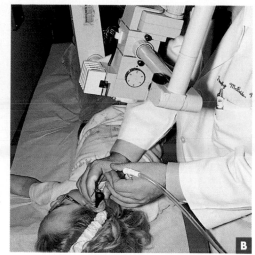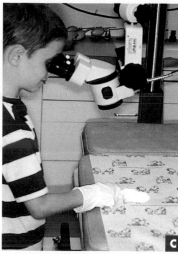

FIG. 22-3 *A,* Equipment for cleaning the external auditory canal. The curette *(1)* is the implement most commonly used to remove cerumen. Use of a surgical otoscope head *(2)* makes the process considerably easier. Additional implements include cotton wicks *(3)* and a suction tip *(4)* for removal of discharge or moist wax, alligator forceps *(5)* for foreign bodies, and an ear syringe *(6)* and motorized irrigation apparatus *(7)* for removing firm objects or impacted cerumen. Lavage is contraindicated when there is a possible perforation of the tympanic membrane. If the motorized apparatus is used for irrigation, it must be kept on the lowest power setting to avoid traumatizing the eardrum. *B,* Use of suction often is necessary when there is copious exudate. *C,* Allowing the child to look through the examining microscope may help him or her cooperate with the examination.

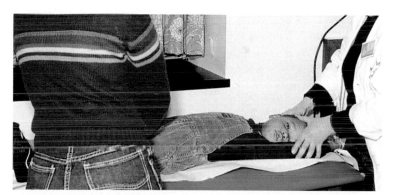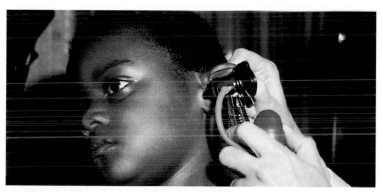

FIG. 22-4 Method of immobilization for cleaning. An assistant holds the child's arms and simultaneously immobilizes the child's head with the thumbs. The parent firmly holds the hips and thighs. This prevents motion by the child during cleaning of the ear canal and is also useful for otoscopy in young children.

FIG. 22-5 Because the external auditory canal usually is angulated in children, lateral traction on the pinna often is required to straighten the canal and improve visualization of the tympanic membrane.

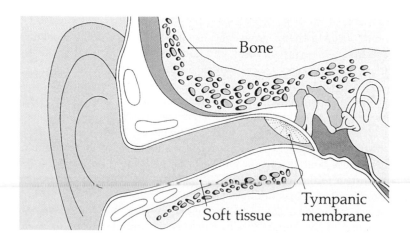

FIG. 22-6 Angulation of the tympanic membrane in infancy. The relationship between the ear canal and eardrum is different in the infant, with the drum being tilted at an angle of 130 degrees. Greater care is required in examining an infant's eardrum because of this angulation and because the landmarks are less prominent.

canal mucosa, being loosely attached, moves readily on insufflation of air, simulating a normally mobile eardrum. To avoid confusion, the canal should be inspected as the speculum is inserted to ensure that the transition between canal wall and tympanic membrane is visualized.

The pneumatic otoscope is the most valuable diagnostic tool when signs or symptoms of otitis media are present. Pediatricians, family practitioners, and otolaryngologists who treat children should be skilled

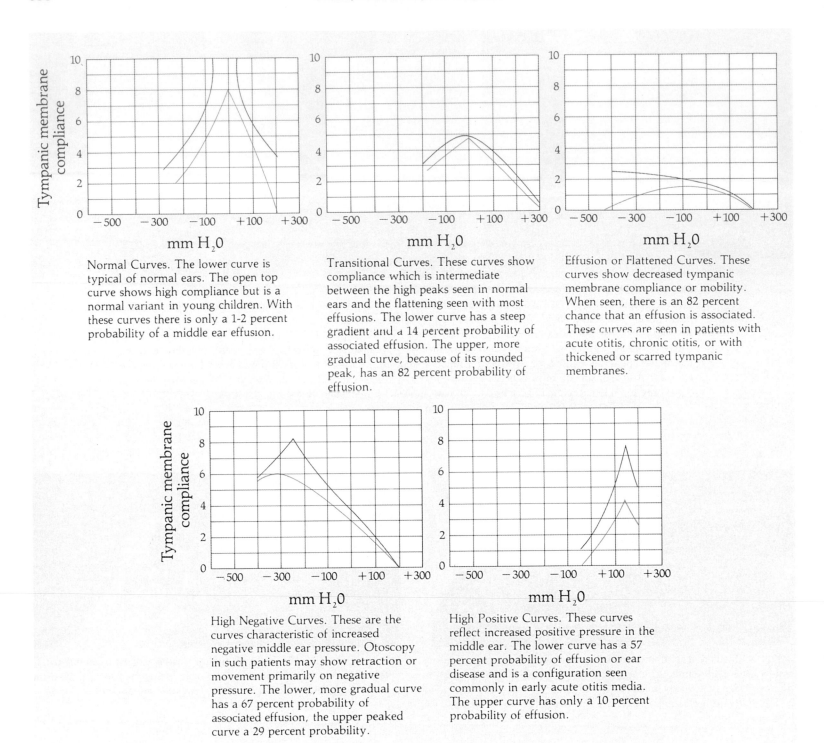

Normal Curves. The lower curve is typical of normal ears. The open top curve shows high compliance but is a normal variant in young children. With these curves there is only a 1-2 percent probability of a middle ear effusion.

Transitional Curves. These curves show compliance which is intermediate between the high peaks seen in normal ears and the flattening seen with most effusions. The lower curve has a steep gradient and a 14 percent probability of associated effusion. The upper, more gradual curve, because of its rounded peak, has an 82 percent probability of effusion.

Effusion or Flattened Curves. These curves show decreased tympanic membrane compliance or mobility. When seen, there is an 82 percent chance that an effusion is associated. These curves are seen in patients with acute otitis, chronic otitis, or with thickened or scarred tympanic membranes.

High Negative Curves. These are the curves characteristic of increased negative middle ear pressure. Otoscopy in such patients may show retraction or movement primarily on negative pressure. The lower, more gradual curve has a 67 percent probability of associated effusion, the upper peaked curve a 29 percent probability.

High Positive Curves. These curves reflect increased positive pressure in the middle ear. The lower curve has a 57 percent probability of effusion or ear disease and is a configuration seen commonly in early acute otitis media. The upper curve has only a 10 percent probability of effusion.

FIG. 22-7   Tympanometric patterns of various conditions of the middle ear. (Courtesy Mrs. Ruth Bachman, Pittsburgh.)

in its use. Practical advice on the use of this instrument is summarized by Schwartz as follows:

1. Use adequate light. A bright halogen lamp is better than an ordinary light bulb. Replace bulbs routinely every 4 to 6 months, and provide for routine battery charging.
2. Choose a speculum of sufficient size to allow adequate penetration (10 to 15 mm) into the external canal for good eardrum visualization.
3. Restrain the patient (on the parent's lap or on the examining table).

When otoscopic findings are unclear or it is difficult to obtain a good air seal for pneumatic otoscopy, tympanometry can be highly useful in evaluating patients over 6 months of age (Fig. 22-7). The procedure is

not of value in young infants because the abundance of loose connective tissue lining the ear canal and the laxity of the cartilage at the entrance increase canal wall compliance and invalidate the results.

Because otitis media can be a reflection of both immunologic and anatomic abnormalities, the practitioner should be suspicious of possible underlying immune or temporal bone defects when seeing patients with chronic or frequently recurrent otitis media. The temporal bone is the bony housing for the auditory and vestibular systems. In addition, it provides bony protection for the facial nerve as it crosses from the brainstem to the facial muscles. The growth and development of this bone is affected in syndromes such as Treacher-Collins syndrome and others that involve altered midface growth (Fig. 22-8). The soft tissues attached to the temporal bone such as the muscles controlling eu-

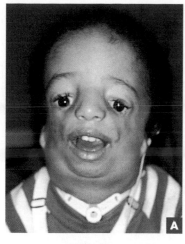
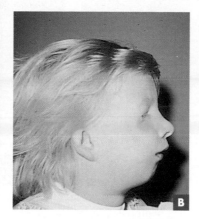
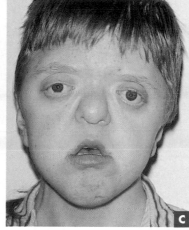
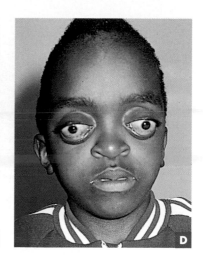

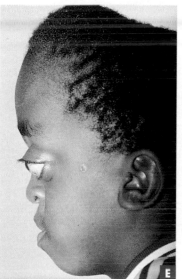
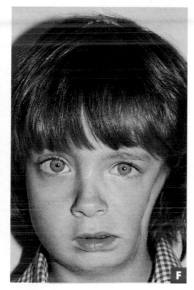

FIG. 22-8 Syndromes affecting the growth of the temporal bone and midface that predispose patients to recurrent or chronic otitis media and chronic recurrent sinus infections. *A* and *B*, Treacher-Collins syndrome. Note the maxillary hypoplasia, micrognathia, and auricular deformity. *C*, Apert syndrome. *D* and *E*, Crouzon syndrome. Both are characterized by severe maxillary and midfacial hypoplasia. *F*, Hemifacial microsomia with unilateral hypoplasia. (*B* to *F*, Courtesy Dr. Wolfgang Loskin, Children's Hospital of Pittsburgh.)

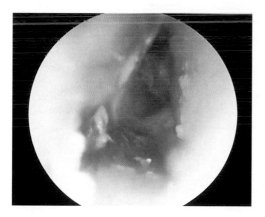

FIG. 22-9 External otitis. Acute bacterial external otitis is characterized by intense pain that is worsened by traction on the ear lobe, purulent exudate, and intense canal wall inflammation.

stachian tube function can be abnormal in children with cleft palates (see section on Palatal Disorders). As a result, children with these disorders tend to have an increased incidence of otitis media and also may be vulnerable to recurrent sinus infections.

Children with chronic effusions who complain of hearing loss, whose parents complain that they do not listen, or those with suspected congenital malformations must have their hearing evaluated by audiometry or brainstem-evoked potentials. Patients with vertigo and/or problems of balance and those with facial weakness or asymmetry warrant testing of both hearing *and* vestibular function. These children, and those suffering from malformations, may require computerized tomography or magnetic resonance imaging studies in select cases to clarify the nature of the problem.

Disorders of the External Ear

The Four "D"s

Examination of every child's ear begins with inspection of the auricle and periauricular tissues for four very important signs—discharge, displacement, discoloration, and deformity (the four "D"s). The canal is normally smooth and slightly angulated anteriorly. Cerumen is often present; it varies in color from yellowish-white to tan to dark brown. It is secreted from glands interspersed among the hair follicles at the entrance to the ear canal, and it may have some bacteriostatic activity. When cerumen obstructs the view, it must be removed to allow adequate visualization of the canal and tympanic membrane. When soft and moist, cerumen is easily removed with a curette. It may be more difficult if the cerumen is dry and flaky and at times may require instillation of drops. In some children, cerumen solidifies, forming a firm plug that impedes sound conduction and necessitates softening and irrigation for removal.

Discharge

Discharge is a common complaint with a number of possible causes. When there is thick, white discharge and erythema of the canal wall, the physician should gently pull on the pinna. If this maneuver elicits pain and the canal wall is edematous, primary otitis externa is the likely diagnosis (Fig. 22-9), although prolonged drainage from untreated otitis media with perforation may present a similar picture (see section on Disorders of the Middle Ear). When the middle ear is the source of otic discharge, the tympanic membrane is abnormal and should show evidence of perforation (Fig. 22-27). The major predisposing condition to

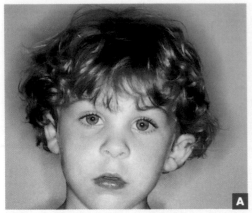
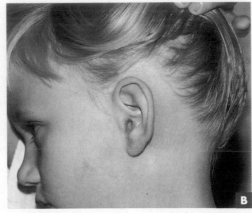
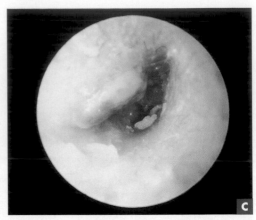

FIG. 22-10　Mastoiditis. *A,* This frontal photo clearly shows the left auricle displaced anteriorly and inferiorly. *B,* In another patient, viewed from the side, erythema can be appreciated over the mastoid process. *C,* On otoscopy, erythema and edema of the canal wall are evident, and the posterosuperior portion of the canal wall sags inferiorly. (*C* courtesy Dr. Michael Hawke, Toronto.)

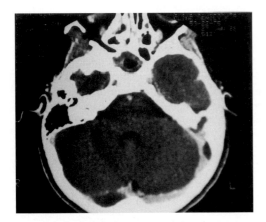

FIG. 22-11　Mastoiditis. This CT image shows acute left-sided mastoiditis with the complication of an associated epidural abscess.

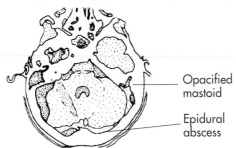

Opacified mastoid

Epidural abscess

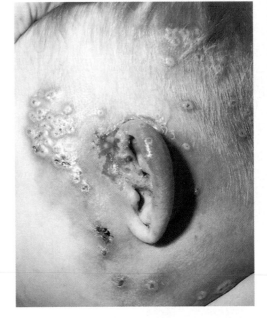

FIG. 22-12　Periauricular and auricular cellulitis. This infant had mild postauricular seborrhea and developed varicella. The vesicular lesions became secondarily infected with group A beta-streptococci, resulting in cellulitis with intense erythema, edema, and tenderness of the auricle and periauricular tissues. In this case the external canal was normal. (Courtesy Dr. Ronald Chludzinski.)

primary otitis externa is prolonged presence of excessive moisture in the ear canal, which promotes bacterial or fungal overgrowth. Thus this is a common problem in swimmers. Another major source is the presence of a foreign body in the ear canal (Fig. 22-19), which stimulates an intense inflammatory response and production of a foul-smelling purulent discharge. Thus when otic drainage is encountered, the discharge must be gently removed under appropriate magnification to assess the condition of the tympanic membrane and rule out the presence of foreign objects. This can be accomplished either by gentle siphoning and wiping with cotton wicks or by careful suctioning (Fig. 22-3).

If the history indicates that the drainage is persistent or recurrent despite therapy, a culture should be obtained to determine both the causative organism and its sensitivity to antimicrobial agents. Treatment consists primarily of topical otic antibiotic/steroid preparations. Systemic antibiotics should be given when pain is severe; when there is evidence of otitis media; or when, despite attempts at cleaning, there

is still uncertainty about an infection of the middle ear. Parenteral antibiotics may be required when the process has extended, producing cellulitis of the periauricular soft tissues.

Displacement

Displacement of the pinna away from the skull is a worrisome sign. The most severe condition causing displacement is mastoiditis, resulting from extension of a middle-ear infection through the mastoid air cells and out to the periosteum of the skull. In addition to displacement, important clinical signs of mastoiditis include erythema and edema of the pinna and the skin overlying the mastoid, exquisite tenderness on palpation of the mastoid process, a sagging ear canal, purulent otorrhea, fever, and usually toxicity (Fig. 22-10). This condition is now considered unusual and is seen mainly in patients with long-standing, untreated or inadequately treated otitis media. Recognition, prompt institution of parenteral antibiotic therapy, and myringotomy are crucial because there is significant risk of central nervous system

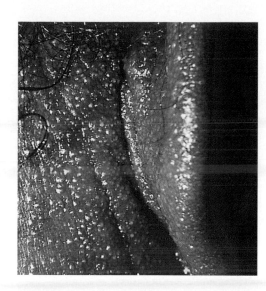

FIG. 22-13 This young girl became sensitive to the nickel posts of her earrings and developed periauricular contact dermatitis. The auricle and periauricular skin are erythematous and covered by a weeping, pruritic microvesicular eruption. (Courtesy Dr. Michael Sherlock.)

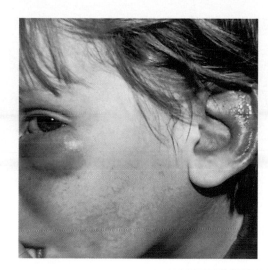

FIG. 22-14 Angioedema. This youngster had pruritic, nonpainful, nontender swelling of his ear and infraorbital region. Close examination of the latter revealed the punctum of an insect bite. This was obscured by the crusting on his ear, which he had scratched. (Courtesy Dr. Michael Sherlock.)

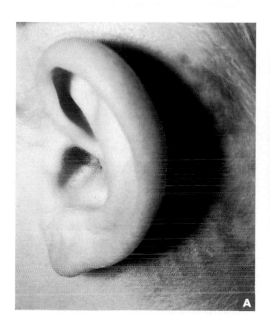

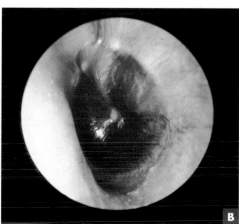

FIG. 22-15 Basilar skull fracture. *A,* The presence of a basilar skull fracture involving the temporal bone is often signaled by postauricular ecchymotic discoloration, termed *Battle sign. B,* The force of the blow may also cause tearing of the ear canal or as shown here middle ear hemorrhage with hemotympanum. Depending on time of examination, this may appear red or blue. (*B* courtesy Dr. Michael Hawke, Toronto.)

(CNS) extension. Radiographs show haziness of the mastoid air cells; a CT scan helps delineate extent of involvement and facilitates surgical approach (Fig. 22-11). Mastoidectomy is indicated in cases complicated by CNS extention and those in which IV antibiotics and myringotomy fail to produce complete resolution.

Other conditions characterized by displacement of the pinna away from the head include parotitis, primary cellulitis of periauricular tissues, and edema secondary to insect bites or contact dermatitis. Parotitis is differentiated by finding prominent induration and enlargement of the parotid gland anterior and inferior to the external ear, together with blunting of the angle of the mandible on palpation (see Figs. 12-25 and 12-26). Primary cellulitis is characterized by erythema and tenderness but can often be distinguished clinically from mastoiditis by the presence of associated skin lesions that antecede the inflammation (Fig. 22-12). In cases secondary to untreated external otitis or otitis media with perforation, the picture may be clinically similar.

Localized contact dermatitis and angioedema may be erythematous, but they are also pruritic and nontender. The former condition is characterized by microvesicular skin changes (Fig. 22-13), whereas in the latter condition, a precipitating insect bite can often be identified on inspection (Fig. 22-14).

Discoloration

Discoloration is another important sign and is commonly a feature of conditions producing displacement. Erythema of the pinna is common when there is inflammation, with or without infection (Figs. 22-10, *B,* and 22-12 to 22-14). Ecchymotic discoloration may be encountered with trauma. When this overlies the mastoid tip, the area immediately posterior to the pinna, it is termed a *Battle sign* (Fig. 22-15, *A*) and usually reflects a basilar skull fracture. In such cases the canal wall should be checked for tears and the tympanic membrane for perforation or a hemotympanum (Fig. 22-15, *B*). These findings are generally more helpful in making the diagnosis than routine skull

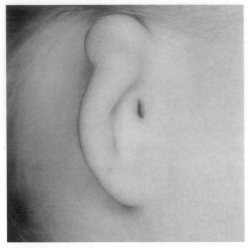

FIG. 22-16 Atresia of the right external ear. In this otherwise normal child, the pinna failed to develop properly, and the external canal was completely stenosed. Audiometric testing revealed a 60-dB hearing loss. Such isolated deformities stem from abnormal development of the first branchial arch.

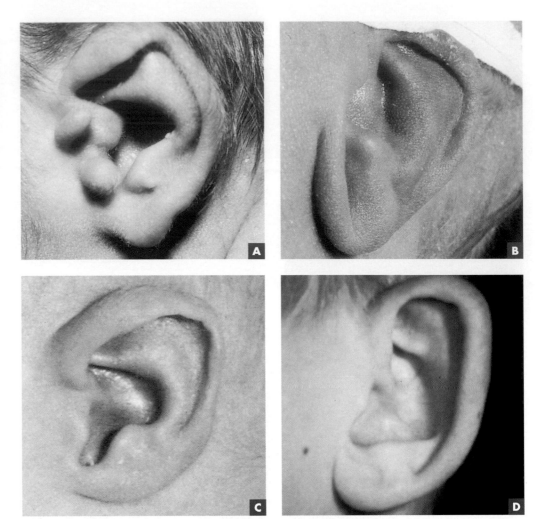

FIG. 22-17 Minor congenital auricular deformities. *A,* In this infant the superior portion of the helix is folded over obscuring the triangular fossa, the antihelix is sharply angulated, and there are three preauricular skintags. *B,* This neonate with orofaciodigital and Turner syndromes has a simple helix and a redundant folded lobule. The ear is low set and posteriorly rotated, and the antitragus is anteriorly displaced. *C,* This infant with Rubinstein-Taybi syndrome has an exaggeratedly elongated intertragal notch. *D,* Lop ear in an otherwise normal child. The auricular cartilage is abnormally contoured, making the ear protrude forward. (*C* courtesy Dr. Michael Sherlock.)

x-rays, which are often inconclusive. Of course, computed tomography can usually confirm the diagnosis of a basilar skull fracture.

Deformity

When the external ear is grossly misshapen or atretic, anomalies of middle- and inner-ear structures are often associated and hearing loss may be profound (Fig. 22-16). Severe deformities stem from developmental anomalies of the branchial arches, which contribute to both the external- and middle-ear structures. Such abnormalities warrant a thorough evaluation in infancy to ensure early recognition and treatment of hearing loss. Deformity of the pinna can be the result of hereditary factors or exposure to teratogens, but at times it is simply produced by unusual intrauterine positioning. Most deformities are minor. In some instances they may be part of a picture of multiple congenital anomalies (Fig. 22-17, *A* to *C*; also see Fig. 22-8 and Chapter 1), but in most cases they represent isolated, minor malformations that are of little significance other than cosmetic (Fig. 22-17, *D*).

Preauricular cysts constitute one of the more common congenital abnormalities. These are branchial cleft remnants located anterior to the pinna with an overlying surface dimple (Fig. 22-18, *A*). These cysts are vulnerable to infection and abscess formation (Fig. 22-18, *B*), which

necessitates incision and drainage in conjunction with antistaphylococcal antibiotics. Once infected, recurrence is common unless the entire cyst is completely excised. This procedure should be undertaken once inflammation has subsided.

Foreign Objects and Secondary Trauma

It is not unusual for children to put paper, beads, and other foreign objects into their ear canals (Fig. 22-19, *A*). Small flying insects also on occasion may become trapped in the external ear (Fig. 22-19, *B*). In some cases small objects may be embedded in cerumen and missed on inspection. As noted earlier, if present for more than a few days, the foreign material stimulates an inflammatory response and production of a purulent discharge that is often foul-smelling and may obscure the presence of the inciting foreign body. Removal of some objects can be accomplished by use of alligator forceps or by irrigation of the ear canal; others—particularly spherical objects—require use of a Day hook or suction (Fig. 22-19, *C* and Fig. 22-3). Foreign objects also may be the source of painful abrasions or lacerations of the external auditory canal or even perforation of the tympanic membrane. Pencils or sticks inserted into the ear canal by the child and parental attempts to

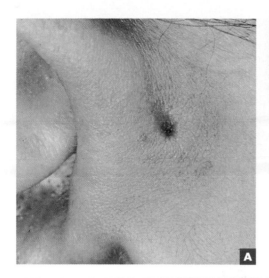
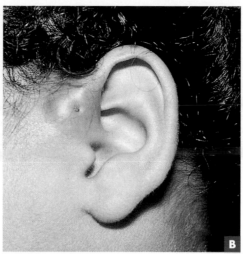

FIG. 22-18 Preauricular sinuses. *A,* These branchial cleft remnants are located anterior to the pinna and have an overlying surface dimple. *B,* In this child the sinus has become infected, forming an abscess. (*A* courtesy Dr. Michael Hawke, Toronto.)

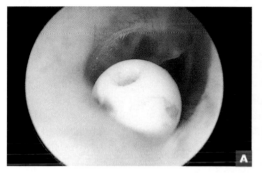
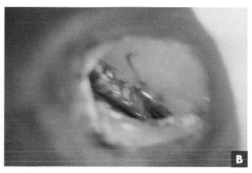
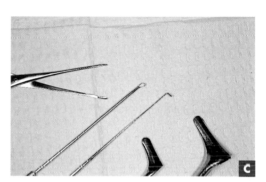

FIG. 22-19 Otic foreign bodies. *A,* This child inserted a bead into her ear. The object must be removed carefully to prevent further trauma. *B,* This patient experienced a period of intense buzzing pain and itching in the ear that abated after a few hours. When the patient was taken to his physician, an insect was found to be the culprit. *C,* A blunt-tipped, right-angled Day hook, smile wire loop currette, Hartman forceps, and an alligator forceps (Fig. 22-3, *A*) are useful instruments for removing foreign bodies from the external auditory canal.

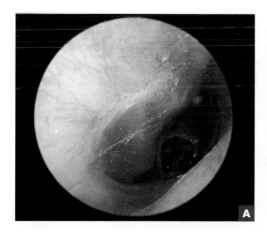
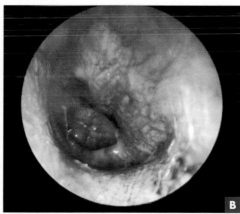

FIG. 22-20 Traumatic perforations of the tympanic membrane. *A,* This 8-year-old boy's tympanic membrane was perforated by a forceful slap on the ear. *B,* Even more severe damage with thickening and hemorrhage is seen in this victim of a blast injury caused by an explosion. (*A* courtesy Dr. Michael Hawke, Toronto.)

clean the canal with a cotton swab are the most common modes of such injury. Exposure to concussive forces such as a direct blow or an explosion can also result in perforation (Fig. 22-20, *A* and *B*). Patients with traumatic perforations must be carefully assessed for signs of injury to deeper structures. If tympanic membrane perforation occurs as a result of penetration by a foreign object or of concussive forces, the physician must be particularly aware of the possibility of middle- or inner-ear damage. Evidence of hearing loss, vertigo, or nystagmus should prompt urgent otolaryngologic consultation because an emergent surgical exploration may be indicated.

Disorders of the Middle Ear

The normal tympanic membrane is thin, translucent, neutrally positioned, and mobile. The ossicles, particularly the malleus, are generally visible through the membrane (Fig. 22-21). Adequate assessment of the

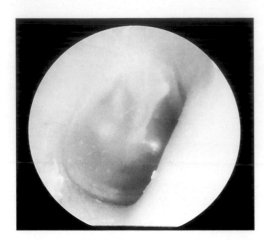

FIG. 22-21 A normal tympanic membrane. The drum is thin and translucent, and the ossicles are readily visualized. It is neutrally positioned with no evidence of bulging or retraction. (Courtesy Dr. Sylvan Stool, The Children's Hospital, Denver.)

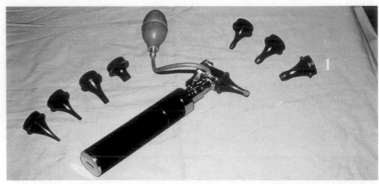

FIG. 22-22 Pneumatic otoscopy. This procedure requires proper equipment, including a pneumatic otoscope head and an appropriately sized speculum, to achieve a good air seal. When a seal is difficult to obtain despite proper speculum size, the head and tubing should be checked for air leaks. If none is found, application of a piece of rubber tubing to the end of the speculum (shown attached to the otoscope) or use of a soft speculum *(1)* may solve the problem.

tympanic membrane requires that the examiner note four major characteristics: (1) thickness, (2) degree of translucence, (3) position relative to neutral, and (4) mobility. Application of gentle positive and negative pressure using the pneumatic otoscope (Fig. 22-22) produces brisk movement of the eardrum when the ear is free of disease and abnormal movement when fluid is present, when the drum is thickened or scarred, or when there is an increase in either positive or negative pressure (Fig. 22-23). An abnormality in any one of the four major characteristics suggests middle-ear pathology.

Acute Otitis Media

Acute otitis media is the term used to describe acute infection and inflammation of the middle ear. Associated inflammation and edema of the eustachian tube mucosa appear to play key roles in the pathogenesis by impeding drainage of the middle-ear fluid. In some children, anatomic or chronic physiologic abnormalities of the eustachian tube predispose to infection. The problem is commonly seen in conjunction with an acute upper respiratory tract infection, and its onset is often heralded by a secondary temperature spike one to several days after the onset of respiratory symptoms. The major offending organisms are bacterial respiratory pathogens. The most commonly isolated organisms and their relative frequency are shown in Fig. 22-24. A small portion of cases constitute an exception to these percentages, that is, those in which otitis is accompanied by conjunctivitis. Here, nontypable *Haemophilus influenzae* is found causative in 70% to 75% of cases. Increasing rates of beta-lactamase positivity in these organisms necessitate use of beta-lactamase–resistant antibiotics whenever this syndrome is seen.

In acute otitis media the classic findings on inspection of the tympanic membrane are erythema and injection; bulging that obscures the malleus; thickening, often with a grayish-white or yellow hue, reflecting a purulent effusion; and reduced mobility (Fig. 22-25, *A*). However, crying rapidly produces erythema of the eardrum, and thus erythema in a crying child is of little diagnostic value. The patient is usually febrile and, if old enough, typically complains of otalgia. However, in many cases this "textbook picture" is not seen. This is probably due in part to time of presentation, the virulence of the particular pathogen, and host factors.

Accuracy in diagnosis necessitates meticulous care on otoscopy and knowledge of the various modes of presentation. Children may have fever of a few hours' duration and otalgia (or if very young, fever and irritability) yet have no abnormality on otoscopy. If reexamined the following day, many of these patients have clear evidence of acute otitis media. Some have erythema and bubbles or air-fluid or air-pus levels (a result of venting by the eustachian tube) without bulging and with nearly normal mobility (Fig. 22-25, *B*). In still other cases the drum may be full and poorly mobile with cloudy fluid behind it but minimally erythematous (Fig. 22-25, *C*). In some patients the drum is retracted, moves primarily or only in response to negative pressure, and shows signs of inflammation and/or a cloudy effusion.

Occasionally the signs and symptoms of otitis media may be accompanied by formation of a bullous lesion on the surface of the tympanic membrane, a condition termed *bullous myringitis* (Fig. 22-26). These children usually complain of intense pain. Whereas this phenomenon is most commonly associated with mycoplasmas in adults, any of the usual pediatric pathogens (Fig. 22-24) can be causative in children. Finally, acute otitis media may, by virtue of increasing middle-ear pressure, result in acute perforation of the tympanic membrane. On presentation the canal may be filled with purulent material; however, tugging on the pinna usually does not elicit pain, and erythema and edema of the canal wall are minimal or absent. Cleansing with a cotton wick usually reveals an inflamed drum with a barely visible perforation (Fig. 22-27).

Just as clinical findings of acute otitis media vary, so do symptoms. Although some patients have severe otalgia, others may complain of sore throat, mild ear discomfort, ear popping, or decreased hearing yet have floridly inflamed eardrums. Fever may be absent.

Radiographic studies generally are of little value in the diagnosis of acute otitis media. When a temporal bone CT scan is obtained of a patient with acute otitis media and fluid in the middle ear, fluid also will be present in the mastoid cavity. This will be interpreted by a radiologist as clouding of the mastoid because it may be difficult to distinguish between the CT findings of acute otitis media and those of acute mastoiditis. In such instances it is important that the physician look at the patient's clinical signs rather than rely on radiographic findings to make the diagnosis.

In addition to treating patients with an appropriate antimicrobial agent and analgesics when needed, follow-up examination is important. This is best done 2 to 3 weeks after diagnosis, when complete resolution can be expected in more than 50% of children. The purpose of

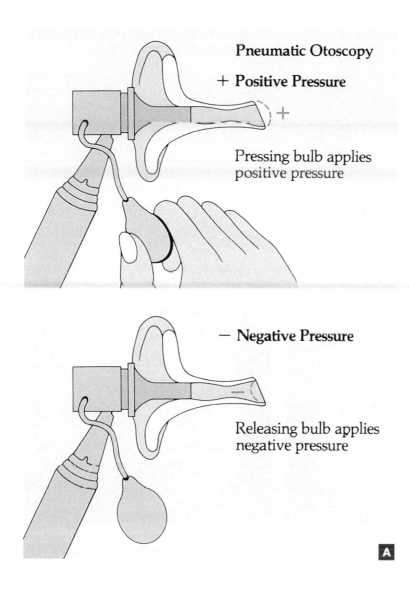

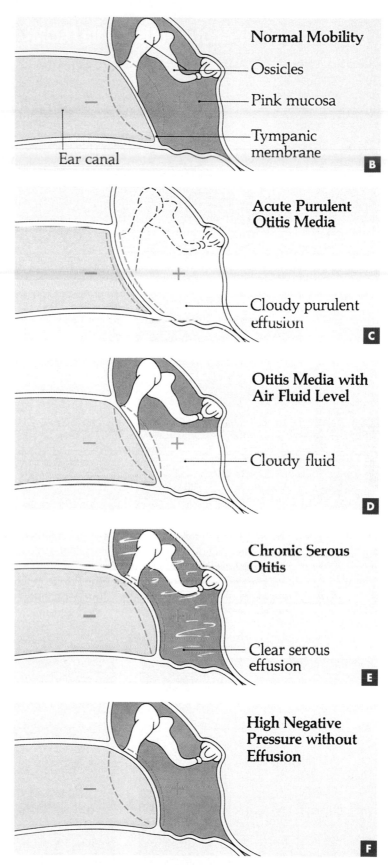

FIG. 22-23 Technique and findings of pneumatic otoscopy. *A,* The speculum is inserted into the ear canal to form a tight seal. The bulb is then gently and slowly pressed and released while the mobility of the drum is assessed. Pressing on the bulb applies positive pressure; letting up applies negative pressure. *B,* A normal drum moves inward and then back. *C,* In cases of acute otitis media in which the middle ear is filled with purulent material, the drum bulges toward the examiner and moves minimally. *D,* In cases of acute otitis media with an air-fluid level, mobility may be nearly normal. In some patients, however, the drum may be retracted, indicating increased negative pressure. If this is the case, mobility on positive pressure may be reduced while movement on negative pressure is nearly normal or only mildly decreased. *E,* This is the same pattern as that seen commonly in children with chronic serous otitis. *F,* In cases of high negative pressure and no effusion, application of positive pressure produces little or no movement, but on negative pressure the drum billows back toward the examiner.

reevaluation is to identify those patients who have persistent serous effusions and require ongoing surveillance.

Otitis Media With Effusion ("Serous Otitis Media")

Serous effusion in the middle ear may result from an upper respiratory tract infection, or it may be the residual of a treated acute otitis. In many instances this effusion is not spontaneously cleared, but instead remains in the middle ear for weeks or months, resulting in a persistent clear gray or yellow effusion behind the eardrum (Fig. 22-28). Persistence appears to result in part from eustachian tube dysfunction. Pneumatic otoscopy often reveals poor mobility of the tympanic membrane, and then primarily on negative pressure. The latter is thought to develop as a result of consumption of middle-ear oxygen by mucosal cells, creating a vacuum that persists with the fluid because of failure

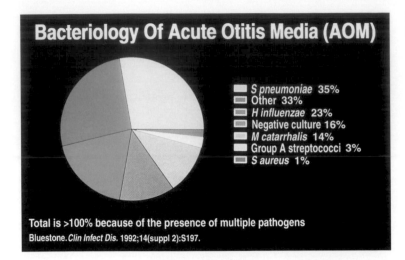

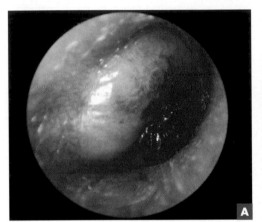
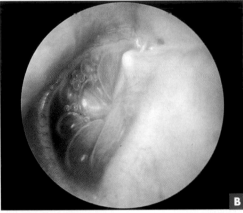
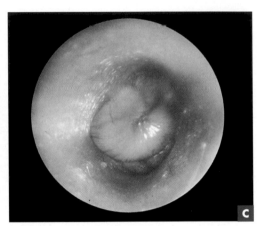

FIG. 22-24 Distribution of pathogens cultured in acute otitis media. (Courtesy Dr. Charles Bluestone, Children's Hospital of Pittsburgh.)

FIG. 22-25 Acute otitis media. *A,* This is the textbook picture: an erythematous, opaque, bulging tympanic membrane. The light reflex is reduced, and the landmarks are partially obscured. Mobility is markedly reduced. *B,* In this acutely febrile child who complained of otalgia, the presence of both air and fluid formed bubbles separated by grayish-yellow menisci. Even though the drum was not injected, this finding, combined with fever and otalgia, is consistent with acute infection. *C,* In this child the tympanic membrane was markedly injected superiorly, and a yellow purulent effusion caused the inferior portion to bulge outward. Mobility was markedly reduced. (*A* courtesy Dr. Michael Hawke, Toronto.)

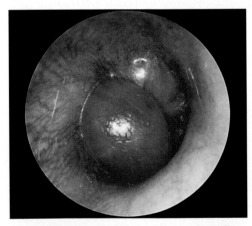
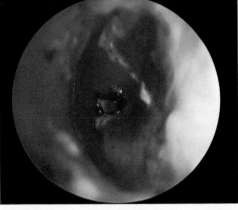
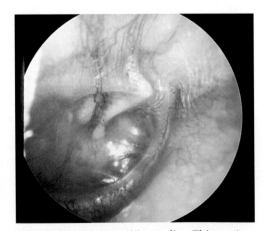

FIG. 22-26 Acute otitis media with bullous myringitis. This patient was febrile and extremely uncomfortable. On otoscopy an erythematous bullous lesion is seen obscuring much of the tympanic membrane. This phenomenon, called *bullous myringitis,* is caused by the usual pathogens of otitis media in childhood. The bullous lesion commonly ruptures spontaneously, providing immediate relief of pain.

FIG. 22-27 Acute otitis media with perforation. In this child, increased middle ear pressure with acute otitis resulted in perforation of the tympanic membrane. The drum is thickened, and the perforation is seen at the 3 o'clock position.

FIG. 22-28 Serous otitis media. This patient has a chronic serous middle ear effusion. The tympanic membrane is retracted, thickened, and shiny. Behind it is a clear yellow effusion. Mobility was decreased and primarily evident on negative pressure. The child was not acutely ill but did have decreased hearing. (Courtesy Dr. Sylvan Stool, The Children's Hospital, Denver.)

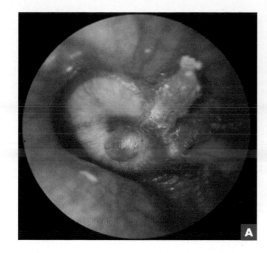
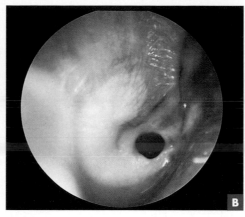

FIG. 22-29 Sequelae of chronic otitis media. *A,* Much of this child's tympanic membrane is scarred and thickened, and a thinned dimeric area balloons out of the anterosuperior portion. *B,* The eardrum is markedly thickened, scarred in an arc from 12 to 5 o'clock, and has a large chronic perforation. (Courtesy Dr. Sylvan Stool, The Children's Hospital, Denver.)

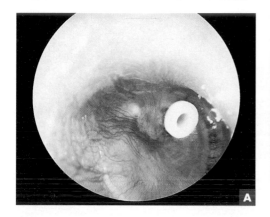
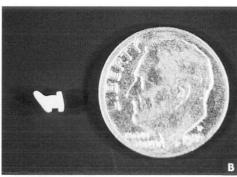

FIG. 22-30 *A,* Tympanic membrane of patient with chronic otitis media, with tympanostomy tube in place. The tubes serve to vent the middle ear, improve hearing, and reduce the frequency of infection. *B,* The tympanic membrane is about the size of a dime. A typical tube takes up approximately 15% of the tympanic membrane's surface area. There are many different types in a variety of shapes, materials, sizes, and colors. Selection is based on specific pathology and surgeon preference. (*A* courtesy Dr. Sylvan Stool, The Children's Hospital, Denver.)

of ventilation by the eustachian tube. Such long-standing effusions impair hearing and are subject to bacterial invasion and thus recurrent middle-ear infection. Persistence of a serous effusion for more than 4 to 6 months is an indication for myringotomy and insertion of tubes (Fig. 22-30, *A* and *B*) to facilitate hearing and reduce risk of recurrent infection.

Chronic–Recurrent Otitis Media

Chronic or chronic–recurrent otitis media with effusion (COME) is common in young children. Patients subject to this condition appear to have significant and prolonged eustachian tube dysfunction. This "otitis-prone" state may be a seemingly isolated phenomenon, or it can be a feature of a number of syndromes characterized by palatal dysfunction or malformation or by facial hypoplasia or deformity. These conditions include cleft palate, Crouzon syndrome, Down syndrome, the mucopolysaccharidoses, and mucolipidoses (Fig. 22-8, and see section on Palatal Disorders). Chronic obstructive tonsillar and adenoidal hypertrophy also may be a predisposing condition. Less commonly, immunodeficiency and the immotile cilia syndrome are identified as underlying etiologic conditions.

Chronic otitis media is associated with significant morbidity in terms of intermittent or chronic hearing impairment, intermittent discomfort, and the ill effects of recurrent infection. Over months or years, the process produces permanent myringosclerotic changes in which the tympanic membrane becomes whitened, thickened, and scarred (Fig. 22-29, *A*). Chronic perforations are common (Fig. 22-29, *B*). Patients with persistent middle-ear infections despite medical therapy and those with frequent recurrences appear to benefit from surgical drainage and insertion of tympanostomy tubes that vent the middle ear (Fig. 22-30). Persistence of a serous effusion for longer than 4 to

6 months is also an indication for myringotomy and insertion of tubes. Once placed, these should be checked at intervals for presence and patency. Spontaneous extrusion generally occurs 6 to 24 months after insertion. It is wise to prevent contamination of the middle ear with water. The need for ear plugs in children with tubes or a perforation is the subject of some controversy, but in general their use is still recommended.

Protection of the Exposed Middle Ear
With Earplugs or Ear Defenders

Earplugs, or ear defenders, come in all shapes and sizes. They vary in cost from inexpensive, premolded earplugs to expensive, custommolded devices. The general purpose of an earplug is to prevent water from entering the external ear canal and contaminating the middle-ear space. There are "wax" earplugs, which act like a putty that can be molded into the particular shape that comfortably blocks the individual's ear canals. There is also a preformed ear defender that is held in place by the conchal bowl and provides quite reasonable protection for children. The ear defenders vary in shape, and a child needs to be fitted for an age-appropriate size. Although custom-made ear plugs are not critical, they do provide a better fit, are more comfortable, and compliance with their use tends to be greater. Children have a propensity to lose or misplace these devices, and it is best to focus on obtaining functional earplugs that are easily replaceable at minimal cost.

Other Middle-Ear Disorders

A number of other disorders involving the tympanic membrane, though considerably less common than otitis media and serous otitis media, are important because of potential seriousness.

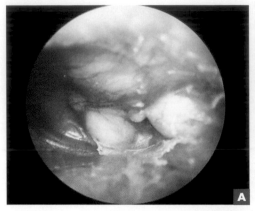
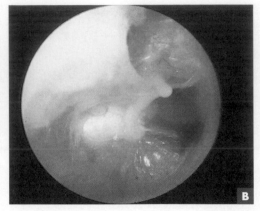
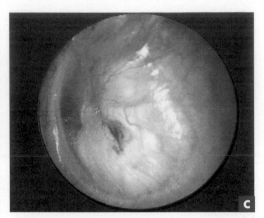

FIG. 22-31 Cholesteatomas. *A,* Congenital cholesteatoma noted in a young child with spontaneous ear drainage. There had been no previous history of ear infections. *B* and *C,* Acquired cholesteatomas, which generally present after a long history of chronic middle ear disease.

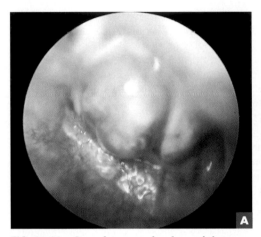
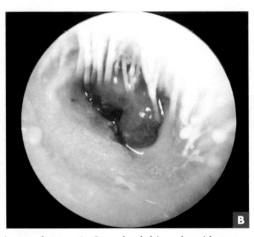
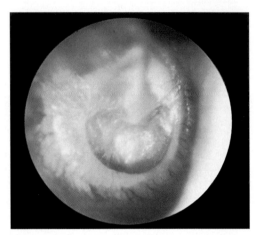

FIG. 22-32 Granulomas and polyps of the tympanic membrane. *A,* Growth of this polypoid granuloma was stimulated by the inflammatory process of chronic middle ear infection. *B,* These polyps, which protrude through a tympanic membrane perforation, have enlarged to entirely fill the external ear canal. Because of the possible attachment of the polyp to the ossicles of the middle ear, removal of polyps requires extreme caution. (*A* courtesy Dr. Sylvan Stool, The Children's Hospital, Denver.)

FIG. 22-33 Dimerism of the tympanic membrane. Otoscopy demonstrates a severely retracted atrophic segment of the eardrum that also has multiple white scars. The thinned portions are the result of abnormal healing of perforations and tend to be hypermobile on otoscopy. (Courtesy Dr. Sylvan Stool, The Children's Hospital, Denver.)

Mass Lesions Involving the Tympanic Membrane

The most common and one of the most serious mass lesions of the eardrum is a **cholesteatoma.** It can present as a defect in the tympanic membrane through which persistent drainage occurs, or it can appear as a white cystic mass behind or involving the eardrum. It consists of trapped epithelial tissue that grows beneath the surface of the membrane (Fig. 22-31). Although many are congenital, some are sequelae of untreated or chronic–recurrent otitis media. If a cholesteatoma is not removed surgically, it continues to enlarge; becomes locally destructive; and can erode the mastoid bone, destroy the ossicles, and even invade the inner-ear structures or cranium. A progressive hearing impairment usually occurs.

Granulomas or **polyps** of the tympanic membrane (Fig. 22-32) can also develop in children with chronic middle-ear infections. The most common cause of aural polyps in children is old, retained PE tubes. Cholesteatomas and chronic infections are other predisposing conditions. These tissues often bleed easily, which can frighten the patient, the parent, and the physician. Left untreated, polyps can enlarge to fill the canal and by expansion can progressively damage the drum and the ossicles. Therefore prompt surgical removal is indicated.

Distortions of the Tympanic Membrane

Thin, dimeric portions of the eardrum also may be observed in patients with chronic middle-ear disease, or they may develop after extrusion of a tympanostomy tube (Fig. 22-33; also Fig. 22-29, *A*). These thinned areas are the result of abnormal healing of perforations and are hypermobile on pneumatic otoscopy. The important points to note on examination are whether the pocket is fully visible or partly hidden, its location with respect to the ossicles, and whether or not it is dry. If the ear canal and drum are not dry, an active infection and/or cholesteatoma is present. In cases of severe deformity, aggressive therapy, including ventilation of the middle ear and excision of the pocket, may be necessary.

Nasal Disorders

A child's nose is examined most commonly for disturbances in external appearance, excessive drainage, or blockage of airflow and interference with breathing. Epistaxis is also frequently encountered.

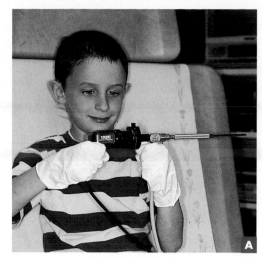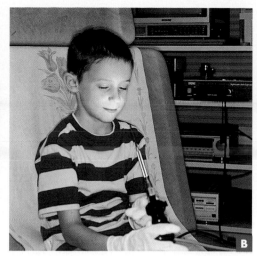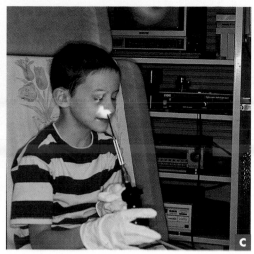

FIG. 22-34   Nasal endoscopic examination. *A,* A child holding and feeling the endoscope. *B,* When he shines the light on himself, the endoscope shows his face on the monitor. *C,* By holding it at the entrance to his nose, he sees that the instrument is neither hot nor painful.

Nasal Examination

The nasal examination can be difficult in younger children. It is best done with the child sitting on a parent's lap or in a chair. The child's head is held in a neutral position, not tilted up. The examiner should try to look toward the back of the nose rather than up into the nose.

An otoscope with a wide speculum (4 mm or greater) is the most practical instrument. The examiner should gently brace his or her free hand on the child's upper lip to prevent sudden head movement from pushing the speculum tip into the nose, which could lead to nasal trauma. If the child is old enough to comply, he or she is asked to breathe through his or her mouth so as not to fog up the lens on the otoscope. If a nasal spreader–type speculum is used, a headlight is desirable. The septum, the anterior edges of the middle and inferior turbinates, and the nasal floor are inspected, and the quality of nasal secretions is noted. With practice and when there is minimal congestion, adenoidal size can be assessed.

A more thorough examination is possible using a nasal endoscope; this enables full visualization of internal nasal structures. Before starting, the nose is sprayed with a decongestant to shrink the nasal mucosa and a topical anesthetic spray. With patience, older children can be coaxed through the insertion and examination. Allowing them to hold and inspect the device, test the light, look at themselves on the monitor, and even insert the tip into their nose facilitates cooperation (Fig. 22-34, *A* to *C*). Most children under 5 years of age require immobilization in a papoose board. If suctioning is necessary, having the patient take a deep breath and hold it before applying suction, reduces discomfort. The nasal endoscope is a useful tool, and this type of examination can be done readily in the otolaryngologist's office.

Nasal Obstruction

Upper Respiratory Infections in Early Infancy

In infancy and early childhood the nasal passages are small and easily obstructed by processes that produce mucosal edema and coryza, whether infectious, "allergic," or traumatic. In the first 1 to 3 months, infants are obligate nose breathers and therefore can have significant respiratory distress from nasal congestion alone. Young infants with upper respiratory tract infections may, in addition to nasal discharge, have tachypnea and mild retractions and often have to interrupt feeding to breathe. This often results in the swallowing of significant amounts of air, which leads to a secondary increase in spitting up after feeding and to intestinal gas pain. These secondary problems can be minimized by instructing parents to hold these infants up on their shoulders and burp them for 10 to 15 minutes after feedings. Instillation of saline nose drops to loosen secretions, followed by nasal suctioning before meals and naps, provides a measure of relief. Oral decongestants are ineffective and often produce marked irritability when given to infants in the first year of life. Fortunately, these upper respiratory tract infections are generally brief and clear within a few days.

On occasion, infants with upper respiratory tract infection go on to have persistent, purulent, or serosanguineous nasal discharge. Culture of discharges persisting longer than 10 to 14 days may disclose heavy growth of a single pathogen. Preliminary studies of empiric antimicrobial therapy in such infants suggest that this produces rapid and effective resolution of symptoms when compared with a placebo. Thus this picture of prolonged nasal discharge probably represents a bacterial ethmoiditis, the infant equivalent of sinusitis.

Congenital Causes of Nasal Obstruction

Congenital causes of nasal obstruction include choanal atresia, choanal stenosis, and mass lesions such as tumors, cysts, and polyps.

Choanal Atresia and Stenosis

Choanal atresia is bony (90%) or membranous (10%), bilateral or unilateral. Newborns with bilateral choanal atresia manifest severe respiratory distress at delivery, with cyanosis that is relieved by crying and returns with rest (paradoxical cyanosis). The true nature of the problem can elude detection if the physician relies solely on passing soft feeding catheters through the nose to determine patency because these can buckle or curl within the nose. The correct diagnosis is best made by using a van Buren urethral sound or a firm plastic suction catheter (both no. 8 French). This is passed gently along the floor of the nose, close to the septum. If bony resistance is encountered, the diagnosis of choanal atresia is suspected (Fig. 22-35, *A*) and can be confirmed by obtaining a computed tomography (CT) scan of the nose and nasopharynx with fine overlapping cuts (Fig. 22-35, *B*).

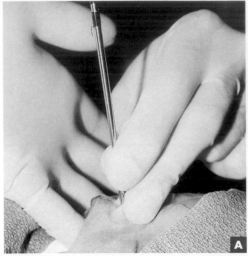

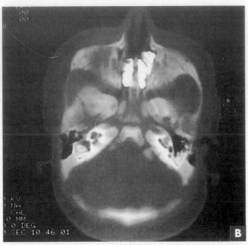

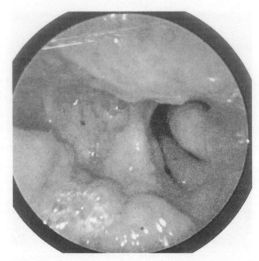

FIG. 22-35 Choanal atresia. *A,* This infant manifested severe respiratory distress at delivery, with paradoxical cyanosis. Attempts to pass a urethral sound revealed bony obstruction of the choanae bilaterally. *B,* A CT scan done after instillation of radiopaque dye reveals pooling of the dye within the nose anterior to the choanae, confirming complete obstruction.

FIG. 22-36 Unilateral choanal atresia. Viewed through the nasopharyngoscope, the left choana is clearly patent whereas the right is atretic.

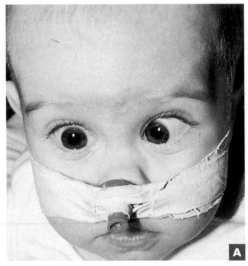

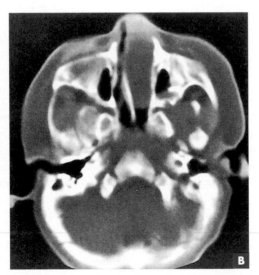

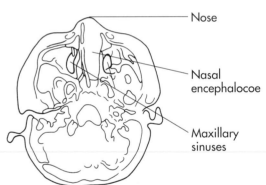

FIG. 22-37 Nasal encephalocele. *A,* This normal-appearing infant had signs of severe nasal obstruction, necessitating insertion of a nasopharyngeal airway to relieve distress. *B,* A CT scan shows a large nasal mass lesion that fills one nostril and pushes the nasal septum into the other. This lesion proved to be an encephalocele extruding through a bony defect in the skull (extrusion seen on another cut).

Immediate relief of respiratory distress may be accomplished by insertion of an oral airway (or a nipple from which the tip has been cut away) into the mouth. Definitive studies can then be performed to aid in planning surgical correction. Infants with unilateral choanal atresia (Fig. 22-36) are usually asymptomatic at birth; however, with time they develop a persistent unilateral nasal discharge.

Choanal stenosis or anterior nasal stenosis also is generally asymptomatic in the newborn period, but acquisition of an upper respiratory tract infection can result in significant respiratory compromise. When suspected, probing with a urethral sound is indicated. If this meets resistance, further evaluation is required. In most cases symptomatic therapy using saline nose drops and nasal suctioning is sufficient to help the infant through the upper respiratory tract infection. With growth, the problem abates.

Congenital Mass Lesions

Congenital mass lesions are another source of nasal obstruction. These are particularly likely to become apparent during the first 2 years of life. The modes of presentation vary; some lesions manifest primarily by symptoms of obstruction and are detected via diagnostic radiography; others become visually evident within a nostril or as a subcutaneous mass located near the root of the nose. Occasionally these patients have recurrent nasal infections and/or epistaxis. All such masses merit thorough clinical and radiographic evaluation, since many have intracranial connections.

An **encephalocele** is an outpouching of brain tissue through a congenital bony defect in the midline of the skull. Some patients have craniofacial deformities and a rounded swelling between the eyes. In other instances the neural tissue prolapses into the nasopharynx, resulting in

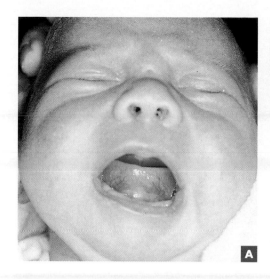

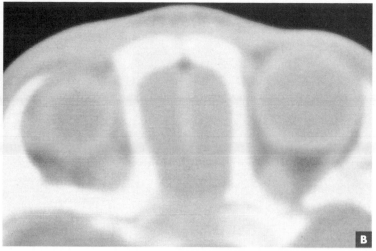

FIG. 22-38 Nasal dermoid. *A,* A firm, round mass with a central dimple is seen over the bridge of this infant's nose. *B,* CT scan demonstrates a bony dehiscence of the nasal bridge with a nasal dermoid extending into the anterior cranial vault in the area of the foramen cecum.

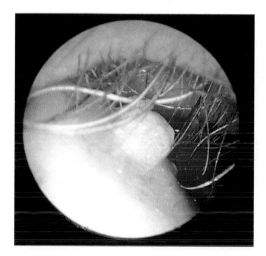

FIG. 22-39 Nasal papillomas present as warty growths at the mucocutaneous junction of the nares. (Courtesy Dr. Michael Hawke, Toronto.)

signs and symptoms of nasal obstruction without obvious external anomalies (Fig. 22-37, *A*). Occasionally a grapelike mass may be seen (via direct nasopharynoscopy) within the nares or protruding into the pharynx. The mass is usually identified by diagnostic radiography. CT (Fig. 22-37, *B*) is particularly helpful in delineating the extent of the mass and the underlying bony defect. Repair requires a collaborative effort by specialists in otolaryngology, neurosurgery, and in some cases plastic surgery.

Nasal dermoids are embryonic cysts containing ectodermal and mesodermal tissue. They present as round, firm subcutaneous masses located on the dorsum of the nose, close to the midline (Fig. 22-38, *A*). Examination of the overlying skin frequently reveals a small dimple, at times with extruding hair. Some of these cysts have deep extensions down to the nasal septum or through the cribriform plate into the cranium. Thorough evaluation using axial and coronal CT scans and magnetic resonance imaging is necessary to determine extent and plan repair (Fig. 22-38, *B*). If such cysts are not removed, secondary infection is common and often results in fistula formation.

Small skintags are frequently seen around the nasal vestibule and should be removed to improve appearance. **Papillomas** (Fig. 22-39) are similar growths that occur on the distal nasal mucosa near the mucocutaneous junction. These growths should be excised to improve appearance and confirm diagnosis; they do not cause obstruction.

Acquired Forms of Nasal Obstruction
Adenoidal and Tonsillar Hypertrophy

The lymphoid tissue that constitutes the tonsils and adenoids is relatively small in infancy, gradually enlarges until 8 to 10 years of age, and then begins to shrink in size. In most instances this normal process of hypertrophy results in mild to moderate enlargement of these structures and does not constitute a problem. A small percentage of children, however, develop marked adenoidal and tonsillar hypertrophy, with attendant symptoms of nasal obstruction and rhinorrhea. A few even have difficulty swallowing solid foods. Recurrent infection appears to be the most common inciting factor, although atopy may play a role in some cases. Occasionally, mononucleosis is the initiating event, resulting in rapid enlargement of adenoidal and tonsillar tissues that is then slow to resolve (see section on tonsillopharyngitis and see also Chapter 12). In most children, progressive adenoidal enlargement appears to be the cumulative result of a series of upper respiratory tract infections. The consequent obstruction to normal flow of secretions then starts a vicious cycle, making the child more vulnerable to recurrent infections of the ears, sinuses, and nasopharynx, which in turn further exacerbate the adenoidal and tonsillar hypertrophy.

Regardless of mode of origin, when adenoidal hypertrophy is marked, blockage of the nasal airway becomes severe and results in mouth breathing, chronic rhinorrhea, inability to blow the nose, and snoring during sleep (Fig. 22-40, *A*). Speech becomes hyponasal and muffled. The child holds his or her mouth open, has little or no airflow through the nares, and his or her tonsils may meet in the midline (Fig. 22-40, *B*). A cephalometric lateral neck x-ray examination reveals a large adenoidal shadow impinging on the nasal airway (Fig. 22-40, *C*). For many patients these features occur primarily in the course of acute illness; however, a number of children have symptoms even when free of acute infection. In a minority of cases obstruction is so severe as to produce sleep disturbance. This is characterized by restlessness and retractions when recumbent, stertorous snoring, and sleep apnea with frequent waking. Some patients begin to sleep sitting up, and many manifest daytime fatigue. Symptoms are worse during sleep because relaxation of the pharyngeal muscles further increases the degree of upper airway obstruction. In severe cases this results in periods of hypoxia and hypercarbia, leading to intermittent apnea and waking. Because a patient may look relatively healthy when awake (with the exception of having to breathe through the mouth), it is important to observe for retractions and pattern of breathing after the child has been recumbent for a period of time or, better still, during a nap. Use of con-

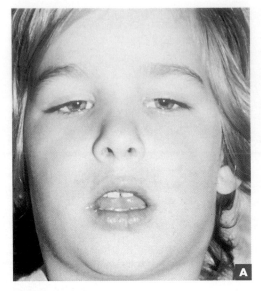

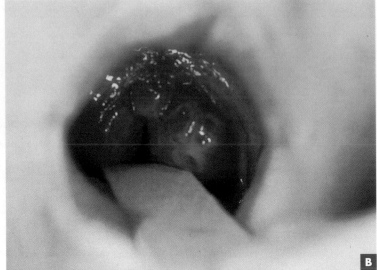

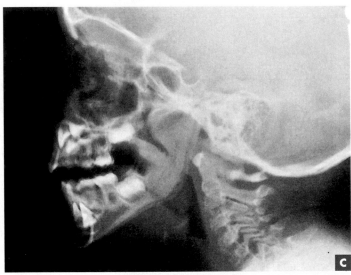

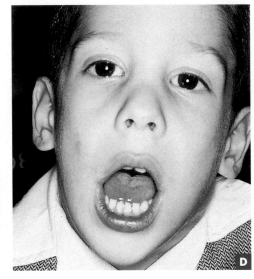

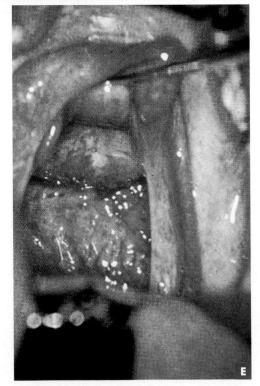

FIG. 22-40   Adenoidal and tonsillar hypertrophy. *A,* External appearance of a child with marked enlargement of tonsils and adenoids. He must keep his mouth open to breathe and shows signs of fatigue as a result of sleep disturbance caused by his upper airway obstruction. *B,* On examination of the pharynx, his tonsils are seen meeting at the midline. *C,* A lateral neck radiograph shows a large adenoid shadow impinging on the nasal airway. *D,* If obstruction is prolonged, cor pulmonale, abnormal facial elongation, and widening of the nasal root may result. *E,* When the palate is retracted before adenoidectomy, the extent of overgrowth of adenoidal tissue is readily appreciated.

tinuous pulse oximetry during this period of observation enables documentation of presence or absence of oxygen desaturation. If obstruction persists for a prolonged period of time, cor pulmonale (with signs of right ventricular hypertrophy on electrocardiogram and chest x-ray) and abnormal facial growth may result (Fig. 22-40, *D*).

Management of patients with adenoidal hypertrophy is dependent in part upon the severity and the duration of the obstruction. In milder cases of short duration or in patients with intermittent symptoms, careful monitoring, prompt institution of antimicrobial therapy for bacterial infections, and treatment of atopy, when present, may bring the problem under control. Children with persistent symptoms despite therapy and those with sleep disturbance or cor pulmonale warrant adenoidectomy, during which the extent of adenoidal overgrowth can be fully ap-

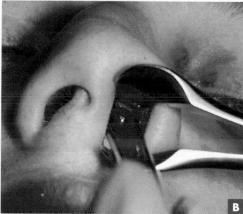
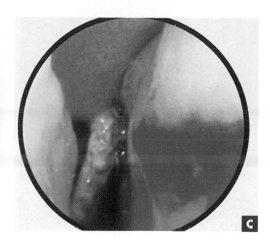
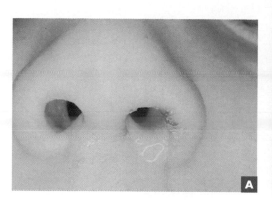
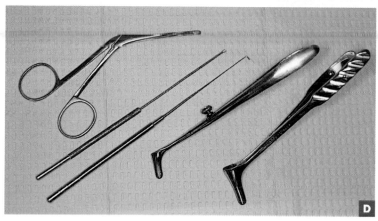

FIG. 22-41 Nasal foreign body. *A*, This child had a unilateral, foul smelling nasal discharge. *B*, Aspiration of the discharge in this patient revealed a red bead that was removed with a Day hook. *C*, A piece of cardboard is seen in this child's nostril. Note the mucosal abrasion from a prior attempt at removal. *D*, Hartman forceps, a small wire loop curette, and a right-angle Day hook are the most commonly used instruments for removal of nasal foreign bodies. Nasal spreaders facilitate visualization and create a wider space for inserting the desired instrument. (*A* Courtesy Dr. Michael Hawke; *C* From Becker W: *Atlas of ear nose and throat diseases,* ed 2, Philadelphia, 1984, WB Saunders.)

preciated (Fig. 22-40, *E*). Children with major orthodontic abnormalities and nasal obstruction also should be considered for adenoidectomy before orthodontic correction.

Nasal Foreign Bodies

As with the external ear, it is not unusual for small children to put beads, paper, pieces of sponge, plastic toys, or other foreign material into their noses. Such foreign objects are irritating to the nasal mucosa and soon incite an intense inflammatory reaction with production of a thick, purulent, foul-smelling discharge that helps to hide their presence. Intermittent epistaxis may accompany the discharge. Because most children below 5 years of age are unable to blow their noses and are afraid or unable to tell their parents what they've done, the object is not expelled and the problem often goes unrecognized until symptoms develop and medical attention is sought. A unilateral nasal discharge and/or a foul smell are the typical chief complaints and should lead the clinician to suspect a foreign body immediately (Fig. 22-41, *A*).

Speculum examination may readily disclose the object (Fig. 22-41, *B* and *C*), but often the purulent discharge obscures the view. Even when visualization is accomplished, removal can be difficult because children are easily frightened at the prospect of instrumentation, and their struggling can result in mucosal injury during attempts at removal (Fig. 22-43, *C*). To minimize problems, topical anesthetic spray and a topical vasoconstrictor can be applied, and the child can be restrained with a papoose board. Older patients or calm young children may do well sitting in a parent's lap, if the examiner is patient, reassuring, and willing to explain each step carefully. The discharge may then be removed by swab or suction. If the object is anterior to the turbinates, removal can be attempted using suction, a small wire loop curette, a right-angled Day hook for spherical objects; or alligator, or Hartman, forceps for material that can be grasped (Fig. 22-43, *D*). Consultation from an otolaryngologist should be sought for removal of objects lo-

cated more posteriorly or those not readily removed on initial attempts. A major concern is that in the attempted removal, a deeply situated foreign body may be dislodged into the nasopharynx, leading to aspiration or worse, laryngeal obstruction. In such cases the best course of action is to remove the object after the airway has been secured with an endotracheal tube in the operating room, under a general anesthetic.

Nasal Polyps

Polyps are thought to be the end result of recurrent infection and/or inflammation, although in a portion of cases, atopy may play a contributing role. Polyps originate in the ethmoid or less commonly the maxillary sinuses and protrude through the sinus ostia into the nasal cavity. The phenomenon is unusual in children under 10 years of age, with the exception of patients with cystic fibrosis, 25% of whom develop polyps, some as early as infancy. Symptoms consist of progressive nasal obstruction, frequently with associated discharge. Recurrent sinusitis is a common complication as a result of impaired sinus drainage. In some cases chronic sinusitis may be the cause of polyp formation. Affected patients with acute infections may also have intermittent epistaxis. Involvement may be unilateral or bilateral. On examination, moist, glistening pedunculated growths that may have a smooth or a grapelike appearance are seen (Fig. 22-42). Bilateral opacification of the ethmoid and maxillary sinuses is commonly found on radiography. Polyps must be distinguished from a nasal glioma or encephalocele, which may have a similar appearance and can produce identical symptoms. These neural mass lesions are more common in infancy but can present in older children. Therefore CT of the nasopharynx should be considered for children under age 10 with polypoid nasal lesions who do not have cystic fibrosis.

Surgical removal of the polyp is indicated to relieve nasal obstruction, reduce the risk of secondary sinusitis, and diminish the possibility of altered facial growth. The latter problem is seen in children with

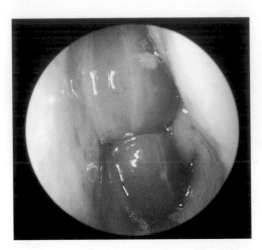

FIG. 22-42 Nasal polyp. This 2-year-old girl with cystic fibrosis was referred because of nasal obstruction and nocturnal snoring of a few months duration. A large grayish polyp was found in the left nostril.

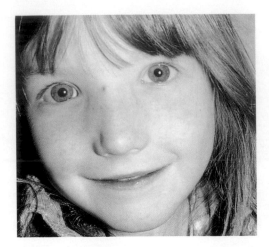

FIG. 22-43 Sequela of chronic nasal polyps. This 7-year-old girl with cystic fibrosis and recurrent nasal polyps shows secondary alteration in facial growth consisting of a broadened nasal dorsum and prominence of the malar areas. This occurred despite several resections.

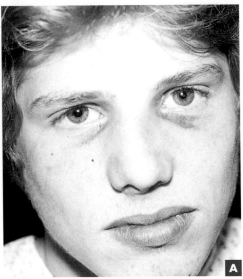

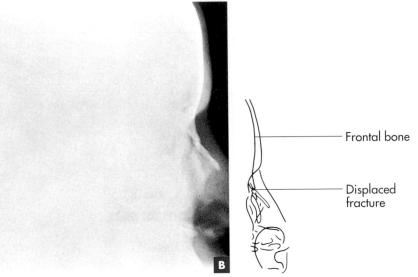

Frontal bone

Displaced fracture

FIG. 22-44 Displaced nasal fracture. *A,* This teenager was hit on the nose while playing football. On external inspection there is obvious deformity, and there are ecchymoses under both eyes. Crepitance was evident on palpation. *B,* A lateral radiograph of another patient shows a displaced fracture of the proximal portion of the nasal bone.

chronic polyps (most frequently those with cystic fibrosis) and consists of widening of the nasal dorsum and prominence of the malar areas of the face (Fig. 22-43).

Nasal Trauma

Blunt nasal trauma is frequently encountered in pediatrics. In the majority of instances it results only in minor swelling and mild epistaxis, which is readily controlled by application of pressure over the nares (see Chapter 2 for nasal trauma incurred during delivery). However, more severe injuries do occur and have a significant potential for long-term morbidity and deformity if not identified and treated appropriately. These injuries include displaced nasal fractures (Fig. 22-44), which, if not reduced, result in permanent deformity; septal deviation or dislocation, with or without an associated fracture (Fig. 22-45), which produces unilateral impairment of airflow; and septal hematomas (Fig. 22-46, *A*), which, if not drained promptly, cause destruction of nasal cartilage resulting in a saddle-nose deformity (Fig. 22-46, *B*). Finally, profuse bleeding that is difficult to stop or recurs readily suggests trauma to deeper structures of the face or frontal bones and warrants prompt stabilization and meticulous clinical and radiographic assessment (see Chapter 20).

In evaluating patients with nasal trauma, the nasal bridge should be inspected for swelling or deformity (the latter may not be apparent if swelling is marked) and the septum palpated for tenderness, crepitus, or excessive mobility. The nares should be cleared of clots and the septum assessed for position and presence of swelling, which would suggest a hematoma. Examination of the oropharynx is also helpful in determining if blood is flowing posteriorly. When marked swelling, severe tenderness, deformity, crepitus, or septal deviation is found, radiography is indicated. However, radiographs should be interpreted with caution because a large portion of the nasal skeleton in children is composed of cartilage rather than bone and serious nasal injuries can be present despite a seemingly normal x-ray film. Septal hematomas, displaced fractures, and bleeding that fails to cease readily with direct pressure necessitate prompt consultation with an otolaryngologist.

Epistaxis

Nasal bleeding in childhood has a number of causes including trauma, infection, mucosal irritation, bleeding disorders, vascular anomalies, and hypertension. Patients with these conditions may have apparently spontaneous bleeding or epistaxis triggered by minor external trauma or by forceful sneezing and blowing. Profuse bleeding that is difficult

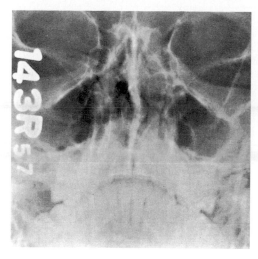

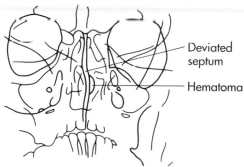

FIG. 22-45 Deviated nasal septum. This patient was punched in the nose, resulting in a leftward deviation of the cartilaginous portion of the nasal septum, which is clearly visible in this radiograph. The small arc of mucosal swelling along the septum proved to be a small septal hematoma. There is no visible fracture. Septal deviation requires correction to prevent deformity and relieve secondary nasal obstruction.

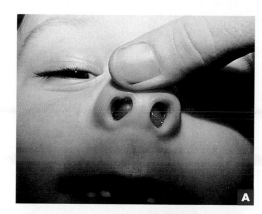

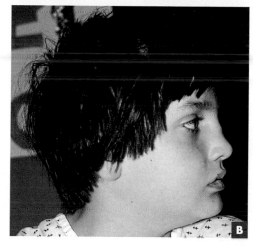

FIG. 22-46 Septal hematoma. This patient incurred facial trauma *(A)* resulting in multiple fractures of the nasal and orbital bones and submucosal bleeding along the nasal septum. Such septal hematomas must be drained promptly to reduce the risk of abscess formation and to prevent cartilage necrosis that ultimately results in *(B)* a saddle nose deformity. (*A* courtesy Dr. Robert Hickey, Children's Hospital of Pittsburgh.)

to stop is most characteristic of acute thrombocytopenia, vascular anomalies, and hypertension. Mild bleeding that is readily controlled by application of pressure suggests mucosal infection or irritation that promotes bleeding from small submucosal veins located on the anterior nasal septum (Fig. 22-47). In all cases the problem should be taken seriously and investigated carefully to correctly diagnose and appropriately treat the primary source of the problem.

In approaching patients with epistaxis, the following historic points should be addressed:

1. Is the problem acute or recurrent?
2. Was external trauma, sneezing, or blowing a triggering event?
3. What is the duration of the current bleed and the approximate volume of blood loss (handkerchiefs soaked, hemodynamic status, etc.)?
4. Is the bleeding unilateral or bilateral?
5. Has the patient been having symptoms suggestive of an upper respiratory tract infection or nasal allergy?
6. Has the child manifested other signs and symptoms of an underlying coagulopathy or of hypertension?
7. Has the patient been taking medication, especially aspirin or ibuprophen?

Physical assessment must address the patient's general well-being in addition to careful examination of the nose. Hemodynamic status is of particular import when hemorrhage has been profuse.

After observation of the external appearance of the nares, the nose is cleared of clots and discharge, if present. Then the septum and mucosa are inspected for possible points of hemorrhage, signs of obstruction, mass lesions, and foreign objects. The oropharynx should also be examined for posterior flow of blood, especially in cases in which no point of bleeding is evident on inspection of the nasal mucosa. Otolaryngologic consultation should be sought in cases involving profuse

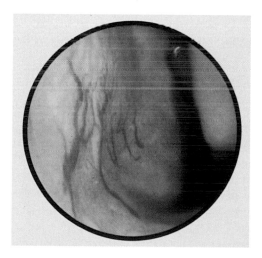

FIG. 22-47 Dilated septal vessels of Kesselbach plexus, which tend to bleed in response to mucosal infection or irritation. (From Becker W: *Atlas of ear, nose, and throat disorders,* ed 2, Philadelphia, 1984, WB Saunders.)

bleeding that does not readily cease upon application of pressure and may require nasal packing or other surgical treatment.

Epistaxis Caused by Infection and Mucosal Irritation

In many patients with nontraumatic epistaxis, examination reveals unilateral or bilateral septal erythema and friability or excoriation (Fig. 22-48). The history given is one of intermittent bleeding, especially with sneezing or blowing the nose or during sleep (the child's pillow is found spotted with blood). The phenomenon is commonly attributed to picking the nose in response to itching. However, in view of the sensitivity of the mucosa to painful stimuli, picking to the point of excoriation is rather unlikely. In many instances these lesions are impetiginous or represent the combined effects of inflammation (the result of nasopharyngitis, sinusitis, or allergic rhinitis) and trauma caused

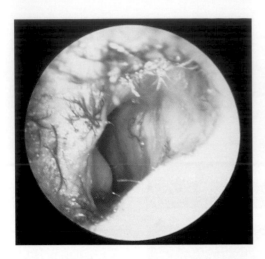

FIG. 22-48 Excoriated nasal septum. This child presented with an upper respiratory tract infection and a history of intermittent epistaxis with nasal blowing during the night. He had a purulent nasal discharge *(lower right)*, and a diffusely excoriated erythematous septum. Cultures of his nose and throat grew group A beta-streptococci.

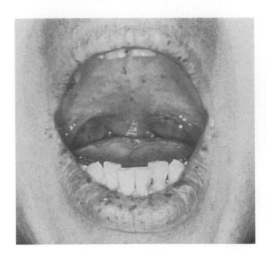

FIG. 22-49 Hereditary hemorrhagic telangiectasia. Numerous telangiectasias dot the lips and palatal mucosa of this boy who had problems with recurrent epistaxis. (Courtesy Dr. Bernard Cohen, Children's Hospital of Pittsburgh.)

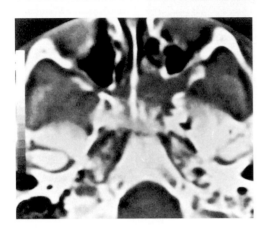

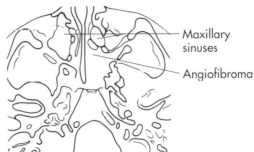

Maxillary sinuses

Angiofibroma

FIG. 22-50 Juvenile nasopharyngeal angiofibroma. CT scan is helpful in assessing the extent of this locally invasive vascular tumor. In this cut, an enhanced mass is seen occupying the posterior portion of the left nostril, deviating the septum and compressing the ipsilateral maxillary sinus.

by forceful sneezing and blowing. When infection is suspected, culturing of the friable area for a predominant bacterial pathogen (especially group A beta-streptococci or coagulase-positive staphylococci) may prove rewarding. In patients with no history of or findings consistent with upper respiratory tract infection, mucosal drying may be responsible. This occurs most commonly in winter, as a result of drying of the air by central heating systems. Although application of topical antibiotic ointment, humidification, and antihistamines (for atopic patients) may provide some relief, oral antimicrobial therapy for bacterial pathogens, when found, is more likely to be successful.

Patients with nasal polyps who have an intercurrent infection and children with nasal foreign bodies with secondary infection and inflammation are also highly prone to intermittent epistaxis and/or blood tinging of their nasal discharge.

Epistaxis Caused by Bleeding Disorders

Despite application of pressure, epistaxis in patients with coagulopathies is more likely to be prolonged and carries a greater risk of significant blood loss. Although many such patients have known bleeding disorders, a few may present with prolonged or recurrent nosebleeds as one of the initial manifestations of their problem. This is most typical of idiopathic thrombocytopenia, aplastic anemia, and acute leukemia. When epistaxis arises in the context of a bleeding disorder, the personal history, family history, and/or other physical findings should point to the diagnosis (see Chapter 11), which can then be confirmed by hematologic studies (CBC and differential, platelet count, prothombin time (PT) and partial thromboplastin time (PTT), and coagulation profile).

Acute management is dependent in part on the source of the coagulopathy (e.g., factor replacement or platelet transfusion) and in part

on severity of bleeding. Topical application of a vasoconstrictor such as epinephrine and insertion of absorbable synthetic material that aids coagulation (Gelfoam or Surgicel) can be very helpful in patients with thrombocytopenia and an anterior point of bleeding. The risks of secondary infection with packing must be given careful consideration when treating patients undergoing immunosuppressive therapy.

Epistaxis Caused by Vascular Abnormalities

In a minority of children with recurrent epistaxis, the history reveals significant bleeding that typically drains from one side of the nose. This suggests a localized vascular abnormality. The most commonly encountered problem is that of a dilated septal vessel or plexus, which may be a sequela of prior inflammation (Fig. 22-47). This may be visible anteriorly but also can be located high on the septum, requiring nasopharyngoscopy for identification. Cauterization is generally curative. In children over 7 years of age, anterior septal lesions can be cauterized in the office with silver nitrate after application of a topical anesthetic. Younger children and many patients with posterior lesions may need general anesthesia for cauterization.

Two relatively rare vascular anomalies may also be the source of recurrent nasal bleeding: telangiectasias and angiofibromas. Patients with **hereditary hemorrhagic telangiectasias** (Osler-Weber-Rendu disease) have an autosomal dominant disorder characterized by formation of cutaneous and mucosal telangiectatic lesions that begin to develop in childhood and gradually increase in number with age. These lesions appear as bright red, slightly raised, star-shaped plexuses of dilated small vessels that blanch on pressure (Fig. 22-49). Mucosal telangiectasias may bleed spontaneously or in response to minor trauma. Recurrent epistaxis is a common mode of presentation in childhood. Multiple

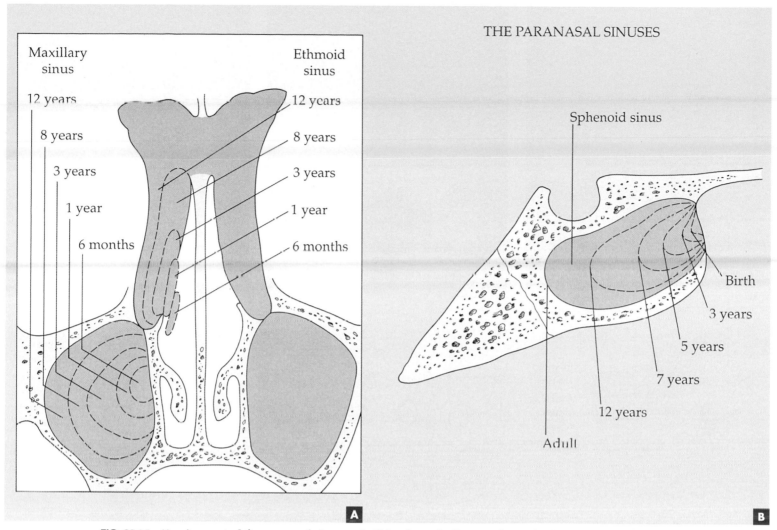

THE PARANASAL SINUSES

FIG. 22-51 Development of the paranasal sinuses. *A,* This schematic diagram shows the development of the maxillary and ethmoid sinuses. Note that development occurs throughout childhood and may not be complete until 12 years of age. *B,* The sphenoid sinus, which sits under the pituitary fossa, develops very slowly, and may not even be well aerated for the first 5 to 6 years of life.

telangiectasias are evident on close examination. Hematuria and/or gastrointestinal bleeding may be seen separately or in combination with epistaxis.

Juvenile nasopharyngeal angiofibroma is a rare vascular tumor seen predominantly in adolescent boys. Although benign, it is locally invasive and destructive and may involve the maxillary sinuses, palate, sphenoid sinus, and anterior portions of the skull. Its most common mode of presentation is profuse, often recurrent epistaxis. Some patients also have symptoms of nasal obstruction with secondary rhinorrhea, and a small percentage may have visual or auditory disturbances. On examination, a purplish soft-tissue mass may be seen through the nares or on nasopharyngoscopy. General radiographs, computerized tomography, and angiography may be needed to assess the extent of the tumor (Fig. 22-50). Carefully planned excision is then the treatment of choice.

Epistaxis Caused by Hypertension

In contrast to the adult population, hypertension is an unusual source of epistaxis in childhood. However, it should be considered, especially in patients with antecedent headache and spontaneous, profuse bleeding that is difficult to stop. It must be remembered that after significant blood loss, blood pressure may drop to normal levels. Patients with such a history may have previously undiagnosed coarctation of the aorta or chronic renal disease, and they should be examined with these possibilities in mind.

Disorders of the Paranasal Sinuses and Adjacent Structures

The paranasal sinuses are air-filled, bony cavities that lie within the facial bones of the skull, adjacent to the nasal passage. They develop through a gradual enlargement of pneumatized cells that evaginate from the nasal cavity. This process occurs over the course of childhood and adolescence; there is a wide normal range in the duration of this process and in the ultimate size of the sinuses and their ostia (Fig. 22-51). In infancy the ethmoid and maxillary sinuses are partially pneumatized, but they are small and not readily demonstrable on x-rays (although they can be readily seen on a CT scan). Therefore radiographs are of little diagnostic value until after the first 2 years of life. The sphenoid sinus is not evident until about 5 to 6 years, and the frontal sinuses are not well developed until after 7 to 8 years of age (Fig. 22-52).

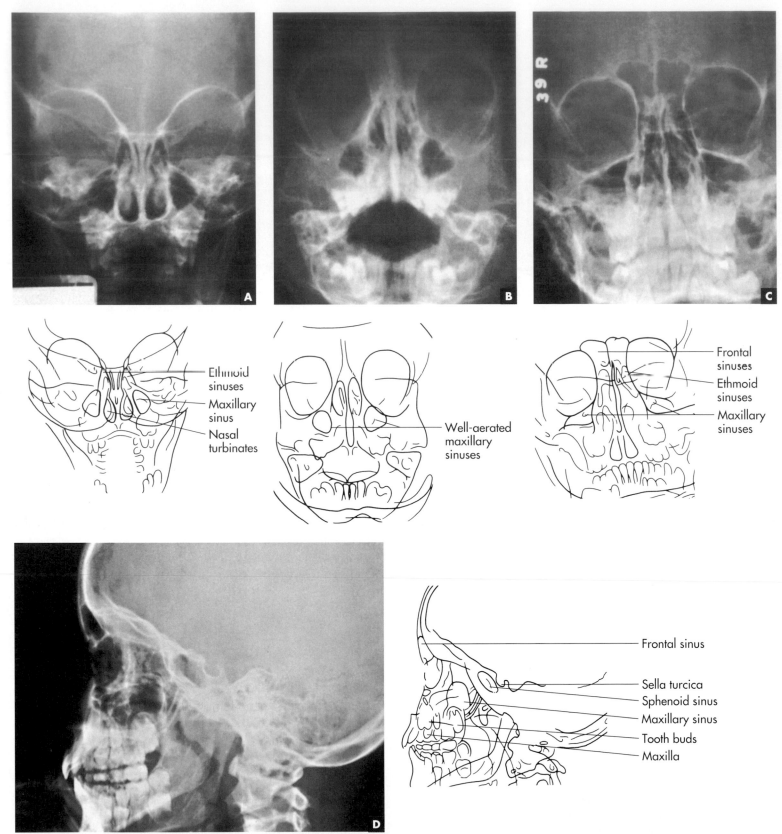

FIG. 22-52 Normal radiography of the sinuses. Radiography is currently the most helpful noninvasive tool for evaluating the paranasal sinuses. Interpretation requires appreciation of the normal pattern of development and the findings seen in health and with disease. *A,* AP or Caldwell view shows clear ethmoid sinuses in an 18-month-old child. The bony margins are sharp and the sinus cavities are dark. *B,* Waters view of the same child shows normal maxillary sinuses with sharply defined bony margins. The cavities appear black. *C,* After age 6 or 7, the Caldwell view is taken PA. In this 8-year-old boy, the bony margins of both the ethmoid and frontal sinuses are sharply defined. Because the calvarium is superimposed, it can be difficult to distinguish frontal sinus clouding on this view alone, particularly with bilateral disease. Therefore evaluation of the frontal sinuses requires close scrutiny of both Caldwell and lateral views. *D,* Lateral view of an 8-year-old child shows pneumatization of the frontal and sphenoid sinuses. Bony margins are sharply defined. The frontal sinuses appear black, but the sphenoid is somewhat gray because there are more overlying structures. Note how the roots of the maxillary teeth are embedded in the floor of the maxillary sinus.

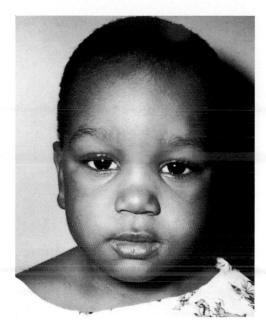

FIG. 22-53 Sympathetic periorbital swelling with sinusitis. This 2-year-old boy was seen late in the afternoon with fever, wet cough, decreased activity, and mild infraorbital puffiness. The latter was neither red, indurated, nor tender and reportedly had been more marked upon awakening in the morning. He also had a scant cloudy nasal discharge. His chest x-ray film was normal, but sinus films showed opacification of the maxillary sinuses.

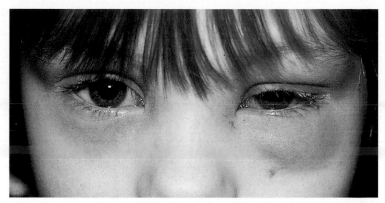

FIG. 22-54 This child with sinusitis had prominent erythematous periorbital edema and signs of purulent conjunctivitis. The redness raised concerns of periorbital cellulitis, but the area was nontender and not indurated. Presence of periorbital swelling is a helpful clue in diagnosing sinusitis in children with other suggestive signs and symptoms. (Courtesy Dr. Ellen Wald, Children's Hospital of Pittsburgh.)

The sinuses are lined by ciliated respiratory epithelium, which produces and transports mucous secretions. They drain into the nasal cavity through various small openings, which are located mainly under the middle and superior turbinates. Several points of clinical importance warrant emphasis. First, the ostia of the sinuses are small and thus easily obstructed by mucosal edema. Further, there are many important structures adjacent to the sinuses that are vulnerable to involvement if a disease process spreads beyond a sinus. These include the orbit, the brain, and the cavernous sinus. The roots of the maxillary teeth lie in the floor of the maxillary sinuses. Therefore dental infections may drain into the maxillary sinuses, resulting in recurrent or chronic sinusitis. Hence the dentition should be thoroughly inspected in evaluating any child with suspected sinus infection (see Chapter 20).

Sinusitis

During the first several years of life, infection of the maxillary and/or ethmoid sinuses is more common than is generally appreciated. Frontal sinusitis becomes important after about 10 years of age. The probable pathogenesis is mucosal swelling (whether the result of upper respiratory tract infection, allergic rhinitis, or chemical irritation), resulting in obstruction of the sinus ostia. This impedes drainage of secretions, promotes mucous plugging, and if prolonged, sets the stage for proliferation of bacterial pathogens with resultant infection. Both bacterial and viral pathogens have been isolated from pediatric patients. The most commonly identified bacteria are *Streptococcus pneumoniae,* nontypable *Haemophilus influenzae,* and *Moraxella catarrhalis.* The viral agents include adenoviruses and parainfluenza viruses. As in adults, there is no good correlation between results of nasopharyngeal and sinus aspirate cultures.

As with otitis media, a number of conditions predispose children to sinus infections by virtue of alterations in anatomy and/or physiology. These conditions include midfacial anomalies or deformities, particularly when maxillary hypoplasia is part of the picture (Fig. 22-8); cleft palate (see section on Palatal Disorders); nasal deformity and/or septal deviation, whether congenital or acquired; mass lesions, including hypertrophied adenoids, nasal foreign bodies, polyps, or tumors; abnormalities of mucus production and/or ciliary action such as cystic fibrosis and the immotile cilia syndrome; immunodeficiency; atopy; dental infection; and barotrauma.

Clinical Presentations

In young children, sinusitis is primarily a disorder of the ethmoid and maxillary sinuses, and the clinical picture differs considerably from that of adolescents and adults. The most common picture is one of a prolonged upper respiratory tract infection that has shown no sign of amelioration after 7 to 10 days. Cough and/or persistent nasal discharge (of any character—thin, thick; clear, cloudy; white, yellow, or green) are the major complaints. The cough is usually loose or wet; it is prominent during the day, but may be worse on waking in the morning and/or on first going to bed at night. Patients tend to clear their throats and sniff or snort frequently. Halitosis or "fetor oris" is commonly noted by parents. In a minority of children, periorbital swelling, most noticeable on awakening, may be reported (Fig. 22-53). A small percentage of patients have a low-grade fever, and a few may complain of headache, facial discomfort, sore throat, or abdominal pain (thought to be due to gastric irritation from swallowing the infected postnasal discharge).

Often, physical examination alone is of little help in distinguishing sinusitis from an upper respiratory tract infection. Findings may include purulent nasal and postnasal discharge with erythema of the nasal mucosa and pharynx; but as noted above this is not uniformly seen. Halitosis may be pronounced and strongly suggests sinusitis in the absence of evidence of dental infection, severe pharyngitis, or nasal foreign body. Sinusitis is also probable when features of the above picture are accompanied by signs of a maxillary dental abscess (see Chapter 20). Tenderness to percussion over the sinuses strongly suggests—but is not seen in the majority of patients with—the "prolonged upper respiratory tract infection" picture. The clinical spectrum is wide; any combination of the above symptoms and signs may be present; and sinusitis should be suspected, even if the course is relatively brief, whenever clinical findings are strongly suggestive.

A less frequent mode of presentation in young children is that of an acute upper respiratory tract infection that is unusually severe, which is characterized by high fever and copious purulent nasal discharge. Facial discomfort and periorbital swelling (nontender, nonindurated, and most marked on waking) are common with this picture. The edematous area may be normal in color or mildly erythematous (Fig. 22-54) and is thought to result from impairment of venous blood flow caused by increased pressure within the infected sinuses. If erythema is intense or the area is indurated or tender, periorbital cellulitis should be suspected. Some of these patients also have conjunctival erythema and

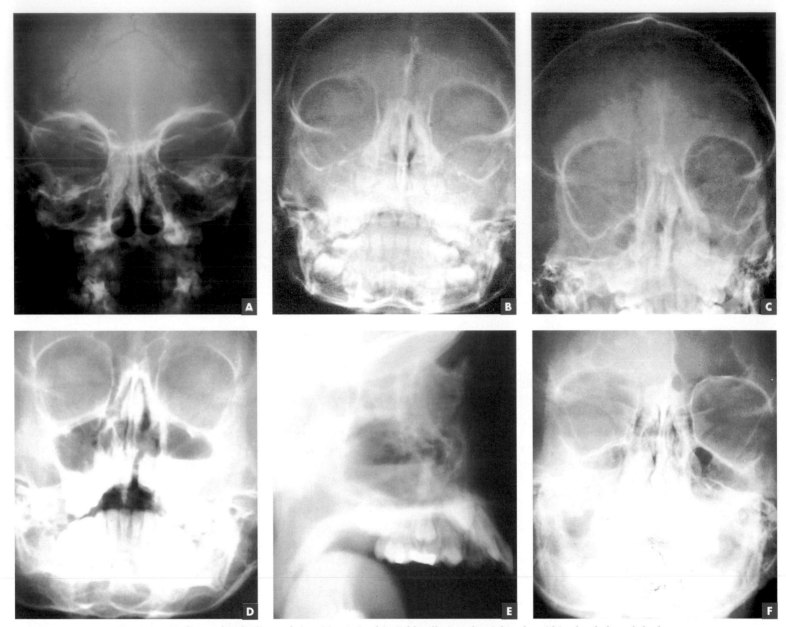

FIG. 22-55 Radiographic findings of sinusitis. *A*, In this Caldwell view the right ethmoid is clouded, and the bony margins are less distinct than on the left. *B*, In this Waters view, complete opacification of both maxillary sinuses is evident. The bony margins are visible but faint. *C*, This child has significant mucosal thickening of the maxillary sinuses. Thickening of greater than 4 mm has a strong association with positive culture on sinus aspirate. *D* and *E*, In another patient an air-fluid level can be seen in the left maxillary sinus on both Waters and lateral views. *F*, Differential opacification of the right frontal sinus is evident in this child who had fever and headache. (*D* and *E* courtesy Dr. J. Ledesma-Medina; *F* courtesy Dr. CD Bluestone, Children's Hospital of Pittsburgh.)

discharge. Occasionally a child with sinusitis has the typical findings of sympathetic edema, but without high fever or the prolonged upper respiratory tract infection picture.

Older children and adolescents with acute maxillary and/or ethmoid sinusitis may have either of the above symptom pictures but are more likely to complain specifically of headache and/or facial pain. The headache may be perceived as frontal, temporal, or even retroauricular. Facial discomfort can be described as malar pain or a sense of pressure or fullness. Occasionally, patients complain that their teeth hurt (in the absence of dental pathology). When the frontal sinuses are involved, frontal or supraorbital headache is prominent, often perceived as dull or pulsating. The sphenoid sinus is rarely a site of isolated sinus infection, but it is often involved in pansinusitis, in which case occipital and postauricular pain may be reported in addition to

other sites of discomfort. Frequently the headache is intermittent. When constant, it varies in severity. This variability appears to be related to degree of drainage. Patients reporting copious "postnasal drip" tend to have less pain. Discomfort and congestion are often most marked on waking, probably as a result of recumbency and lack of gravity-promoted drainage. Some patients also report aggravation of pain with head movement, particularly bending down and then straightening up. Swallowed discharge often produces significant abdominal discomfort as well. Coughing is often a feature but tends to be less prominent than in younger children. Physical findings include purulent (often bloodstreaked) nasal and postnasal discharge, erythema of the nasal mucosa, and halitosis. Tenderness on sinus percussion is common. As with younger children, the clinical spectrum is wide and highly variable.

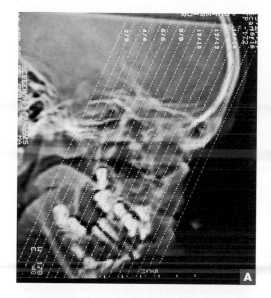

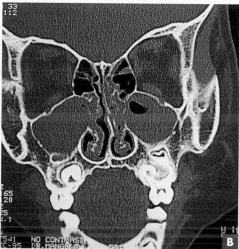

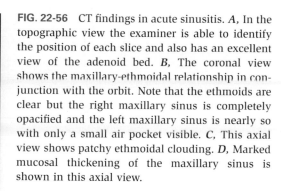

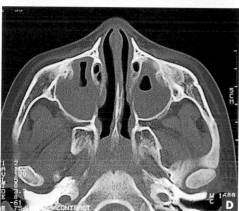

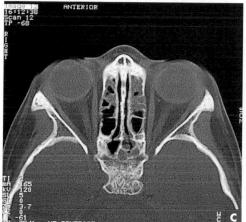

FIG. 22-56 CT findings in acute sinusitis. *A,* In the topographic view the examiner is able to identify the position of each slice and also has an excellent view of the adenoid bed. *B,* The coronal view shows the maxillary-ethmoidal relationship in conjunction with the orbit. Note that the ethmoids are clear but the right maxillary sinus is completely opacified and the left maxillary sinus is nearly so with only a small air pocket visible. *C,* This axial view shows patchy ethmoidal clouding. *D,* Marked mucosal thickening of the maxillary sinus is shown in this axial view.

Ancillary Diagnostic Methods

When patients have most of the signs and symptoms of sinusitis, the diagnosis can be made on clinical grounds and treatment started empirically. This is particularly true for the younger child with the prolonged upper respiratory tract infection picture. Amoxicillin remains the drug of first choice for patients who are not allergic to penicillin. If there is no clear clinical improvement in 3 to 4 days, switching to amoxicillin/clavulanate or a comparable antimicrobial is indicated. If this also fails to produce clinical improvement in 3 to 4 days, radiographs should be obtained. If they show findings of sinusitis, resistant pneumococci are the likely culprits, and clindamycin is indicated. In less clear-cut cases, ancillary tools and tests are often needed. The usefulness of the various diagnostic methods in evaluating suspected sinusitis is still under study. Radiography appears to be the most helpful noninvasive tool in children over 2 years of age. Radiographs are most useful in patients in whom the clinical picture is not distinct enough to distinguish between sinusitis and allergic rhinitis and in patients who fail to respond to antimicrobial therapy as noted above. Findings of complete opacification, mucosal thickening greater than 4 mm, or an air-fluid level on standard radiography (Fig. 22-55) are strongly associated with positive findings on sinus aspiration. However, the wide range of variability in development and configuration of the sinuses can make interpretation difficult. The CT scan (Fig. 22-56) is the most sensitive modality for diagnosis, but it can be falsely positive in patients with viral upper respiratory tract infections, is expensive, and requires sedation of the younger patient for an adequate examination. Thus,

perhaps it should be reserved for patients with possible complications of sinusitis, underlying anatomic abnormalities, or suspected chronic sinusitis who fail to respond to a prolonged course of antimicrobial therapy. Needle aspiration of the sinuses is conclusive but invasive and not without risk. It is, however, justified in patients with very severe symptoms, patients with central nervous system or orbital extension, those not responding to treatment, and those who are immunocompromised or immunosuppressed.

At minimum, therapy consists of a 10- to 14-day course (or until symptom free for 7 days) of an antimicrobial agent suitable to the likely spectrum of organisms. If the causative organism is sensitive to the agent selected, a definite clinical response is seen in 3 to 4 days. If this does not occur, a broader spectrum agent should be considered and/or radiographs obtained to check the accuracy of the clinical diagnosis. Analgesia is given as needed for discomfort and perhaps an oral antihistamine in patients known to have allergic rhinitis. Some children with intense headaches or facial pain experience symptomatic relief by using topical nasal vasoconstrictors and warm compresses during the first 1 or 2 days of therapy. Patients with sinusitis should be instructed to avoid swimming underwater or diving until completion of therapy because the resultant barotrauma aggravates symptoms and may promote intracranial spread of infection.

Complications of Sinusitis

Infectious sinusitis is important not only because of the discomfort it causes, but also because there is a significant risk of extension of in-

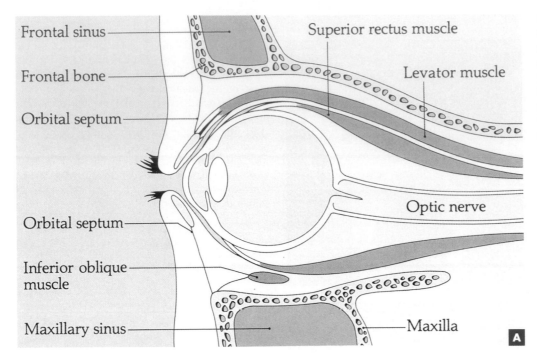

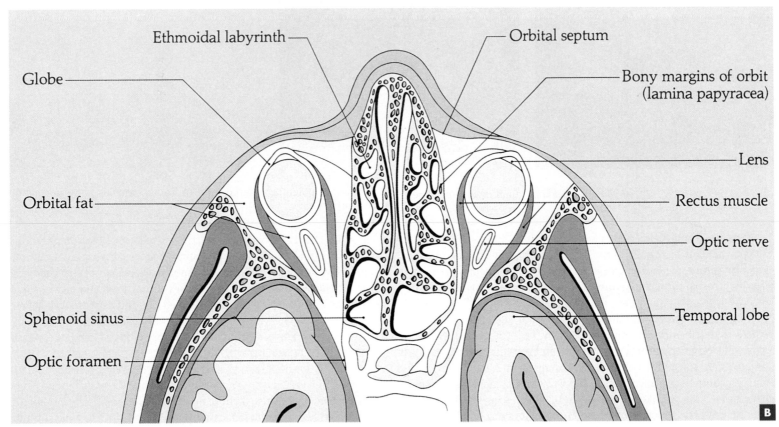

FIG. 22-57 The anatomy of the orbit. *A*, Sagittal section shows the relationship of the orbit to the maxillary and frontal sinuses, and the position of the orbital septum within the eyelid. The latter structure appears to serve as an anatomic barrier, helping to prevent the spread of infection from periorbital tissues into the orbit. *B*, In this horizontal section, the close relationship of the orbit to the ethmoid sinuses is apparent.

fection and secondary complications. This risk stems from several anatomic factors. First, the sinuses surround the orbits superiorly, medially, and inferiorly. The bony plates that make up the sinus walls are very thin and porous, and their suture lines are open in childhood. This is especially true of the lamina papyracea, which separates the ethmoid air cells from the orbits (Fig. 22-57). Increased sinus pressure as a result of ostial blockage and fluid collection can cause separation of portions of these bony septa and can compromise their blood supply. The resultant necrosis promotes extension of infection. Facial vascular anatomy also contributes to the spread of infection. The veins of the face, nose, and sinuses drain in part into the orbit, then into the ophthalmic venous system, which is in direct continuity with the cavernous sinus. The ophthalmic veins are valveless and thus may present less defense against spread of infection. The orbit is also devoid of lymphatics, which helps explain the ease of periorbital edema formation when there is increased sinus pressure. The relative looseness of the subcutaneous tissues of the face augments this and may also aid in spread of infection. As a result of these factors, direct extension of infection can occur: (1) into the periorbital soft tissues, producing periorbital cellulitis; (2) through the bony walls into the orbits, resulting in

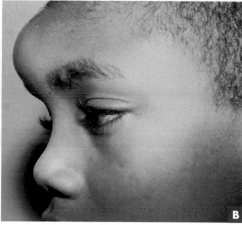

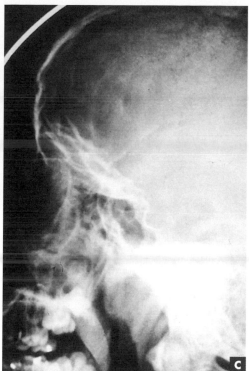

FIG. 22 58 Pott's puffy tumor. *A* and *B*, This patient had fever, headache, and an erythematous swelling over the forehead that was exquisitely tender and had a doughy consistency. *C*, A lateral radiograph shows frontal sinus clouding, irregularity of the frontal bone, and marked soft-tissue swelling that is highlighted by a wire placed over the forehead and scalp. (*C* courtesy Dr. Kenneth Grundfast, National Children's Medical Center.)

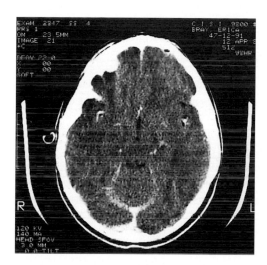

FIG. 22-59 Epidural abscess. This patient had lethargy, high fever, left eye pain, and periorbital swelling after 1 week of severe nasal congestion. A CT scan, obtained to rule out orbital involvement, revealed a small epidural abscess behind the left frontal sinus. Note the small central air pocket.

subperiosteal abscess, classically known as *Pott's puffy tumor.* This is seen as an erythematous frontal swelling that has a doughy consistency and is exquisitely tender (Fig. 22-58). Affected patients tend to be toxic, febrile, and extremely uncomfortable. Prompt surgical drainage is of utmost importance. A CT scan should be obtained before surgical drainage to evaluate the extent of the abscess and identify other sites of spread.

Epidural Abscess

Another potential complication of frontal sinusitis is the formation of an epidural abscess as the result of erosion through the posterior wall of the frontal bone. This should be suspected in patients with frontal sinusitis who have unusually high temperature, unusually severe headache, signs of toxicity, or altered sensorium. Diagnosis is best confirmed by CT scan (Fig. 22-59). Although intravenous antimicrobial therapy and careful monitoring may suffice in management of small lesions, larger abscesses necessitate surgical intervention.

Periorbital and Orbital Infections

Periorbital Cellulitis Caused by Spread From Adjacent Sinusitis

Periorbital cellulitis is the mildest of the complications of infectious sinusitis. The cellulitis is confined to tissues outside the orbit, with spread blocked in part by the orbital septum (Fig. 22-57, *A*). When sinusitis is the underlying condition, the ethmoid or maxillary sinuses are the structures primarily affected. Typically, patients are under 4 or 5 years of age and have an antecedent history of upper respiratory tract infection with or without conjunctivitis, otitis, or sinusitis. This is superseded by the sudden appearance of lid and periorbital swelling. In contrast to the uncomplicated sympathetic edema seen in some patients with sinusitis, the swelling in these children is usually unilateral and definitely erythematous, indurated, and tender (Fig. 22-60). Conjunctival injection and discharge also may be seen. In many patients a secondary increase in temperature accompanies the onset of swelling, but although most patients appear uncomfortable, toxicity is unusual. The course of periorbital cellulitis resulting from extension of sinus infection is milder and characterized by much slower progression than is true of cases resulting from hematogenous spread.

orbital cellulitis; (3) via erosion outward through the frontal bone, producing Pott's puffy tumor; or (4) via erosion inward through the frontal bone, resulting in an epidural abscess. On rare occasions, hematogeneous seeding of bacteria may occur.

Fortunately, improved recognition of sinus infection and early use of antimicrobial therapy, whether before or early in the course of recognized extension, have reduced the frequency, severity, and morbidity of these disorders.

Pott's puffy tumor and epidural abscess, being direct complications of frontal sinusitis, are discussed below. Periorbital and orbital cellulitis, stemming at times from sinusitis and at times from other predisposing conditions, are covered in the section following.

Pott's Puffy Tumor

Frontal sinusitis assumes importance after 8 to 10 years of age (once the frontal sinuses have begun to form) and has the potential for serious complications, particularly when neglected or inadequately treated. Erosion anteriorly through the frontal bone results in formation of a

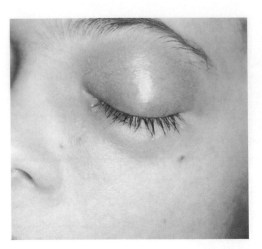

FIG. 22-60 Periorbital cellulitis. Intense erythema and edema of the lids are evident. The swollen tissues were indurated and very tender on palpation. Ocular motion was normal. Underlying ethmoid sinusitis was confirmed by CT scan.

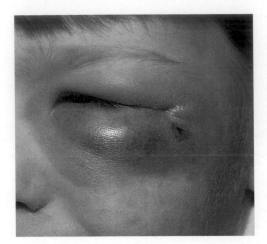

FIG. 22-61 Periorbital cellulitis caused by spread of an adjacent facial infection. This child developed fever and erythematous, tender periorbital swelling a few days after incurring an abrasion as a result of a fall.

Periorbital Cellulitis Caused by Hematogenous Spread

When periorbital cellulitis is the result of hematogenous seeding, the organisms tend to be more virulent, the onset more explosive, and the course more fulminant. Typically the patient experiences sudden onset of high fever (often after a mild upper respiratory tract infection) accompanied by the appearance of erythematous, indurated and tender periorbital swelling, which progresses rapidly and is accompanied by signs of systemic toxicity. The majority of these patients are under 1 year of age or only slightly older, and bacteremia with *Haemophilus influenzae* type b or *Streptococcus pneumoniae* is usual. Widespread use of the *H. influenzae* b vaccine has dramatically reduced the incidence of *H. influenzae* b–induced cellulitis.

Periorbital Cellulitis Caused by Spread From Adjacent Facial Infection3

More than 50% of periorbital cellulitis cases have neither sinusitis nor bacteremia as a predisposing condition. Rather, the patients appear to suffer from extension of nearby facial infections to periorbital tissues. They tend to have a history of antecedent trauma to the orbit or nearby facial structures often with a break in the skin (Fig. 22-61) or primary skin infection (impetigo, a pustule, a chalazion, or infected dermatitis or insect bite). They subsequently experience a temperature spike and evolution of periorbital and eyelid edema. This group tends to be somewhat older, generally over 5 years of age. *Staphylococcus aureus* and group A beta-hemolytic streptococci are the predominant offending organisms.

Diagnostic Studies

A number of cultures are often obtained in an attempt to isolate the causative pathogen in cases of periorbital cellulitis. Needle aspiration of the leading edge of the cellulitis has perhaps the highest yield but requires caution. It is perhaps best avoided when the inflamed area does not extend well beyond the orbital rim because of the risk of eye injury if the patient moves suddenly despite efforts to immobilize his or her head. Cultures of adjacent skin wounds, when present, are also commonly positive. Nasopharyngeal and conjunctival drainage reveals the offending organism in about one half to two thirds of cases, respectively. Blood cultures are positive in about one third of patients overall, with the highest incidence found in cases caused by hematogenous spread. Sinus x-rays show opacification in more than two thirds of patients without antecedent trauma or skin lesions and in about 40% to 50% of patients with such a history. Ethmoid opacification is the predominant finding. Radiographic interpretation can be difficult, however, because overlying edema may give a false impression of clouding.

In addition, x-rays are relatively useless in most cases of hematogenous origin because the patients are typically under 1 year of age. CT, however, is an excellent tool for assessing the extent of infection and the presence or absence of sinus opacification and for detecting evidence of early orbital involvement.

Because of the severity and the potential for further extension and hematogenous spread, aggressive intravenous antimicrobial therapy is urgently required. This necessitates empiric selection of agents to cover likely pathogens, pending culture results. Patients also require close monitoring for signs of complications.

Orbital Cellulitis

In orbital cellulitis, infection extends into the orbit itself. It may take the form of undifferentiated cellulitis, or it may evolve into a subperiosteal or orbital abscess. Patients tend to have a history similar to those with periorbital cellulitis but are generally more ill, toxic, and lethargic. The most common source of spread is an adjacent, infected ethmoid sinus, although extension from a nearby facial infection occasionally occurs. Causative organisms are the same as those in periorbital cellulitis. Patients old enough to be articulate describe intense, deep retroorbital pain aggravated by ocular movement. Edema and erythema of the lid and periorbital tissues are often so marked that it is impossible to open the eye without use of lid retractors (Fig. 22-62, *A* and *B*). Tenderness is exquisite. If the lid can be retracted, the clinician may find proptosis, conjunctival inflammation with chemosis and purulent discharge, decreased extraocular motion, and some loss of visual acuity.

Aggressive intravenous antimicrobial therapy and close monitoring for evolution and central nervous system complications are vital in the management of orbital cellulitis. CT is proving exceptionally useful for determining the presence or absence of abscesses (Fig. 22-62, *C*). When a subperiosteal abscess is present or the clinical ocular examination shows deterioration, surgical drainage combined with an ethmoidectomy is indicated. Optimal management necessitates a team approach involving pediatrics, otolaryngology, ophthalmology, and at times neurosurgery.

Local complications of orbital cellulitis include abscess formation, optic neuritis, retinal vein thrombosis, and panophthalmitis. Central nervous system complications may result from direct extension or spread of septic thrombophlebitis. Meningitis, epidural and subdural abscesses, and cavernous sinus thrombosis have been described. All are characterized by marked toxicity and alteration in level of consciousness. Cavernous sinus thrombosis is heralded by sudden, bilateral, pulsating proptosis in association with increased toxicity and obtundation.

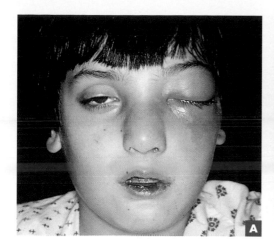 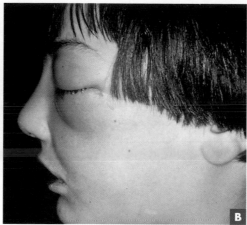 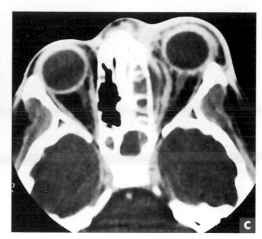

FIG. 22-62   Orbital cellulitis. *A* and *B,* This child had a fever, severe toxicity, and marked lethargy. He experienced intense orbital and retroorbital pain, and showed a limited range of ocular motion. *C,* This CT scan shows preseptal swelling, proptosis, and lateral displacement of the globe and orbital contents by a subperiosteal abscess.

Atopic Sinus Disorders

Allergic Sinusitis With Postnasal Discharge

Patients with allergic rhinitis appear to be more susceptible to infectious sinusitis than nonatopic individuals, probably as a result of mucosal swelling in response to allergen exposure and alterations in ciliary action. They can also have symptoms mimicking sinusitis in the absence of infection, and this can be a source of confusion. Two major clinical pictures are seen. In the first, nasal congestion, nighttime cough, and morning throat clearing are prominent. Some patients may complain of morning nausea, and a few may have morning emesis containing large amounts of clear mucus. Fever is absent, and in contrast to infectious sinusitis, nasal discharge is never purulent, there is no halitosis, and daytime cough is not prominent. Patients may complain of itching of the nose and eyes, and some have frequent sneezing. On examination, the nasal mucosa is edematous but does not appear inflamed. Discharge, if present, is clear. Patients also tend to have the typical allergic facies (see Chapter 4) with Dennie lines, allergic shiners, and cobblestoning of the conjunctivae. Environmental control and antihistamines provide symptomatic relief for most of these children.

Vacuum Headache

The second potentially confusing clinical picture is that of the allergic sinus headache, or vacuum headache. In this condition, older atopic individuals complain of intense facial or frontal headache, without fever or other evidence of infection. This occurs during periods in which patients are having exacerbation of allergic symptoms or after swimming in chlorinated pools. The phenomenon appears to be caused by acute blockage of sinus ostia by mucosal edema, with subsequent creation of a vacuum within the sinus as a result of oxygen consumption by mucosal cells. The resultant negative pressure pulls the mucosa away from the walls of the sinus, producing the pain. In these patients the nasal mucosa tends to be pale and swollen but without discharge. Sinuses may be tender to percussion but are clear radiographically. Symptoms respond promptly to application of a topical vasoconstrictor and warm compresses over the face. Improvement is maintained by antihistamines.

Oropharyngeal Disorders

Oropharyngeal Examination

Adequate examination of the pharynx is very important in pediatrics because of the frequency of pharyngeal infections. However, the procedure can be challenging at times. The small size of the mouth and difficulty of depressing the tongue in infancy, lack of cooperativeness in toddlers, and fear of gagging with use of tongue blades in older children can impede efforts. These problems can be minimized with a few simple techniques. Infants and young children, when placed supine with the head hyperextended on the neck, tend to open their mouths spontaneously, enabling visualization of the anterior oral cavity and facilitating insertion of a tongue blade to depress the tongue and inspect the posterior palate and pharynx. When examining older children, asking them to open their mouths as wide as possible and pant "like a puppy dog" or say "ha ha" usually results in lowering of the posterior portion of the tongue, revealing posterior palatal and pharyngeal structures. Because conditions involving the lips, mucosa, and dentition are presented in Chapter 20, this section concentrates on palatal and pharyngeal disorders.

Palatal Disorders

Palatal malformations range widely in severity and can significantly impact feeding, swallowing, and speech. In addition, by altering normal nasal and oropharyngeal physiology, they place affected patients at increased risk for chronic recurrent ear and sinus infections.

Cleft Palate

Palatal clefts are among the most severe abnormalities encountered. They stem from a failure of fusion during the second month of gestation and have an incidence of about 1 in every 2000 to 2500 births. They are usually but not always associated with a cleft lip. The defect is often isolated in an otherwise normal child. In many cases there is a positive family history for the anomaly. A number of teratogens have also been linked to the malformation. In a small percentage of cases the

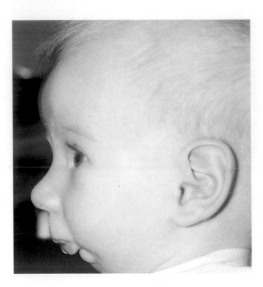

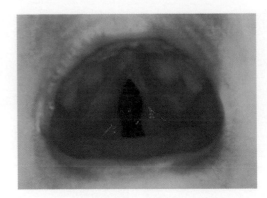

FIG. 22-63 Pierre-Robin syndrome, characterized by severe micrognathia and cleft palate. In this infant the micrognathia produced posterior displacement of the tongue, resulting in airway obstruction that necessitated a tracheostomy. (Courtesy Dr. Wolfgang Loskin, Children's Hospital of Pittsburgh.)

FIG. 22-64 Cleft palate. This child has a midline cleft of the soft palate. The hard palate, alveolar ridge, and lip are spared. (Courtesy Ms. Barbara Elster, Cleft Palate Center, Pittsburgh.)

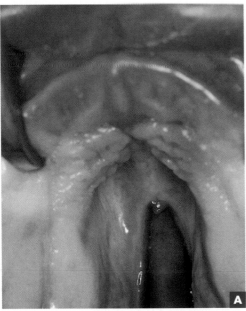

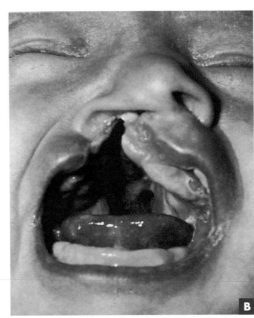

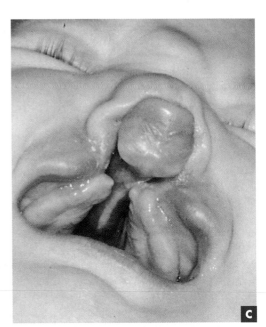

FIG. 22-65 Cleft palate. *A*, Cleft of the hard and soft palate, sparing the alveolar ridge. Complete clefts of the palate, alveolar ridge, and lip may be unilateral *(B)* or bilateral *(C)*. (*A* and *C* courtesy Dr. William Garrett, Children's Hospital of Pittsburgh; *B* courtesy Dr. Michael Sherlock.)

cleft palate is one of multiple congenital anomalies in the context of a major genetic syndrome such as the Pierre-Robin anomaly (Fig. 22-63) and trisomies 13 and 18 (see Chapter 1).

The extent of the cleft varies: some involve only the soft palate (Fig. 22-64), others extend through the hard palate but spare the alveolar ridge. Still others are complete (Fig. 22-65). The defect may be unilateral or bilateral. The four major types of congenital cleft palate are:

Type I	Soft palate only (Fig. 22-64)
Type II	Unilateral cleft of soft and hard palate (Fig. 22-65, *A*)
Type III	Unilateral cleft of soft and hard palate extending through the alveolar ridge (Fig. 22-65, *B*)
Type IV	Bilateral cleft of soft and hard palate extending through the alveolar ridge (Fig. 22-65, *C*)

These anomalies create a number of problems beyond the obvious cosmetic deformity. In infancy a cleft palate prevents the child from

creating an effective seal when nursing and hampers feeding. In addition, formula tends to reflux into the nasopharynx with resultant choking. This necessitates patience during feeding and careful training of parents in feeding techniques that facilitate nursing and prevent failure to thrive. Eustachian tube function is uniformly abnormal, and before repair, all patients have chronic middle ear effusions that are frequently infected. Even after repair, recurrent middle ear disease (characterized by negative pressure and effusions) remains a problem. Hearing loss, with its potential for hampering language acquisition, ultimately occurs in more than 50% of patients. Despite corrective surgery, palatal function is never totally normal, and many patients continue to have hypernasal speech and difficulties in articulation, necessitating long-term speech therapy. Secondary dental and orthodontic problems are routine as well.

The multitude of problems and the need for frequent medical visits and multiple operations, in combination with the oft-associated cos-

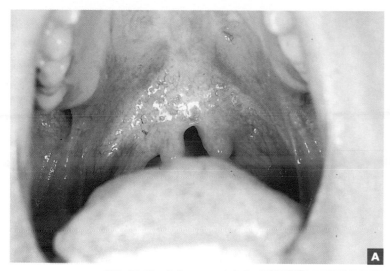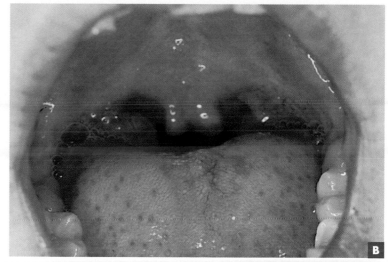

FIG. 22-66 Submucous cleft of the palate. *A,* This girl shows failure of normal midline fusion of the palatal muscles, resulting in midline thinning of the soft palate. Palpation confirms the area of weakness. A U-shaped notch can also be felt in the midline at the junction of the hard and soft palate. She also has a bifid uvula. *B,* This child was found to have a notched uvula on pharyngeal examination. This may serve as a clue to the presence of a submucous palatal cleft, or it may be an isolated anomaly.

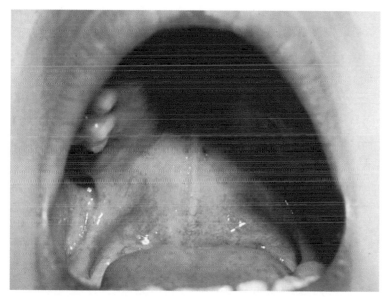

FIG. 22-67 High-arched palate. This is a common minor anomaly, usually isolated, but occasionally associated with genetic syndromes.

metic deformity, can have significant psychologic impact on the child and family. Optimal management necessitates a multidisciplinary team, preferably coordinated by a primary care physician who is aware of the patient's individual needs and those of his or her family. Timing of corrective surgery remains somewhat controversial. Cleft lips are repaired at about 3 months, but scheduling of palatal repair must be individualized depending on the size and extent of the cleft. Defects of the soft palate are generally repaired at about 8 months, and the hard palate is either closed surgically or by use of a prosthetic plate. Most patients also require early myringotomy with insertion of tubes to help manage the chronic middle ear disease. Tonsillectomy and adenoidectomy are contraindicated because of adverse effects on palatal function.

Another disorder of clinical importance, **submucous cleft of the palate,** is often overlooked in infancy. The condition is characterized by a U-shaped notch, palpable in the midline, at the juncture of the hard and soft portions of the palate (Fig. 22-66, *A*). There also may be pal-

pable midline thinning of the soft palate. The anomaly results from a failure of the tensor veli palatini muscle to insert properly in the midline. Some children have an associated double or notched uvula that, when present, serves as a clue to the existence of the palatal abnormality (Fig. 22-66, *B*). The latter may be an isolated anomaly, however. Although not subject to the feeding difficulties seen in children with overt clefts, children with submucous clefts have similar problems with eustachian tube dysfunction and recurrent middle ear disease. Speech is often mildly hypernasal. Recognition is particularly important when considering tonsillectomy and adenoidectomy for recurrent tonsillitis and otitis because surgical removal of the adenoids in these children can result in severe speech and swallowing dysfunction; hence these procedures may be contraindicated.

High-Arched Palate

High-arched palate, a minor anomaly, is a common clinical finding (Fig. 22-67). Although usually an isolated variant of palatal configuration, it occasionally occurs in association with congenital syndromes. Long-term orotracheal intubation of premature infants creates an iatrogenic form of the problem. Although generally clinically insignificant, the high arch can be associated with increased frequency of ear and sinus infections and hyponasal speech in severe cases.

Tonsillar and Peritonsillar Disorders

Tonsillitis/Pharyngitis

As noted earlier, the tonsils and adenoids are quite small in infancy, gradually enlarge over the first 8 to 10 years of life, then start to regress in size. When evaluating the tonsils, particularly during the course of an acute infection, or when monitoring patients for chronic enlargement, it is helpful to use a standardized size-grading system, as shown in Fig. 22-68. Inspection of the palate is also important in assessing patients with tonsillopharyngitis because lesions characteristic of particular pathogens are often present on the soft palate and tonsillar pillars (see Chapter 12).

The tonsils appear to serve as a first line of immunologic defense against respiratory pathogens and are frequently infected by viral and

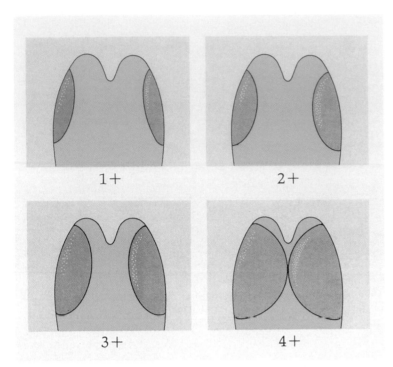

FIG. 22-68 Grading of tonsillar size for children with acute tonsillopharyngitis and those with chronic tonsillar enlargement. This grading system is particularly useful in serial examinations of a given patient. (Modified from Feinstein AR, Levitt M: Role of tonsils, *N Engl J Med* 282:285-291, 1970.)

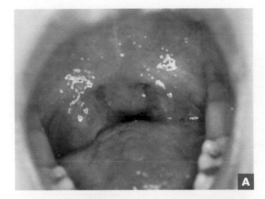

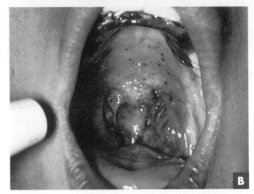

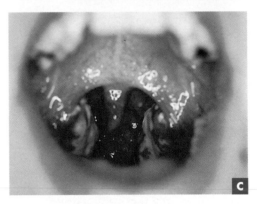

FIG. 22-69 Tonsillopharyngitis. This common syndrome has a number of causative pathogens and a wide spectrum of severity. *A*, The diffuse tonsillar and pharyngeal erythema seen here is a nonspecific finding that can be produced by a variety of pathogens. *B*, This intense erythema, seen in association with acute tonsillar enlargement and palatal petechiae, is highly suggestive of group A beta-streptococcal infection, though other pathogens can produce these findings. *C*, This picture of exudative tonsillitis is most commonly seen with either group A streptococcal or EB virus infection. (*B* courtesy Dr. Michael Sherlock.)

bacterial agents. The most commonly identified organisms are group A beta-hemolytic streptococci, adenoviruses, coxsackieviruses, and the Epstein-Barr (EB) virus. There is a wide range of severity in symptoms and signs, regardless of the pathogenic organism. Sore throat is the major symptom, and it may be mild, moderate, or severe. When severe, it is typically associated with dysphagia. Erythema is the most common physical finding and varies from slightly to intensely red (Fig. 22-69). Additional findings may include acute tonsillar enlargement, formation of exudates over the tonsillar surfaces, and cervical adenopathy. In a small percentage of cases the findings suggest a given pathogen. Patients with fever; headache; bright red, enlarged tonsils (with or without exudate); palatal petechiae (Fig. 22-69, *B*); tender and enlarged anterior cervical nodes; and perhaps abdominal pain are likely to have streptococcal infection. Patients with marked malaise, fever, exudative tonsillitis, generalized adenopathy, and splenomegaly are probably suffering from EB virus mononucleosis (Fig. 22-69, *C*; see Chapter 12). Those with conjunctivitis, nonexudative tonsillar inflammation, and cervical adenopathy may have adenovirus. Yellow ulcerations with red halos on the tonsillar pillars strongly suggest coxsackievirus infection, whether or not other oral, palmar, or plantar lesions are present (see Chapter 12). Unfortunately, the majority of patients with tonsillopharyngitis do not have such clear-cut clinical syndromes. Patients with streptococcal infection may have only minimal erythema; in its early stages, mononucleosis may consist of fever, malaise, and nonexudative pharyngitis without other signs; and although streptococci and

EB virus are the most common sources of exudative tonsillitis and palatal petechiae, other pathogens produce these findings as well.

Because of the variability in the clinical picture and the importance of identifying and treating group A beta-streptococcal infection to prevent both pyogenic (e.g., cervical adenitis, peritonsillar, retropharyngeal and parapharyngeal abscesses) and nonpyogenic (e.g., rheumatic fever) complications, a screening throat culture is advisable for patients with even mild signs or symptoms of tonsillopharyngitis. In obtaining this culture, the clinician swabs both tonsils and the posterior pharyngeal wall to maximize the chance of obtaining the organism. In the first 3 years of life, when streptococcal infection is suspected (because of history of exposure, signs of pharyngitis, or scarlatiniform rash), it is helpful to obtain a nasopharyngeal culture as well. For reasons as yet unclear, the nasopharyngeal culture is often positive when the throat culture is negative in this age group.

Treatment is symptomatic for all forms of tonsillopharyngitis except that caused by group A beta-streptococci, which requires a 10-day course of penicillin or erythromycin. Follow-up is also important. As noted earlier, the tonsillitis of mononucleosis may appear mild early in the course of the illness, yet tonsillar inflammation and enlargement may progress over a few to several days to produce severe dysphagia and even airway obstruction. Thus parents should be instructed to notify the physician if such signs develop. Follow-up is also important in monitoring for other complications and for frequent recurrences.

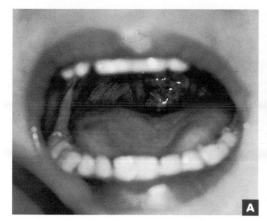
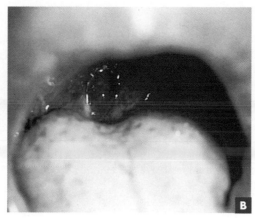
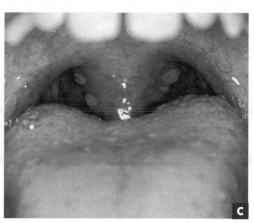

FIG. 22-70 Uvulitis. *A,* The uvula appears markedly erythematous and edematous, with pinpoint hemorrhages, in this case caused by beta-streptococci. *B,* In this child with mononucleosis the tonsils are enlarged and covered with a gray membrane and the uvula is edematous and erythematous. The patient had respiratory compromise because of the severity of his tonsillar and adenoidal hypertrophy. *C,* The vesicular lesions on the swollen, painful uvula of this patient suggest a viral etiology, probably an enterovirus.

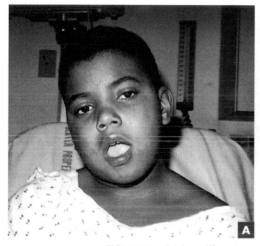
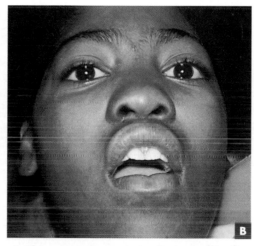
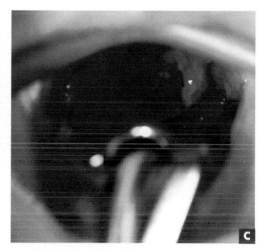

FIG. 22-71 Peritonsillar abscess. *A,* This patient demonstrates the torticollis often seen with a peritonsillar abscess in an effort to minimize pressure on the adjacent, inflamed tonsillar node. *B,* Sympathetic inflammation of the pterygoid muscles causes trismus, limiting the patient's ability to open the mouth. *C,* This photograph, taken in the operating room, shows an intensely inflamed soft palatal mass that obscures the tonsil and bulges forward and toward the midline, deviating the uvula.

Recurrent Tonsillitis

Frequent recurrences of tonsillitis, despite antibiotic therapy when indicated, must be handled on an individual basis. In some cases frequent recurrences of streptococcal infection can be traced to other family members. When they are treated along with the patient, the cycle of recurrences often ends. In other instances frequent recurrent tonsillar infections have no traceable source within the family, and they are significantly debilitating. In children with six or more episodes in any one year or three episodes per year for three consecutive years, tonsillectomy has a favorable outcome in reducing both frequency and severity of sore throats.

Uvulitis

Uvulitis is characterized by inflammation and edema of the uvula. In addition to throat pain and dysphagia, affected patients commonly complain of a sense of having "something in their throat" or a gagging sensation. The phenomenon has been reported in association with pharyngitis caused by the group A beta-hemolytic streptococcus, in which cases the uvula was bright red and often hemorrhagic (Fig. 22-70, *A*). The condition also has been noted in association with mononucleosis, in the presence and in the absence of exudative tonsil-

litis (Fig. 22-70, *B*) and other viral agents as well (Fig. 22-70, *C*). Uvulitis has also been reported in a patient with concurrent epiglottitis. In this case the child was anxious, toxic, febrile, and drooling, a more severe clinical picture than that seen with streptococcal or EB virus infection. Culture of the uvular surface grew *Haemophilus influenzae* type B.

Peritonsillar Abscess or Cellulitis

A peritonsillar abscess is an abscess that surrounds the tonsil and extends onto the soft palate. Patients are usually school age or older, and they typically have a history of an antecedent sore throat a week or two earlier, which was not cultured or treated, or the patient took an incomplete course of antimicrobial therapy. The patient may experience initial improvement but then has a sudden onset of high fever and severe throat pain, which is worse on one side. The pain usually radiates to the ipsilateral ear and is associated with marked dysphagia, such that the patient spits out saliva to avoid swallowing. On examination, the child often appears toxic and has obvious enlargement of the ipsilateral tonsillar node, which is exquisitely tender. Many patients have torticollis, tilting the head toward the involved side to minimize pressure of the sternocleidomastoid muscle on the adjacent tonsillar lymph node (Fig. 22-71, *A*). Speech is thick and muffled because of splinting

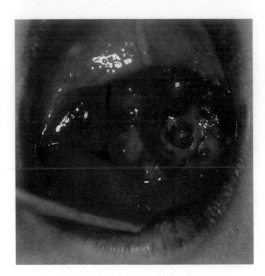

FIG. 22-72 Tonsillar lymphoma. This adolescent had painless dysphagia. Examination revealed marked unilateral tonsillar enlargement. The asymmetry and degree of enlargement prompted tonsillectomy. Pathologic examination confirmed a tonsillar lymphoma.

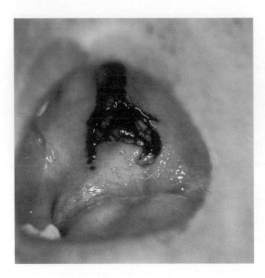

FIG. 22-73 Palatal laceration. This large, complex laceration occurred when this boy fell with a piece of metal tubing in his mouth. A flap of palatal tissue has retracted away from the tears, warranting surgical approximation.

of the tongue and pharyngeal muscles. Trismus, or limitation of mouth opening, is often noted as a result of sympathetic inflammation of the adjacent pterygoid muscles (Fig. 22-71,. *B*). If visualization of the pharynx is possible (despite the trismus), a bright red, smooth mass is seen in the supratonsillar area projecting forward and medially, obscuring the tonsil, and deviating the uvula to the opposite side (Fig. 22-71, *C*). Group A beta-streptococci and *Staphylococcus aureus* are the most common pathogens. Patients with mononucleosis, concurrently infected with group A streptococci and treated with steroids, are reportedly at risk for developing a rapidly evolving peritonsillar abscess as well.

If fluctuance is evident on palpation, operative drainage is needed in addition to antibiotic therapy to prevent spontaneous rupture and secondary aspiration. When fluctuance is not present, the patient is in a cellulitic stage and management consists of intravenous antimicrobial therapy and serial reexamination. Because of the risks of rupture, prompt otolaryngologic consultation is suggested from the outset.

Tonsillar Lymphoma

The majority of children, whether well or acutely ill with tonsillitis, have tonsils that are symmetrical in size. When a child has an asymmetrically enlarged tonsil without evidence of infection, the possibility of a lymphoma should be considered (Fig. 22-72). Thorough history of recent health and meticulous regional and general examination are in order. Particular attention should be paid to cervical and other nodes and to the size and consistency of abdominal viscera. Hematologic studies may be helpful as well. In the absence of other evidence, a brief period of observation may be justified. If other findings are suggestive or enlargement continues during observation, excisional biopsy is indicated.

Penetrating Oropharyngeal Trauma

Penetrating oral injuries are fairly common in childhood and are usually the result of falling with a stick, pencil, or lollipop in the mouth. Gunshot wounds and external stab wounds are unusual occurrences in the pediatric population, but the incidence begins to increase in adolescents.

The majority of intraoral injuries involve the palate and consist of simple lacerations. Many of these injuries heal spontaneously and require no repair. Large lacerations producing mucosal flaps must be sutured (Fig. 22-73). Prophylactic penicillin is also indicated because of the high risk of secondary infection.

Penetration of the posterior pharyngeal wall may result in a number of complications. Therefore these patients merit careful clinical evalua-

tion of the oropharynx and neck; neck radiographs also should be obtained. Whenever an object penetrates the pharyngeal wall, it introduces oral flora into the retropharyngeal soft tissues, setting the stage for development of infection and abscess formation (see section on Retropharyngeal Abscess). This complication is seen predominantly in patients who failed to seek care immediately after the injury. However, it can develop even in treated patients. Symptoms generally begin a few to several days after the initial trauma. Fever, pain, dysphagia, and signs of airway compromise predominate.

In a number of patients with posterior pharyngeal tears, penetration results in dissection of air through the retropharyngeal soft tissues (Fig. 22-74). Such children may complain of throat and neck pain. Subcutaneous emphysema may be noted clinically. Occasionally, signs of airway compromise develop with this complication. Therefore hospitalization for observation is advisable when this sequela is encountered.

When penetration involves posterolateral structures (e.g., the tear is located near the tonsil or tonsillar pillar), the possibility of vascular injury must be considered. Deep penetration in this area can puncture or nick the internal carotid artery or nearby vessels, resulting in hemorrhage or more commonly gradual hematoma formation. Clues to vascular injury are lateral pharyngeal or peritonsillar swelling and fullness or tenderness on palpation of the neck on the side of the wound. Radiographs should confirm soft-tissue swelling. Patients with peritonsillar tears should be admitted for observation even in the absence of these signs. Those with findings that suggest vascular involvement warrant angiography.

Upper Airway Obstruction

Acute Upper Airway Obstruction

Few conditions in pediatrics are as emergent and potentially life threatening as those causing acute upper airway obstruction. In these conditions, expeditious assessment and appropriate stabilization are often lifesaving. In contrast, underestimation of severity of distress, overzealous attempts at examination or invasive procedures, and efforts by the unskilled to intervene may have catastrophic results.

The major causes are severe tonsillitis with adenoidal enlargement (see section on Tonsillar Disorders and Fig. 22-70, *B*), retropharyngeal abscess, epiglottitis, croup or laryngotracheobronchitis, foreign body aspiration, and angioedema (see Chapter 4). All are characterized by stridor and retractions that are primarily suprasternal and subcostal (unless distress becomes severe and retractions generalize) and mild to

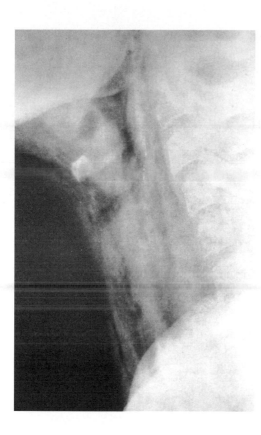

FIG. 22-74 Retropharyngeal air dissection. This lateral neck radiograph of a child with a puncture wound of the posterior pharyngeal wall reveals extensive air dissection through the retropharyngeal soft tissues. Subcutaneous air has tracked anteriorly as well.

T A B L E   2 2 - 1

Clinical Features of Acute Upper Airway Disorders

Clinical finding	Supraglottic disorders	Subglottic disorders
Stridor	Quiet and wet	Loud
Voice alteration	Muffled	Hoarse
Dysphagia	+	−
Postural preference*	+	−
Barky cough	−	+ Especially with croup
Fever	+	+ Usually with croup
Toxicity	+	
Trismus	+ Usually with peritonsillar abscess	−
Facial edema	−	+ Usually with angioedema

From Davis HW, et al: Acute upper airway obstruction: croup and epiglottitis, *Pediatr Clin North Am* 28:859-880, 1981.
*Epiglottitis—patient characteristically sits bolt upright, with neck extended and head held forward; retropharyngeal abscess—child often adopts opisthotonic posture; peritonsillar abscess—patient may tilt head toward affected side.

T A B L E   2 2 - 2

Estimation of Severity of Respiratory Distress

Clinical finding	Mild	Moderate	Severe
Color	Normal	Normal	Pale, dusky, or cyanotic
Retractions	Absent to mild	Moderate	Severe and generalized with use of accessory muscles
Air entry	Mild ↓	Moderate ↓	Severe ↓
Level of consciousness	Normal or restless when disturbed	Anxious, restless when undisturbed	Lethargic, depressed

From Davis HW, et al: Acute upper airway obstruction: croup and epiglottitis, *Pediatr Clin North Am* 28:859-880, 1981.

moderate increases in heart and respiratory rates. For purposes of assessment, it is helpful to classify the disorders into two categories—supraglottic and subglottic—based on major signs and symptoms listed in Table 22-1.

The key to appropriate management is a brief history detailing the course and associated symptoms, followed by rapid assessment of clinical signs to determine the approximate level of airway involvement and the degree of respiratory distress (Table 22-2). This can be done for the most part through visual inspection, without ever touching the patient. It is particularly important to avoid upsetting a child with upper airway obstruction who shows signs of fatigue or cyanosis or meets any of the other criteria for severe distress. Such disturbances can serve only to worsen distress and may precipitate complete obstruction. Therefore when a child has signs of moderately severe or severe obstruction, his or her parents should be allowed to remain with him; any positional preference (if manifested) should be honored; and oral examination, venipuncture, IVs, and x-rays should be deferred until the airway is secure. Once the initial assessment is done, the most skilled personnel available are assembled to stabilize the airway. This procedure is best accomplished under controlled conditions in the operating room.

Retropharyngeal Abscess

A retropharyngeal abscess usually involves one of the retropharyngeal lymph nodes that run in chains through the retropharyngeal tissues on either side of the midline. Because these nodes tend to atrophy after 4 years of age, the disorder is seen primarily in children under 3 or 4 years. The major causative organisms are group A beta-streptococci, although *Staphylococcus aureus* is found in some cases.

The child with a retropharyngeal abscess generally has a history of an acute, febrile upper respiratory tract infection or pharyngitis beginning several days earlier, which may have improved transiently. Suddenly, the child's condition worsens with development of a high spiking fever, toxicity, anorexia, drooling, and dyspnea. On examina-

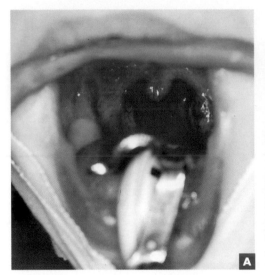

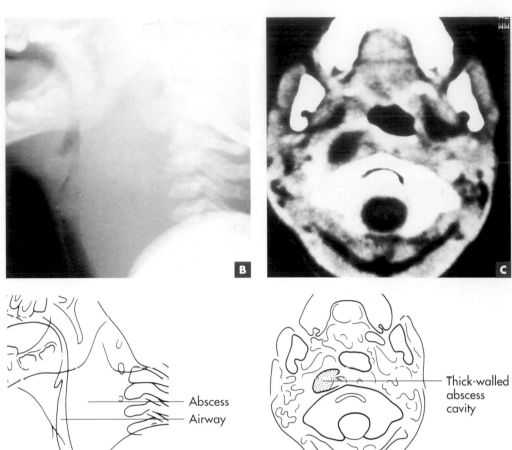

FIG. 22-75 Retropharyngeal abscess. A young child presented with high fever, drooling, quiet stridor, and an opisthotonic postural preference. *A,* Pharyngeal examination in the operating room revealed an intensely erythematous, unilateral swelling of the posterior pharyngeal wall. *B,* A lateral neck radiograph shows prominent prevertebral swelling that displaces the trachea forward. *C,* On CT scan, a thick-walled abscess cavity is evident in the retropharyngeal space. The highly vascular wall enhanced with contrast injection.

Abscess
Airway

Thick-walled abscess cavity

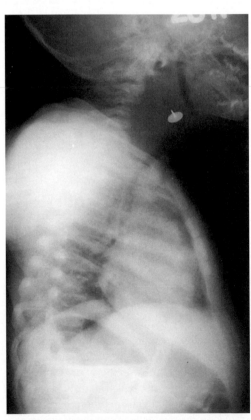

FIG. 22-76 Retropharyngeal abscess after a puncture wound. This child tried to swallow a tack that punctured and became lodged in the posterior pharyngeal wall. The incident was unwitnessed, and he came to medical attention only when he developed fever and began drooling. (Courtesy Dr. Robert Gochman, Schneider Children's Hospital, Long Island Jewish Medical Center.)

tion, the patient is restless and irritable and tends to lie with his or her head hyperextended, simulating opisthotonus. Quiet gurgling stridor is heard. If respiratory distress is not severe, the pharynx can be examined, and a fiery red asymmetrical swelling of the posterior pharyngeal wall may be observed pushing the uvula and ipsilateral tonsil forward (Fig. 22-75, *A*). Even with direct examination, this swelling can be difficult to appreciate at times. A portable lateral neck x-ray taken (with a physician in attendance) on inspiration shows marked widening of the prevertebral tissues (Fig. 22-75, *B*), which are normally no wider than a vertebral body. When diagnosed, prompt otolaryngologic consultation should be sought to determine if the mass is fluctuant, necessitating surgical drainage, or if it is in an early cellulitic phase, requiring serial reexamination. A CT scan can be helpful in this regard (Fig. 22-75, *C*). High-dose intravenous antimicrobial therapy is needed whether or not drainage is required.

As noted earlier, a retropharyngeal abscess may occasionally form in an older child after a puncture wound of the posterior pharyngeal wall (Fig. 22-76). Signs of infection develop acutely a few days later. In these cases oral flora are found on culture.

Parapharyngeal Abscess

Lateral neck space abscesses can also occur in infants and young children. Most patients are toxic with high spiking fevers. The history and clinical picture are nearly identical to those of children with retropharyngeal abscess. However, these patients have torticollis, bending toward the affected side, and examination of the neck reveals diffuse anterolateral swelling that is exquisitely tender (Fig. 22-77, *A*). Oral inspection may reveal medial displacement of the tonsil or lateral pharyngeal wall. A CT scan is essential to confirm the diagnosis (Fig. 22-77, *B*). Prompt drainage is important to prevent extension into the mediastinum.

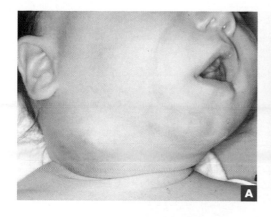
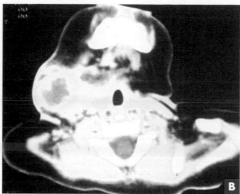

FIG. 22-77 Parapharyngeal abscess. *A,* This child had high fever, toxicity, and marked, exquisitely tender anterolateral neck swelling with overlying erythema. These manifestations followed a week of upper respiratory tract infection symptoms and decreased feeding. *B,* His CT scan reveals an encapsulated abscess in the right parapharyngeal area.

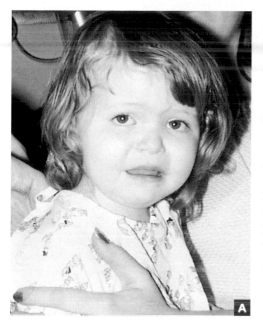
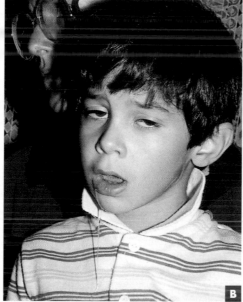

FIG. 22-78 Epiglottitis. *A* to *C,* These three patients with acute epiglottitis demonstrate the varying degrees of distress that may be seen, depending on age and time of presentation. *A,* This 3-year-old seen a few hours after onset of symptoms was anxious and still, but had no positional preference or drooling. *B,* This 5-year-old, who had been symptomatic for several hours holds his neck extended with head held forward, is mouth breathing and drooling and shows signs of tiring. *C,* This 2-year-old was in severe distress, and was too exhausted to hold his head up. *D* and *E,* In the operating room the epiglottis can be visualized and appears intensely red and swollen. It may retain its omega shape or resemble a cherry.

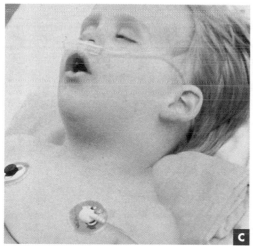
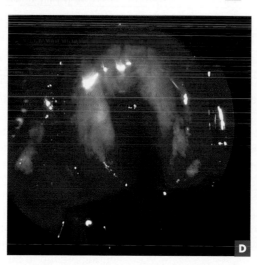
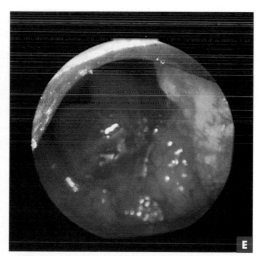

Epiglottitis

Epiglottitis, perhaps the most acutely emergent form of acute upper airway obstruction, is an infection caused by *Haemophilus influenzae* type B. Its incidence has dropped precipitously since introduction of the *H. influenzae* b vaccine. Hence many younger practitioners have never seen a case, increasing the risk of delayed diagnosis. Epiglottitis is characterized by marked inflammation and edema of the pharynx, epiglottis, aryepiglottic folds, and ventricular bands. The peak age range is 1 to 7 years, but infants and older children may be affected. Onset is sudden and progression rapid; most patients are brought to medical attention within 12 hours of the first appearance of symptoms. Generally the child is entirely well until several hours before presentation, when he or she abruptly spikes a high fever. This is rapidly followed by severe throat pain with dysphagia and drooling, and soon thereafter by dyspnea and anxiety.

On examination, the child is usually toxic, anxious, and remarkably still, sitting bolt upright with neck extended and head held forward (unless obstruction is very mild or fatigue has supervened) (Fig. 22-78, *A* to *C*). Quiet gurgling stridor and drooling are evident, along with dyspnea and retractions. If the child will talk, which is unusual, the voice

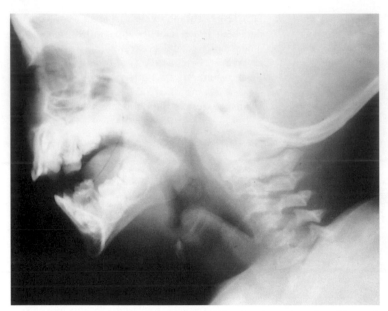

FIG. 22-79   Mild epiglottitis or supraglottitis. The lateral neck radiograph demonstrates mild epiglottic swelling and thickening of the aryepiglottic folds.

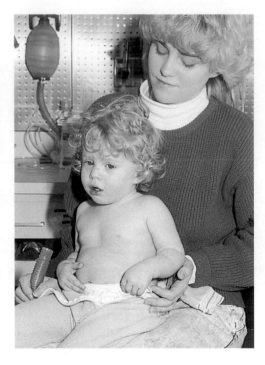

FIG. 22-80   Croup. This toddler with moderate upper airway obstruction caused by croup had suprasternal and subcostal retractions. Her anxious expression was the result of mild hypoxia confirmed by pulse oximetry.

is muffled. This clinical picture is so typical that when seen the best course of action after initial assessment is prompt airway stabilization, usually intubation under controlled conditions by experienced personnel in the operating room. At this time, the epiglottis is found to be markedly swollen and erythematous (Fig. 22-78, *D* and *E*). After airway stabilization, cultures can be obtained and intravenous antimicrobial therapy initiated. Obtaining an x-ray before transfer to the operating room is contraindicated; it adds nothing and may precipitate decompensation.

On occasion, children present with a similar history but milder symptoms and signs. In these cases, presentation is very early or the child is older than average. Respiratory distress is minimal, and visualization of the pharynx can be attempted (without use of a tongue blade) if the child will voluntarily open his or her mouth. In some instances a swollen epiglottis is seen projecting above the tongue. When the history suggests epiglottitis but clinical findings are mild and the diagnosis is not confirmed by attempted noninvasive visualization, a portable lateral neck x-ray examination (done in the emergency room with physician in attendance) can be useful. It may reveal mild epiglottic enlargement (Fig. 22-79) or merely swelling of the aryepiglottic folds and ventricular bands: a condition called *supraglottitis.* If either is found, the diagnosis is confirmed. Intubation is generally advisable in the former instance despite mild symptoms, but close observation on intravenous antibiotic therapy (covering for *H. influenzae* type B) may suffice when supraglottitis is the only finding.

Croup or Laryngotracheobronchitis

Croup, an acute respiratory illness, is characterized by inflammation and edema of the pharynx and upper airways, with maximal narrowing in the immediate subglottic region. There is probably a component of laryngospasm as well. The majority of cases are caused by viral pathogens, with parainfluenza, respiratory syncitial virus, adenoviruses, influenza viruses, and echoviruses being the agents most commonly identified. The peak season is between October and April in the Northern Hemisphere. The disorder primarily affects children between the ages of 3 months and 3 years. This is probably because their airways are narrower, and the mucosa is both more vascular and more loosely attached than in older children, enabling greater ease of edema collection. Older children can be affected, however.

Typically the child has had symptoms of a mild upper respiratory tract infection with rhinorrhea, cough, low-grade fever, and perhaps a sore throat for 1 to 5 days before developing symptoms of croup. The change is generally sudden and usually occurs at night or during a nap. The child awakens with fever, loud inspiratory stridor, a loud "barky" or "seal-like" cough, and hoarseness. The severity of symptoms and the course vary widely and are highly unpredictable. Duration averages 3 days but can be as brief as 1 day or as long as a week. Most patients have a waxing and waning course, with symptoms more severe at night, but it is impossible to predict which night will be the worst. Some patients remain relatively mild throughout the course, while others progress either slowly or rapidly to severe distress. Airway drying, probably in part as a result of mouth breathing necessitated by nasal congestion (especially while sleeping), appears to aggravate the cough and possibly the element of laryngospasm.

Physical findings are highly variable, depending on degree of distress at the time of presentation. Most affected children are moderately febrile but not toxic and have a loud barky cough and loud inspiratory stridor, with suprasternal and subcostal retractions (Fig. 22-80) and a mild decrease in air entry. A small percentage of patients with more extensive airway inflammation may have wheezing on auscultation. Many improve substantially as a result of exposure to cool night air during the trip to the emergency room. Some have restlessness or agitation reflecting hypoxia, and a few have severe distress. In these more severely affected patients, stridor may be both inspiratory and expiratory, with generalized retractions. If impairment of airflow is extreme, fatigue supervenes, stridor abates, and retractions diminish. **This must not be mistaken for clinical improvement.** A clinical scoring system that helps in grading severity of distress is presented in Table 22-3. In mild to moderate cases the pharynx can be visualized and reveals only mild erythema. **Oral examination should be deferred in severe cases until the airway is secure.** Radiography can be helpful in demonstrating subglottic narrowing—the "steeple sign" (Fig. 22-81, *A*). However, this is not necessary for patients with mild disease, and it is contraindicated for those with severe distress.

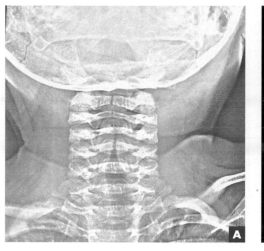
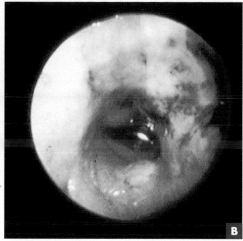

FIG. 22-81 Croup. *A,* This radiograph reveals a long area of narrowing extending well below the normally narrowed area at the level of the vocal cords. The finding is often termed the *"steeple sign."* *B,* In this patient, direct visualization revealed sub-glottic narrowing that was so severe, only tracheostomy would enable establishment of an adequate airway. (*A,* Courtesy Dr. Sylvan Stool, The Children's Hospital, Denver.)

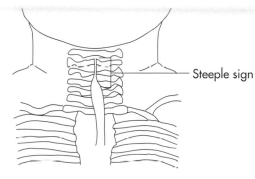
Steeple sign

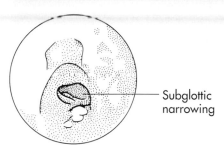
Subglottic narrowing

TABLE 22-3

Croup Scoring System

Clinical finding	0	1	2	3
Stridor	None	Mild	Moderate at rest	Severe, on inspiration and expiration, or none with markedly decreased air entry
Retraction	None	Mild	Moderate	Severe, marked use of accessory muscles
Air entry	Normal	Mild decrease	Moderate decrease	Marked decrease
Color	Normal	Normal (0 score)	Normal (0 score)	Dusky or cyanotic
Level of consciousness	Normal	Restless when disturbed	Anxious, agitated; undisturbed	Lethargic, depressed

Modified from Taussig LM, et al: Treatment of laryngotracheobronchitis (croup): use of intermittent positive pressure breathing and racemic epinephrine, *Am J Dis Child* 129:790-793, 1975.

Management depends largely on severity of distress when seen and on clinical response to mist therapy. Most patients have mild disease, improve considerably on mist alone, and can be managed at home with humidification. Parents must, however, be instructed to watch for signs of increasing distress, which would warrant return to the hospital. Aerosolized racemic epinephrine is effective in reducing airway obstruction caused by croup. It is particularly useful for children with moderate obstruction who do not show marked improvement on mist alone, and it can provide significant relief for children with severe distress. This agent, though effective, is short acting, and rebound tends to occur. Thus patients requiring racemic epinephrine should generally be admitted for further observation. Administration of dexamethasone IM (sometimes followed by a 2 to 3 day course of oral prednisone) appears to reduce severity of symptoms and thereby the need for hospitalization.

Patients in severe distress who do not improve dramatically after treatment with racemic epinephrine, and those who steadily worsen in the hospital despite mist and aerosol treatments warrant airway stabilization, via intubation or tracheostomy under controlled conditions in the operating room. The choice of procedure remains controversial and is perhaps best made in accordance with the skills of the personnel and facilities available at the individual institution. In some instances, subglottic narrowing is so severe as to necessitate tracheostomy (Fig. 22-81, *B*). Attempts at emergency tracheostomy in the emergency department are fraught with hazard and should be avoided at all costs.

Bacterial Tracheitis

In a small percentage of cases, children with a crouplike picture are atypically toxic and markedly febrile and have rapidly progressive air-

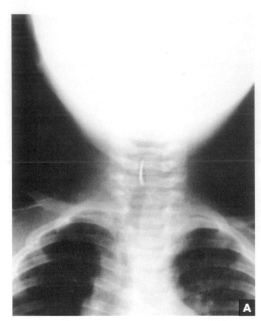
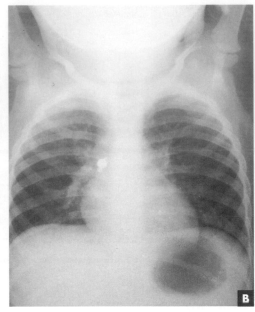
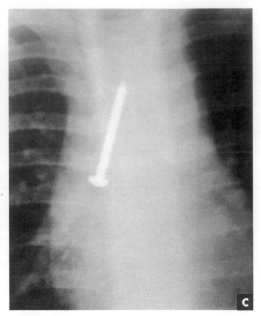

FIG. 22-82   Foreign body aspiration. Radiopaque objects and those well outlined by air are readily visualized on x-rays. *A,* A piece of eggshell is seen in the subglottic portion of the trachea, clearly outlined by the air column. *B,* An earring lies in the entrance of the right mainstem bronchus. *C,* A screw is seen lodged in the right mainstem bronchus and projecting into the trachea. (*A* courtesy Dr. Mananda Bhende, Children's Hospital of Pittsburgh; *B* and *C* courtesy Dr. Robert Gochman, Schneider Children's Hospital, Long Island Jewish Medical Center.)

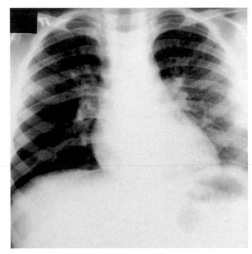
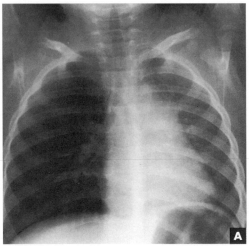
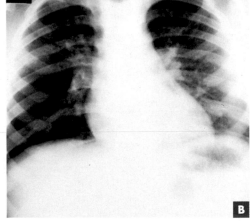

FIG. 22-83   Foreign body aspiration with ipsilateral hyperinflation. This 18-month-old child was eating popcorn when he suddenly began choking. Within a few hours, he developed significant respiratory distress and his chest x-ray revealed massive hyperinflation of the right lung caused by the ball-valve effect of the popcorn lodged in the right mainstem bronchus. (Courtesy Department of Radiology, Uniontown Hospital, Uniontown, Pennsylvania.)

FIG. 22-84   Foreign body aspiration, inspiratory and expiratory radiographs. *A,* This inspiratory film taken during fluoroscopy suggests hyperinflation of the right lower and middle lobes. *B,* This becomes much more evident on expiration when the hyperinflation persists, and the mediastinum shifts to the opposite side. (Courtesy Dr. Robert Gochman, Schneider Children's Hospital, Long Island Jewish Medical Center.)

way obstruction necessitating urgent intubation. Bronchoscopy before airway stabilization reveals severe inflammation, edema, and a copious, purulent subglottic exudate that contains large numbers of bacteria. Most of these patients appear to have a history of viral croup with sudden worsening. It is thus thought that the disorder may represent secondary bacterial infection. However, there is still some speculation that this disorder may represent an unusually virulent form of viral laryngotracheobronchitis.

Foreign Body Aspiration

Foreign body aspiration is seen for the most part in older infants and toddlers. The story is usually one of a sudden choking episode while the child was eating material that the immature dentition is ill equipped to chew. Such foods include nuts, seeds, popcorn, raw vegetables such as carrots and celery, and hot dogs. Occasionally the episode occurs when the child is chewing on a small object, a toy, or a detachable portion of a toy. If the object lodges in the larynx, asphyxiation results un-

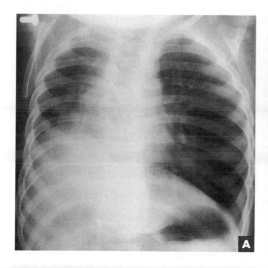
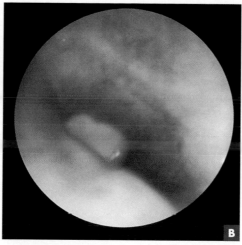

FIG. 22-85 Foreign body aspiration—delayed presentation. *A*, With delay in presentation of partial obstruction or with complete obstruction of a bronchus, radiographic findings consist of atelectasis and a mediastinal shift toward the side of the foreign body. *B*, In this case a peanut was found completely obstructing the bronchus. (Courtesy Dr. Robert Gochman, Schneider Children's Hospital, Long Island Jewish Medical Center.)

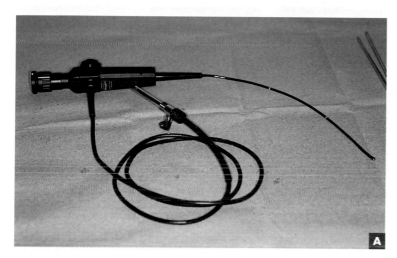

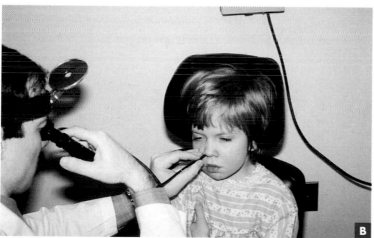

FIG. 22-86 Fiberoptic laryngoscopy. *A*, The flexible fiberoptic laryngoscope. *B*, With careful preparation the patient can tolerate insertion of the flexible fiberoptic tubing and the examination.

ated with decreased breath sounds. Later, diffuse wheezing may be heard simulating asthma or bronchiolitis. Lateral neck and chest radiography reveal aspirated objects that are radiopaque or outlined by the air column (Fig. 22-82, *A* to *C*), enabling localization before endoscopy. However, most cases involve materials not visible on x-rays, although other radiographic clues may be present. Partial obstruction of a bronchus creates a ball-valve effect, allowing air in during inspiration but preventing its egress on expiration. This produces hyperinflation of one or more lobes of the lung on the same side as the foreign body (Fig. 22-83), which may be evident on the plain chest film. In subtler cases, chest fluoroscopy may highlight the differential inflation and deflation, showing mediastinal shift away from the side of the foreign body or exhalation (Fig. 22-84). These findings are particularly likely if the patient is seen fairly soon after the aspiration episode. When there is a delay in seeking medical attention (usually because the aspiration episode was unwitnessed and onset of symptoms is insidious), the patient may have cough and fever. In these instances, atelectasis and a mediastinal shift toward the side of the foreign body may be found on chest radiograph (Fig. 22-85). This finding also may be seen acutely when the bronchus is totally obstructed. Many patients presenting acutely have no detectable radiographic abnormality after foreign body aspiration. Hence, when clinical suspicion is high, given the history and physical findings, endoscopic examination is indicated despite normal plain films. Conversely, when physical findings and x-ray films are normal and the history is questionable, a period of close observation may be indicated.

Unfortunately, in up to 50% of cases the aspiration episode is not reported, because the parent does not relate it to the child's symptoms or did not witness the choking spell. For this reason, this diagnosis should be considered and specific questions asked regarding possible aspiration whenever a young child has acute onset of cough and stridor or experiences a first episode of wheezing.

Chronic Upper Airway Obstructions

Laryngeal Examination

In children with a subacute or chronic airway disorder a laryngeal examination is necessary to arrive at a definitive diagnosis. If a child is in distress or has acutely decompensated, this examination should be done in an operating room where rigid ventilating bronchoscopes and anesthesia are available as backup. When the airway has been stable, laryngoscopy can be performed by an otolaryngologist in the office or emergency department using a flexible fiberoptic laryngoscope (Fig. 22-86, *A*). These are now available in a range of diame-

less the Heimlich maneuver or backslaps are performed promptly. In the majority of cases the foreign material clears the larynx and lodges in the trachea or a bronchus (more commonly, the right mainstem). After the choking spell, there is a silent period usually lasting a few to several hours (occasionally days or weeks), after which the child develops cough, stridor (lodged in trachea) or wheezing (lodged in a bronchus), and respiratory distress. In this acute phase, when the object is situated in a bronchus, wheezing may be unilateral and associ-

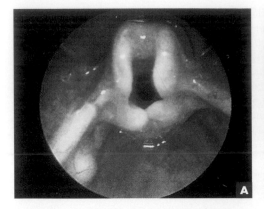
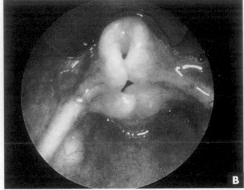

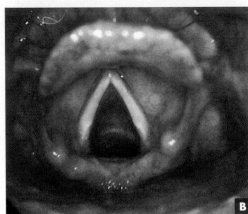

FIG. 22-87 Laryngomalacia. *A,* Note the omegoid shape of the epiglottis, and the elongation of the arytenoid cartilages. *B,* This is the larynx during inspiration. Note that the forces of the inspired air lead to collapse of the laryngeal inlet. Infolding of the epiglottic surfaces and the arytenoid cartilages causes partial airway obstruction.

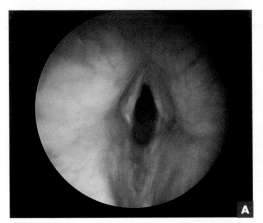
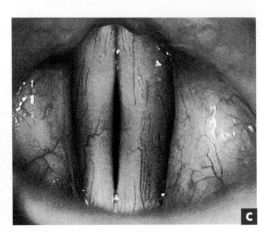

FIG. 22-88 Bilateral vocal cord paralysis. *A,* The marked narrowing of the aperture between the cords stems from loss of ability to abduct on inspiration. This is in contrast to normal opening and closing on inspiration and expiration as seen in *B* and *C.*

ters suitable for pediatric patients. Letting the older child handle the scope (with close supervision) and look through the lens facilitates cooperation. The child is then prepared by spraying the nasal mucosa with a decongestant and topical lidocaine. With careful preparation, most patients can be examined in the parent's lap or an examination chair, but the toddler usually requires immobilization in a papoose board. The fiberoptic tube is then gently inserted into the nose and guided through past the palate (Fig. 22-86, *B*). If the child is exclusively mouth breathing, the soft palate may be apposed to the posterior pharyngeal wall. Asking the child to try to breathe through the nose a few times moves the palate forward, facilitating passage. Anatomic abnormalities and dynamic motion of the supraglottic and glottic structures are easily seen with this device. Asking the child to phonate by saying the letter *e* enables observation of cord movement. In infants, cord movement is generally observed with crying. Although less well seen, the subglottic space can generally be viewed as well.

Subglottic Stenosis

Subglottic stenosis is a disorder in which the subglottic region of the trachea is unusually narrow in the absence of infection. In some instances the stenosis is the result of abnormal cricoid development and is therefore congenital. In other cases narrowing is the long-term result of injury and scarring from prior intubation. Regardless of the source, these children tend to develop stridor and respiratory distress with every upper respiratory tract infection. A few are identified by virtue of having an atypically prolonged episode of croup. Some also have stridor with crying, even when well. Neck x-rays may present a similar appearance to that seen with croup. The problem generally improves with

growth, but up to 40% of these children develop such severe distress with colds that tracheostomy is required.

Laryngomalacia

Laryngomalacia, a congenital condition, accounts for greater than 70% of cases of persistent stridor in infants. The problem is the result of unusual flaccidity of the laryngeal structures, especially the epiglottis and the arytenoid cartilages. The etiology is uncertain, but it is thought to be caused by lack of neural coordination of the laryngeal muscles, with the result that supraglottic structures hang over the airway entrance like a set of loose sails over a sailboat (Fig. 22-87).

Clinically these infants tend to have mild inspiratory stridor that is worse when lying supine and tends to improve when they are placed in the prone position or their necks are slightly hyperextended. The condition is usually benign and rarely interferes with feeding or respiration. The diagnosis can be confirmed only by direct visualization of the larynx during active respiration. This is important in that it is necessary to document that the stridor is not the result of a more dangerous condition. Once the examination has been completed, the parents can be reassured that the condition is benign and that with growth the stridor usually abates by the end of the first year and a half of life. Management consists of observation, with particularly close monitoring during upper respiratory tract infections.

Vocal Cord Paralysis

Paralysis of the vocal cords may be present at birth, or it may develop in the first 2 months of life. It may be bilateral or unilateral. The underlying problem generally is located somewhere along the vagus

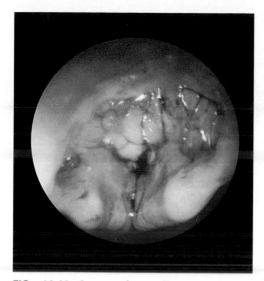

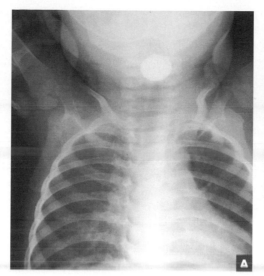

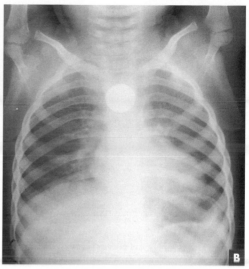

FIG. 22-89 Laryngeal papillomas. Multiple smooth, warty growths are seen nearly occluding the larynx in this child who had a history of chronic hoarseness.

FIG. 22-90 Esophageal foreign bodies. *A,* This youngster accidentally swallowed a coin. He complained of throat pain and refused oral intake. When initially seen, the coin was lodged high in the esophagus. *B,* After observation overnight, repeat radiography revealed that the coin had moved but was still lodged in the esophagus. The patient underwent endoscopic removal. Note that asymmetric objects in the esophagus are oriented in the coronal plane, whereas in the trachea they lie in the saggital plane. (Courtesy Dr. Robert Gochman, Schneider Children's Hospital, Long Island Jewish Medical Center.)

nerve and may be found in the central nervous system or in the periphery. Even though many paralyses are idiopathic, a thorough evaluation must be done to locate the lesion and identify its source. Ten percent of stridor cases in neonates is thought to be due to this condition.

Infants with unilateral cord paralysis have stridor, hoarseness, and a weakened voice. The airway diameter is generally adequate for respiration, and unless a secondary lesion is present, it is rarely necessary to perform a tracheotomy. This lesion is most often caused by a cardiac abnormality because the recurrent laryngeal nerve is looped around these structures as it passes through the chest.

In contrast, bilateral vocal cord paralysis is a life-threatening condition because the vocal cords are unable to abduct on inspiration, and there is concomitant stridor and cyanosis caused by severe narrowing of the aperture between the cords (Fig. 22-88). This condition usually is associated with a depressed laryngeal cough reflex, and therefore aspiration is common. A tracheotomy is essential to secure the airway. Hydrocephalus and Arnold-Chiari malformations often are the underlying problem, because they cause compression of the vagus nerve as it leaves the brainstem. Neurosurgical intervention may correct the problem and allow eventual decanulation.

Juvenile Laryngeal Papillomatosis

Juvenile laryngeal papillomatosis is a condition in which multiple benign papillomas develop and grow on the vocal cords. In a few patients they may extend to involve the pharyngeal walls or tracheal mucosa. They are apparently of viral origin, and there is some evidence of transmission during delivery to children born to mothers with condyloma accuminata. The main symptom is hoarseness, but stridor may develop in children with large lesions or tracheal extension. Radiographs are usually normal. The diagnosis should be considered in patients with chronic hoarseness and in those with atypically prolonged croup. On laryngoscopy, irregular warty masses are seen (Fig. 22-89). Biopsy is required to confirm the diagnosis. Excision can be attempted using forceps or a laser, but it is often followed by regrowth. Tracheostomy should be avoided if at all possible because this often promotes seeding further down the tracheobronchial tree.

Esophageal Foreign Bodies

Ingestion of foreign objects is relatively common in older infants and toddlers, who are prone to putting almost anything they can pick up into their mouths. Coins, small toys, and pieces of toys are the objects most frequently found. Most traverse the esophagus, stomach, and intestines without incident and are of little concern. A small percentage of swallowed foreign bodies, being too large to pass through to the stomach, become lodged in the esophagus (usually at the level of the cricopharyngeus [C6] and less commonly at the level of the aorta [T4], or the diaphragmatic inlet [T11 to T12]). With mild obstruction, the child may refuse solid foods (although 17% of patients are asymptomatic); with moderate obstruction, liquids often are refused as well, or the child may appear to choke with drinking. When obstruction is nearly complete, the child may begin drooling. If the object is particularly large, it may compress the trachea as well, producing signs of upper airway obstruction. Older patients may complain of neck or substernal pain or discomfort, especially with swallowing.

Patients who have significant symptoms of esophageal or respiratory obstruction, and those who have ingested sharp, potentially toxic, or caustic objects should undergo prompt endoscopic removal. Those who have ingested smooth objects and have mild symptoms can be observed for 12 hours and then have a repeat x-ray examination. If the object has passed into the stomach, then endoscopy can be avoided. Otherwise, such intervention is indicated.

Although in many cases there is a clear history of ingestion, in a significant percentage the ingestion was not witnessed. A high level of suspicion is often required to make the diagnosis, and the possibility of an esophageal foreign body should be considered in evaluating any young child for a sudden change in eating pattern. Plain radiographs detect metallic and other radiopaque objects (Fig. 22-90). Most objects are plastic, however, and require barium swallow or in some cases endoscopy for detection. Delays in diagnosis can result in stricture formation or more rarely esophageal perforation with secondary pneumomediastinum, mediastinitis, pneumonia (Fig. 22-91), and/or large vessel hemorrhage.

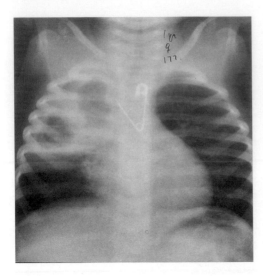

FIG. 22-91 Esophageal foreign body. An unwitnessed ingestion of this safety pin led to a period of anorexia followed by fever and respiratory distress. The point of the pin had perforated the esophageal wall and pleura, causing a secondary right upper lobe pneumonia. (Courtesy Dr. Robert Gochman, Schneider Children's Hospital, Long Island Jewish Medical Center.)

NOTE

Neck disorders, including adenitis, congenital cysts, vascular and lymphatic masses and tumors, are commonly managed by otolaryngologists. Limitations of space have required us to be selective in presenting disorders in this chapter. The reader is referred to Chapter 12 for a discussion of cervical adenitis and to Chapter 17 for a description of mass lesions.

ACKNOWLEDGMENTS

The authors would like to acknowledge and thank Children's Hospital of Pittsburgh, Department of Radiology, and University Health Center of Pittsburgh, Department of Neuroradiology, for providing many of the radiographs and CT scans in this chapter.

BIBLIOGRAPHY

Bluestone CD, Stool SE, eds: *Pediatric otolaryngology*, ed 2, Philadelphia, 1990, WB Saunders.

Bluestone CD: Recent advances in the pathogenesis, diagnosis, and management of otitis media, *Pediatr Clin North Am* 28:727-755, 1981.

Bluestone CD, Wald ER, Shapiro GC: The diagnosis and management of sinusitis in children: proceedings of a closed conference, *Pediatr Infect Dis J* 4:549-555, 1985.

Bowen AD, Ledesma-Medina J, Fujioka M, Oh KS, Young LW: Radiologic imaging in otorhinolaryngology, *Pediatr Clin North Am* 28:905-939, 1981.

Davis HW, Gartner JC, Galvis AG, Michaels RH, Mestead PH: Acute upper airway obstruction: croup and epiglottitis, *Pediatr Clin North Am* 28:859-880, 1981.

Gellady AM, Shulman ST, Ayoub EM: Periorbital and orbital cellulitis in children, *Pediatrics* 61.272-277, 1978.

Lim DJ, Bluestone CD, Klein JO, Nelson JD, eds: *Recent advances in otitis media with effusion,* Toronto, 1988, BC Decker.

McGuirt WF, ed: *Pediatric otolaryngology case studies*, Garden City, NY, 1980, Medical Examination.

Wald ER: Acute sinusitis in children, *Pediatr Infect Dis J* 2:61-68, 1983.

Wald ER, Milmoe GI, Bowen A'D, Ledesma-Medina J, Salamon N, Bluestone CD: Acute maxillary sinusitis in children, *N Engl J Med* 304:749-754, 1981.

Index